PERSPECTIVES IN

Athletic Training

evolve

ELSEVIER

To access your free Student Resources, visit:

http://evolve.elsevier.com/Cummings/athletic/

Evolve® Student Resources to accompany ***Cummings/Stanley-Green/Higgs: Perspectives in Athletic Training,*** offers the following features:

Resources

- **Illustrated Case Studies**
  15 written scenarios with accompanying photographs and follow-up questions for practice provide realistic situations involving diagnosis and management of injuries to encourage critical thinking.
- **Self-Test Questions**
  Approximately 350 practice questions with instant feedback serve as an excellent study tool.
- **Glossary Exercises**
  Chapter key terms are reproduced within a game of hangman for fun vocabulary practice.
- **Labeling Exercises**
  Key illustrations from anatomy chapters form the basis for an interactive drag-and-drop labeling exercise.
- **Anatomical Video Clips**
  Segments offer a unique look at human dissection and highlight key areas of common athletic injuries.
- **Internet Assignments**
  Written exercises encourage online research to reinforce chapter content and help put it into a realistic context for the practice of athletic training.
- **Quick-Reference Card**
  The HIPS/HOPS assessment information provided on the inside cover of the book is available in full color online for printing and handy reference on the go.

http://evolve.elsevier.com/Cummings/athletic/

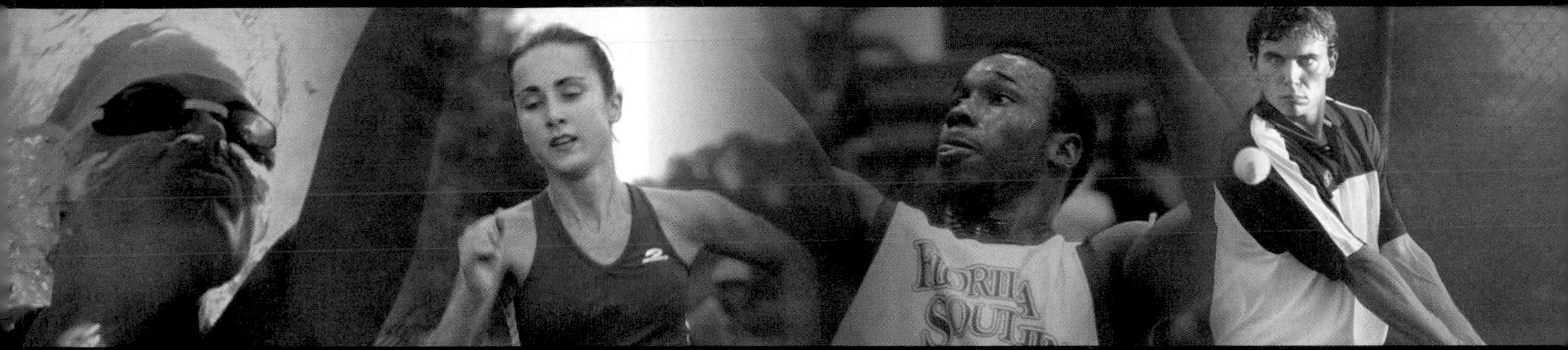

PERSPECTIVES IN

Athletic Training

Nancy H. **CUMMINGS**
EdD, ATC, LAT, CSCS

Assistant Professor
Physical Education and
Athletic Training Departments
Divisions of Education
and Health Sciences
Florida Southern College
Lakeland, Florida

Sue **STANLEY-GREEN**
MS, ATC, LAT

Director
Athletic Training
Education Program
Associate Professor
Athletic Training Department
Division of Health Sciences
Florida Southern College
Lakeland, Florida

Paul **HIGGS**
MEd, ATC, LAT, CSCS

Head Athletic Trainer
Department of Athletics
Georgia College
& State University
Milledgeville, Georgia

MOSBY
ELSEVIER

MOSBY
ELSEVIER

11830 Westline Industrial Drive
St. Louis, Missouri 63146

PERSPECTIVES IN ATHLETIC TRAINING ISBN: 978–0–323–03385–5

978-0-323-03385-5

Vice President and Publisher: Linda Duncan
Senior Editor: Kathy Falk
Managing Editor: Kristin Hebberd
Publishing Services Manager: Patricia Tannian
Project Manager: John Casey
Design Direction: Reneé Duenow

Printed in China

Last digit is print number: 9 8 7 6 5 4 3 2 1

Contributors

Michael R. Dillon, MA, ATC, CSCS, EMT-I
Associate Athletic Trainer
Department of Athletics
Adjunct Instructor
Department of Kinesiology
University of Georgia
Athens, Georgia

Denise M. Fandel, MS, CAE
Executive Director
National Athletic Trainers' Association Board of Certification, Inc.
Omaha, Nebraska

Michael S. Ferrara, PhD, ATC
Professor and Program Director
Department of Kinesiology
University of Georgia
Athens, Georgia

Thomas V. Gocke III, MS, ATC, PA-C
CEO, Co-Founder
GIZMO Educational Enterprises, Inc.
Cary, North Carolina

Pat Graman, MA, ATC
Director, Athletic Training Program
Department of Health Promotion and Education/Athletic Training
University of Cincinnati
Cincinnati, Ohio

Valerie W. Herzog, EdD, LAT, ATC
Graduate Athletic Training Program Director
Department of Health Promotion and Human Performance
Weber State University
Ogden, Utah

Kathleen M. Laquale, PhD, ATC, LAT, LDN
Associate Professor
Department of Movement Arts, Health Promotion, and Leisure Studies
Bridgewater State College
Bridgewater, Massachusetts

Karen M. Lew, MEd, ATC, LAT
Athletic Training Program Director
Department of Kinesiology and Health Studies
Southeastern Louisiana University
Hammond, Louisiana

James M. Lynch, MD
Professor
Athletic Training Education Program
Department of Physical Therapy
Florida Southern College
Lakeland, Florida

Robert C. Manske, PT, DPT, SCS, ATC, CSCS
Associate Professor
Department of Physical Therapy
Wichita State University
Staff Physical Therapist/Athletic Trainer
Department of Physical Therapy/Sports Medicine
Via Christi Medical Center
Teaching Associate
Department of Family Medicine
Via Christi Sports Medicine Fellowship Residency Program
University of Kansas Medical School
Wichita, Kansas

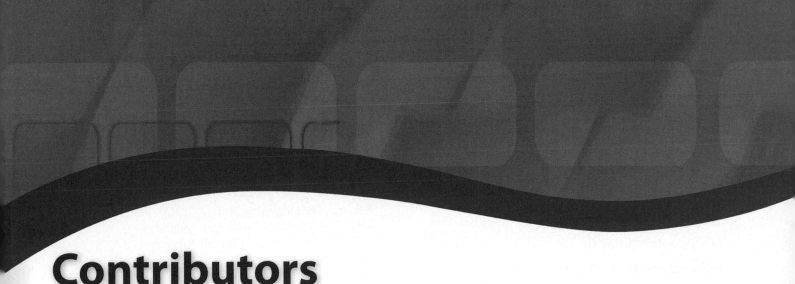

James W. Matheson, PT, DPT, SCS, OCS, CSCS
Clinical Research Director and Physical Therapist
Therapy Partners, Inc.
Burnsville, Minnesota

William N. Miller, DPE, ATC, LAT
Associate Professor
Director, Athletic Training Education
Department of Movement Science
Westfield State College
Westfield, Massachusetts

Robert Moss, PhD, ATC, FOT
Professor and Director
Athletic Training Education Program
Department of Physical Education
Albion College
Albion, Michigan

Gretchen D. Oliver, PhD, ATC, LAT
Clinical Coordinator
Graduate Athletic Training Education Program
Department of Health, Kinesiology, Recreation, and Dance
University of Arkansas
Fayetteville, Arkansas

Michael P. Reiman, PT, MEd, ATC, CSCS, USAW, USATF
Assistant Professor
Department of Physical Therapy
Wichita State University
Clinician
Department of Physical Therapy
Via Christi Sports and Orthopedic Physical Therapy
Wichita, Kansas

Kathy Taylor Remsburg, MS, LAT, ATC
Director, Athletic Training Education Program
Assistant Professor of Athletic Training
Education Division Head
Department of Athletic Training
Franklin College
Franklin, Indiana

Chad Starkey, PhD, LAT
Athletic Training Education
School of Recreation and Sport Sciences
College of Health and Human Services
Ohio University
Athens, Ohio

Gary B. Wilkerson, EdD, ATC
Professor
Graduate Athletic Training Education Program
Department of Health & Human Performance
University of Tennessee at Chattanooga
Chattanooga, Tennessee

Reviewers

Eva Beaulieu, MEd, ATC, LAT
Assistant Athletic Trainer
LaGrange College
LaGrange, Georgia

Jim Buriak, MS, ATC
Associate Professor
Chairperson
Department of Education, Health, and Human Performance
Roanoke College
Salem, Virginia

Shannon Courtney, MA, ATC
Lecturer
Curriculum Director
Head Athletic Trainer
School of Sport & Exercise Science
College of Natural and Health Sciences
University of Northern Colorado
Greeley, Colorado

David Florkowski, MEd, ATC, LAT, CEAS, CSCS
Assistant Professor
Department of Kinesiology
Georgia College & State University
Milledgeville, Georgia

Suzanne Gushie, MA, ATC
Instructor,
Curriculum Director
Athletic Training Program
Sportsmedicine Department
Mercyhurst College
Erie, Pennsylvania

Sharon Menegoni, MS, ATC
Program Director
Athletic Training Education
Department of Health, Recreation, & Kinesiology
Longwood University
Farmville, Virginia

Jamie L. Musler, MS, ATC
Associate Clinical Specialist
Program Director
Athletic Training Education Program
School of Health Professions
Bouvé College of Health Sciences
Northeastern University
Boston, Massachusetts

Kimberly S. Peer, EdD, ATC, LAT
Coordinator
Assistant Professor
Athletic Training Education Program
School of Exercise, Leisure, and Sport
College of Education, Health, & Human Services
Kent State University
Kent, Ohio

Charles J. Redmond, MEd, MSPT, LATC
Associate Professor
Department Chair
Department of Exercise Science and Sport Studies
School of Health, Physical Education, and Recreation
Springfield College
Springfield, Massachusetts

Donna M. Ritenour, EdD, ATC
Assistant Professor
Director
Athletic Training Program
Salisbury University
Salisbury, Maryland

Kristen C. Schellhase, MEd, ATC, LAT, CSCS
Program Director
Program in Athletic Training
College of Health and Public Affairs
University of Central Florida
Orlando, Florida

James R. Scifers, DScPT, PT, SCS, LAT, ATC
Program Director
Athletic Training Education Program
Associate Professor
Department of Health Sciences
College of Applied Sciences
Western Carolina University
Cullowhee, North Carolina

Thomas F. West, PhD, ATC
Associate Professor
Department of Health Science and Sport Studies
College of Education and Human Services
California University of Pennsylvania
California, Pennsylvania

To my family and loved ones who have always supported and encouraged me
and who sacrifice so much in allowing me to pursue my dreams.
Daddy, Ann, Dale, Karen, Susan, and Tayler—
you have loved me, believed in me, supported me, encouraged me,
motivated me, and celebrated me. Because of you, this journey called
"the book" is successfully finished. I love you so much!

Momma and Granddaddy, your unconditional love and passion for life
inspire me to continue the legacies you have left behind.
Even though your footprints are large, I will attempt to follow in them.
I pray that I can humbly complete the paths we are so blessed you began…

NHC

To Al, my husband and best friend,
and to Logan, our daughter and light of our lives,
thank you for your love, patience, and support
through a very chaotic time of our lives.
I am only complete with both of you by my side. I love you!

To my family and "forever friends," thanks for always caring
and for constantly being there for me.
My special thoughts go to Linda Daniel, who left us too early
but who brought so many of us together and started us on the adventure
of athletic training. Linda, we love you and miss you.

My mom was my inspiration and my hero.
Every day I try to imitate her incredible patience and total unconditional love
for everyone in her life. She empowered me with the strength and courage to
take the road less traveled.
Thanks, Mom!

SSG

To the three most important people in my life—
my wife, Karen, and my two favorite redheads, Mary Helen and Matthew—
who bring me joy and remind me daily what is truly important in life
and whose ongoing support, encouragement, and confidence
throughout this project made it worthwhile.

PH

Preface to the Instructor

Perspectives in Athletic Training is the first of its kind—a full-color text that provides just the right amount and level of content to best introduce students to the profession of athletic training. This textbook is written in a conversational style that engages learners and entices them to want to learn more. With a holistic approach to injury evaluation and management and a number of related topics and developmentally appropriate instructional strategies, issues facing today's athletic training students are brought to the forefront. These instructional strategies encourage critical thinking, assimilation, innovation and problem-solving skills to enable your students to fully mature from a beginner to a competent and successful athletic trainer.

The underlying premise to *Perspectives in Athletic Training* is to create intentional learning opportunities—to integrate core cognate concepts into workable units, or clusters that are reinforced with a variety of pedagogical features. If we present the information in a way that the student will both use it and learn it, then we have created a successful learning environment. The novelty, then, becomes how we present the information and features in a student-centered manner. For learning to take place, the student must be engaged. All of the pedagogical features promote just that—an interaction between the learner and the information at hand.

AUDIENCE

The primary audience for this textbook is the student enrolled in the introductory course in undergraduate athletic training education programs. Due to the comprehensive coverage of the profession of athletic training as a whole, this textbook serves well as a tool for students to truly grasp what athletic training really is.

The secondary audience is the student who is a non-athletic training major studying exercise science, care and prevention of injuries, general physical activity, sport and fitness, athletic administration, kinesiology, or recreation. Also, students who are enrolled in the pre-major courses for athletic training, sport and fitness, and exercise science would benefit from the holistic approach of this textbook. High school athletic training students would find this book to be an invaluable resource for attending to their current athletes, as well as for preparing for entry into the undergraduate athletic training program.

ORGANIZATION

Focused and thoughtful coverage is the hallmark of *Perspectives in Athletic Training*. The chapters and units follow a logical organization, introducing students to foundational information about the profession and the body's reaction to injury before moving into functional anatomy and the diagnosis and management of specific injuries. The book concludes with chapters on nutrition, psychosocial concerns, pharmacology, and prevention and protection of injuries. Intentional learning is what prompted the design of the table of contents.

Unit I, Introduction to the Profession of Athletic Training, introduces the student to the broad issues surrounding this career choice. Chapter 1 provides an overview of the role of the certified athletic trainer and the vast career possibilities currently available. Chapter 2 presents a unique exploration of the history of athletic training, the individuals who shaped its inception and growth, and the expanding role of the certified athletic trainer. Chapter 3 supplies a practical working model of recordkeeping and documentation, plus an effective emergency action plan, as an introduction into organization and administration within athletic training.

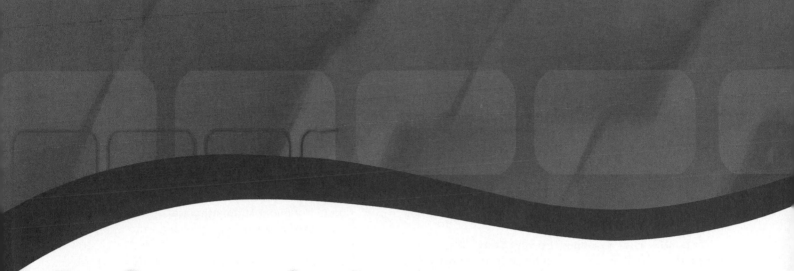

Unit II, The Body's Reaction to Injury, discusses basic concepts involving the how the body operates. Chapter 4 offers a unique and easy-to-understand explanation of the body's repair process or healing cycle within a discussion of general evaluation and diagnosis. Chapter 5 teaches a common-sense approach to the identification and management of the signs and symptoms of injury and illness in each of the basic body systems. Chapter 6 explores the various environmental illnesses and injuries that can hamper an individual's performance on any level. The unit concludes with Chapter 7 on managing emergency situations in athletics and, Chapter 8, which identifies a safe and progressive method for the development and progression of therapeutic rehabilitation programs.

Unit III, The Amazing Lower Body, begins the regional study of body regions—the heart and soul of the book. Chapter 9 provides a well-illustrated anatomical review, from the toes up through the hip and pelvis. All the anatomy chapters are written in a conversational yet in-depth style that enhances understanding and describes the ways in which movement within the body affects anatomy. The following three chapters discuss the diagnosis and management of lower leg, foot, ankle, and toe injuries (Chapter 10); knee and thigh injuries (Chapter 11), and hip and pelvis injuries (Chapter 12). These chapters address common acute and chronic injuries in athletics within a templated format that identifies the mechanism of injury, the signs and symptoms, appropriate special tests necessary to diagnose injury, and the immediate and intermediate care recommended to manage it.

Unit IV, The Remarkable Head and Trunk, and Unit V, The Complex Upper Body, are set up in the same way as Unit III to provide a consistent and logical progression of information among all the body regions. Anatomical discussions focus on the skull, spine, thorax, and abdomen (Chapter 13), the sense organs (Chapter 16), and the lower body (Chapter 18) Unit IV is rounded out with chapters on the diagnosis and management of sports-related concussion (Chapter 14), injuries to the spine (Chapter 15), and injuries to the sense organs (Chapter 17). Unit V concludes with chapters on the diagnosis and management of neck and shoulder injuries (Chapter 19) and elbow, wrist, hand, and finger injuries (Chapter 20).

In Unit VI, Balancing It Out, discussions move beyond injuries to focus on broader, surrounding issues. Chapter 21 covers nutrition in the athlete, and Chapter 22 deals with the psychosocial concerns unique to athletics. Chapter 23 provides an overview of pharmacology and the most commonly used medications in the treatment of illness and injury. Chapter 24 concludes with a highly illustrated look at taping and bracing for injury prevention and protection.

DISTINCTIVE FEATURES

- *Complete, balanced coverage* strikes a perfect balance in what and how much information to provide for the introductory student.
- *A clear, conversational style* engages the student and makes them want to read more and continue to learn.
- *Vivid, full-color photos and illustrations* create excitement and enthusiasm for the students.
- *A holistic, clustered approach* to the topics integrates knowledge of the body as a whole in a way that the student will learn it and use it.
- *The unique history chapter* provides an overview of the profession through words and pictures.
- *Points to Ponder* supply thought-provoking questions posed to encourage relevance and application of knowledge.
- *Issues & Ethics* boxes assists the student in problem-solving potential ethical and related situations that confront athletic trainers.
- *The "Age Group Athlete" sections* within diagnosis and management chapters provide information on injuries that are specific to certain age populations.
- *Concept maps* visually summarize the main ideas within each chapter, providing a concise summary of the key content.
- *A quick reference card* for HIPS/HOPS evaluation on the inside front cover provides a systematic approach to diagnosing acute and chronic injuries

LEARNING AIDS

A variety of pedagogical features throughout each chapter enhances the learning experience:

- *Opening Scenario:* Chapters begin with realistic cases that introduce chapter concepts.
- *Revisiting the Opening Scenario:* This end-of-chapter discussion asks the student to refer back to the beginning case study and examine the issues in light of the content presented.
- *Issues & Ethics:* This feature box at the end of each chapter calls attention to difficult situations and decisions students may face as athletic trainers.
- *Key vocabulary:* Throughout each chapter, key terms appear in boldface purple within their discussion and are then followed by a definition box at the bottom of that same page, ensuring that definitions are always at hand.
- *Related terminology:* Chapters on anatomy and diagnosis and management provide a wealth of terminology in boldface green type. These terms are then defined in an expanded glossary at the end of the book.
- *Points to Ponder:* Questions are interspersed throughout the chapters to challenge students to think critically about topics within and beyond the chapter's coverage.
- *Diagnosis and management chapter design:* The discussion within these chapters is presented consistently for each body region, with acute and chronic injuries broken down into sections covering for each the mechanism of injury, the signs and symptoms, appropriate special tests, and immediate and intermediate care.

- *Age group icons:* This symbol appears throughout the book to highlight material that is specific to certain age populations.
- *Concept maps:* These illustrations visually and succinctly summarize the key issues within that chapter, providing a broad overview.
- *Learning Goals:* A list of objectives highlights significant topics covered in each chapter.
- *Design:* An engaging full-color design brings the content to life.
- *Summary boxes, tables, and lists:* Chapters summarize key content in eye-catching features used liberally throughout the book.
- *Web Links:* This end-of-chapter feature provides the students with additional sources of information for further exploration on any given topic.
- *Expanded glossary:* The back of the text contains alphabetized listings not only of the key terms defined in each chapter but also separate listings of related anatomical and special tests terminology, providing an excellent reference tool.
- *Inside front cover:* The inside cover of the book contains a quick-reference card that serves as a handy on-the-go tool for diagnosis and management, outlining HIPS/HOPS.

ANCILLARY MATERIALS

An Evolve website has been created specifically to accompany this textbook and can be accessed via the following link: http://evolve.elsevier.com/Cummings/athletic/. A wealth of resources is provided to enhance both teaching and learning, as follows:

For the Instructor

- **Test Bank:** Nearly 1800 objective-style questions—multiple-choice, true/false, short answer, and matching—accompanied by rationales for correct answers and page-number references to where the content can be found within the textbook
- **Instructor's Manual:** A file for each chapter containing a summary, learning goals, key terms, a detailed chapter outline, and discussion questions
- **Image Collection:** All the textbook's artwork and tables reproduced online for download into PowerPoint or other presentations
- **PowerPoint Presentations:** Approximately 35 slides per chapter containing a mixture of text and images to assist in classroom lecture
- **Animations:** High-quality, three-dimensional animations of the anatomy and physiology of the various body systems, along with musculoskeletal and orthopedic conditions and injuries

For the Student

- **Illustrated Case Studies:** 15 written scenarios with accompanying photographs and follow-up questions for further realistic practice situations in athletic training diagnosis and management
- **Self-Test Questions:** Approximately 350 practice questions with instant feedback for examination preparation
- **Glossary Exercises:** Chapter key terminology in the form of a game of hangman for fun and interactive practice
- **Labeling Exercises:** Key illustrations from the book's four anatomy chapters presented in the form of a drag-and-drop labeling exercise
- **Anatomical Video Clips:** Segments from a series of dissections on fresh cadavers highlighting key areas of athletic injury, such as the knee and shoulder
- **Internet Assignments:** Exercises that require online research to introduce students to the growing body of literature in athletic training
- **Quick-Reference Card:** The HIPS/HOPS summary located inside the book's cover is reproduced on the website as a printable PDF file for easy use on the go.

We hope you find in this textbook all of the information and resources you need to instruct students entering the new era of athletic training!

Nancy H. Cummings
Sue Stanley-Green
Paul Higgs

Preface to the Student

Perspectives in Athletic Training was written for you! As the profession of athletic training evolves, so do you, the learner. This textbook centers on the specific needs of today's learner. From studying this textbook, you will obtain a keen understanding of the profession of athletic training and the various roles and settings to explore for employment. Because *Perspectives in Athletic Training* uses a conversational writing style focusing on a whole-body approach to both evaluating and managing injuries and illnesses, you walk away with a unique and practical skill set—the ability to think critically and problem-solve in real-world situations that athletic trainers commonly face. Embedded within the book are multiple instructional strategies that enable you to acquire the foundational knowledge necessary to become a competent and successful athletic trainer.

To optimize your learning, engage yourself in all the activities within each chapter. For example, read the *Opening Scenario* and spend some time to really consider how you would respond. After finishing the chapter, compare your answer with the information provided in *Revisiting the Opening Scenario*. How did the answers compare? How did they differ? Why did they differ? Challenge yourself to elevate your own thinking to the next level with the resources we provide. You will find not only the content in each chapter but the tables, boxes, illustrations, and *Points to Ponder* to be so valuable you will want to keep this book as a reference source for years to come!

Nancy H. Cummings
Sue Stanley-Green
Paul Higgs

- **Opening Scenarios** present realistic situations that help set the stage and provide relevance to the chapter content.
- **Chapter Summary** sections bring closure and help highlight the key concepts presented, serving as a check to help you ascertain whether you have grasped the content.
- **Revisiting the Opening Scenario** at the end of the chapter provides differential diagnosis and related information to demonstrate the way in which a competent athletic trainer might handle that particular case.

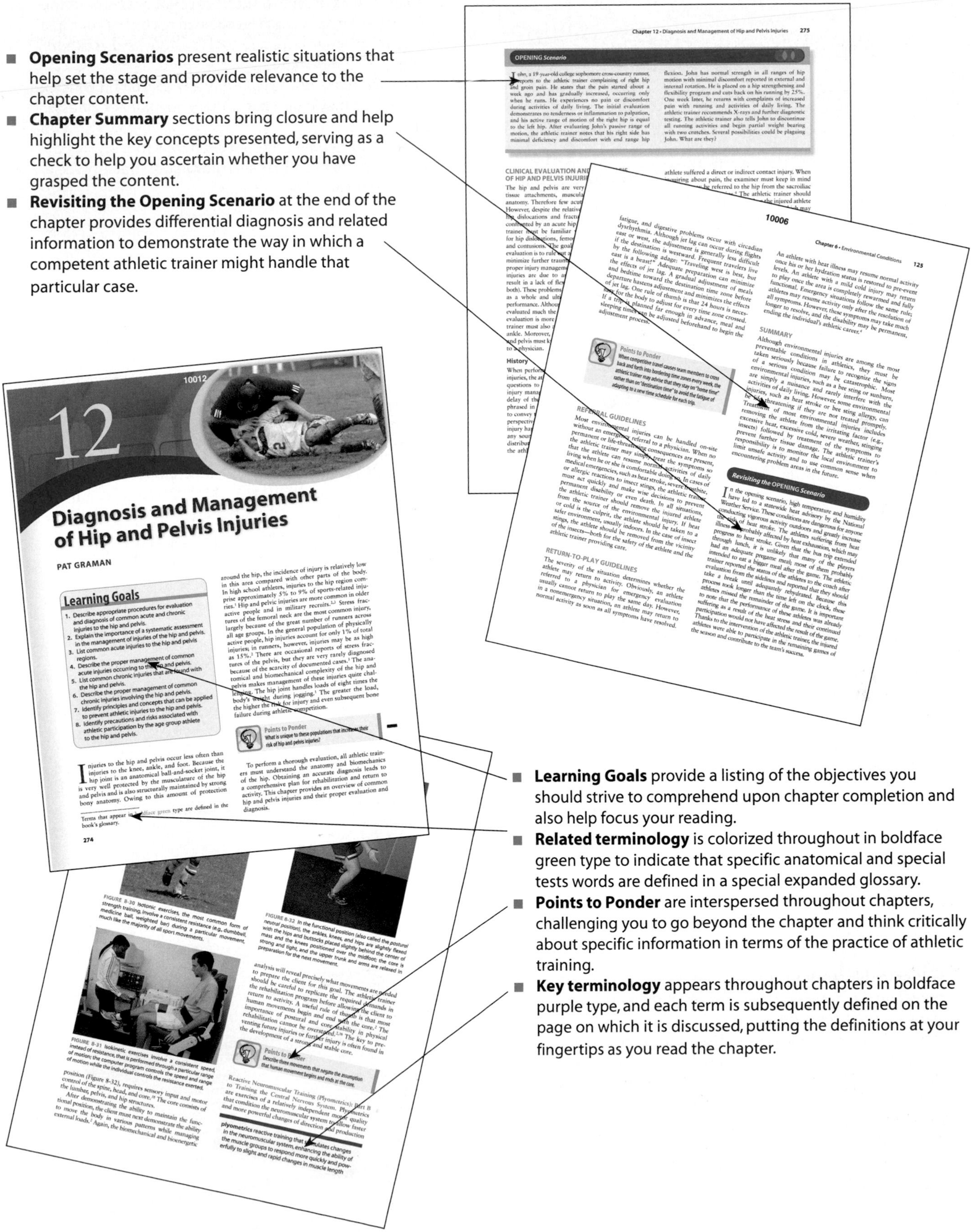

- **Learning Goals** provide a listing of the objectives you should strive to comprehend upon chapter completion and also help focus your reading.
- **Related terminology** is colorized throughout in boldface green type to indicate that specific anatomical and special tests words are defined in a special expanded glossary.
- **Points to Ponder** are interspersed throughout chapters, challenging you to go beyond the chapter and think critically about specific information in terms of the practice of athletic training.
- **Key terminology** appears throughout chapters in boldface purple type, and each term is subsequently defined on the page on which it is discussed, putting the definitions at your fingertips as you read the chapter.

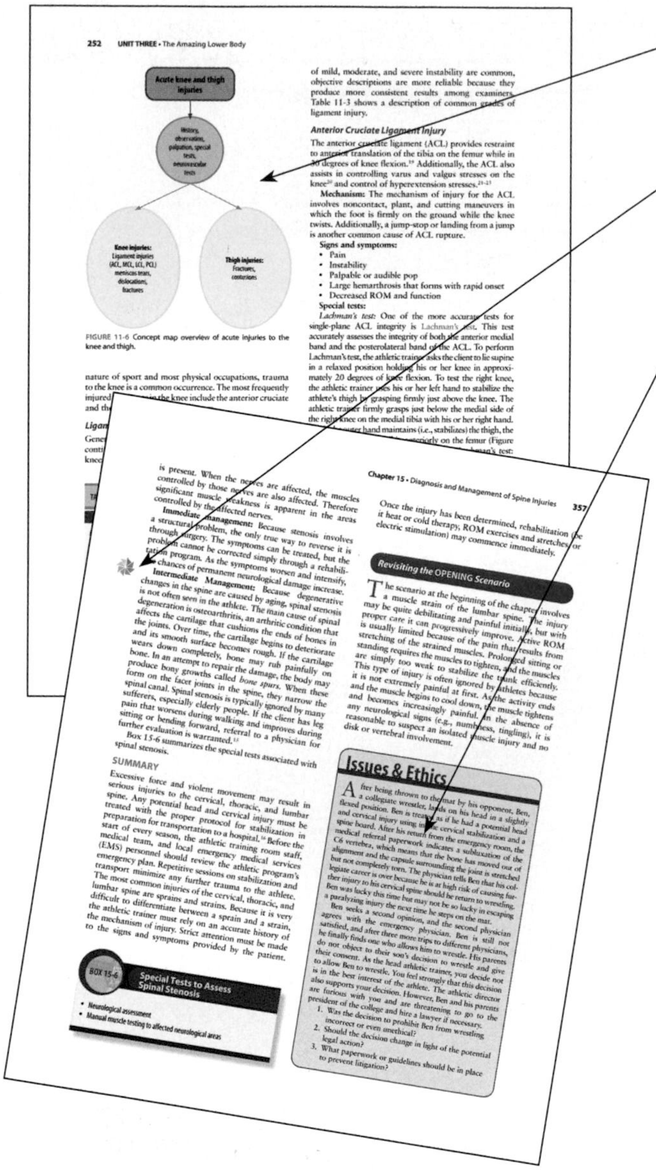

- **Concept maps** provide a succinct visual overview of the main issues and concepts involved in each chapter topic, providing another summary tool for study and content mastery.
- **Age group icons** quickly identify any content in which an athlete's age may play a part in how an injury or illness is managed.
- **Issues & Ethics** boxes present situations that involve the types of ethical dilemmas and gray issues that athletic trainers confront each day.

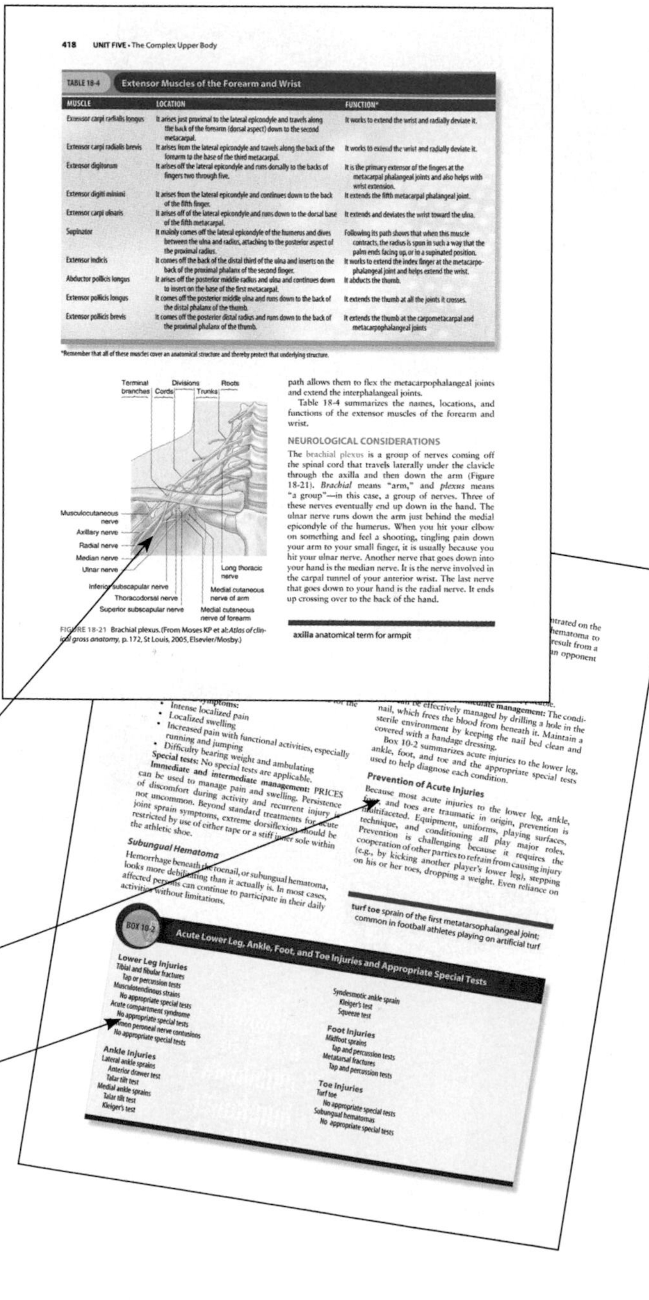

- **Full-color illustrations** supplement the text throughout, providing the necessary visual accompaniment to help clarify difficult concepts.
- **Diagnosis and management discussions** are presented consistently throughout, detailing first the acute and then the chronic injuries, and spelling out for each the mechanism of injury, signs and symptoms, appropriate special tests, and immediate and intermediate care.
- **Summary boxes** within the anatomy and diagnosis and management chapters provide a quick reference to the key areas covered.

Acknowledgments

So many people contributed on various levels to the overall success of this project. We would like to thank Elsevier, first and foremost, for believing in both the concept of the project and in us as authors. Numerous resources were allocated on a "first-time" basis to our textbook and ancillary materials. Thank you for the trust and opportunity that provided the recipe for success for this edition.

Marion Waldman, we must start with your name, as it was with you that this project evolved from discussion to reality. Transitioning with you as an Executive Editor at Elsevier managing our project to Founder of ContentConcepts Publishing, Inc., continuing as a strong editorial presence, you maintained the steady pace and rigor of our work. Through your humor and patience, you successfully guided us down the right path, even though we inadvertently swerved a few times. Thank you for your passion, dedication, and enthusiasm for advancing the profession of athletic training.

The Elsevier team deserves special thanks as well. Kathy Falk, Senior Editor, maintained a watchful eye on the project as it continued to take on new life. Her confidence in the editorial team provided a calming presence during challenging times. Kristin Hebberd, Managing Editor, replaced Marion toward the end of the project. Kristin assumed the daunting task of keeping the book as well as the authors on track. Her keen attention to detail and her cheerful countenance provided wonderful stability to the project. John Casey, Senior Project Manager, propelled the book into its final state. His ability to creatively influence words and visually represent our thoughts took the book to new heights. Reneé Duenow, Senior Book Designer, amazed us with how she could listen to our ideas, see our sketched attempts, and literally transform things into works of art through her handiwork. The cover, concept maps, illustrations, and so much more make this project stand out in a truly unique way. Thank you, all!

Micki Cuppett, Associate Professor and Director of Educational Design and Technology for the College of Medicine at the University of South Florida, tackled the ancillary materials that helped make this project a high-quality, user-friendly tool for both students and instructors. Her passions for technology and instructional strategies combined beautifully to provide very impactful learning experiences for our students. Her ongoing commitment to the profession of athletic training is to be commended!

Thank you to all the contributing authors. Their expertise and shared knowledge will be revered by the students reading their works. The time they invested was definitely well spent, as the next generation of athletic trainers will benefit from their contributions and generosity.

We need to thank Florida Southern College and Georgia College & State University. Our co-workers, students, and athletes allowed us to tape them, pose them, and photograph them. Special thanks to Kathy Benn, Physical Education Program Coordinator, and Lois Webb, Athletics Director, both at Florida Southern College, and to Stan Aldridge, Athletics Director at Georgia College & State University, for granting us the time and resources for completing this project. A note of appreciation to Wayne Koehler, photographer extraordinaire at Florida Southern College, who offered exciting action shots of our athletes; Tracy Green, who captured incredible photographs for the taping and emergency care sections; and to SkyHawk Sports Photography for generously sharing artwork used in the book. Thanks are also extended to former co-workers at the National Training Center, a part of South Lake Hospital, for supporting efforts in the early phases of this project.

Our athletic training students at both schools deserve to be recognized. Their enthusiasm and support of this project has been unwavering. Their questions, comments, and feedback helped tailor the chapters to our true audience—them! Thank you for reading, reviewing, and providing such candid and honest recommendations. Sharon J. Elliott and John R. Bennett stand out, as they lived "on call" throughout this project and contributed countless hours in the acquisition of figures, illustrations, and resources and also provided feedback on most chapters.

Collectively, we represent diversity in our own areas of expertise, professional backgrounds, courses taught, teaching styles, passions, and interests. In the midst of this great diversity, common ground was always found—the need to improve the learning experiences of our students. Embracing this desire to provide a quality tool for our students to use, new friendships were fostered and old ones were strengthened. As the book evolves and our students move on, may we never lose sight of how precious we all are.

Nancy H. Cummings
Sue Stanley-Green
Paul Higgs

Contents

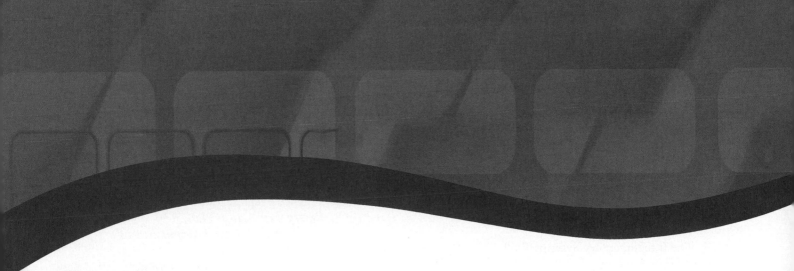

PERSPECTIVES IN

Athletic Training

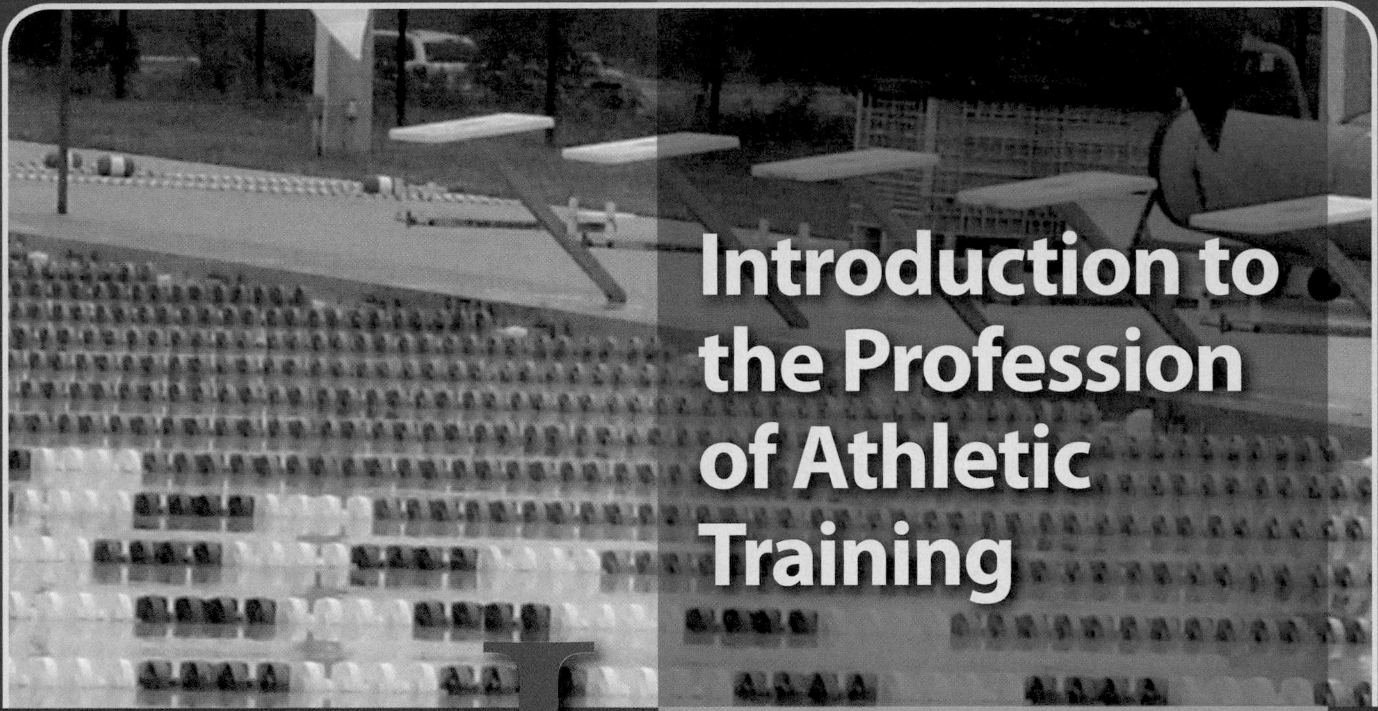

Introduction to the Profession of Athletic Training

UNIT ONE I

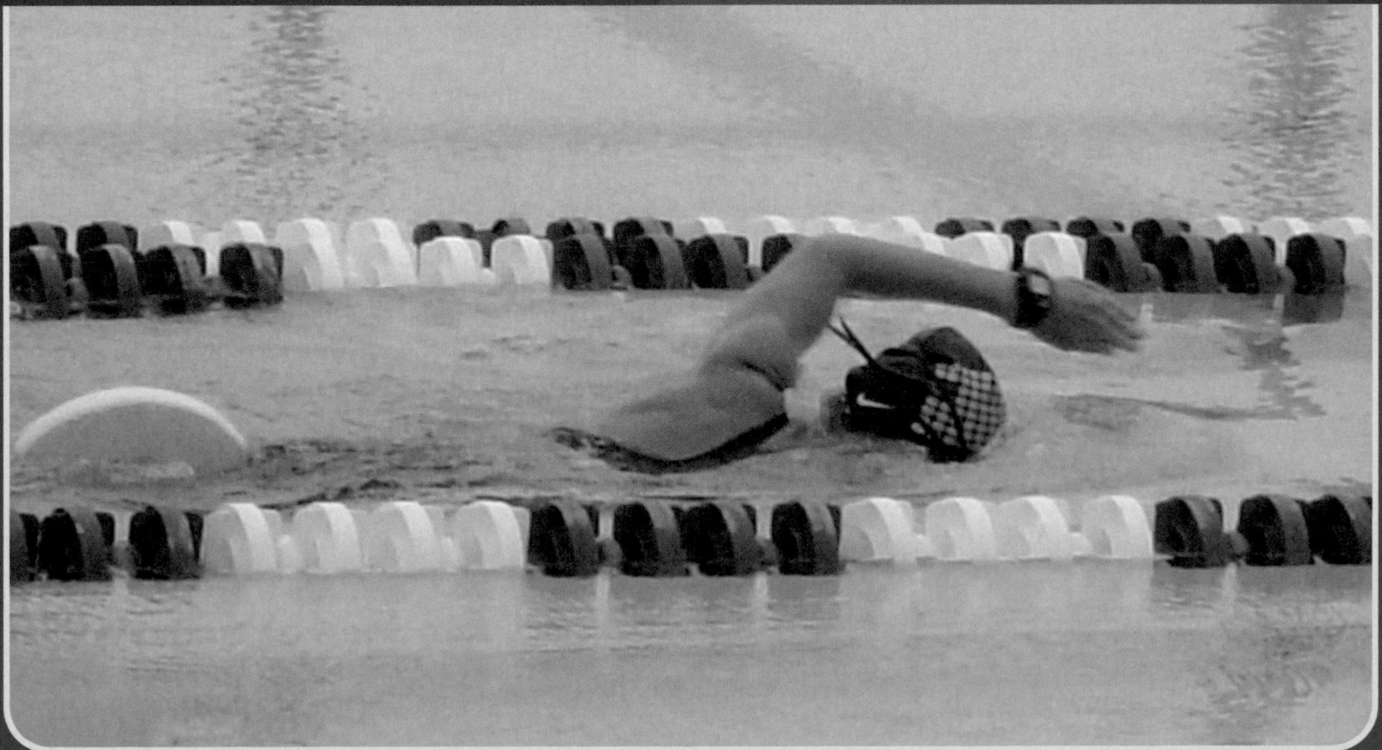

1

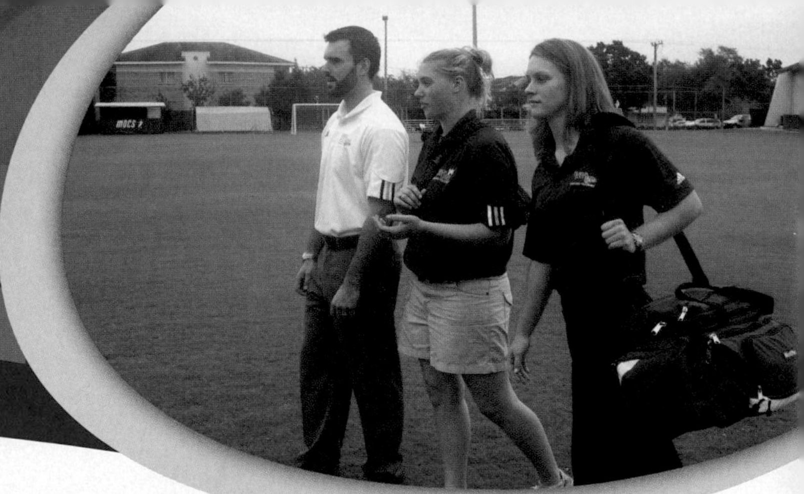

Welcome to the Field

NANCY H. CUMMINGS, SUE STANLEY-GREEN, AND DENISE FANDEL

Learning Goals

1. Describe the roles and responsibilities of an athletic trainer.
2. Identify various career opportunities that are of interest within the scope of the athletic training profession.
3. Discuss the educational process required to become an athletic trainer.
4. Explain the responsibilities of the various agencies associated with different aspects of the athletic training profession.
5. Describe the role of continuing education in the profession of athletic training.
6. Understand the importance of research in the field of athletic training.

Athletic training is a rewarding and exciting profession, with a variety of employment settings. You could be working in an outpatient clinical setting, at a high school or college, on-site with a major corporation, or in your own business. More athletic trainers are graduating and finding opportunities outside of the traditional settings. The athletic trainers of previous years who dreamed of working for the "pros" have been replaced with those who value freedom and flexibility. Graduates are able to consider multiple work settings other than high schools, colleges, and professional sports leagues.

Who would have thought an athletic trainer would be in the pit of a NASCAR race or in the ring with an angry, charging bull? Who could have thought that athletic trainers would be working around the clock to rehabilitate and recondition astronauts before a mission to the space station? Could you have imagined an athletic trainer assisting in surgery or managing a physician's office? When did we dare to think that an athletic trainer could be on the battlefields with our troops helping to maintain the peak condition of their bodies? Did you ever think an athletic trainer could have his or her own business helping athletes regain elite levels of fitness and function?

Daily routines are also diverse and depend on your work setting. Some athletic trainers work evenings and weekends, some work a typical workday schedule similar to that of most professions, and others commit to work hours that vary dramatically according to the sport or season. Similarly, the populations and communities that you serve will change depending on where you work. You may be working with mostly older athletes participating in senior games or competing in the Master's championships, you may be employed in a factory with hundreds of workers, or you may work in a college setting with many student athletes. The athletic trainers that have come before you have forged many different paths and given you numerous options to consider.

Your hours will differ dramatically from those of your athletic trainer friends who have chosen a direction that is different from yours. Travel schedules can either attract you to a specific job or drive you away. Do you need the certainty of a set schedule? Does the excitement of constant change and different locales appeal to you? You could ask 10 athletic trainers what they do for a living, and you will most likely get ten different responses. All of their answers, though, will have several things in common. The following are some of

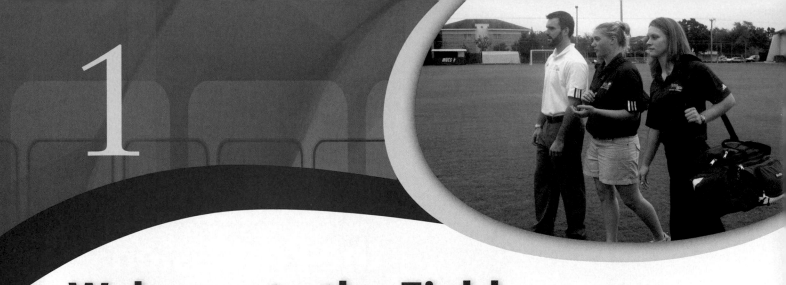

OPENING *Scenario*

Years of taking classes, writing papers, and taping body parts has finally found you rushing to your mailbox. You are anxiously waiting for a letter, any letter, to come back with a job offer inside. Looking back at your clinical rotations, you find that you really enjoyed the clinical outpatient setting as well as the collegiate environment. So, you applied for four jobs, two in each setting. All four of the jobs are in different parts of the country. Any of these locations would, in your view, be a great change of pace. Knowing that you are possibly moving out of state for this job, you should give serious consideration to your professional credentialing and relevant local regulations.

When you see that there is no offer letter in the mail today, you begin to reminisce about your football experiences at the university. One injury in particular stood out because it occurred during the play-off game just this year. The center went down on a snap unexpectedly. After what seemed like an eternity, the shouts from the crowd tapered off and a quiet hush descended as everyone realized that the center was not getting up anytime soon. He was obviously hurt and in a tremendous amount of pain. You remember the grimace on his face. His teammates frantically gathered around him. From the sidelines, you carried the appropriate medical supplies and sprinted out onto the field. After asking his teammates to give him some space, you began to talk with the center and move his leg in various directions. What incredible pressure you were feeling at that moment with the whole audience watching! Good thing the game was not on television that week! You remember one of the coaches reminding you that he had a tryout with a professional football team after the season, which seemed inappropriate given the seriousness of the center's injuries. An all-too-familiar situation arose as you remembered that the coach and the athlete did not agree as to whether he could play the rest of that game. The pressure of an NFL tryout is huge, and the center would need to be healthy for that weekend. Winning the play-off game was just as important for the school and the coach. Do you potentially sacrifice the center's future career for the game today? What would you do in this situation?

the athletic trainer's responsibilities that are common to all settings:

- They are involved in the prevention of injuries. Many times, athletic trainers are intimately involved in the strength and conditioning programs of teams and also in preshift stretching and warm-up routines in various work settings (Figure 1-1).[1,2]
- They perform **evaluation** and **diagnosis** of injuries as well as design rehabilitation programs combining **therapeutic exercises** and **therapeutic modalities.**
- They educate athletes, clients, and patients in ways to safely and properly return to their pre-injured status and previous activities (Figure 1-2).
- They educate various populations in ways to prevent future injuries of a similar nature.

evaluation a systematic process that enables the athletic trainer to determine what is wrong with the injured person

diagnosis the end result of the evaluation specifically identifying the exact cause of the injury or illness

therapeutic exercises exercises that are used in a preventive or prescriptive manner to either prevent injury or to rehabilitate an injured athlete

therapeutic modalities any type of device, mechanical or manual, that aids in the healing process of an injury or illness

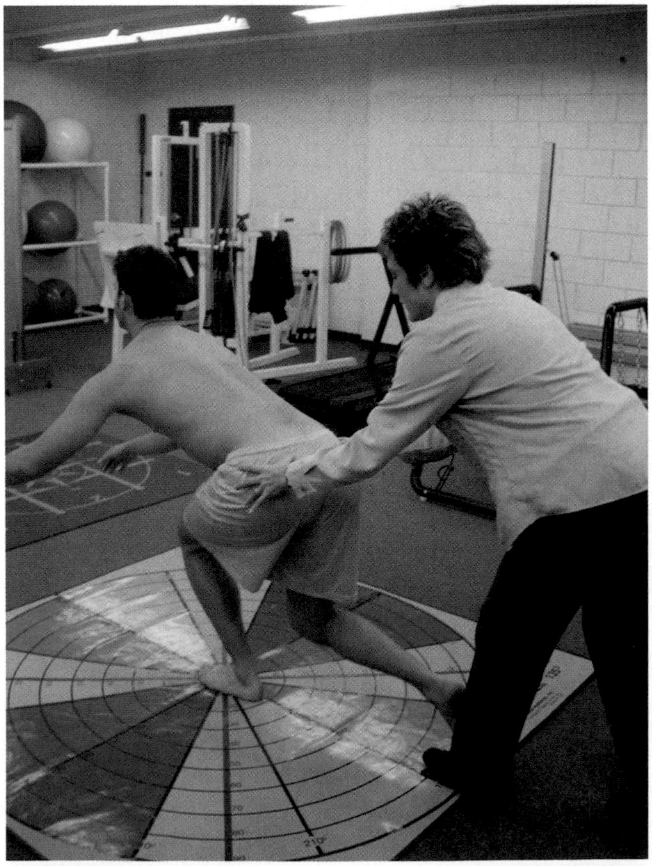

FIGURE 1-1 All athletic trainers are involved in injury management, which includes the design and execution of strength and conditioning, warm-up, and stretching routines.

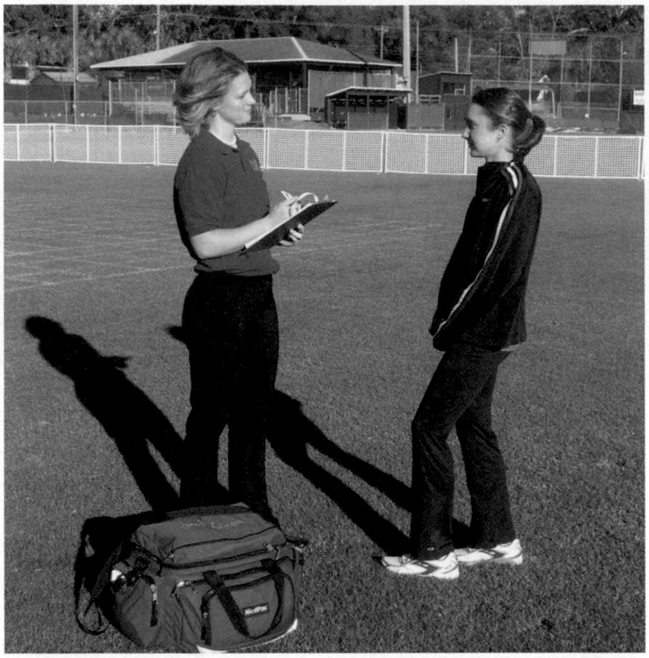

FIGURE 1-2 Another aspect of injury management and return to activity in athletic training is education—of athletes, clients, patients, and various other populations.

All of the preceding responsibilities allow us to be involved in **injury management.** But is that all we do? And where do all of these injured people come from? Athletic trainers work only with athletes, right? Look at the athletic training career decisions concept map in Figure 1-3. Starting in the middle of the figure, work your way around the map. Spend some time evaluating your responses to each of these topics. Where do you see yourself in your first job after you graduate and pass the Board of Certification Exam?

Points to Ponder
I prefer to be inside (or outside) most of the day. What workplace setting(s) would allow me this freedom?

DEFINING AN ATHLETIC TRAINER

According to the U.S. Department of Labor, the American Medical Association (AMA), and the National Athletic Trainers Association (NATA), the national membership organization for athletic trainers, an athletic trainer is an allied health care professional with primary practice areas in physical medicine and rehabilitation.[1] Athletic trainers work diligently to gain specialized skills to care for various populations with acute and chronic injuries and illnesses. These skill sets are used to help manage and rehabilitate injured people whose populations can be found in myriad settings: elementary schools, secondary schools, and colleges; factories and industrial settings; research institutions; outpatient and inpatient rehabilitation clinics and hospitals; physician's offices and operating rooms; Olympic training facilities; military posts; and professional sports venues. Most athletic trainers still work in the traditional settings, such as schools, colleges, and professional sport teams. However, the innovative, entrepreneurial athletic trainer of today is finding it quite rewarding to step outside of the box and create his or her own niche setting (Figure 1-4). As an athletic training student, you should seek experiences in as many settings as you can. The diversity of your clinical education will help determine the direction of your career path.

THE EDUCATIONAL PROCESS

Before you consider the vast number of career opportunities available to the athletic trainer, you should start at the beginning: How do you become an athletic trainer? Athletic trainers must hold at least a bachelor's degree from a university or college accredited by the Commission on Accreditation of Athletic Training Education (CAATE)[3] CAATE has established standards that define the educational experiences and requirements of all entry-level athletic training educational programs. The ultimate goal is to ensure that the student is competent to enter the workforce after graduation. Of interest to most parents, athletes, and coaches is the fact that over two thirds of all athletic trainers today have obtained some form of advanced degree.[1]

The undergraduate athletic training education programs are designed to provide specialized knowledge and training in the prevention, assessment, treatment, and rehabilitation of injuries and illnesses. These areas of knowledge are set by the NATA Educational Council and are called *educational competencies*[4] (Box 1-1). Clinical proficiencies are also a part of the accredited undergraduate curriculum and are the experiential component supporting the competencies. The competencies and proficiencies combine to help guide the educational experience.

Pursuing graduate and doctorate programs in athletic training, education, or other related fields allows the student to expand on specific areas addressed in the undergraduate programs. Some students may want to focus their work on the application of modalities (e.g., ultrasound, lasers, cryotherapy) and wound healing, some may want to focus on rehabilitation techniques and outcome studies, and others may prefer to focus their advanced training on areas such as hydration and heat illness. Still other students may choose

injury management a comprehensive approach to providing care to an individual that includes immediate care and treatment of the current injury while providing pertinent education to prevent further or future injuries from occurring

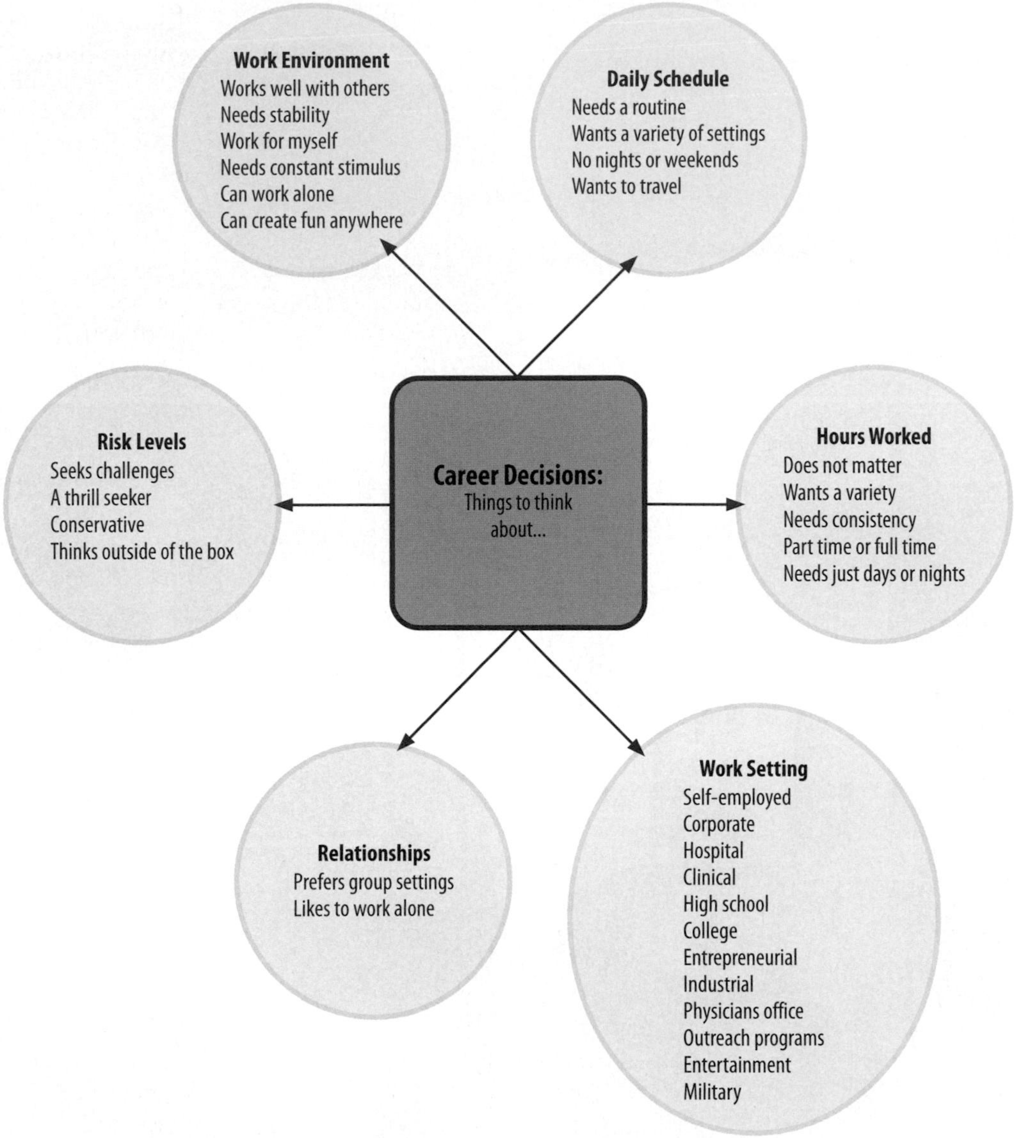

FIGURE 1-3 Athletic training career decisions concept map.

to concentrate on pedagogical, research-oriented areas such as curriculum planning and instructional strategies. These are but a few examples of the many choices athletic training students may make during their graduate studies.

Yet another alternative you have in becoming an athletic trainer is to graduate from an entry-level master's degree program. In these programs, your athletic training studies actually begin in your graduate-level coursework. Regardless of which type of educational program you select, the basic tenets or competencies that each program covers will be the same.

Certification

Once you, the athletic training student, have graduated from a CAATE-accredited undergraduate athletic training education program and meet all requirements

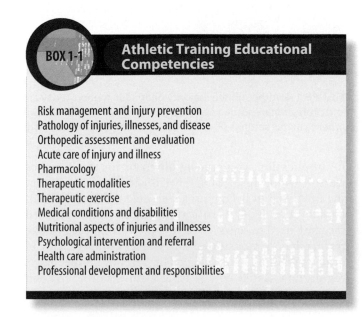

BOX 1-1 Athletic Training Educational Competencies

- Risk management and injury prevention
- Pathology of injuries, illnesses, and disease
- Orthopedic assessment and evaluation
- Acute care of injury and illness
- Pharmacology
- Therapeutic modalities
- Therapeutic exercise
- Medical conditions and disabilities
- Nutritional aspects of injuries and illnesses
- Psychological intervention and referral
- Health care administration
- Professional development and responsibilities

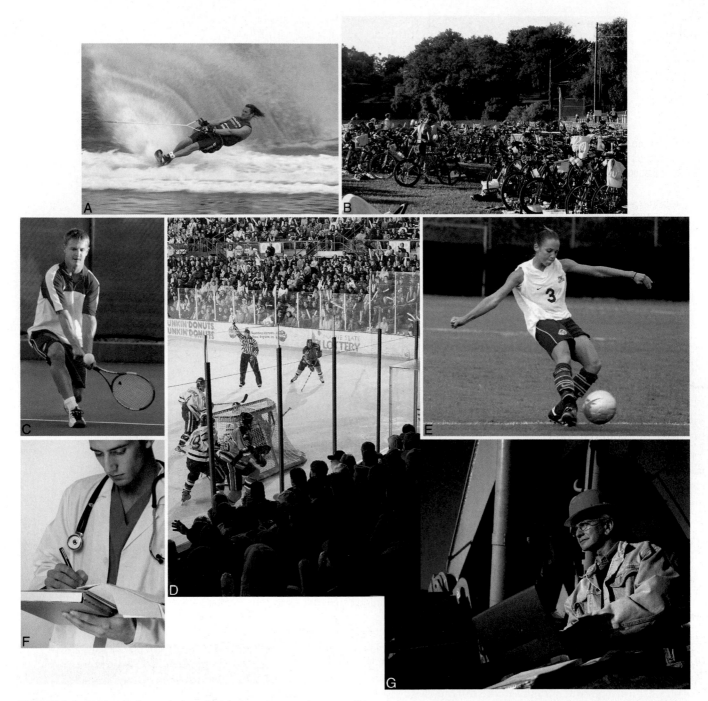

FIGURE 1-4 Although the majority of athletic trainers today are still employed in traditional settings such as in colleges, high schools, and professional sporting venues (**A-D**), as the profession continues to evolve, more athletic trainers are seeking employment in various other dynamic settings (**F, G**). (**F, G,** Copyright 2007 JupiterImages Corporation.)

for application, you are eligible to sit for the Board of Certification, Inc. (BOC) certification examination, the next step in becoming a Certified Athletic Trainer. Passing the BOC certification exam is a standard measure used to represent to the public that the athletic trainer has demonstrated entry-level competencies in athletic training knowledge. This level of knowledge is regularly assessed with a Role Delineation Study—in essence, an analysis of what practicing athletic trainers really do.[4] This analysis results in professional domains that are then used as a blueprint for developing the exam (Box 1-2).

Thus a check and balance has been established to make sure the tasks that working athletic trainers really perform are assessed and incorporated into the undergraduate curriculum. This ensures that beginning athletic trainers are educated and trained in the requisite content.

TABLE 1-1 **Forms of Athletic Training Regulation**

TYPE OF REGULATION	CHARACTERISTICS REQUIRED	VOLUNTARY	TITLE PROTECTION	SCOPE OF PRACTICE	STANDARDS OF PRACTICE	INDIVIDUAL OR INSTITUTIONAL	BENEFICIARIES OF REGULATION
Licensure	✓		✓	✓		Individual	Public
Certification	*		*		*	Individual	Public and profession
Registration	✓		?			Individual	Public and profession
Accreditation	✓	✓				Institution	Student

* States can use "certification" as a level of regulation.

State laws govern the practice standards and acts for health care professionals. **Regulation** pertaining to the practice of athletic training currently exists in almost every state in this country. The purpose of regulatory agencies is to license, certify, and discipline health care professions. This process helps to ensure that athletic trainers are practicing according to the letter and intent of the law and upholding requisite standards to achieve the highest quality of health care. It is the responsibility of the athletic trainer to learn the specific laws of his or her state because such legislation varies dramatically across the country. Table 1-1 summarizes the various types of regulations.

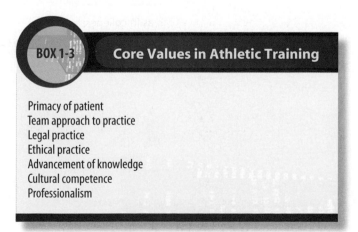

BOX 1-2 **Athletic Training Domains**

- Prevention
- Clinical evaluation and diagnosis
- Immediate care
- Treatment, rehabilitation, and reconditioning
- Organization and administration
- Professional responsibility

BOX 1-3 **Core Values in Athletic Training**

- Primacy of patient
- Team approach to practice
- Legal practice
- Ethical practice
- Advancement of knowledge
- Cultural competence
- Professionalism

Along with the athletic training educational competencies, core values have been defined to help elevate the standards and daily practices of the athletic trainer. Box 1-3 lists these core values that provide a foundational model and guide for every athletic trainer to emulate in their daily practice. To round out all of these foundational principles, the NATA has also established a Code of Ethics (Appendix A),[5] and the Board of Certification has defined the Standards of Practice (Appendix B),[6] which all certified athletic trainers must respect and follow. Taking the time to review these documents, which represent the foundation of our profession, will help you in your quest to become a great athletic trainer.

Points to Ponder

What agency do you contact to find out how you can enter the next exciting phase of your career as you transition from a student to a full-time athletic trainer? What will you have to do to maintain your certification in your new setting?

Continuing education is the ongoing pursuit of professional knowledge that is both current and timely in nature. As the field advances, the need for lifelong professional training becomes obvious. Upon certification, athletic trainers are expected to regularly seek educational growth opportunities throughout their careers. These opportunities are required to assure consumers that their athletic trainers maintain an ongoing commitment to the practice of athletic training. Box 1-4 provides examples of continuing education opportunities. The Board of Certification requires documentation of ongoing continuing competency, or continuing education that assists the athletic trainer in their professional growth and development, while ensuring a level of general knowledge common to all

regulation a process that provides laws to define expected professional behaviors as well as methods to address unacceptable behaviors

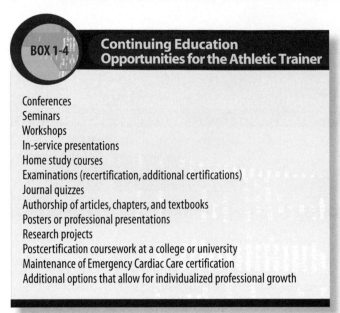

BOX 1-4 Continuing Education Opportunities for the Athletic Trainer

Conferences
Seminars
Workshops
In-service presentations
Home study courses
Examinations (recertification, additional certifications)
Journal quizzes
Authorship of articles, chapters, and textbooks
Posters or professional presentations
Research projects
Postcertification coursework at a college or university
Maintenance of Emergency Cardiac Care certification
Additional options that allow for individualized professional growth

athletic trainers. According to the Board of Certification,[7] continuing education serves the following purposes:

- Learn current information relevant to the field.
- Explore and acquire new knowledge in various content areas.
- Master new professional skills and techniques.
- Expand on effective known practices in the field.
- Enhance professional decision making and judgment abilities.
- Implement and abide by the Code of Ethics and Standards of Practice.

As previously discussed, several organizations are involved in the process of becoming a certified athletic trainer (ATC) and maintaining your credential as a certified athletic trainer. Three professional organizations that most athletic trainers will confront during some point in their careers are the NATA, the BOC, and CAATE. Each of the following organizations has a unique mission or focus establishing the need for their involvement in your professional life:

1. The mission of the NATA is to enhance the quality of health care provided by certified athletic trainers and to advance the athletic training profession.[8]
2. The mission of the BOC is to certify athletic trainers and, through a system of certification, adjudication, standards of practice and continuing competency programs, to identify for the public quality health care professionals.[9]
3. The mission of the CAATE is to provide accreditation services to institutions that house athletic training degree programs and verify that all accredited programs meet the minimal acceptable educational standards for entry-level athletic trainer education.[10]

Together, they provide the broadest service and protection to athletic trainers, the public, and our profession as a whole. Table 1-2 lists the primary responsibilities of each of these organizations.

DIVERSITY WITHIN THE PROFESSION

Of the more than 30,000 members in the NATA, the vast majority are certified athletic trainers, with most holding master's-level and terminal degrees.[1] Our profession sees a fairly even representation of men and women. Athletic trainers can now be found in so many different work venues that it is quite difficult to track and define all of the new and prospering settings. Globally, athletic trainers are experiencing incredible career opportunities in Asia, Europe, Canada, and Africa. The World Federation of Athletic Training and Therapy was

TABLE 1-2 Professional Responsibilities of Each Organization

PROGRAMS AND AREAS OF RESPONSIBILITY	BOC	CAATE	NATA
Exam eligibility	✓		
Exam development	✓		
Exam administration	✓		
Professional practice/discipline	✓		
Standards of professional practice	✓		
State regulation	✓		✓
Accreditation site visits		✓	
Accreditation standards and guidelines		✓	
Accreditation recommendations		✓	
Training and evaluation of site visitors		✓	
Educational competencies		✓	✓
Code of ethics			✓
Membership			✓
Advanced graduate education			✓

BOC, Board of Certification; *CAATE,* Commission on Accreditation of Athletic Training Education; *NATA,* National Athletic Trainers' Association.

established to support international athletic trainers in their endeavors around the world. Other professional settings are allowing the athletic trainer to organize to help prevent and treat injuries. Wherever there are athletes, industrial jobs, colleges, or military posts, the athletic trainer has the opportunity to find employment.

Numerous professional groups (e.g., the American Academy of Orthopedic Surgeons, American Academy of Pediatrics, National Federation of State High School Activities Associations, and the President's Council on Physical Fitness) have partnered with the NATA to promote the effectiveness of athletic trainers within their respective settings. Several position statements and consensus statements have been created from these collaborative partnerships. For example, two important consensus statements resulting from these joint ventures are "Appropriate Medical Care for Secondary School-Age Athletes" and "Prehospital Care of the Spine-Injured Athlete." Everyone recognizes the need for appropriate and timely care. However, these dedicated organizations have taken their commitment to the next level and aligned themselves with not only the NATA but others who share a common goal: to both prevent injury and subsequently rehabilitate the injured person as quickly and safely as possible. Keeping people healthy and active is what this profession is all about.

TODAY'S SPORTS MEDICINE TEAM

The sports medicine team of today looks markedly different than it did 50 years ago and even 10 years ago. The efficient yet small and intimate team used to consist of the team physician, the athletic trainer, the equipment manager, the coach, and possibly the parents. As we have diversified and new medical subspecialties have evolved, the need to enlarge our team and recruit additional members from other areas of expertise has become more apparent with each event that we cover.

Key contributors that represent the cornerstone of our sports medicine team still include the coach, athletic trainers, medical doctors, orthopedic surgeons, physician assistants, emergency medical personnel, physical therapists, nutritionists, psychologists, and strength and conditioning specialists. The coach assumes the ultimate responsibility for the welfare of his or her athletes. The medical doctor, or team physician, is responsible for the medical decisions and outcomes of the team. Protocols that you as the athletic trainer will follow will be developed and managed by the team physician. The orthopedic surgeon will most often be your resource for musculoskeletal injuries requiring surgical interventions. Nutritionists and psychologists frequently are consulted to round out the team with holistic approaches that address concerns that are more far-reaching than merely the injured body part. The strength and conditioning specialist works to enhance performance outcomes and prevent injuries through appropriate conditioning programs throughout the year.

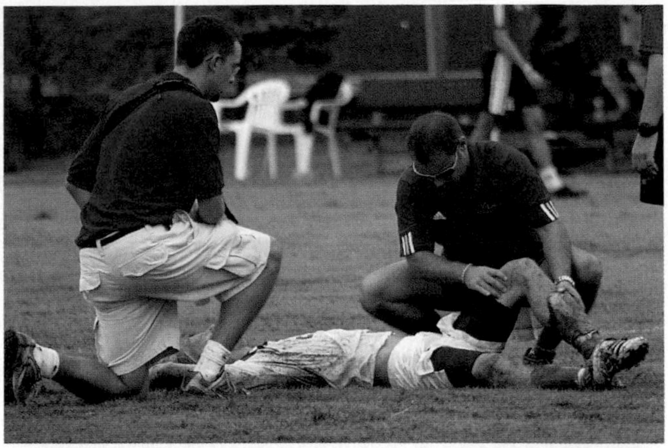

FIGURE 1-5 The small sports medicine team of 50 years ago has grown in size to include not only the physician, athletic trainer, equipment manager, coach, and parents of the athlete (if applicable) but also members of medical subspecialties such as physician assistants and orthopedic surgeons.

Other professionals that might round out the comprehensive sports medicine team of today include a biomechanist, podiatrist, orthotist, exercise physiologist, cardiologist, internist, pharmacologist, radiologist, engineer, computer analyst or programmer, and maybe even an ergonomist, to name a few. These professions bring a diversified perspective to the comprehensive plan of care as well as a unique base of knowledge and a varied span of experiences from which to draw. The team of today is innovative and is always striving to find the answer to the following question: How do we keep people healthy and active so they can perform at their required or desired level of activity without unnecessarily compromising their bodies? Once you define what the particular required or desired level of activity is, you can begin to assemble your appropriate sports medicine team (Figure 1-5).

> **Points to Ponder**
> If you could partner with any organization and create a position statement that would transform the ways in which clients are rehabilitated and reconditioned, what area would you most want to affect positively? Why did you choose this particular area?

ATHLETIC TRAINING RESEARCH

Research in any field is the backbone that keeps the profession abreast of cutting-edge topics, impending issues, and concerns. It modifies or corrects older theories and sometimes puts to rest antiquated ideas. Research seeks to validate what we do by finding specific answers and sharing those findings. We conduct research because there is a burning question that needs to be addressed. It may be in athletic training education, instructional strategies, or curriculum and program

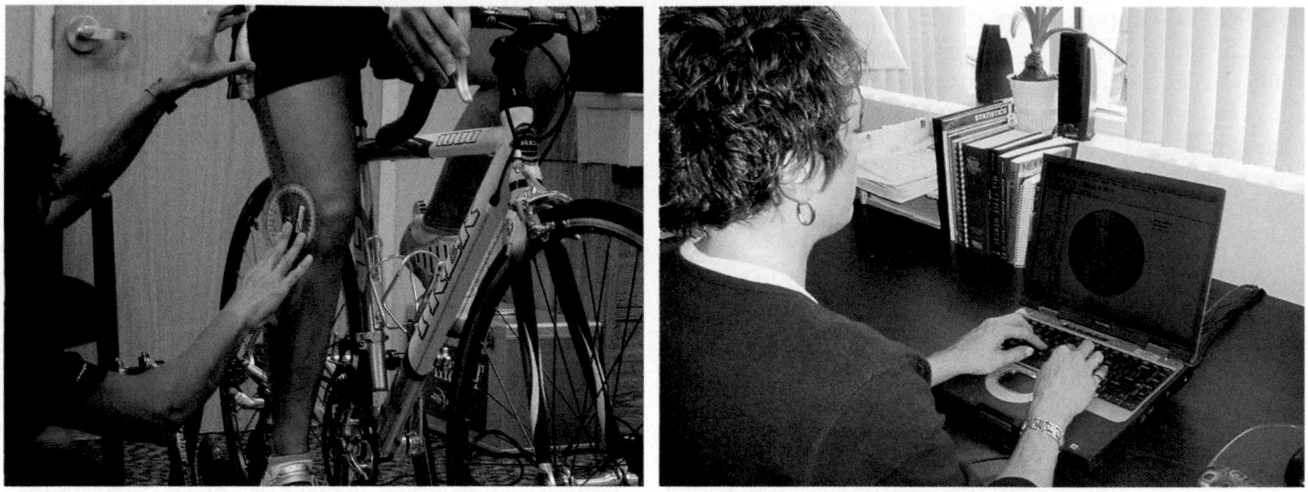

FIGURE 1-6 Research provides the backbone to help advance the profession of athletic training.

design. Concepts related to cellular responses to training; new hydration and recovery strategies; clinical outcomes assessments; and the creation of new products with technologically advanced materials that are lighter, stronger, and heat resistant are all current research projects. Developing safety equipment that can decrease injuries, assist in performance, and allow ongoing activity are exciting paths being forged. Having the forethought to envision a device that could help prevent a common career-ending injury for certain athletes is a welcome development for some athletic trainers. Being part of a multidisciplinary team that helps develop a novel assistive prosthetic device allowing an amputee to walk or run a marathon is even more gratifying.

A focus on relevant research allows the profession of athletic training to continue to move forward (Figure 1-6). Dedicating time and resources to advancing our field—be it through educational studies, patient outcomes, best practices in modalities, or rehabilitation protocols—will only make us better. By pushing the envelope, stepping outside of your comforts zone, and riding this wave of intellectual creativity, you will lay the foundation for your future endeavors.

You may find it difficult to imagine yourself performing research. What does it mean? How do you do it? Who really does research? All of these are great questions. The answers are right in front of you and all around you. Every day, every one of us performs research of some kind, be it anecdotal or empirical. **Anecdotal research** is what you do daily as you watch the ways in which people respond to the new postoperative rotator cuff repair protocol you wrote. You take the time to write the protocol, you have several clients perform the protocol, you monitor their responses, and you determine whether the protocol is effective on the basis of these responses. **Empirical research** follows a strict protocol monitored by an Institutional Review Board (IRB) whose sole purpose is to protect human subjects and patient health information (PHI). A study design delineating research methods such as data collection, data analysis, enrollment and protection of human subjects, and statistical procedures to be employed are required components. The gathering, documenting, analyzing, and presenting of the subjects and data uncovered in the research process should conform to the scientific method. Regardless of the type of research you perform, your goal is to document that what you do is both safe and effective for the population that you serve.

TOMORROW'S ATHLETIC TRAINER

As you ponder your place in the profession of athletic training, you are probably starting to get excited. You are tomorrow's athletic trainer! Where will you be? What will you be doing? With whom will you work? What kind of academic background will you need? Refer to Figure 1-7, and walk through the career decision concept map. Notice that the map has nothing but questions in it. These questions should spark some simple but provocative personal decisions that you will have to make before you find your place in the athletic training profession. Taking the time to think about these options now will help you choose the right career opportunity for you. Keep in mind, though, that your niche as an athletic trainer can be anywhere you want it to be.

SUMMARY

People from all walks of life rely on athletic trainers, whose specialized skills and techniques help clients accomplish their rehabilitation goals and resume their

anecdotal research research that is based on experiences

empirical research research that is based on documented observations and experimental designs

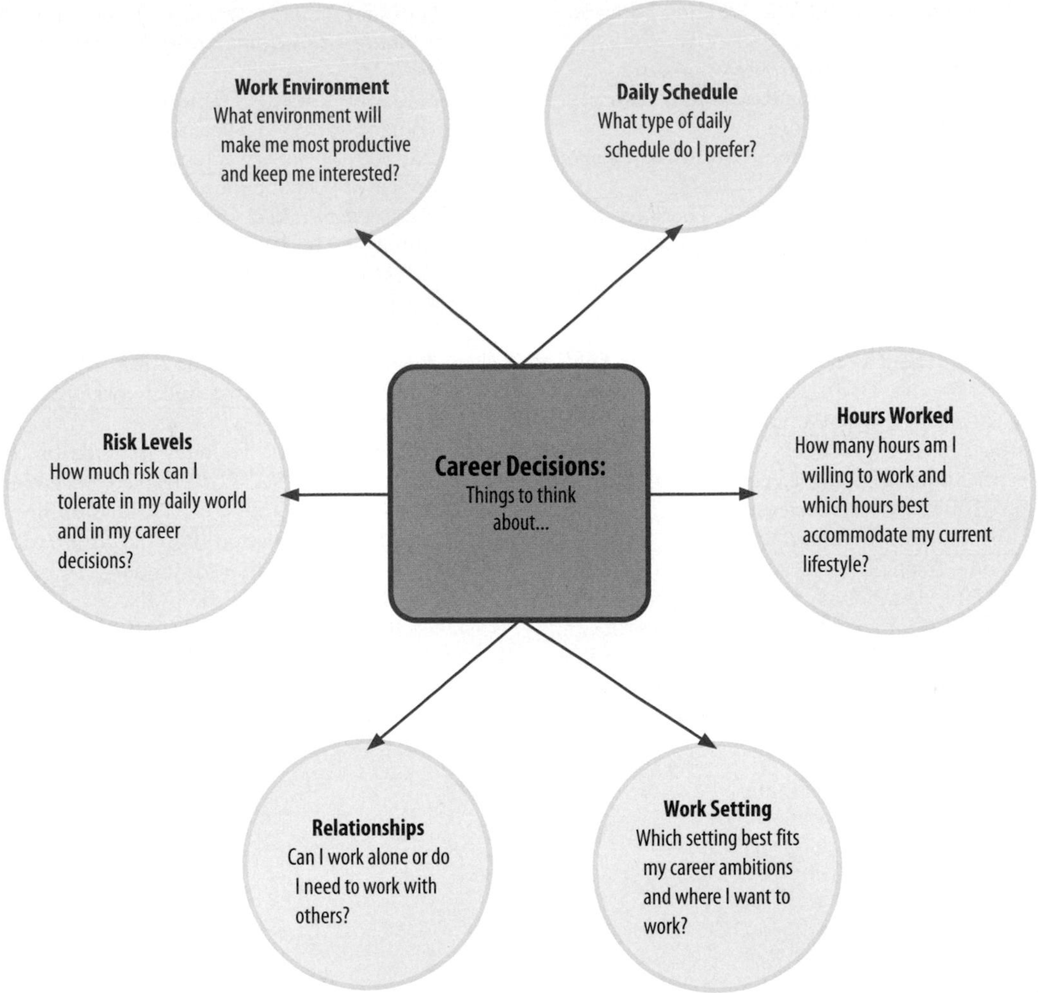

FIGURE 1-7 Personalized athletic training career decision map.

active, healthy lifestyles. Being part of a team that helps other people achieve their goals and dreams is extremely rewarding. Pulling together with the sports medicine team to rehabilitate an injury, return a worker back to the job site, or create a conditioning program that prevents a costly career-ending injury is very gratifying. If you are wondering whether you can do this, wonder no more. You too can become an athletic trainer and have a positive impact on the lives of your clients while pursuing an exciting and fulfilling career. By reading the rest of this textbook, you are taking the first step toward accomplishing your goal of becoming an athletic trainer.

Revisiting the OPENING *Scenario*

The team physician has the final decision as to whether an athlete is capable of returning to play. Once the doctor makes that decision, the coach, athlete, and athletic trainer must respect it. Any actions taken that are in conflict with the medical decision leave the injured athlete in an unfortunate situation. If the athlete sustains another injury or worsens the current injury, not only does he miss his NFL tryout, but also legal actions could be taken against the person or parties who ignored the team physician's advice.

Issues & Ethics

You are torn. It is time to make a decision. Most of your peers are members of the National Athletic Trainers' Association. You know you do not have to be a dues-paying member to practice athletic training. However, there are significant professional advantages in being a member of this organization. What do you do and why?

Web Links

American Medical Association www.ama-assn.org
Athletic Training Education Journal: www.nataej.org
Board of Certification: www.bocatc.org

Commission on Accreditation of Athletic Training Education: www.caate.net
National Athletic Trainers' Association: www.nata.org
National Athletic Trainers' Association Research & Education Foundation: www.natafoundation.org
National Athletic Trainers' Association Education Council: www.nataec.org
World Federation of Athletic Training and Therapy: www.wfatt.org

References

1. National Athletic Trainers' Association (NATA): *Public information documents*, Dallas, 2006, NATA. Retrieved January 25, 2007, from www.nata.org/publicinformation/index.htm.
2. Board of Certification (BOC): *Defining athletic training*, Omaha, Neb, 2004, BOC. Retrieved January 5, 2007, from www.bocatc.org/athtrainer/DEFINE/.
3. Commission on Accreditation of Athletic Training Education (CAATE): *Standards for the accreditation of entry-level athletic training education programs*, Round Rock, Texas, 2005, (updated June 2006), CAATE. Retrieved January 25, 2007, from http://caate.net/ss_docs/standards.6.8.2006.pdf.
4. National Athletic Trainers' Association (NATA): *Athletic training educational competencies*, ed 6, Dallas, 2006, NATA.
5. National Athletic Trainers' Association (NATA): *NATA code of ethics*, Dallas, 2005, NATA, Retrieved January 25, 2007, from www.nata.org/codeofethics/index.htm.
6. Board of Certification (BOC): *BOC standards of professional practice*, Omaha, Neb, 2006, BOC,Retrieved January 25, 2007, from www.bocatc.org/BOCATC_Files/bocweb/_Items/SI-R-TAB4-355/Docs/Stds_of_Practice.PDF.
7. Board of Certification (BOC): 2003–2005 Guidelines & reporting, Omaha, Neb, 2005, BOC. Retrieved January 25, 2007, from www.bocatc.org/atc/Docs/SI-MR-TAB4-153.htm.
8. National Athletic Trainers' Association (NATA): *Mission*, Dallas, 2007, NATA, Retrieved December 7, 2006, from www.nata.org/about_NATA/mission.htm.
9. Board of Certification (BOC): *Our mission*, Omaha, Neb, 2004, BOC, Retrieved January 25, 2007, from www.bocatc.org/aboutus/MISSION.
10. Commission on Accreditation of Athletic Training Education (CAATE): *Mission*, Round Rock, Texas, 2007, CAATE, Retrieved January 25, 2007, from www.caate.net/documents/OverviewDocument-CAATE.pdf.

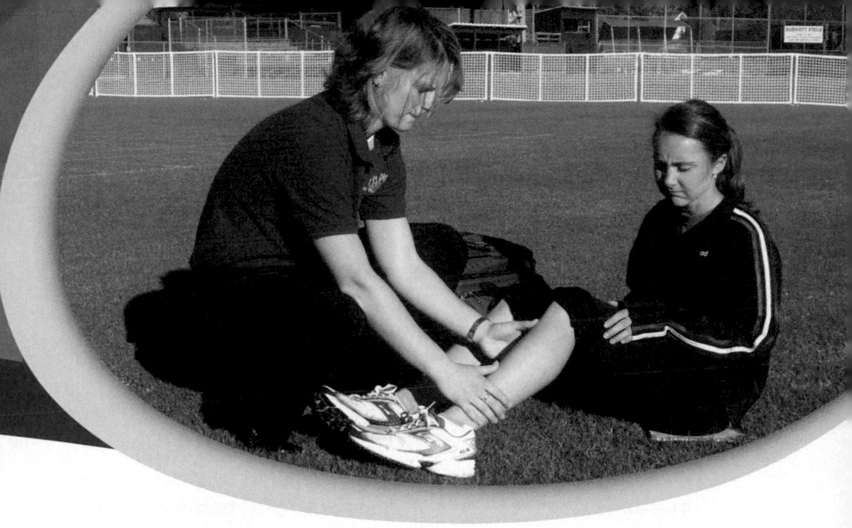

2

Evolution of the Profession

NANCY H. CUMMINGS AND SUE STANLEY-GREEN

Learning Goals

1. Understand and describe athletic training as it existed before the formation of the National Athletic Trainers' Association (NATA).
2. Describe the formation and demise of the first incarnation of NATA.
3. List the significant events that allowed the subsequent formation of the current NATA.
4. Describe how and when women entered the athletic training profession.
5. Identify the relevant historical events leading to the current state of our profession.
6. Describe the rich tradition and legacy of the NATA.

For a true sense of identity, athletic trainers must reflect on both their own origins and those of their profession. The opportunities that athletic trainers enjoy today may be credited to the tireless efforts of their predecessors. Knowing and appreciating this reality is part of the culture of the athletic training profession. This chapter will provide a historical account of the origins of athletic training and how it evolved into today's diverse profession.

HISTORICAL PERSPECTIVES

The ancient Greeks are famous for their athleticism, having founded the games that eventually became our modern Olympics. There are many fascinating stories and fables recounting the accomplishments of these early athletes. There are also stories of the men who cared for these athletes when they were injured. They were call *paidotribes*, or "boy rubbers," which was appropriate in that only male athletes were allowed to compete in the ancient Olympic games. Others were termed *aleittes,* or "anointers," which suggests that massage with oils was an important part of athlete care. The most famous of the ancient Greek athletic trainers was Herodicus of Megara, a physician who studied under Hippocrates.[1]

The athletic training profession began in the late 1800s as sports began to flourish in the colleges and universities around the United States. In 1869, Rutgers and Princeton introduced a new sport called *football.* By 1905, football was associated with so many deaths and serious injuries that President Theodore Roosevelt threatened to abolish it as an intercollegiate sport.[1] Motivated by the president's warning and the welfare of their student athletes, many school administrators realized the need for someone other than the coach to treat the athletes. Schools began seeking people with more medical training to treat their injured athletes (Figure 2-1).

Two brothers, Chuck and Frank Cramer, from Gardner, Kansas, were intrigued by this opportunity and answered the call. These brothers were instrumental in taking the profession of athletic training to the next level. Chuck Cramer was a pharmacist who concocted a liniment for injuries and sore muscles that he sold to various athletic teams. The great Knute Rockne, who coached at Notre Dame from 1918 to 1930, was one of the Cramer brothers' customers. He was convinced that Cramer products would help heal his injured

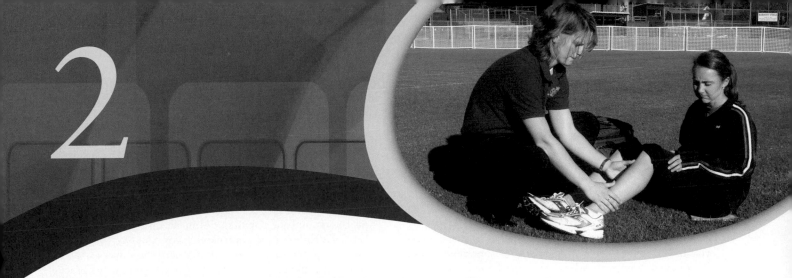

OPENING *Scenario*

Imagine yourself sitting at the front table onstage in a room filled with hundreds of people. Some members of the crowd are family, friends, former athletes, former students, and colleagues. You look around and see people of many generations, representing many work settings. It is hard to believe that you and the profession have evolved this far and this quickly over these past 25 years.

With the realization that this is your retirement dinner, you have recently spent a great deal of time reflecting on your career. Your memories have carried you back to when you sat for the certification exam, accepted your first job, and joined the faculty of the university where you worked for 20 years. Throughout this time, you have witnessed many changes in the profession, changes that have been both sudden and slow. Overall, though, all of the changes have been for the betterment of the profession. You feel fortunate to have been personally involved in many of these changes.

As you approach the podium to address the crowd, one final moment of reflection is warranted. Service to the profession and the communities in which you worked has been the hallmark of your career. You want to impart to the next generation of athletic trainers the same sense of dedication and responsibility. You want them to embrace this legacy and be brave enough to move the National Athletic Trainers' Association and the profession of athletic training to the next level. What is it that you could say to create such a meaningful call to action?

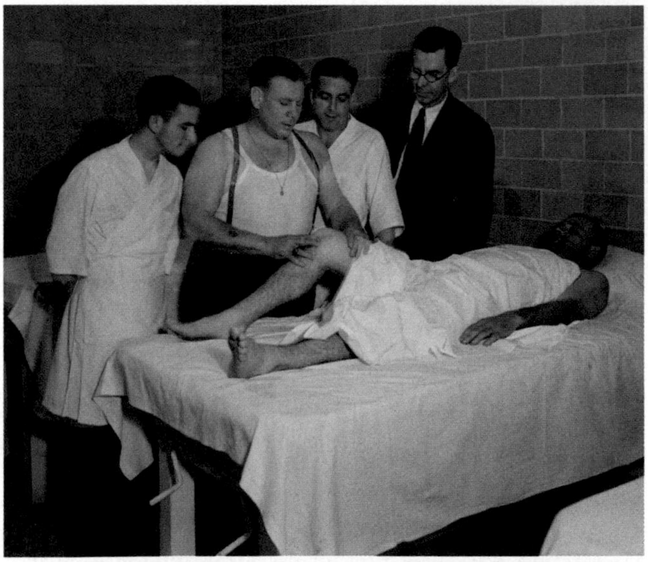

FIGURE 2-1 In the early part of the twentieth century, athletic-related deaths and serious injuries forced college administrators to recognize the need for qualified medical personnel to care for their athletes. (Courtesy Cramer Products Inc., Gardner, Kan.)

athletes. With Rockne's endorsement, the Cramer Chemical products became a hit, and the brothers supplied athletic training supplies all over the country (Figure 2-2).

The Cramer brothers traveled with the U.S. Olympic Team in 1932 and had the opportunity to learn different techniques to care for injured athletes (Figure 2-3). After returning, they shared these new ideas and techniques with their colleagues in workshops and in their publication, ***The First Aider***, which is still produced by Cramer Products, Inc. Over the years, many athletic trainers got their start in this profession by attending a Cramer Workshop or by taking a Cramer Home Study Course[2,3](Figure 2-4).

Although a few textbooks on athletic training began to emerge, most information and new skills were passed on by athletic trainers at sporting events. As they gathered to provide coverage for the events, the athletic trainers would meet and share new ideas and techniques. The first **National Athletic Trainers' Association (NATA)** was formed in 1939. The Drake Relays and the Penn Relays provided the ideal location for the first meetings. Both were large invitational track meets located in two geographical regions of the country.[2] The meetings were held at these large track meets because head athletic trainers traditionally traveled with their track teams to the meets. Shortly after its formation, the NATA had problems with communication and finances.[4] With many of the men leaving

The First Aider a classic athletic training publication written and published by the Cramer brothers after they traveled with the U.S. Olympics Team in 1932 and had the opportunity to learn different techniques to care for injured athletes; still in print today

National Athletic Trainers' Association (NATA) based in Dallas, Texas, the membership association for certified athletic trainers and others who support the athletic training profession

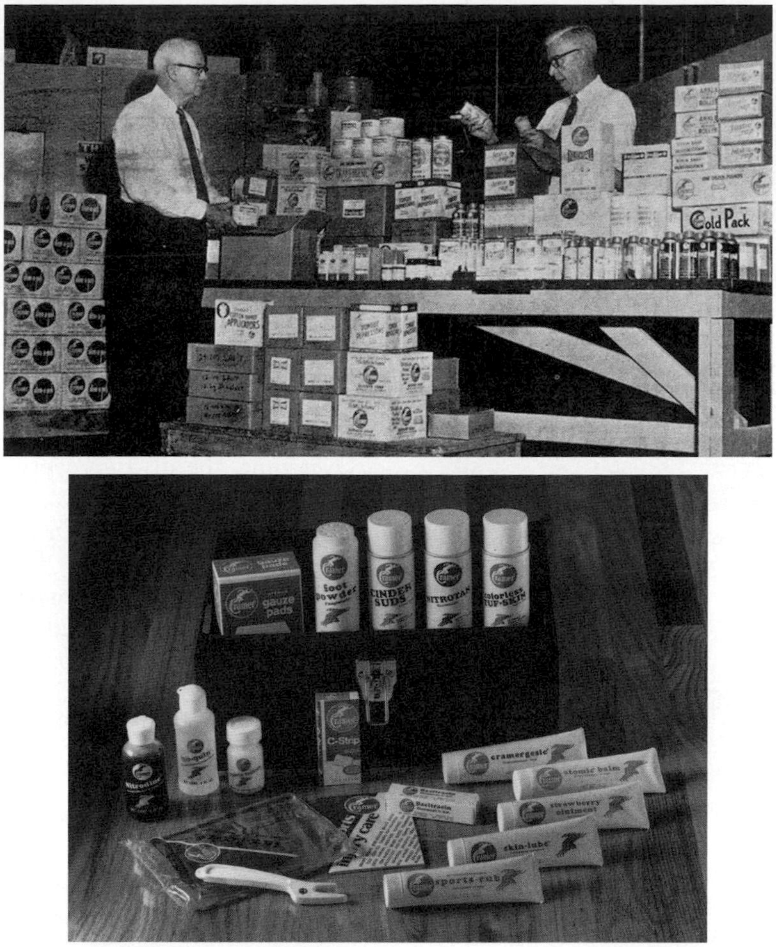

FIGURE 2-2 In the early 1900s, the pharmacist Chuck Cramer concocted a liniment to help heal injuries and sore muscles. It quickly gained popularity with coaches, including well-known Notre Dame coach Knute Rockne, and launched the Cramer Chemical Co., which still operates today as Cramer Products Inc. (Courtesy Cramer Products Inc., Gardner, Kan.)

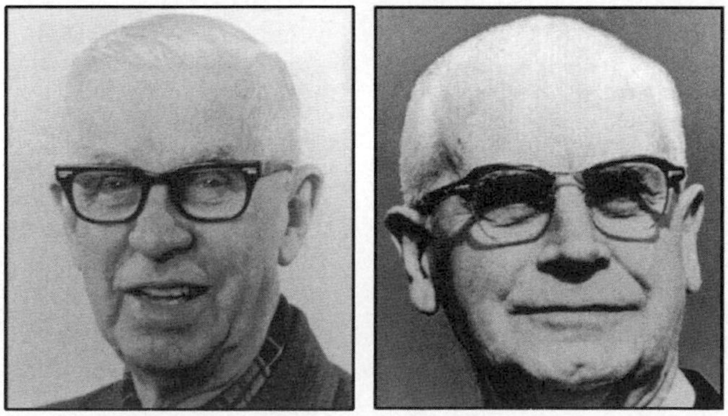

FIGURE 2-3 Brothers *(left to right)* Chuck and Frank Cramer were instrumental in the development of the National Athletic Trainers' Association (NATA). (From Ebel RG: *Far beyond the shoebox*, New York, 1999, Forbes Custom Publishing. Copyright National Athletic Trainers' Association.)

their homes and schools to fight in World War II, the first NATA eventually dissolved in 1944. Although the war put an end to the NATA, it forced athletic trainers to improvise and develop new skills that would eventually shape the future of the profession. Frequently, athletic trainers were the ones who helped train and condition troops who were going overseas to fight. Later, as many wounded soldiers came home, the athletic trainer was responsible for performing post-injury rehabilitation.[1]

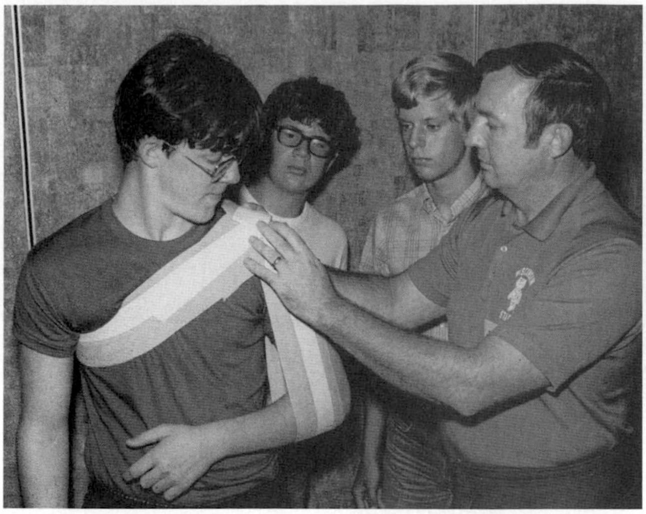

FIGURE 2-4 Many students jump-started their careers in athletic training by attending a Cramer workshop. (Courtesy Cramer Products Inc., Gardner, Kan.)

BEGINNING OF THE NATIONAL ATHLETIC TRAINERS' ASSOCIATION

After World War II, athletic trainers once again felt the need to form an organization that would allow them to share ideas and improve their skills. They had the foresight to realize that this was necessary if athletic training were to become a profession that would be recognized by other health care professions. On June 24 and 25 of 1950, the Cramer Chemical Company, the company founded by Chuck and Frank Cramer, hosted the first National Athletic Training Clinic, considered to be the first annual NATA Convention (Figure 2-5). There were about 100 attendees, all male athletic trainers. With guidance from Chuck and Frank Cramer, the group formed the second National Athletic Trainers' Association. This was the beginning of the organization that still governs athletic trainers today. The association's goal was "to build and strengthen the profession of training by the exchange of ideas, knowledge, and methods of the art."[5]

The founding fathers of the NATA established a model of governance that included a national organization. This new organization was divided into 10 districts. Over time, the districts were set up geographically by college athletic conferences. For example, the Southeastern Conference became District 9, the Big Ten Conference became District 4, and The PAC Ten became District 8. Box 2-1 summarizes members of each district, and these are mapped in Figure 2-6. The state athletic training organizations also became part of the District Governance. The NATA at that time was run by a **board of directors**, with each director selected from each of the 10 districts and afforded an equal vote.

board of directors organization within NATA made up of the 10 district directors; also included are NATA's president, vice president, and secretary/treasurer

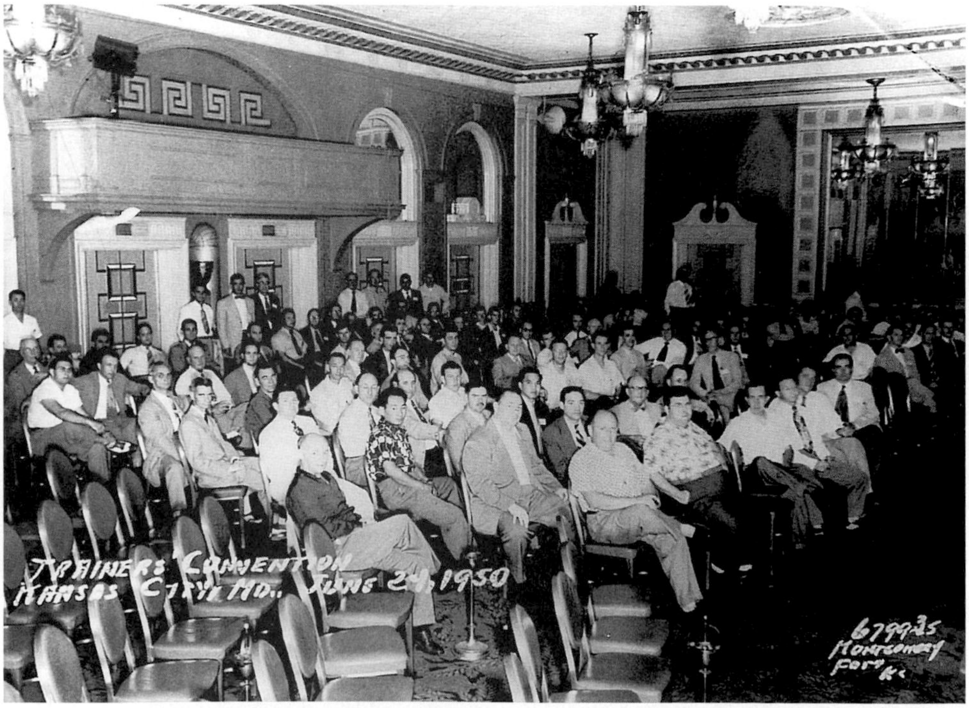

FIGURE 2-5 The first meeting of the National Athletic Trainers' Association was held in Kansas City, Missouri, in 1950. (Courtesy National Athletic Trainers' Association, Dallas.)

BOX 2-1 Districts of the National Athletic Trainers' Association

District 1: Eastern Athletic Trainers' Association
Connecticut
Maine
Massachusetts
New Hampshire
Rhode Island
Vermont
In Canada: New Brunswick, Nova Scotia, and Quebec

District 2: Eastern Athletic Trainers' Association
Delaware
New Jersey
New York
Pennsylvania

District 3: Mid-Atlantic Athletic Trainers' Association
District of Columbia
Maryland
North Carolina
South Carolina
Virginia
West Virginia

District 4: Great Lakes Athletic Trainers' Association
Illinois
Indiana
Michigan
Minnesota
Ohio
Wisconsin
In Canada: Manitoba and Ontario

District 5: Mid-America Athletic Trainers' Association
Iowa
Kansas
Missouri
Nebraska
North Dakota
Oklahoma
South Dakota

District 6: Southwest Athletic Trainers' Association
Arkansas
Texas

District 7: Rocky Mountain Athletic Trainers' Association
Arizona
Colorado
New Mexico
Utah
Wyoming

District 8: Far West Athletic Trainers' Association
California
Hawall
Nevada

District 9: Southeast Athletic Trainers' Association
Alabama
Florida
Georgia
Kentucky
Louisiana
Mississippi
Tennessee
Puerto Rico
Virgin Islands

District 10: Northwest Athletic Trainers' Association
Alaska
Idaho
Montana
Oregon
Washington
In Canada: Alberta, British Columbia, andSaskatchewan

During these years, each district was responsible for screening its own members and the dues for each member were $2[1,2,5] (Figure 2-7).

In 1952, the Board of Directors decided to elect a leader, and Dean Nesmith, of the University of Kansas, became the first Chairman of the Board of Directors of the NATA. This year also marked the first time that athletic trainers from professional sports were allowed to join this organization, which was initially founded by college and university athletic trainers. An official NATA logo was adopted. The second attempt at founding the NATA, an organization for the advancement of the profession of athletic training, proved to be a success (Figure 2-8).

During the first 5 years, the new NATA was predominantly funded by the Cramer Chemical Company. Eventually, the board of directors and the membership recognized the need to free the NATA from corporate funding and allow it to stand on its own. This independence led to the formation of the new position of executive secretary. The NATA board filled the executive secretary position with the athletic trainer from Purdue University, William "Pinky" Newell (Figure 2-9).[6] The profession thrived under

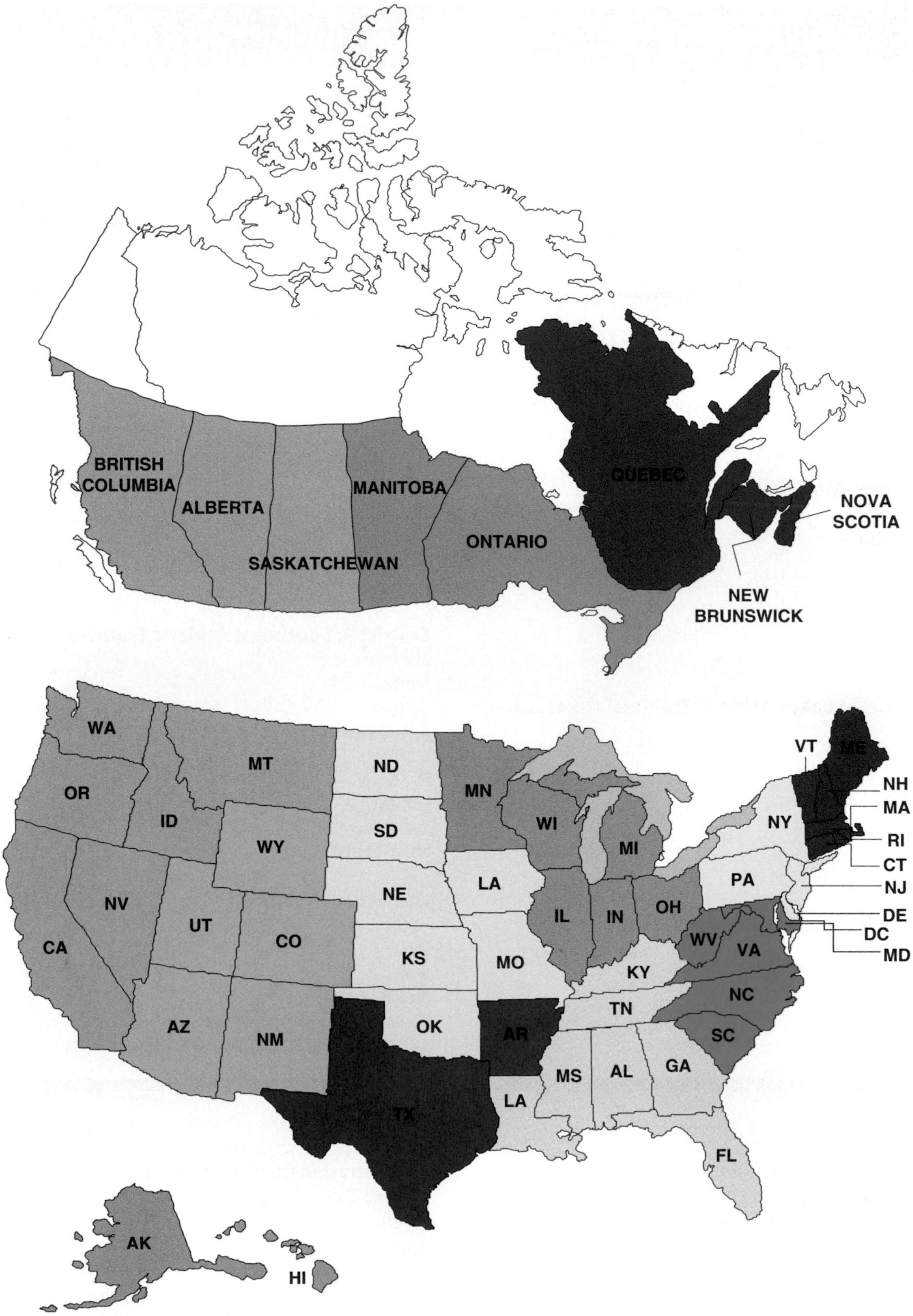

FIGURE 2-6 The National Athletic Trainers' Association today is divided into 10 districts *Not pictured*: Puerto Rico and Virgin Islands.

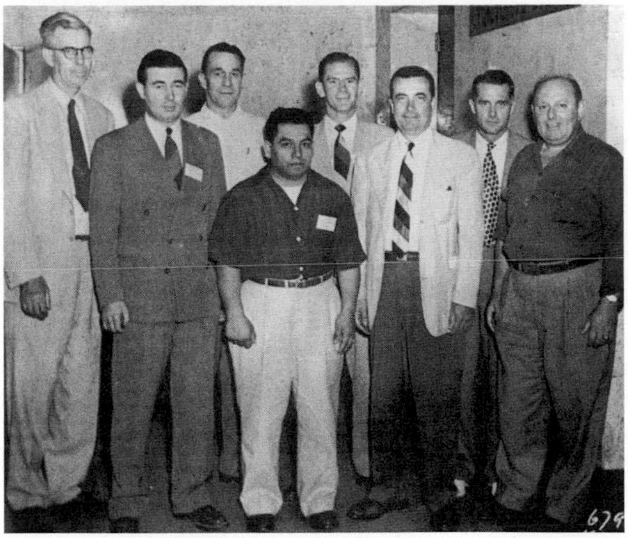

FIGURE 2-7 Members of the first National Athletic Trainers' Association board of directors in 1950. *Back row, from left:* Chuck Cramer, Al Sawdy, Buck Andell, and Joe Glander. *Front row, from left:* Fred Peterson, Frank Medina, Duke Wyre, and Henry Schmidt. Not pictured: Frank Kavanaugh and Richard Wargo. (From Shoop J: *The Southeast Athletic Trainers' Association: A historical review,* p. 44, 1987, Southeast Athletic Trainers' Association.)

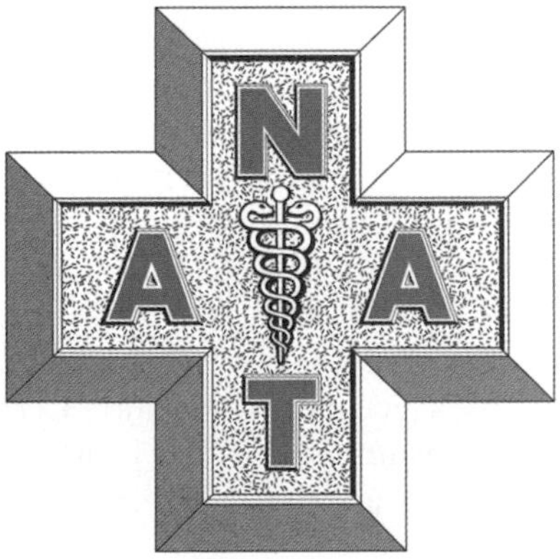

FIGURE 2-8 The first logo of the National Athletic Trainers' Association. (Courtesy National Athletic Trainers' Association, Dallas.)

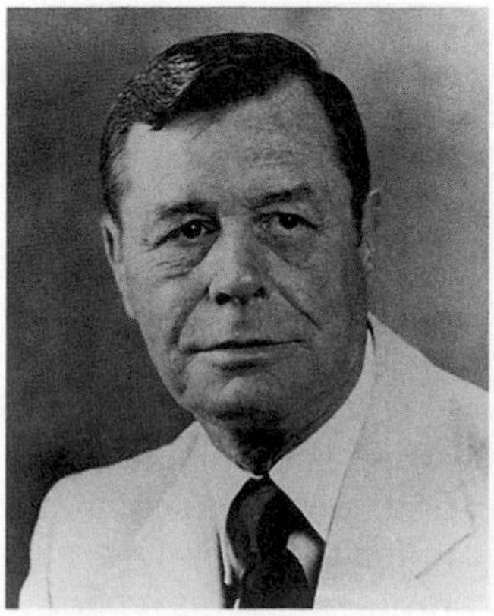

FIGURE 2-9 Pinky Newell served as the first executive director of the National Athletic Trainers' Association. (Courtesy National Athletic Trainers' Association, Dallas.)

Newell's guidance. During his tenure, the NATA established a journal of scholarly research, adopted a code of ethics, and began to align with outside organizations, including the National Collegiate Athletic Association (NCAA), the U.S. Olympic Committee, and various medical groups. One important goal that Newell set for the NATA was to be recognized in the medical field as an allied health profession. In 1961, the American Medical Association (AMA) paid tribute to the NATA for conducting itself as an ethical, professional unit. In 1967, the AMA recognized the role of the professionally prepared athletic trainer. How proud it would have made Newell to know that in 1990, the AMA recognized athletic training as an allied health profession. Newell was executive secretary for 12 years and garnered a great deal of respect for the NATA.

REORGANIZATION: THE 1970s AND 1980s

The 1970s brought the need for a structural reorganization of the NATA. As its membership grew, the needs of the organization were changing and expanding. In the reorganization plan, the board of directors remained as the main decision-making entity. The chairman of the board was replaced by the election of an NATA president. Bobby Gunn, of Lamar University, became the NATA's first president. Jack Rockwell replaced Pinky Newell as the interim executive secretary but stayed on for several years to oversee the restructuring of the NATA. The permanent replacement was Otho Davis, the athletic trainer at Duke University. He was named the **executive director** of the NATA in 1971, went on to become the head athletic trainer with the Philadelphia Eagles, and remained as the NATA executive director for the next 19 years (Figure 2-10). Around the same time, committees within the NATA began to expand, providing valuable input and information to the board of directors regarding current issues facing athletic training.

One of the most significant events in the history of the NATA was the initiation of the Corporate Sponsorship Program. For the first time, the NATA partnered with **corporate sponsors**, allowing them to assist with funding and support the vision of the organization. The money generated through this sponsorship program allowed the leadership of the NATA to earn more recognition and respect as an allied health care profession. In 1989, Gatorade and Johnson & Johnson were the first companies that signed on as corporate sponsors. They have remained

executive director individual in charge of leading the day-to-day operations of the NATA organization

corporate sponsors businesses that serve as funding sources for an organization by paying an agreed-upon fee to the organization for a certain amount of publicity

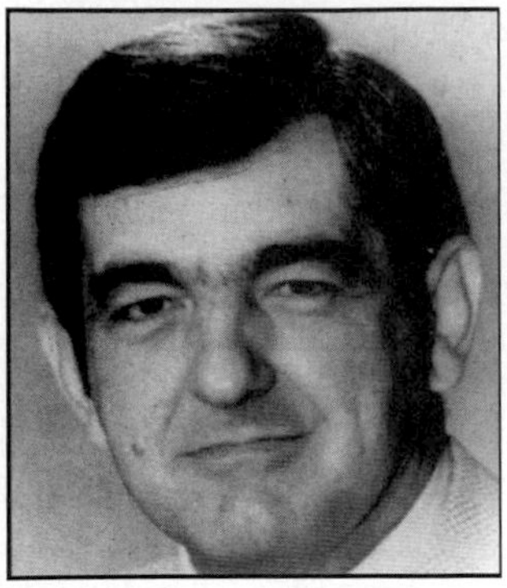

FIGURE 2-10 Otho Davis served as a longtime executive director of the National Athletic Trainers' Association and as head athletic trainer for the Philadelphia Eagles. (From Ebel RG: *Far beyond the shoebox,* p. 15, New York, 1999, Forbes Custom Publishing. Copyright National Athletic Trainers' Association.)

the leading corporate sponsors of the NATA and the athletic training profession. Every year, Gatorade and Johnson & Johnson have increased their support and expanded their partnership with the NATA.

THE TWENTY-FIFTH ANNIVERSARY OF THE NATIONAL ATHLETIC TRAINERS' ASSOCIATION

In 1974, the NATA celebrated its twenty-fifth anniversary in Kansas City, Missouri, at the Mulenburg Hotel, where the first NATA convention was held. At this meeting, the board of directors approved the first **Professional Education Committee** and made a resolution defining athletic training as "the art and science of prevention and management of injuries at all levels of athletic activity." The athletic trainer was defined as "one who is a practitioner of athletic training."[1] In 1977, the NATA National Office relocated to Greenville, North Carolina, from West Lafayette, Indiana, where it had been since Pinky Newell became the first executive secretary.

ATHLETIC TRAINING EDUCATION AND CERTIFICATION

One of the most important charges before the NATA board of directors was to establish educational standards for the Athletic Training Education Programs. The establishment of voluntary standards for entry into practice is not a concept created by athletic trainers. For example, before there were schools of medicine and law, a student would study with a mentor for a period of years, similar to an apprenticeship. When the older, more learned colleague decided that the student was sufficiently prepared to practice independently, the student was released to begin independent practice. The student then became the teacher and passed on the acquired knowledge and skills to another generation of students. Athletic training education followed this internship model of education. The classroom was the athletic training room, and the assignments were the injured athletes. As the profession's body of knowledge increased, a formalized curriculum was established. As the profession of athletic training grew, more formal instruction of athletic training became necessary, leading to the creation of accreditation, or educational and certification standards. Today, education is governed by the Commission on Accreditation of Athletic Training Education (CAATE), which provides accreditation guide-lines; the NATA **Education Council**, which provides content areas for the accredited programs; and a **Board of Certification** (BOC), which determines entry-level standards for athletic trainers and coordinates the certification examination. Even now, reform in the athletic training education programs is considered a pressing issue.[7]

Points to Ponder

Were there advantages to an internship program? How do today's athletic training education programs incorporate on-the-job training?

The Professional Advancement Committee was formed by the board of directors and given the charge to pursue the areas of Athletic Training Education and Certification. From this committee, the Professional Education and the Certification Committees were formed.[6] In 1969, the NATA approved its first Education Program.[6] The need to prove professional competency, along with the rapid growth in membership,[8] helped move the organization toward a certification exam. Certification of athletic trainers was initiated in the 1960s primarily as a

Professional Education Committee organization responsible for issues pertaining to precertification education; also a resource for existing and developing accredited programs at the undergraduate and graduate levels.

Education Council organization that represents NATA in all educational matters; facilitates continuous quality improvement in entry-level, graduate, and continuing athletic training education and coordinates the delivery of educational programming for the profession of athletic training

Board of Certification (BOC) a certification program incorporated in 1989 for entry-level athletic trainers intended to provide standards for entry into the profession; also sets recertification standards for certified athletic trainers means to enhance the recognition of the athletic trainer by the national professional association, the NATA. The Certification Committee, which subsequently became the BOC, was created to oversee the certification process for the athletic training profession. In 1982, the BOC exam program was initially accredited by what is now the National Commission for Certifying Agencies.

The purpose of the BOC certification exam is to provide a valid and reliable assessment tool by which to ensure that the credential holder has demonstrated entry-level knowledge and skills. The BOC exam is based on the **Role Delineation Study (RDS)**. The RDS is sometimes called a "job analysis." This document is constantly reviewed and revised when necessary to provide a blueprint for the development of the exam. The first Certification Examination was given in 1970, in Waco, Texas.

Athletic training education continued to become more formal and systematic. For many years, there were two routes to take the Certification Exam. To be eligible to sit for the Certification Examination, students had to graduate from either a recognized accredited program or an internship program, in which the student learned mostly on the job. As of January 1, 2004, the NATA and BOC recognize only one route of eligibility to sit for the Certification Exam: graduation from a CAATE-accredited program.

WOMEN JOIN THE PROFESSION

With the advent of Title IX in 1972, opportunities for girls and women in athletics increased significantly. Commensurate with the increased involvement of female students in sports at the high-school and collegiate levels, women began to join the heretofore all-male profession of athletic training. In 1966, Dotty Cohen became the first female member of the NATA. Later, in 1972, Sherry Kosek Babagian became the first woman to take and pass the NATA Certification Examination. In 1974, a survey showed that of the 23 NATA-approved undergraduate education programs, 15 schools accepted women into their programs. Both of the approved graduate programs also accepted women. Although it was difficult for women to enter the profession through the traditional internship programs, they were able to join the profession by being accepted into the academic programs.

Points to Ponder
Do male athletes feel comfortable being treated by a female athletic trainer? Are female athletes comfortable with a male athletic trainer covering their sport?

The NATA Board of Directors established a Special Committee on Women in Athletic Training in 1974. This committee was chaired by Holly Wilson, and its charge was to examine the challenges women face in the profession and identify ways in which the NATA could help them address these challenges. The women who were consulted shared their feelings of exclusion and their suspicions that they had been denied positions of leadership within the organization. Others in the profession felt the women weren't aggressive in trying to get involved. Despite the early challenges and frustrations, by the mid-1980s, it was obvious that women were ready to take an active role in the leadership of the administration of the NATA. In 1984, Janice Daniels from California and District 8 was the first woman to be elected to the board of directors (Figure 2-11). In 1993, Eve Becker-Doyle was hired as the second full-time executive director of the NATA (Figure 2-12). Julie Maxx was elected as the first female vice president of the NATA and then made history again as the first female president of the NATA in 1991 (Figure 2-13). Today, women hold leadership roles in every aspect of governance in the NATA, and the numbers of women and men in the athletic training profession are now almost equal.

A NEW BEGINNING: THE 1990s

The NATA and the profession of athletic training enjoyed significant growth in the late 1980s and the 1990s. Athletic trainers were traditionally employed in athletic settings, predominantly in colleges, universities, and professional sports franchises. In recognition of the benefit to collegiate and professional athletes, high-school administrators began to hire athletic trainers to care for their sports teams. The unique and aggressive

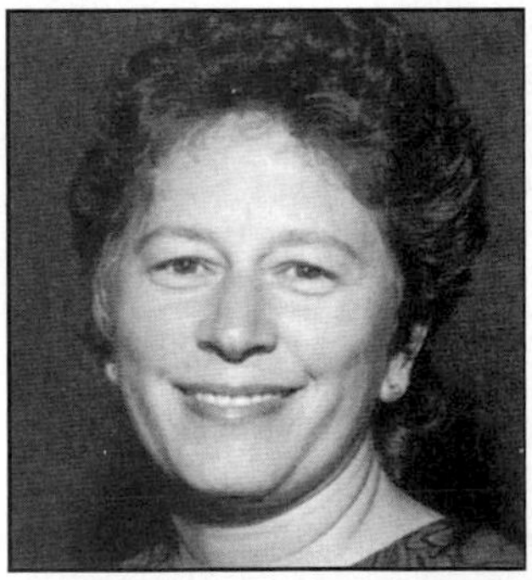

FIGURE 2-11 In 1984, Janice Daniels, from District 8 (Far West Athletic Trainers' Association), was named the first female member of the National Athletic Trainers' Association board of directors. (From Ebel RG: *Far beyond the shoebox*, p. 71, New York, 1999, Forbes Custom Publishing. Copyright National Athletic Trainers' Association.)

Role Delineation Study (RDS) a job analysis performed by the Board of Certification every 5 years to formulate the blueprint for the certification examination

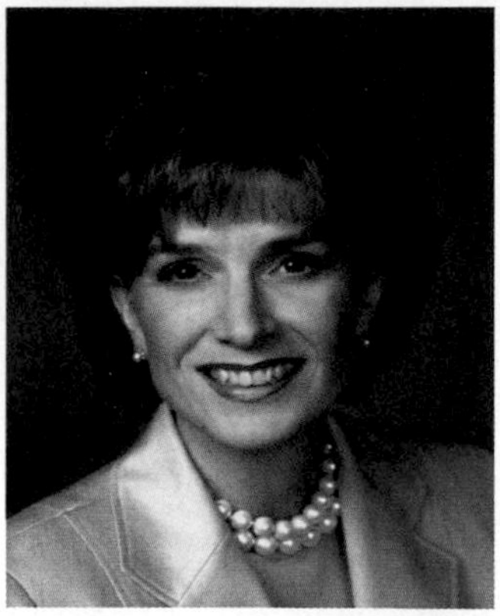

FIGURE 2-12 Eve Becker-Doyle was hired as the first woman and the first non–athletic trainer executive director of the National Athletic Trainers' Association. (Courtesy National Athletic Trainers' Association, Dallas.)

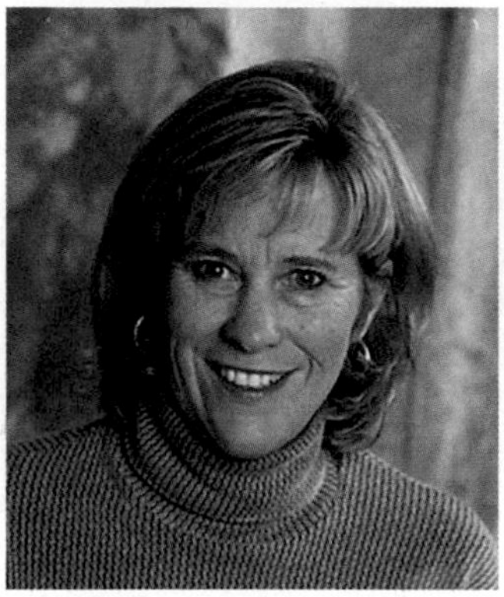

FIGURE 2-13 Julie Max, from District 8 (Far West Athletic Trainers' Association), has the distinction of being the first female vice president and president of the National Athletic Trainers' Association board of directors. (Courtesy National Athletic Trainers' Association, Dallas.)

skill sets that athletic trainers used in treating athletic injuries for accelerated return to play also became attractive in other, nontraditional settings. Sports medicine clinics and physical therapy clinics began to hire athletic trainers as part of the sports medicine team. Many athletic trainers started outreach programs for the clinics to provide coverage for high schools and small colleges.

As the skills of the athletic trainer became more widely known, job opportunities in industrial settings (e.g., General Motors, General Electric) emerged. Many factories and even NASA copied the athletic model of care in which the on-site physician, such as the team physician, evaluates and refers the injured workers to athletic trainers for treatment and rehabilitation. The positive result was less time loss for employees, which was credited to immediate and aggressive treatment and rehabilitation.

The NATA responded to the expansion of the profession by creating committees, task forces, and councils to meet the needs of its members by addressing their specific issues and concerns. With athletic trainers in clinics, hospitals, and physician offices, third-party reimbursement moved to the top of the list of priorities for the NATA leadership. The NATA worked to teach state legislators, other medical professionals, and the public that athletic trainers should treat people with athletic injuries and illness and be reimbursed for those services. The NATA and BOC share the goal of having 50 states with strong and consistent regulation for athletic trainers. In light of these efforts, the NATA will undoubtedly continue to face and meet new challenges in the coming years.[9]

THE FIFTIETH ANNIVERSARY OF THE NATIONAL ATHLETIC TRAINERS' ASSOCIATION

The fiftieth anniversary of the NATA was celebrated in 1999 at the site of both its first meeting and the twenty-fifth anniversary celebration in Kansas City, Missouri. The NATA had undergone many changes over the past half century. It had 101 members at the first meeting in 1950; 50 years later, it had over 27,000 members, with close to 9000 people attending its annual convention (Figure 2-14). Although there were no female members of the NATA at the first meeting, by 2000 the numbers of males and females were just about equal. The only diversity at the first meeting in 1950 was in geographical locations. Now, the Ethnic Diversity Advisory Council supports and encourages diversity in all work settings. To celebrate the fiftieth anniversary, the NATA commissioned Richard Ebel to write a book detailing the history of the NATA. The book, *Far Beyond the Shoe Box*, was given as a registration gift to all attendees of the convention.

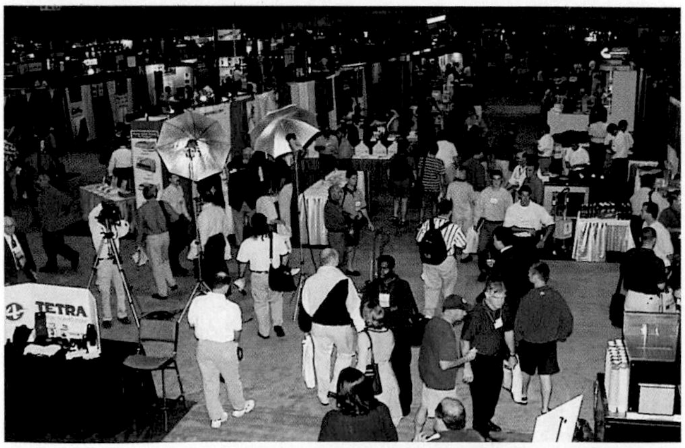

FIGURE 2-14 The annual meeting of the National Athletic Trainers' Association has grown tremendously since the first meeting in 1950. (Courtesy National Athletic Trainers' Association, Dallas.)

SUMMARY

It is exciting to imagine where athletic training is heading at the beginning of the twenty-first century. Athletic trainers are flourishing in a variety of practice settings and assuming a wide range of responsibilities. These diverse practice settings have brought about a new set of challenges for the profession's leaders, who are aggressively addressing these issues by studying them and carefully formulating plans to address them. The need for high-quality, uniform state regulation is a lofty but necessary goal. Third-party reimbursement, which establishes appropriate pay for services rendered, must be addressed for the profession to work in tandem with other allied heath care professionals. For the first time, the NATA hired a national lobbyist and created a **political action committee (PAC)** to aggressively pursue the rights of its members to be considered valued members of the health care team and to be recognized by leaders in the insurance companies. The NATA Public Relations Committee strives to educate the medical community; the local, state, regional, and national legislators; and the general public about the profession of athletic training. Women and minorities continue to take leadership roles to promote equality and fair hiring practices in all settings (Figure 2-15). Quality of life issues must be addressed to allow for the important balance of our professional and personal lives. The NATA is committed to providing support and resources for its members to address these issues and more. With the strong leadership of the NATA and its unparalleled volunteer spirit, the future is bright for the athletic training profession.

political action committee (PAC) a committee formed by business, labor, or other special-interest groups to raise money and make contributions to the campaigns of political candidates whom they support

Revisiting the OPENING *Scenario*

To inspire young athletic trainers and the next generation of athletic trainers to respond to your call to action, you must instill in them a sense of belonging and ownership. Having a good understanding of the history of the NATA is a great start. Most people want to know where they came from so that they can know where they are headed. Impressing on your up-and-coming peers the hard work and efforts that others have expended to make this profession what it is today is paramount.

Athletic training as an organized profession is very young, just over 50 years old. The evolution of the profession has been closely linked with the changes in education and the expansion of the practice settings. What has remained consistent is the nurturing nature of the athletic trainer, the volunteer spirit of the members of the NATA, and the dedication to improving care for the wide variety of individuals who benefit from this unique profession.

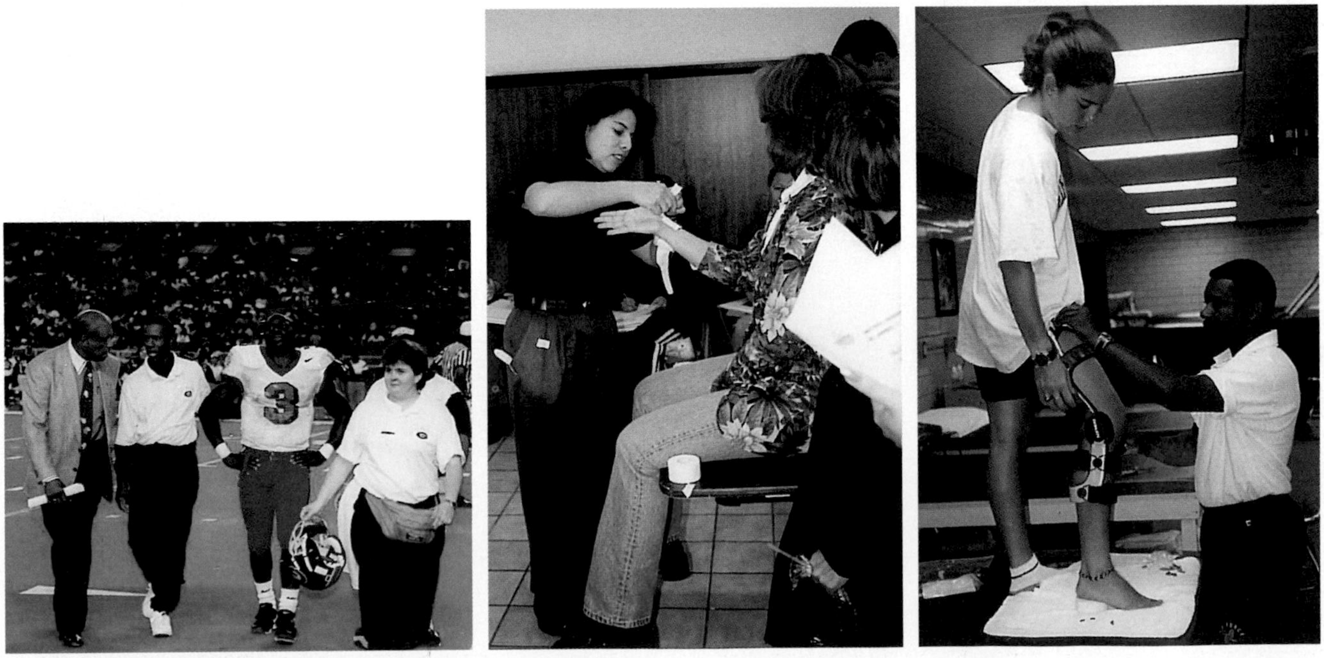

FIGURE 2-15 The National Athletic Trainers' Association is a diverse membership organization. (Courtesy National Athletic Trainers' Association, Dallas.)

Issues & Ethics

Athletic trainers learn to evaluate, treat, and rehabilitate injuries and illnesses common to athletes. Many of the skills they learn and use overlap with skills used by other allied health professions. It is widely accepted that athletic trainers use these skills to treat athletes at the professional, college, and high-school levels. In some cases, athletic trainers are not allowed to treat individuals in physical therapy or sports medicine clinics who have the same conditions but were not injured on the playing field. Therefore athletic trainers are working to be recognized for their skills and not for the patient population they treat. Should athletic trainers be able to treat only people who are called *athletes,* or should they be able to use their expertise on anyone who suffers from a condition that they have been trained to treat?

Web Links

Board of Certification (BOC): www.bocatc.org
Commission on Accreditation of Athletic Training Education (CAATE): www.caate.net
Cramer Products Inc.: www.cramersportsmed.com
Gatorade Sports Science Institute: www.gssiweb.com
Johnson & Johnson: www.jnj.com
National Athletic Trainers' Association (NATA): www.nata.org
National Athletic Trainers' Association Education Council: www.nataec.org

References

1. Ebel RC: *Far beyond the shoe box,* New York, 1999, Forbes Custom Publishing.
2. O'Shea M: The National Athletic Trainers' Association twenty-fifth annual convention, *Athletic Training* 9(2): 83–88, 1974.
3. Shoop J: *The Southeast Athletic Trainers' Association: A historical review*, 1987, The Southeast Athletic Trainers' Association.
4. Hillman SK: *Introduction to athletic training*, Champaign, Ill, 2000, Human Kinetics.
5. O'Shea M: *A history of the National Athletic Trainers' Association*, Dallas, 1980, National Athletic Trainers' Association.
6. Delforge GD, Behnke RS: The history and evolution of athletic training education in the United States, *JAT* 34(1): 53–61, 1999.
7. Platt LS, Turocy PS, McGlumphy BE: Preadmission criteria as predictors of academic success in entry-level athletic training education programs and other allied health education programs, *JAT* 36(2): 141–144, 2001.
8. Grace P. Milestones in athletic trainer certification, *JAT* 34(3): 285–291, 1999.
9. Peer KS, Rakich JS: Accreditation and continuous quality improvement in athletic training education, *JAT* 35(2): 188–193, 2000.

3

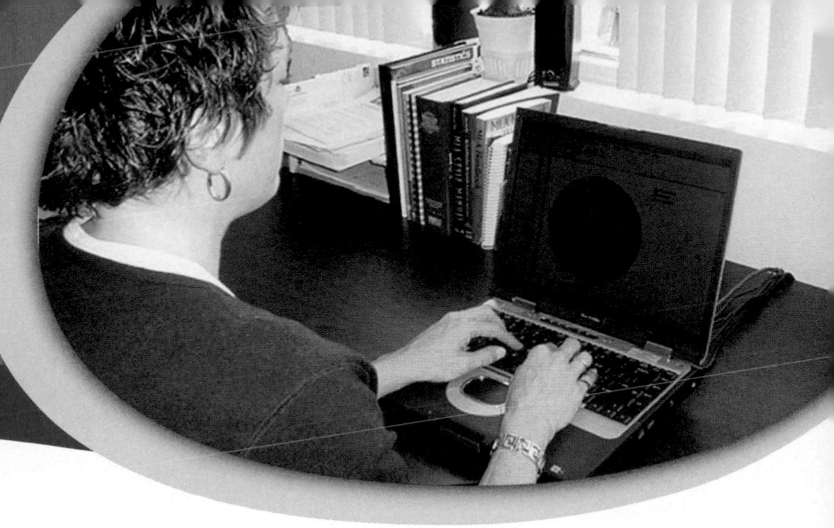

Organization and Administration

CHAD STARKEY AND GRETCHEN D. OLIVER

Learning Goals

1. Identify forms of risk management.
2. Distinguish among the different types of liability.
3. Describe ways to prevent negligence and decrease risk.
4. Design an emergency action plan.
5. Recognize types of medical disqualifications.
6. Discuss and use various forms of medical records documentation.
7. Describe the importance of the Health Insurance Portability and Accountability Act (HIPAA).

Athletic trainers are intimately involved in the numerous facets of their job. Many of their responsibilities are related to organization and administration (Figure 3-1). Organizational duties include maintaining accurate inventories, keeping appropriate documentation records, and filing insurance claims. Administrative components may include tasks that range from documenting an injury to filling out a purchase request form for a new piece of athletic equipment to creating an emergency action plan for a venue. Although this chapter covers a diverse sampling of possible activities in a variety of athletic training settings, it cannot cover every organizational and administrative concept. After completing this chapter, students will have a strong sense of how organization and administration affect their day-to-day choices and responsibilities as athletic trainers.

LIABILITY AND RISK REDUCTION

In the broadest sense, *risk management* describes the steps taken to eliminate, reduce, or share the risk and liability associated with athletic participation.[1] The administrative aspect of athletic training entails two facets of risk management: decreasing the likelihood of injury or reducing the severity and decreasing the risk of liability. In other words, a primary administrative responsibility for athletic trainers is to prevent injuries from occurring and decrease personal and institutional liability that may be incurred in the unfortunate event that an injury happens.[1]

Although any athletic endeavor carries a certain amount of risk, some sports are riskier than others. For example, the risk of injury is much greater in football and ice hockey than it is in golf or tennis. Some sports are associated with a higher risk of injury because of the gender of the athlete playing the sport. Female soccer and basketball players are more likely than their male counterparts to sustain an anterior cruciate ligament (ACL) injury. After careful study of the frequency and severity of injuries, the National Athletic Trainers' Association (NATA) has classified sports according to their potential injury risk (Box 3-1).

liability legal responsibility to do something

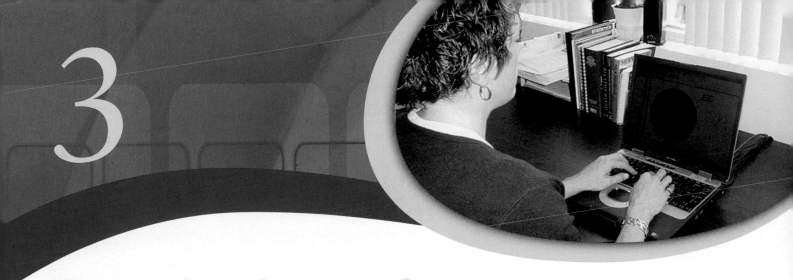

OPENING *Scenario*

Your star player is injured during the final moments of the game. The press is going crazy because he is a top recruit with the possible option of playing overseas in an All-Star tournament this summer. After escorting him back to the locker room, you return to the field and begin packing up all of your supplies and equipment. A reporter with whom you are acquainted approaches you and begins a casual conversation about the game. Before you know it, you are discussing the player's injury and future. How much information can you share with the reporter, and when do you need to stop talking?

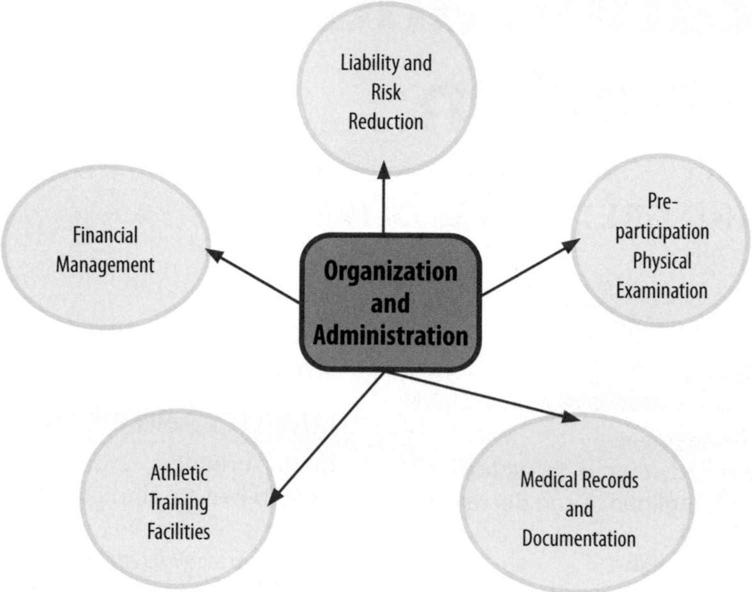

Liability and Risk Reduction
Financial Management
Organization and Administration
Pre-participation Physical Examination
Athletic Training Facilities
Medical Records and Documentation

FIGURE 3-1 Organization and administration responsibilities concept map.

Athletic trainers are expected to comply with standards of care that take into consideration any legal documentation required to perform services. Failure to maintain proper documentation for services may result in legal action if a procedure or activity is questioned later. Likewise, not providing proper care may lead to charges of negligence. Disregarding these legal concerns could leave the athletic trainer liable (i.e., legally bound or responsible by law) for anything that might happen to the individual in his or her care.

Many unforeseen events can occur in the athletic trainer's various work settings; subsequently, certain legal ramifications go along with these incidents. Typically, the legal sanctions imposed on those involved in the medical care of athletes are classified into two categories. These two categories are called *torts* and *negligence*. Although they are discussed separately here, they often overlap in most real-life work environments.

A **tort** is loosely defined as an intentional or unintentional civil wrong. An example of an unintentional tort common in athletic training involves use of an electrical stimulation modality on an athlete who turns out to be allergic to the adhesive on the electrodes. To prevent this type of tort from occurring, athletic trainers should always have on file a signed medical consent form and medical history form stating all known allergies of each athlete or worker being treated (Figure 3-2). Another common tort is the defamation of character by a verbal or written release (slander and libel, respectively) of medical information when the individual's explicit approval has not been obtained.

tort an intentional or unintentional civil wrong

BOX 3-1 NATA Classification of Sports Based on the Relative Risk of Injury

Low-Risk Sports
Baseball
Crew (M, W)
Cross country (M, W)
Fencing (M, W)
Golf (M, W)
Outdoor track (M, W)
Softball
Swimming (M, W)
Tennis (M, W)
Water polo (M, W)

Moderate-Risk Sports
Basketball (W)
Diving (M, W)
Field hockey
Indoor track (M, W)
Lacrosse (M, W)
Soccer (M, W)
Volleyball (M, W)

Increased-Risk Sports
Basketball (M)
Football
Gymnastics (M, W)
Ice hockey (M. W)
Skiing
Wrestling

Data from National Athletic Trainers' Association: *Recommendations and guidelines for appropriate medical coverage of intercollegiate athletics,* Dallas, 2000 (revised 2003), National Athletic Trainers' Association. Retrieved March 21, 2007, from www.nata.org/statements/support/AMCIARecsandGuides.pdf; and Mueller FD, Cantu RC: *Twenty-third annual report,* Chapel Hill, NC, 2002, National Center for Catastrophic Sport Injury Research.
M, Men; W, women.

Negligence is the failure to provide the standard of care that otherwise would have been deemed appropriate for that particular circumstance. The standard of care is based on the actions that a reasonable and prudent person would have taken if faced with the same situation. Frequently, this determination is based on the testimony of expert witnesses (e.g., other athletic trainers), professional position papers, state practice acts, and professional standards. Assume that a worker sprains his ankle. The standard of care would be to evaluate, treat, and send the patient back to work if possible. Applying ice or a compression wrap and possibly administering crutches would be a minimal expectation, along with education on what to do at home. If the athletic trainer allows the patient to return to work without providing any of these services and his condition worsens, the athletic trainer is negligent.

Both the lack of action (omission) and improper actions taken (commission) can be deemed negligent (Box 3-2). **Omission** occurs when an athletic trainer does nothing about a particular injury. For example, an outside hitter on the volleyball team falls down and twists his knee while attempting to block a spike. If the athletic trainer evaluates the knee injury but fails to diagnose the torn ACL and allows the athlete to return to play, this could be an act of omission. **Commission** is responding incorrectly to a situation. For example, if the same outside hitter dislocates his shoulder falling to the ground and the athletic trainer decides to reduce it without first identifying the presence of a fracture, this is an act of commission.

In the event that a charge of negligence is brought against the athletic trainer or another member of the staff, the plaintiff (i.e., the person bringing the charges) must make the case that negligence on the part of the defendant (i.e., the athletic trainer) did indeed occur. Negligence is established on the provision of the following four arguments:

1. The defendant had the duty to respond.
2. The defendant breached that duty.
3. The plaintiff must have suffered physical, emotional, or financial harm (or some combination thereof).
4. The defendant's negligence caused that harm.

If any one of the aforementioned points is ruled to be nonexistent, then it is deemed that negligence could not have occurred.

Not all injuries result in a lawsuit. Remember, however, that an athletic trainer or the institution with which he or she is affiliated can be sued for either negligence or tort. The institution is most often sued through **vicarious liability,** which means that the institution did not commit an act of wrongdoing but

negligence failure to provide the standard of care that would otherwise have been deemed appropriate for that particular circumstance
omission lack of action by an athletic trainer to take appropriate and necessary steps to render care
commission incorrect response to a situation
vicarious liability perceived wrongdoing of an individual who is acting on behalf of an institution

Georgia College & State University
Athletic Department
Student-Athlete Medical Information Form

Name: ____
Sport: ____________________ SS# ______________________________
Date of Birth: ____________________

Home Information:

____
Home Street Address

____
City State ZIP Country Phone#

GCSU/Local Information:

____
School/Local Address

____
City State ZIP Phone#

Preferred Email address: ____

I, ______________________, hereby give my consent to the Sports Medicine staff of GC&SU's Athletic Department to perform emergency and first aid treatment to my person relative to injuries occurring during practices for and participation in various athletic contests and events, as well as injuries occurring during transportation to or from such practice or contest sessions.

I hereby further authorize and consent to the release of any pertinent medical information and records regarding the treatment, diagnoses, and/or examination relative to injuries or illnesses that may affect my participation in GC&SU athletics programs to the GC&SU Athletic Department and Medical Staff as is necessary for the appropriate treatment of those injuries/illnesses. Medical information may also be released to my parents/legal guardians. I also acknowledge tha certain details of my injuries or illnesses may be used in the athletic training education programs in the Kinesiology Department as long as these facts are not personally identifiable as related to me. This authorization shall be in force for one year from the date of my signature given below.

I further understand that there are risks of injury or death arising form my participation in intercollegiate sports and that even though proper coaching techniques are used, rules are adhered to, and protective equipment is used, the possibility of an accident still exists. To decrease the risk of injury, I understand that equipment must be worn properly and that I must adhere to all instructions and all rules applying to the sport. I agree to do so. I further agree to report to the Equipment Managers, Athletic Trainers, or Coaches any defects, or change of fit, in my athletic equipment. However, I acknowledge that proper use of equipment, proper training, and adherence to the rules may not prevent all risks of injury and I assume those risks.

In consideration of my being permitted to participate in GC&SU's Intercollegiate Athletic Program, I hereby release GC&SU, its Trustees, employees, agents, and those volunteering in the course of my medical care together with all persons assisting with any phase of the program, from all liability and responsibility for any loss or injury related to my participation in the GC&SU athletic program. I further agree to indemnify and hold harmless said parties from all claims hereafter made by me or on my behalf by my parents, guardians, heirs, executors, or assigns.

I have read and understand the above contents and releases.

______________________ ___/___/___ ______________________
Athlete's Signature Date Parent or Guardian (if athlete is a minor)

FIGURE 3-2 Sample medical consent form. (Courtesy Georgia College & State University, Milledgeville, Ga.)

Box 3-2 Types of Negligence

Malfeasance: Performance of an unlawful or improper act
Misfeasance: Improper performance of an otherwise lawful act
Nonfeasance: Failure to respond when there is a duty to do so

that the athletic trainer, acting as a representative of the institution, was perceived to have done wrong. Thus the lawsuit can name both the athletic trainer and the place of employment as defendants. Following certain practices, such as functioning within the athletic trainer's scope of practice and maintaining proper documentation, can reduce the likelihood of legal liability being found against the athletic trainer and the institution.

Points to Ponder

Kristen, an athletic trainer, was covering a large event for a national age-group championship. At her site, eight teams were practicing and preparing for the beginning of the tournament. As she was taping a player on one court, two players collided on the court farthest from her while her back was to the court. One of the players in the collision was transported to the emergency room, where he remained hospitalized for 3 days. His parents are now suing Kristen for negligence. According to the previously mentioned four steps, was Kristen negligent and responsible for any part of the hospitalization of the injured player?

Athletes who participate in organized athletics are recognized as having an **assumption of risk** associated with participation in their sport. In other words, athletes should know and be informed that injury is a risk inherent to sports participation. Football players know that there is a strong probability, because of the nature of their sport, that they may incur injury while they are playing. Hockey players know that if they do not wear full padding and equipment, they will most likely sustain an injury. Assumption of risk covers most injury situations but does not apply to faulty equipment, poor facilities, or negligent behavior on the part of the athletic training staff. Athletes may also be asked to sign an informed consent form or a release of liability form indicating that he or she has been warned of the risks associated with the activity and has received proper instruction in safe performance. Ultimately, the safety of the athlete rests with the head coach of the team.

Points to Ponder

Think of two ways to prevent any legal action from being taken during an injury situation that involves activation of the emergency action plan and transportation of an athlete.

Policies and Procedures Manual

All athletic training staff members, physicians, athletic training students, and departmental administrators should receive a policies and procedures manual that details the standard operating procedures performed in the athletic training facility. All involved parties must also be educated on the contents in the manual. **Policies** are written rules used to guide decision making or a course of action. **Procedures** are documented steps taken to comply with a policy.

The policies and procedures manual is used as an operational guide and a reference tool to ensure the consistent implementation of the policies and procedures. All information pertaining to the athletic training program should be contained in the manual. This may include, but is not limited to, the examples in Box 3-3.

The policies and procedures manual should be regularly updated. When the manual is updated, new copies should be supplied to all involved parties. When warranted, an educational or training session should be held to bring everyone up to date on the changes.

assumption of risk informed decision based on knowledge and information of dangers involved, as in a decision to participate in athletics
policies written rules used to guide your decision-making or a course of action
procedures documented steps taken to adhere to a policy

BOX 3-3 Examples of Information in a Policies and Procedures Manual

- All personnel with their contact information
- Expectations of the staff and students
- Dress code
- Operating hours of the athletic training facility and satellite facilities
- Daily operations
- Emergency action plan (EAP)

Emergency Action Plans

Emergency action plans (EAPs) are established for all athletic venues where practices or games are held, as well as athletic training facilities. The basic contents of an EAP are similar, but each plan is specific to the venue (Box 3-4).[2] The EAP must be communicated to all persons who may be associated with the venue, including coaches and administrators. Communication plans must become an integral part of the athletic department's EAP.

Personnel includes all persons who could be accessible during any event at which an incident might happen, such as the athletic training student, the employee nurse, and institutional safety officers. Emergency communication plans within the EAP should ensure that at least two of the following forms of communication are available at all times: landline telephone, radio, or cell phone. Athletic trainers should make a point to check the batteries and connections often so that they have the means to contact the necessary support services when an emergency arises.

Emergency equipment such as an automated external defibrillator (AED), spine board, airway, bag-valve mask, and splint kit should be easily and readily accessible. Emergency personnel who will be using this equipment must be properly trained in the safe use of each apparatus. All emergency personnel must be knowledgeable regarding directions to the venue and be able to describe them to emergency medical services (EMS) personnel if needed. Keys to gates and doors that may impede the transportation of the ambulance to the injured person must be readily accessible. Ideally, staff members will be designated in the EAP as responsible for unlocking any closed gates or doors and meeting the ambulance crew upon arrival.

Liability Insurance

Liability insurance is recommended for all heath care professionals. However, it does not reduce the risk of being sued; it merely provides health care professionals with some measure of financial protection in the event that they are found negligent. It should be noted that most malpractice insurance policies do not provide coverage in cases in which gross negligence has occurred.

Many institutions provide liability insurance coverage as part of the employee contract. This coverage applies to all events sponsored or hosted by the institution. If the employer does not provide liability insurance or if the individual athletic trainer is employed in a venue outside of the employer's responsibility (e.g., providing coverage to a local high school), then the athletic trainer should purchase a separate individual liability policy. These policies are available for purchase through several reputable vendors associated with the NATA.

BOX 3-4 Components of an Emergency Action Plan

- Emergency personnel
- Means of communication and chain of communication
- Emergency equipment
- Personnel roles
- Facility/venue directions
- Emergency phone numbers (e.g., emergency medical services)
- Staff phone numbers

PREPARTICIPATION PHYSICAL EXAMINATION

The **preparticipation physical examination (PPE)** is one of the most important aspects of the athletic training medical model because it prevents injury by identifying people who may be at increased risk. This type of medical examination should be tailored to each setting and used to determine the individual's physical capability to undertake the intended physical activity. As is the case in colleges and high schools, most employers have a medical screening form or physical examination that is tailored to the specific work site.

In the early years of the athletic training profession, most athletes were considered to be in optimal physical condition, in part because athletes with medical conditions that are considered manageable by today's standards were often disqualified from participating in physically demanding sports. As medicine and technology have improved, so has the physician's ability to correct, manage, or control a wide range of musculoskeletal conditions and diseases that would otherwise disqualify the individual. Therefore we cannot assume that today's athletes are all in perfect health. However, as demonstrated later in this chapter, some conditions can disqualify a person from participating or at least influence the types of activity that are allowed. The physical examination is the first line of defense in making some of these important decisions, which ultimately protect the participant.

emergency action plan (EAP) a written emergency plan identifying key personnel, equipment, and communications involved in order to safely address all possible emergencies

preparticipation physical examination (PPE) document used to determine an individual's capacity to undertake the intended physical activity involved in athletics

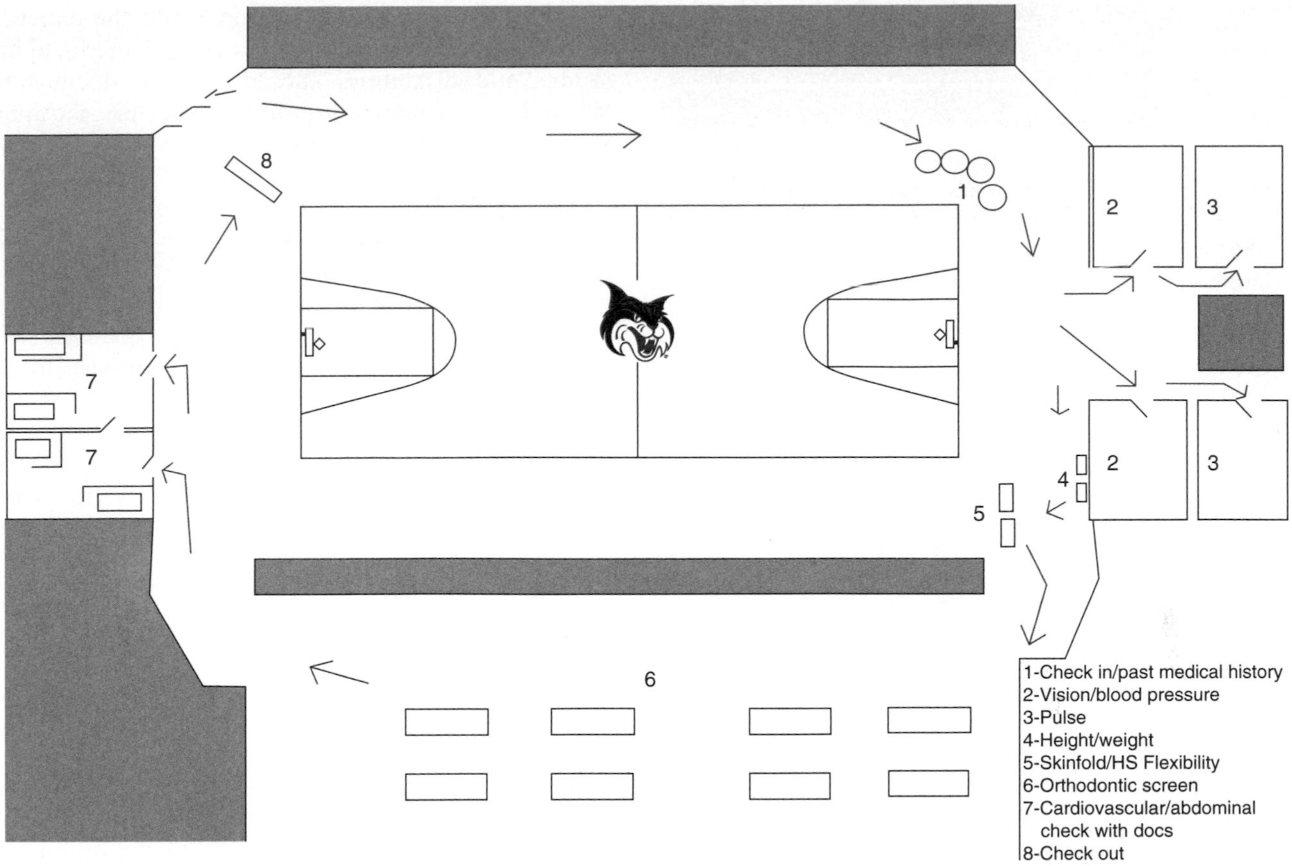

FIGURE 3-3 Flow chart depicting a station examination system. (Courtesy Georgia College & State University, Milledgeville, Ga.)

The athlete's family physician or personal physician sometimes administers the PPE. Because these physicians may not have a sports medicine background, they may not be familiar with the specific rigors of the given sport, which can create inconsistencies in the depth and breadth of the findings. Ideally, the PPE should be administered by a team of physicians, athletic trainers, and other medical and health care personnel. This medical team can be created to fully understand and identify the specific physiological needs of the athletes using a station system (Figure 3-3). This approach helps standardize the examination, creates a system of efficiency, and ensures consistency in the exam.

Regardless of the type of PPE used, a common set of information should be collected (Table 3-1). A pre-established PPE document standardizes the data collected during physical examinations, especially in those cases in which an outside physician performs the PPE (Figure 3-4). The information obtained in the PPE should be updated annually in the athlete's medical file, although a full examination is not always needed. Release forms and other pertinent forms of documentation should be distributed and collected at the time the PPE is administered or updated.

Medical Disqualifications

Some medical conditions disqualify an individual from participation in certain types of sports or jobs. The participation level is determined on a case-by-case basis, but according to the NCAA Sports Medicine Guideline 2a, "The team physician has the final responsibility to determine when a student-athlete is removed or withheld from participation due to an injury, an illness, or pregnancy."[3]

Examples of disqualifying conditions pertaining to various sports include the absence or decreased function of a paired organ (e.g., eye, kidney, testicle), neurological diseases, cardiovascular dysfunction (e.g., arrhythmia, valve defect), sickle-cell anemia (as opposed to sickle-cell trait, which may not be a disqualifier), and an enlarged spleen. Other limiting medical conditions can exist; this is not an exclusive or exhaustive list. In athletic conditions in which a vital organ is at risk, collision and contact sports are strongly discouraged. In certain situations, such as the absence of a paired organ, special protective equipment, such as extra padding, may be required.

THE MEDICAL RECORD AND DOCUMENTATION

The Board of Certification's Standards of Professional Practice (Appendix B) identifies adequate documentation as an integral part of the health care services delivered by athletic trainers. Medical records serve several functions in the delivery of athletic health care (Box 3-5).

TABLE 3-1 Components of the Preparticipation Physical Examination

COMPONENT	PURPOSE
Personal medical history	Identifies congenital or acquired disease states that may hinder athletic participation Establishes a history of prior orthopedic injury
Family medical history	Identifies patients who may be at increased risk for cardiovascular disease or other sudden death conditions by demonstrating a family history of these conditions
Cardiovascular and respiratory	Establishes baseline vital signs: pulse, blood pressure, respiration Identifies the presence of conditions such as high blood pressure, irregular heartbeat, or asthma
General medical examination	Includes baseline height and weight information Contains results of laboratory blood work, urinalysis, and other laboratory tests used to identify illness, disease, or at-risk populations Screening of the genitalia may be performed as needed; males are usually screened for an inguinal hernia and testicular cancer at this time
Orthopedic evaluation	Identifies prior musculoskeletal injury Confirms normal strength and range of motion Identifies predisposing conditions to further orthopedic injury
Vision	Identifies baseline vision and the need for corrective lenses Determines adequate visual acuity needed to play the athlete's sport and position
Physical maturity (for youth sports)	Determines the athlete's physical maturity to compete in organized athletics

Computer-based record-keeping systems are rapidly making the traditional paper-based systems obsolete. A computer-based system allows for the rapid transfer of an athlete's or patient's medical record among providers, increased consistency and accuracy of documentation, quick recall and analysis of data, and the electronic storage of radiographs and other diagnostic test results. Innovations such as PDAs and Tablet PCs allow the athletic trainer to carry this important information to any event venue and into the athletic training facility.[4]

From a medical perspective, proper documentation improves patient care by enhancing the communication among caregivers, identifying the patient's functional limitations, noting primary complaint(s) and subsequent care rendered to date, and listing the short- and long-term rehabilitation goals. The medical record should contain as much quantifiable (i.e., measurable) information as possible to demonstrate the patient's strength, range of motion, function, and pain. These measurable data allow both the athletic trainer and the patient to accurately assess and monitor progress. Functional limitations and disabilities should also be documented. When this information is gathered over time, the appropriateness of responses to the treatment plan can then be determined.

From a legal perspective, medical records serve as a record of the services provided to the individual. The documentation should present the details of the individual's health status and minimally include the following:[5]

- Patient's name and identification number
- Referral source
- Date(s) of service
- Initial evaluation
- Rehabilitation program plan and estimated length of service
- Rehabilitation program methods, results, and revisions
- Date of discontinuation
- Summary of program
- Athletic trainer's signature and any other medical team members involved

As athletic trainers become more involved in third-party reimbursement (i.e., billing insurance companies for their services rendered), medical records assume a new level of importance in the billing process. Because billing for services can be a tedious and complicated process, detailed, measurable, and goal-based medical records serve as the foundation for obtaining reimbursement. Ideally, in the quest to further establish the necessity of the athletic trainer's role in the provision of these services, medical records provide leverage to this claim. Proper documentation can also add to the professional body of knowledge by identifying injury rates and trends (i.e., epidemiology) and assisting in determining the effectiveness of the care provided (i.e., outcome studies).

Confidentiality Concerns

In 2003, the United States federal government instituted the **Health Insurance Portability and Accountability Act (HIPAA)**. This critical piece of legislation was originally intended only to ensure the confidentiality of electronically transmitted medical records. However, the bill was amended to cover most forms of oral and written communication contained in medical records.

Health Insurance Portability and Accountability Act (HIPAA) federal legislation designed to ensure the confidentiality of electronically transmitted records and of oral and written communication contained in medical records

Georgia College & State University
Athletic Department
Preparticipation Physical Exam

Name__________________________________ Team____________________

SS#________-________-________ Date of Birth _____/_____/_____

Academic Year 200______-200______ GC&SU Class: F So Jr Sr 5th Grad

---

Have you had a history of any of the following?
(Check all that apply)

☐ Concussion/ Knocked Out
☐ Heart Murmur
☐ Kidney Problem
☐ Asthma
☐ Diabetes
☐ Head Injury
☐ Neck Injury
☐ Shoulder Injury
☐ Elbow Injury

☐ Wrist/Hand Injury
☐ Back/Spine Injury
☐ Hip Injury
☐ Knee Injury
☐ Ankle Injury
☐ Foot Injury
☐ Dislocation
☐ Chronic Cough
☐ Dizzy After Exercise

☐ Mononucleosis
☐ Surgery
☐ Overnight Hospital Stay
☐ Seizures/Convulsion
☐ Allergies
☐ Wear Contacts/Glasses
☐ Missing Body Part/Organ
☐ Broken Bone

☐ Other Medical Condition(s):

• Do you take *any* medications or supplements on a regular basis?	YES	NO
• Have you seen a physician for *any* reason in the past 6 months?	YES	NO
• Has a physician ever limited your athletic participation?	YES	NO
• Have your mother, father, brothers, or sisters ever had any heart problems prior to age 50?	YES	NO

Explanations/Details/Dates: ________________________________

PHYSICIAN CERTIFICATION

In review of the above information and following the limited examination, I certify the student:

☐ Passes without restriction

☐ Passes with restriction:________________________.

☐ Fails the examination due to ________________________

Physician Signature:______________________ Date:____________

Revised Fall 2006

FIGURE 3-4 Sample preparticipation physical examination (PPE). (Courtesy Georgia College & State University, Milledgeville, Ga.)
Continued

GC&SU Athletics
Preparticipation Physical Exam

Name ______________________________ **Year 200**___ **- 200**____

Height __________ **Weight** __________ **Body Fat** ________% **Blood Pressure**_____ /_____

Resting Pulse______ **Vision Screening** Rt. 20/_____ Lt. 20/_____ Corrected / Uncorrected

Flexibility Hamstring Flexibility: Lt._______ Rt._______

Heel Cord Flexibility: Lt._______ Rt._______

Examination	WNL		Comments	Needs Referral or Follow-up	Clinician
	Yes	No			
Ears-Nose-Throat					
Lungs					
Heart					
Abdomen					
Spine/Neck					
Shoulder					
Elbow					
Wrist/Hands/Fingers					
Hip					
Knee					
Ankle					
Foot/Toes					

WNL, Within normal limits.
The examination performed for this participation certificate is limited and designed to identify conditions or infirmities that would limit or prevent a student from participating in athletic activities. This exam is NOT intended to be comprehensive and may not detect some types of latent or hidden medical conditions. All athletes should receive periodic comprehensive medical examinations.

Revised Fall 2006

FIGURE 3-4 Cont'd.

BOX 3-5 Functions of Medical Records

- Improves communication among caregivers
- Demonstrates the patient's response to treatment
- Provides a legal record of the services provided
- Aids in reimbursement
- Facilitates research

Records that contain individually identifiable health information—meaning the individual's name, social security number, or any other unique identifier—are considered to be protected health information (PHI) under HIPAA regulations.[6,7] In the college or university setting, the student-athlete's medical records are also protected by the **Family Education Rights and Privacy Act,** better known as the Buckley Amendment.

Institutional protocol and athlete release of information forms may restrict the type of medical information that is provided to the media and the coaching staff, thereby requiring a signed **release of medical information form** (Figure 3-5). In this case, the athlete may grant a blanket release statement, to be signed annually, that permits the release of information regarding his or her medical conditions to the media and coaching staff. These conditions are those that occur as a direct result of athletic participation while at that institution. The document may restrict or prohibit the release of information regarding nonathletic general medical conditions such as illnesses or pregnancy, in which case a specific release of information must be signed by the student-athlete. As with all minors, if the individual is younger than 18, the release form must also be signed by a parent or legal guardian. Even in settings outside of the college/university, the release of information must conform to the regulations set forth in the HIPAA guidelines. The athletic trainer's institution should provide specific training on HIPAA guidelines because the implications of this legislation are very broad.

Medical Records

As previously discussed, the preparticipation physical examination is the foundation of the medical file. Updated at least annually or as needed, this document provides baseline information regarding the patient's health status and serves as a frame of reference during the evaluation, rehabilitation, and return to play/work phases of injury management. Other records, however, make up an integral part of the documentation folder maintained for all athletes. Without proper documentation, the objective description of injuries, treatment plans, length of treatment, or specific responses to treatment would be impossible, making insurance reimbursement unlikely.

Injury Report

The injury report should document the onset of the condition, the pathology involved (e.g., left medial collateral ligament sprain), any functional limitations (e.g., inability to bear weight), disabilities of any kind (e.g., inability to walk), disposition, and the identity of the professional who performed the initial evaluation (Figure 3-6). Several types of medical records are used, but one of the most popular is the SOAP note, which includes subjective and objective findings of the patient's level of function, an assessment (i.e., clinical diagnosis) of the condition, and a plan for restoring health (Table 3-2).

Follow-up notes regarding progress, adjustments in long- and short-term goals, and physician notes should be updated and documented as needed. Injury reports are also used for insurance and liability-reduction purposes.

Physician Referral

Documentation of patients who are referred to or from a physician requires another layer of record keeping. The physician's subsequent diagnosis and recommendations for treatment and rehabilitation are needed to demonstrate the ongoing plan of care (Figure 3-7). These recommendations by the physician should serve as the foundation for the medical plan of care provided to the patient and followed by the athletic training staff.

Treatment and Rehabilitation Records

Daily treatment and rehabilitation logs are used to record when a patient reports for care, what services were provided, and who provided those services (Figure 3-8). These records are useful in a number of ways. Most important, they demonstrate consistency in the performance of the rehabilitation plan. Additionally, the compliance (or lack thereof) in following through with the prescribed rehabilitation program will become obvious through review of the logs. When practical, the treatment log should also document the response to each treatment session.

Computer-based treatment logs can be useful in scheduling medical staff and personnel. Identifying the

Family Education Rights and Privacy Act a provision that protects athletes' medical records; also known as the *Buckley Amendment*

release of medical information form paper restricting the type of medical information that is provided to the public outside of the athlete and family

Georgia College & State University
Athletic Department

Authorization for release of medical information and/or x -rays

I hereby authorize: ______________________________
____
____
____

to furnish full details of the medical care and treatment of:
____
____

Date of Birth: ______________________

Social Security Number: ______________

Please send this information to the following address:

Paul Higgs, ATC
Head Athletic Trainer
Georgia College & State University
Campus Box 65
Milledgeville, GA 31061
(478) 445-1787
Fax (478) 445-1790

Signature: ______________________________

Witness: ______________________________

Date: ______________________________

FIGURE 3-5 Sample medical release form. (Courtesy Georgia College & State University, Milledgeville, Ga.)

trends in treatment care hours allows staff to be increased during peak times and patients to be scheduled for treatments in slots when the overall caseload is reduced. Looking at the analysis of the number and types of treatments rendered can be used to help justify the purchase of new equipment, the addition of new staff members, and even the future expansion of facilities.

Although not normally part of the daily treatment log, any home care treatment and home-based exercises prescribed to the patient should be documented. If the daily log does not provide space for this information, the athletic trainer should note it in the individual medical record. Home care programs are used to maximize the healing cycle while the patient is away from the athletic training facility. The patient should receive detailed instructions in how to provide the self-treatment and perform selected exercises.

Medication Logs

All physician-prescribed and over-the-counter (OTC) medications should be recorded in the patient's medical file. In addition to the patient's name, the athletic trainer should include the condition being treated, other prescription and OTC medications that the patient is currently taking, and any known allergies. Specific to the medication being used, the medication log should provide documentation of the drug name, dosage, usage information (e.g., number of times per day the patient is to take the medication), method of administration (e.g., oral, injection), the amount of the medication dispensed, the lot number of samples where it was

Georgia College & State University
Injury/Illness Report

Name ______________________________

Injury Date ______________________ Sport ______________________

Report Date ______________________ Onset Acute Chronic Re-injury

History:

Observation:

Palpation:

Strength: ______________________ ROM: ______________________

Special Tests: ______________________

Functional Tests: ______________________

Initial Treatment: ______________________ Referral: ______________________

Clinical Impression: ______________________

Comments:

Student Signature ______________________ Staff Signature: ______________________

FIGURE 3-6 Sample injury report form. (Courtesy Georgia College & State University, Milledgeville, Ga.)

TABLE 3-2 Content of a SOAP Note

COMPONENT	DESCRIPTION
S (Subjective)	Information provided by the patient such as the history of injury (when it happened, mechanism of injury) and other patient complaints
O (Objective)	Observable and measurable findings from the physical examination such as strength, range of motion, girth, and the results of orthopedic tests
A (Assessment)	The athletic trainer's or physician's clinical diagnosis
P (Plan)	Short-term management (e.g., level of activity, ambulatory aids) and, if applicable, the long-term rehabilitation goals

Florida Southern College Physician Referral

Athlete's **Home** Address and Phone Number: ____________________

Physician's Name: ____________________

Address: ____________________

Campus Phone Number: ____________________

Appointment Date: ____________________

Athlete's Name: ____________________ Sport: ____________________

SS#: ____________ DOB: ____________ WC#: ____________

Date of injury/symptoms beginning: ____________________ Is this a follow up visit? Yes / No

Complaint: ____________________

Physician's diagnosis: ____________________

Treatment plan: ____________________

Refer to PT? Yes / No Duration: ____________________

Medication prescribed: ____________________

Restrictions, activity level, etc.: ____________________

Athlete is cleared to ***FULLY*** participate: Yes / No As of (date): ____________

Follow-up appointment: Yes / No Office / ATR Date: ____________

____

Physician/ARNP Signature and Date

I give permission to the treating physician, the athletic training staff, health center staff and all necessary billing departments to release information regarding this injury/illness for the purposes of treatment and payment of any bills incurred.

____________________ ____________________

Name Date

FIGURE 3-7 Sample physician referral form. (Courtesy Florida Southern College, Lakeland, Fla.)

Georgia College & State University

Daily Treatment Log

Date ____________________

	Name	Team	Injury Site	Taping	Ice Pack	Ice Massage	Compression Pump	Electrical Stimulation	Hot Pack	Cryocuff	Iontophoresis	Massage	Ultrasound	Whirlpool	Laser	Paraffin Bath	Stairmaster/Bike/UBE	Rehabilitation Exercises	**Treatment By**	**Time**
1																				
2																				
3																				
4																				
5																				
6																				
7																				
8																				
9																				
10																				
11																				
12																				
13																				
14																				
15																				
16																				
17																				
18																				
19																				
20																				

MBK=Mens Basketball	MCC=Men's Cross Country	MTN=Men's Tennis	BSB=Baseball	CHR=Cheerleading	GLF=Golf
WBK=Women's Basketball	WCC=Women's Cross Country	WTN=Women's Tennis	SFB=Softball	SCR=Soccer	

FIGURE 3-8 Sample treatment and rehabilitation record. (Courtesy Georgia College & State University, Milledgeville, Ga.)

Florida Southern College Athletic Training Medication Log

Name	Sport	Symptoms	Current Medications	Allergies	Medication Administered	Lot #	Expiration Date	Quantity	Usage	Date and Time

FIGURE 3-9 Sample medication log. (Courtesy Florida Southern College, Lakeland, Fla.)

dispensed, and the date and time the patient received it (Figure 3-9). The roles, responsibilities, and abilities of athletic trainers to dispense prescription and OTC medication are defined by both the state's athletic training practice act and the state's pharmacy laws. Athletic trainers must become familiar with the specific regulations of the state in which they are practicing. When working with athletes, medical staff members must be aware of any possibility that the medication is listed as a banned substance. As previously mentioned, these substances are published by the organization(s) that govern the individual sports, as well as the NCAA and the USOC and the International Olympic Committee (IOC). Many medications may be on the banned substance list, even when used for legitimate medical conditions.

Coach's Injury Report

A coach's report helps identify those athletes who are participating at less than 100% capacity on any given day. Although the information contained in the report can be modified to meet individual needs, this document lists the player's name, injury, level of participation, special considerations and notes, and anticipated date of full participation (Figure 3-10). The descriptors for the level of participation must be established and defined in the athletic department's policies and procedures manual. In this way, the medical staff and the coaching staff have the same understanding of what the athlete can and cannot do during activity (Table 3-3).

Discharge Notes

Upon discharge from formal medical care, the levels of function and activity must be documented in the medical file. The discharge notes should also contain quantifiable measures of the patient's physical function, including strength, range of motion, and pain. The discharge notes provide an opportunity to demonstrate and document successful completion of the short- and long-term goals established in the initial evaluation. Any prescribed preventive measures such as bracing and any ongoing maintenance such as home treatments or exercises should also be recorded in the discharge notes.

Discharge notes offer a level of protection from liability should a player be cut from the team and later file a claim or suit related to an injury. Discharge notes are particularly important in the reimbursement process. When an insurance company receives a discharge note, the current case is closed and no further payments are made.

Insurance Records

The documents submitted to receive reimbursement from an insurance provider are different from those

Florida Southern College
Daily Coaches Injury Report

Sport: **Date:**

NEW INJURIES

Name	Injury/Illness

NO PRACTICE/GAME

Name	Injury/Illness

LIMITED

Name	Limitations

REHAB/TREATMENT

Name	Condition

APPOINTMENTS (MD, x-rays, MRI, etc.)	

OTHER/COMMENTS

FIGURE 3-10 Sample coach's injury report. (Courtesy Florida Southern College, Lakeland, Fla.)

used for the day-to-day documentation described in this section. Although most clinical medical records use written descriptors of the condition (e.g., calcaneofibular ligament sprain of the left ankle), those submitted for insurance purposes use prescribed numerical coding. The description of the condition is recorded using International Classification of Disease (ICD) terminology. The care rendered, including evaluation, treatment, and rehabilitation, is recorded in the medical file using the common procedural terminology (CPT) coding system.

Depending on state insurance laws, a physician referral is usually required to initiate the reimbursement process. Once the patient sees the physician and

TABLE 3-3 Sample Participation Levels for Athletes

DESCRIPTOR	DEFINITION
Full go	Participation with no restrictions. This is often used to identify players who will no longer be on the injured list.
Practice as tolerated	The athlete may participate within his or her limits of pain, stamina, and comfort. The athlete, coach, or medical staff member can reduce (or stop) the athlete's participation. This classification usually means that the athlete is unable to participate in games.
Practice: light contact	The athlete practices in partial pads and does not participate in full-contact drills, especially those that place the injured body part at risk.
Practice: no contact	The player may participate in conditioning or walk-through activities but should not be placed in an "at risk" position.
Out	The athlete is withheld from practice and game competition. The medical staff may use this time for general or sport-specific rehabilitation.

receives a referral or prescription for services, the insurance company will verify coverage. If the patient's coverage is adequate, the insurance company will then permit the necessary medical services to be rendered. Frequently, the number of visits allowed or the number of billable units will be mandated and policed by the insurance carrier. If the last visit approved does not coincide with the athlete's ability to return to play, he or she may be released to an independent exercise program. This program may be performed in the strength complex at school or at the patient's home gym. Periodic follow-up appointments may then be scheduled to manage the remainder of the rehabilitation program.

FINANCIAL MANAGEMENT

Athletic trainers play a crucial part in the financial management of their program, although this is primarily the responsibility of the sports medicine program administrator or athletics director. Financial management is mainly performed through the maintenance of accurate inventory records. Misuse of supplies and equipment can seriously alter the overall inventory as well as the next fiscal budget. The amount of supplies that remain available serves as the basis for ordering future supplies. In general, supplies are classified as expendable (i.e., equipment that must be replaced annually), general (i.e., equipment with a life span of 3 to 5 years), and capital (i.e., equipment that costs more than a certain amount, usually in excess of $500).

Budgeting

Budgets represent the amount of money allocated to specific areas within the department. Each budget should reflect the financial priorities, goals, and objectives of the department. The budgeting process requires that prudent decisions be made regarding the amount of money that will be spent on certain supplies; these decisions are based on the specific funds designated. A useful tool to guide the purchasing process, the budget also ensures accountability with respect to true purchasing needs.

Over the span of many years and through trial and error, several budgeting systems have been established. The budgeting system ultimately selected is often determined by the specific work setting. The following budgeting systems are commonly used by athletic departments:

- *Zero-based budgets:* A new budget is developed each fiscal year that is independent of those from previous years. The budget must be tightly aligned with the mission, goals, and objectives of the department. In most cases, incorporating these into a financial justification ensures the successful procurement of equipment and capital.
- *Line-item budgets:* This budgeting system focuses on a budget that is divided among common categories such as expendable supplies, operational expenses, and capital equipment. Each of these sample areas could contain multiple sublines. For instance, expendable supplies could have sublines of athletic tape, bandages, and sports drinks. Capital sublines could be modalities, flooring, or rehabilitation equipment.
- *Program budgets:* This budgeting system includes all of the costs associated with a particular program. Whether the costs are expendable, capital, or operational, they will all appear within the same program budget.

These budgets can be modified to a performance-based budget by incorporating programmatic goals similar to those in a zero-based budget system.

Ordering Process

Ordering supplies for the department is not as simple as running to the grocery store to buy food for dinner. Spending institutional finances, which often come from state and federal sources, requires fiscally prudent habits supported by operational documentation. Maintaining an accurate and current inventory of all items used is a prerequisite to knowing what to buy and when.

The purchasing process begins when the athletic trainer submits bids to prospective vendors. The bid should describe the item desired and its quantity. The vendor will return the bid with a firm price. In most situations, the purchase must be awarded to the vendor who responds with the lowest bid. In this case, a purchase order is written, again describing the equipment needed and the quantity needed. Attached to the order is a promise that the institution will pay the balance of the account in 30 days.

THE ATHLETIC TRAINING FACILITY

The design of the athletic training facility should promote the safe and effective use of therapeutic modalities, rehabilitation equipment, and supplies. The facility must allow for maximal function and be designed with the safety of everyone in mind. The physical location of the athletic training facility significantly influences its overall functionality and usage. Providing a safe working environment is also critical.

The athletic training facility should have an outside entrance from the athletic fields and unencumbered access from the playing area or work setting. All doorways should be free of obstacles and wide enough to allow an ambulance squad to transport injured athletes or workers to and from the facility. If the athletic training facility is not located on the ground floor, an elevator should be nearby and accessible. Ideally, the facility should have designated areas for the various duties required of the athletic training staff and, except for private areas, provide for line-of-sight supervision of the activities occurring within the facility.

Physical Examination Area

The physical examination area is used primarily by the athletic trainer or physician while examining the patient's condition and determining a clinical diagnosis. The nature of the physical examination sometimes requires privacy. At least one of the examination stations should have privacy screens or be located in a separate room, such as the physician's examination room. The physical examination area is equipped with diagnostic supplies, such as goniometers (used to measure joint range of motion) and tape measures (used to measure limb girth, swelling, and leg length), and any other supplies that may be used to manage the injury, such as splints and crutches.

Treatment and Rehabilitation Area

The treatment and rehabilitation area is used to restore the patient's function to the pre-injury level. This space requires treatment tables (plinths), open floor space for exercise, and therapeutic modalities and rehabilitation equipment (Figure 3-11). The number of plinths is determined by the space available and the number of patients seen during the facility's peak hours. Having one or more adjustable-height

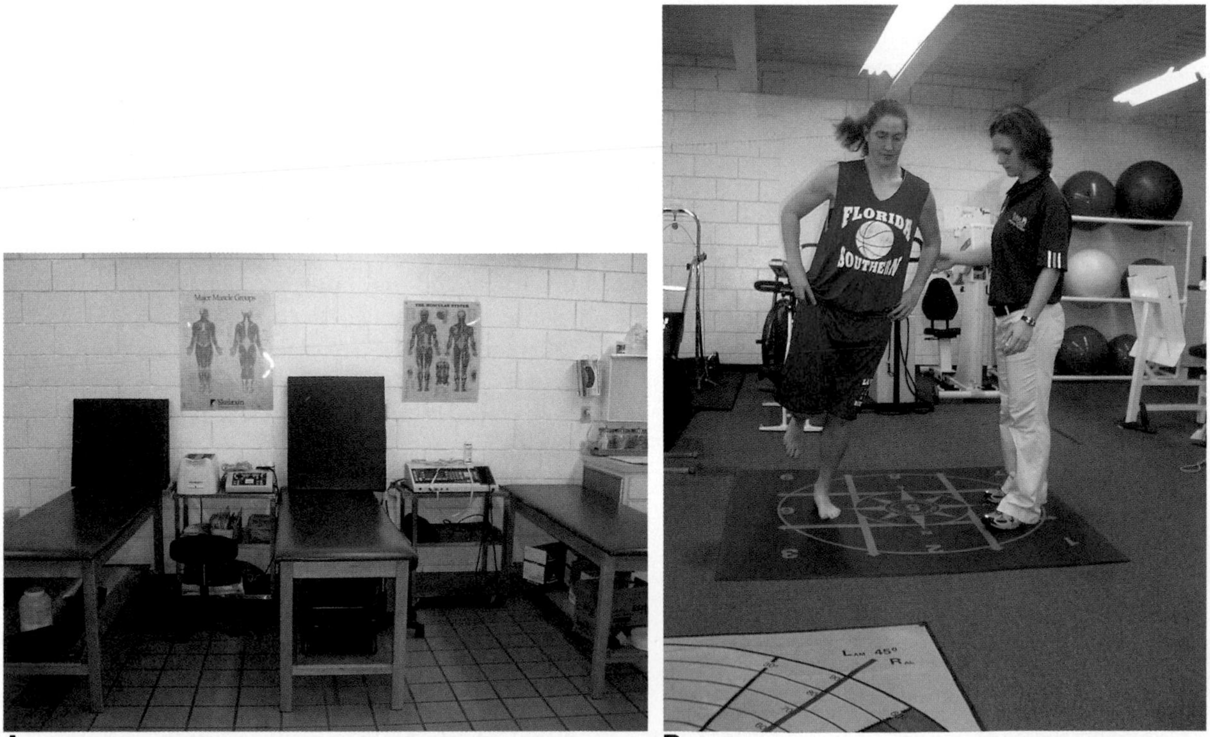

FIGURE 3-11 The athletic training facility should have areas designed for treatment **(A)** and rehabilitation **(B)**.

tables is useful when administering manual therapies such as stretching, proprioceptive neuromuscular facilitation (PNF), massage, or joint mobilization techniques. Several tables are located next to therapeutic modalities such as electrical stimulation or ultrasound devices for early- and late-stage treatments.

Although some therapeutic exercise programs may be performed on a plinth, a large open area is needed for many rehabilitation exercises. Programs may also be conducted in the weight room, basketball court, field, and swimming pool. The various types of rehabilitation equipment depend on the athletic trainer's rehabilitation philosophy but typically include a stationary bike, exercise balls, rubber tubing, and weights.

Hydrotherapy Area

Whirlpool baths, the ice machine, and stations for filling coolers are located in the hydrotherapy area (sometimes called the "wet room"; Figure 3-12). To contain moisture, humidity, and noise, the hydrotherapy area should be in a separate room of the sports medicine facility with a glass wall facing the rest of the facility. This configuration allows the proper monitoring of individuals receiving treatment. Special ventilation is needed to control humidity in the hydrotherapy area.

Several styles of whirlpools are available, including above-ground tanks and in-ground pools, which are maintained at warm (105°F to 110°F) or cool (50°F to 60°F) temperatures. Some specialized pools include a treadmill

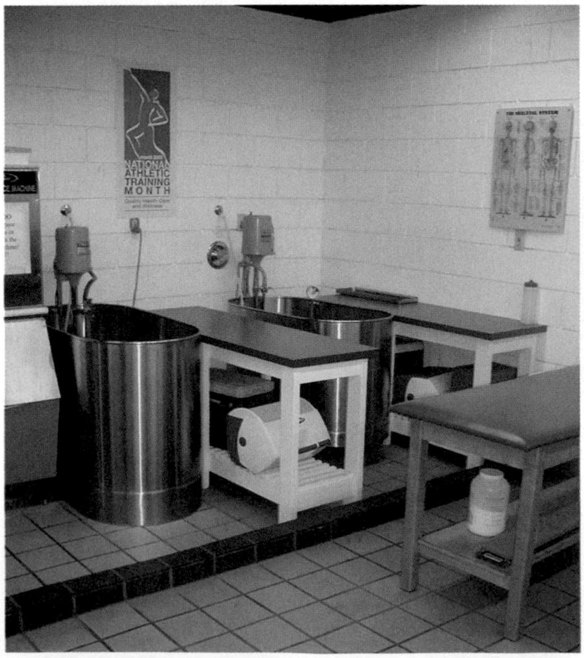

FIGURE 3-12 Another area of the athletic training facility, often referred to as the "wet room," provides hydrotherapy equipment such as whirlpools and ice machines.

to allow the patient to walk, jog, or run while immersed in water. Because of the potential for accidents, the hydrotherapy area must be monitored when being used.

Taping Stations

To expedite the taping, bracing, and wrapping of athletes before practice, specialized taping tables are used. These tables are higher than standard treatment tables and allow the athletic trainer to tape athletes without undue strain on his or her back. Athletes can sit upright with their knees extended, making taping a relatively comfortable process for all. Taping tables are usually located near the doorway to ease the traffic flow.

Administrative Area

Administrative responsibilities, such as completion of injury reports, budgets, insurance claims, and schedules, make up a large part of the athletic trainer's workload. The administrative area (i.e., office) should be equipped with a computer, telephone, and lockable file cabinets for medical records. Offices should be separate from the main area of the athletic training facility to help ensure patient confidentiality and allow for individual patient counseling sessions.

SUMMARY

An athletic trainer's role as an administrator and manager plays a large part in preventing injuries and ensuring legal compliance. Processes such as the preparticipation physical examinations and accurate record keeping are important in keeping athletes safe and facilitating the efficient management of the department or athletic training program. The culture and norms of the particular employment setting dictate the types of management skills required for success. More advanced skills, such as properly managing inventory and obtaining competitive bids from vendors, ensure that the athletic training program will operate efficiently within a budget. As athletic trainers mature professionally, they will develop the administrative and managerial style that most effectively helps them achieve their goals and those of the athletic training program.

Revisiting the OPENING *Scenario*

Both HIPAA and the Family Education Rights and Privacy Act strictly limit the information that athletic trainers may disclose regarding the player's injury and career. You cannot discuss anything pertaining to the player's injury or ability to play again. Since the previously described player's future overseas depends on the outcome of his injury, none of this can be discussed with your reporter friend. Only the player can discuss his condition with the media, unless he has signed forms allowing others to discuss his medical condition.

Issues & Ethics

Code 2 in the BOC Standards of Professional Practice[5] states that an athletic trainer must be involved in continuing educational activities and comply with the BOC requirements for recertification. You know that several of your friends have developed a system whereby they create false reporting records. In essence, they are signing forms for people who either did not attend the particular sessions or did not even attend the meeting. Sometimes, we all get in a bind and need help fulfilling our continuing education requirements. But you have noticed that the members of this group always seem to sign off on one another's forms. Is this acceptable? Where does the responsibility lie in this situation?

Web Links

Board of Certification, State Regulatory Agency Contacts: www.bocatc.org/atc/STATE/

National Athletic Trainers' Association: www.nata.org

NCAA Sports Medicine Handbook: www.ncaa.org/library/sports_sciences/sports_med_handbook/

U.S. Department of Health & Human Services, Office for Civil Rights—HIPAA: www.hhs.gov/ocr/hipaa/

References

1. Rankin JM, Ingersoll CD: Risk management. In Rankin JM, Ingersoll CD, editors: *Athletic training management, concepts and applications,* ed 3, pp. 106–121, New York, 2006, McGraw-Hill.
2. Anderson JC, Courson RW, Kleiner DM, McLoda TA: National Athletic Trainers' Association position statement: emergency planning in athletics, *J Athl Train* 37: 99–104, 2002.
3. National Collegiate Athletic Association: *NCAA sports medicine handbook 2005–06*, ed 18, Indianapolis, 2006, NCAA. Retrieved February 6, 2007, from www.ncaa.org/library/sports_sciences/sports_med_handbook/2005–06/2005–06_sports_medicine_handbook.pdf
4. Stengel D et al: Comparison of handled computer-assisted and conventional paper chart documentation of medical records: a randomized, controlled trial, *J Bone Joint Surg* 86A: 553–560, 2004.
5. Board of Certification: *Standards of professional practice,* Omaha, Neb, 2006, BOC. Retrieved February 6, 2007, from www.bocatc.org/athtrainer/STDS/.
6. News briefs. Sports medicine braces for HIPPA impact, *Physician and Sportsmedicine* 31(1): 13, 2003.
7. U.S Department of Health & Human Services, Office for Civil Rights—HIPPA, *Medical privacy: National standards to protect the privacy of personal health information*, Washington, DC, [no date], USDHHS. Retrieved February 6, 2007, from www.hhs.gov/ocr/hipaa/.

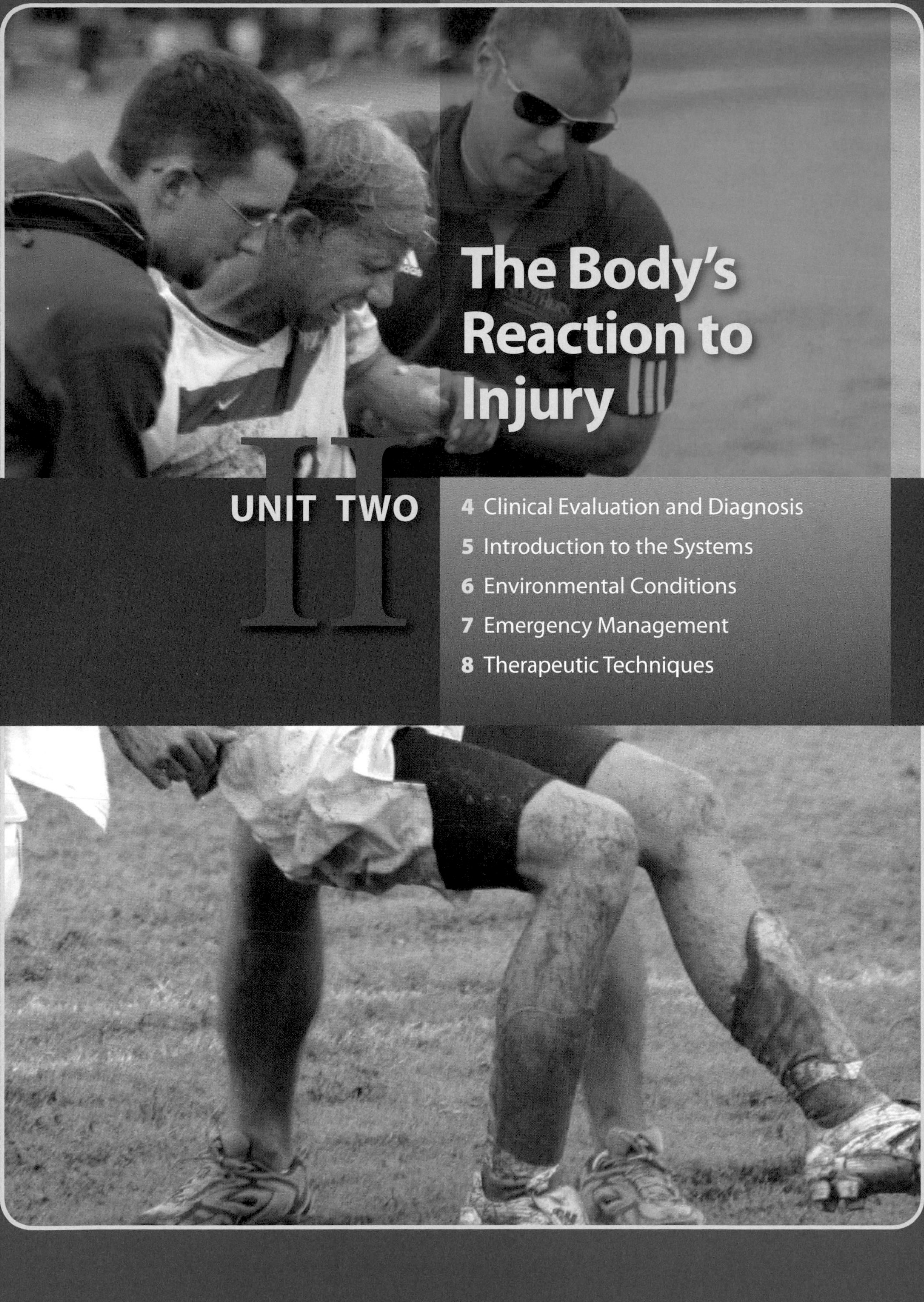

The Body's Reaction to Injury

UNIT TWO II

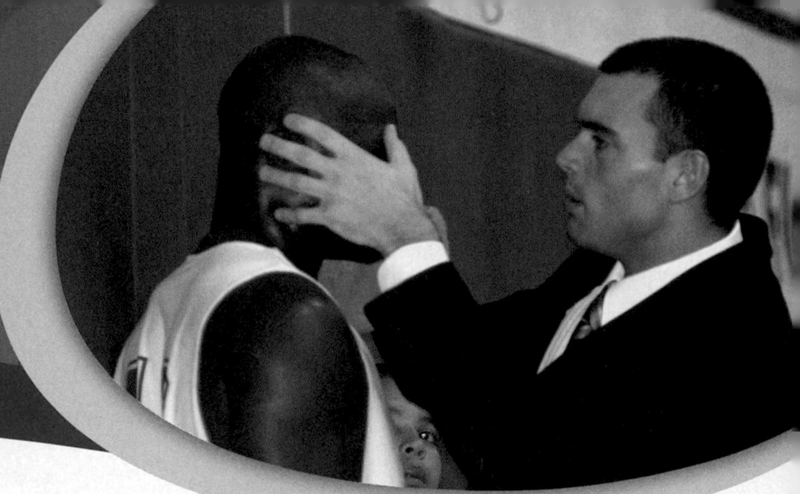

4 Clinical Evaluation and Diagnosis

VALERIE W. HERZOG

Learning Goals

1. Explain why determining the mechanism of injury is critical in the prevention and treatment of injuries and illnesses.
2. Define the various factors that contribute to an understanding of mechanisms of injury and illness.
3. Explain the relationship between the mechanism of injury or illness and the body's response to that injury and the subsequent repair process.
4. Describe the three stages of the body's repair process.
5. Apply knowledge related to the mechanism and pathology of injury or illness to potential injury management decisions.
6. Describe how to care for a superficial open wound incorporating universal precautions as defined by Occupational Health and Safety Administration (OSHA) standards.

One of the most exciting aspects of being an athletic trainer is returning an individual to play or work after an injury. Watching an athlete progress through the phases of healing and return to activity without limitations is wonderful. The truly rewarding part is when all of the pieces fall into place; the history leads to an accurate diagnosis. Once an athletic trainer obtains the correct diagnosis, the plan of care flows smoothly and the injury progresses like clockwork through the phases of injury healing and repair. Not all injuries will follow a predictable path, however. Therefore an athletic trainer must employ a systematic process to help determine the mechanism of injury, diagnosis, and phase of injury repair. An understanding of the injury pathology is necessary to accomplish the common goal—that is, returning the injured person back to play or work as quickly and as safely as possible (Figure 4-1).

MECHANISM OF INJURY

Imagine the following scenarios: A patient complains to the athletic trainer of dull knee pain deep in the joint. While providing on-site coverage for a game, an athlete drops to the ground holding her ankle. The athletic trainer is called out to a basketball practice because an athlete fell and is bleeding. The athletic trainer's actions, which begin with his or her initial questions, help in the proper diagnosis and treatment of these injuries. Whether the athletic trainer asks verbal questions or makes observations while approaching the athlete, the first response to every injury situation will likely be "What happened?" The goal of the questions are to determine the **mechanism of injury** (**MOI**). The MOI or mechanism of illness details specifically how the injury or illness

mechanism of injury (MOI) the way an athlete was injured

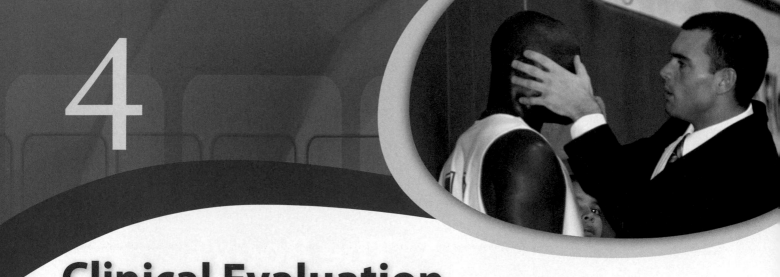

OPENING *Scenario*

At the state gymnastics meet, an athlete misses his hand grip on the high bar and immediately falls to the mat. After hitting his face on the bar, he lands on his side, holding both his cheek and his left knee. As you approach him, you can see blood coming out of the laceration on his cheek. Although you can't immediately tell what is causing the pain in his knee, it does appear as if he sprained his medial collateral ligament when he made his awkward landing on the mat. Before you can determine the exact cause of injury and make the appropriate diagnosis, you need to question and evaluate the athlete in a systematic manner. What do you ask him, and how do you move through the evaluation? How do you protect yourself while you are also attempting to provide quick and thorough care to him?

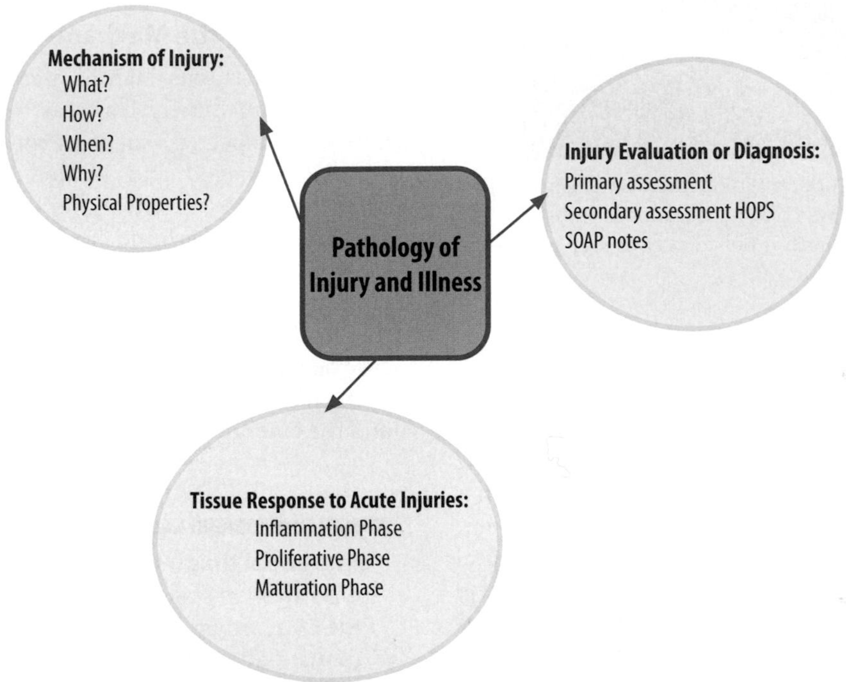

FIGURE 4-1 The systematic process that helps determine the mechanism of injury, injury diagnosis, and phase of injury repair.

occurred. In other words, it identifies the main cause of the injury. Initially, this information will be in lay terms: "I jumped up to catch the basketball and then landed on someone else's foot. I rolled my right ankle out a lot!" The athletic trainer will then translate this into medical terminology: "The athlete's right ankle inverted severely" (Figure 4-2).

The MOI should also provide clues as to whether the injury is **acute**, of recent onset, or **chronic**, with symptoms that persist longer than a few weeks. Right away, the athletic trainer will want to ask how long the injury has been bothering the athlete. The injuries presented in the previous scenarios are acute injuries—acute because they just occurred. A statement such as "It always hurts when I walk up and down stairs" points to a long-term injury. If the pain has been present for several weeks, with a gradual onset, the injury would be labeled as chronic.

It is very important to understand and establish an accurate MOI. The MOI guides the evaluation for both emergency and nonemergency situations regardless of the setting. It can provide clues as to the nature and severity of the injury or illness. For example, even before the physical examination begins, the severe inversion sprain would lead the athletic trainer to suspect possible injury to the lateral ankle ligaments, distal fibula, and the peroneal

acute describes a rapid onset
chronic describes a long progression

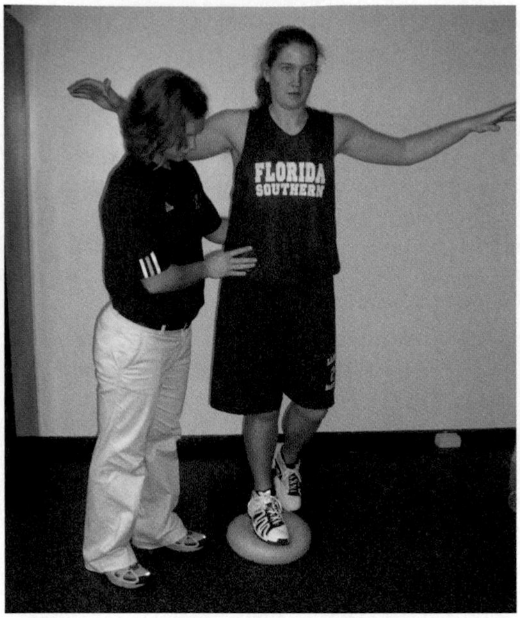

FIGURE 4-2 After properly determining the mechanism of injury, this athlete's ankle injury was diagnosed and her rehabilitation program was designed to return her to play as well as prevent future injuries.

tendons. All these structures are located on the lateral side of the ankle and can be damaged in an inversion injury.

The MOI helps lead to the **differential diagnosis**. The differential diagnosis includes all of the injuries that might be present after the initial evaluation. At this point, the differential diagnosis would be sprain of the lateral ankle ligaments, fibular fracture, and strain of the peroneal tendons. The evaluation would then shift to focus on confirming or ruling out these injuries. On completion of the evaluation, multiple injuries may still remain in the differential diagnosis. The clinical tests performed may have been inconclusive, requiring further diagnostic tests such as X-rays or a magnetic resonance imaging (MRI) scan to confirm the diagnosis.

The MOI can also guide immediate treatment of the injury. Because the athletic trainer already knows that the fibula could be fractured in this injury, he or she would immediately rule out the fracture before proceeding to other parts of the examination. If the initial exam shows positive signs for a fracture, the ankle should be splinted and the patient referred for X-rays. However, if the athletic trainer is able to determine that the injury is a sprain, a more thorough evaluation would typically follow, with an appropriate treatment of participation, rest, ice, compression, elevation, and stabilization (**PRICES**), as discussed in Chapter 8.

Knowledge of MOI also drives change and improvement in sport- and work-related rules, techniques, equipment, surfaces, policies, and procedures (Box 4-1). For example, extensive research has indicated that **spearing** is an MOI for cervical spine fractures and cervical spinal cord trauma. Spearing occurs when a football player tackles another athlete using his head or helmet as the point of contact. This technique can cause serious injuries to both players involved. In 1976, these findings resulted in the strict enforcement of the rules regarding spearing.[1] Another example of MOIs driving change involves the evolution of turf. The shorter, older style of artificial turf used for playing fields was found to increase the risk of tearing a major knee ligament called the anterior cruciate ligament (ACL). Knowledge of numerous injuries with the same MOI resulted in many teams eventually returning to grass playing fields or upgrading their old turf to the newer, thicker type.

Determining the Mechanism of Injury

The athletic trainer should ask questions to determine the MOI immediately. If a catastrophic or life-threatening injury is suspected, such an injury must take priority and be managed and treated right away. Once the situation is under control, the athletic trainer should ask questions to determine how the injury occurred. For example, if a football player makes a hard tackle, lies motionless, and says that he has numbness in both legs, the head and neck should be stabilized immediately in case he had suffered a spinal injury. A discussion related to the MOI would not ensue until after he was stabilized and the emergency medical system (EMS) was activated.

differential diagnosis a list of diagnoses being considered after an evaluation

PRICES acronym for the appropriate treatment path (participation, rest, ice, compression, elevation, and stabilization)

spearing a football tackle in which the tackler uses the helmet (including face mask) to butt or ram an opponent

BOX 4-1 Importance of the Mechanism of Injury

- Details how the injury occurred
- Determines when the injury occurred (acute versus chronic)
- Guides evaluation
- Determines level of severity
- Leads to a differential diagnosis
- Guides treatment plans
- Helps prevent future injuries
- Drives policy changes for injury prevention

At this point, the MOI is secondary to stabilizing the athlete and providing acute care.

After arriving on the scene of an emergency, the athletic trainer should immediately begin asking questions to determine what happened and how it happened. The athletic trainer may ask these questions while surveying the scene for victims and signs of inherent danger. Some situations require special caution. For example, the athletic trainer should not provide physical assistance to a victim who is in contact with an active power line. Caution must also be exercised when the victim appears to have fallen a distance greater than his or her own height. In this case, the athletic trainer should immediately suspect a spinal injury and treat the individual accordingly.

When the situation is not an emergency, the athletic trainer may ask questions to determine the MOI while taking the patient's medical history (Box 4-2). Examples of appropriate questions include the following: "What is your primary complaint?" and "How did you hurt yourself?" If the patient does not remember exactly how the injury occurred, the athletic trainer may need to probe deeper by asking questions such as "What activities seem to aggravate the injury most?" or "What activities are most difficult to do?" Determining whether the pain began suddenly (an acute onset) or gradually over time (an insidious onset or chronic injury) is also important.

Physical Properties Related to Mechanism of Injury

The athletic trainer must have a solid understanding of the physical principles or forces that can act on the body to help determine the MOI. A strong basis in kinesiology, the study of human movement, and specifically biomechanics, the application of both physics and mechanical models to describe human movement, will help the athletic trainer determine whether the individual's body movements and posture are normal or abnormal. An understanding of how different body tissues, such as tendons, ligaments, and bone, respond to the various stresses placed on them during activity is equally important.

Several factors determine whether a given force results in injury. Forces can act at different angles, over large or small surfaces, and over varying periods of time. For example, **hypermobility** in an ankle can cause repeated compression of the medial deltoid ligaments. This condition occurs because excessive movement at the joint results in an instability of the soft tissue, which can lead to injury. If the force is of a small magnitude, such as that which might occur during jogging, the patient probably will not develop pain or have an apparent injury on the first day or even during the first week of training. However, over time, this repeated **microtrauma** may result in chronic inflammation of the ligaments, swelling, and pain. A small lesion can subsequently develop as a result of the repetitive force applied to the tissues. If the patient rests adequately between bouts of exercise, he or she might be able to heal and make a full recovery. However, if the trauma is substantial and the athlete repeats the activity with sufficient frequency, damage to the ligaments may result in pain and swelling.

In an acute injury, a single traumatic event can be isolated as the cause of injury. This event is caused by a single, large force that results in a larger lesion, or **macrotrauma**. For example, a soccer player may tell the athletic trainer that her knee buckled when another player kicked her on the outer part of her knee. She now has a great deal of pain and swelling on the medial aspect of the knee, which suggests that she suffered a severe valgus force to her medial collateral ligament (Figure 4-3). Depending on the intensity of the force, the ligament could have minor tears (a Grade I sprain), have moderate tears (a Grade II sprain), or be completely ruptured (a Grade III sprain). Table 4-1 differentiates each type of grade.

Tissue Type

The type of tissue involved can also affect the type of injury that results from a particular force. Some tissues are more **extensible** than others and simply increase in length, or elongate, with repeated tension (Box 4-3). For example, muscles can readily elongate with rapid or sustained forces and are more extensible than tendons,

BOX 4-2 Questions to Determine Mechanism of Injury

- What is your primary complaint?
- What happened?
- How did it happen?
- Where do you hurt?
- What makes your symptoms worse?
- What makes your symptoms better?
- When did it happen?
- Was the pain sudden, or did it gradually appear?
- What activities can you do?
- What activities are challenging right now?

hypermobility excessive motion in a joint that can result in injury and instability
microtrauma very small lesion caused by small amounts of force over time
macrotrauma a larger lesion caused by a single large force
extensible describes a tissue that elongates in response to repeated tension

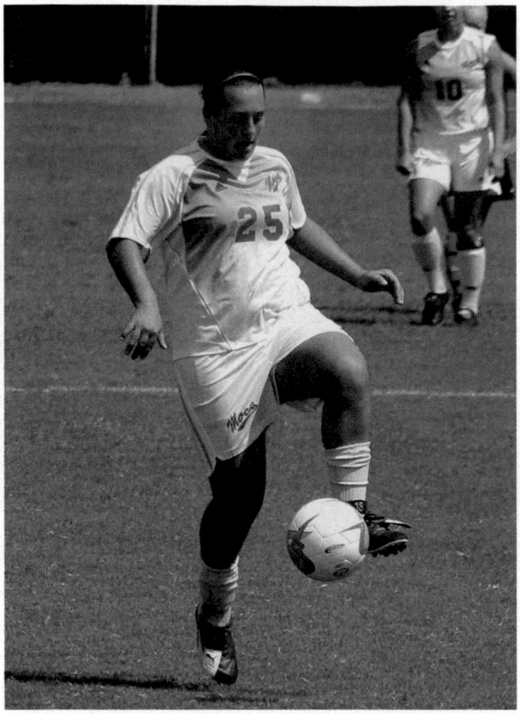

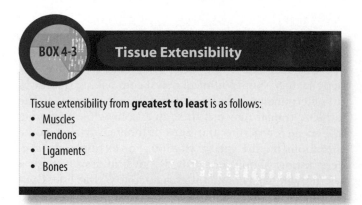

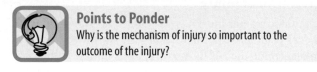

FIGURE 4-3 Depending on the amount of force producing the injury, this soccer player could sustain a Grade I, II, or III sprain. The laxity in the ligament is the deciding factor in determining the correct level of trauma.

TABLE 4-1 Grading Scale for Forces Resulting in Acute Injuries

GRADE	DESCRIPTION
Grade I sprain	Minor tissue tears
Grade II sprain	Moderate tissue tears
Grade III sprain	Complete tissue tear or rupture

which in turn are more extensible than bone. Forces applied to these tissues typically do not result in injuries or tears. With gentle repeated stretching over time, the length of the muscles can increase without causing pain or decreased strength or function. On the other hand, bones cannot be stretched without resulting in damage. Repeated forces on bones, even if minor, can lead to stress fractures over time.

Types of Forces

The type of force determines both the injury itself and the severity of the injury. Forces that can cause damage in the body include tension, compression, bending, shearing, and rotational forces (Figure 4-4). Tension is a longitudinal force, such as a muscle stretch. Compression forces squeeze or crush tissues, such as in a direct blow that causes a contusion (i.e., bruise). A bending force results in tension on one side and compression on the opposite side. In a severe inversion ankle sprain, the tissues on the lateral side (i.e., lateral ligaments and peroneal tendons) are stretched and the tissues on the medial side (i.e., deltoid ligaments and posterior tibialis tendon) become compressed. Another type of force that can damage tissues is a shearing force. Shearing forces occur in a direction that is perpendicular to the tissue fibers involved, as when the tibia translates anteriorly on the femur, resulting in an anterior cruciate ligament (ACL) tear. Shearing can also result in friction blisters or abrasions. Rotational forces are often a combination of both tension and shearing forces. Spiral fractures as well as ACL tears are frequently the product of rotational forces that act on the specific tissues. Table 4-2 summarizes the various types of forces and potential resulting injuries.

BOX 4-3 Tissue Extensibility

Tissue extensibility from **greatest to least** is as follows:

- Muscles
- Tendons
- Ligaments
- Bones

Points to Ponder

Why is the mechanism of injury so important to the outcome of the injury?

Stress Produced by Force

Some forces result in injury, whereas others do not. This variability occurs because the amount of damage caused by a particular force is determined in part by the amount of surface area affected by the force. If a large force is applied over a small area, such as when someone is hit by a baseball at a high velocity, great stress is applied to the area and significant trauma, in the form of contusions or fractures, can be expected. However, being hit by a soccer ball in the same forearm at the same speed would result in less stress and thus less trauma. Because the force of the impact is distributed over the soccer ball's larger surface area, the opportunity for injury lessens dramatically.

Examples of intrinsic factors that determine the extent of injury caused by any particular force are the strength and extensibility of the tissue (Box 4-4). Weaker tissues are injured more easily and more often. This increased vulnerability becomes apparent in older people as their bones, muscles, and ligaments become less dense and more brittle and therefore more prone to injury. The

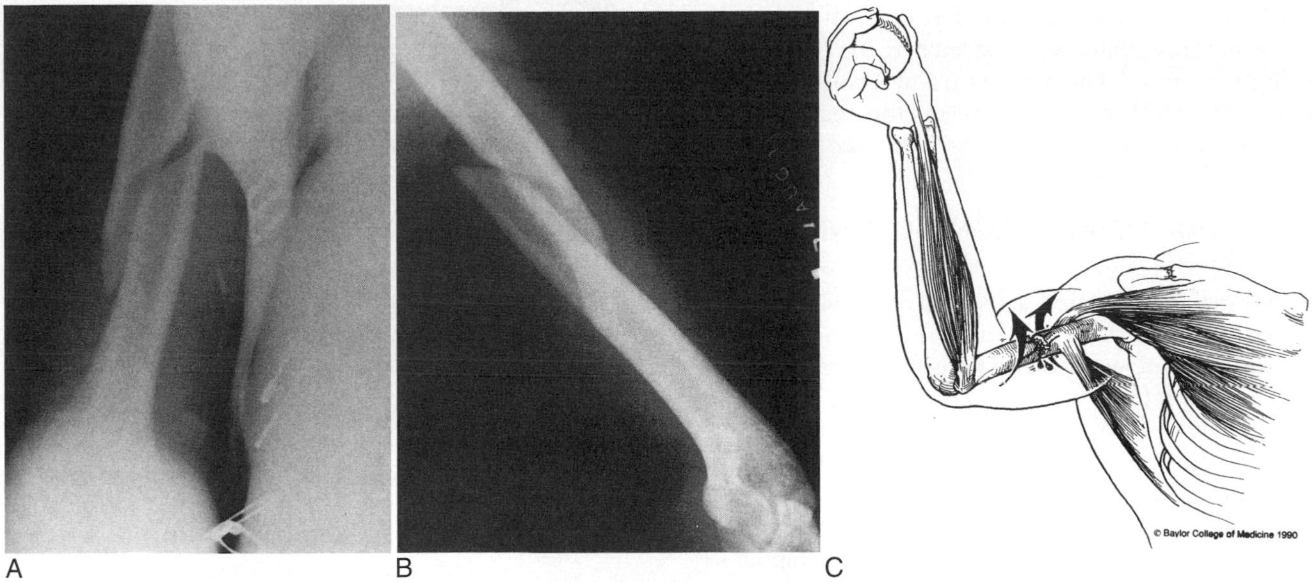

FIGURE 4-4 Forces such as tension, compression, bending, shearing, and rotational forces can cause various injuries. Rotational forces caused this spiral oblique fracture of the humerus. **A**, Anteroposterior view. **B**, Lateral view. **C**, Muscular rotational and biomechanical forces produced this spiral fracture of the humerus. (From DeLee JC, Drez J Jr, Miller MD: *DeLee &Drez's orthopaedic sports medicine,* ed 2, Philadelphia, 2003, Elsevier/Saunders.)

TABLE 4-2 Forces and Resulting Injuries

FORCE	RESULTING INJURY
Tension force: longitudinal force or stretching	Soft-tissue stretching: strains
Compression force: squeeze or crush	Squeezing or crushing tissue: contusions, tearing, direct blows
Bending force	Tension and compression forces on opposite sides: ligament tears, fractures
Shearing force	Forces occur perpendicular to the tissue fibers: ligament tears, blisters, abrasions
Rotational force	Combined tension and shearing forces: ligament tears, spiral fractures

BOX 4-4 Factors Affecting Injury

Intrinsic
- Tissue strength
- Tissue extensibility
- Fitness levels
- Nutrition
- Disease

Extrinsic
- Protective equipment
- Playing surfaces
- Training regimen
- Footwear
- Environment

same trauma that causes minimal to no injury at age 18 might result in a complete ligament rupture at age 60. The strength and extensibility of tissues also can be affected by both the fitness level and the nutritional status of the individual. On average, the healthier and more fit someone is, the less likely he or she is to sustain an injury.

Extrinsic factors that can affect the extent of the injury include protective equipment, playing surfaces, training regimen, and even footwear (see Box 4-4). Although helmets protect the head from direct compression forces by distributing that force throughout the entire helmet, an improperly fitted helmet can focus that force on one small area, resulting in a concussion or skull fracture. Shoes designed for normal feet and arches with flexible support can reduce the impact forces of running on hard surfaces; the same shoe, however, can allow excessive pronation in runners with high medial longitudinal arches, resulting in unnecessary injuries such as medial tibial stress syndrome (MTSS), or shin splints.

Understanding the mechanism of injury and illness is an important part of the evaluation process. Athletic trainers must be able to use the information gained to determine which tissues may have been damaged. If an

MOI can be visualized, it should be possible to visualize the structures that were stretched or compressed during the injury. The athletic trainer must be able to express the MOI in technical terms for documentation purposes and also in lay terms to better explain the injury to the athlete.

BASIC INJURY EVALUATION: OBTAINING THE DIAGNOSIS

Performing an evaluation may seem quite overwhelming at first. Where does the athletic trainer start? How does the athletic trainer know whether to activate EMS? Should the athletic trainer perform the evaluation immediately at the site of injury or move the patient to another location? Although no two situations are identical, it is best to use a systematic approach to the injury evaluation similar to the process for determining the MOI. Consistent technique helps ensure that all key areas are methodically addressed and nothing that could possibly lead to an accurate diagnosis and treatment plan is overlooked.

Primary Assessment

The most important step to take in any injury situation is first to rule out life- and limb-threatening conditions (Figure 4-5; see also Box 4-5). As discussed in detail in Chapter 7, this is referred to as the *primary assessment*. The athletic trainer always begins by assessing consciousness and then the airway, breathing, and circulation (**ABC**). Other examples of life-threatening conditions that the athletic trainer must assess and monitor include severe bleeding, head injury, and shock. The priority is to assess thesc potential situations and then methodically move through the rest of the evaluation.

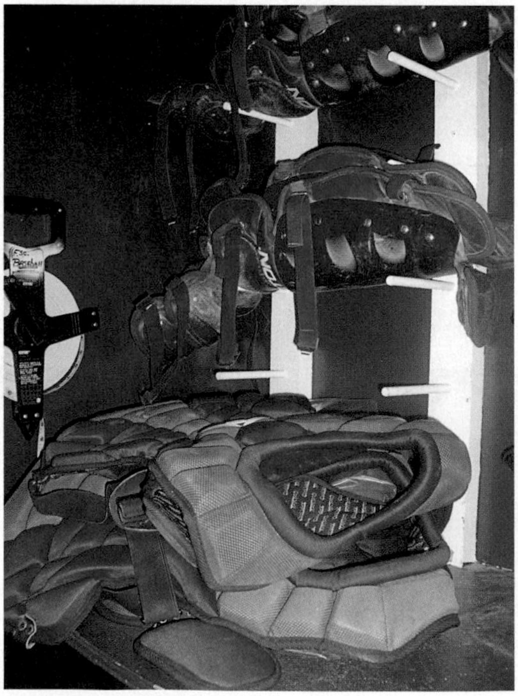

FIGURE 4-5 Extrinsic factors can easily affect the outcome of an injury, especially if these items are improperly fitted, worn, or inappropriate for the activity.

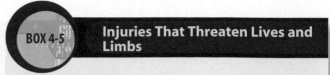

BOX 4-5 Injuries That Threaten Lives and Limbs

Life-Threatening Conditions
- Obstructed airway
- Severe bleeding
- Head injury
- Shock

Limb-Threatening Injuries
- Major fractures
- Dislocations
- Severe bleeding

Limb-threatening injuries, though not life-threatening at first, can rapidly deteriorate (see Box 4-5). Before doing anything else, the athletic trainer must perform a thorough assessment to determine the severity of injury to the extremities. Examples of limb-threatening injuries include major fractures (open or closed), dislocations, and severe bleeding. Once the status of the limbs is determined, the injury evaluation can progress. Remember, the primary assessment is ultimately determining if a situation requires emergency transportation.

Secondary Assessment

Once life- and limb-threatening conditions have been ruled out, the secondary assessment can begin. The acronym HOPS (sometimes referred to as HIPS) is a useful guide in completing the nonemergency portion of the evaluation. The acronym *HOPS* stands for history, observation/inspection, palpation, and stress tests and special tests. This information is obtained through questions and the visual and physical inspection of the body. Box 4-6 summarizes the four steps of the **HOPS/HIPS** process, each of which is described in greater detail in the following sections.

ABC acronym used in primary assessment (airway, breathing, circulation)

HOPS/HIPS acronym used to guide secondary assessment (history, observation/inspection, palpation, stress)

BOX 4-6 Steps in the HOPS Evaluation

History
- Previous injury to the affected body part?
- If yes, what was it and how was it treated?
- Has it happened more than once?
- Mechanism of injury?
- Acute: where, how, when, what, why, and fully describe the pain
- Chronic: where, how, when, what, why, and fully describe any changes in the pain over time
- Comments from family, spouse, or guardians
- Systemic conditions or disease?
- Medications?
- Pregnancy?

Observation

Body Position and Movement
- Gait
- Posture
- Carrying angle and technique of injured body part
- Position of comfort
- Pain gestures or grimaces
- Other contributing factors

Injured Body Part
- Swelling
- Discoloration
- Deformity
- Muscle atrophy
- Blisters or calluses
- Redness, open wounds, or infection

Palpation
- Palpation of noninvolved side first, followed by the involved side
- Palpation away from the injured site first, then toward the injury
- Palpation superficially and gently, with progression to deeper and firmer
- Palpation for possible deformities in the following:
  Bony landmarks
  Ligaments
  Tendons
  Muscles
  Joint capsules
  Menisci
- Palpation of nerves for sensitivity irregularities
- Palpation of blood vessels for presence and strength of pulses

Stress Tests and Special Tests
- Range of motion—active first, then passive, then resisted
- Strength testing
- Injury-specific special tests
- Functional testing
- Diagnostic testing

History

The history is mostly subjective information, meaning that it cannot be objectively verified in its entirety. When taking a history, the athletic trainer should ask questions that rely solely on the memory of the athlete (Figure 4-6). Though similar to determining the mechanism of injury, completing the history portion of the evaluation prods more deeply to provide conclusive information on the diagnosis, not just information on how the injury may have happened. The athletic trainer should find out whether the athlete has previously injured the affected area of the body. If so, the athletic trainer should ask what kind of injury it was, how it was treated, and if it healed completely. The athletic trainer should determine whether the previous diagnosis was made through a physical examination or if previous diagnostic testing such as X-rays, MRI scans, or blood work was performed. It is also helpful to find out whether the athlete has experienced similar injuries in the **contralateral**, or opposite, limb.

The next set of questions in the history will help determine the MOI, as previously discussed (see Box 4-6). Did the athlete trip over something? Did someone push him or her? Did the leg just seem to give way suddenly? If so, was he or she running straight or changing directions at the time? Did the athlete receive a blow to the lateral portion of the knee (a valgus force) or get stepped on (a crushing force)? Unless the athletic trainer saw the injury occur or can review a videotape, verifying the MOI will be impossible.

If the injury is acute, the injured person probably will have already described the pain; the key is to get the patient to describe the pain in detail. Where does it hurt most? Can the athlete point to one spot on the body that is most painful? Is it sharp or dull? Is it throbbing or aching? Does the athlete feel the pain only at the site of injury, or does it seem to radiate beyond that site? How would the athlete rate the pain on a scale of 0 to 10 (with 0 being no pain and 10 being the worst pain imaginable)? If the injury did not just happen, the athletic trainer should ask questions about the athlete's previous pain. What did it feel like when it happened? How long ago did it

contralateral opposite

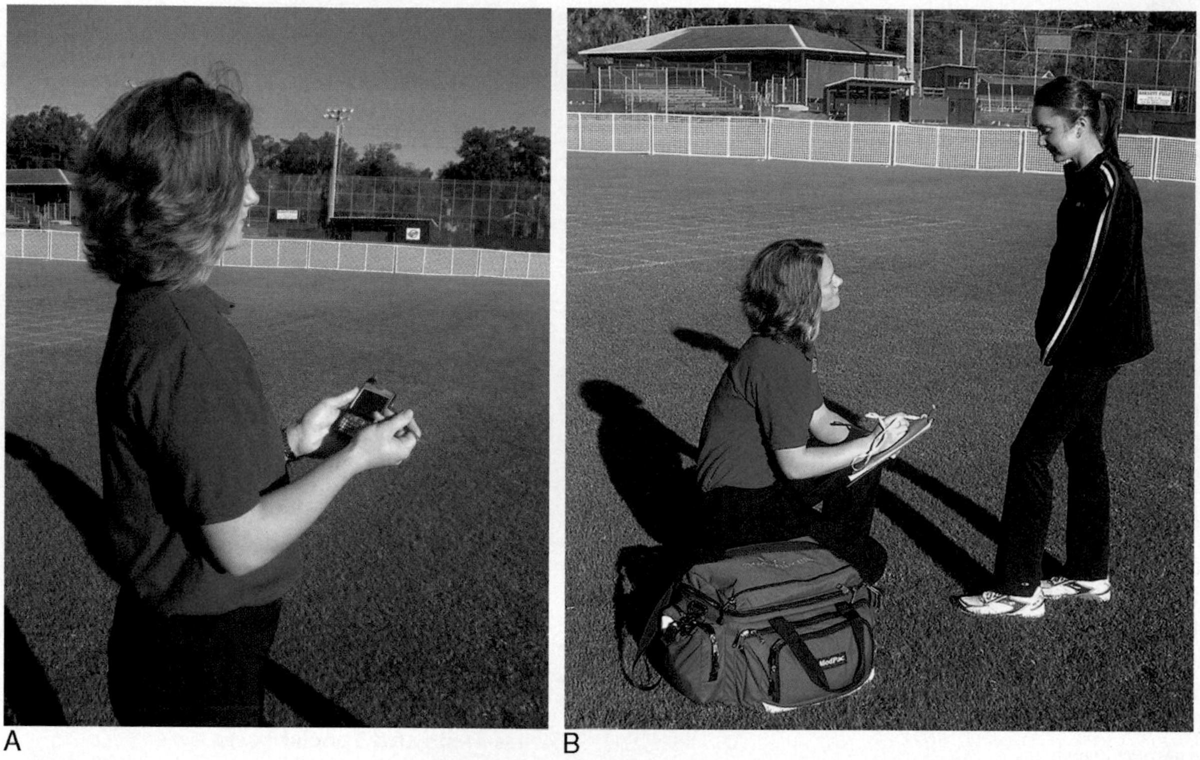

FIGURE 4-6 Subjective injury being recorded with newer electronic devices **(A)** and the traditional way, with paper and pen **(B)**.

happen? Did the onset of symptoms occur suddenly or gradually over time? Between then and now, has the pain increased or decreased? What time of day does it seem to be most or least intense? What seems to reduce or increase the pain? Are there any daily activities that are difficult or impossible because of this injury? Have any changes occurred in the athlete's daily routine, such as beginning a new workout routine, adding more stair-walking at work, or wearing new shoes? A thorough history often leads the athletic trainer 80% to 90% of the way toward making an accurate diagnosis.

The history may include subjective statements from the patient or other involved parties. Often, important information is not disclosed by the injured person but instead comes from his or her companions. The fear of not being able to compete or return to work frequently interferes with the clear communication of important information. The athletic trainer should ask other general questions to determine additional mitigating factors as well as conditions that may affect the course of treatment. For example, has the athlete had any systemic conditions such as diabetes or pregnancy? Documenting any medications that the patient is currently taking is important in preventing dangerous drug interactions, in the event that medications are involved in the course of treatment.

Observation or Inspection

During the observation or inspection portion of the examination, the athletic trainer looks at the injured athlete to uncover clues that may further assist in determining an accurate diagnosis (see Box 4-6). Although it is listed second (after the history), the observation should begin as soon as the patient enters the room or the athletic trainer approaches him or her. Observe the way in which the athlete is holding the body. Is he or she lying down in pain or walking into the examination/training room calmly? Is the athlete's arm hanging at the side, or is he or she cradling it with the other arm? Can the athlete walk with a normal gait, or is there a noticeable limp? How is the posture? The athletic trainer should also look for other signs that might contribute to the injury, such as obesity, equipment issues, surfaces, or general poor health.

The second level of observation or inspection is more specific to the injured body part. Is there swelling, discoloration, or deformity present? How does the body area look compared with the contralateral limb (bilateral comparison)? Does one side appear to have muscle atrophy (muscle wasting) when compared with the other? Does the athlete have blisters or calluses? Are there any signs of infection, such as redness of the skin or pus oozing from an open wound?

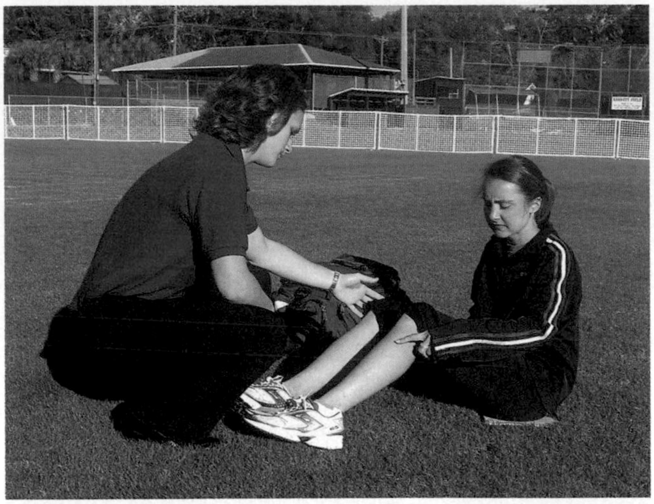

FIGURE 4-7 Observation of the injury provides critical information in the determination of the correct diagnosis.

It may be necessary to remove certain clothing, protective equipment, or shoes to thoroughly observe the injured body part (Figure 4-7).

Palpation

Palpation involves physically touching the injured athlete. To establish normal standards for the patient, the athletic trainer begins by palpating the uninjured side first. This approach helps put the patient at ease and allows him or her to know what to expect when the athletic trainer palpates the injured side. The athletic trainer should begin by palpating away from the location of most intense pain and work toward the injured area. Palpation should be superficial and gentle at first and then progress to deeper, firmer palpation. The athletic trainer should attempt to locate and feel each bony landmark, ligament, and tendon as well as other structures, such as joint capsules and menisci. The goal is to determine what specific areas are painful or physically different (deformed) compared with those of the uninjured side. The athletic trainer should locate and palpate nerves to determine hyposensitivity or hypersensitivity and palpate prominent blood vessels to establish the presence and strength of the pulse (Figure 4-8).

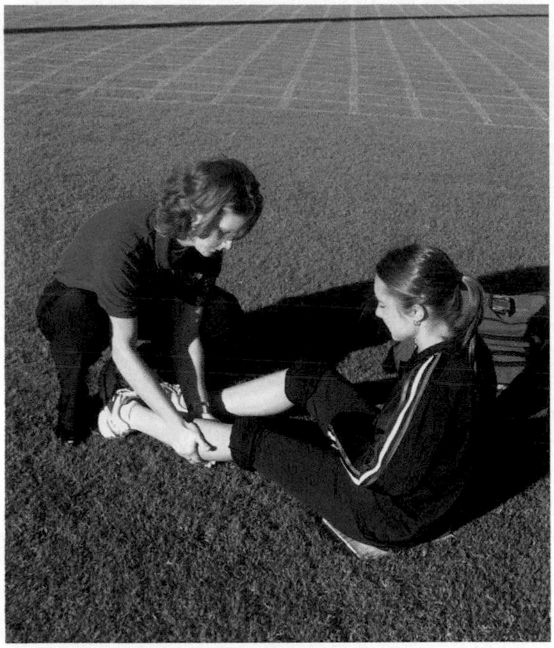

FIGURE 4-8 Palpation of an injury allows detection of abnormalities that might otherwise go undetected.

Stress Tests and Special Tests

The stress test part of the evaluation includes a variety of assessment tools such as range of motion (ROM), strength, injury-specific special tests, and functional tests based on the demands of the particular activity. Assuming that any obvious fractures have been ruled out through the initial evaluation, ROM testing can be performed. The athletic trainer asks the patient to move the affected body part through the appropriate ROM on his or her own; this is known as **active range of motion (AROM)**. AROM provides a good idea of how far the patient is comfortable moving the involved body part. AROM assessment also provides a baseline for subsequent passive ROM and resisted ROM testing. Next, the athletic trainer asks the athlete to relax while motion is initiated, and the limb is moved through the same movement patterns, known as **passive range of motion (PROM)**. PROM identifies elements like quality of movement and joint end points or end feel. The next step is to assess strength through resisted ROM (RROM). This means that the athletic trainer has the athlete move through the motions while the athletic trainer manually resists the motion, looking to establish strength deficits, pain, muscle spasm, and so on.

A great number of injury-specific special tests are available to confirm or rule out certain diagnoses (Figure 4-9). In the case of the twisted ankle in the runner, the bump test and squeeze tests can rule out fractures. The talar tilt and anterior drawer tests evaluate the integrity of the ligaments supporting the joint. In the following chapters, special tests will be presented for each injury. Some conditions can be diagnosed through multiple injury-specific special tests.

active range of motion (AROM) movement possible when an individual actively moves a joint

passive range of motion (PROM) movement possible when another person moves an individual's joint

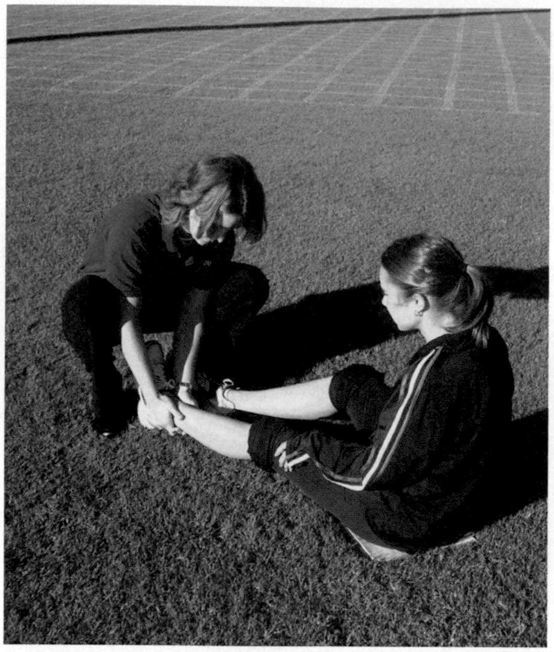

FIGURE 4-9 Injury-specific tests are performed as soon as possible to help rule out specific diagnoses. The possibility of fractures should always be ruled out before any special tests are attempted.

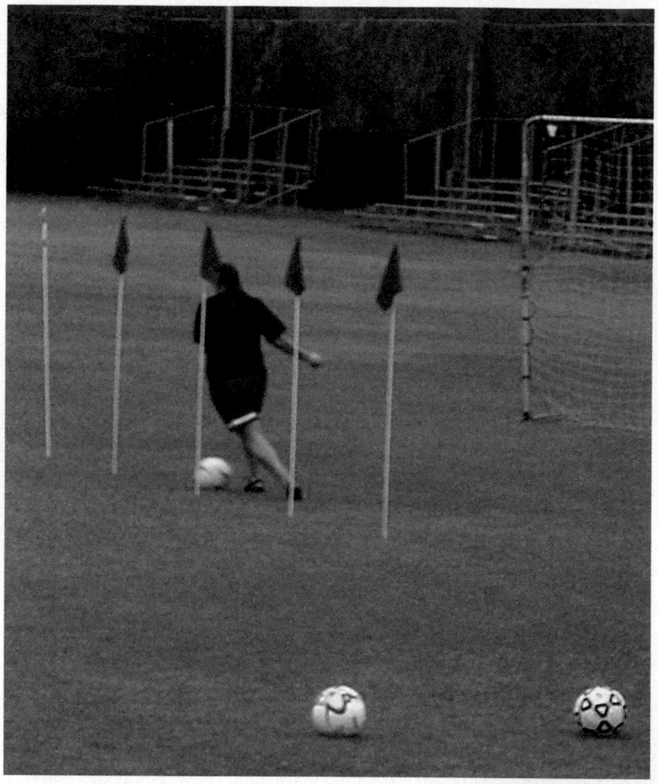

FIGURE 4-10 Functional clearance tests should be used to provide the final verification that the patient is ready to return to his or her chosen activity.

It is also prudent to include functional testing in the comprehensive stress test section. Functional testing helps determine whether the athlete can walk, run, hop, jump, or perform specific activities that are required to perform the sport or job (Figure 4-10). Other activities that could be included in the functional test are assessments such as lifting a box, pulling a heavy item, or kicking a ball—all activities that the athlete would perform regularly.

The final elements in the comprehensive stress tests are not necessarily stress inducing. The remaining assessment tools include any special diagnostic testing such as X-rays, MRI tests, bloodwork, diagnostic ultrasounds, and computed tomography (CT) scans. Also included are a range of prescriptive and invasive neurological testing tools, from the simple evaluation of deep tendon reflexes to nerve conduction velocity testing, balance testing, and cranial nerve assessments.[2]

Although the athletic trainer should never risk further injury by moving an athlete off the field too soon, the game cannot stop for 20 to 30 minutes to allow for a complete assessment. As discussed previously, the first duty of the athletic trainer is to rule out life- and limb-threatening injuries. The athletic trainer should monitor the patient's airway, breathing, and circulation (ABCs), evaluate for spinal and head injuries, look for severe bleeding, check for fractures or dislocations, and then move the athlete from the area of activity. Once the athlete has been moved elsewhere, such as the athletic training room, the athletic trainer will have more time to complete a thorough evaluation. This procedure will vary somewhat depending on the circumstances of the case. For example, the runner who fell on the course may suffer only a moderately sprained ankle but still be so distressed about her injury that she refuses to be moved at first. In this instance, the athletic trainer would first have to calm the athlete, despite the lack of harm that would be caused by gently moving her off the course.

Documentation: SOAP Notes

Once the evaluation is completed and the athletic trainer has made an accurate diagnosis, the findings must be recorded either on paper or in a computer using injury tracking software. The format typically used to document the evaluation is referred to as a **SOAP note** (Figure 4-11). Some choose to write these notes in paragraph form, whereas others prefer a bulleted format. SOAP notes consist of the following components:[3]

SOAP note acronym for documentation in an evaluation (subjective, objective, assessment, plan)

- S = Subjective (includes the *H* from HOPS)
- O = Objective (includes the *OPS* from HOPS)
- A = Assessment (the diagnosis, short-term goals, and long-term goals)
- P = Plan (course of treatment and/or referral)

When writing the subjective portion of the SOAP note, the athletic trainer should include all the items discussed and discovered in the history section. The athletic trainer should also include the patient's name, age, sex, sport or activity (if applicable), date of injury,

FLORIDA Mocs SOUTHERN

Daily Progress Note

Name:__________________________ Date:__________

Sport:____________________ Position:________________

Body part injured:________________________ R L N/A

Subjective:________________________________

Objective:

Observation:____________________________

Palpation:______________________________

ROM:__________________________________

Strength:_______________________________

Injury-specific special tests:____________________

Functional tests:__________________________

Diagnostic tests:__________________________

Assessment:______________________________

Diagnosis:______________________________

Short-term goals:__________________________

Long-term Goals:__________________________

Plan:___________________________________

Referral to whom:__________________________

Treatment time:______ ATS/AT signature:____________________

FIGURE 4-11 A sample SOAP note form showing the necessary information that assists in developing the diagnosis and documents the plan of care.

date of examination, and name and credentials of the clinician. This information is sometimes included in the "subjective" section but more often summarized as a header at the top of the page.

The objective portion of the SOAP note includes all the information obtained from the remainder of the examination: observation, palpation, and stress tests (ROM, strength, special tests, functional tests, and diagnostic tests). Remember, subjective items generally cannot be verified because they are generated from the patient's memory or feelings. Objective items, conversely, are verifiable and reproducible by athletic trainers and other practitioners.

The assessment section includes the diagnosis or the differential diagnosis. A differential diagnosis includes several possible diagnoses that are still being considered. For example, after the examination of the runner's ankle, a Grade II sprain of both the anterior talofibular ligament and the calcaneofibular ligament may be suspected. It may also be possible that the runner has strained her peroneal muscles. Completing a full assessment immediately after the injury is sometimes difficult because of the patient's high levels of pain, spasm, or anxiety. Athletes may not allow the athletic trainer to assess ROM with any accuracy because they may be too frightened to move the injured body part.

The assessment section of the SOAP note should also include short- and long-term goals. These may be listed in the plan section as well. The goals must reflect what was discovered in the subjective and objective portions of the examination. Short-term goals, such as reducing pain and swelling and increasing ROM, should be benchmarks for the next week or so. Long-term goals are generally more functionally oriented and include items such as walking with a normal gait or returning to full activity. However, if the patient has undergone surgery and the recovery period is expected to last several months, long-term goals might be more modest, such as restoring full ROM or achieving strength equal to 80% of the uninjured side.

The plan in the final portion of the SOAP note describes ways to achieve the goals established in the assessment. If swelling is found and the goal is to reduce swelling, then the plan should include treatments designed to do so. It is vital for the plan to include specific details for every treatment and rehabilitation exercise. If the athletic trainer is not available to work with the patient on any subsequent visit, the plan should ensure that another clinician could continue with the treatment plan and rehabilitation program without delay or disruption. Also, all modality parameters must be listed, including time, waveform, phase duration, intensity, pad placement, and type of heat source. Rehabilitation exercises should specify the amount of weight used, the number of sets and repetitions, and any other relevant instructions. If the athlete has been referred to another practitioner for further evaluation, the following should be included: the name of the new practitioner, his or her credentials, and the date and time of the appointment. The final portion of the plan should be devoted to any instructions regarding the patient's daily home exercise program. Specific details, such as ongoing cardiorespiratory training, the rigor of the athlete's routine, instructions regarding elevation of the injured body part, and exercises to perform at home, should be included.

TISSUE RESPONSE TO INJURY OR ILLNESS

Healing is a matter of time but is sometimes also a matter of opportunity.

—Hippocrates

The human body is an amazing entity that can heal itself after almost any form of trauma. This section explains the way in which tissues heal as well as the time frame of the healing process. Inflammation, the first stage in the healing process, must occur for healing to take place.[4] However, the effects of excessive inflammation can cause secondary cell death. This secondary injury may be mitigated by prompt and efficacious treatments performed primarily with the use of PRICES, as previously discussed. *Inflammation* is often used as an umbrella term encompassing physical findings at the clinical, physiological, cellular, and molecular levels.[5] The inflammatory process is affected by both the type of tissue that is injured and the extent of the injury. Tissues with greater blood supply, such as muscles, heal better and more quickly than those with limited blood supply, such as ligaments.

Understanding the **pathology** of injury and the healing process is foundational for athletic trainers. The term *pathology* refers to the study of the nature, causes, and development of abnormal conditions that result in changes to the tissues' structure and function.[6] This knowledge helps determine the specific treatments chosen for the different phases of the healing process. Pathology affects decisions in the rehabilitation program and provides information that is useful in deciding when and how an athlete is ready to return to activity. Understanding pathology is also important when educating athletes about what is going on in their bodies and why.

The goal immediately after injury is to identify the extent of the injured area by reducing blood flow via vasoconstriction. The next step is to rid the area of waste products such as the fluids that have leaked out of cells and vessels as well as any dead cells that may have accumulated. Finally, the body takes steps to facilitate healing and return the tissue to its normal state.

Although no one can accelerate the healing process, the athletic trainer can ensure that optimal conditions

pathology the study of the nature, causes, and development of abnormal conditions, involving changes in structure and function exist for healing to occur by localizing and minimizing acute inflammation with cryotherapy and other steps in the PRICES process. Limiting the development of scar tissue can be accomplished in two steps: minimizing swelling and initiating early motion. Friction massage may be helpful in separating tissues (e.g., the skin and an underlying ligament) from one another when they are joined by scar tissue. Ultimately, the goal is to return the patient to play or work as quickly and as safely as possible.

Soft Tissue Response to Acute Injury

After an acute injury, such as an ankle sprain, various types of tissues suffer injury. The ligament that is torn suffers obvious damage, but the vascular tissue (e.g., the capillaries) may also be harmed. Damage to the tissue triggers a systematic and well-defined response by the body. The healing process follows a typical three-phase path: (1) inflammation; (2) proliferation, or repair; and (3) maturation, or remodeling (Figure 4-12). The inflammatory phase can last as long as 6 days after an acute injury. The proliferation phase lasts between 2 and 21 days and involves the formation of new tissue or the repairing of damaged tissue (or both). The final phase, maturation, can last up to a year or longer. During the last phase, the tissues realign along the lines of tensile force. Even though the time line is predictable, duration of each stage of repair can vary, and overlapping stages are also possible.

Inflammation Phase

The first event in the inflammation phase is the actual injury, which occurs when the tissue undergoes some sort of trauma, such as overstretching or a direct blow. The normal physiology of the tissue can be disrupted not only by these mechanical forces but also by chemical, thermal, or infectious agents. Immediately after the disruption, the tissue bleeds as a result of disruption of the vascular structures—namely, the capillaries. Fluids from damaged cells may also leak out into the **interstitial space** (i.e., the space between the cells), contributing to the local swelling. The body responds with vasoconstriction in an attempt to decrease the local bleeding and contain the extent of the injury. This initial phase lasts approximately 10 seconds to 10 minutes after the injury.

During the next phase of the inflammatory process, an initial wave of chemical mediators such as serotonin, adrenaline, noradrenaline, and histamine are released, which attracts various cells to the area and initiates healing. Initially, the locally circulating platelets respond to the injury by coming into contact with collagens in the blood vessel walls. Specific receptors on the platelet surface bind to collagen and trigger platelet adhesion and activation. The platelets release adenosine diphosphate (ADP) and serotonin to attract other platelets to the area, and together they combine with fibrin to form a platelet plug that seals tears in the vessels. This process is called **margination**. The second surge of platelet action involves the release of growth factors that influence other cells to repair tissue. These factors include transforming growth factor (TGF), platelet-derived growth factor (PDGF), and endothelial growth factor (EGF).

Once the clot is formed and bleeding has been mitigated, another wave of chemical mediators are released by the mast cells, basophils, and a local axon reflex, inducing **vasodilation**. This vasodilation brings white blood cells and other types of healing cells to the area. One such cell activated during the inflammatory phase is the endothelium. Endothelial cells regulate pain, aid in **coagulation**, improve vascular tone, and participate in the recruitment and passage of white blood cells. Induced by chemical mediators, endothelial cells proliferate and remodel their surrounding extracellular matrix, laying the groundwork for the early formation of scar or granulation tissue (Figure 4-13).

The third type of cell, **neutrophils**, are informally known as the "smart bomb" of inflammation. These cells are highly destructive and attack any injury as if it were an infection. The main functions of neutrophils are killing bacteria and performing **phagocytosis**, which is the engulfing of dead cells and tissue. The problem lies in the fact that neutrophils often attack and destroy

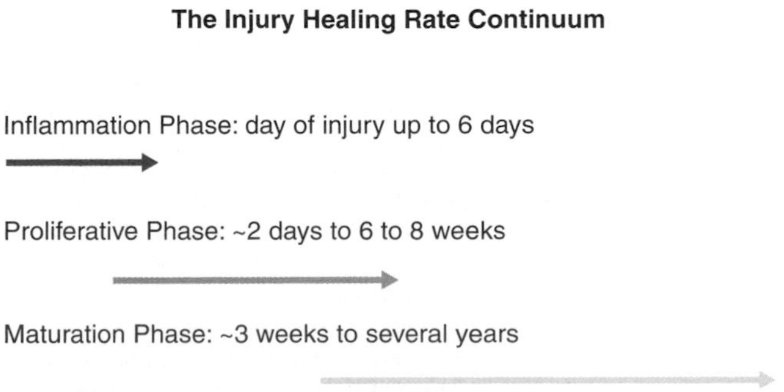
The Injury Healing Rate Continuum
Inflammation Phase: day of injury up to 6 days
Proliferative Phase: ~2 days to 6 to 8 weeks
Maturation Phase: ~3 weeks to several years

FIGURE 4-12 Approximate time line showing the injury healing rate continuum. This time line varies with each injury and each athlete.

interstitial space space between elements
margination initial response of platelets in early phase of inflammation
vasodilation opening or widening of a blood vessel
coagulation clotting, or changing blood from a liquid to a solid state
neutrophils white blood cells that destroy bacteria during inflammation; "smart bombs" of inflammation
phagocytosis the process of ingestion and digestion of solid substances by other cells

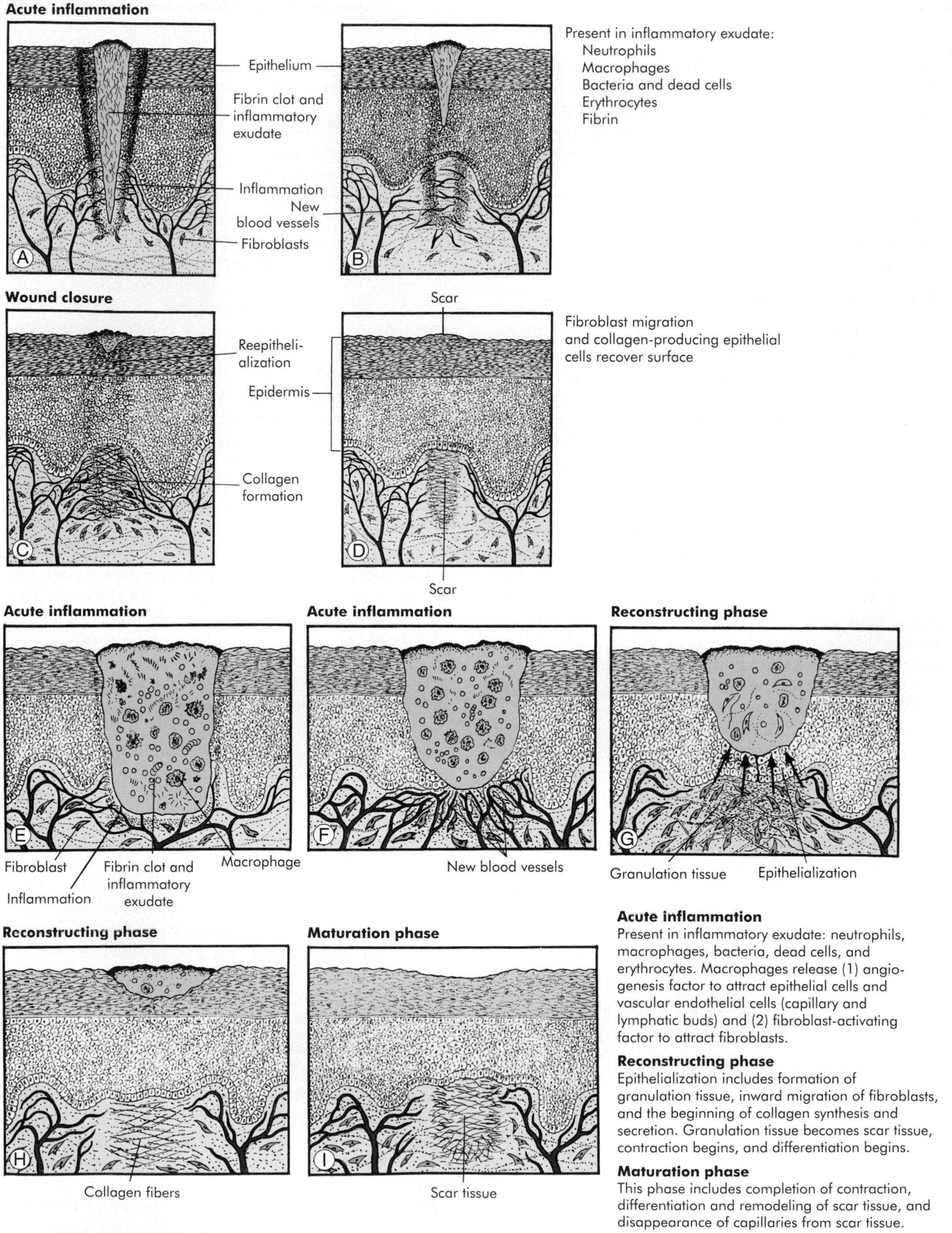

FIGURE 4-13 The phases of wound repair by primary or secondary intention. **A** to **D**, Healing by primary intention, which is when tissue is incised and reapproximated and healing occurs without complications. **E** to **I**, Healing by secondary intention, which is when open wound edges are not approximated and healing occurs through the formation of granulation tissue, contraction, and epithelialization. (From McCance KL, Huether SE: *Pathophysiology: the biologic basis of disease in adults and children,* ed 5, p. 202, St Louis, 2006, Mosby/Elsevier.)

not only the surrounding injured cells but also the healthy cells, treating them as if they were harmful bacteria. These destructive cells become active at the site of the injury within 24 hours. The purpose of phagocytosis is to debride tissues and reabsorb clots.[7] Without the presence of infection, neutrophils are not seen as vital for the successful repair of injuries. Therefore one therapeutic goal is to reduce their recruitment into the injured areas after injury by administering various anti-inflammatory drugs and using rest, ice, compression, and elevation (RICE).[8,9]

During the later phases of inflammation (i.e., between 24 and 48 hours), **macrophages** and **monocytes** become the most prominent cell types. Macrophages release additional chemical mediators in response to local hypoxia (i.e., lack of oxygen). The monocytes aid in coagulation and phagocytosis. Later, they will also secrete growth factors that attract the fibroblasts required during the repair phase of the healing process. The fibroblasts form and deposit collagen fibers that strengthen the nascent scar.[7]

Another effect of the second wave of chemical mediators is increased blood vessel permeability, which allows for a greater exchange of the healing cells described previously and also aids in the removal of waste products. Unfortunately, vasodilation and increased vascular permeability also lead to effusion, or edema. Combined with the effects of several chemical mediators, effusion can increase pain perception and decrease function.

Table 4-3 summarizes the response of the body's tissue at various times during the inflammation phase.

During the inflammation phase, five cardinal signs of inflammation can be identified: (1) swelling (tumor); (2) pain (dolore); (3) redness (rubor); (4) warmth (calor); and (5) loss of function (functio laesa). Evaluating the injury can be challenging because not all signs are present during the inflammation phase. Some symptoms may be present well into the repair and remodeling phases. One sign to monitor is any decrease or increase in symptoms. If the symptoms seem as if they are decreasing, the injury is most likely passing into the next phase, the proliferative phase. If the symptoms appear to be increasing, a re-injury or some other setback may have occurred that is prolonging the inflammation phase. Treatment and rehabilitation in the inflammation phase is relatively conservative, given that the scar or repaired tissue remains weak. Too much tissue stress in this phase can result in chronic injuries that do not move beyond the inflammatory process. This persistent inflammation results in a repetitive stress injury that never progresses adequately to the repair and remodeling phases.[10]

The first cardinal sign of inflammation is often the most obvious—swelling. Initially, swelling occurs because blood from torn vessels seeps into the interstitial space. Later, the increase in cell and vessel permeability allows more fluids and other cells to flood the area in an attempt to initiate healing. Cells die as a result of the initial trauma and the subsequent action of the neutrophils, which in turn causes intracellular fluid, proteins, and other cellular debris to leak out. As the extracellular pressure increases, the venous and lymphatic networks become blocked, trapping the swelling in the area. This fluid in the interstitial space becomes less fluid (transudate) and more thick and protein rich (exudate). It becomes more difficult to remove this fluid from the area because of its greater viscosity, or thickness.[11,12]

Pain, the second cardinal sign of inflammation, can be a friend and sometimes a foe. It tells the body to refrain from certain activities, such as running with a fractured tibia or touching a hot stove. Unfortunately, the body sometimes overreacts, generating pain even after an injury has healed. Pain is the result of mechanical

macrophages phagocytes involved in later phases of inflammation; cell that releases chemical mediators in response to hypoxia

monocytes phagocytes involved in later phases of inflammation; cell that aids in coagulation and phagocytosis

TABLE 4-3 Tissue Response During the Inflammation Phase

TIME	BODY'S RESPONSE	MAIN PURPOSE(S)
10 seconds to 10 minutes after injury	Tissue bleeding from capillaries; local swelling	Vasoconstriction; localization of injury
Within minutes after injury	Platelets binding together with fibrin to form plugs; beginning of tissue repair as serotonin, adrenaline, noradrenaline, histamine, and growth factors are released	Margination: clot formation and cessation of bleeding; beginning of healing process
Once the clot is formed	White blood cells appearing and activating endothelial cells	Vasodilation, formation of scar or granulation tissue
Within 24 hours of the injury	Release of neutrophils	Phagocytosis
24 to 48 hours after injury	Emergence of macrophages and monocytes	Coagulation and phagocytosis; increased blood vessel permeability

or chemical irritation of nerve endings. After an injury, pain is caused both by the trauma of the injury and the irritation caused by the release of chemical mediators, especially histamine, bradykinin, and prostaglandins. The swelling can also cause secondary pressure on the nerve endings, resulting in a residual dull ache.

Redness and warmth, the third and fourth cardinal signs of inflammation, are mainly a result of increased blood flow to the injured area. When the blood vessels dilate, the capillary beds may become engorged. Increased skin temperature may also be caused by the increase in metabolic activity related to tissue healing. The word *inflammation* is actually derived from the Latin term *inflammare,* which means to set on fire.[5] Although some redness and warmth are normal after an acute injury, prolonged signs of redness and warmth can indicate that an infection is present or the patient is still suffering from acute inflammation.

The fifth and last cardinal sign of inflammation, loss of function, is a combined result of the four previous signs. Pain and swelling, in particular, can inhibit function. Swelling increases pain, which causes local muscle spasms. The spasm causes more pain, which results in a vicious pain-spasm-pain cycle. The loss of function may also be a result of instability caused by the damage to support structures such as ligaments and bones. In summary, inflammation is a vital stage in the healing process. However, through the use of PRICES, the amount of secondary injury to the area can be limited and a favorable environment for healing can be created. To accomplish this task, athletic trainers must understand the inflammatory process and communicate this knowledge to the patient, parents, and coaches.

Box 4-7 summarizes these cardinal signs of inflammation.

Proliferative (Repair) Phase

The second stage in the healing process is the proliferative, or repair, phase. It can begin as early as 48 hours after the initial injury and last as long as 6 to 8 weeks. The body is now replacing damaged or dead cells and extracellular matrices with new cells and matrices. This process begins with endothelial cells, myofibroblasts, and fibroblasts accumulating at the injury site.

The repair process can occur in any of the following three ways, and often all three are occurring to some degree at the injury site:

1. *Resolution:* Dead cellular material and debris are removed by macrophages through the process of phagocytosis. In this case, the tissue suffered minimal damage and is left with its original architecture intact. The cells grow and return to their pre-injured state after inflammation resolves.
2. *Granulation, or fibroplasia:* **Fibroplasia** allows the lost tissues to be replaced with a fibrous scar produced from granulation tissue. The purpose of the scar is to form a bridge between the portions of tissue that became separated or torn as a result of the injury. The larger the gap between the disrupted tissues, the larger the scar will be. This process also begins with phagocytosis to clear away dead tissues and other debris. Proliferation of new capillaries, or angiogenesis, begins to establish blood flow in the healing area. Fibroblasts also migrate to the area to form a loose connective tissue framework within the exudate, similar to a spiderweb. These fibroblasts then produce collagen to provide mechanical strength to the new scar. Although the scar provides a necessary junction between separated tissues, it generally lacks the same vascularity and neurological feedback of the tissue it replaced. For this reason, it sometimes forms a barrier that prevents oxygen and nutrients from reaching nearby tissues. The maximal strength of this new tissue is approximately 70% of the original tissue (see Figure 4-13).
3. *Regeneration:* The third way that tissues repair themselves following injury is through regeneration. In regeneration, dead or damaged cells are replaced by new cells. These cells are of the same type as the damaged cell, as opposed to the scar tissue deposited in granulation. Several factors affect a tissue's ability to regenerate, including age, nutritional status, the amount of tissue loss, and the local blood supply.

The primary role of the athletic trainer during the repair phase is to assist the involved structures in gaining strength through moderate stress. Collagen fibers align along the lines of tensile force and increase in number and size in response to the appropriate stresses, such as movement and weight-bearing and strengthening exercises. The most important point to remember is not to re-injure the area by inducing too much stress, such as by allowing the athlete to run

BOX 4-7 Five Cardinal Signs of Inflammation

1. Swelling
2. Pain
3. Redness
4. Warmth
5. Loss of function

fibroplasia formation of granulation, or fibrous, tissue in healing a mile while he or she still has an antalgic gait pattern, or a limp. Athletic trainers should re-evaluate the injury regularly to look for signs of new inflammation indicating excessive stress. Inducing new inflammation will delay the total healing process as well as the return to full activity.

Maturation (Remodeling) Phase

The third and final stage of the healing process is referred to as *maturation,* or remodeling. This phase can last a year or more, but it generally peaks within 6 to 8 weeks after the initial injury. The maturation phase typically is not completed before a return to full activity. As mentioned previously, this phase overlaps on the time line with the repair phase. During this stage in the healing process, a reduced number of macrophages and fibroblasts are present at the wound site. The definitive scar is formed, and its tensile strength increases in response to the stresses applied. Blood flow returns to normal levels in the surrounding capillaries, and those capillaries with minimal flow are reabsorbed[11] (see Figure 4-13).

The goal for the athletic trainer during the remodeling phase is to assist the injured structure(s) in regaining flexibility and strength through controlled motion and stress. It should be noted that this was also a goal during the repair phase. However, in this phase the patient may be expected to tolerate an increase in stress and motion during the remodeling phase. Rehabilitation focuses on increasing functional activities, such as performing a layup and agility drills. The key is to functionally progress the patient by slowly attempting to maximize conditioning while minimizing the risk of re-injuring the tissue.

Several factors can impede the healing process, despite the amount of initial trauma. Any local infection or embedded foreign material can interfere with the process. Other local factors include an inadequate blood supply or locally applied drugs such as corticosteroids. Too much movement in the acute stage can damage the fragile collagen bridgework and new capillaries. During the aging process, the body's ability to heal itself diminishes. Nutritional deficiencies in vitamin C, zinc, and protein can also limit the body's ability to repair itself. Other systemic issues affecting healing include metabolic diseases such as renal failure or diabetes mellitus. Ingested and injected corticosteroids can also adversely affect healing.[13,14]

Points to Ponder
What can you do to facilitate the healing process?

Nature of Specific Soft Tissue Healing

Different types of soft tissues heal at different rates because of their cellular makeup and blood supply and the level of support provided by adjacent structures. Tendons, ligaments, and joint capsules are composed primarily of collagen fibers with a very limited direct blood supply. These tissues are designed to be somewhat elastic and are able to absorb stretching forces. However, if the load on the tissue exceeds approximately one third of the maximum load, tears occur. When these microtears become sufficiently numerous, gross tissue disruption, or macrotears, may occur. The tissue may also be chronically weakened, making it susceptible to a complete rupture or chronic inflammation. When the tears are incomplete, the tissue attempts to heal itself by forming a scar, as described in the previous section on healing. Regeneration is typically limited, and repair is often slow because of the limited blood supply to these types of tissues.

Contractile muscle tissue is quite different from that of ligaments, tendons, and joint capsules (Figure 4-14). Muscles may also be injured by overstretching, but this is not the only way they are torn. Unlike connective tissue, musculoskeletal tissue can become fatigued as a result of activity. It can also be weakened by overuse, as is often the case with distance runners. Fortunately for muscles, they have a strong blood supply, as manifested by their rich red color. This vascularity increases the muscle tissue's capacity for healing. If blood vessels become torn as a result of the injury, healing may not proceed as expected. This pooled blood that leaks beneath the skin can sometimes be seen as bruising under the skin subsequent to a muscle strain that did not involve a direct blow. The ability to return to full function after a muscular injury is also affected by the size of the tear and subsequent scar formation. The scar tissue is noncontractile and often stiff and can form adhesions that limit movement and function in an otherwise healthy muscle.[15]

Nerves are thought to heal more slowly than all of the other tissues discussed in this section. Nerves are the electrical wires that connect our brain to the systems that it controls (e.g., muscles, organs). These nerves must remain intact if the electrical signal is to pass from the brain to its target area. When nerves become torn, the edges must physically touch for functional healing to occur. If the gap between the torn portions becomes filled with a scar, the electrical impulses cannot be transmitted; the scar acts as a permanent road block. If nerve healing is successful, it is typically very slow because of the nerve's limited blood supply and its inability to utilize scar tissue effectively.

Bone healing is primarily mitigated by two types of cells: osteoblasts and osteoclasts. **Osteoblasts** lay down new bone cells at sites of injury repair, bone growth, or increased bone stress. **Osteoclasts** remove bone cells that are no longer needed because of decreased local

osteoblast cell responsible for bone formation
osteoclast bone cell that removes bone tissue

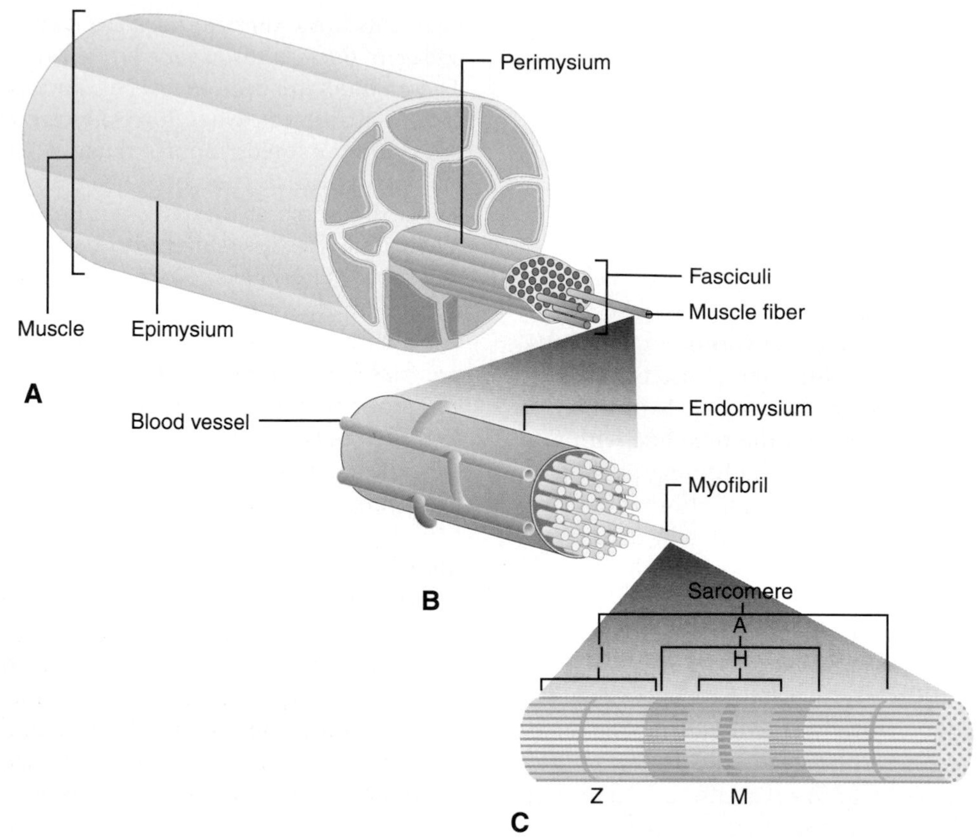

FIGURE 4-14 Muscle fiber. **A**, The epimysium runs continuously with the endomysium and the perimysium. **B**, The arrangement of fasciculi varies among muscles. **C**, The banding pattern apparent on microscopic inspection of a muscle cell results from the organized structure of the proteins (myofibrils) of the contractile apparatus. (From Copstead-Kirkhorn L-E C, Banasik JL: *Pathophysiology,* ed 3, p. 1245, Philadelphia, 2005, Elsevier/Saunders.)

stress or inactivity, aging, or the maturation phase of the healing process. When a bone is fractured, the site is initially supported by a collagenous scar, similar to what is seen in soft tissue. This soft callus is slowly calcified and hardens to form the hard callus, which can be seen as a small bulge in the area of the fracture on an X-ray. As described in Wolff's Law, the bony tissue will realign along the lines of tensile force over time.[16] Although the fracture site may be stable enough to resume activity within 4 to 8 weeks, the hard callus may remain to some extent for more than a year (Figure 4-15).

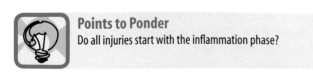

Points to Ponder
Do all injuries start with the inflammation phase?

OCCUPATIONAL HEALTH AND SAFETY ADMINISTRATION STANDARDS

Because of their working knowledge of the injury healing process, athletic trainers are highly skilled in treating and rehabilitating a wide variety of musculoskeletal injuries. However, one of the more common acute injuries with which athletic trainers have to deal is an open skin wound. These wounds require a great deal more than simply sticking on a bandage. Athletic trainers must know whether they can treat the wound themselves or whether they need to refer the athlete to a physician. As part of this process, athletic trainers must know how to care for these wounds while also protecting themselves from bloodborne pathogens.

The safety of the athletic training staff and those using the athletic health care facility is always a concern. Human tissue, blood, saliva, synovial fluid, and other secretions (other than perspiration) may contain bloodborne pathogens such as hepatitis B (HBV), hepatitis C (HBC), or the human immunodeficiency virus (HIV). These bodily specimens are collectively referred to as **biohazards**.

Universal Precautions

The most important concept for those who deal with bodily fluids is universal precautions. Adherence to universal precautions means treating *all* human blood and bodily fluids as if they were known to be infected with HIV, HBV,

biohazards bodily specimens or conditions that pose harm to humans

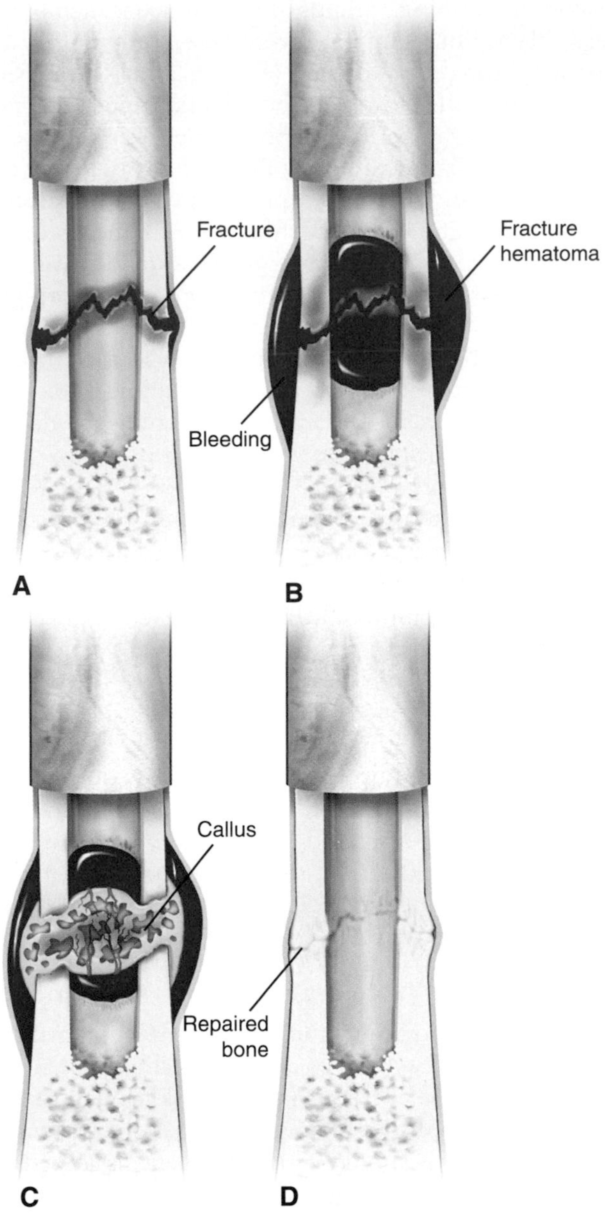

FIGURE 4-15 The steps that take place during repair of a fractured (i.e., broken) bone. **A,** Fracture of the femur. **B,** Hematoma has formed. **C,** Callus has formed; this callus is initially composed of fibrocartilaginous tissue and then later calcifies to create a bony callus. **D,** Bone repair is complete. A remnant of the bony callus is still evident and would likely be palpable as a bump at the site of the fracture. (From Thibodeau GA, Patton KT: *Anatomy & physiology,* ed 6, p. 243, St Louis, 2003, Mosby.)

or other bloodborne pathogens. Individuals with these illnesses cannot always be identified easily. They may not even list these conditions on their medical history form. Moreover, many people do not even know that they are infected and therefore cannot notify health professionals. The athletic trainer's goal is to minimize exposure to bodily fluids and therefore bloodborne pathogens.

In 1991, the Occupational Safety and Health Administration (OSHA) established standards to protect medical workers, including athletic trainers, from bloodborne pathogens. The standards related to bloodborne pathogens (OSHA 29 CFR, Chapter XVII 1910.1030) applies to all employees who have occupational exposure to blood or **other potentially infectious materials** (OPIM). These standards, summarized in Box 4-8, apply just as much to an athletic trainer as they do to an emergency room physician.[17]

Having and maintaining an exposure control plan is the first requirement of the OSHA standards. The exposure control plan, as its name suggests, is designed primarily to eliminate or minimize exposures. This plan must be accessible to all employees (and students) and must be reviewed and updated annually (see Box 4-8).[17]

Bloodborne Diseases

As mentioned earlier, the major bloodborne diseases of occupational concern are HBV, hepatitis C, and acquired immunodeficiency syndrome (AIDS, which is caused by HIV). Hepatitis B, caused by the HBV, primarily affects the liver and can lead to cirrhosis and liver cancer. The symptoms of HBV, such as loss of appetite and stomach pain, are similar to those associated with a mild flu. Other symptoms, such as **jaundice** and dark urine, indicate many conditions affecting the liver. After infection with the virus, symptoms may not appear for

other potentially infectious materials (OPIM) defined by the Occupational Safety and Health Administration (OSHA) as all human body fluids and unfixed tissues, excluding intact skin

jaundice yellowing

BOX 4-8 OSHA Standards Related to Bloodborne Pathogens

- Develop and maintain an exposure control plan containing the following:
  - Plans for exposure prevention
  - Determination of exposure incidences
  - Action steps to take if exposure occurs
  - Education regarding bloodborne pathogens and their signs and symptoms
- Maintain accurate records to every occupational exposure
- Train employees annually

Data from Occupational Safety and Health Administration: *Regulations (standards – 29 CFR). Bloodborne pathogens – 1910.1030,* Washington, DC, 1992, U.S. Department of Labor. Retrieved March 16, 2007, from www.osha.gov/pls/oshaweb/owadisp.show_document?p_table=STANDARDS&p_id=10051.

1 to 9 months, possibly not at all. Although there is no cure for the disease, it can be prevented with a three-shot vaccine series. Many medical facilities already require this series. The vaccine can also be given after exposure and can be effective in preventing the transmission of this disease. Employers are required to provide the HBV vaccination series to their qualified employees at no cost to the employee. HBV is extremely hardy and can survive in a drop of dried blood, outside of a host or the body, for up to 7 days. In the context of athletic training, HBV could be on your treatment tables, taping tables, or even inside your medical kit.

Hepatitis C, caused by the hepatitis C virus (HCV), may not be as well known to the public, but it is still a cause for concern. No known vaccine for this disease exists. The symptoms are very similar to those of hepatitis B, but 80% of infected individuals show symptoms within the first 2 weeks to 6 months after infection. The liver is also affected in the same way. Chronic infections occur in 55% to 85% of infected persons.

Several other types of hepatitis exist, but most are less common in the United States than in other parts of the world. Hepatitis D is also a bloodborne pathogen, but it can be duly prevented by the HBV vaccine. The other two types of hepatitis, A and E, are not bloodborne pathogens. These are both transmitted through fecal and oral routes, generally because of absent or ineffective handwashing after use of the bathroom. Hepatitis A outbreaks are particularly associated with restaurants, the result of contamination by food handlers who touch food with soiled hands. Although there is a vaccine for hepatitis A, none exists for hepatitis E.

AIDS is caused by HIV. It is a fatal disease with no known cure or vaccine. HIV attacks the body's immune system, making it difficult for the body to fight off other viruses and bacteria. Because the virus cannot survive for long outside the human body, the occupational transmission rate is very low. However, through sexual intercourse and the sharing of intravenous needles, infection rates are on the rise around the world.

After infection with HIV, the progression is fairly typical. In the first stage, the infected person exhibits few or no symptoms. Most people have no idea that they have contracted the virus in this stage. In the second stage, the person may experience swollen lymph glands and have trouble fighting off other bugs as the immune system begins to weaken. During the third stage, the infection develops into full-blown AIDS, whereupon the body is completely unable to fight off life-threatening diseases and infections, such as pneumonia.

Personal Protection

To reduce the risk of contracting a contagious disease, the athletic trainer should undertake self-protection measures. The typical routes of occupational exposure are through contaminated sharps (e.g., needles and scalpels), splashing of fluids into the mucous membranes (e.g., those found in the eyes, nose, or mouth), and contact through broken skin (e.g., an abrasion or even a small hangnail). However, the athletic trainer can take precautions against these opportunities for exposure.

Before dealing with bodily fluids of any kind, the athletic trainer should always put on **personal protective equipment (PPE)**. How much is needed depends on the situation. At the very least, gloves should always be worn. A resuscitation mask, an apron or lab coat, goggles or a face shield (or both, depending on the amount of blood or bodily fluids that are involved with the specific injury situation) may also be required (Box 4-9). The athletic trainer should practice donning and doffing the PPE before being faced with a situation that requires quick action (Figure 4-16).

One of the issues in emergencies and acute situations is the pressure to begin providing care as soon as possible. The athletic trainer should remember that in most situations, injured athletes can usually place and hold sterile gauze on their own wounds. While direct pressure is being applied by the athlete, the athletic trainer can then gather the necessary PPE and begin donning it. Also, this is a good time to secure any other wound-care supplies that may be required. One of the worst mistakes athletic trainers make is to begin treating an open wound and then needing to dig through a medical kit. At this point, everything in the medical kit has been contaminated with the body fluids from the gloves.

Biohazardous Waste Disposal

Sharp objects should be immediately placed in a sharps container after use. Sharps containers should be within reach so that it is not necessary to walk around or near other people with potentially infectious sharps (Figure 4-17). A needle should *never* be bent, crimped, or

personal protective equipment (PPE) clothing or gear used to shield the wearer from hazard or contamination

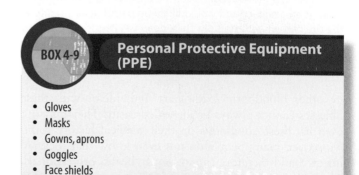

BOX 4-9 Personal Protective Equipment (PPE)

- Gloves
- Masks
- Gowns, aprons
- Goggles
- Face shields

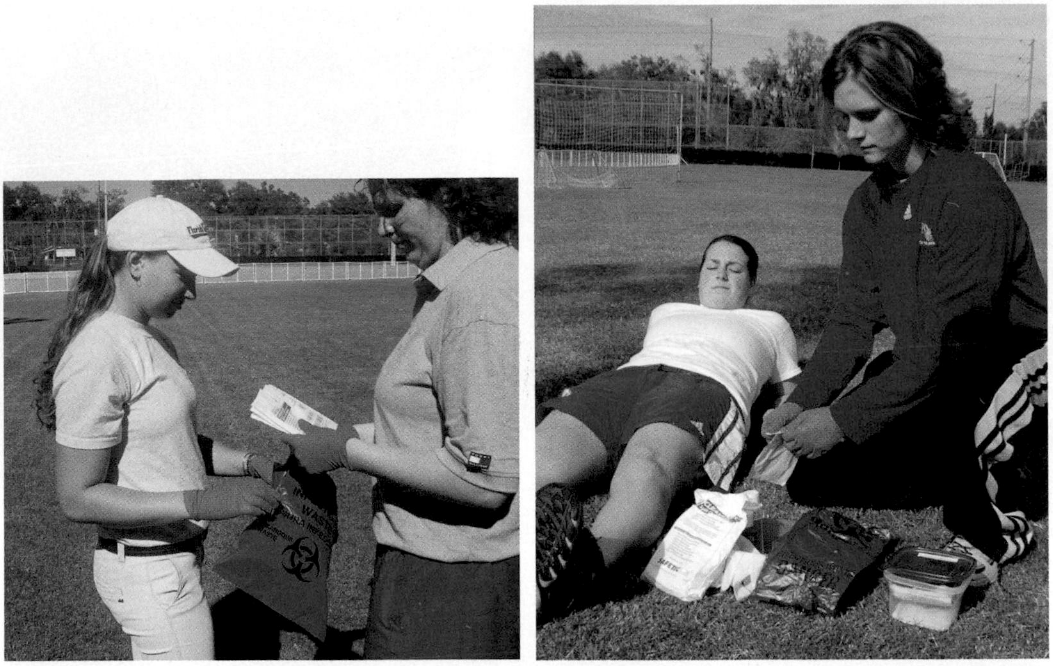

FIGURE 4-16 These athlete trainers and athletic training students are donning appropriate personal protective equipment (PPE) for their setting and level of injury.

recapped. Sharps must be properly discarded as soon as possible after use to minimize the risk of exposure. The athletic trainer should always work in a well-lit area to avoid self-injury or harm to others.

Several other important measures should be taken to minimize the risk of exposure. All disposable waste contaminated with blood must be placed in a properly labeled biohazardous waste container. This waste includes towels and uniforms that have become contaminated. It is not always necessary to throw them away, but laundry handlers must receive adequate warning to don their own PPE. Other containers, such as refrigerators and freezers containing blood or OPIM, must also be properly labeled to protect anyone who may use them. The receptacles for disposable wastes should be emptied regularly—more frequently if the wastes are **putrescible**.

While treating a wound, athletic trainers must keep their hands away from their own faces. Otherwise, the mucous membranes of the eye, nose, or mouth may be inadvertently exposed to bloodborne pathogens. After caring for the wound, athletic trainers should remove PPE without touching any body parts with the contaminated gloves. All PPE should be removed while gloves are still on. Then, the gloves can be removed without the risk of contaminating or touching clothes or skin. After removing PPE, athletic trainers should wash their hands thoroughly with soap and water.

If exposure does occur, the athletic trainer should perform the following steps to minimize exposure:[17]

- Immediately cleanse the wound area with soap and water.
- Inform a supervisor about the exposure incident.
- Seek medical care within 2 hours as designated in the exposure control plan.
- Request medical information or testing from the involved source person.

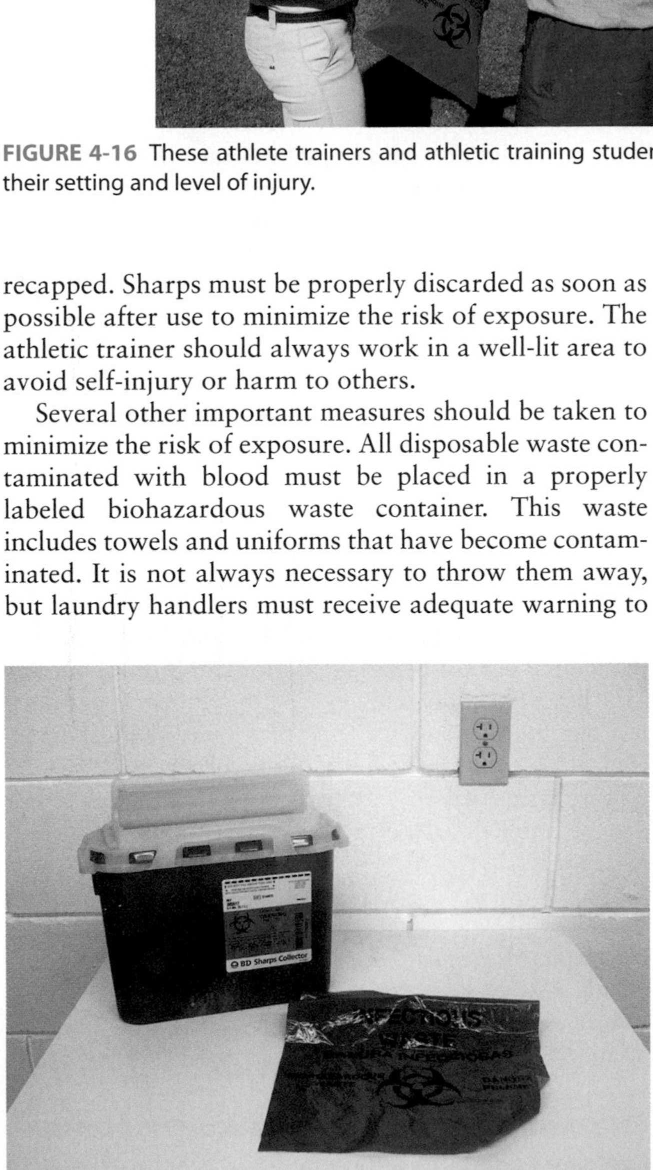

FIGURE 4-17 Sharps container and biohazard bag used to dispose of sharps and contaminated items.

putrescible subject to decomposition by microorganisms that produce a foul odor

- Notify other pertinent departments (e.g., Environmental Health and Safety Office), and complete all necessary documentation.

If blood or bodily fluids have been spilled, only those who have received the HBV vaccination should clean them up. PPE must always be worn, even after vaccination. Before any attempt is made to clean up the spill, an approved absorbent material should be placed on it to minimize splashing. After the materials have been placed in a biohazard-specific leak-proof container, the area should be disinfected with a 1:10 solution of bleach to water.[17]

Points to Ponder

Do you know how to gain access to the exposure control plan at your school?

Do you know what steps to take if you think you may have been exposed to blood or OPIM?

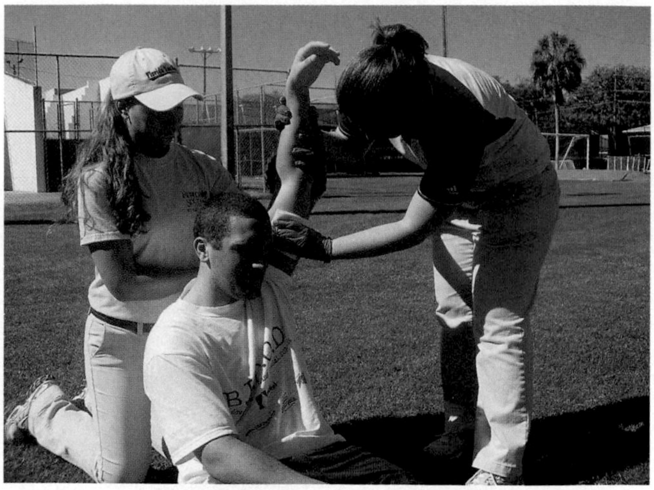

FIGURE 4-18 Gloved direct pressure technique with elevation used to control bleeding.

WOUND CARE

Whether the wound is an abrasion, laceration, open blister, or puncture wound, the first goal is to stop the bleeding. The second goal is to clean the wound and apply a sterile dressing, and the final goal is to secure the dressing with a bandage. Athletic trainers should keep in mind that their response to any injury determines how quickly and efficiently the wound or injury will advance through the injury healing process.

The first method used to stop the bleeding is simply the application of direct pressure over the wound with a sterile dressing. Athletic trainers should refrain from lifting the dressing every 5 seconds to see whether the bleeding has stopped because this will interfere with the clotting process. (Peeking every minute or two is fine for smaller wounds.) While continuing to apply direct pressure, the athletic trainer should elevate the body part above the level of the heart unless a fracture, dislocation, or spinal injury is suspected or an impaled object is present. Adding a cold pack over the dressing may also discourage blood flow to the area and help stop the bleeding. If the dressing becomes saturated with blood, the athletic trainer should apply additional dressings over it and continue to apply direct pressure. The first dressing should not be removed. If direct pressure and elevation are not effective in stopping the bleeding, arterial bleeding can be controlled by applying pressure with the thumb or finger to a **pressure point** (Figure 4-18).

Once the bleeding has been controlled, the wound should be cleaned. Superficial wounds should be cleaned with either saline or soap and water[18] or a combination of soap and water.[17] Cleansing of the wound with hydrogen peroxide, iodine, or alcohol may harm healthy tissues, which results in a longer healing time for the wound.[19–21] Vigorous scrubbing of the wound should also be avoided because it may damage the involved tissues.[22]

Wounds that are kept moist will heal more quickly and with less scarring than wounds that are allowed to dry and scab over.[23] Wounds should be covered and kept moist for about 5 days. After the wound has been cleaned, an antibiotic ointment or petroleum jelly can be applied to maintain the moist environment. However, these products may cause allergic reactions in some individuals.[24]

It may be necessary to close larger wounds or lacerations before applying dressing and bandaging. Closure can be accomplished with small adhesive strips, skin adhesives, stitches, or staples (Figure 4-19). Care should always be exercised when using skin adhesives because these seal the wound closed and if an infection develops, the wound cannot be irrigated, nor can it drain out pus as it heals naturally. However, skin adhesives are much less painful than stitches or staples and do not require a return trip to the physician's office for removal. Wound closure strips are an excellent alternative because they can be applied by the athletic trainer and removed if necessary.[25]

SUMMARY

Developing a systematic approach to both query the injured person and evaluate the injury often allows the athletic trainer to determine the correct diagnosis. Obtaining an accurate diagnosis requires a basic understanding of the

pressure point a location where the artery is close to the skin surface or overlies a bone (e.g., brachial artery on medial upper arm, femoral artery on anterior hip)

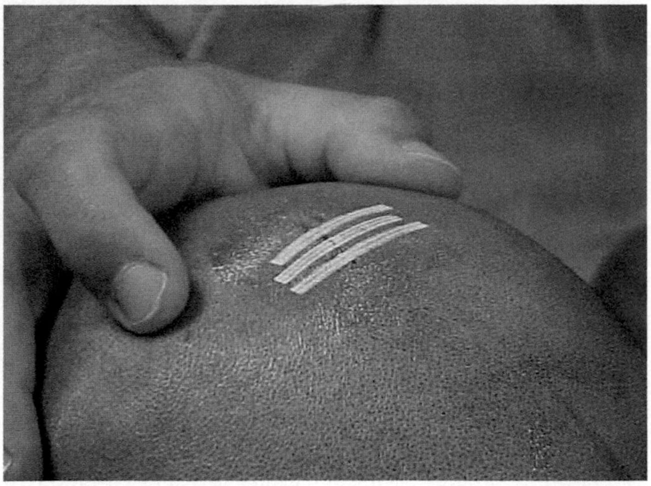

FIGURE 4-19 Wound closed with Steri-Strips applied on the field.

mechanism of injury and the tissues' response to the injury. With injury or trauma, the body moves through distinct phases of healing and repair. Ultimately, decisions on modalities, exercises, and return to play or work stem from where and how the injury is passing through these phases. Returning someone to activity too soon can create a new inflammatory response and cause a relapse to Phase One, thus delaying healing and repair. Proper documentation through a SOAP note demonstrates progress in the rehabilitation program and will likely prevent unnecessary setbacks in the program.

Caring for superficial skin wounds is more than simply applying a bandage. The wound must be properly treated and the patient referred to a physician for further treatment if necessary. At all times, the athletic trainer must minimize his or her risk of exposure to bloodborne pathogens. A seemingly simple task can have devastating consequences if not properly performed.

Revisiting the OPENING Scenario

Depending on what you saw, your initial questions to the gymnast would most likely include some of the following: What happened? How did it happen? Where exactly does it hurt? Did you hear or feel a snap or pop in your face or knee? Can you move your jaw and mouth? Do you have a headache? Can you see clearly? Was your foot planted on the ground when you landed? What do you feel now? Can you feel your toes?

If you did not see the injury, your first round of questions will help you determine what really happened after the gymnast's impact with the bar and the mat. Once you get enough information about how the injury occurred, you can move on to the rest of the evaluation process.

To protect yourself, you should don the appropriate PPE for this situation: gloves. Keep in mind that you do not want to touch bodily fluids. Once you have completed the evaluation, you should properly discard your gloves and any other PPE in a biohazardous waste bag, which should then be removed according to local regulations.

Issues & Ethics

Should you treat an individual with more caution if you know that he or she engages in high-risk behavior such as having multiple sexual partners or sharing needles? If you learn that one of your patients is HIV or HBV positive, should you alert the other members of your staff? What are the reasons to do so? With what privacy issues are you obligated to comply?

Web Links

Acute inflammation (Department of Pathology, University of Birmingham, UK): http://medweb.bham.ac.uk/http/mod/3/1/a/acute.html

Bloodborne pathogens (OSHA Regulations, Standards – 29 CFR, Section 1910.1030): www.osha.gov/pls/oshaweb/owadisp.show_document?p_table=STANDARDS&p_id = 10051

Bone and fracture healing (Duke University, *Wheeless' Textbook of Orthopaedics*): www.wheelessonline.com/ortho/bone_healing

Inflammation and repair (Ed Friedlander, MD, Pathologist): www.pathguy.com/lectures/inflamma.htm

Ligament injury recovery: after straining, spraining, or partially tearing a ligament, 'loading' can improve recovery (*Sports Injury Bulletin*): www.sportsinjurybulletin.com/archive/ligament-injury.html

Questions and answers about strains and sprain: (National Institute of Arthritis and Musculoskeletal and Skin Diseases, National Institutes of Health): www.niams.nih.gov/hi/topics/strain_sprain/strain_sprain.htm

Skin closure application (3M): http://solutions.3m.com/wps/portal/3M/en_US/SH/SkinHealth/solutions/skin-closures/

Web MD

Are stitches, staples, or skin adhesives necessary?: www.webmd.com/hw/health_guide_atoz/sid42906.asp?navbar

How to clean a skin wound: www.webmd.com/hw/health_guide_atoz/sig51564.asp

Skin adhesives: www.webmd.com/hw/health_guide_atoz/tm7002.asp?navbar=

World wide wounds: www.worldwidewounds.com/1997/july/Thomas-Guide/Dress-Select.html

References

1. Heck JF et al: National Athletic Trainers' Association position statement: Head-down contact and spearing in tackle football, *Journal of Athletic Training* 39(1): 101–111, 2004.
2. Shultz SJ, Houglum PA, Perrin DH: *Examination of musculoskeletal injuries*, ed 2, Champaign, Ill, 2005, Human Kinetics.
3. Konin JG, Frederick MA: *Documentation for athletic training*, pp. 26–29, Thorofare, NJ, 2005, Slack.
4. Scott A et al: What is "inflammation?" Are we ready to move beyond Celsius? *Br J Sports Med* 38(3): 248–249, 2004.
5. Scott A, et al: What do we mean by the term "inflammation?" A contemporary basic science update for sports medicine, *Br J Sports Med* 38(3): 372–380, 2004.
6. *Stedman's medical dictionary for the health professions and nursing*, pp. 300, 1093, 1118, Philadelphia, 2005, Lippincott Williams and Wilkins.
7. Butterfield T, Best T, Merick T: The dual roles of neutrophils and macrophages in inflammation: a critical balance between tissue and repair, *Journal of Athletic Training*, 41(4): 457–465, 2006.
8. Toumi H, F'guyer S, Best TM: The role of neutrophils in injury and repair following muscle stretch, *J Anat* 208: 459–470, 2006.
9. Toumi H, Best TM: The inflammatory response: friend or enemy for muscle injury? *Br J Sports Med* 37(4): 284–286, 2003.
10. Nathan C: Points of control in inflammation, *Nature* 420(6917): 846–848, 2002.
11. University of Birmingham: *School of Medicine pathology teaching pages*, Birmingham, UK, [no date], Author. Retrieved March 16, 2007, from http://medweb.bham.ac.uk/http/depts/path/Teaching/teachdir.html.
12. Starkey C: *Therapeutic modalities*, ed 3, pp. 11–27, Philadelphia, 2004, FA Davis.
13. Stovitz SD, Johnson RJ: NSAIDs and musculoskeletal treatment, *The Physician and Sports Medicine* 31(1): 35, 2003.
14. Harvey C: Wound healing, *Orthopaedic Nursing* 24(2): 143–157, 2005.
15. Best TM, Hunter KD: Muscle injury and repair, *Scientific Principles of Sports Rehabilitation* 11(2): 251–266, 2000.
16. Huiskes R: If bone is the answer, then what is the question?, *Journal of Anatomy* 1979 (Part 2): 145–156. 2000.
17. Occupational Safety and Health Administration: *Bloodborne pathogens (OSHA regulations, standards – 29 CFR, section 1910. 1030)*, Washington, DC, 1992, U.S. Department of Labor. Retrieved March 16, 2007, from www.osha.gov/pls/oshaweb/owadisp.show_document?p_table=STANDARDS&p_id=10051
18. Beam J: Wound cleansing: water or saline? *Journal of Athletic Training* 41(2): 196–197, 2006.
19. D'Acampora AJ et al: Morphological analysis of three wound-cleaning processes on potentially contaminated wounds in rats, *Acta CirArgica Brasileira* 21(5): 332–340, 2006.
20. Myles J: Woundcare: assessment and principles of healing, *Practice Nurse* 32(8): 62–67, 2006.
21. Rees JE: Where have all the bubbles gone? An ode to hydrogen peroxide, the champagne of all wound cleaners, *Accident and Emergency Nursing* 11(2): 82–84, 2003.
22. Gwynne B, Newton M: An overview of the common methods of wound debridement, *British Journal of Nursing* 15(19 suppl): S4–S10, 2006.
23. Thompson J: A practical guide to wound care, *RN* 63(1): 48–52, 2000.
24. Rubin A: Managing abrasions and lacerations, *Physician and Sports Medicine* 26(5): 45–48, 51–55, 1998.
25. Web MD/Healthwise, *Skin adhesives (liquid stitches)*, Boise, Idaho, 1995–2006, Author. Retrieved March 16, 2007, from www.webmd.com/hw/health_guide_atoz/tm7002.asp?navbar=

5

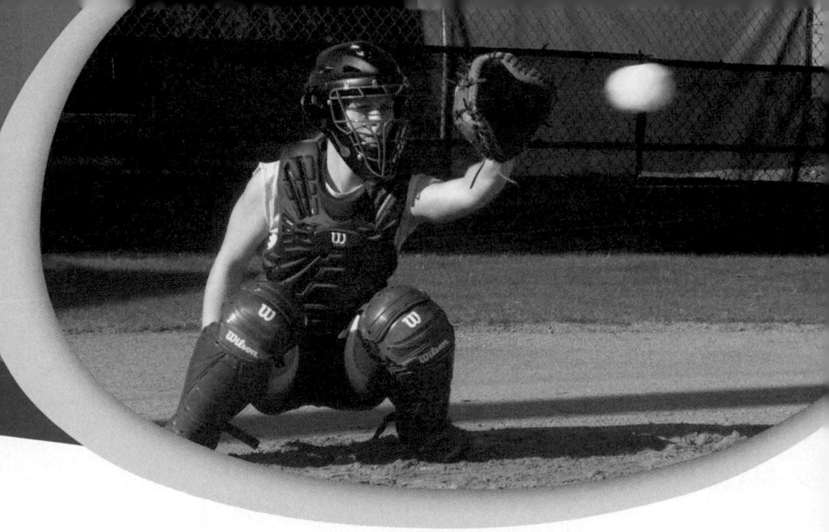

Introduction to the Systems

JAMES M. LYNCH

Learning Goals

1. List and describe the major organ systems of the human body.
2. Identify key anatomical structures and their primary function in each system.
3. Discuss potential diagnoses associated with each organ system, and suggest initial steps for treatment.
4. Explain the common infectious diseases found in various community settings.
5. Describe supportive treatment for several of the common infectious diseases.

The human body is composed of many intricately linked systems. Each system has one or more functions that interrelate with the other systems. Understanding the anatomy and physiology of any one system within the human body will aid in the understanding of other systems and allow health professionals to make informed medical decisions. This chapter discusses each of the major organ systems that may be involved in various nonorthopedic medical diseases and disorders and the means by which these diseases and disorders may affect an individual's performance or activity level (Figure 5-1).

THE INTEGUMENTARY SYSTEM

The skin, also known as the **integument**, is the exterior system of the human body. It has the largest surface area of any system in the body, covering 21½ square feet in the average adult. The major functions of the skin are to serve as a protective barrier and aid in sensation and regulation of body temperature. Normal skin is an elastic, sheetlike layer that varies in appearance, depth, and thickness depending on the specific anatomical site. Because skin is the body's external barrier, it is populated by bacteria found in the environment. Human skin has a pH level between 4.5 and 5.5; pH measures the levels of the skin's acidity or alkalinity. This range of 4.5 to 5.5 decreases the ability of normal bacterial flora to cause infections. Therefore normal skin maintains good health.

Physical activity puts a great deal of stress on the skin. In the workplace, stress may include working in a factory with heavy machinery, working in hot or cold environments such as those common in restaurant kitchens, or even working as a crossing guard day after day in inclement weather. In athletics, the skin may be stressed during competition or even during daily practice. Likewise, physical activity can exacerbate or increase susceptibility to some skin conditions.

Common skin diseases or disorders are caused by external stimuli, such as the weather or, in the case of a swimmer, daily exposure to chlorinated water. Other common causes of skin disorders include mechanical factors such as a traumatic blow or blunt force; infectious organisms; environmental factors such as wind, rain, heat, and cold; and allergic reactions. Correctly diagnosing the cause of the skin disorder or disease rather than just treating the symptoms is essential for reducing the effects of skin disorders.

integument the skin of the human body

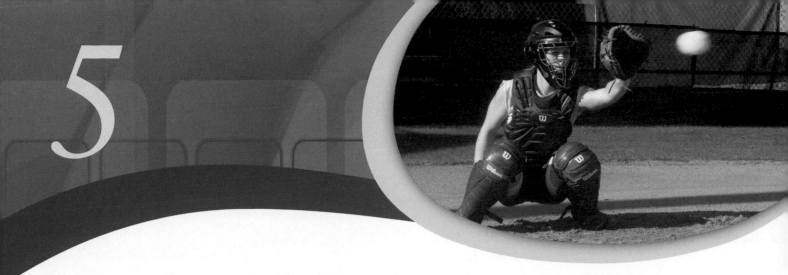

OPENING *Scenario*

The center midfielder on the high-school soccer team has asthma, or reactive airway disease. She takes daily medication to control her shortness of breath and coughing. She comes to you with an abrupt onset of fatigue and malaise that began 1 hour ago during class. She is beginning to feel hot and is also developing nausea. The state play-offs start in 3 days. What should you do? What are you going to tell the coach?

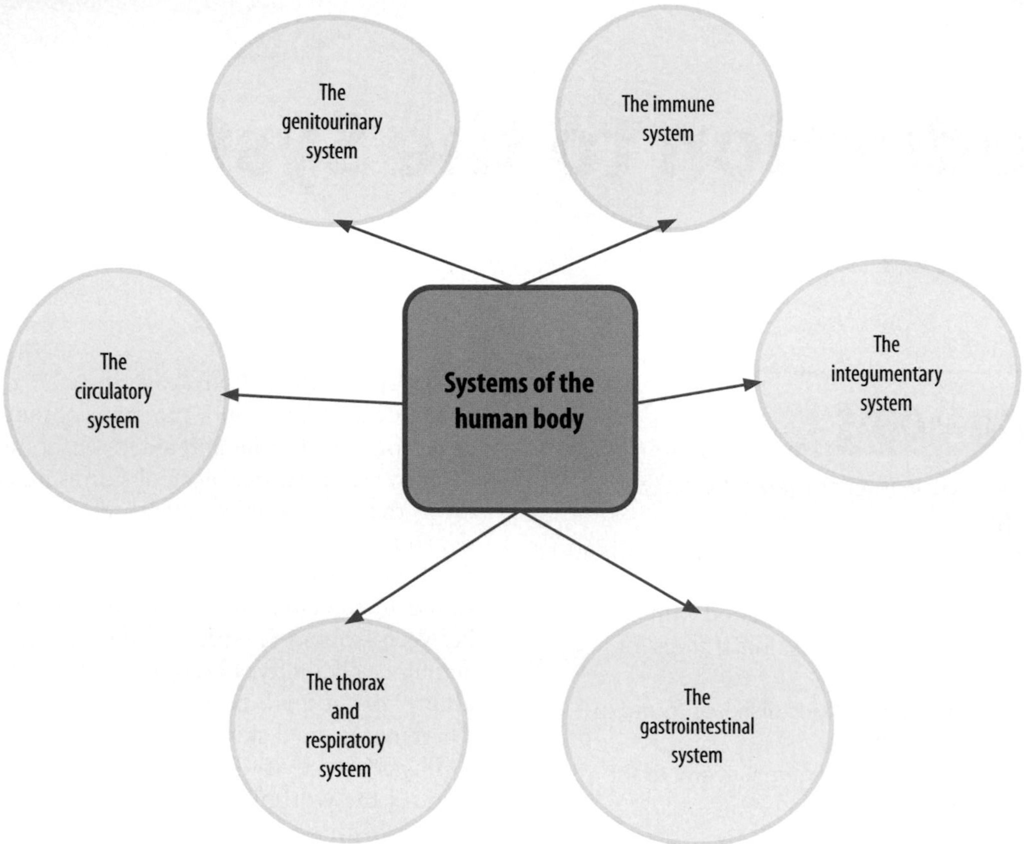

FIGURE 5-1 Concept map outlining the systems of the human body.

Skin Anatomy

Skin has three layers. The first layer is the epidermis, which is the outer protective barrier containing three major cell types and five layers. The second layer is the dermis, which provides the skin's strength and elasticity and contains hair follicles and sweat glands with an extensive blood and nerve supply. The third layer, the subcutaneous layer, lies under the dermis. The subcutaneous layer, or hypodermis, is a supportive structure that serves as a receptacle for the formation and storage of fat. Here the blood supply for the skin originates and extends upward into the dermis (Figure 5-2).

The three types of cells in the epidermis are (1) keratinocytes, (2) melanocytes, and (3) Langerhans cells. Table 5-1 outlines the specific function each type of cell has in the overall protection and structure of the integument.

The actual epidermis has five layers: (1) the basal cell layer, (2) the stratum spinosum, (3) the stratum granulosum, (4) the stratum lucidum, and (5) the stratum cor-

epidermis the outer protective layer of the skin
dermis the middle layer of the skin
hypodermis the subcutaneous layer that lies under the dermis
keratinocytes cells that produce a protein called keratin that provides the waterproofing of the body
melanocytes cells that release a pigment that provides the myriad of skin tones
Langerhans cells cells that ingest foreign, or antigenic, particles to prevent allergic reactions

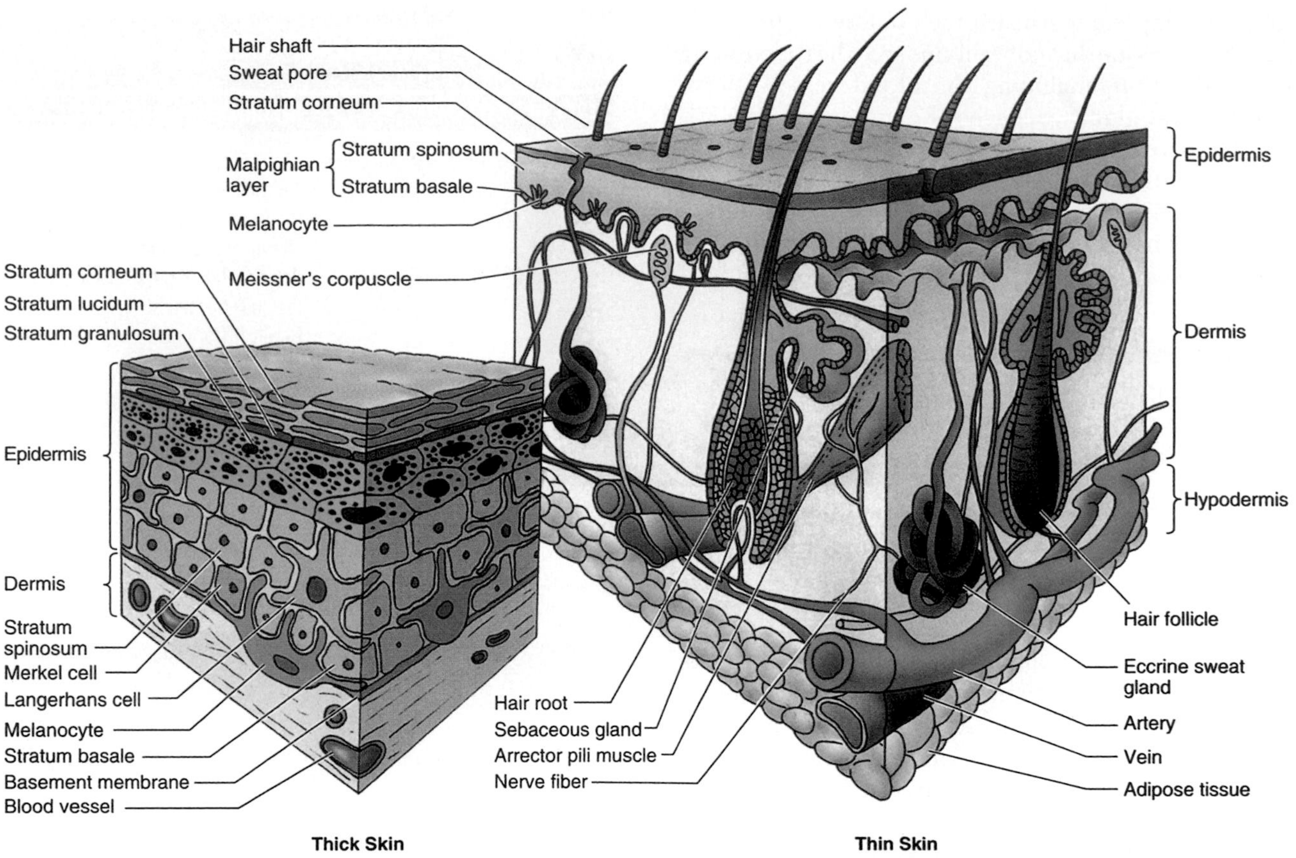

FIGURE 5-2 Anatomy of normal skin. (From Gartner LP, Hiatt JL: *Color textbook of histology,* ed 2, p. 326, Philadelphia, 2001, Saunders.)

TABLE 5-1 Cells of the Epidermis

CELL TYPE	DESCRIPTION
Keratinocytes	Keratinocytes produce a protein called *keratin* to provide the waterproof covering for the body.
Melanocytes	Melanocytes release a pigment that creates a variety of skin tones. All humans have approximately the same number of melanocytes. Changes in size and activity of the melanocytes determine the differences in human skin color.
Langerhans cells	Langerhans cells are part of the skin's immune system. These cells ingest foreign or antigenic particles to prevent allergic reactions.

neum. Each of these layers is necessary in the function, vitality, and performance of your skin, as outlined in Table 5-2.

Between the epidermis and the dermis lies the basement membrane. This membrane is a wavy junction that provides support and allows for the exchange of fluids and cells between the two layers. The dermis is

TABLE 5-2 Layers of the Epidermis

LAYER	DESCRIPTION
Stratum corneum (horny layer)	The exterior layer of the epidermis; primarily composed of dead keratinized cells; provides the body's major mechanical and chemical barrier
Stratum lucidum	Below the stratum corneum; a thin, translucent layer found in the thickened areas of the palms of the hand and soles of the feet
Stratum granulosum	The middle layer of the epidermis that contains the Langerhans cells
Stratum spinosum	Lies just above the basal cell layer and has spinelike extensions to the basal layer that provide some stability to the skin
Basal cell layer (also called *stratum germinativum*)	A single layer of cells; the only layer of the epidermis capable of mitosis and regeneration; constantly produces cells that are moved to the surface and eventually sloughed off

an irregular layer underneath the epidermis composed of connective tissue that contains most of the functioning parts of the skin, including the blood vessels, nerve endings, sweat glands, sebaceous glands, and hair follicles. The irregular form is caused by projections of the dermis into the epidermis, which prevent the epidermis from slipping off the dermis. This configuration is especially important in areas that require a grip, such as the palms of the hands and soles of the feet.

Remember the kid in third grade who used to stick a needle through his finger in a feeble attempt to make the girls squirm? He could do that because the epidermis does not contain nerve endings. If he directed the needle too deep and entered the dermis, his grin would quickly disappear.

TABLE 5-3 **Assessment of Skin Disorders**

TYPE OF ASSESSMENT	INFORMATION NEEDED
History	Time of onset Symptoms Duration of lesion Size or color change Relationship to physical agents Previous treatment Family history Social history
Physical exam	Type of lesion Distribution Surface features Border Site Shape Color Arrangement

Skin Pathology

Skin disorders are among the most common reasons that people see a physician. A recent study in Florida showed that 21% of patients seen by a family medicine physician had at least one skin complaint.[1] Similar studies suggest that approximately one in four people goes to a physician for skin disorders.[2]

Lesions are among the most common skin conditions. Discovery of a skin lesion requires a detailed description, which may be done over the phone to the team physician or through a SOAP note or other documentation format. The athletic trainer must take a concise history that includes time of onset, type of symptoms, size of lesions, color change, and duration of the symptoms (Table 5-3). The relationship of symptoms to physical agents (e.g., chemicals, irritants, trauma) and the success of previous treatment must be documented. Details regarding family and social history are also important.

Mechanical Trauma

Mechanical trauma refers to the application of an external force to the skin or tissue. The force may range from the rubbing of a shoe on the heel to a violent collision during a tackle in a football game. The skin undergoes a great deal of mechanical trauma or friction during athletics and certain work occupations. The amount of friction incurred over a specified period of time determines the response of the skin. In general, the harder the rubbing, the bigger the problem. Various kinds of dysfunction can occur if the barrier of the skin is disrupted, and these often lead to infection. Several skin disorders are common to the athlete and active worker.

Calluses

A small amount of friction over a bony area with subsequent pressure on the skin causes hypertrophy of the epidermis. This condition results in **keratosis**, or the formation of calluses.

Signs and symptoms: Calluses generally appear over bony prominences in weight-bearing or contact areas and serve in a protective function to prevent further injury. Without proper care, these calluses may become overly thick with rough edges. Rough calluses may be torn away during many types of movements or endeavors. One common example is a rip sustained by a gymnast, in which a rough callus on the palm of the gymnast's hand catches on the bar during a swing and tears off. Torn calluses also occur in many occupations that require significant use of the hands. Factory workers, landscapers, rowers, and carpenters frequently complain of such rips.

Calluses may also occur in non–weight-bearing areas as a result of excessive friction. Such a callus is usually called a corn, or clavus. Corns frequently occur on the superior surface of the toes and are often the result of toe deformities or poorly fitting shoes (or both). Over time, the skin and underlying tissues conform to the stresses placed on them. The result can often be disfiguring and uncomfortable (Figure 5-3).

Treatment: The thickness of both calluses and corns can be managed by using a pumice stone or other abrasive material to sand the skin smooth. Soaking the foot in warm water before using the pumice stone usually makes the treatment more effective and less uncomfortable.

lesion an injury to the skin
keratosis the formation of calluses

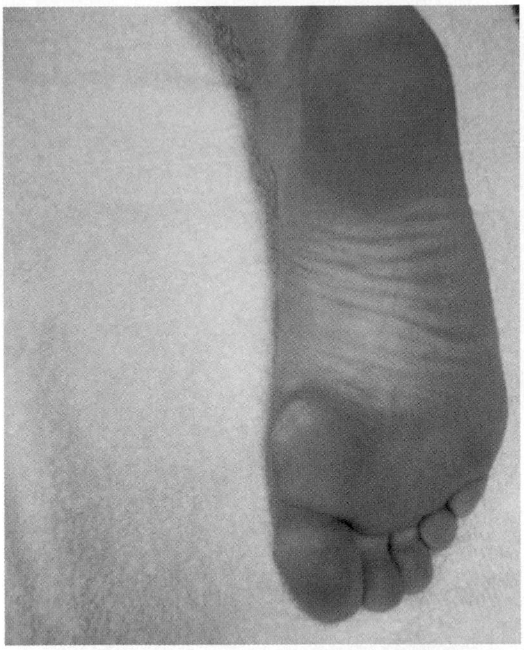

FIGURE 5-3 Callus.

Chafing

If excessive friction occurs between folds of skin, chafing or **intertrigo** will take place.

Signs and symptoms: Overlapping folds of skin sometimes trap moisture, which in turn breaks down the skin and leaves it vulnerable to infection. This type of chafing is more common in heavier individuals because of their increased skin surface. Another more common and less severe form of chafing occurs when shorts rub on thighs or thighs rub together. This type of chafing is often seen in runners or cyclists. Male runners may suffer from chafed nipples because of the constant rubbing of their T-shirt or racing singlet. Chafed nipples may lead to bleeding and extreme discomfort, sometimes causing the athlete to forgo the activity altogether.

Treatment: Any type of skin lubrication or protective balm may be applied to these areas to prevent chafing. Allowing the area to air dry and form a scab often alleviates the pain from the chafing. Tape or adhesive bandages may be placed over the nipples to keep the chafing from worsening or recurring.

Blisters

A greater amount of friction applied over a shorter time span may result in shearing forces in or under the epidermis. This friction causes fluid accumulation and blister formation.

Signs and symptoms: Hot spots are often palpable before the formation of the actual blister. These provide the athlete with adequate warning to decrease the friction. Redness is also present at the site. Typically, blisters become very tender and can also adversely affect performance if they are severe.

Treatment: If the possibility of keeping the blister roof intact remains in doubt, puncturing the side of the blister to allow the roof to fall over the ulcer bed is a reasonable option. To accomplish this, the athletic trainer should pop the blister on an edge near the normal, healthy skin to allow the fluid to drain out. The top of the blister will fall down, providing a natural bandage underneath the dressing. Athletic trainers should be careful to watch the top layer's response to draining; the top layer may begin to slide back and forth over the ulcer bed, aggravating the blister condition even more. Creating a padded dressing with a cut-out for the actual blister eases the discomfort directly over the blister. The athletic trainer should apply a balm over the blister inside the cut-out and then apply tape or an adhesive dressing to hold the doughnut cut-out in place (Figure 5-4). Numerous forms of protective skins or films that can be applied over the blister without the bulk of the padded cut-out are currently available. These skins are sometimes medicated to help prevent infection of the open blister.

Prevention: Methods to prevent undue friction around the feet include wearing an additional pair of socks; applying lubrication to the skin or covering the hot spot with a dressing are also effective. The roof of the blister is the epidermis, which forms a natural protective barrier. Leaving the roof intact is the best method to promote healing while reducing the risk of infection.

Abrasions, Lacerations, and Avulsions

An even greater amount of friction in a shorter period of time results in an abrasion. An **abrasion** (Figure 5-5) occurs when the skin is scraped against a rough surface, as in road rash sustained from a fall off a bicycle. Trauma in a smaller or more restricted area will result in a **laceration** (Figure 5-6), better known as a scratch or cut. An **avulsion** (Figure 5-7) is a wound in which a portion of the tissue is torn away. This tearing effect leaves a tissue defect of varying depths that must be corrected through the healing process.

---

intertrigo inflammation caused by folds of skin rubbing together

abrasion an injury that occurs when the skin is scraped against a rough surface

laceration trauma in a smaller or more restricted area that results in jagged edges around the wound

avulsion a wound in which a portion of the tissue is torn away

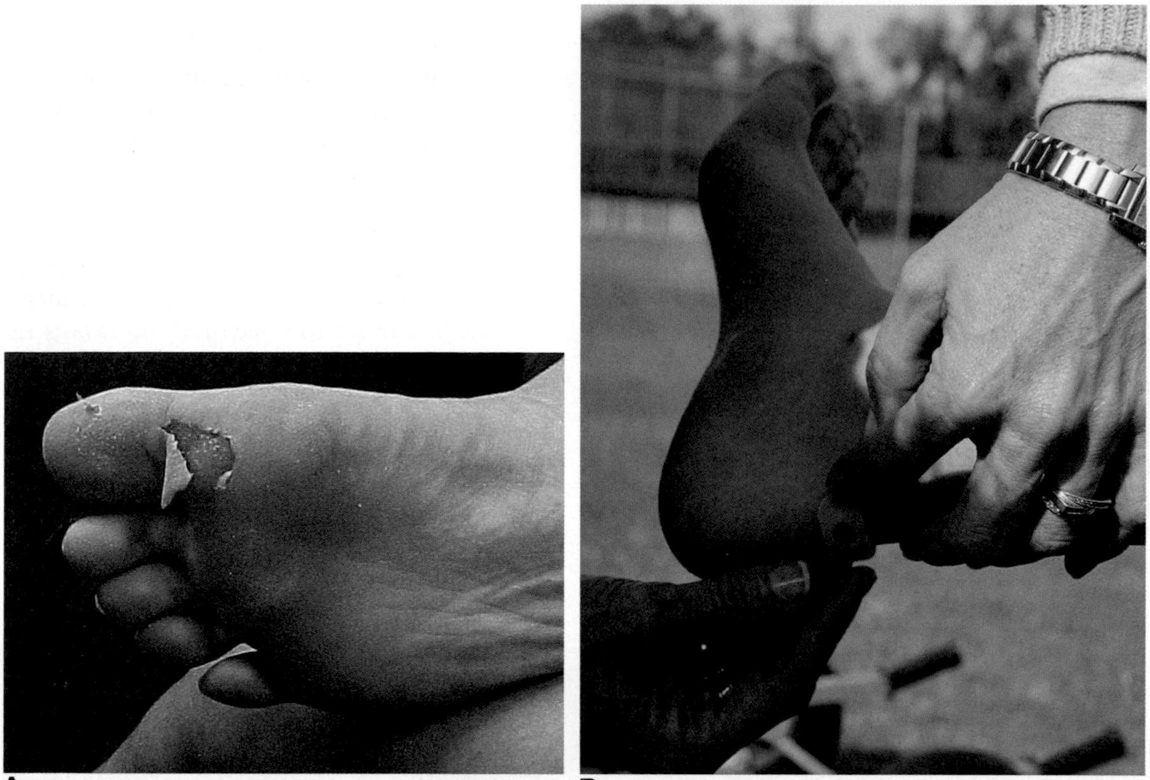

A B

FIGURE 5-4 **A,** Skin blister. **B,** Cut-out pad used to treat blister.

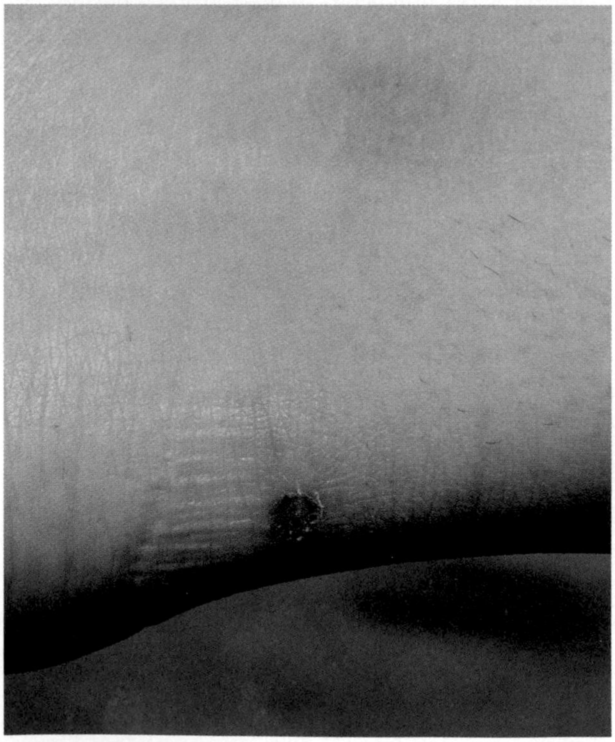

FIGURE 5-5 Skin abrasion.

Treatment: Treatment is generally the same for abrasions, lacerations, and avulsions. The wound should be thoroughly cleansed first. If necessary, the edges of the wound should be sealed by use of Steri-Strips, glue, or stitches. Then, a protective layer or bandage should be applied to prevent further damage to the area and possible infection.

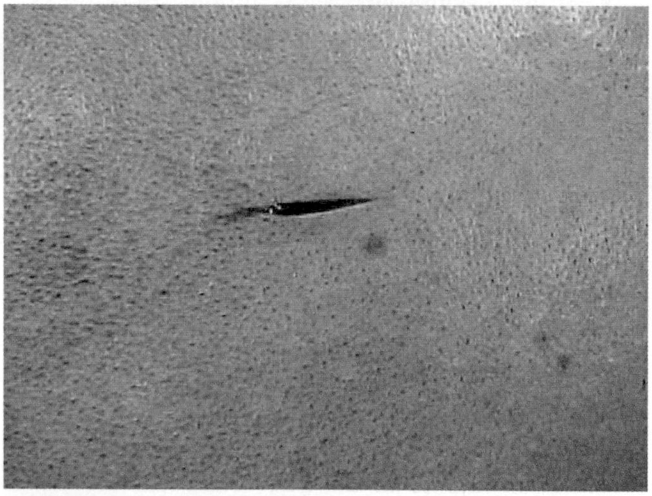

FIGURE 5-6 Laceration.

Points to Ponder

Your star cross country runner comes to you with a huge blister on the ball of her right foot. She is running in new shoes and is having difficulty pushing off of the affected foot. The conference championships are in 3 days. How do you treat her blister?

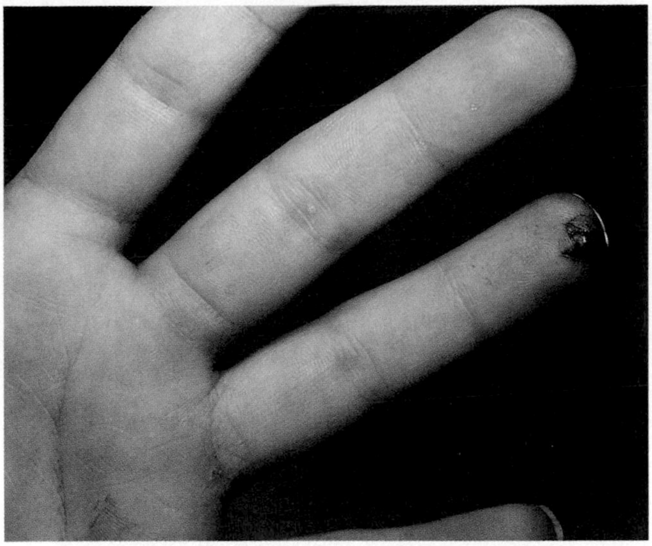

FIGURE 5-7 Avulsion.

Punctures

Puncture wounds are very serious. Whenever a foreign object penetrates the skin or other body parts, the risk of infection is great. Most puncture wounds are traumatic and require medical intervention for removal and treatment.

Treatment: Treatment for puncture wounds involves keeping the penetrating object in place by stabilizing the object with whatever resources are available. Once the object is stabilized, the injured person should be transported for further medical intervention. For example, if a pencil got stuck in someone's eye, the athletic trainer would cut a small hole in the bottom of a paper cup, place the cup over the pencil, and slide it down until the open end of the cup rests on the cheekbone. The cup would then be taped in place to keep the pencil from moving. Once the penetrating object appears to be stable, the patient is transported to the nearest emergency room. The other eye will need to be covered (since eyes move together) to minimize damage to the punctured eye.

Contusions

The sudden impact of an object on the body causes traumatic hemorrhaging or bleeding under the skin. Broken capillaries create an opportunity for blood to ooze into the surrounding tissues. **Contusions** vary in severity, ranging from the mild contusion that merely looks bad to severe **hematomas** that limit activity by restricting motion and increasing pain (Figure 5-8). Repeated trauma to the same injured area can cause an advanced form of hematoma. This condition, called **myositis ossificans**, results in calcification within the muscle tissue.

Signs and symptoms: Most contusions in the body are manifested by skin discoloration, slight discomfort, and edema or swelling; in more serious cases, deformity may occur because of excessive swelling. Myositis ossificans is manifested by a palpable lump in the injured or discolored area, pain and tenderness, limitations in muscle strength and flexibility, and swelling.

Treatment: Treatment for acute hematomas that are not serious can be comfortably managed with ice, compression, elevation, pressure, and rest if needed. More serious contusions may require electrical modalities to minimize pain and swelling. If a case of myositis ossificans does not appear to be healing properly and reabsorbing back into the body, surgical excision or debridement may be necessary.

Infectious Diseases of the Skin

Trauma to the skin occurs constantly. Macrotrauma results in visible breaks in the skin, whereas microtrauma causes tiny abrasions that may even be invisible. If the protective barrier of the skin is injured, infectious organisms can enter the body and cause infections. Infections are usually caused by microorganisms such as bacteria, viruses, fungus, and yeast (Table 5-4). These organisms can enter the body through even the slightest disruption of the skin. An infection results if the infectious organisms are sufficiently numerous to overcome or invade the body's immune defenses. When arthropods or mites enter the body through the skin, infestations such as scabies or lice may occur.

An old adage in the treatment of skins lesions states, "If it is dry, wet it. If it is wet, dry it." This simplistic formulation gains its truth from the fact that all organisms require a particular environment in which to live and grow. Changing the environment to a hostile one, or at least a different or aggravating one, makes growing and reproducing more difficult for the infecting organism. Therefore these measures help keep the infection from spreading within the individual or to other persons.

Bacterial Infections of the Skin

Bacteria are found throughout the human body. Infections do not typically occur unless the bacteria find a lesion on the skin through which to enter the body. Some bacteria cause a range of diseases, however. With management, most infections remain localized, but some may spread throughout the body and cause a major

puncture a serious wound resulting in a small hole caused by a sharp object

contusion a wound that causes bleeding in the tissue but does not break the skin

hematoma a contusion that is very swollen and discolored

myositis ossificans repeated trauma to the same injured area that causes an advanced form of hematoma with calcification

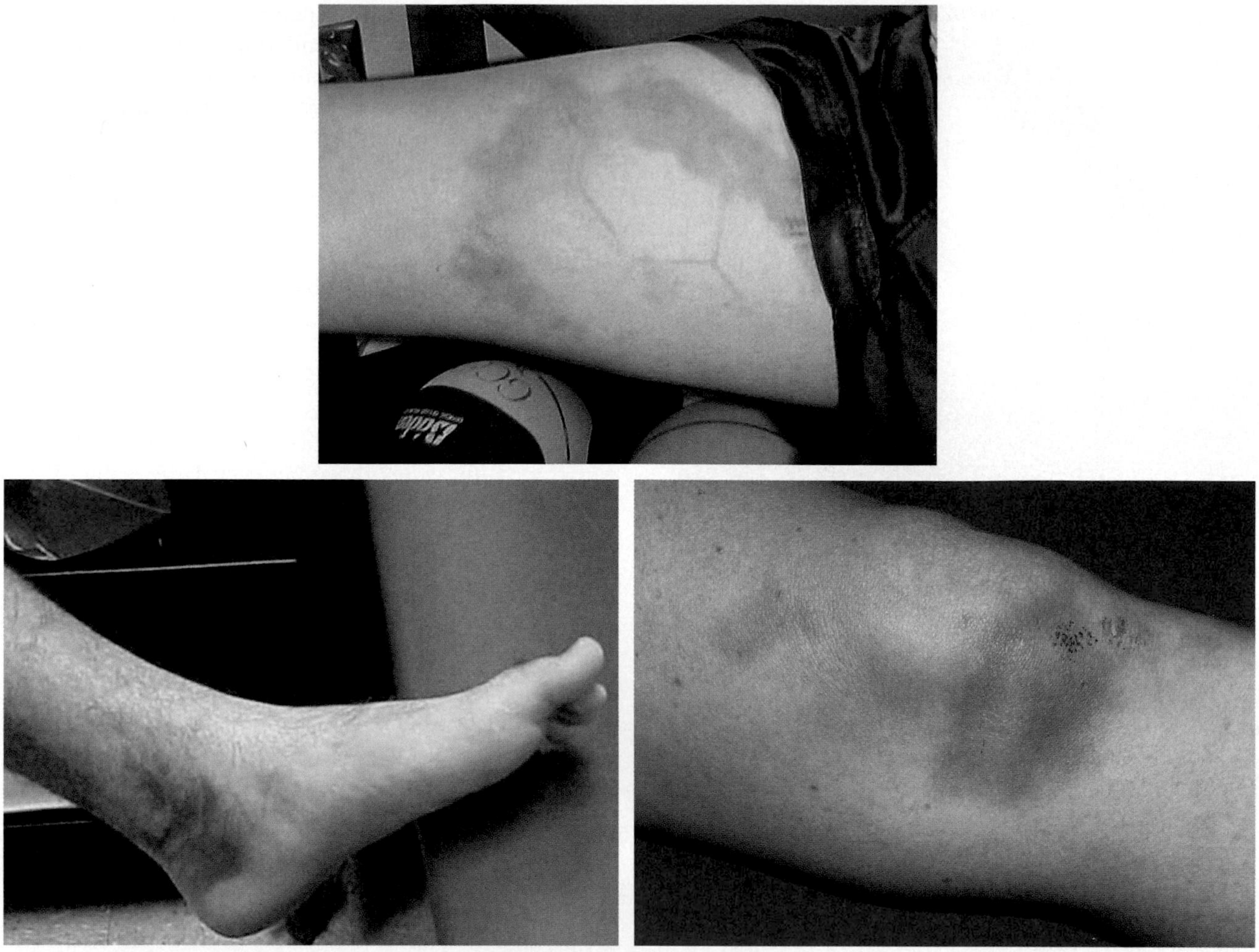

FIGURE 5-8 Examples of contusions.

infection. Unfortunately, bacteria eventually develop resistance to medications through frequent exposure. Because bacteria reproduce at a rapid rate, new genetic characteristics (i.e., mutations) can develop quickly. Bacteria that are resistant to an antibiotic continue growing during the administration of a course of medication. If the antibiotic regimen is discontinued too early, the resistant bacteria repopulate the infected area, causing a more serious infection.

Community-Associated Methicillin-Resistant Staphylococcus aureus *(CA-MRSA)*

The occurrence of **community-associated methicillin-resistant** *Staphylococcus aureus* (CA-MRSA) infection has increased markedly in athletics. CA-MRSA is one of

community-associated methicillin-resistant *Staphylococcus aureus* (CA-MRSA) a community-acquired bacterial infection ("super bug"); difficult to treat because of its resistance to a strong cousin of penicillin

TABLE 5-4 Common Organisms That Cause Infection

ORGANISM	DESCRIPTION
Bacterium	Single-celled microorganism that contains a nucleus and various organelles: Bacteria come in 3 shapes: cocci (spherical), bacilli (rod), spirochetes (corkscrew).
Virus	Protein shell encapsulating either a DNA or an RNA molecule: The virus attaches to a host cell and injects the DNA or RNA molecule with the viral DNA, much in the way that a needle and syringe inject medication. The viral molecule then latches onto the host cell to take over its functions and create new virus particles.
Fungus	A slow-growing organism that will establish itself most often in warm moist environments: Fungi are similar to plants but lack chlorophyll and rigid cell walls.
Yeast	Yeast infections are caused by *Candida*, which is a small, circular organism that can be considered a cousin to the fungus. Yeast also thrive in moist, humid environments. Yeast infections of the skin are characterized by beefy-red (erythematous) areas with surrounding small dots of redness.

the more recent so-called super-bugs in a long list of problem infections that have emerged over the last several decades. Methicillin-resistant *Staphylococcus aureus* implies that the bacterium is no longer susceptible to methicillin, a strong cousin of penicillin. As bacteria develop resistance to more antibiotics, only a few expensive medications remain to treat infections. Because of the difficulty in treating CA-MRSA, new strategies, especially preventive strategies, must be used to treat these cases.[3]

Signs and symptoms: CA-MRSA begins inauspiciously as a skin lesion. Any lesion, regardless of mechanism, can provide an opportunity for CA-MRSA to thrive. Once infection with CA-MRSA occurs, a cascade of events begins that usually results in the athlete's being barred from activity until medically cleared as noncontagious. CA-MRSA infections can also travel deep into other tissues and disperse throughout the body. In many cases, afflicted individuals feel a general malaise and localized discomfort in the infected area.

Treatment: Curing a CA-MRSA infection requires extensive medical intervention, long-term expensive antibiotic treatment, and complicated wound management with frequent dressing changes. In some cases, surgical removal of infected tissue is recommended. Prevention of CA-MRSA infections demands frequent cleaning of all facilities (e.g., athletic training rooms and playing areas), use of disposable towels, strict attention to body fluid precautions, and proper cleansing of wounds with special soaps. Additional detailed information about CA-MRSA and similar infections may be viewed at the Web site of the Centers for Disease Control and Prevention: www.cdc.gov/ncidod/dhqp/ar_mrsa_ca.html. (See Appendix C for the official statement on CA-MRSA from the National Athletic Trainers' Association [NATA]).

Points to Ponder

All the members of the wrestling team have been trying to combat a strange infection. You realize that it might be CA-MRSA. What are your responsibilities to your team members and to the other teams with which they compete?

Impetigo

Signs and symptoms: Impetigo is an oozing lesion. It often has a honey-colored crust and may be accompanied by large blisters. This highly contagious condition may be caused by *Staphylococcus* or *Streptococcus* bacteria.

Treatment: A culture of the fluid is often obtained to determine which organism is causing the infection. Once the exact organism is identified, the appropriate antibiotic may be administered for the most effective outcome. Treatment requires a thorough cleansing of the lesion, a topical antibiotic, and in some cases an oral antibiotic.

Paronychia and Onychia

Paronychia and onychia are infections of the fingernails and toenails.

Signs and symptoms: An **onychia** occurs at the nail bed, whereas **paronychia** affects the side nail fold, usually at the proximal aspect of the nail. Swelling and edema of the nail fold traps the infectious material, creating a functional abscess, or accumulation of pus.

Treatment: Treatment consists of warm soaks several times a day to soften the skin so that it can be manually pushed off the nail edge to allow drainage of the pus. An antibiotic ointment is also useful. Oral antibiotics are sometimes necessary if the infection persists (Figure 5-9).

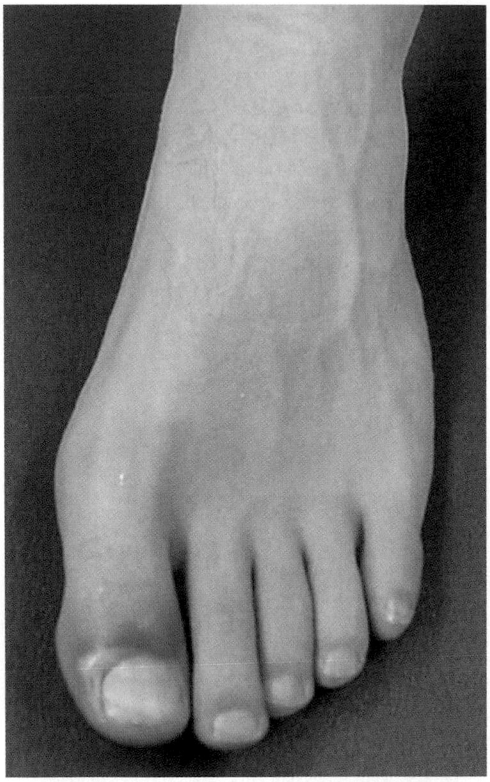

FIGURE 5-9 Paronychia surrounding the great toe. (From Cuppett M, Walsh KM: *General medical conditions in the athlete*, p. 330, St Louis, 2005, Elsevier/Mosby.)

impetigo an oozing lesion sometimes accompanied by large blisters that may be caused by the bacteria *Staphylococcus* or *Streptococcus*
onychia an infection that occurs at the nail bed
paronychia an infection that happens mostly in the side nail fold

Ingrown Toenail

An ingrown toenail usually occurs at the distal edge of the nail. If the trimming of a nail is incomplete, a sharp shard may lacerate the skin fold overlying the nail edge.

Signs and symptoms: The skin disruption becomes infected and painful. Sometimes, the affected area turns red and becomes **febrile.**

Treatment: The nail must be prevented from continuing to cut the skin. Steri-Strips are placed underneath the nail edge to lift the nail above the laceration and facilitate healing of the wound edges. Cleansing of the wound is mandatory, and ointment may be necessary to resolve an infection.

Prevention: Prevention is simple: proper nail trimming, frequent changing of socks, and regular washing of the toes and feet.

Folliculitis

Folliculitis is an infection of the base of a hair follicle. It is often the result of *Staphylococcus* bacteria found on the skin that penetrate lesions and cause infections.

Signs and symptoms: These lesions start as **erythematous** (reddish) papules, which eventually become filled with pus (Figure 5-10). Frequently, scratching or shaving irritates the hair follicle and provides an entry for the infection.

A **furuncle** is a progression of the follicle infection into an abscess (Figure 5-11). If several furuncles coalesce, a carbuncle, or large abscess, develops.

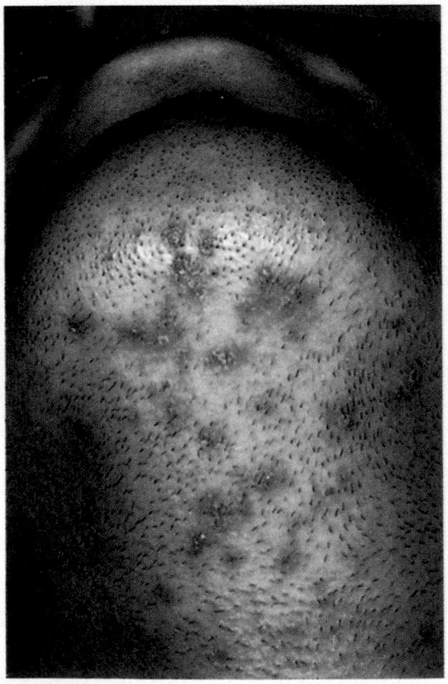

FIGURE 5-10 Folliculitis in a beard. (From Cuppett M, Walsh KM: *General medical conditions in the athlete,* p. 328, St Louis, 2005, Elsevier/Mosby.)

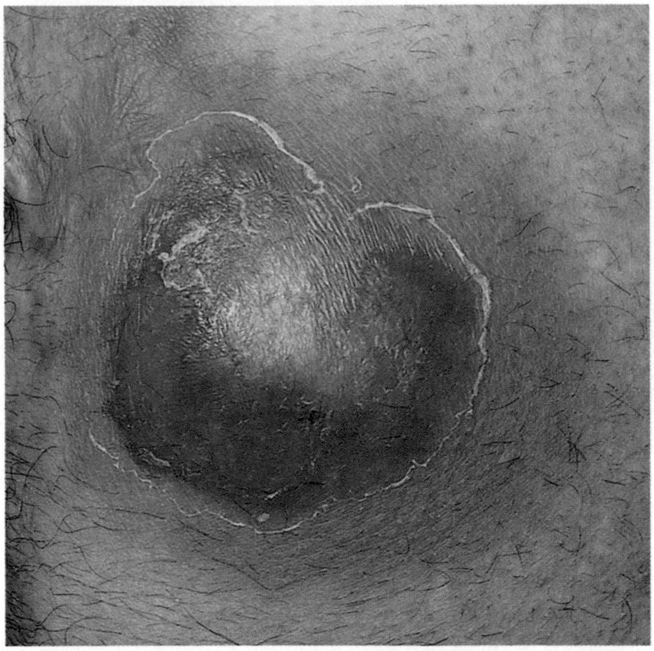

FIGURE 5-11 Furuncle. (From Cuppett M, Walsh KM: *General medical conditions in the athlete,* p. 329, St Louis, 2005, Elsevier/Mosby.)

Treatment: Treatment for folliculitis depends on the severity of the infection. Warm compresses can soften the hardened plugs of pus at the follicle. It may be necessary to drain infected abscesses for a culture to ascertain the particular bacteria. Topical or oral antibiotics are usually required for the infection to clear. Anything that irritates the skin is prohibited until the condition heals.

Viral Infections of the Skin

Like other skin infections, viral infections of the skin are relatively common in athletes. By performing occasional skin checks, the athletic trainer can limit the athlete's risk of developing more serious conditions or spreading the virus to other athletes.

Herpes Simplex

Herpes simplex is a virus that affects the skin and mucous membranes. Herpes Type I tends to infect above the waist, whereas herpes Type II tends to involve the genitalia. According to recent research, approximately one fifth of American adults have Type II herpes, although most are unaware of it.[4] There is a great deal of overlap between the two types of herpes. An initial

febrile possession of a fever
folliculitis an infection of the base of a hair follicle
erythematous reddish
furuncle a progression of the follicle infection into an abscess

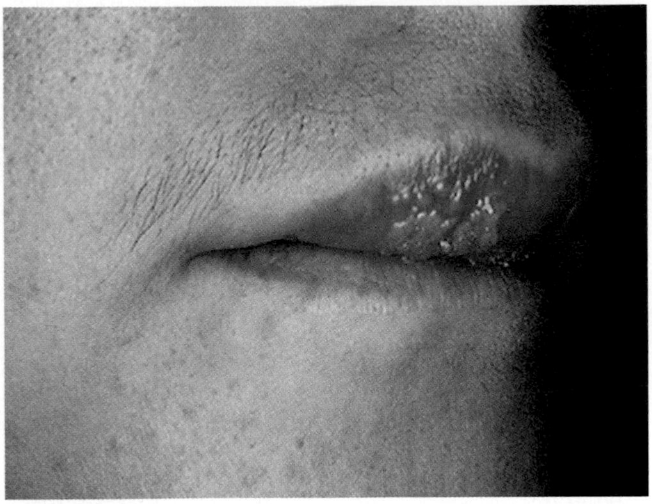

FIGURE 5-12 Herpes simplex or cold sore. (From Cuppett M, Walsh KM: *General medical conditions in the athlete,* p. 331, St Louis, 2005, Elsevier/Mosby.)

infection allows the virus to establish a chronic presence in nerve structures. Reactivation of the virus occurs as a result of stress, regardless of the stimulus or the type.

Signs and symptoms: The most common example of Type I is a cold sore or fever blister (Figure 5-12). The presenting symptoms of an infection initially are tingling or mild burning in an area that turns red. Then, small blisters or vesicles erupt on the red, erythematous patch. These vesicles evolve into larger blisters that often break, leaving a sore that is commonly seen in winter. These symptoms are true of Type II herpes as well. The difference is determined by the location of the lesions.

Treatment: Moist lesions are contagious, which means that direct physical contact with others should be limited. Treatment consists of drying agents, mild **analgesics**, and antiviral agents in the more severe outbreaks. These treatments, however, merely reduce symptoms. No cure for herpes is available at this time.

Warts

Warts, or **verrucae**, are overgrowths of skin caused by several types of the human papillomavirus. Approximately 15% of sexually active adults are infected with the human papillomavirus.[4]

Signs and symptoms: Common warts, called *verruca vulgaris,* have rough, irregular surfaces that grow outward and can appear anywhere on the skin. Warts that grow on the plantar surface of the feet are called *plantar warts.* These warts usually grow inward because the affected tissue cannot push out and up against the body's weight. Plantar warts can invade deeply into the tissues of the foot, resulting in lesions that are very painful during weight-bearing activities, even walking. It may be difficult to distinguish between large calluses and plantar warts. The difference is that warts disrupt the normal whorl of the foot's pattern, and calluses do not. Warts in the genital area are called *condylomata acuminata.* The moist environment in this region often leads to softened skin, leaving the warts with a smooth, dome-shaped appearance.

Treatment: Warts are treated through several destructive methods, including the following: chemical cautery, electrocautery (burning through electric current), freezing with liquid nitrogen, or excision with a scalpel to remove the involved tissue.

Fungal Infections of the Skin

Most fungal infections can be diagnosed merely by their outward appearance. Prevention of fungal infections includes proper personal hygiene and isolation of infected body parts as permitted (e.g., not reusing or sharing clothing or towels and uniforms). Likewise, proper cleansing and storage of equipment, towels, and uniforms can help prevent fungal infections.

General Tinea Infections

Tinea infections are caused by several types of fungi. Topical, or surface, fungi are found everywhere on the body, but most people do not become infected with daily exposure. Fungal skin infections occur with the introduction of the fungus through a lesion or breakdown of the skin.

Signs and symptoms: External signs include scaling and itching accompanied by redness.

Tinea Pedis

Tinea pedis, commonly known as *athlete's foot,* is the most common site for tinea infections.

Signs and symptoms: Athlete's foot is an infection of the foot with a dry, scaling formation in a moccasin pattern and white macerated skin between the toes (Figure 5-13). This infection may cause uncomfortable itching and inflammation.

Treatment: Antifungal cream and powder on clean, dry feet typically clear up this infection.

Tinea Cruris

Tinea cruris, an infection of the groin, is informally referred to as "jock itch." It is common in the summer

analgesic a pain reliever

verrucae warts caused by the human papillomavirus (HPV)

tinea pedis athlete's foot; infection characterized by patterned scaling and macerated skin between the toes

tinea cruris an infection of the groin frequently referred to as "jock itch"; commonly characterized by red patches that itch, blister, and ooze

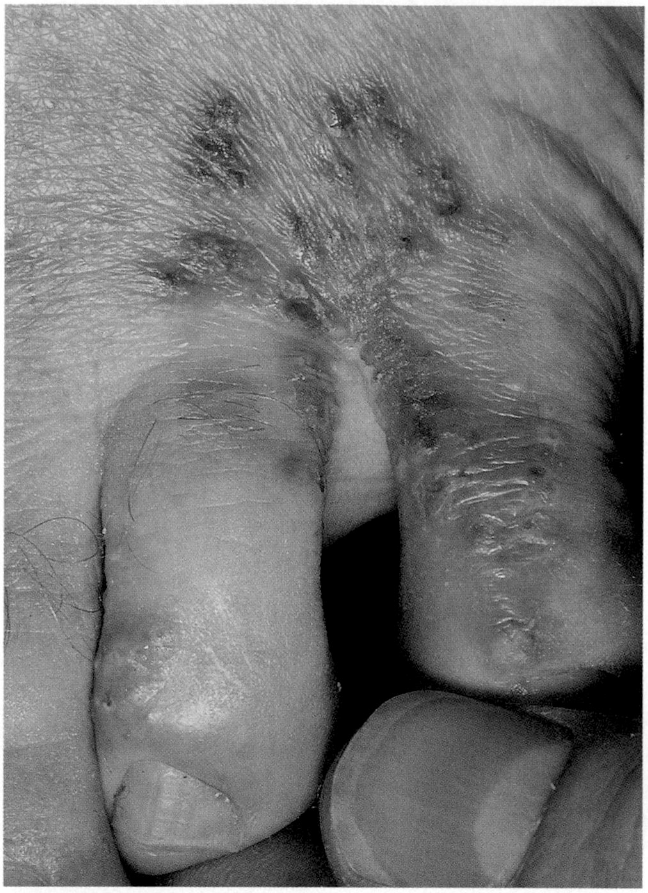

FIGURE 5-13 Tinea pedis of athlete's foot. (From Cuppett M, Walsh KM: *General medical conditions in the athlete,* p. 337, St Louis, 2005, Elsevier/Mosby.)

months because of hotter temperatures and is often associated with tinea pedis because fungal hyphae are transported to the groin when undergarments are pulled over the feet.

Signs and symptoms: Red patches that may blister and ooze and itching in the groin area are very common. As the term "jock itch" implies, itching is a common symptom in many people.

Treatment: Over the counter antifungal creams and powders are usually recommended.

Tinea Unguium

Tinea unguium is an infection of the nails that occurs in both fingernails and toenails.

Sign and symptoms: Discoloration, scaling, and destruction of the nail in severe cases are common.

Treatment: Combined topical and oral treatments may be used.

Tinea Corporis

Tinea corporis, a type of ringworm, is spread by direct contact with infected skin. Tinea corporis is grouped with the other tinea infections, but it is actually categorized as a yeast infection.

Signs and symptoms: Tinea corporis often results in variations in skin color depending on the normal coloring of the person and the season of the year in which the infection is contracted.

Treatment: Topical antifungal creams and possibly oral antifungal medications may be applied if the case is severe.

Candidal Infections

Candidal infections are caused by the yeast *Candida albicans.*

Signs and symptoms: Candidal infections usually occur in the groin or armpits with an intense, beefy-red inflammatory reaction. Small satellite lesions are often seen at the edges of candidal infections.

Treatment: Topical creams and occasionally oral medication are necessary to eradicate the infection.

THE THORAX AND RESPIRATORY SYSTEM

The thorax is also called the *thoracic cavity* or *chest cavity.* It extends from the clavicle down to the diaphragm. The major organs of the thoracic cavity are the heart and lungs. These organs are not commonly injured in athletics, but immediate attention is required when they are (Figure 5-14).

Thorax and Respiratory System Anatomy

The anatomy of the thorax and respiratory system includes those structures responsible for breathing (Figure 5-15). As such, the structures of the thorax and respiratory system have an enormous impact on overall health as well as sports-specific issues such as endurance and stamina.

Throat

The entry point to the thorax is the throat. Between the base of the skull and the sixth cervical vertebrae is the pharynx, which connects the mouth and nasal cavity to the larynx above and esophagus below. The larynx, also known as the *voicebox* or *Adam's apple,* is a cartilaginous tube connecting the throat and trachea. The larynx contains two vocal cords separated by an opening called the *glottis.* As expired air passes over the vocal cords,

tinea unguium an infection of the nails characterized by discoloration and sometimes by scaling and nail destruction

tinea corporis more commonly known as ringworm; spread by direct contact with infected skin; often results in variation in skin color

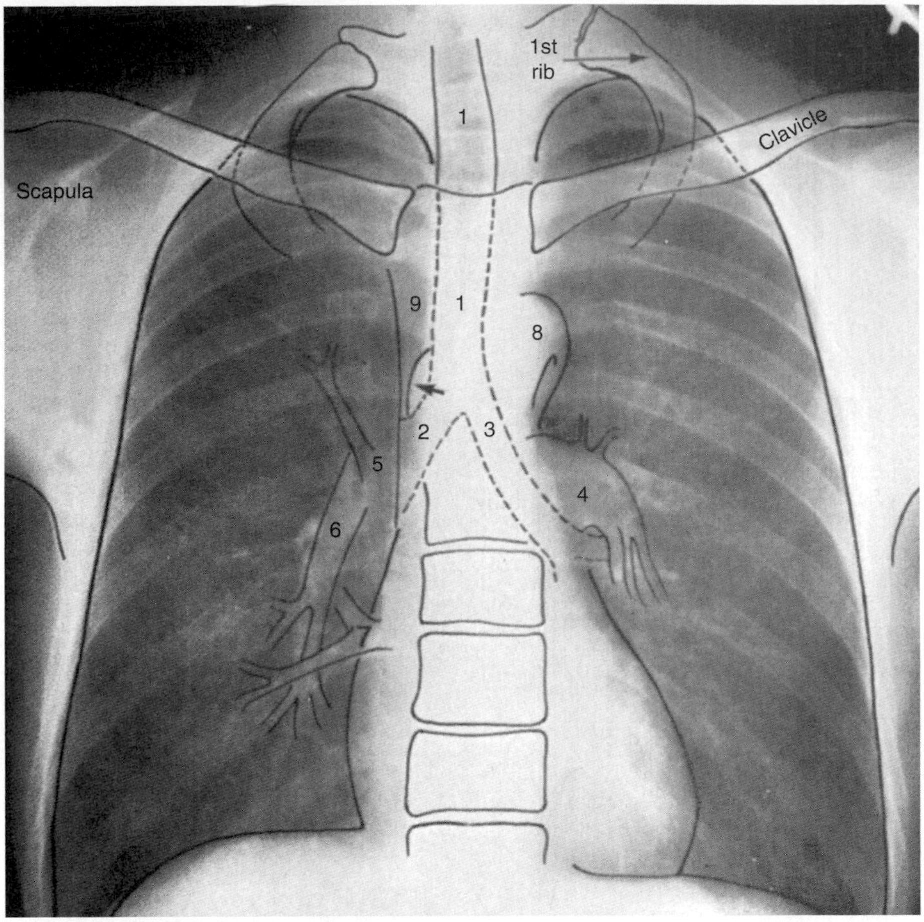

FIGURE 5-14 Normal radiograph of the chest. *1,* Trachea; *2,* right main bronchus; *3,* left main bronchus; *4,* pulmonary artery; *5,* right upper lobe vein; *6,* right pulmonary artery; *7,* right lower and middle lobe veins; *8,* aortic arch; *9,* superior vena cava. (From Fraser RS et al, editors: *Fraser and Paré's diagnosis of diseases of the chest,* ed 4, Philadelphia, 1970, Saunders.)

laryngeal muscles manipulate the length of the vocal cords and the size of the glottis to vary the pitch and volume of the voice. If the vocal cords become so swollen that they cannot move, the voice disappears until the swelling resolves. In the condition singer's throat, or cheerleader's throat, nodules develop on the vocal cords, producing a raspy voice. Protecting the larynx is a spoon-shaped dense covering called the *epiglottis* that blankets the opening of the trachea during the process of swallowing. If food or liquids do slip past the epiglottis, a cough reflex is initiated to expel the foreign material and prevent choking. If the cough reflex fails and a foreign object becomes lodged in the trachea, the Heimlich maneuver must be initiated to dislodge the object.

Trachea

The trachea is a C-shaped ring of cartilage extending downward from the larynx through the neck into the midthorax (Figure 5-16). The open side of the C is covered by the smooth muscle of the trachealis. Contraction of the trachealis during coughing reduces the size of the trachea to dramatically increase the pressure and assist with mucus clearance. The trachea divides into two bronchi; the left main bronchus divides into two segmental bronchi, and the right divides into three (the heart takes up the space a third left segmental bronchus would occupy) to supply the lobes of the lungs. Each segmental bronchus then divides into bronchioles, which continue to divide into smaller passageways. There are approximately 23 levels of branching before the alveoli of the lungs are reached. The cross-sectional area of the bronchioles is controlled by smooth muscle tissues in the bronchiolar walls.

Esophagus

The esophagus is a tube made of muscle that runs from the pharynx, behind the trachea to the stomach, and in

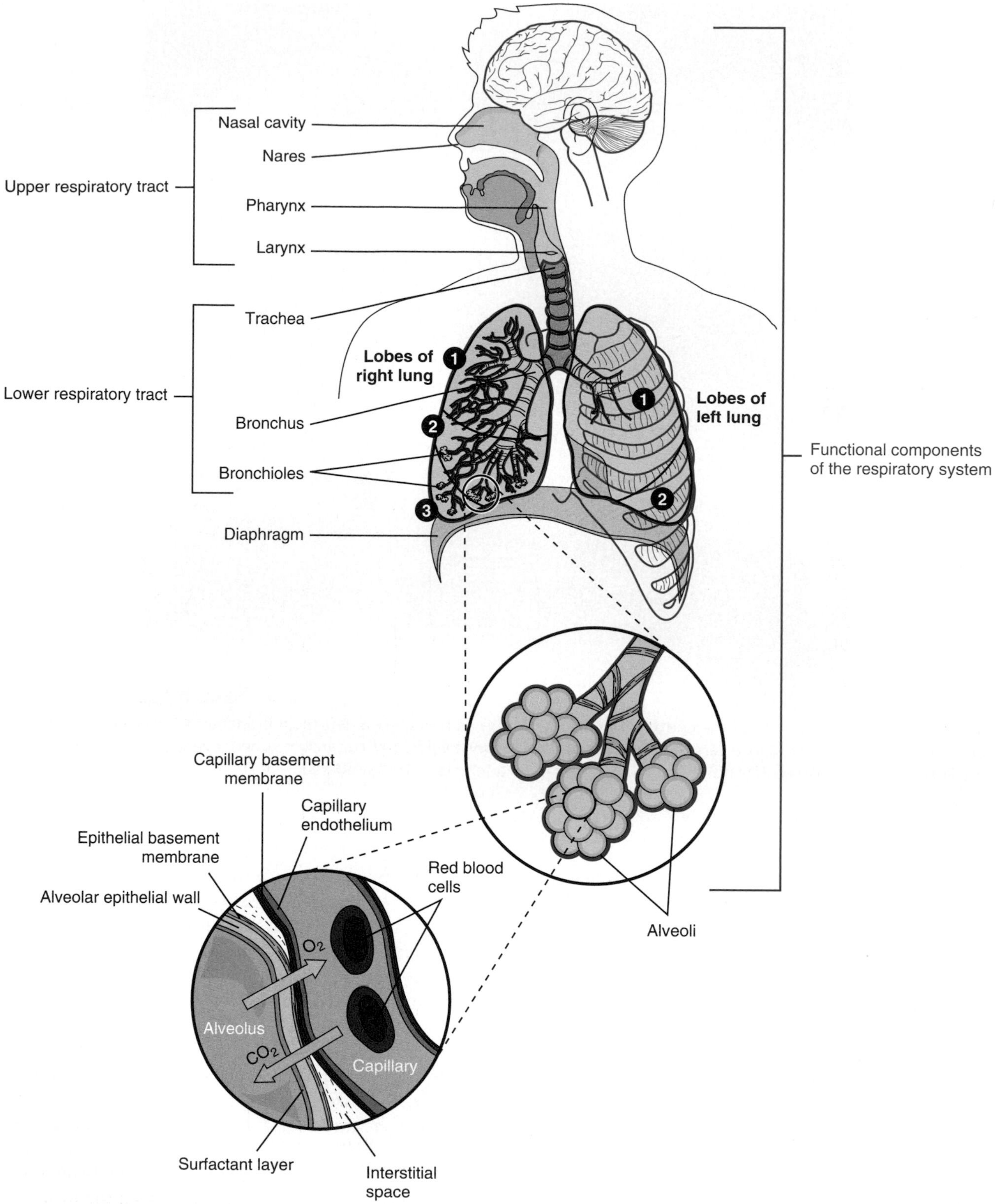

FIGURE 5-15 Organs of the respiratory system with a detailed view of the alveolar site. (From Mahan LK, Escott-Stump S: *Krause's food, nutrition, & diet therapy,* ed 11, p. 939, Philadelphia, 2004, Elsevier/Saunders.)

front of the spine. Several major blood vessels also course through the thorax. Common carotid arteries run on each side of the neck lateral to the trachea and divide into the internal and external carotid arteries at the level of the larynx. These proceed superiorly to supply blood to the face and brain.

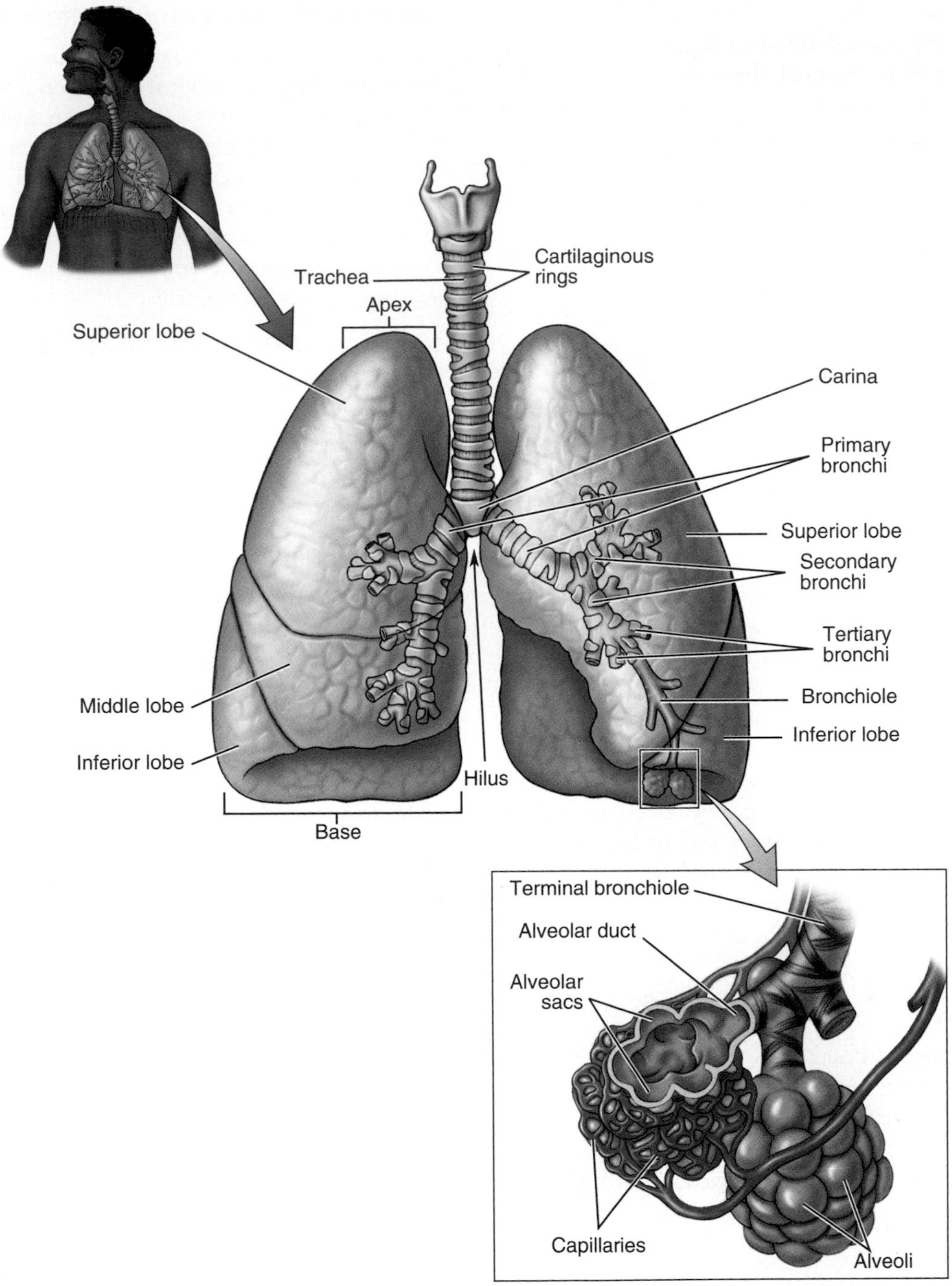

FIGURE 5-16 The trachea and bronchial tree of the lungs. (From Herlihy B: *The human body in health and illness,* ed 3, p. 375, Philadelphia, 2007, Saunders/Elsevier.)

Note that there are three lobes in the right lung and three parts to the right-sided tricuspid valve, two lobes to the left lung and two cusps of the left-sided bicuspid valve. There are only two lobes of the left lung because the heart occupies space on the left side.

Thoracic Cage

The thoracic cage is formed by the sternum, ribs and costal cartilage, and the thoracic vertebrae. The function of the thoracic cage is to provide protection for the internal organs housed in this area of the body. The sternum, which consists of the manubrium, sternal body, and xiphoid process, resembles a short sword with the manubrium, or handle of the sword, in the superior portion that connects with the first and second ribs. Connecting to the second through seventh ribs is the body, or the blade of the sword. The xiphoid process, the sharp sword tip, is a trapezoidal projection off the lower portion of the sternum. There are twelve pairs of ribs fastened in the back at the thoracic vertebrae. In the front, the costal cartilage of the first seven ribs joins directly to the sternum. The eighth through tenth ribs connect to the costal cartilage of the rib directly above, whereas the eleventh and twelfth are called *floating ribs* because no anterior connection to any bony or cartilaginous structure exists. The clavicle is an integral part of the thoracic cage with important functions in stability and mobility. The clavicle articulates with the sternum just above the first rib. On the distal portion of the clavicle, it articulates with the acromion process and aids in shoulder movement and structure.

Diaphragm

The lower border of the thoracic cavity is the diaphragm. The diaphragm has several portal holes to allow passage of the esophagus and large blood vessels into the abdominal cavity. In a relaxed state, the diaphragm is dome shaped and pushes air up and out of the lungs, causing exhalation, or expiration. The diaphragm contracts and flattens down with inhalation, or inspiration, to increase the size of the thoracic cavity. This activity creates a negative pressure while decreasing intrathoracic pressure so as to pull air into the lungs. The diaphragm is activated by the phrenic nerve. Irritation of the phrenic nerve is one of several theoretical causes for singultus, commonly known as the hiccups.

Thoracic Cavity

The thoracic cavity is lined with a thin double-layered membrane called the *pleura*. The visceral pleura lines the lungs, and the parietal pleura lines the interior of the thoracic wall. The pleural cavity is the nominal space between these two layers and is lubricated with fluid to allow the lungs to move along the thoracic wall without undue friction.

The Respiratory System

The organs of respiration, the lungs consist of an elastic network of air spaces and passageways bound together by connective tissue. The lungs are comparable to sponges, occupying most of the space of the thoracic cavity but weighing less than 2 pounds. Air is pulled into the alveoli, which are small clusters of sacs at the ends of the terminal bronchioles. The walls of the alveoli contain capillaries. Carbon dioxide is exchanged for oxygen across the alveolar membranes, releasing carbon dioxide from the deoxygenated blood to the alveoli and absorbing oxygen from the alveoli into the blood. The oxygen attaches to hemoglobin in the red blood cells for transport throughout the body.

Thorax and Respiratory System Pathology

The most common problems encountered in the respiratory system are due to viral or bacterial infectious agents. Typically, these agents are airborne and easily transmitted through coughing or sneezing. Because of the nature of transmission, they tend to be highly contagious and are hard to avoid in certain environments. The best measures of prevention are getting regular vaccinations, covering the mouth when coughing or sneezing, and washing hands frequently.

Infectious Diseases of the Respiratory System

Most viral infections are self-limited illnesses, meaning symptoms often resolve in due course regardless of whether medical care is rendered. Individuals may continue daily activities according to their perception of their own symptoms.

The Common Cold

The common cold begins with a gradual onset of symptoms that last a few days. The most prevalent infectious disease of the respiratory system, it is caused by a wide variety of viruses. The increase in temperature is mild, approximately 1 degree. Symptoms usually affect the body from the neck upward and, though annoying, are rarely debilitating.

Signs and symptoms: Sore throat, sneezing, and runny nose are frequently associated with the common cold. Cough, fatigue, malaise, weakness, and chest discomfort are generally mild and short-lasting symptoms. Headaches are less common but also mild.

Treatment: Treatment of viral illnesses is entirely supportive and aimed at keeping the person comfortable while the infection takes its natural course.

Influenza

Influenza is a distinct entity caused by a different family of viruses than those associated with the common cold (Table 5-5). Prevention of influenza is accomplished through annual vaccinations.

Signs and symptoms: The onset of influenza is quite abrupt. A fever of 100.4° to 104°F is common and a strong distinguishing factor in the diagnosis. Joint pain, muscle pain, and weakness are common and significant. A severe dry cough, headache, and lack of appetite are frequent components of this illness. Fatigue often lasts 2 to 3 weeks. Chest discomfort is common with influenza.

Treatment: Presence of a fever warrants the administration of an **antipyretic**, or fever-reducing medication.

---

influenza a viral infection typically referred to as flu; much more serious than the common cold
antipyretic fever-reducing medication

TABLE 5-5 Comparison of the Symptoms of Influenza and the Common Cold

CHARACTERISTIC	INFLUENZA	COMMON COLD
Onset	Abrupt	More gradual
Fever	Common: 37.7° to 40° C (100° to 104° F)	Increase of only approximately 0.5°C (1° F)
Myalgia	Severe, common	Uncommon
Arthralgia	Severe, common	Uncommon
Anorexia	Common	Uncommon
Headache	Severe, common	Mild, uncommon
Cough (dry)	Common, severe	Mild to moderate
Malaise	Severe	Mild
Fatigue, weakness	More common, lasting 2 to 3 weeks	Very mild, short duration
Chest discomfort	Common, severe	Mild to moderate
Stuffy nose	Occasional	Common
Sneezing	Occasional	Common
Sore throat	Occasional	Common

Data from National Institute of Allergy and Infectious Diseases, National Institutes of Health: Is it a cold or the flu, Bethesda, Md, 2005 (September), U.S. Department of Health & Human Services. Retrieved February 14, 2007, from www.niaid.nih.gov/publications/cold/sick.pdf.

Normal human body temperature is approximately 98.6° F, with a range of 97° to 99° F. A temperature above 100.4° is considered a fever. A dry cough calls for the use of a cough suppressant (**antitussive**), and a productive cough might benefit from an expectorant. Headache, **arthralgia, myalgia,** and **malaise** lessen with administration of an analgesic, or pain reliever. Use of single-ingredient medications aimed at a particular symptom is more effective from both a therapeutic and financial standpoint than are the combination preparations prevalent in local pharmacies. Some form of caloric intake should be encouraged and maintained despite a lack of appetite. The old adage "starve a cold and feed a fever" is not applicable (Box 5-1).

BOX 5-1 Symptoms and Treatment for the Common Cold and Influenza

SYMPTOM	TREATMENT
Runny nose	
Cold (virus)	Decongestant
Allergy	Antihistamine
Cough	
Dry	Antitussive (suppressant)
Productive	Expectorant
Sore throat	
Viral	Salt water gargles, lozenges
Bacterial	Antibiotics

Bronchitis

Bronchitis involves an inflammatory process in the bronchial passages leading to the lungs. It is associated with several etiologies but usually is secondary to either a viral or a bacterial infection.

Signs and symptoms: The hallmark symptom of bronchitis is a productive cough. Fever and malaise sometimes accompany bronchitis, but not always.

Treatment: Presence of a fever or sputum increases the likelihood of a bacterial etiology and prompts the addition of antibiotics to the supportive therapeutic regimen.

Pneumonia

Pneumonia, or pneumonitis, is an inflammatory process in the substance of the lungs. It is usually caused by an infectious agent, generally a virus or bacteria. Pneumonia caused by bacteria is more serious and requires treatment with antibiotics.

Signs and symptoms: Symptoms of pneumonia progress gradually and often mimic an upper respiratory infection. So-called walking pneumonia, a milder form of pneumonia, is commonly thought to be of viral etiology. People who are affected by walking pneumonia do not require hospitalization and are often able to continue participating in school or work functions.

antitussive a cough suppressant
arthralgia joint pain
myalgia muscle pain
malaise nonspecific feeling of discomfort or being ill

Mononucleosis

Infectious mononucleosis, also called *mono* or the *kissing disease,* is seen most commonly in adolescents and young adults. Mononucleosis is caused by the Epstein-Barr virus (EBV). It is usually transmitted through saliva, blood, eating utensils, or needles among individuals who appear to have no symptoms. The virus may also be transmitted through airborne means such as coughing or sneezing. Researchers have recently found that mononucleosis is not as contagious as previously believed. It is estimated that 90% of the adults in the world have EBV-antibodies, having been infected with EBV at some point in their lives.[5] Most infections do not result in the development of mononucleosis.

Signs and symptoms: Mono is characterized by a fever, sore throat, and debilitating fatigue. A person may be infected with the virus for a long time before any symptoms appear. Symptoms typically appear 4 to 7 weeks after the initial infection and may resemble strep throat or other bacterial or viral respiratory infections. The first signs of the disease are commonly confused with cold and flulike symptoms. Frequently, an enlarged spleen is also apparent, a finding that helps in making a conclusive diagnosis of mononucleosis.

Treatment: Treatment involves treating the symptoms and may include consumption of a lot of fluids, bed rest, and analgesics. Corticosteroids may benefit patients with compromised respiratory systems. Generally, patients should not go back to athletics or work for approximately 4 weeks and should receive medical clearance. The duration of symptoms varies from weeks to months, with some cases lasting even longer. Even after the initial symptoms are gone, there may be a risk of rupturing the enlarged spleen, a condition known as *splenomegaly.*[5,6]

Points to Ponder

You have been battling what could be the cold or influenza. You have a great deal of work to finish, and yet you know you might be contagious. Do you tough it out and go into work, or do you stay home and try to recover in isolation? How do you decide when it is safe to go to work when you are ill?

Asthma

A more accurate term for **asthma** is *reactive airway disease.* Given a sufficiently noxious stimulus (i.e., poisonous fumes), anyone's airways react by wheezing. People with asthma have airways that react easily to a variety of stimuli. The size of the bronchiolar passages is controlled by the smooth muscle. A triggering stimulus, often considered an allergen, causes the smooth muscles to react, decreasing the size of the airway as a protective mechanism. The decrease in cross-sectional area causes an obstruction in the exhalation of air and results in wheezing if the hindrance is significant.

The lungs can be compared to a squeaker toy. Squeezing air out of the toy is analogous to the exhalation of the lungs and results in a squeak or wheeze. Releasing the grip on the toy allows air to rush back into the toy, as with inhalation.

Signs and symptoms: Several stimuli can function as triggers for reactive airway disease; any individual may be susceptible to one or more. Pollen, dust mites, animal dander, candle or cigarette smoke, smog, perfume, and exercise are a few common triggers.

Exposure to a trigger results in reactivity of the airway, or bronchospasm. A mild exposure or mild reactivity on the individual's part results in narrowing of the airway with a decrease in available oxygen. A more significant exposure causes wheezing, considered a mid to late manifestation of the reactive airway disease process.[7] Note, however, that decreased air flow occurs long before wheezing occurs. A more accurate measure of airway reactivity is expiratory flow rate, which is measured with a spirometer. A simple hand-held spirometer measures peak expiratory flow rate when a subject forcefully exhales through a small tube. The peak velocity of the air flow is measured and recorded. More sophisticated spirometers record air velocity throughout exhalation, generating a graph of volume versus elapsed time. Either measure may be compared with normal values or previous recorded values for the individual. A decrease in either of the measures indicates a worsening of the reactive airway disease and suggests the need for more aggressive treatment.

Treatment: A key component of successful treatment of reactive airway disease is identification of offending factors with avoidance of those triggers. Individuals with reactive airway disease often have accompanying postnasal drainage and gastro-esophageal reflux disease (GERD). These symptoms may require simultaneous treatment for successful resolution. Treatment of reactive airway disease involves avoidance of identified triggers, maintenance medications, and rescue medications. Maintenance medications are taken daily and are usually administered by oral or inhaled routes. The aim is a decrease of bronchiolar inflammation to lessen the reactivity of the smooth muscle. Rescue medications are

asthma a chronic disease in which the respiratory system becomes inflamed and constricts as a result of external triggers; also known as reactive airway disease administered by the inhalation route to disrupt an episode of acute bronchospasm, or what is commonly referred to as an *asthma attack*. Rescue medications, such as bronchodilators, should be available at all times for individuals with significant reactive airway disease[7] (Box 5-2).

Exercise-Induced Asthma

Exercise-induced asthma (EIA) is synonymous with exercise-induced bronchospasm. Physical activity is the triggering stimulus for the acute bronchoconstriction. The mechanism remains unknown, although several theories have been proposed.

Signs and symptoms: The classic description involves the onset of shortness of breath, fatigue, and possible wheezing 5 to 8 minutes into physical activity. Before diagnosis, many people simply assume that they are unable to get into shape. Afflicted athletes also require a greater recovery period after exercise to return to normal resting values.

Special tests: People with exercise-induced bronchospasm routinely have additional triggers that may induce bronchoconstriction. Diagnosis is best obtained by use of spirometer testing. A baseline value is obtained before the subject is asked to exercise on a treadmill. A repeat spirometer value is obtained immediately after exercise. If the repeat value is significantly decreased, exercise-induced bronchospasm is present.

Treatment: Treatment of exercise-induced bronchospasm usually involves the use of a rescue inhaler 20 to 30 minutes before the onset of exercise. Maintenance medications may be necessary if significant disease or numerous other triggers are present. Exercise-induced bronchospasm is also notable for the presence of a refractory period. Following the cessation of the exercise bout, the bronchioles become less susceptible to triggering stimuli. A competitive athlete may experience difficulty during a match but may get a second wind during an overtime period by entering a refractory period between the end of the game and the start of an overtime period.[7]

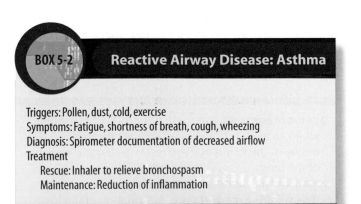

BOX 5-2 Reactive Airway Disease: Asthma

Triggers: Pollen, dust, cold, exercise
Symptoms: Fatigue, shortness of breath, cough, wheezing
Diagnosis: Spirometer documentation of decreased airflow
Treatment
- Rescue: Inhaler to relieve bronchospasm
- Maintenance: Reduction of inflammation

Hyperventilation

Hyperventilation is the state of breathing faster or deeper than is necessary. It reduces the carbon dioxide concentration of the blood to levels that are below normal.

Signs and Symptoms: Hyperventilation causes a range of symptoms such as numbness or tingling in the hands, feet and lips, lightheadedness, dizziness, headache, chest pain, slurred speech, and sometimes fainting. Stress or anxiety are typical reasons for hyperventilation, sometimes referred to as hyperventilation syndrome. Hyperventilation also results from various lung diseases, head injury, stroke, or lack of oxygen in the body (hypoxia). Hyperventilation may also occur as a result of sepsis.

Treatment: The common treatment of breathing into a paper bag is no longer recommended because it can cause the carbon dioxide levels to rise too rapidly. Instead, treatment should center on relieving the underlying condition, such as anxiety.[8] Often, talking calmly with the individual helps address the situation causing the unexpected stimulus. The athletic trainer's focus should be on helping the hyperventilating person resume a normal breathing pattern as quickly as possible.

Traumatic Injuries of the Thorax and Respiratory System

The thorax and respiratory system can sustain traumatic injuries. When such an injury occurs, it usually results in a medical emergency. Being prepared to properly diagnose the injury and respond is critical to a successful outcome.

Fractures

A significant blow to the chest can result in fractures of the ribs, most commonly in the fifth through ninth ribs. Fractures of the eleventh and twelfth ribs are much less common because these are floating ribs that have only a posterior attachment. Thus they can bend to absorb forces more effectively.

Signs and symptoms: The chief complaint with rib fractures is usually pain directly over the site of the fracture. Pain may increase with physical effort and inspiration and may also radiate with coughing, sneezing, and movements of the torso.

Fractures of the sternum are not common in sporting events or most activities. The sternum or breastbone is a sturdy structure that can tolerate the application of large forces. Sternal fractures are more likely to be seen in motor vehicle accidents when the chest wall comes into contact with the steering wheel. Forces large enough to fracture the sternum are likely to be transmitted to underlying structures. A cardiac contusion must also be considered whenever a sternal fracture is discovered. A severe blow to the sternum can subsequently transmit these same violent forces to the heart.[9]

Flail Chest

A flail chest occurs when multiple rib fractures isolate a segment of the chest wall. This isolated segment can no longer move in concert with the chest wall, limiting air intake and ventilatory capacity.

Special tests: Rib fractures may be assessed with a rib compression test (Figure 5-17). The thorax is compressed from the sides and is quickly released. A positive test occurs with pain directly at the site of the fracture. A rib compression test should not be performed if there is an obvious fracture, damage to the lung, or wheezing.

Pneumothorax

A **pneumothorax** (Figure 5-18, *A*) is an emergency situation that occurs when air leaks into the pleural cavity located between the lining of the chest wall and the covering of the lungs (i.e., visceral and parietal pleura). A pneumothorax can be open or closed. An open pneumothorax suggests that the chest wall and lung has been damaged, allowing air to leak from the chest cavity as it escapes from the lung. A closed pneumothorax suggests an intact chest wall, which means that the leaking air stays enclosed in the thoracic cavity. Other variations of a pneumothorax include tension pneumothorax and spontaneous pneumothorax. A tension pneumothorax occurs when continued accumulation of trapped air begins to force one of the lungs to collapse.

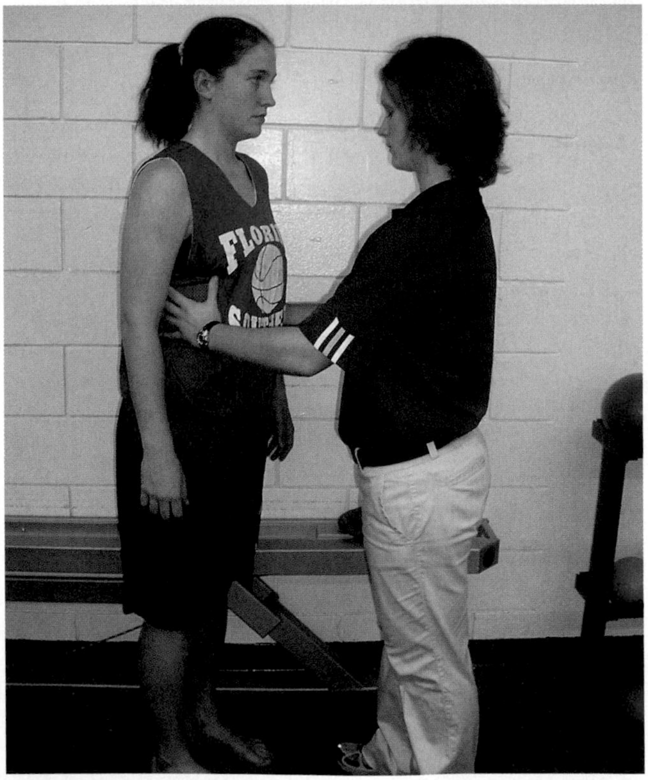

FIGURE 5-17 Rib compression test.

Signs and symptoms: Respiratory distress, pain, cyanosis (i.e., blueness of lips and fingers), and decreased blood pressure are common manifestations of a pneumothorax. A tension pneumothorax may further cause displacement of the trachea and larynx to one side as the pressure inside the chest cavity forces the other lung to collapse. A spontaneous pneumothorax can occur with an idiopathic rupture of an alveolar sac, causing an air leak; this often happens in the absence of any identifiable trauma.

Treatment: Emergency medical care should be sought if any type of rib fracture or pneumothorax is suspected.

Hemothorax

A **hemothorax** (see Figure 5-18, *B*) results from blood entering the pleural cavity and prevents inflation of the lung, which is unable to expand with the chest wall. The necessary volume of air cannot be pulled into the lung with inspiration. As with a pneumothorax, any suspicion that a hemothorax exists should result in an immediate activation of the emergency medical team.

THE CIRCULATORY SYSTEM

The circulatory system is analogous to pipework in that it transports the blood to and from the heart. This system of vessels carries not only the blood but also vital nutrients and oxygen necessary for organs and muscles to function properly. Without this conduit of vessels, the body would not be able to maintain even its most basic functions.

Circulatory System Anatomy

The circulatory system consists of a pump connecting two series of vessels. Arteries are the vessels that allow blood to course away from the heart while veins travel and carry blood back to the heart. The heart is a four-chambered pump consisting of two atria and two ventricles (Figure 5-19). Each atrium serves as a lobby or antechamber for the ventricle that it supplies with blood. Each ventricle is the major pump for the right and left sides of the heart. The right side of the pump (i.e., the right ventricle) supplies a short series of vessels, collectively termed the *pulmonary circuit,* that

pneumothorax an emergency condition occurring when air leaks into the pleural cavity located between the lining of the chest wall and the covering of the lungs

hemothorax condition occurring when blood enters the pleural cavity and prevents inflation of the lung

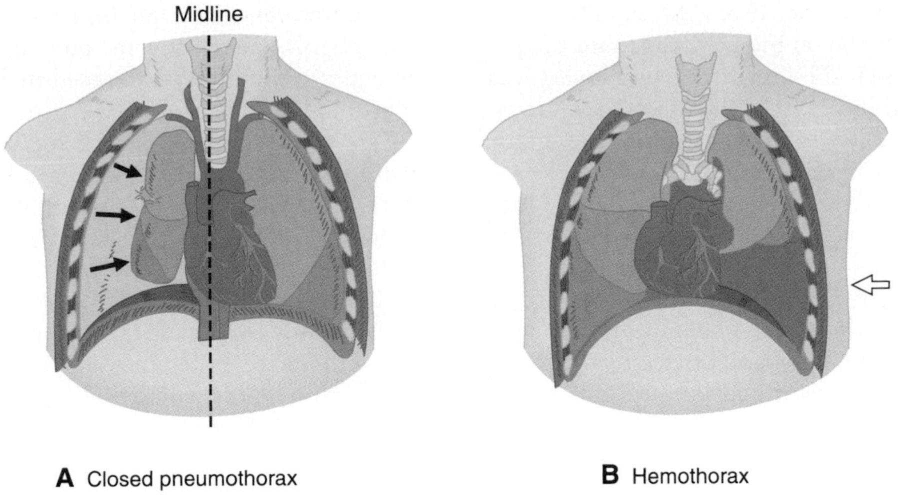

FIGURE 5-18 **A,** Pneumothorax. **B,** Hemothorax. (From Black JM, Hawks JH: *Medical surgical nursing: Clinical management for positive outcomes,* ed 7, p. 1903, St Louis, 2005, Mosby.)

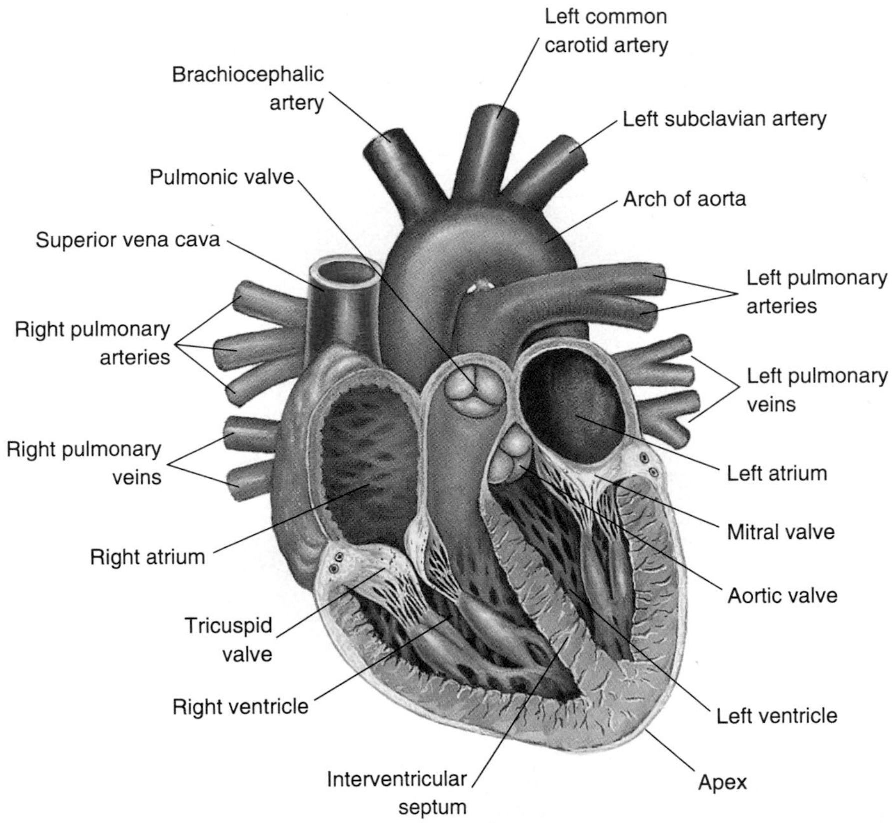

FIGURE 5-19 Anatomy of the chambers of the heart. (From Seidel HM et al: *Mosby's guide to physical examination,* ed 6, p. 415, St Louis, 2006, Mosby/Elsevier.)

travel to the lungs to oxygenate the blood. The left side of the pump (i.e., the left ventricle) connects to a series of vessels (called the *systemic circuit)* that supply the remainder of the body. Between each chamber is a passive valve that allows blood to flow forward but not backwards.

As an example of this process, blood reaches the heart from the body through the vena cava. The superior vena cava drains blood from the head and upper extremities while the inferior vena cava transports blood from the trunk and lower extremities. Blood then travels by entering the right atrium, passing through the tricuspid valve into the right ventricle. From the right ventricle, blood travels through the pulmonary valve into the pulmonary artery to reach the lungs. The pulmonary vein channels oxygenated blood from the lungs back toward the left atrium. Blood leaves the left atrium through the bicuspid (mitral) valve to enter the left ventricle. The aortic valve connects the left ventricle to the aorta. The aorta supplies blood to the rest of the body via the systemic circuit.

The heart is stimulated by an electrical circuit with the electrical impulse starting in the sinoatrial (SA) node (Figure 5-20). The action potential, or electrical impulse, travels through both the right and left atria to activate the cardiac muscle and pump the blood located in each atria into the ventricles. The electrical impulse is collected in the atrioventricular (AV) node and transferred down the right and left branches of the bundles of His to the apex (bottom tip) of the heart. The bundle of His is a cluster of cardiac muscle fibers that conducts the electrical impulses regulating the heartbeat. The impulse then travels up the Purkinje fibers, which are specialized conductive fibers located within the walls of the ventricles. They are responsible for relaying cardiac impulses to the cells of the ventricles, allowing the ventricles to contract. The impulse next activates the ventricular musculature to squeeze the blood contained in the chamber out the top of the heart.

The electrical heartbeat is measured by the electrocardiogram (EKG or ECG; Figure 5-21). The EKG consists of the P, QRS, and T waves, which are described in Table 5-6. Note that the repolarization of the atria is hidden by the QRS complex.

Cardiac muscle, or intercalated muscle, is anatomically distinct from skeletal and smooth muscle. The cell membranes are more integrated to allow better electrical conduction. Electrical activity can travel in any direction through the cardiac muscle, whereas in skeletal muscle the signal travels in one direction along a pathway. When the electrical impulse travels through the normal pathways, the atrial muscle activates and contracts from the top down, propelling blood into the ventricles. After being collected by the A-V node, the electrical impulse travels to the apex of the heart to contract the ventricular muscle from the bottom up and squeeze blood out of the top through the pulmonary artery and into the aorta.

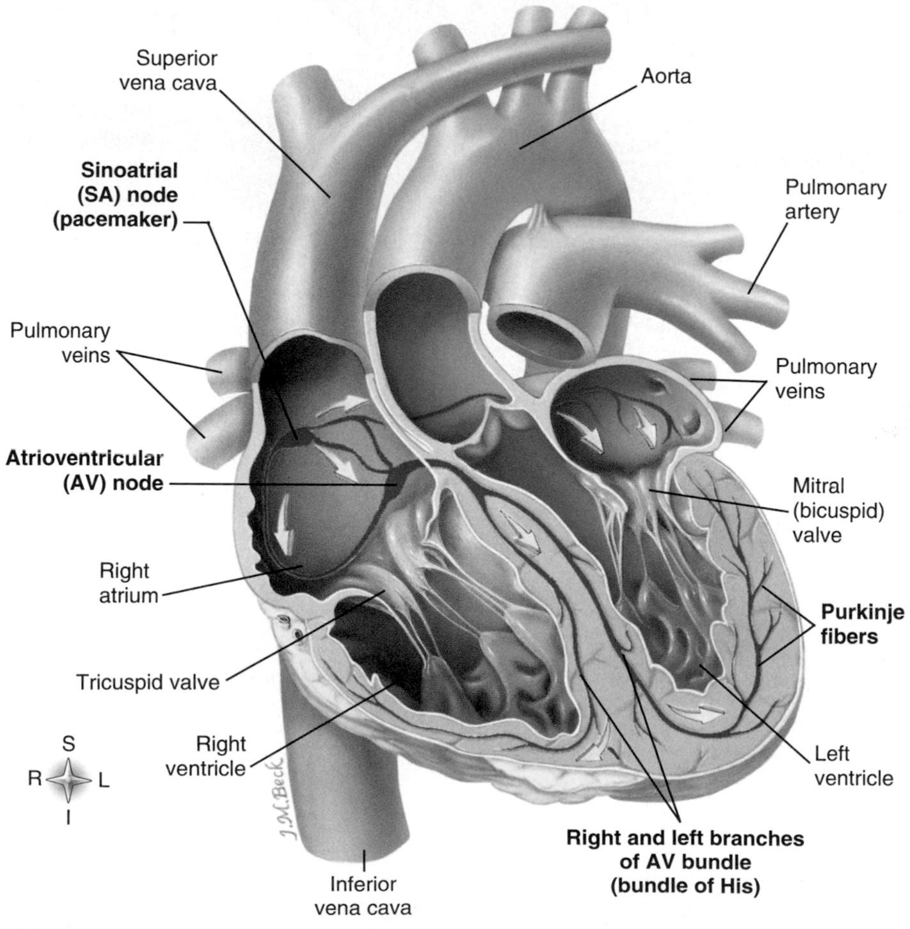

FIGURE 5-20 Course of the electrical activity of the heart. (From Thibodeau GA, Patton KT: *Anatomy & physiology,* ed 6, p. 690, St Louis, 2007, Mosby/Elsevier.)

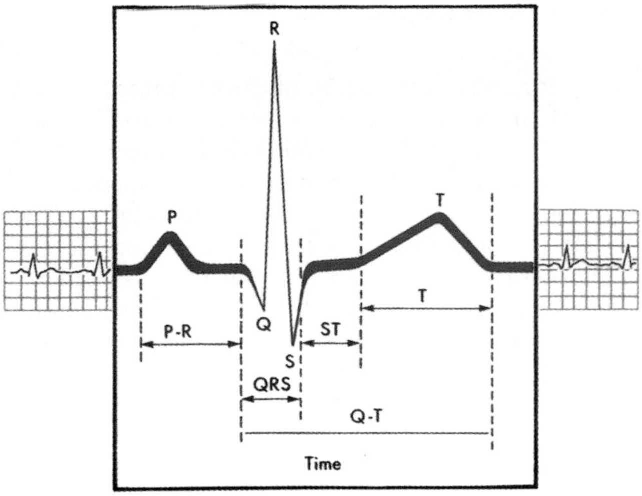

FIGURE 5-21 Electrocardiogram. (From Berne RM, Levy MN: *Cardiovascular physiology,* ed 7, St Louis, 1996, Mosby.)

TABLE 5-6 P, QRS, and T Waves

WAVE TYPE	DESCRIPTION
P waves	P waves mark the depolarization and activation of the atria.
QRS complex	The QRS complex signifies the depolarization and activation of the ventricles.
T waves	T waves mark the repolarization of the ventricles.

The cardiac muscle receives its blood supply through the coronary artery system. Two coronary arteries, the right and left, exit the initial segment of the aorta near the top of the heart. They are the only branches of the ascending aorta. The right coronary artery travels down the right side of the heart and provides blood to the right and left sides of the heart. The initial portion of the left coronary artery is called the *left main coronary artery.* The left main divides into the left anterior descending coronary artery and the left circumflex coronary artery. The left anterior descending artery travels the front of the heart to supply the left ventricle. The left circumflex coronary artery traverses the left edge of the heart to supply the posterior aspect of the left ventricle.

Pressure from contraction of the cardiac muscle drives blood flow throughout the body. Heart sounds are caused by turbulence created in the blood, which vibrates the tissue. As the ventricles contract, the bicuspid and tricuspid valves are first forced shut, preventing any regurgitation of blood back into the atria. As pressure continues to rise, the pulmonic and aortic valves are forced open to allow ejection of the blood from the ventricle into the pulmonary artery and the aorta. The turbulence and vibration caused by the closing of the bicuspid and tricuspid valves generates the first audible heart sound (S1). The opening of the pulmonic and aortic valves generates the vibration that produces the second audible heart sound (S2).

Blood pressure is measured in millimeters of mercury (mm Hg) and listed as two numbers. The average blood pressure is considered to be 120/80. The first, or top, number represents the **systolic blood pressure,** and the bottom number represents the diastolic blood pressure. The systolic pressure, which occurs as the ventricles contract to force blood into the arteries, is the maximum pressure the blood vessels will experience. **Diastolic blood pressure** is the force exerted by the volume of blood on the artery walls when the heart is not actively contracting. Blood pressure that is consistently too high puts too much strain on the cardiovascular system, causing heart disease. Blood pressure increases and decreases transiently with exercise. Table 5-7 summarizes the two types of blood pressure.

Blood pressure is measured using a sphygmomanometer (blood pressure cuff) and a stethoscope. The cuff is an inflatable air bladder controlled by a manual valve. Larger arms require wider cuffs. The cuff is inflated to a high pressure—usually 180 to 200 mmHg—while the stethoscope head is placed over the brachial artery located in the antecubital fossa of the elbow. This cuff pressure exerts pressure on the blood vessels and prevents blood from flowing through. As the manual valve is slowly released and the cuff pressure lowers, blood is able to squirt through the blood vessels with each ventricle contraction. The turbulence caused by the intermittent blood flow causes the sounds heard through

systolic blood pressure the pressure of blood into the arteries resulting from ventricular contractions

diastolic blood pressure the force exerted by the volume of blood on the artery walls when the heart is not actively contracting

TABLE 5-7 Normal Blood Pressure

TYPE OF PRESSURE	AVERAGE PRESSURE	DESCRIPTION
Systolic	120 mmHg	Pressure of blood into arteries via ventricular contraction
Diastolic	80 mmHg	Amount of force, or pressure, exerted on arterial walls via blood volume passing through the arteries while the heart is at rest (not contracting)

the stethoscope. These sounds are called *Korotkoff's sounds*. They are audible until the diastolic blood pressure exceeds the cuff pressure.

Circulatory System Pathology

Any of the organs or vessels within the circulatory system can malfunction. The most dramatic dysfunctions are those that cause sudden death, defined as death within 1 hour of the onset of symptoms from a nontraumatic cause. The incidence of sudden death in high-school athletics is approximately 1 in 200,000 and is five times higher in males than females. The most common causes of sudden death are cardiac related. Hypertrophic cardiomyopathy accounts for one third of these deaths, whereas coronary artery abnormalities account for one fifth and an increased cardiac mass for one tenth. The remainder of sudden death cases result from an assortment of noncardiovascular and cardiovascular causes.[10] Sudden death presents no warning signs in a vast majority of cases. A history of fainting during exercise and a family history of death before age 50 on account of cardiovascular causes are the best predictors of risk for sudden death.[11]

Hypertrophic Cardiomyopathy

Hypertrophic cardiomyopathy and increased cardiac mass is the leading cause of sudden death in the United States.[12] Hypertrophic cardiomyopathy deals with the size of the chamber walls and subsequently the chamber size itself. Several malfunctions may occur in the presence of hypertrophic cardiomyopathy and increased cardiac mass. The decreased chamber size may prevent normal amounts of blood from being ejected from the ventricles. Decreased wall distensibility and incomplete myocardial relaxation can adversely affect blood flow to the cardiac musculature. The combination of these malfunctions can lead to arrhythmia and sudden death.[5]

Coronary artery abnormalities deprive the cardiac muscles of blood and therefore necessary nutrition and oxygen. Such anomalies occur in approximately 1% of the total U.S. population and 4% to 15% of young people who experience sudden death.[11] Myocardial bridging occurs when a portion of the coronary vasculature is surrounded by myocardium. Activation of the surrounding myocardium can constrict the vessel just as blood should be flowing through.

Signs and symptoms: Chest pain occurring at rest and after meals, dizziness, and palpitations may appear. In many cases, no symptoms precede these episodes.

Treatment: Beta blockers, antiarrhythmics, and calcium channel blockers are used to control arrhythmias. Surgery may be required. Some people may be advised to stop strenuous activities. Being overweight, smoking, and consuming too much alcohol are also risk factors that should be addressed.[13]

Myocardial Infarction

A **myocardial infarction** is commonly known as a heart attack. It results in the death of cardiac muscle because of a lack of blood supply to the affected area. The muscle loss can happen in any section of the heart.

Signs and symptoms: Crushing substernal chest pain, sweating, shortness of breath, and pain radiating down the left arm or both arms are the classic symptoms of a heart attack in men. Women frequently have different symptoms, such as profuse sweating, cold and clammy skin, pain in the upper back or shoulder blade region, and nausea.

Treatment: Ingestion of an aspirin and prompt activation of EMS are mandatory with any suspicion of a myocardial infarction. The resulting amount of impairment that will occur depends on the location and the amount of the lost muscle. Muscle loss in the left ventricle causes more problems than the same amount in the atria or in the right ventricle.[14]

Commotio Cordis

Direct blows to the chest can result in blunt force trauma to the heart. When this trauma happens during a vulnerable period of the cardiac electrical cycle just before the T wave, an abnormal rhythm can ensue that ultimately results in death. As stated in the NATA official statement on **commotio cordis**[9] (see Appendix D), teaching individuals how to avoid direct blows to the chest and providing protective equipment that fits properly are first steps in preventing this situation from occurring. If commotio cordis is suspected, the emergency action plan must be activated at once.

Arrhythmias

Arrhythmias occur when the normal electrical patterns of the heart become disrupted. Most arrhythmias are benign, but a few are pathological and dangerous. The resultant abnormal patterns are divided into supraventricular and ventricular arrhythmias. Ventricular fibrillation is an arrhythmia involving disorganized activation of the ventricles, preventing any significant blood flow away from the heart. Atrial fibrillation is not as problematic because the atria contribute smaller amounts to the total blood flow.[14]

Viral infections sometimes cause myocarditis. The enteroviruses (usually coxsackievirus B) are the most

myocardial infarction a heart attack resulting from a lack of blood supply in a portion of the heart

commotio cordis disturbance of the heart rhythm caused by a blunt, nonpenetrating impact to the chest

arrhythmia abnormal heart rhythm occurring when the normal electrical patterns of the heart become disrupted common cause of this inflammatory process. The inflamed cardiac musculature is easily irritated, also producing irregular heart beats, or arrhythmias.

With increased understanding of the true frequency of heart-related anomalies, the severity and subsequent consequences of these conditions becomes glaringly apparent.

Signs and symptoms: Identification of individuals at risk for sudden cardiac death is uncommonly difficult. The most useful tests are expensive, unwieldy, and inappropriate for preparticipation examinations or prework screenings. The best way to screen for risk in athletes is through identification of episodes of fainting during exertion and the death of a relative younger than 50 as a result of cardiac causes.[11]

Treatment: Automated external defibrillation (AED) devices are commonplace today and are a great adjunct in the care of on-site cardiac emergencies. These machines use a computerized algorithm to detect electrical abnormalities of the heart. Electrodes packaged with the device are easily applied to the chest according to the manufacturer's instructions. Once applied, the AED device reads the electrical rhythm of the subject's heart. If an abnormality is detected, a message appears indicating whether a shock should be applied. Some abnormal electrical rhythms are reversible with the AED device and can be reset to restore normal rhythm and function immediately. The AED device can sense an abnormal rhythm and suggest continued cardiopulmonary resuscitation or continued monitoring of the individual. Whenever the use of an AED device is required, the athletic trainer should take immediate steps to activate the emergency action plan.

Heart Murmurs

Heart murmurs are much more common and less dramatic manifestations of circulatory pathologies. These extra heart sounds, known as murmurs, result from excessive turbulence of blood flow and are often caused by abnormalities of the valves. Most murmurs are benign. Many children have a flow murmur at some point in their early lives that typically disappears within a few years. Obviously, valve abnormalities that decrease blood flow are problematic. A scarred pulmonic or aortic valve may not open to the fullest extent, causing excessive turbulence and a decreased volume of blood flow. Any of the four valves can allow back flow (i.e., regurgitation) if the cusps do not fit tightly together. Past studies estimated mitral valve prolapse in 5% to 17% of the general population, although recent studies suggest the percentage is actually lower.[15] A cusp or leaf of the bicuspid valve is too large, allowing blood to regurgitate into the right atrium as ventricular pressure increases.

Signs and symptoms: The symptoms of mitral valve prolapse include, but are not limited to, palpitations and chest pain. An integral portion of the preparticipation physical examination or prework screening is the cardiac auscultation. Murmurs are sometimes identified during preseason exams. Previous unknown murmurs require thorough medical follow-up but usually are found to be benign.

Treatment: The American College of Cardiology and the American Heart Association do not recommend follow-up appointments for patients with no current symptoms or even mild symptoms. If symptoms change, an echocardiography procedure with Doppler ultrasonography is recommended as a functional assessment for more detailed inspection of the heart. Risk factors that could exacerbate the condition include hypertension and high body mass index. Athletes who have survived sudden cardiac death or experienced other serious symptoms should be restricted from competitive sports. Individuals with palpitations should avoid caffeine, alcohol, nicotine, and certain drugs.[15]

THE IMMUNE SYSTEM

A network of cells, tissues, and organs, the immune system is a complex mechanism intended to protect the human body from invasion by foreign organisms. The foundation of the immune system is the ability to recognize self from nonself. There are two main mechanisms within the immune system: innate immunity and acquired immunity. The innate mechanism is used when an invading foreign particle is detected for the first time. The acquired system relies on a mechanism analogous to memory that is used if repeated exposure to the same foreign entity occurs. Invaders are usually infectious organisms such as bacteria, viruses, and fungi. Like any complex system, the immune system can be overloaded or fail, resulting in infection (i.e., not recognizing an invader), an allergy (i.e., recognizing a harmless substance as an invader), a cancer (i.e., not recognizing a defective cell), or autoimmune disease (i.e., mistaking the body's own tissues as a foreign invader).[16] The presence of the immune system is the basis for the success of vaccines. Fragments of an infecting organism are injected to initiate a memory immune response so that future exposure to a complete organism will allow the body to fight off the infection.

Immune System Anatomy

The structure of the immune system is distributed throughout the body in the lymphatic system (Figure 5-22), a system of tubes that are comparable to the arteries and veins of the circulatory system. Lymph nodes are small way stations that house lymphocytes. The lymph nodes are stationed along the lymph vessels throughout the entire body to provide quick access whenever a foreign particle is detected. These lymphoid organs are the distributing system for lymphocytes, the white blood cells that are the key components of the immune system. Bone marrow is

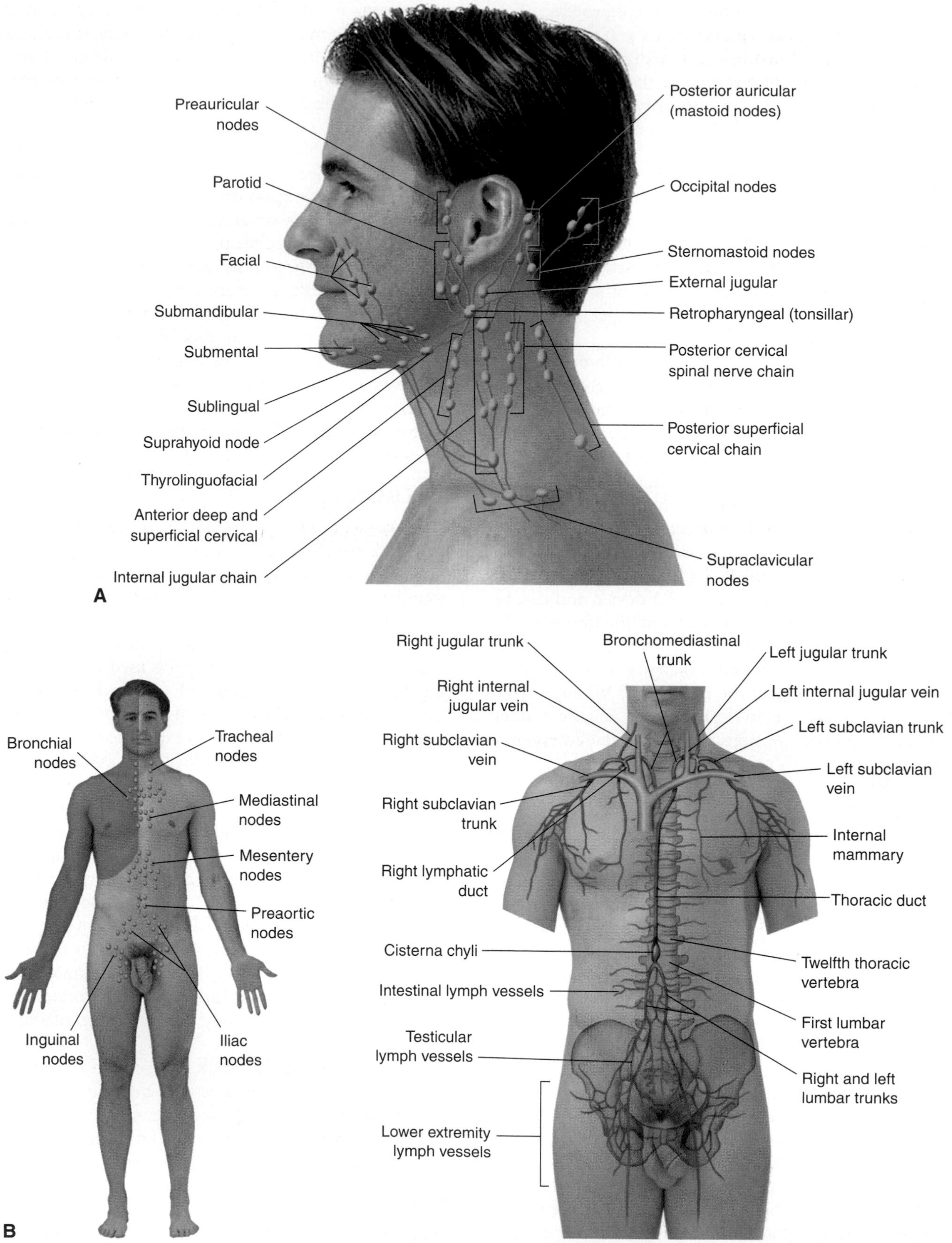

FIGURE 5-22 The lymphatic system is the core of the body. Shown here are the complete lymphatic drainage pathways from the head and neck (**A**) through the trunk and extremities (**B**). (From Seidel HM et al: *Mosby's guide to physical examination,* ed 6, pp. 232, 236, St Louis, 2006, Mosby/Elsevier.)

the ultimate source of all blood cells, including the white blood cells. The thymus is an organ in the neck in which the lymphocytes that become T cells mature. These T cells become the regulators of the acquired immune response.

Immune System Pathology

The effectiveness of the immune system hinges on a communication network among the many cell types. When a foreign particle is detected, several chemicals are released to activate components of the immune system. These chemicals, or cytokines, stimulate cells to differentiate and initiate a variety of processes to combat the offending agent.

Just a few of each immune cell type are distributed throughout the body in normal situations. If a foreign particle is detected, mass production of immune cells begins in response to the cytokine messages. Once the invader is overcome, the cells fade away, leaving a few watchdogs behind. The components of the immune system communicate with one another through the cytokines in the bloodstream. Mild to moderate exercise is beneficial to the immune system.[17,18] It is thought that exercise improves the ability of the immune system to adapt.[19]

The skin and linings of the body provide a mechanical barrier to infectious organisms. Participation in athletics often causes disruption in the skin, allowing entry of infectious particles. The linings of the body's passageways also produce secretions that provide additional defense against foreign particles; for example, an infection with a cold virus produces increased nasal secretions, or a runny nose. If these initial defenses are overcome, then more complicated mechanisms of the immune system are activated.

Remember how you get tender enlarged knots in your neck when you have a sore throat? Those are the lymph nodes, which swell in response to increased immune activity. The lymph nodes closest to any site of infection routinely become tender, enlarged, and painful.

Human Immunodeficiency Virus and Acquired Immunodeficiency Syndrome

An immunodeficiency disorder results when components of the immune system stop working. Currently, the best-known immunodeficiency is acquired immunodeficiency syndrome (AIDS), which is caused by the human immunodeficiency virus (HIV). AIDS is a progressive disease that leads to immune suppression and the development of opportunistic infections and malignancies. These infections and malignancies are eventually fatal, but the course often lasts a long time. At present, there is no cure or vaccination for this viral infection.

The transfer of the HIV virus occurs through intimate sexual contact, the placenta between mother and fetus, or direct blood contamination. The virus is present in several body fluids, but only blood poses a risk for transmission. Occupation-related transmission has been documented only in cases in which prolonged exposure to large amounts of blood occurred through some portal of entry. Data indicate that the risk of transmission during athletic contests is very low.[19]

Signs and symptoms: AIDS results after infection with the HIV virus. The immune system becomes compromised, leading to an unusually small number of cells that are capable of fighting off the HIV virus. Common opportunistic infections include, but are not limited to, pneumonia, skin cancer, and *Candida* infections.

Treatment: As the prevalence of AIDS increases worldwide, more athletes will be diagnosed as HIV positive. However, given improved treatment methods, participation in athletics will remain possible for long periods. The most important goal for an HIV-infected athlete is to remain under the care of a knowledgeable physician. The decision to continue athletics depends on several variables, including the athlete's current state of health, nature and intensity of training, potential contribution of stress from athletics, and potential risk of HIV transmission.[19] Physical activity of moderate intensity is beneficial for HIV-infected people and should be encouraged with appropriate monitoring.[19] HIV infection alone is insufficient grounds to prohibit athletic competition.[19] Medical information is the property of the patient. Therefore only the patient (or the parent or guardian in the case of a minor) has the right to decide who is informed of his or her HIV status.

Prevention: Because the protracted course of AIDS affords many years of good health, participation in sport and exercise is possible. An athlete is much more likely to contract HIV through sexual activity or drug use than in the sporting arena. But the risk of HIV transmission is not zero in collision sports, which present opportunities for significant blood exposure to open wounds. Therefore preventive actions, such as adherence to universal blood precautions and exclusive individual use of medical supplies, should be implemented whenever possible.

THE GASTROINTESTINAL SYSTEM

The gastrointestinal (GI) system, also called the *alimentary canal* or *digestive tract,* is a long tube that is approximately 9 meters (30 feet) in length, with numerous accessory organs attaching to the sides. The major organs of the alimentary canal are the mouth, pharynx, esophagus, stomach, small intestine, and large intestine (Figure 5-23). The accessory organs are the teeth, tongue, salivary glands, liver, gallbladder, pancreas, and appendix. The tube starts in the mouth, coils through the abdomen, and ends at the anus. The various organs of the abdomen are often termed the *viscera.* The function

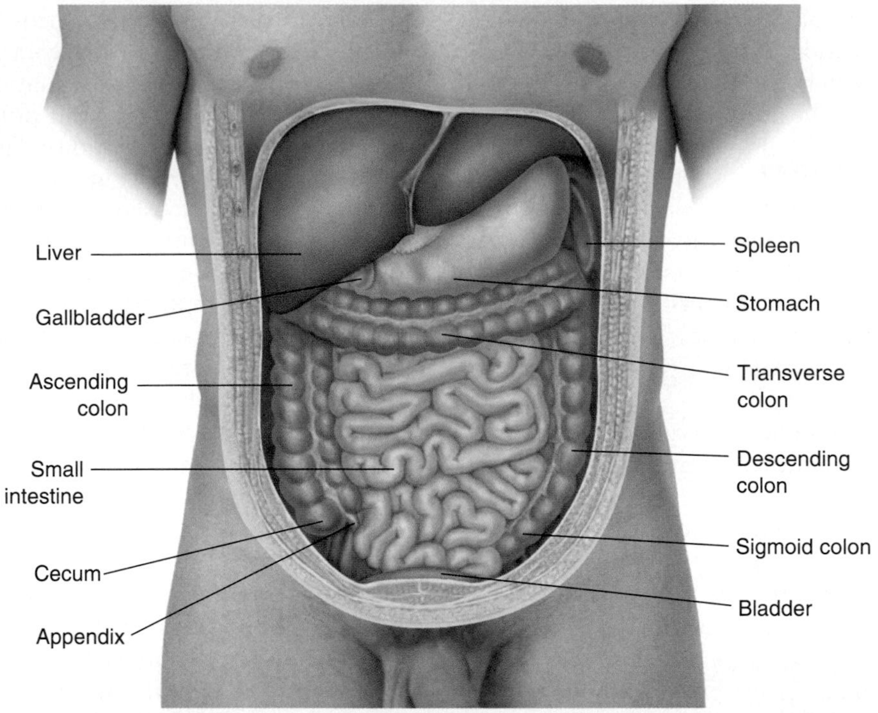

FIGURE 5-23 Anatomical structures of the abdomen. (From Seidel HM et al: *Mosby's guide to physical examination,* ed 6, p. 522, St Louis, 2006, Mosby.)

of the GI system is primarily transportation, digestion, and absorption of nutrients along with expulsion of unused material.

Gastrointestinal System Anatomy

The abdominopelvic cavity, lying below the thorax, is lined by a peritoneum. The peritoneum is a serous membrane that forms the lining of the abdominal cavity and is composed of a layer of simple squamous epithelium called the *mesothelium.* This membrane is supported and held in place by connective tissue. The parietal peritoneum lines the inner walls of the abdominopelvic cavity while the visceral peritoneum literally covers the organs. The peritoneum contains large folds that weave between the organs and the cavity walls to bind the organs into place. Serous membranes are also associated with the heart (pericardium), lungs (pleura), and other thoracic organs.

The abdominopelvic cavity reaches down from the undersurface of the diaphragm to the bottom of the bowl of the pelvis. The abdomen and pelvis are divided by an arbitrary line along the top rim of the pelvis. The GI tract and the genitourinary systems are contained within the abdominopelvic cavity. The abdomen is clinically divided into four sections to ease description of the location of pathology: right and left upper and lower quadrants (Figure 5-24). The right upper quadrant is home to the liver, the left upper quadrant contains the spleen, the right lower quadrant houses the appendix, and the left lower quadrant shelters the colon.

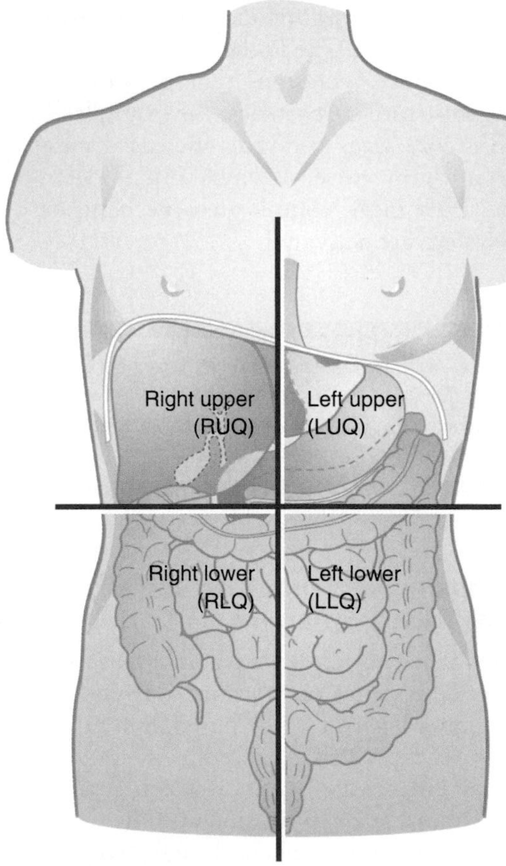

FIGURE 5-24 Abdominal quadrants. (From Black JM, Hawks JH: *Medical surgical nursing: clinical management for positive outcomes,* ed 7, p. 681, St Louis, 2005, Elsevier.)

Box 5-3 summarizes the most common causes of abdominal pain by location.

Esophagus

Food and liquids enter the digestive tract through the mouth and pharynx to enter the esophagus, a muscular collapsible tube that lies behind the trachea and larynx. The esophagus passes anterior to the vertebral column and pierces the diaphragm through an opening called the *esophageal hiatus*. It eventually ends at the upper portion of the stomach. Food passes through the esophagus and the remainder of the GI tract with the assistance of smooth muscle contractions called **peristalsis.** The bottom of the esophagus contains the lower esophageal sphincter (LES). It is a muscular valve that prevents the backflow of stomach contents into the esophagus. This sphincter relaxes momentarily when food or liquid is swallowed. Dysfunction of the sphincter allowing backflow is commonly called *gastroesophageal reflux disease (GERD)*.

Have you ever tried to cure hiccups (singultus) by drinking a glass of water upside down? How does an astronaut eat in a gravity-free environment? The synchronous activation of the smooth muscle in the alimentary canal pushes material through with or without the aid of gravity. The synchronous activation results in smooth muscle contraction called peristalsis.

Stomach

The stomach is a J-shaped enlargement of the digestive tract located directly below the diaphragm. The size of the stomach varies with the volume of contents present. Churning ingested food and liquid with gastric acid produced by the stomach, the key function of the stomach, is an early step in the process of breaking down food into nutrients that the body is capable of absorbing through the membranes of the GI tract. The stomach empties into the small intestine by way of the pyloric valve, which is another sphincter that controls passage of food through the alimentary canal.

Small Intestine

The small intestine is the location of absorption for most ingested nutrients. The small intestine is divided into three segments: the duodenum, jejunum, and ileum. Gastric contents enter the small intestine through the duodenum, the area in which several digestive

peristalsis the undulating contraction and relaxation of the smooth muscles in the GI tract that aid in digestion and transportation of food through the system

BOX 5-3 Common Causes of Abdominal Pain in Different Anatomical Locations

Right Upper Quadrant (RUQ)
- Cholecystitis
- Duodenal ulcer
- Hepatitis
- Pneumonia

Left Upper Quadrant (LUQ)
- Abdominal aortic aneurysm
- Gastric ulcer
- Pneumonia
- Splenic laceration or rupture

Periumbilical
- Abdominal aortic aneurysm
- Diverticulitis
- Early appendicitis
- Intestinal obstruction

Right Lower Quadrant (RLQ)
- Appendicitis
- Ectopic pregnancy
- Hernia
- Ovarian cysts
- Pelvic infection
- Renal stone

Left Lower Quadrant (LLQ)
- Constipation
- Diverticulitis
- Ectopic pregnancy
- Hernia
- Ovarian cysts
- Pelvic inflammation

Modified from Seidel HM et al: *Mosby's guide to physical examination,* ed 6, p. 551, St Louis, 2006, Mosby/Elsevier.

enzymes are added to the mix of foods to assist in nutrient breakdown and absorption. Between the duodenum and the ileum lies the jejunum, which is lined with projections called *villi* that offer yet another means to absorb more nutrients. Next, the ileum attaches to the large intestine at the ileocecal valve, a third sphincter that controls the passage of GI contents into the large intestine.

Large Intestine

The large intestine consists of the cecum, ascending colon, transverse colon, descending colon, sigmoid colon, and rectum. The cecum is a pouch that also attaches to the ileocecal valve along with the ileum. Attached to the cecum is the vermiform appendix, a coiled loop. The open end of the cecum merges with a long tube called the *colon*. The ascending colon traverses up the right side of the abdomen and, just below the liver, turns to travel across the upper aspect of the abdomen. The turn of the colon toward the horizontal is termed the *hepatic flexure*. The transverse colon travels across the abdomen and then turns at the splenic flexure (another right turn) to become the descending colon. An S-shaped curve in the colon designed to bring the colon back to the midline is referred to as the *sigmoid colon*.

Liver

The liver is located under the diaphragm on the right side and is the largest organ in the abdomen. The liver has the following major functions:

- Stores glycogen and several vitamins and minerals
- Serves as a filtering system to metabolize toxins and chemicals
- Absorbs old red blood cells
- Manufactures bile and several plasma proteins

Gallbladder

Located beneath the liver, the gallbladder is a sac that stores bile produced by the liver. As food passes into the duodenum, the gallbladder squeezes to empty bile into the small intestine. Bile emulsifies fat in the diet, aiding in the digestion and absorption of food and nutrients.

Pancreas

An oblong gland nestled behind the stomach near the duodenum, the pancreas is composed of small clusters of two types of cells scattered throughout the gland, with each cluster type having a different function. The exocrine portion of the gland is composed of groups of cells called *acini* that produce digestive enzymes. These enzymes also empty into the duodenum to help with digestion and absorption of nutrients. The endocrine portion of the pancreas contains the islets of Langerhans, which secrete insulin directly into the bloodstream. Insulin regulates the amount of glucose in the bloodstream by driving blood glucose into cells. The islets of Langerhans function by way of a negative feedback loop. If blood glucose is high, insulin is secreted into the bloodstream to drive the excess glucose into cells for utilization and storage. If blood glucose is low, insulin levels will eventually decrease.

Spleen

The spleen, a soft elastic organ that is analogous to a sponge in a capsule, is located high in the left upper corner of the abdomen. It is the largest mass of lymphatic tissue in the body, measuring about 5 inches in length. The spleen functions as a blood reservoir and filtering system for nutrients and wastes. Easily damaged by trauma, the spleen is particularly susceptible if the organ is distended secondary to splenic dysfunction.

Gastrointestinal System Pathology

The most common problems encountered in the GI system stem from infections, usually caused by either virus or bacteria. Viral illnesses are more common, do not respond to antibiotics, and are usually self-limiting. Treatment of viral illness is primarily supportive and includes fluids to prevent dehydration, antipyretics as needed for fever or myalgias, rest, and foods as tolerated. Bacterial infections also require supportive treatment, but the course of action differs in that antibiotics may be required for complete resolution of the symptoms.

Gastritis

Gastritis is an inflammatory condition localized in the upper GI tract.

Signs and symptoms: Presenting symptoms include nausea, vomiting, dyspepsia (heartburn), and fever.

Treatment: Blood in the vomit suggests a more serious condition and should prompt an urgent medical referral. For typical cases of gastritis, however, supportive treatment such as administration of fluids to prevent dehydration, rest, and antipyretics for fever is adequate.

Gastroenteritis

Gastroenteritis involves both the upper and the lower GI tract.

Signs and symptoms: Symptoms include diarrhea and abdominal cramping in addition to the symptoms present with gastritis.

Treatment: Various medications usually ease symptoms of gastroenteritis. Fluid replacement is essential because of dehydration caused by diarrhea and vomiting.

Traveler's Diarrhea

Although traveler's diarrhea is more common in developing countries, it occurs in all regions of the world. The underlying cause is food or water that has been contaminated by either bacterial or viral agents.

Signs and symptoms: Fever and abdominal cramping accompany frequent loose or watery stools.

Treatment: Traveler's diarrhea is usually a self-limiting illness that often requires only supportive treatment to replace fluid losses. Medications that decrease the cramping and frequency of stools are often withheld with this condition. The goal, then, is to evacuate the infectious agent as quickly as possible so that the course of the disease is not prolonged. High fevers or bloody diarrhea should be closely monitored and may require further treatment with antibiotics.

Appendicitis

Appendicitis is an urgent medical condition involving inflammation of the vermiform appendix.

Signs and symptoms: Fever, nausea, and vomiting usually accompany abdominal pain, which is the hallmark symptom of this condition. Pain often starts in the periumbilical region (i.e., the area surrounding the navel, or belly button) before migrating to McBurney's point—halfway between the right anterior superior iliac spine (ASIS) and the navel (Figure 5-25). Patients often prefer to lie on their back with their right leg flexed at the hip and knee to alleviate painful sensations. The absence of bowel sounds and a rigid abdomen with marked rebound tenderness are classic physical examination findings. Because the colon has shut down as a result of inflammation, diarrhea is not a symptom of appendicitis. The greatest danger in appendicitis is rupture. A ruptured appendix can allow spillage of the intestinal contents and wastes into the abdominopelvic cavity.

Treatment: Appendicitis requires immediate surgical intervention.

Hepatitis

Inflammation of the liver is associated with several etiologies, or causes. Infections are the most common cause of inflammation, but several chemicals and toxins can also damage the liver. Hepatitis A is a liver condition that is caused by a virus from contaminated food or water. The route of transmission is fecal-oral. One of the most famous outbreaks of hepatitis A was the Chi Chi's restaurant outbreak in 2003, when 601 cases were recorded in 3 weeks.[20] Hepatitis B is a bloodborne illness in the liver caused by a different virus.

The body fluid precautions mandated by the Occupational Safety and Health Association (OSHA) are aimed at protection from hepatitis, a highly contagious disease. The liver may also become inflamed as a result of infectious mononucleosis caused by the Epstein-Barr virus. Viral hepatitis (A, B, and C combined) affects 20% of the population. Approximately 5% of those affected develop liver disease, and half of those with liver disease require a transplant. Although most cases are mild or go away on their own, severe cases result in liver failure, in which case patients ultimately require a liver transplant.[20]

Signs and symptoms: Abnormally high levels of liver enzymes, a history of intravenous drug use, blood transfusions occurring before 1992, emigration from a third-world country, and participation in high-risk behavior increase the risk for contracting hepatitis.

Treatment: Both hepatitis A and infectious mononucleosis are self-limiting illnesses from which afflicted persons take a long time to recover. Hepatitis B may become a chronic infection, and no cure exists at the present time. However, there is an effective vaccination for hepatitis B that may be administered before initial exposure to the virus. This vaccine is safe, and everyone involved in community health care should receive it. It is a three-part vaccination, with the second and third injections being administered 3 and 6 months after the initial injection.

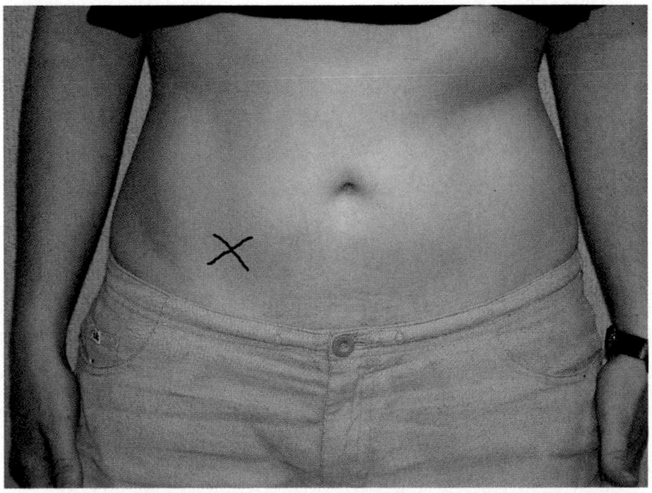

FIGURE 5-25 McBurney's point. Tenderness at this point (*X*), halfway between the umbilicus and the anterior superior iliac spine (ASIS), generally indicates appendicitis when accompanied by fever and nausea. (From Cuppett M, Walsh KM: *General medical conditions in the athlete,* p. 141, St Louis, 2005, Mosby/Elsevier.)

Splenic Rupture

The spleen can become enlarged as a consequence of infectious mononucleosis or exposure to several of the blood diseases. Blunt force trauma to the abdomen, such as from a hockey or lacrosse stick or even an automobile accident, may cause the spleen to rupture. Such an occurrence is more likely if the splenic capsule is distended or enlarged for any reason. **Hypovolemic shock** may ensue because of the large amounts of blood loss associated with the rupture.

Signs and symptoms: Kehr's sign occurs when the tip of the shoulder is acutely painful because of the presence of blood or other irritants in the peritoneal cavity while a person is lying down and the legs are elevated. Kehr's sign is a classic sign indicating splenic rupture. Symptoms may be aggravated by movement, and nausea might also occur.

hypovolemic shock a state of shock that follows large amounts of blood loss

Treatment: Kehr's sign is an emergency situation that requires urgent care.

Diabetes Mellitus

The endocrine portion of the pancreas that secretes hormones can fail, resulting in **diabetes mellitus**. Diabetes mellitus is a disorder of the body's ability to properly metabolize carbohydrates. Diabetes is divided into two types: Type I and Type II. Type I generally occurs in younger individuals. Approximately 1.3 million Americans have Type I diabetes, and 13,000 new cases are diagnosed each year.[21] Type II is more common in older people and those with risk factors, such as obesity. The incidence of Type II diabetes mellitus in young overweight people has been rising greatly in recent years. Approximately 25 million people in the United States have diabetes mellitus.[22] Older, less precise terminology refers to Type I diabetes mellitus *as juvenile-onset* or *insulin-dependent* diabetes and to Type II as *adult-onset* or *noninsulin-dependent*. Sufficient overlap exists in the pathology of both types to make the older terms confusing.

Type I diabetes involves the failure of the islets of Langerhans to produce insulin. Individuals with Type II diabetes have either abnormal insulin receptors in the end organ cells or islets of Langerhans that produce an abnormal insulin. This disorder of insulin metabolism disrupts the body's ability to get glucose from the bloodstream and into the cells. Individual cells therefore starve in the midst of plenty. If untreated, diabetes mellitus is a uniformly fatal disease.[22]

If insulin is not functioning properly, glucose from food is absorbed into the bloodstream but cannot enter the cells of the body. The **hyperglycemia**, or increased glucose, that occurs causes numerous vascular and neurological problems in addition to the lack of proper nutrition available to the body.

Signs and symptoms: The hallmark symptoms of diabetes mellitus are polyphagia, polyuria, and polydipsia. Polyphagia is a constant hunger caused by the inability of glucose to penetrate cells. Polydipsia is a constant thirst, and polyuria is frequent, copious urination caused by the large osmotic load resulting from the hyperglycemia.

Treatment: Treatment for Type I and Type II diabetes mellitus requires strict attention to the amount and timing of carbohydrate ingestion. Type I diabetes also requires the additional administration of insulin via injections into the body. The use of an insulin pump to provide a constant subcutaneous infusion of insulin is an increasingly popular method of treatment in individuals with diabetes mellitus. Individuals with Type II diabetes mellitus often do not require insulin. Reduction of weight to normal values and strict control of carbohydrate intake may be enough to return the glucose levels to normal. Whether they have Type I or Type II diabetes, patients should check their blood sugar values several times daily to monitor their specific glycemic levels.[22,23] Two acute problems, with similar symptoms, may arise in people with diabetes mellitus.

Hypoglycemia is a low blood glucose level that can quickly become fatal if levels drop too low. This can occur with improper insulin administration and inadequate carbohydrate intake. Hyperglycemia results from an excessive amount of carbohydrate intake. Disorientation, lethargy, and tremor can occur with either condition. Without the ability to test blood glucose values, differentiating between hypoglycemia and hyperglycemia in a disoriented or unconscious patient is difficult. When the patient's status is in doubt, the patient should be treated for hypoglycemia because this condition is more serious. A conscious person should receive oral glucose in the form of hard candy, sport gels, popsicles, or juices, whereas an unconscious person should receive an injection with a glucagon pen. If the preparticipation physical examination reveals that an athlete has diabetes mellitus, an emergency action plan must be devised, one that includes the proper storage, instruction, and use of a glucagon pen or other medications or natural treatments.

THE GENITOURINARY SYSTEM

The genitourinary system is composed of the urinary tract and the reproductive organs. Analogous to plumbing, the urinary tract functions to remove metabolites and wastes that cannot be utilized within the human body. The kidneys serve as the filtering system, with the ureters and urethra acting as conduit pipes and the bladder acting as a storage reservoir (Figure 5-26). The reproductive system differs according to the subject's sex. The male reproductive system consists of testicles, epididymis, spermatic cord, prostate, and the penis. The female reproductive system comprises the ovaries, fallopian tubes, uterus, cervix, and vagina.

Urinary System Anatomy

One kidney is located on each side of the vertebral column. Because the kidneys are housed behind the abdominal cavity, they are considered retroperitoneal. The right kidney is slightly lower than the left as a result of the large space occupied by the liver (Figure 5-27).

diabetes mellitus a disorder of the body's ability to properly metabolize carbohydrates
hyperglycemia increased glucose level in the blood
hypoglycemia a low blood glucose level that can quickly become fatal if levels drop too much

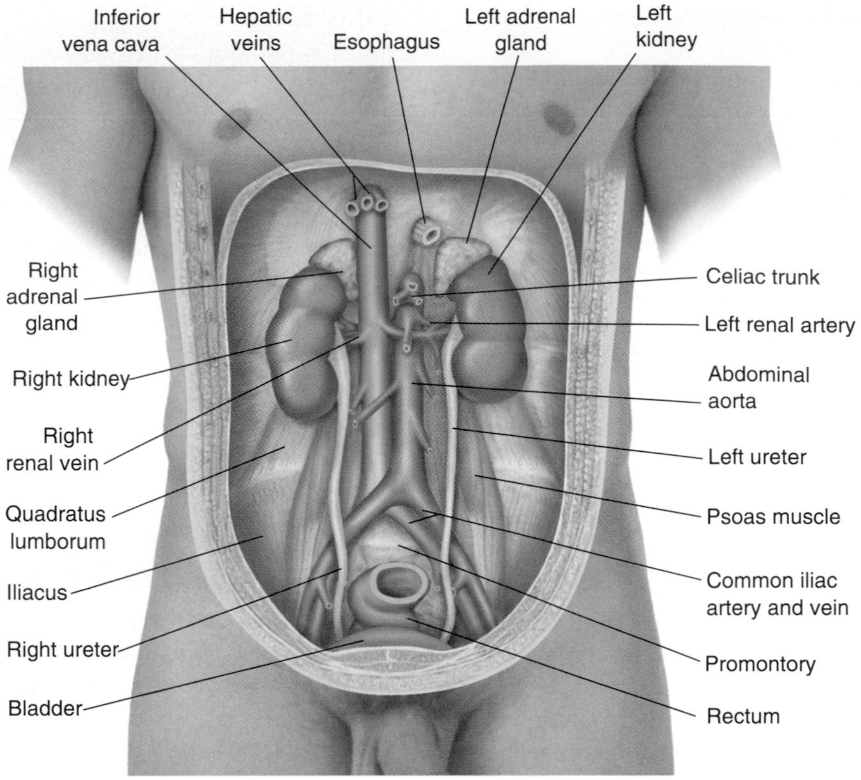

FIGURE 5-26 Organs of the urinary system. (From Seidel HM et al: *Mosby's guide to physical examination,* ed 6, p. 523, St Louis 2006, Mosby.)

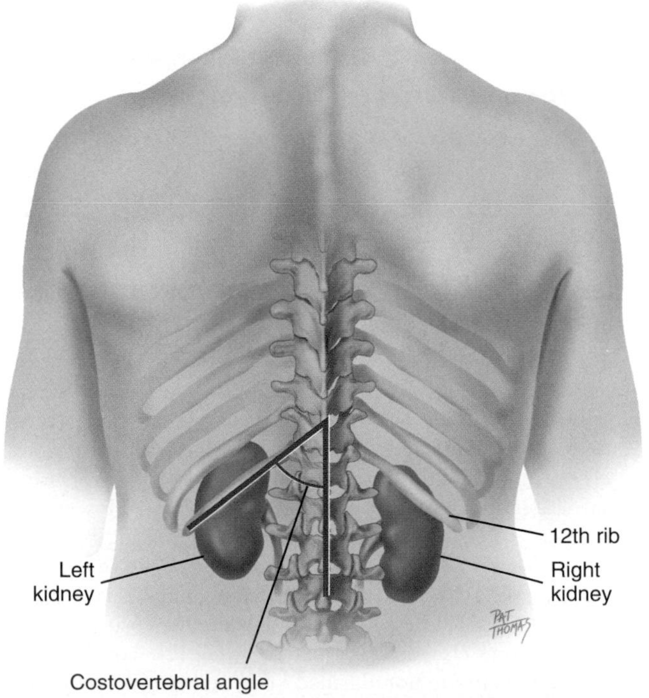

FIGURE 5-27 Posterior view of the kidneys. (From Jarvis C: *Physical examination and health assessment,* ed 4, p. 564, Philadelphia, 2004, Elsevier/Saunders.)

Blood reaches each kidney by way of the renal artery, where it is then filtered through the functional unit of the kidney, termed the *nephron*. Urine is collected from each kidney and flows down the respective ureters eventually to be stored in the bladder. The location of the bladder is anterior in the midline, posterior to the pubis of the pelvis. The urethra is the outlet of the bladder providing passageway to the external environment.

Urinary System Pathology

Urinary system pathology includes common infections as well as more serious conditions such as kidney stones.

Bladder Infections

Problems within the urinary tract are usually infectious. Bladder infection, or **cystitis**, is the most common infection of the urinary tract. Cystitis is more common in women because of their shorter urethras and is due to an overgrowth of bacteria in the bladder. Bacteria from the skin or the external environment traverse the urethra to establish abnormal growths in the bladder. Urinary tract infection is usually confined to the bladder. Urethritis

cystitis bladder infection

can be caused by several different organisms and is often sexually transmitted.

Signs and symptoms: Symptoms may include dysuria (i.e., burning on urination), frequency of urination (i.e., the need to urinate often), urgency of urination, and oliguria (small volumes at any single episode). Hematuria, or blood in the urine, is a common manifestation and should precipitate a referral to a physician.

Treatment: Definitive treatment of cystitis and urethritis requires antibiotics. Increased fluid intake may also help lessen the symptoms. Altering the environmental conditions of the bladder (i.e., changing the pH) to inhibit bacterial growth is an additional treatment technique and can be accomplished with the oral ingestion of cranberry juice.

Pyelonephritis

An infection of the kidney, termed *pyelonephritis,* may result if an infectious agent continues to track upward and ascends into one of the ureters. Because of the nature of the infection and its repercussions, a kidney infection is much more serious than a bladder infection.

Signs and symptoms: Pyelonephritis results in high fever, chills, nausea, painful vomiting, backache, and marked malaise.

Treatment: Successful treatment often requires intravenous antibiotic treatment and hospitalization.

Nephrolithiasis

Nephrolithiasis is more commonly known as a *kidney stone.* Deposits of minerals coalesce in the kidney because of a supersaturation of urine. The excess solute precipitates from the solution (i.e., the urine) to form a stone. If the deposits break off and move into the ureter, a great deal of pain results. As the deposit moves further into the ureter, smooth muscle spasms will result. This condition is one of the most painful medical conditions commonly seen.

Signs and symptoms: A hallmark of the malady is an inability of the patient to find a comfortable position. A person in the midst of passing a kidney stone suffers waves of excruciating pain as the stone is moved toward the bladder by smooth muscle spasms. The pain may subside for short periods of time as the spasm releases. However, once the stone begins to move again, the pain returns. Once the stone reaches the bladder, the pain abates.

Treatment: Protocol dictates straining urine through a filter until the stone is passed through the urethra. If the stone is obtained, a laboratory analysis is performed to determine its chemical structure. Dietary recommendations may then be given to decrease the chance of recurrence. Although people often attempt to ignore a kidney stone, the condition typically benefits from medical or surgical intervention to alleviate the pain and limit bleeding. On occasion, the stone can be passed in the privacy of the patient's own home.

SUMMARY

The human body consists of many interrelated systems, each of which includes many components that play a specific role in the maintenance and preservation of the human body. The skin is the first line of defense, protecting the body from infections, external trauma, or other events that may compromise its ability to defend against external dangers. Various systems within the body allow it to perform at its best. Once one of these systems is compromised, injury or illness may ensue. The key to being a great athletic trainer is knowing the subtle differences in each system, how the various systems rely on one another, and how to identify and diagnose the medical conditions that affect our daily activities.

Revisiting the OPENING *Scenario*

The list of problems that the soccer center midfielder might have includes asthma exacerbation, flare up of allergy symptoms, viral infection, and bacterial infection. The abrupt onset and the presence of fever and nausea decrease the likelihood that this episode is merely the result of asthma or allergy symptoms. An infection is a strong consideration because of the athlete's nausea and fever. Viral infections are most common, but there is not yet enough information to rule out a bacterial infection. A thorough history is always a key tool in providing medical care.

nephrolithiasis presence of kidney stones

Issues & Ethics

You are on the bus on the way to the girls' basketball playoff. The starting center has Type I diabetes. The coach and team physician know that you are well prepared to handle any type of diabetic emergency; you always carry a glucagon pen as well as hard candy, sports gels, and juices. You check with the player to make sure that she monitors her glucose level regularly. However, you notice that she seems sluggish and lethargic on the bus. Although her blood sugar reading appears normal, you are still concerned that something may be wrong. When you get to the game, you ask the coach if he can find someone else to start just in case. The coach and team physician are not alarmed because her glucose level seems normal. They attribute her lethargy to staying up late studying for an exam. What action should you take?

Web Links

American Academy of Allergy, Asthma & Immunology: www.aaaai.org
American College of Sports Medicine: www.acsm.org
American Diabetes Association: www.diabetes.org
American Heart Association: www.americanheart.org
American Orthopaedic Society for Sports Medicine: www.sportsmed.org
Centers for Disease Control and Prevention: www.cdc.gov
National Athletic Trainers' Association: www.nata.org
National Institutes of Health: www.nih.gov

References

1. Fien S, Berman B, Magrane B: Skin disease in a primary care practice, *Skin Med* 4(6): 350–353, 2005.
2. Goodman C, Boissonnault B, Fuller K: *Pathology: implications for the physical therapist*, ed 2, St Louis, 2003, Elsevier/Saunders.
3. Romano R, Lu D, Holtom P: Outbreak of community-acquired methicillin-resistant *Staphylococcus aureus* skin infections among a collegiate football team, *J Athletic Train* 41(2): 141–145, 2006.
4. Rosen T: Sexually transmitted diseases 2006: a dermatologist's view, *Cleveland Clinic Journal of Medicine* 73(6): 537–538, 2006.
5. Centers for Disease Control and Prevention: *Epstein-Barr virus and infectious mononucleosis*, Atlanta, [no date], CDC. Retrieved February 13, 2007, from www.cdc.gov/ncidod/diseases/ebv.htm.
6. Ebell M: Epstein-Barr virus infectious mononucleosis, *American Family Physician* 70(7): 1279–1287, 2004.
7. Miller MG et al: National Athletic Trainers' Association position statement: management of asthma in athletes, *Journal of Athletic Training* 40(3): 224–245, 2005.
8. Stocchetti N et al: Hyperventilation in head injury: a review, *Chest* 127(5): 1812–1827, 2005.
9. National Athletic Trainers' Association: Official statement from the National Athletic Trainers' Association on commotio cordis, Dallas, 2004 (May), NATA. Retrieved February 13, 2007, from www.nata.org/statements/official/ASTFstmt.pdf.
10. Cheitlin M, Douglas P, Parmley W: 26th Bethesda Conference: Recommendations for determining eligibility for competition in athletes with cardiovascular abnormalities. Task force 2: Acquired valvular heart disease, *Medicine & Science in Sports & Exercise* 26: S254–S260, 1994.
11. Maron BJ et al: Cardiovascular preparticipation screening of competitive athletes: a statement for health professionals from the Sudden Death Committee and Congenital Cardiac Defects Committee, American Heart Association, *Circulation* 94: 850–856, 1996. [Addendum published in *Circulation* 97:2294, 1998.]
12. Ali S., Antezano ES: Sudden cardiac death, *Southern Medical Journal* 99(5): 502–510, 2006.
13. Bruce J: Getting to the heart of cardiomyopathies, *Nursing* 35(8): 44–49, 2005.
14. Van Camp SF et al: American College of Sports Medicine position stand: exercise for patients with coronary artery disease, *Medicine & Science in Sports & Exercise* 26(3): i–iv, 1994.
15. Mulumudi MS, Vivekananthan K: Mysteries of mitral valve prolapse, *Postgraduate Medicine*, 110(2): 5432–5481, 2001.
16. National Institutes of Health: *Understanding the immune system*, NIH Pub. No. 03–5423, Washington, DC, 2003 (September), U.S. Department of Health & Human Services.
17. Woods JA, Viera VJ, Keylock KT: Exercise, inflammation, and innate immunity, *Neurol Clin* 24: 585–599, 2006.
18. Weber TS: Environmental and infectious conditions in sports, *Clin Sports Med* 22: 181–196, 2003.
19. American Medical Society for Sports Medicine: Human immunodeficiency virus (HIV) and other blood-borne pathogens in sports: Joint Position Statement by the American Medical Society for Sports Medicine and the American Orthopedic Society for Sports Medicine, Overland Park, Kan, [no date], AMSSM. Retrieved February 13, 2007, from .www.newamssm.org/hiv.html.
20. Stonsifer E, Burke A, Simwale O: Hepatitis in primary care: What NPs can do to save lives, *The Nurse Practitioner* 31(6): 53–55, 2006.
21. Habich M: Establishing a standard for pediatric inpatient diabetes education, *Pediatric Nursing* 32(2): 113–115, 2006.
22. Zinman B et al: American Diabetes Association/American College of Sports Medicine joint statement: Diabetes mellitus and exercise, *Medicine & Science in Sports & Exercise* 29(12): 1–6, 1997.
23. Albright A, et al: American College of Sports Medicine position stand: exercise and type 2 diabetes, *Medicine & Science in Sports & Exercise* 32(7): 1345–1360, 2000. Retrieved February 13, 2007, from www.acsm-msse.org/pt/pt-core/template-journal/msse/media/0700.pdf.

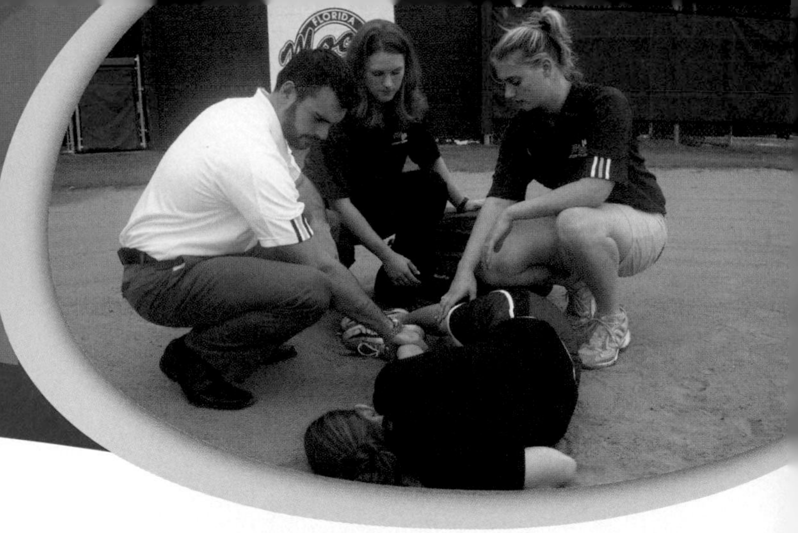

6

Environmental Conditions

PAUL HIGGS AND JAMES M. LYNCH

Learning Goals

1. Recognize the effects of extremes in heat, cold, and humidity on the human body during physical activity.
2. Describe the methods of heat gain and loss caused by environmental conditions.
3. Describe the effects of pollen allergies and insect stings on the body.
4. Define the effects of travel (jet lag) on the human body.
5. Comprehend the dangers of lightning and list strategies to decrease those risks.

This chapter focuses on the conditions that occur not because of an opponent or even overtraining but because of effects of the environment on the body. The environment is the physical place or surroundings in which we choose to be active, whether indoors or outdoors, and the associated conditions of those surroundings such as air temperature, **humidity**, and altitude. Some of the conditions, such as heat exhaustion, are relatively uncommon and mostly preventable, whereas others, such as bee stings or jet lag, are unpredictable and sometimes even unavoidable. Figure 6-1 presents an overview of the major areas of environmental injuries, each of which is discussed in more detail later in this chapter.

Just as a runner prepares in advance through training to avoid injury in an upcoming marathon, the impact of most environmental injuries can be prevented or lessened through wise decision making and pre-event preparation. Environmental injuries should not be taken lightly. Although most of the life-threatening conditions are rare, every reaction of the body to the environment must be monitored to ensure that the response does not signify an emergency. It is the responsibility of the athletic trainer to monitor these reactions and responses and effectively manage the resulting conditions to prevent them from becoming life threatening whenever possible.

Points to Ponder

An orthopedic injury can prevent activity for several days or even weeks. What is the impact on an athlete's training or performance of an environmental illness or acclimatization issue that is left untreated?

THERMOREGULATORY CONDITIONS

Metabolism, a normal body function, causes heat production that must be dissipated to prevent damage to the tissues of the body. Physiological processes function properly only when body temperature is maintained in a normal range, approximately 37° C (98.6° F, with a range of 97° F to 99° F). Body temperature consists of **shell temperature**, the temperature of the skin, and **core temperature**, the internal temperature of the

humidity amount of water vapor in the air
metabolism normal working processes of the body systems
shell temperature the temperature of the body's skin
core temperature the internal temperature of the body

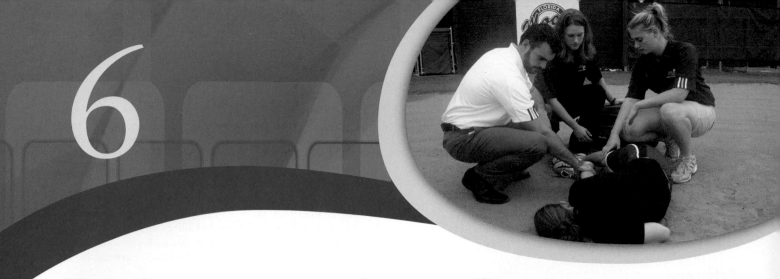

OPENING *Scenario*

The women's soccer team is playing in early August. The National Weather Service has issued a statewide heat advisory, meaning that all outdoor activity should be limited because of the risk of heat-related illness owing to the high temperature and high humidity. The game began at 2 PM after a pregame warm up that started at 12:45 PM. The team left the campus at 10:30 AM and drove straight to the game site. Players were instructed to bring a snack to eat on the bus and plan for a bigger meal after the game. Most of the players are from the southern states and are generally accustomed to playing in this environment, but today even some of them are complaining of excessive fatigue, dizziness, headache, and occasional blurred vision. Two of your players tell you privately that they need a break from the game. The coach notices their diminished performance but has no one of comparable talent to use in their place. What do you tell the coach?

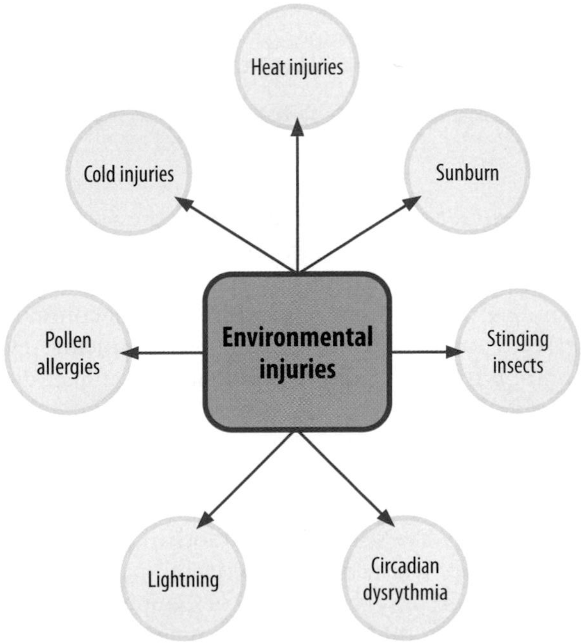

FIGURE 6-1 Concept map overview of environmental injuries.

body. Monitoring core temperature is more important because it indicates the circumstances inside the body and whether the temperature is in a range that allows the internal organs to function effectively and efficiently. Under normal circumstances, the body is remarkably proficient at regulating a stable core temperature, but this regulation may be altered by factors such as outside temperature and workloads. If the core temperature increases or decreases without regulation, an environmental heat illness results.

Heat Injuries

When the internal organs overheat, they begin to function erratically or even shut down. Fortunately, the body's general efficiency in maintaining a stable core temperature ensures that the emergency situation of total internal system failure is not especially common given the number of people who are active in hot and humid environments every year. However, even minor heat illnesses can escalate to a more severe and life-threatening level if not promptly identified and treated. A responsible athletic trainer will identify the athlete's potential for injury by noting the dangerous characteristics of the hot and humid environment and also monitor the athlete for signs of intolerance to these conditions.

Methods of Heat Gain and Loss

The body uses four primary means for heat gain or loss: (1) conduction, (2) convection, (3) radiation, and (4) evaporation (Table 6-1). Each method is effective, depending on the circumstances, in increasing or decreasing heat in the body. Rarely is only one method working at a time.

In **conduction,** heat is transferred by direct physical contact. For example, sitting on a cold metal bench radiates heat away from the body and sitting on a hot metal bench radiates heat into the body. An object feels cool to the touch not because it is emitting cold but because it is absorbing heat. In the athletic training room, ice packs melt during use not because they lose their coldness but because they gain heat from the body through conduction. Heat always moves from an area of higher temperature to an area of lower temperature.

Transfer of heat from the body by circulation of a medium such as wind or water current is **convection.** A breeze can cool, and a whirlpool can warm or cool.

conduction the transfer of heat through physical contact
convection the transfer of heat from the body by the circulation of a medium (e.g., wind, water current)

TABLE 6-1 Methods of Heat Gain and Loss in the Body

METHOD	HEAT TRANSFER	EXAMPLE OF HEAT LOSS	EXAMPLE OF HEAT GAIN
Conduction	An object transfers heat to a cooler item through direct contact.	An ice bag used to treat a sprained ankle absorbs heat from the body, melting the ice.	The heating element on a stove warms a pot of water placed on it through direct contact with the pot.
Convection	Heat transfers by way of a current (i.e., flowing air or water).	A car's air conditioning system cools the car's interior by absorbing the heat from the surfaces as the blowing cool air passes by.	Heated air swirling around inside a grill helps cook food placed on the cooking surface.
Radiation	Heat transfers from an object directly into the surrounding environment.	Waves of heat energy can be seen as they radiate from the asphalt of a parking lot on a hot summer day.	Heat from the sun enters the body when a person stands outside in an open unshaded area such as a soccer field or outdoor basketball court.
Evaporation	Heat transfers as water vapor dissipates, taking heat from the source into the surrounding air.	Heat is transported from the body as sweat evaporates into the air, pulling the heat away with it.	The air picks up heat from the body as sweat turns to vapor, moving from an area of high humidity (the skin) to lower humidity (the air); the heat moves in the same direction, from an area of higher temperature to an area of lower temperature.

Convection is helpful in dissipating heat from the body, but in land-based athletics the only available current is from the air and the athlete must stay in constant motion to create that current (i.e., creating more body heat to dissipate through increased activity) or wait for unpredictable wind currents (which are not present in most indoor sports). Simple immersion into cooler air or water does not create convection. The movement of the air or water removes the heat from an object.

A sunny day is the best example of **radiation**. Standing in the shade is cooler than standing in the sun. Heat energy radiates from a source to an object. Heat is transferred without direct contact and without assistance from a current of air or water. In the body, radiation is quite effective for heat gain and very ineffective for heat loss. Consider how hot a black car becomes when it is sitting in a paved parking lot on a cloudless summer day—this is a result of the heat radiating from the sun. A stove becomes hot when it is turned on, and its heat can be detected without directly touching any of the surfaces.

The fourth method, **evaporation**, is generally the most effective means to dissipate heat from the human body during physical activity. The evaporation of fluid, in the form of sweat, removes large quantities of heat from the body. As the sweat pouring from the human body is converted to vapor, heat is pulled away with it. However, evaporation is effective only when environmental humidity, or moisture in the air, is significantly lower than the humidity on and near the skin.

Of the four methods of heat gain and loss, evaporation is the most readily used by the human body for heat loss in hot environments. Therefore evaporation is the primary, and most productive, form of heat dissipation from the body.

Simple rules of diffusion dictate that the sweat vapor will move from an area of high concentration (on the skin) to an area of low concentration (off the skin). If the air surrounding the skin is very humid, which is commonly the case in many outdoor athletic environments, even evaporation is stifled as an efficient method of heat dissipation. Evaporation is also limited by the amount of skin exposed to that lower humidity environment. An athlete with very little exposed skin—such as football or lacrosse players—is even more unlikely to achieve efficient evaporation. Consider the scenario of a football player during summer afternoon practice session in full pads: Much of his body is covered by the uniform or equipment, and the local environment often has a high temperature and high humidity. Because his core body temperature will elevate steadily, the limited amount of exposed skin must act very efficiently to cool the body. Given that a great deal of heat is lost through the head, athletes involved in a sport that requires a helmet are often at a slightly greater risk of heat illness because this pathway of heat loss is blocked.

Heat Regulation

Body temperature is regulated by the autonomic nervous system. The hypothalamus is located in the brain and serves as the thermostat. Skin and blood temperature are the stimuli for the hypothalamus. As the core

radiation the transfer of heat from a source to an object without direct contact or assistance from a current

evaporation the dissipation of heat from the body through conversion of water to vapor temperature rises (i.e., hyperthermia), blood flow is shifted to the skin to allow more transference of core heat to the surface and initiate the process of evaporation. If core temperature lowers (i.e., hypothermia), blood is shifted to the core to decrease heat transference, which triggers the process of shivering. Even at rest in normal environmental conditions, body heat escapes through unnoticed perspiration.

The following three factors determine the net heat loss or gain, and therefore the heat stress, of an environmental situation:

1. Air temperature
2. Air humidity
3. Air movement

All three factors act independently, but all are related in the means by which they increase heat stress in the body. If the air temperature is high but the humidity is low, the net effect is a minimal increase in heat stress. If the air temperature and the air humidity are both high but the air movement is constant, the net effect is reduction of heat stress because proper evaporation can still take place. The situation becomes dangerous when the air temperature and air humidity are high with low or only occasional air movement. Evaporation cannot be effective, and the heat in the body soars quickly.

The **heat index** combines air temperature with relative humidity to determine how hot it feels, or the apparent temperature. It acts much like the chill factor as an indication of a person's subjective perception of temperature in cold weather. The higher the heat index, the more uncomfortable the outdoor activities will be for the athlete. When the heat index increases, the risk of heat illness also increases (Figure 6-2).

The most commonly used instrument to assess heat stress is the **sling psychrometer**, a device that measures air temperature and humidity. Knowing these measures allows the athletic trainer to calculate the relative heat stress for the local environment (Figure 6-3). Another method to assess relative heat stress is with a **wet bulb globe temperature (WBGT) device** (Figure 6-4). This type of device is used in athletic and industrial settings to assess the air temperature, humidity, and radiant heat in the local environment. These three measures combine to give an estimate of the relative heat stress for a given setting and the consequent risk of heat illness for those active in that setting.

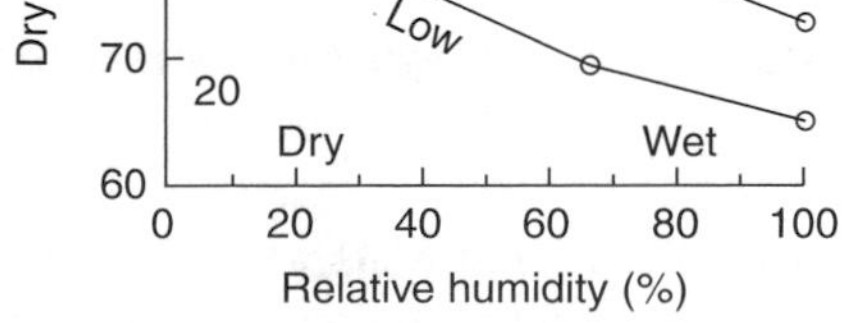

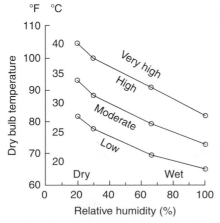

FIGURE 6-2 Estimation of heat injury risk can be based on air temperature and humidity, also used to determine the heat index. (Redrawn from Convertin VA, Armstrong LE, Coyle EF: American College of Sports Medicine. Position stand on exercise and fluid replacement, *Med Sci Sports Exerc* 28(1): i, 1996.)

Points to Ponder

In light of regional differences in temperature and humidity, why is it difficult for school boards or other governing bodies to create a standard whereby no one in any part of the country should participate in sports activity at a given heat index? How would such a standard affect most traditional outdoor athletic seasons?

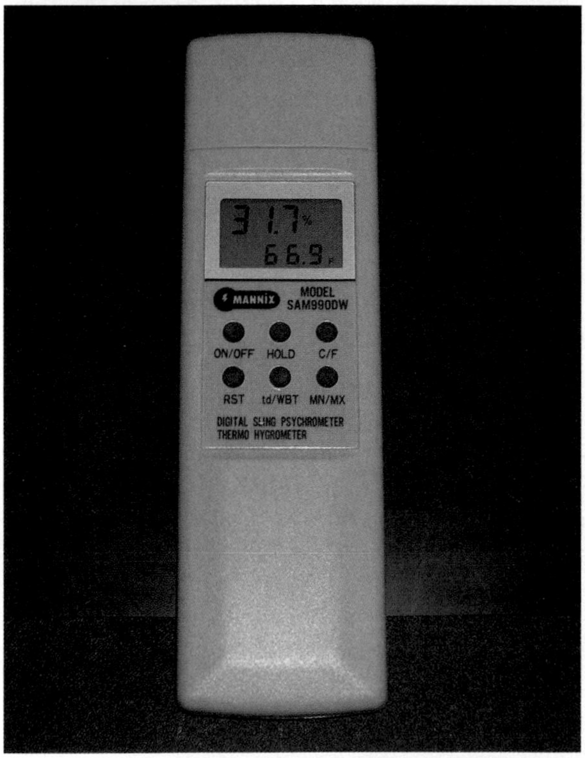

FIGURE 6-3 Psychrometers assess air temperature and humidity.

heat index scale used to predict the level of heat stress placed on the body during activity in a given temperature and humidity

sling psychrometer device used to measure air temperature and humidity

wet bulb globe temperature (WBGT) a device used to assess relative heat stress

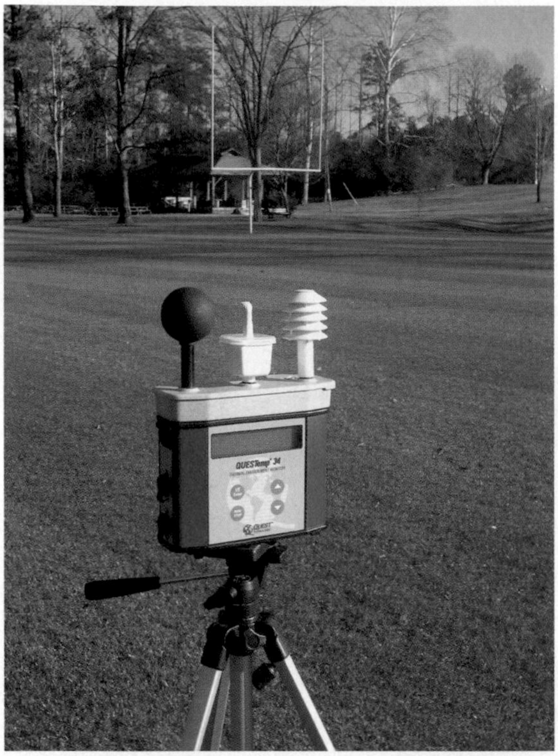

FIGURE 6-4 Wet bulb globe temperature (WBGT) device used to measure air temperature, humidity, and radiant heat.

Specific Heat Illnesses

Hyperthermia. **Hyperthermia** is an increase in the core temperature of the body and can occur regardless of the level of fitness or conditioning. Exercise accentuates these factors because it accelerates heat production. During exercise, part of the energy production converts to mechanical energy and the remainder becomes heat energy. To dissipate this heat and take it away from the core of the body, blood flow to the skin is increased.

Profuse sweating can occur at a rate of 2 to 3 liters per hour and may cause dehydration. Athletes involved in weight-restricted sports often elect to limit fluid intake to remain in a designated weight class. One liter of sweat weighs one kilogram, or 2.2 pounds. Sweat consists primarily of water, with approximately 2.6 grams of salt per liter of sweat. The **electrolytes** in sweat are mainly sodium and chloride.[1,2] With dehydration, blood flow decreases because blood volume decreases. Decreased blood volume results in less efficient sweating and heat dissipation.

This chapter presents a spectrum of heat injuries. Although heat injuries range from those that are merely annoying to those that are catastrophic, the following list of problems is not a progression of symptoms but rather a ranking of catastrophic impact. The most minor injury does not always appear first and lead to the next most dangerous problem. An athlete may enter the spectrum at the milder level or at the most dangerous level without showing any overt symptoms of something less dangerous. Fortunately for athletic trainers, the life-threatening problems are relatively rare compared with the less severe problems. Athletic trainers should not assume that heat illness occurs only outdoors, in the summer, during preseason practice. These problems can occur whenever the environmental temperature or humidity is high and the body cannot adequately cool itself or replace lost fluids.

Heat Cramps. Most of the time, **heat cramps** occur in the calf or abdomen, but they may affect any muscle. Immediate fluid replacement and gentle stretching usually relieve the pain of these cramps, which are by no means catastrophic but can nevertheless be quite painful and disruptive to athletic performance.

Mechanism: Heat cramps also occur because of slow dehydration over several days or sessions of intense workouts in a hot and humid environment. In this scenario, an athlete loses a significant amount of fluid volume in several successive practices or workout sessions without replacing the lost volume between sessions. Eventually, the loss of fluid and electrolytes triggers an involuntary muscular contraction known as a cramp.

Signs and symptoms: The muscles stricken with heat cramps are involuntarily contracted. The force of the contraction can be quite painful, and relief comes through stretching to break the tension. At times, the muscle is so tightly contracted that stretching it will present a challenge for the athletic trainer. Heat cramps may occur in one muscle group at a time, such as the hamstring group, or they may occur in several muscle groups simultaneously. This assault may even occur in opposing muscle groups—such as the hamstrings and the quadriceps simultaneously—making it very difficult to stretch one muscle without shortening and worsening the opposing cramping muscle group. Pregame anxiety can also increase the risk of altered eating habits, robbing the body of vitally needed fluids and electrolytes such as potassium and sodium. Athletic trainers should emphasize to their athletes the need for proper nutrition before and on competition days.

hyperthermia abnormal increase in core body temperature

electrolytes minerals in the blood that are important for the regulation of the amount of water in the body, blood pH, muscle action, and other important functions

heat cramps heat-related painful muscle contractions that often involve the calf or abdomen

When a hot, humid environment is combined with decreased fluid intake and pregame jitters, heat cramps are likely. Often, they occur long after an activity session ends, in which case return to play that day is not an issue.

Immediate management: The affected muscle must be stretched (Figure 6-5). Therefore the athletic trainer must understand the underlying muscular anatomy to determine which muscles are affected and which motions will stretch that particular muscle. Ice packs may also be applied to the affected muscle to decrease pain, thereby decreasing the spasm as well.

Intermediate management: Long-term treatment and prevention of heat cramps include increasing fluid intake before, during, and after an event to maintain normal fluid and electrolyte reserves for proper muscle activity. Return to play is determined by function; as the athlete feels better, activity may be resumed. If the cramping prevents normal participation, the athlete must refrain from playing until normal function and ability are regained.

Heat Syncope. **Heat syncope** is the next most severe heat illness. As with any form of heat illness, victims may enter the spectrum at any point and not necessarily progress from the least severe to the most severe. Heat syncope is also known as heat collapse and is a form of fainting. Although not as painful as heat cramps, the condition should be thoroughly evaluated and not dismissed as a minor incident.

Mechanism: Heat syncope occurs with excessive vasodilation. Blood vessels expand to move more blood (and heat) from the core to the surface, but the decreased volume from excessive fluid losses and the wider diameter of the vessels cause a decrease in blood pressure with associated dizziness and fainting.

Signs and symptoms: A momentary sudden drop in blood pressure decreases the amount of oxygenated blood serving the brain, and the body uses its energy to shut down less immediately critical functions such as consciousness to maintain the vital functions of pulse and respiration. As a result of this drop in oxygen flow to the brain, the person faints.

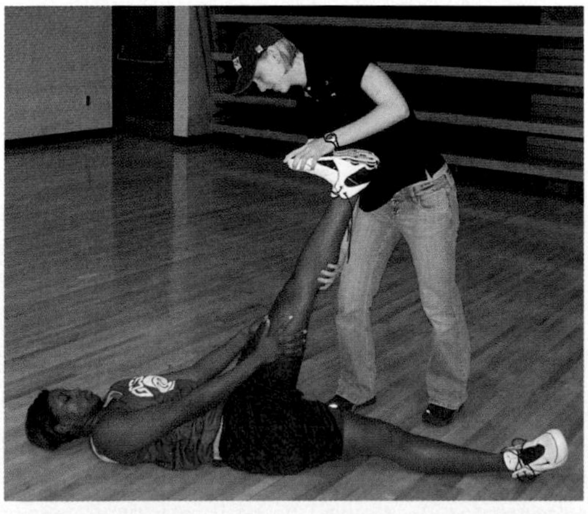

FIGURE 6-5 Heat cramps are not catastrophic, but they can cause the individual significant pain and disrupt athletic participation.

Immediate management: Treatment measures for heat syncope take place after the victim has been moved to a safer, cooler place. The victim should be made to lie down in a cool environment with the feet elevated so that normal amounts of oxygenated blood can return to the brain. After regaining consciousness, the victim should drink cool fluids such as water, juice, or sports beverages. The victim should also be assessed for any injuries that occurred from the fall (e.g., contusions, lacerations, head injury).

Intermediate Management: Because syncope can also be a symptom of serious systemic problems such as diabetes, hypertension, stroke, aneurysm, or even the more serious heat illness of heat stroke, all cases of syncope should be assessed and not explained away as a product of the environment.

Heat Exhaustion. **Heat exhaustion** is common and occurs most often in individuals who are not acclimatized. The condition can also occur as a result of several consecutive sessions of intense activity in a high temperature or high humidity environment.

Mechanism: Victims of heat exhaustion have exhausted the surplus fluid in the body that would normally have been converted to sweat for evaporation. Excessive sweating, a routine precursor to heat exhaustion, may be an acute situation, occurring in one session, or a cumulative condition, in which the athlete has a net loss in total fluid volume over the course of several successive activity sessions.

Signs and symptoms: Individuals with heat exhaustion experience fatigue and nausea, are pale and covered with sweat, and may have a decreasing sweat rate. The athlete is usually sweating profusely or reports sweating more than usual. The athlete remains conscious during heat exhaustion but will have significantly altered performance. The core temperature generally remains stable, but if the condition is left untreated, the body's inability to cool itself through sweat evaporation could cause the temperature to rise to a dangerous level.

Immediate management: Fluid replacement and cooling procedures are critical to a prompt recovery. Fluid intake before, during, and after activity, especially in

heat syncope heat-related fainting; also known as *heat collapse*

heat exhaustion heat-related condition characterized by excessive sweating and dehydration high-risk environments, can significantly decrease the incidence of heat exhaustion. Without proper intervention, heat exhaustion can progress quickly to heat stroke. Treatment of heat exhaustion requires first moving the person to a cooler environment. As long as the victim is conscious, he or she may be allowed to drink cool fluids, sipping several ounces over time rather than gulping large quantities. Cool water may be poured over the body to encourage heat loss through convection. Ice packs may be applied to various spots on the body. However, application of cool or cold fluids on the body should never be substituted for ingestion of cool or cold fluids in the body. The victim of heat exhaustion should refrain from activity until all symptoms are resolved, which includes replacement of lost fluids (Figure 6-6).

Intermediate management: The victim of heat exhaustion should be monitored for symptoms that indicate a worsening of the situation. With proper treatment, the person stabilizes and then recovers. Anyone suffering from heat exhaustion should refrain from strenuous activities in the heat until fully recovered. Full recovery is demonstrated by a full return of any weight lost during the session as well as full resolution of any symptoms. Without proper treatment, the person may progress to a much worse condition, heat stroke.

Heat Stroke. **Heat stroke** is a true medical emergency that must be identified and treated quickly. It is the most severe condition in the continuum of heat illnesses and can be deadly if left untreated. Fortunately, in light of the total number athletes exposed to hot and humid settings, the condition is much less common than the other heat illness conditions.

Mechanism: Heat stroke involves a major and life-threatening breakdown of the **thermoregulatory** mechanism. For whatever reason, the body cannot efficiently remove excess heat, which builds internally to a life-threatening level.

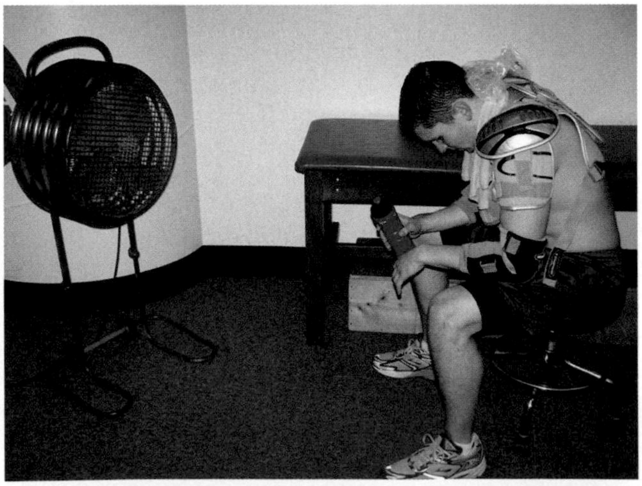

FIGURE 6-6 Effective treatment for heat exhaustion involves the effective distribution of as much fluid as possible in, on, and through the body.

Signs and symptoms: The victim experiences mental disorientation or severe confusion. The skin is warm and red, there is often very little sweating, and core temperature is often markedly increased. Heat stroke often renders the victim unconscious. If conscious, the athlete may complain of chills—this response indicates a severely failing thermoregulatory system in which heating and cooling mechanisms and perceptions are altered.

Immediate management: Lowering core temperature is of prime importance. The brain and other major organs are literally cooking as they overheat because of a significant breakdown in the body's cooling system, and death can occur in 20 minutes if treatment is delayed.[3] Treatment of heat stroke must be immediate and efficient. The athlete must be removed from the area to a cooler, safer environment. Any previously mentioned cooling measures, as well as full-body immersion into a cold water bath, may be initiated while transportation by ambulance is being arranged. Unconscious athletes must be monitored carefully and, because they might choke, should not receive anything orally. Obviously, submersion is not a wise choice for an unconscious athlete.

Intermediate management: In an athletic setting, treatment for most other heat-related illnesses can take place on or near the sidelines. However, victims of heat stroke must be transported to a medical center as soon as possible. All treatment methods described earlier are intended to be implemented only while waiting for emergency medical personnel to transport the athlete to a hospital.

Prevention of Heat Illness

Heat illness is generally preventable.[4] At the very least, its progression to a more severe illness can be prevented if the warning signs are identified and the athletic trainer intervenes quickly. Poor physical fitness is a major risk factor, but failure to maintain a proper fluid surplus can also increase the risk of injury and accelerate tissue damage (Table 6-2).

Fluid replacement is essential. Athletes must have unlimited access to water during heat stress, and even then replacement may not be adequate. A surplus fluid

heat stroke heat-related medical emergency resulting from the body's inability to efficiently remove excess heat

thermoregulatory describes an involuntary system of the body that controls heating and cooling

TABLE 6-2 Factors That Increase the Risk of Heat Illness

FACTOR	DESCRIPTION
Larger body mass	Heat production is greater with increased muscle mass; increased layers of adipose tissue slow the release of excess heat.
Age	Thermoregulation is not efficient in the very young or the elderly.
Conditioning level	Poorly conditioned individuals generate more internal heat during activity and dissipate the heat less efficiently.
Hydration	Decreased amounts of excess fluid in the body hinder the availability of fluid for evaporation.
History of heat illness	A previous history may indicate a chronically inefficient thermoregulatory system; recent dehydration requires adequate time to rehydrate if recurrence is to be avoided.
Medication	Certain medications may promote fluid retention or release, which may increase heat transfer through evaporation.

Data from Starkey C, Ryan J: *Evaluation of orthopedic athletic injuries,* ed 2, p. 658, Philadelphia, 2002, FA Davis.

Points to Ponder

The ingredients and temperature of the drink are what dictate its physiological benefit. However, if the taste is not acceptable to the team, what good is it in preventing heat illness? Find a drink that is beneficial to the body as well as acceptable to the palate—even if that drink is plain water.

amount is optimal to allow for heat loss evaporation. As little as a 2% loss in total body weight can lead to a decrease in aerobic performance.[2] This deficit is primarily attributable to fluid loss, which compromises the thermoregulatory function of the circulatory system and the brain. Cold fluids empty from the stomach more rapidly. Drinks with glucose concentrations in the 5% range are absorbed more rapidly than those with a higher glucose content.[2]

Recording body weight before and after practice is a simple way to monitor fluid loss and replacement. A loss of 5% of body weight that is not regained before the next practice is problematic.[5,6] An athlete commonly loses 3% in one outdoor session of moderate activity, but this deficit can be easily erased by consuming one nutritious meal before the next session of high-risk activity (Table 6-3). Athletes who do not replace enough fluid to put themselves within the 3% window should not be allowed to return to their given activity. Once the athlete is within this window, activity may resume.

Whether worn to dissipate heat in a warm environment or conserve heat in a cold climate, clothing should be appropriate. Darker clothing tends to absorb or retain heat, and lighter colored clothing tends to repel heat. When active in high-risk environments, athletes should expose as much skin surface as possible to allow the greatest area for evaporation to occur. When exercising in very humid environments, athletes may even need to put on different clothes (e.g., dry jerseys, new undershirts, dry socks) during breaks in activity; sweat-saturated clothing actually interferes with evaporation and heat loss. Also, breathable, loose-fitting fabrics dissipate heat more efficiently than tighter-weave, form-fitting garments. Because the head and neck make up 10% of body surface area, 10% of heat loss occurs through the head region. Therefore heat loss can be increased simply by removing the athlete's hat or helmet during rest periods (Figure 6-7).

Heat Illness as a Brain Injury

Because of the many individual variances among athletes, it is vitally important for athletic trainers to recognize the individual tolerances of the athletes under their care when assessing the risk of heat illness. Although the common symptoms (e.g., high core temperature, fatigue, profuse sweating) are usually the cardinal signs to assess, it is

TABLE 6-3 Effect of Fluid Loss on Participation in Athletics*

FLUID LOSS	EFFECTS	RECOMMENDATION
1%-2%	Minimal negative effects on performance	Additional fluid intake between activity sessions
3-4%	Common loss during moderate activity in high temperature/humidity; Noticeable negative effect on performance (e.g., recovery time, fatigue, endurance, aerobic performance)	High risk of heat illness if not corrected before next activity session; normally reversed through good diet and additional fluid intake
5%-7%	Significant effect on performance and serious risk of heat illness	Important to lower deficit to less than 3% before return to activities

*As determined through the percentage of body weight lost during activity.

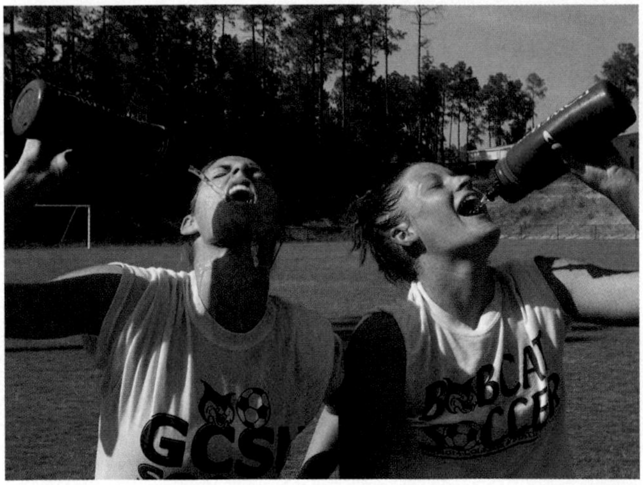

FIGURE 6-7 Proper clothing, an adequate water supply, and frequent breaks can greatly decrease the risk of heat illness.

very possible, if not common, to encounter athletes who are suffering a significant heat stress episode without the typical symptoms. Conversely, athletes with classic signs of heat illness may have no discomfort and may not suffer any decrease in athletic performance.

Consider the wide variability among healthy athletes. Some athletes break into a profuse sweat during pregame warm-up sessions. Some athletes even begin to sweat when getting dressed for a game. Does that level of sweating indicate acute heat exhaustion? Also consider the athlete who, whether because of favorable genetics or proper conditioning, can finish an intense workout session and sweat minimally with no heat stress or significant loss of performance. Does this lack of sweating indicate heat stroke? The local environment can make it difficult to assess heat stress as well. In a high-humidity environment, an athlete may sweat excessively, soaking his uniform. Later, when he complains of blurred vision and fatigue, the athletic trainer may mistakenly interpret the sweat on his skin and uniform as recent and not as something that occurred several minutes earlier. What was incorrectly interpreted as "profuse sweating" and labeled "heat exhaustion" was actually "no sweating" and should have been labeled "heat stroke," a medical emergency.

Extreme heat stress is a brain injury, with all of the symptoms that normally accompany other brain injuries, such as stroke, concussion, or even drug or alcohol abuse. Although it is important to note the cardinal symptoms of heat stress, the greatest indicator of heat stress in the body is brain function. As long as brain function is normal, the body has a fighting chance of cooling itself and staying alive. The athletic trainer's intervention can increase those odds (Figure 6-8). Once brain function is altered, the thermoregulatory system is compromised and death can occur rapidly. Altered brain function is a medical emergency that calls for immediate referral to a physician. Examples of altered brain function include the following: unconsciousness, memory

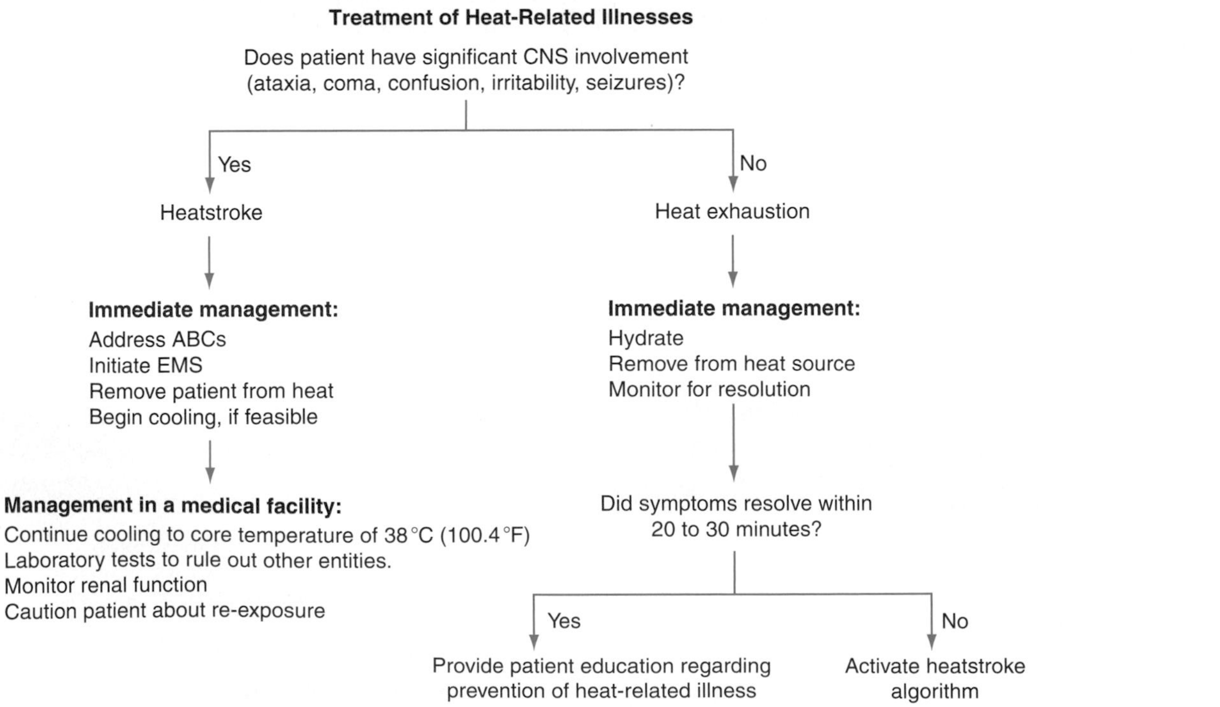

FIGURE 6-8 Assessment of brain function reveals the severity of heat stress. (Redrawn from Glazer JL: Management of heatstroke and heat exhaustion, *American Family Physician* [online serial] 71(11): 2133–2140, 2005. Retrieved February 15, 2007, from www.aafp.org/afp/20050601/2133.pdf.)

loss, visual disturbances, abnormal sensitivity to light or sound, and inappropriate emotional states. If any of these symptoms accompany signs of heat stress (e.g., cramps, syncope, extreme fatigue, dizziness), as well as any other sign that indicates a problem with the central nervous system, the athlete should be rushed to a medical facility. All measures to cool the body quickly are acceptable while transportation is being arranged.

General Treatment of Heat Injuries

Although heat injuries are generally preventable in most athletic settings, they happen every season. Prevention is the ideal treatment, but in the event that a heat illness occurs, the first objective, as with any injury, is to remove the injured athlete from the source of harm and prevent further injury. In the case of heat illness, moving the athlete to a cooler location—preferably indoors, but at least somewhere that is shaded—will achieve this goal. The next goal in the treatment of heat injuries is to limit or reverse the damage that has already occurred. If the athlete is not showing any signs of neurological instability, simple measures to quickly cool the body are effective in reversing the damage of the heat illness: giving the athlete water to drink, removing excess or restrictive clothing, applying ice packs to the body, and so on. Finally, if neurological damage is evident (e.g., unconsciousness, confusion, amnesia, visual disturbances), the athlete should be referred immediately to a physician and transported by ambulance if possible. The athlete must be cooled quickly by any means possible while awaiting the next phase of care (Table 6-4).

Cold Injuries

Like heat injuries, cold injuries fall along a continuum of severity. The least severe problems are generally the most common. Fortunately, the worst cases of cold injury occur less frequently. However, all cold injuries must be evaluated and treated to prevent progression to a more severe condition.

Specific Cold Injuries

Hypothermia. The most common cold injuries include some form of **hypothermia**, or abnormally low core body temperature. Low air temperatures, cold wind, and excess moisture may exacerbate the problem. In a cool environment, the majority of heat is lost through radiation because the body is warmer than the surrounding environment and the heat travels from hotter areas to cooler areas. Some heat is additionally lost through evaporation, mostly from the skin and partially from the respiratory tract. Even a small drop in core temperature can induce shivering and adversely affect neuromuscular coordination (Table 6-5).

Just as the circulatory system increases blood flow to the surface from the core to dissipate heat during activity in hot climates, the circulatory system constricts blood flow to the surface to conserve heat in the body's core. The core heat is preserved to protect the central nervous system and internal organs, compromising the extremities and causing the temperature in these tissues to drop quickly. Decreased blood flow to the extremities prevents these areas from rewarming effectively, which means that less oxygen is going to the tissues and cells, making them sluggish and clumsy at times. The tissues and cells die quickly if they are not fed by this life-preserving flow of oxygenated blood. As the tissue temperature drops, so does the sensitivity of the nerves

hypothermia abnormally low core body temperature

TABLE 6-4 Ways to Cool the Body

WHAT TO DO	WHY IT WORKS
Consumption of cool fluids (e.g., water, sports, drink, juice, etc) *only* if victim is conscious	Replaces fluid lost in sweat; conduction of heat into blood stream on its way to skin surface to be eliminated via evaporation
Total immersion of body into tub of cool water	Reduces core body temperature quickly through conduction of body heat into the cool water; may or may not include ice; core temperature monitored so that it does not drop too much
Cool water poured over the body (via water hose, shower, etc.)	Elimination of excess heat from the body through convection or conduction
Removal of excess clothing—anything that can reasonably be removed	Exposes more skin surface for evaporation or convection to occur
Removal of restrictive clothing	Allows normal blood flow to occur, moving heat from the core to the surface
IV fluids (by physician)	Replaces fluid lost in sweat; conduction of heat into blood stream on its way to skin surface to be eliminated via evaporation; convection current created in blood vessels, which cools surrounding tissues
Transportation of athlete indoors or to shady area	Reduces heat gain of radiation
Placement in front of fan	Increases evaporation; increases convection of heat from the body into air current

TABLE 6-5 Wind Chill Calculation

WIND SPEED (MPH)	TEMPERATURE READING (°F) 50°	40°	30°	20°	10°	0°	−10°	−20°	−30°	−40°	−50°	−60°
Calm	50	40	30	20	10	0	−10	−20	−30	−40	−50	−60
5	48	37	27	16	6	25	−15	−26	−36	−47	−57	−68
10	40	28	16	4	−9	−24	−33	−46	−58	−70	[illegible]	[illegible]
15	36	22	9	−5	−18	−32	−45	−58	−72	[illegible]	[illegible]	[illegible]
20	32	18	4	−10	−25	−39	−53	−67	[illegible]	[illegible]	[illegible]	[illegible]
25	30	16	0	−15	−29	−44	−59	−74	−88	−104	[illegible]	[illegible]
30	28	13	−2	−18	−33	−48	−63	[illegible]	[illegible]	[illegible]	[illegible]	[illegible]
35	27	11	−4	−20	−35	−51	−67	[illegible]	[illegible]	[illegible]	[illegible]	[illegible]
40	26	10	−6	−21	−37	−53	−69	[illegible]	−100	−116	[illegible]	[illegible]
Little danger					Moderate danger Skin freezes within 1 minute				Skin freezes < 1min			

MPH, Miles per hour; *°F,* degrees Fahrenheit.
From Starkey C, Ryan J: *Evaluation of orthopedic athletic injuries,* ed 2, p. 663, Philadelphia, 2002, FA Davis.

in the area, blocking the pain message to the brain and masking the damage.

Wind chill is the relative temperature in light of the wind speed. In other words, the wind chill is an indicator of what the body feels when outside in a given wind and temperature scenario. If wind increases or temperature decreases, the wind chill drops. A temperature above freezing (32° F) with a high wind speed may make the air seem as if it is much colder than freezing. *Wind chill* describes a cold environment in the same way that *heat index* describes a hot environment. An outdoor activity with a cold air temperature, approximately 40° F, may not be very uncomfortable for participants when there is no significant wind to lower the wind chill. However, that same temperature coupled with just a 10-mph wind would produce a wind chill of 30° F, making it very uncomfortable for the participants.

Frostnip. **Frostnip**, the least severe form of cold injury, involves ears, nose, cheeks, chin, fingers, or toes. Frostnip is a very mild form of frostbite, and although it is certainly not a catastrophic condition, it indicates a severe cold environment that must be respected. A sign of risky environmental conditions that can lead to more severe damage, frostnip should serve as warning to increase protection of exposed skin.

Mechanism: This condition occurs with extreme cold, high wind, or both. The length of exposure contributes to the risk as much as the factors of exposure; in other words, severe problems with a short period of exposure may result in only minor frostnip, whereas a longer exposure to lesser environmental risks may result in a severe case.

Signs and symptoms: Frostnip sufferers complain of pain and eventually numbness in the affected area, which has a reddened appearance. The skin appears firm, with cold painless areas that peel and blister within 24 hours.

Immediate management: Treatment measures include going inside to a warmer environment or, if that is not possible, adding more layers to insulate the body from the cold environment. Gloves, hats, extra socks, and heavier coats are all possible solutions to treat frostnip and should adequately protect the body from further damage.[7]

Chilblains. **Chilblains** result from prolonged and constant exposure to cold air or moisture for several hours and usually affect the fingers and toes. The condition may also strike the face and ears. Again, thc longer the exposure to cold, the greater the symptoms and the lengthier the recovery.

Mechanism: The condition is caused by an abnormal constriction in the peripheral blood supply during exposure to cold; the tissue does not actually freeze,

wind chill scale used to predict the level of cold stress placed on the body during activity in a given temperature and wind speed

frostnip cold-related injury describing a mild form of frostbite to the ears, nose, cheeks, chin, fingers, or toes

chilblains cold-related irritation of the skin resulting from prolonged and constant exposure to cold air or moisture; usually affecting the fingers and toes but it is extremely irritated by the cold environment. The condition is more common in children than adults and more common in women than in men.

Signs and symptoms: The skin will be reddened, with swelling, tingling, itching, and pain. After prolonged exposure to cold, painful nodules can form in the skin and may open, or rupture, causing still more pain. The skin may not show symptoms for several hours after exposure. Areas that have suffered from chilblains in the past are more prone to recurrence with future cold exposures.[6,7]

Immediate management: Treatment of chilblains includes the use of antiinflammatory medications, gradual rewarming, and elevation. These measures, if taken when symptoms are first recognized, should prevent the progression to a more serious cold illness.

Intermediate management: Intermediate management includes prevention of subsequent episodes by layering clothes in a more protective fashion when returning to a high-risk cold environment.

Frostbite. Frostbite results as ice crystals form in and around the cells of the chilled tissue. Frostbite worsens with prolonged exposure to cold, and the depth of the tissue damage worsens as well. If unchecked, the frostbite may even reach the bone and destroy all tissue layers along the way.

Mechanism: Prolonged exposure to cold air and humidity may result in frostbite. This condition is triggered by mechanisms similar to those causing other cold injuries, although its consequences are more severe.

Signs and symptoms: Frostbite (Figure 6-9) can be subdivided into two categories: superficial and deep. Superficial frostbite involves the skin and subcutaneous tissue. The skin appears pale, hard, cold, and waxy. The affected area feels hard when palpated, with underlying yielding tissue. The area stings and burns with rewarming and then blisters and feels painful for several weeks. Deep frostbite is a serious injury that involves frozen tissue. During rewarming, tissue becomes blotchy red, swollen, and very painful. Deep frostbite often requires surgical excision or amputation of the tissue for definitive treatment.

Immediate management: Cold injury requires rapid rewarming and prevention of further cold exposure. It is better not to rewarm tissue if it is only going to refreeze later. Treatment of frostbite is more difficult than other cold injuries because damage to the involved tissues is greater. With frostbite, a more severe condition than other cold stress problems, rapid rewarming is indicated to prevent the death of tissue in the area. Rewarming at any speed is usually uncomfortable as the nerves "wake up" and begin to pass along news of the tissue damage to the brain. However, slow or delayed rewarming may lead to cell death. Massaging

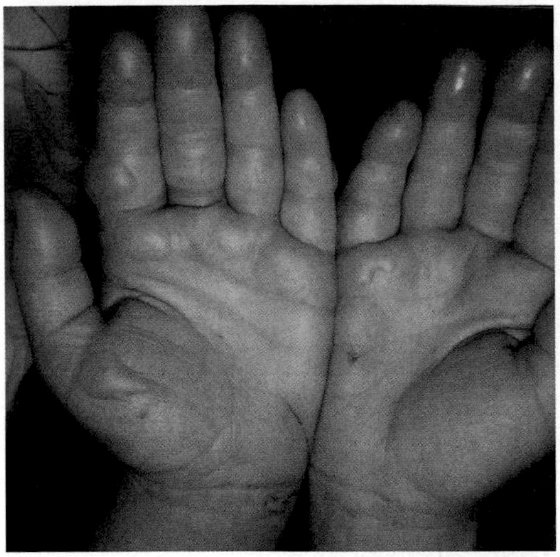

FIGURE 6-9 Frostbite. (From Marx J, Hockberger R, Walls R: *Rosen's emergency medicine,* ed 6, St Louis, 2006, Mosby/Elsevier.)

the affected tissue is not warranted and may be dangerous because the chilled tissue is fragile and prone to breaking or tearing. Table 6-6 outlines the degrees of severity in cold injuries.

Intermediate management: Intermediate treatment is to facilitate transportation to a hospital for further care. Because frostbite can affect very deep layers of tissue, the damage could be irreparable if ignored. Rewarming the affected area is most important, but this measure will be of little benefit if the area is lost as a result of extensive untreated tissue damage.

General Treatment of Cold Injuries

Initially, the athletic trainer may find it difficult to assess the level of cold injury. All levels of cold injury have

TABLE 6-6 Degrees of Cold Injury*

DEGREE	DESCRIPTION OF DAMAGE
First degree	Damage to superficial skin layers only
Second degree	Damage to dermis and subdermal fat cells
Third degree	Damage to underlying tissues, including muscle and bone

* Based on tissue damage developed through rewarming.
Data from Howard TM, Butcher JD: *The little black book of sports medicine,* ed 2, Sudbury, Mass, 2006, Jones and Bartlett.

frostbite potentially severe cold-related injury resulting from ice crystals that form in and around the cells of tissue exposed to cold air and humidity for prolonged periods varying degrees of numbness, redness, coldness, and pain. Confirmation comes as the tissue rewarms. The greater the length of exposure to the cold, the greater the risk of permanent damage in the form of tissue death and related permanent loss of sensation and function. Because the damaged tissues may involve open wounds resulting from ruptured blisters, topical or oral antibiotics may be indicated to decrease the chance of infection in the injured tissue.[6]

Prevention of Cold Injuries

Apparel should be appropriate for the weather (Figure 6-10). It should be windproof but allow free passage of moisture from the body. Multiple thin layers of clothing are most effective in cold environments to provide insulation, which can be added or removed as needed. For exposure to temperatures below 0° C (32° F), it is advisable to add a layer of protective clothing for every 5 mph of wind. Improper clothing, inadequate warm-up exercises, and a high wind-chill factor form a triad that can lead to cold injuries.[8]

Proper hydration is also important in cold weather, just as it is in hot weather. Adequate hydration maintains normal blood circulation, which improves temperature regulation.

Acclimatization

Acclimatization, the gradual adaptation to activity in a new environment, helps the athlete avoid a decrease in performance. Ideally, this process takes several days, even as long as 2 weeks, depending on the individual's current heat tolerance and environmental temperature and humidity conditions. Activity, whether in cold or hot conditions, should be increased gradually to decrease the risk of injury. The body needs approximately 2 hours of daily activity, either in a single activity session or divided into 2 sessions of 1 hour each, to bring about efficient acclimatization.[9] The duration and intensity of activity may be increased gradually with each session, progressing from short bouts of recreational activities to more intense bouts of training activities.

Fluid intake should never be restricted. Fluid restriction will not make athletes tougher or stronger; it will only increase the risk of deadly injury.[10] In fact, acclimatization actually increases the need for fluid intake as the body begins to regulate itself to avoid extremes in core temperature. Sweating occurs more quickly than usual, and this increased fluid output must come from a surplus created by adequate fluid intake. Thirst is a poor indicator of fluid depletion because it occurs long after the body experiences a fluid deficit. Athletes attempting to acclimatize to a new environment should drink before, during, and after activity without regard to perceived thirst.[9]

Although acclimatization can take 2 weeks to complete, some physiological changes are apparent after only 2 days. Physiological changes occur before performance changes, and individuals with better cardiovascular/aerobic conditioning acclimate more quickly than those with decreased conditioning. With proper acclimatization, the risk of injury is minimized through improved efficiency of the body's thermoregulatory system (Box 6-1). Acclimatization remains in force for about a week after removal from the hot environment, declining to about 25% after about 3 weeks. An occasional cool day during the acclimatization process, therefore, does not significantly delay the acclimatization process.[9]

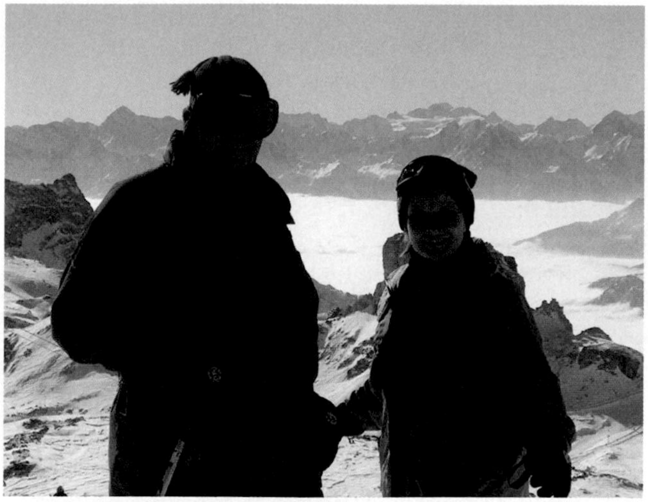

FIGURE 6-10 Proper clothing is an easy defense against cold injury. Note the caps, clothing, and gloves worn to maintain proper body temperature.

LIGHTNING

Electrical storms are consistently one of the top three causes of weather-related deaths in the United States. Lightning kills approximately 100 people every year in the United States.[11] Most lightning casualties occur between June and August, with the greatest incidence in July. The most common time for lightning strikes is between 2:00 PM and 6:00 PM, which is also the most popular time for athletic and recreational activity. The most common sites of fatalities are open fields.[11]

Wind, updrafts in particular, cause the collision of rising and descending ice and water particles, generating positive and negative charged particles. The positive charges collect in the top of the cloud, and negative charges accumulate in the bottom of the cloud. A lightning flash is the result of the buildup and subsequent discharge of static electricity between charged regions. A cloud-to-ground

acclimatization process by which the body gradually adjusts from one environment to another

BOX 6-1 **Advantages of Proper Acclimatization**

Reduction of Heat Stress

Slower increase in core temperature during activity
Earlier sweating
Greater volume of sweat
Reduced heat production during exercise
Improved protection of internal organs

Improved Performance

Decreased heart rate at a given activity level
Improved thirst
Reduced sodium loss (in sweat and urine)
Decreased fatigue

Data from U.S. Army Center for Health Promotion and Preventive Medicine: *Ranger and airborne school students heat acclimatization guide: 2003,* Aberdeen Proving Ground, Md, 2003, U.S. Army.

lightning flash is the discharge of static electricity between charged regions of the cloud and the earth. Objects on the ground such as trees, chimneys, and people can produce positively charged upward streamers that connect with the negatively charged lower layer in a cloud. A lightning flash is a brief spark, similar to the shock a person receives when touching a doorknob after walking across carpet. The electrical potential between cloud and ground can be between 10 million and 100 million volts. The lightning channel is approximately 2.54 cm (1 inch) wide and averages between 3 and 5 miles in length. Thunder occurs as lightning superheats the surrounding air. The rapidly heated air explodes, creating the sound. The audible range of thunder is approximately 16 kilometers (10 miles). Thunder never occurs without lightning[11] (Figure 6-11).

A flash-to-bang count of 30 seconds (i.e., time in seconds from the appearance of lightning to the sound of thunder) should be considered a minimal criterion for suspending activity. The flash-to-bang method is the easiest and most convenient way to determine the distance to a lightning flash. This rule of thumb is based on the fact that light travels faster than sound. Counting the time between flash and sound and dividing the sum by 5 provides an estimate of the distance in miles from the lightning flash. A flash-to-bang ratio of 30 seconds suggests a distance of 6 miles from the lightning.[11]

Several lightning detection systems are currently on the market. Some monitor the environmental conditions (e.g., humidity, air temperature, wind speed) to predict the likelihood of lightning activity. Other detectors monitor the same conditions and report the occurrence of lightning as it happens to inform the user of lightning activity in the area. Both technologies give false positives and false negatives at times—that is, they sometimes

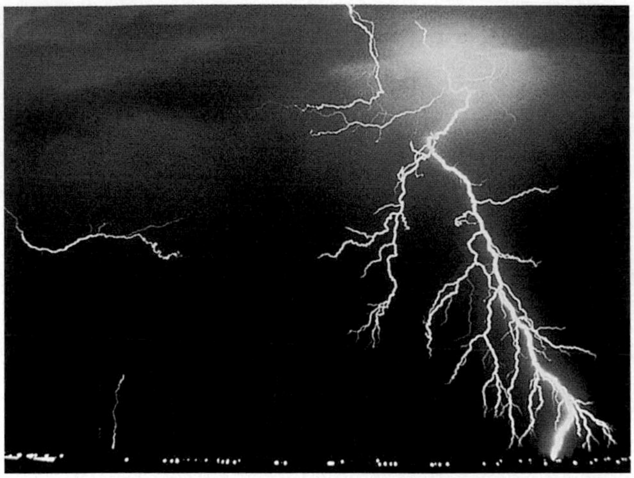

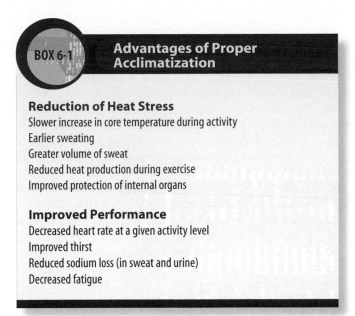

FIGURE 6-11 Lightning occurs in nearly every environment and can cause severe injury. (From Auerbach PS: *Wilderness medicine,* ed 4, St Louis, 2001, Mosby.)

sound a warning unnecessarily and sometimes do not sound a warning when danger is in the area. However, both types of systems are quite accurate at times (Figure 6-12). Another type of lightning detection system is tied into the National Weather Service or other reputable weather reporting service. Some allow the user to see the actual radar screen, whereas others send warnings through text message, voice mail, e-mail, or another method to alert the user to dangerous weather in the area. Whatever technology is selected, these devices can only supplement common sense, not replace it. Having the common sense to avoid dangerous weather situations remains the most accurate method of preventing lightning injury. An accurate flash-to-bang count is low tech, easily mastered, and user friendly.

Height above ground plays a prominent role in determining strike probability. Minimizing vertical height is critical in decreasing the risk of becoming a victim of a lightning strike. The warning signs of an impending lightning strike include hair that stands on end and sizzling sounds. After witnessing these signs, the potential victim should immediately crouch in the lightning-safe position: feet together, weight on the balls of the feet, and head lowered with ears covered.

Height above ground also determines areas of safety, which explains why trees are not safe cover. When the

Points to Ponder

Lightning detectors that report the distance to or from a nearby storm may actually increase the time a team is allowed to practice or compete; if the detector indicates that the storm is moving away or even stalling, the athletic trainer has a clearer idea of the risk.

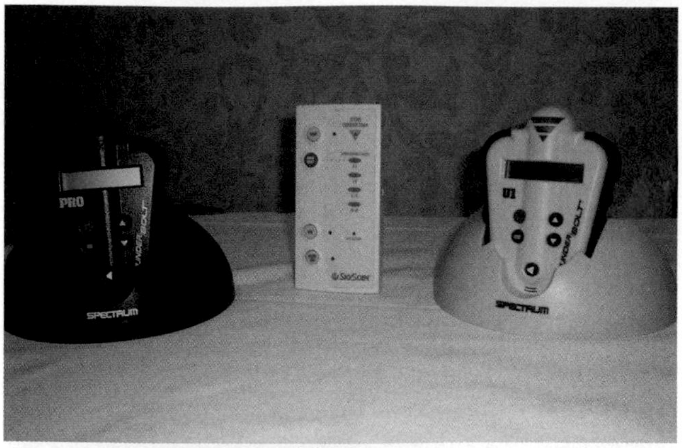

FIGURE 6-12 Lightning detectors can be very useful in determining the proximity of lightning and the associated risk of continued activity.

flash-to-bang ratio decreases below 30 seconds, potential victims should be evacuated to a safe area, preferably a fully enclosed nonmetal building with plumbing, electrical wiring, and telephone service. Although moving to a building encased in so many electricity-conducting materials may seem counterintuitive, this network of pipes and wires actually helps direct any lightning strike *around the building* rather than *through the building* to the ground beneath it. If a substantial building is not available, a fully enclosed vehicle with the windows closed is a reasonable alternative. Small structures such as picnic shelters and storage sheds are usually not properly protected and may even increase the risk of a lightning strike. The excellent conductivity of water makes it a risk whether inside or out. In an indoor swimming pool or locker room shower area, lightning current may travel through the pipes.[11]

Resumption of activity should not occur until 30 minutes after the last lightning flash or clap of thunder.[11] The average thunderstorm travels 40 kilometers (25 miles) per hour. Waiting 30 minutes should put the storm outside the range of a lightning strike. Because victims of a lightning strike are not connected to a power source, they do not carry an electric charge and are therefore safe to assess. Unless the victim suffers a cardiopulmonary arrest, he or she is unlikely to die. A cardiopulmonary arrest could involve a primary and secondary event. The electrical jolt of the lightning temporarily short circuits the heart, causing it to stop. The diaphragm and other muscles responsible for breathing are also overwhelmed, and breathing stops. An organized series of contractions usually resumes within a short time, but damage to the brain's respiratory center may induce respiratory paralysis that lasts much longer than the cardiac arrest. Unless the victim receives respiratory support, the prolonged hypoxia may induce a secondary cardiac arrest.[11,12]

Treatment of Lightning Injuries

As in any emergency situation, the athletic trainer's initial concerns should be Check, Call, and Care with the ABCs (airway, breathing, and circulation). When the lightning strike involves multiple persons, **triage** must be instituted. The athletic trainer should assess the areas and systems that are affected and work to restore function as indicated with cardiopulmonary resuscitation or rescue breathing. Victims of lightning strike should be referred to a physician for further evaluation. It is completely safe to touch someone recently struck by lightning; the current is eliminated as quickly as it appeared. Although the lightning strike can be quite painful and cause serious burns, the primary concern is to limit or reverse any damage caused by cardiac or respiratory arrest. Without efficient circulation of oxygenated blood throughout the body, permanent disability or death can occur quickly.

STINGING INSECTS

The environment also contains many highly annoying pests. The most common pests affecting athletic participation are the stinging insects of the Hymenoptera order, which includes bees, wasps, and fire ants. Although these creatures are just a nuisance for most athletes, others are deeply allergic to the stings of these insects. In the United States, about 40 deaths each year are attributed to insect stings, most of them in adults over age 45.[13] The risk of serious reaction increases with the number of stings received. Multiple stings usually occur because a nest was disturbed; the first insect releases alarm pheromones that incite aggressive behavior in the rest of the colony.

Stings occur in exposed areas of skin, usually on the head and neck, followed by foot, leg, hand, and arms. A single sting can cause instant pain, swelling, and itching at the site of penetration. Large local reactions spreading several inches beyond the sting site and lasting longer than 24 hours are common. Multiple stings in an unsensitized person may result in vomiting, diarrhea, and generalized edema.

Allergic reactions are by far the most serious consequence of hymenoptera stings. Up to 4% of the U.S. population exhibit some degree of clinical allergy to hymenoptera stings.[10] Allergic sting reactions occur away from the sting site. Typical symptoms resemble those typically seen in nonallergic individuals—itchiness (pruritus), hives (urticaria), and swelling (edema)—but may also include respiratory difficulties and nausea.

triage process by which care is prioritized according to the severity of injury or illness in those seeking treatment

Life-threatening situations include hypotension, loss of consciousness, and marked respiratory distress. Roughly one half of severe reactions occur within 10 minutes and all occur within 6 hours. Most of the fatalities happen within 1 hour. Children are less likely than adults to have severe reactions.

Treatment of Insect Stings

Application of ice packs affords relief for mild stings. Honeybees and yellow jackets may leave stingers in the wound; these should be scraped or brushed off. Forceps should not be used because more venom may be squeezed into the wound. Because the toxin is injected under the surface of the skin, topical anesthetics are not generally effective, but oral antihistamines, which circulate through the bloodstream to reach the tissues affected by the sting, may be of benefit. Large local reactions may be minimized by the use of oral corticosteroids. Multiple stings may require hospitalization. Anaphylactic reactions result from airway obstruction or hypotension and are treated with epinephrine injected under the skin through an Epi-pen. Individuals with known sensitivity should have such a device readily available, especially in the late summer and early fall, when insect populations are greatest.[10]

POLLEN ALLERGIES

Pollen is almost always present in the atmosphere, but it is more of a problem for those sensitive to it in the summer and spring. These seasons are generally drier and windier than other times of the year, making it easier for the small grains of pollen to circulate in the air rather than drop quickly to the ground, as they do in a humid, still environment.

Sensitivity, or allergy, to inhaled pollen is referred to as *allergic rhinitis,* or more commonly *runny nose* or *hay fever.* A runny nose can be a symptom of other conditions, such as a viral infection or an occupational exposure (e.g., chemical fumes, dust, smoke, mold), but allergic rhinitis always involves an irritation to the lining of the upper respiratory system by inhaled pollen (Figure 6-13). In reaction to these irritants, the lining of the nasal passages becomes inflamed and produces more mucus to flood out the irritants. The same process occurs when the eyes produce additional tears to cleanse the surface of the eye when it is irritated by environmental pollen; some of these tears empty into the nasal passages and increase the rhinitis. Other common symptoms include sneezing and coughing, clear or discolored nasal discharge, headache, sore throat, and itchy and watery eyes.[14] The primary difference between allergic rhinitis and nonallergic rhinitis is the causal relationship with environmental pollen. Moreover, pollen allergies do not produce a fever, whereas viral conditions often do.[15] When the pollen count in the air is high, the symptoms worsen; when the pollen count is low, the symptoms improve or even disappear.[3]

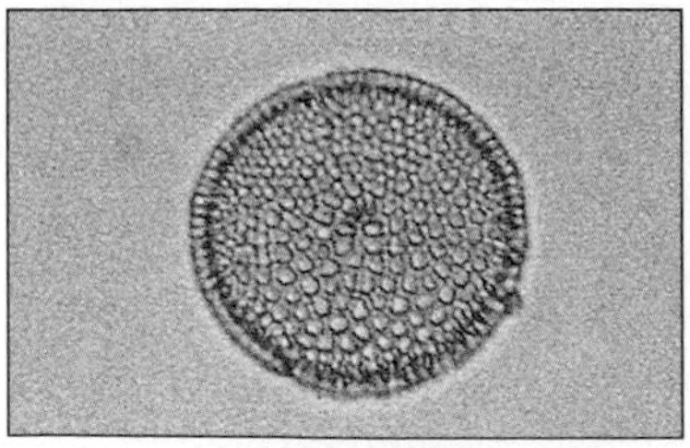

FIGURE 6-13 Pollen is the cause of many seasonal allergies. It is easy to see how the rough grains of pollen can irritate the sensitive nasal lining. (From McPherson RA, Pincus MR: *Henry's clinical diagnosis and management by laboratory methods,* ed 21, Philadelphia, 2006, Saunders/Elsevier.)

Treatment of Pollen Allergies

Treatment of pollen allergies resembles that of other environmental injuries: Avoid exposure to the irritating condition to reduce the risk of injury. At times, activities in high-pollen environments cannot be avoided, and the use of over-the-counter or prescription antihistamine medications before or after activity can help decrease the severity of symptoms. Increasing fluid intake can also help decrease the symptoms by giving the body a surplus of fluid to use in flushing out the irritated respiratory system. Symptoms that last a week or longer should be evaluated by a physician.[15,16]

SUNBURN

Sunburn is damage caused by ultraviolet radiation. This exposure to ultraviolet radiation may be natural and incidental, the result of being outdoors in the sun, or it may be intentional, the result of using a tanning bed. Acute sunburn can be very painful and often affects activities of daily living. The degree of damage caused by the sun is directly proportional to the length of exposure to ultraviolet radiation and is easily prevented by simply covering the skin while outdoors. However, doing so can increase the risk of heat illness in certain climates and situations, so the safest alternative in high-risk heat scenarios is to use a good sunscreen.

As with other burns, sunburn is described by degrees, with first degree being the mildest form and third degree being the most severe. Initially, the degree may be difficult to assess because the symptoms develop slowly. Most symptoms have fully developed within 24 to 48 hours of exposure. First-degree sunburn produces redness, hypersensitivity, and increased temperature in the affected area. Second-degree sunburn has all of the symptoms of first-degree sunburn as well as fluid-filled blisters on the surface of the skin. With third-degree burns, the skin exhibits all of the previous symptoms in addition to some areas of ulceration, or open wounds. Pain increases with each level of sunburn severity. As the skin is damaged, nerve endings are exposed and the pain level increases. As the skin is dehydrated from the burn, it cracks and increases the risk of infection.

An isolated occurrence of sunburn is generally not a long-term concern. However, repeated sunburns—even minor ones—have a cumulative traumatic effect and significantly increase the risk of skin cancer. Repeated sunburns as a child correlate to a higher risk of skin cancer as an adult (Table 6-7). Sun sensitivity, or the tendency to burn rather than tan, is a primary indicator of skin cancer risk.[17] People with lighter skin have a higher risk of developing skin cancer after multiple sunburns than those with darker skin. Although people with lighter skin often have lighter eyes and hair as well, sun sensitivity and risk of skin cancer development correlate most closely with skin color.[18]

Treatment of Sunburn

As with many environmental injuries, prevention is the best solution. Liberal amounts of sunscreen decrease the risk of a damaging burn. Sunscreens are rated with a sun protection factor (SPF) that indicates their relative ability to protect the skin from a burn. The higher the SPF rating, the greater the protection. Sunscreens with an SPF of 15 or higher are best and should be re-applied often, before and during outdoor activities, to maintain a high level of protection (Box 6-2). If possible, outdoor activities in the sun should be limited during hours of the most intense ultraviolet radiation (i.e., between 10 AM and 4 PM). If activity during these peak hours cannot be avoided, the use of hats, sunglasses, and long-sleeved shirts will help to minimize ultraviolet exposure.[18]

If sunburn does occur, many over-the-counter topical medications are available to moisturize the dry skin and alleviate the pain until the skin can heal. With severe burns (i.e., second or third degree), prescription medications may be necessary to protect the damaged skin and prevent infection. Aspirin or a nonsteroidal antiinflammatory medication can also be beneficial in decreasing the pain of sunburn. For maximal benefit, the aspirin must be taken immediately after sun exposure.[18]

BOX 6-2 Proper Application of Sunscreen

- Apply sunscreen at least 20 to 30 minutes before exposure.
- Use a waterproof sunscreen with a high SPF.
- Apply liberally to all exposed areas, including ears, back of the neck, and posterior aspects of the legs.
- Reapply often (at least every hour) and after drying off from water activities.
- Realize that the sun does not have to be shining to create dangerous UVA or UVB light, so make using sunscreen a daily habit.
- Use sunscreen even when in the shade; sunlight reflected off water can also damage the skin.

From Cuppett M, Walsh KM: *General medical conditions in the athlete,* p. 326, St Louis, 2005, Elsevier/Mosby.
SPF, Sun protection factor; *UVA,* ultraviolet A; *UVB,* ultraviolet B.

TABLE 6-7 The ABCDs of Skin Cancer

DESCRIPTOR	PARAMETERS
A: Asymmetry	A melanoma lesion cannot be "folded in half"; in other words, the lesion does not have equal right and left sections or top and bottom sections.
B: Border	Benign lesions have a sharp, distinct border that can easily be traced, whereas malignant lesions may have indeterminate borders, making them difficult to trace.
C: Color	Benign lesions have a uniform tan, brown, or black color, whereas malignant lesions may have variegated or multiple (e.g., red, white, and blue) color patterns. In addition, a sudden darkening in color or spreading into normal skin suggests a malignant lesion.
D: Diameter	Benign lesions usually have a diameter of less than 6 mm, whereas malignant lesions usually have a diameter greater than 6 mm.

From Cuppett M, Walsh KM: *General medical conditions in the athlete,* p. 325, St Louis, 2005, Elsevier/Mosby.

CIRCADIAN DYSRHYTHMIA

Jet lag, the common name for **circadian dysrhythmia,** occurs with travel across time zones and is not exclusively reserved for those who travel by air in jets. The human body maintains many metabolic cycles that follow a daily pattern; these are termed *circadian rhythms.*

The physiological stress is cumulative as additional time zones are crossed. The various metabolic processes adjust to time changes at varying rates. Protein metabolism adjusts quickly, but the rise and fall of body temperature takes up to eight days. Headaches,

circadian dysrhythmia condition commonly known as jet lag in which the body is placed under physiological stress after crossing multiple time zones fatigue, and digestive problems occur with circadian dysrhythmia. Although jet lag can occur during flights east or west, the adjustment is generally less difficult if the destination is westward. Frequent travelers live by the following adage: "Traveling west is best, but east is a beast!" Adequate preparation can minimize the effects of jet lag. A gradual adjustment of meals and bedtime toward the destination time zone before departure hastens adjustment and minimizes the effects of jet lag. One rule of thumb is that 24 hours is necessary for the body to adjust for every time zone crossed. If a trip is planned far enough in advance, meal and sleeping times can be adjusted beforehand to begin the adjustment process.

Points to Ponder

When competitive travel causes team members to cross back and forth into bordering time zones every week, the athletic trainer may advise that they stay on "home time" rather than on "destination time" to avoid the fatigue of adapting to a new time schedule for each trip.

REFERRAL GUIDELINES

Most environmental injuries can be handled on-site without an emergency referral to a physician. When no permanent or life-threatening consequences are present, the athletic trainer may simply treat the symptoms so that the athlete can resume normal activities of daily living when he or she is comfortable doing so. In cases of medical emergencies, such as heat stroke, severe frostbite, or allergic reactions to insect stings, the athletic trainer must act quickly and make wise decisions to prevent permanent disability or even death. In all situations, the athletic trainer should remove the injured athlete from the source of the environmental injury. If heat or cold is the culprit, the athlete should be taken to a safer environment, usually indoors. In the case of insect stings, the athlete should be removed from the vicinity of the insects—both for the safety of the athlete and the athletic trainer providing care.

RETURN-TO-PLAY GUIDELINES

The severity of the situation determines whether the athlete may return to activity. Obviously, an athlete referred to a physician for emergency evaluation usually cannot return to play the same day. However, in a nonemergency situation, an athlete may return to normal activity as soon as all symptoms have resolved. An athlete with heat illness may resume normal activity once his or her hydration status is restored to pre-event levels. An athlete with a mild cold injury may return to play once the area is completely rewarmed and fully functional. Emergency situations follow the same rule; athletes may resume activity only after the resolution of all symptoms. However, these symptoms may take much longer to resolve, and the disability may be permanent, ending the individual's athletic career.[4]

SUMMARY

Although environmental injuries are among the most preventable conditions in athletics, they must be taken seriously because failure to recognize the signs of a serious condition may be catastrophic. Most environmental injuries, such as a bee sting or sunburn, are simply a nuisance and rarely interfere with the activities of daily living. However, some environmental injuries, such as heat stroke or bee sting allergy, can be life threatening if they are not treated promptly. Treatment of most environmental injuries includes removing the athlete from the irritating factor (e.g., excessive heat, excessive cold, severe weather, stinging insects) followed by treatment of the symptoms to prevent further tissue damage. The athletic trainer's responsibility is to monitor the local environment to limit unsafe activity and to use common sense when encountering problem areas in the future.

Revisiting the OPENING *Scenario*

In the opening scenario, high temperature and humidity have led to a statewide heat advisory by the National Weather Service. These conditions are dangerous for anyone conducting vigorous activity outdoors and greatly increase the risk of heat stroke. The athletes suffering from heat illness are probably affected by heat exhaustion, which may progress to heat stroke. Given that the bus trip extended through lunch, it is unlikely that many of the players had an adequate pregame meal; most of them probably intended to eat a bigger meal after the game. The athletic trainer reported the status of the athletes to the coach after evaluation from the sidelines and reported that they should take a break until adequately rehydrated. Because this process took longer than the time left on the clock, these athletes missed the remainder of the game. It is important to note that the performance of these athletes was already suffering as a result of the heat stress and their continued participation would not have affected the result of the game. Thanks to the intervention of the athletic trainer, the injured athletes were able to participate in the remaining games of the season and contribute to the team's success.

Issues & Ethics

The athletic trainer is responsible for monitoring the risk of environmental injury to the team and informing those in charge of the need to reschedule the event or move it to a safer area. Although coaches often want their athletes to become tougher by competing in harsh environments, this desire must be balanced against the need to practice safely without risking injury or even death.

Interactions between a coach who wants a competitive team and an athletic trainer who wants the athletes to stay healthy and avoid risks can be challenging. Achieving these competing goals requires creativity. In environments that present heat-related dangers, the athletic trainer should advise the coach to schedule frequent water breaks. When the athletes have unrestricted access to fluids, they have better endurance and sharper reactions, which promote stable performance. Some water breaks should be scheduled when no other activity or instruction is taking place. Other breaks should be ongoing, which means that the athletes may get a drink whenever doing so is not disruptive to the ongoing drill or instruction.

Another area of possible contention is enforcement of a site's lightning policy. Although lightning fatalities are relatively rare, the risk must be taken seriously. Athletic trainers often feel intimidated when informing a coach or administrator that an event must be suspended until a lightning threat has passed. Often, thunder and lightning are evident, but the absence of rain means that the greater public does not perceive a risk. One duty of a responsible athletic trainer is to be proactive in preventing injury as well as treating those that have already occurred. Informing a coach or administrator about an impending danger is entirely appropriate in the case of an oncoming thunderstorm. To avoid confrontation during the game, the athletic trainer should strive to discuss the lightning policy with the coach and administrative staff ahead of time. Many of these policies are set by the sport's governing body and are not negotiable.

Although most people agree that the policies are warranted, suspending a very competitive game because of a potential risk is often difficult. If that decision is made ahead of time, when cooler heads prevail, the likelihood of conflict decreases; the scenario becomes one in which one professional simply informs another professional that it is time to enforce a predetermined policy. Consider the best strategies for approaching a coach or administrator regarding these policies, which allow a competitive season without compromising the health of the athletes involved.

Web Links

American Academy of Allergy, Asthma, and Immunology: www.aaaai.org/

Gatorade Sports Science Institute: www.gssiweb.com/

Lightning and Atmospheric Electricity at the Global Hydrology Climate Center of the National Aeronautics and Space Administration: http://thunder.nsstc.nasa.gov/

National Climatic Data Center: www.ncdc.noaa.gov/oa/ncdc.html

National Lightning Safety Institute: www.lightningsafety.com/

National Severe Storms Laboratory: www.nssl.noaa.gov/

National Weather Service, National Oceanic and Atmospheric Administration: www.nws.noaa.gov/

U.S. Army Research Institute of Environmental Medicine: www.usariem.army.mil/

References

1. Convertino V, et al: American College of Sports Medicine position stand: exercise and fluid replacement, *Medicine & Science in Sports & Exercise* 28(1): i–vii. 1996.
2. Casa DJ, et al: National Athletic Trainers' Association position statement: fluid replacement for athletes, *Journal of Athletic Training* 35(2): 212–224, 2000.
3. Starkey C, Ryan J: *Evaluation of orthopedic and athletic injuries*, ed 2, Philadelphia, 2002. FA Davis.
4. Binkley HM, Beckett J, Casa DJ: National Athletic Trainers' Association position statement: exertional heat illness, *Journal of Athletic Training* 37(3): 329–343, 2002, Retrieved February 15, 2007, from www.nata.org/statements/position/exertionalheatillness.pdf.
5. National Athletic Trainers' Association: *NATA age specific task force issue on youth football & heat related illness*, Dallas, 2005, NATA Retrieved February 15, 2007, from www.nata.org/statements/official/youth_football.pdf.
6. Howard TM, Butcher JD: *The little black book of sports medicine*, ed 2, Sudbury, Mass, 2006, Jones and Bartlett.
7. Mellion MB, Putukian M, Madden CC: *Sports medicine secrets*, ed 3, Philadelphia: 2003, Hanley & Belfus.
8. Armstrong L, et al: American College of Sports Medicine position stand: heat and cold injuries during distance running, *Medicine & Science in Sports & Exercise*, 28(12): i–x, 1996.
9. U.S. Army Center for Health Promotion and Preventive Medicine: *Ranger and airborne school students heat acclimatization guide: 2003*, Aberdeen Proving Ground, Md, 2003, U.S. Army.
10. Maughan RJ, Shirreffs SM: Gatorade Sports Science Exchange: Preparing athletes for competition in the heat: developing an effective acclimatization strategy, *SSE#6510*(2) 1997. Retrieved February 15, 2007, from www.csmfoundation.org/GSSI_-_Preparing_Athletes_for_Competition_in_the_Heat.doc.
11. Walsh KM, et al: National Athletic Trainers' Association position statement: lightning safety for athletics and recreation, *Journal of Athletic Training* 35(4): 471–477, 2000.
12. Auerbach PS: Wilderness medicine: management of wilderness and environmental emergencies, ed 4, St Louis, 2001, Mosby.

13. Golden DBK: Stinging insect allergy, *American Family Physician* [serial online] 67(12):2541–2546 2003. Retrieved February 15, 2007, from www.aafp.org/afp/20030615/ 2541.html.
14. Quillen DM, Feller DB: Diagnosing rhinitis: allergic vs. nonallergic, *American Family Physician* [serial online] 73(9), 2006. Retrieved February 15, 2007, from www.aafp.org/afp/20060501/1583.html.
15. Cuppett M, Walsh KM: *General medical conditions in the athlete*, St Louis, 2005, Elsevier/Mosby.
16. Anderson MK, Hall SJ, Martin M: *Sports injury management*, ed 2, Philadelphia, 2000, Lippincott Williams & Wilkins.
17. Goldstein BG, Goldstein AO: Diagnosis and management of malignant melanoma, *American Family Physician* [serial online] 63(7), 2001. Retrieved February 15, 2007, from www.aafp.org/afp/20010401/1359.html.
18. Jerant AF, et al: Early detection and treatment of skin cancer, *American Family Physician* [serial online] 62(2), 2000. Retrieved February 15, 2007, from www.aafp.org/afp/20000715/357.html.

7

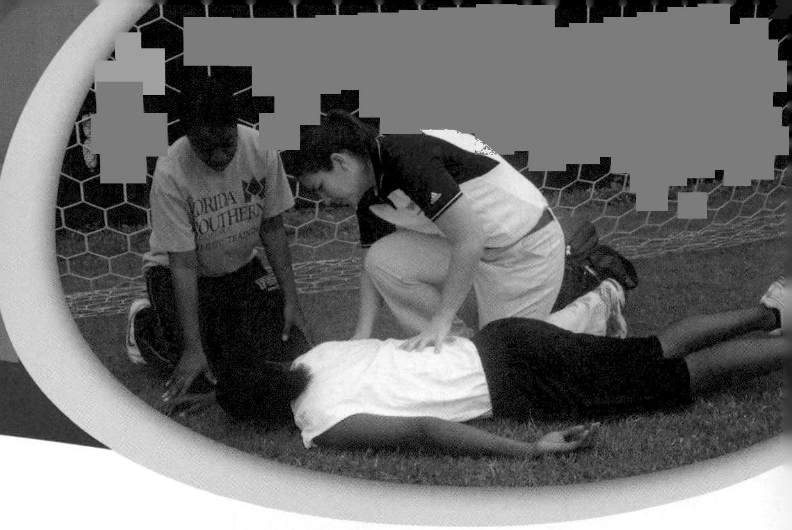

Emergency Management

MICHAEL R. DILLON

Learning Goals

1. Develop an emergency action plan for various venues.
2. List and perform the steps in a primary emergency assessment.
3. List and perform the steps in a secondary emergency assessment.
4. Identify basic types of emergency equipment needed in various athletic settings.
5. Describe the essential emergency skills used for typical injury situations seen by athletic trainers.
6. Document injury management strategies for emergency situations.

At some point, nearly every athletic trainer is called on to handle a potentially catastrophic injury or illness. How the athletic trainer identifies and manages the situation may save a life, prevent paralysis, or reduce the severity of the injury. Preventing a potentially dangerous situation by early recognition of signs and symptoms is paramount to the job of the athletic trainer. Whether it is recognition of a diabetic episode, heat illness, or a potentially serious asthma attack, prevention and early recognition are crucial. Unfortunately, not all emergencies can be prevented in the athletic environment, and because they may happen at any given moment, it is of utmost importance that the athletic trainer be prepared. An athletic trainer who has the knowledge and skill to recognize potentially serious conditions can provide immediate care and make the critical decision to refer the athlete or patient to the appropriate medical facility.

A certified athletic trainer has a duty to act and an obligation to provide emergency care in a wide variety of situations.[1] The recognition and treatment of emergency skills and the standards of care for acute injuries and illnesses are clearly defined in the National Athletic Trainer's Association (NATA) Educational Competencies [2] and the Board of Certification (BOC) Role Delineation Study.[3] Emergency skills discussed in this chapter include designing and activating an emergency action plan, implementing emergency techniques and procedures for life-threatening injuries and illnesses, and initiating appropriate first aid techniques for nonlife-threatening injuries or conditions. Expedient action must be taken to provide the best possible care of the athlete with an emergent or life-threatening condition. Being prepared and properly trained increases the likelihood of a positive outcome for the athlete. Figure 7-1 is a concept map outlining the various issues surrounding emergency management, including emergency preparation and the assessment and management of emergency situations.

Points to Ponder

If the booster club has agreed to pay for one piece of equipment for the athletic training room, should you purchase an AED or a modality? You may never use the AED, but you will use the modality unit daily on multiple athletes.

EMERGENCY PREPARATION

Emergency situations can occur at any time during an athletic practice or event. The various skills and standard

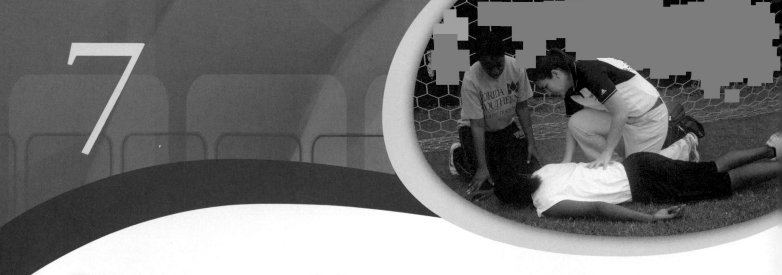

OPENING *Scenario*

It is early fall, and the baseball team has just begun workouts to prepare for the upcoming season. All team members have received thorough physical examinations before the fall workouts. This season, all reporting players have been cleared to participate without any restrictions. Today's conditioning session started with an easy jog to the track followed by a series of flexibility and warm-up exercises. The head athletic trainer and you, an athletic training student, are on the baseball field along with the strength and conditioning coach. Earlier today, the athletic trainer brought out the usual supplies, including water, ice, towels, an athletic training kit, an automated external defibrillator (AED), and a cell phone.

After the athletes run a series of form-running drills, one of the infielders appears to be in distress. He bends over in an attempt to catch his breath, possibly trying to force himself to vomit. As you and the athletic trainer approach the athlete, he stands up very quickly and then collapses. Suddenly, he is unconscious and face down on the ground. You look up and notice that the temperature on the track is 106° F and it is already 6:00 PM. The players have been working out for less than 15 minutes, and that was spent mostly on their stretching routine. What should you and the athletic trainer do first?

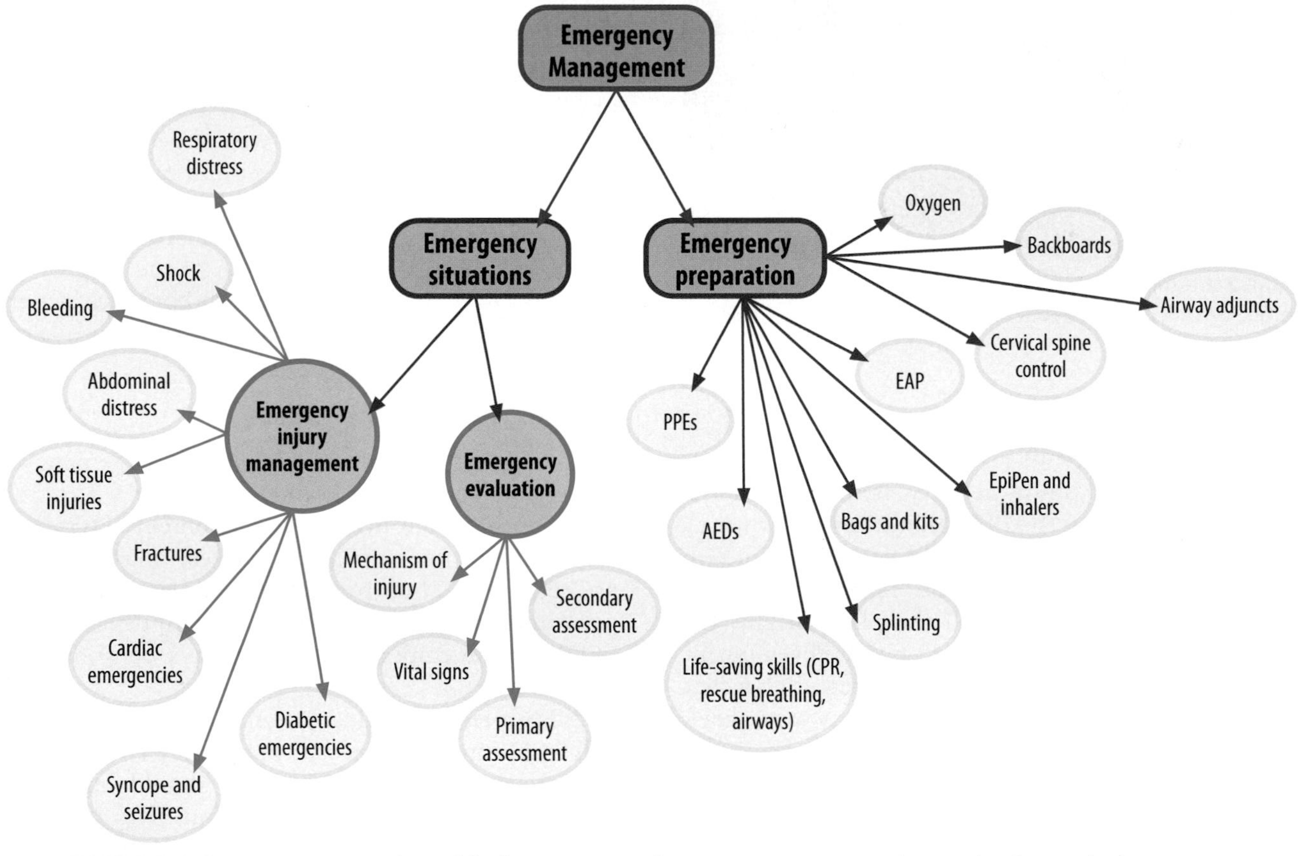

FIGURE 7-1 Concept map overview of the issues surrounding emergency preparation, evaluation, and management.

of care that make up emergency care provided by the athletic trainer are detailed in the Board of Certification's Role Delineation Study.[3] The skills include but are not limited to first aid and emergency care, rescue breathing, cardiopulmonary resuscitation (CPR), and the use of bag-valve-masks, pocket masks, primary surveys, secondary surveys, inspection, palpation, cervical stabilization, splinting, and spine boarding.[3] These skills may be the most important ones an athletic trainer possesses. The athletic trainer is often the first person at the athlete's side after an injury and frequently the only trained medical professional available. It is vital for the athletic trainer to know and *practice* these emergency skills. Having access to the necessary equipment is only part of the solution. Having the appropriate emergency equipment on-site, combined with the requisite skills to use the equipment, is what makes the situation turn out well for all parties concerned (Figure 7-2).

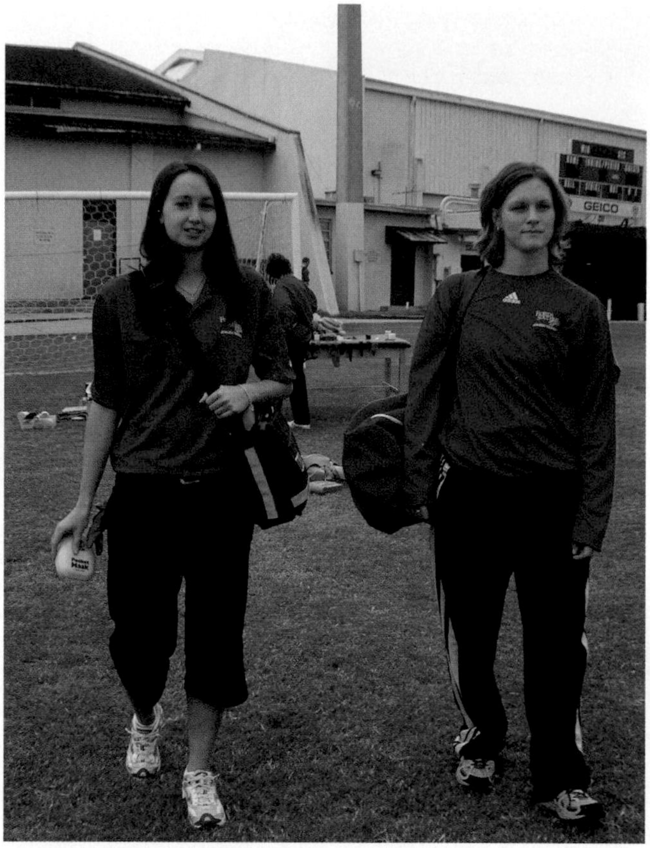

FIGURE 7-2 Athletic trainers must always come prepared for an emergency, which can occur at any time.

Emergency Action Plan

The athletic trainer must be very familiar with the **emergency action plan** (EAP) at all of the sites at which he or she provides care and should be instrumental in ensuring that coaches, administrators, and other staff members are also familiar with the plan. Ideally, the athletic trainer should be involved in the development and review of the EAP. The EAP is a detailed plan that addresses the following areas: emergency personnel, communication, equipment, preparation, and transportation. The written emergency plan is a detailed document that describes the roles of involved personnel, emergency equipment available at the site (and the exact location of this equipment), a list of emergency numbers and modes of communication, a venue or site map, and detailed directions to that venue. Each venue should have its individual EAP posted in several locations. Figure 7-3 is a sample EAP.[4] The EAP is the cornerstone of an athletic trainer's emergency preparation.

A copy of the EAP should be made available to all visiting teams. Its details should be reviewed with the team's athletic trainer or coach before the beginning of any contest. The plan must cover the treatment and transportation of any injured parties, including those from visiting teams. On rare occasions, spectators or bystanders fall victim to accidents or illnesses beyond their control and will need to be treated according to the EAP.

The plan should be discussed and reviewed with the local emergency medical services (EMS) personnel who are covering each venue. It is especially important to review the responsibilities of the various medical professionals who might be involved with the care of the athlete. The EAP should be rehearsed, at the very least, before the beginning of each sport season and should involve all parties that might be involved in a real-life emergency, including, but not limited to, the following individuals: athletic trainers, athletic training students, team physicians, local EMS personnel, coaches, event management staff members, local emergency room personnel, and campus police. The rehearsal should include worst-case scenarios and should be taken very seriously. Rehearsals should include the use of emergency equipment and physical transportation to the local emergency room. Appropriate communication with the local emergency room director is very important and can help ease the transition to the emergency medical model. Ongoing rehearsal in every venue using numerous scenarios is critical to the successful execution of the EAP. A well-planned EAP with regular review and practice is a great way to ensure that everyone is prepared for a serious injury or illness.

Personal Protective Equipment

In practicing sound emergency management and protection, the athletic trainer first should have ready access to **personal protective equipment** (PPE; Figure 7-4). These items include gloves, masks, gowns, pocket mask, and protective eyewear. All medical personnel should be trained in the appropriate use of PPE, and the equipment must always be immediately accessible.

PPE protects the athletic trainer from any body fluid that may transmit disease or present the risk for disease or infection. The athletic trainer should immediately dispose of gloves in a biohazardous bag after making contact with a patient. Steps for glove removal are described in Box 7-1. A new pair of gloves must be worn

emergency action plan (EAP) detailed crisis plan that addresses emergency personnel, communication, equipment, preparation, and transportation

personal protective equipment (PPE) articles such as gloves, masks, and eyewear designed to protect health care personnel from disease or infection

BASEBALL EAP: Foley Field

Emergency Personnel: Certified athletic trainer, _____ _____ (___-___-____) and athletic training student(s) on site for practice and competition; additional sports medicine staff accessible from **Butts-Mehre athletic training facility** (across street from stadium).

Emergency Communication: Fixed telephone line in **Baseball satellite athletic training room** (___-____)

Emergency Equipment: Supplies (AED, trauma kit, splint kit, spine board) maintained in baseball satellite athletic training room; additional emergency equipment accessible from **Butts-Mehre athletic training facility** (across street from stadium **(___-____ and ___-____)**.

Roles of First Responders:

1. Immediate care of the injured or ill student athlete
2. Activation of emergency medical system (EMS)
   a. **9-911** call (provide name, address, telephone number (of individual injured), condition of injured, first aid treatment, specific directions, other information as requested)
   b. Notify **Campus Police** at ___-____
3. Emergency equipment retrieval
4. Direction of EMS to scene
   a. Open appropriate gates
   b. Designate individual to "flag down" EMS and direct to scene
   c. Scene control: limit scene to first aid providers and move bystanders away from area

Venue Directions: Foley Field baseball stadium is located on the corner of Pinecrest Street and Rutherford Street; adjacent to Butts-Mehre Hall. Two gates provide access to the stadium:

1. Pinecrest Street (1st base side): drive leads to field as well as rear door of complex (locker room, athletic training room)
2. Rutherford Street (3rd base side): drive leads to the outfield and visitors' dugout

GPS Coordinates (in the event of the need for a medical helicopter transport): 33 56.44/83 22.81

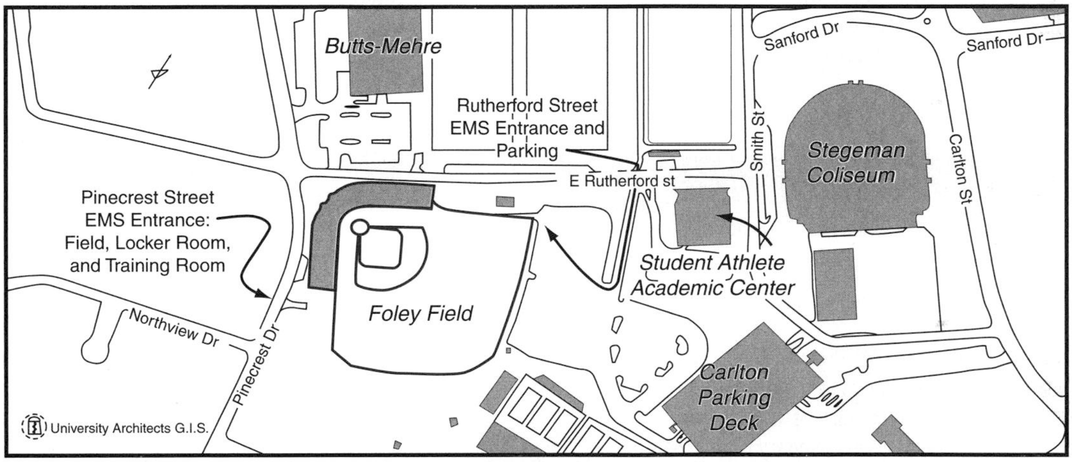

Baseball: Foley Field

FIGURE 7-3 Sample emergency action plan (EAP). (From University of Georgia: *University of Georgia emergency plan—Baseball: Foley Field,* Athens, Ga, 2007, Author.)

while treating each person in situations in which contact with body fluids is possible.

Another piece of equipment that must be readily available is the **Pocket Mask,** which is used for performing rescue breaths during cardiopulmonary resuscitation (CPR; see Figure 7-4). These masks contain a one-way valve that allows air to be passed through to the victim but does not allow body fluids to exit back through the valve. The athletic trainer should periodically inspect the mask for potential malfunctions or other flaws that would necessitate replacement. As with gloves, most pocket masks are designed to be discarded after each use, although some masks may be sterilized and used multiple times. It is imperative to remember that athletic trainers must always protect themselves before assisting others.

Trauma Bag

A **trauma bag** is simply a comprehensive kit in which emergency equipment is stored. The trauma bag is usually an addition to the typical athletic training kit

Pocket Mask hand-held device containing a one-way valve that is used to perform rescue breaths

trauma bag kit containing all the emergency equipment

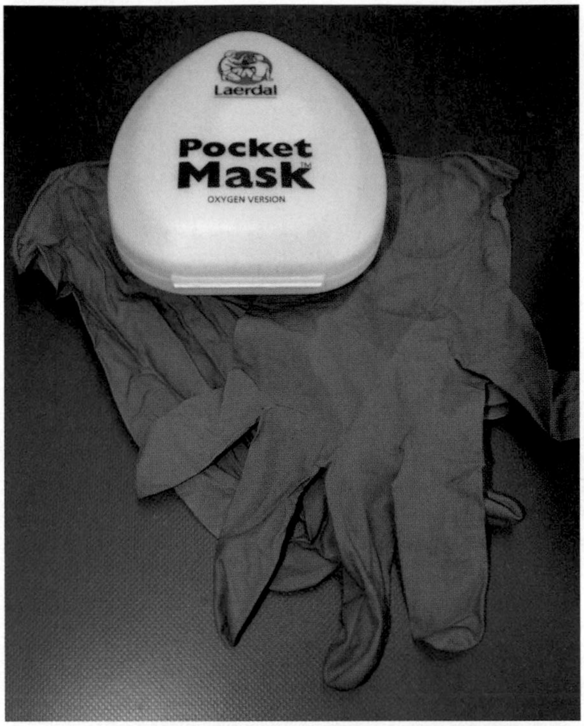

FIGURE 7-4 Personal protective equipment (PPE) is one of the first items to consider when preparing for sound emergency management.

BOX 7-1 Steps for Proper Glove Removal

1. Pull the edge of one glove at your wrist towards your fingertips so the glove folds over.
2. Carefully grab the edge that is folded over, and pull it down to your fingertips. This will turn the glove inside out.
3. Continue pulling the edge until the glove is almost off your fingertips.
4. While still holding the glove, completely remove your hand from the glove. Maintaining control of the glove and not letting it fall will decrease the risk of spreading any contaminants that may be on the glove.
5. Slide your now-ungloved fingers under the edge of the glove still on your other hand. Slide your fingers under the glove until about half of the glove is covering those fingers. Your gloved hand is still holding the glove that you just removed.
6. Turn your fingers so the pads are facing away from the gloved hand, and pull the glove towards your gloved fingertips. This motion will encase the removed glove in the now partially removed glove. The second glove will now be inside out as well.
7. Carefully grab the gloves with the area that was touching your skin (the uncontaminated surface), and pull your second hand completely free of the gloves. Dispose of the gloves in the appropriate container.

and contains only those supplies that are needed in an emergency. Typically, the trauma kit contains at minimum an assortment of splints, PPE, and cervical collars. The team physician may also choose to keep in the trauma kit some of the emergency equipment that might be necessary. This bag should be taken to each practice, game, and conditioning session. In other settings, the trauma kit remains on location in an easily accessible and visible location. Either in addition to the trauma bag or inside the kit, an AED should also always be available at the scene (Figure 7-5). All of this emergency equipment should be checked at least weekly to ensure that everything is in proper working order and ready to use in case of an actual emergency.

Cardiopulmonary Resuscitation, Rescue Breathing, and Airway Obstruction

The Board of Certification (BOC) requires all certified athletic trainers, as a condition of holding athletic training certification, to maintain certification in emergency cardiac care.[3] This certification includes adult, child, and infant **cardiopulmonary resuscitation** (CPR), rescue breathing, obstructed airways, two-rescuer CPR, AED administration, barrier devices, and oxygen administration.

Several providers, including the American Red Cross, American Heart Association, and the National Safety Council, provide the certifications to satisfy the BOC continuing education requirement. It is very important that athletic trainers renew their emergency cardiac care and first aid certifications on the required regular basis to ensure that they stay abreast of any changes in the procedures and have the opportunity to practice the skills. Many schools, conferences, and leagues also require their coaches and strength and conditioning staff to be certified in CPR and first aid.[2] Having more than just one staff member certified in these important skills is another step in providing appropriate levels of proper emergency care. In many cases, athletic trainers provide coverage for multiple sports in several sites. Because coaches spend the most time with the athletes, they must be able to activate the EAP, carry out immediate first aid,

cardiopulmonary resuscitation (CPR) procedure used to support and maintain breathing in an emergency

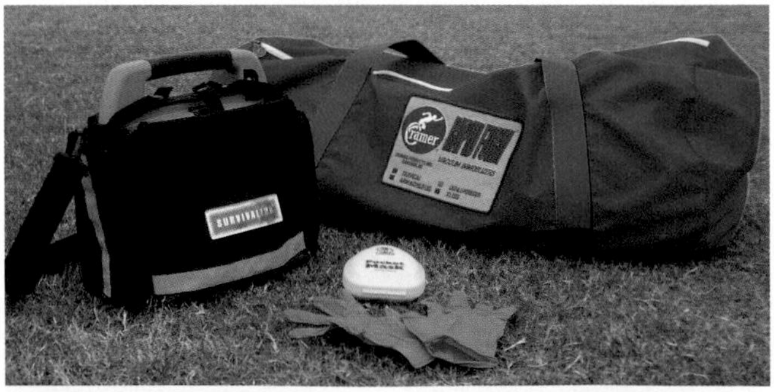

FIGURE 7-5 Athletic trainers should be prepared with the trauma bag and automatic external defibrillator (AED) at every practice, game, and conditioning session.

and perform emergency cardiac care in the event that the athletic trainer is at another venue. It is often the athletic trainer's role and responsibility to certify the coaches in first aid and CPR and to ensure that they know and understand the steps to carry out in an emergency. Athletic trainers and coaches also may be the first to provide first aid or CPR for a fan or spectator at an event until EMS personnel arrive on the scene.

Obstructed Airway

Obstructed airways present a serious concern for obvious reasons. Without adequate oxygen, the body and its systems will eventually shut down. If the airway is not obstructed, rescue breathing can be performed. With obstruction, however, rescue breathing becomes irrelevant and the athletic trainer must resort to other means to establish an open airway. The most common object that obstructs a person's airway is the tongue itself. When a person becomes unconscious, the tongue falls back and blocks the airway. The athletic trainer can open the airway by using the head-tilt chin-lift method (Figure- 7-6). If a neck injury is suspected, the jaw-thrust method must be used (Figure 7-7). These techniques are taught in the emergency cardiac care course required of all athletic trainers. EMS personnel often use an oral pharyngeal or nasal pharyngeal airway to maintain an airway in an unconscious person.

Automatic External Defibrillator

The public is beginning to recognize both the need for and the benefit of equipping facilities with **automatic external defibrillators** (AEDs). These units attach externally to the patient's chest and deliver an electrical shock that will correct the firing of the heart's internal electrical circuits when they are damaged. All persons who may be called upon to use an AED should be properly trained in its use and know where it is located.

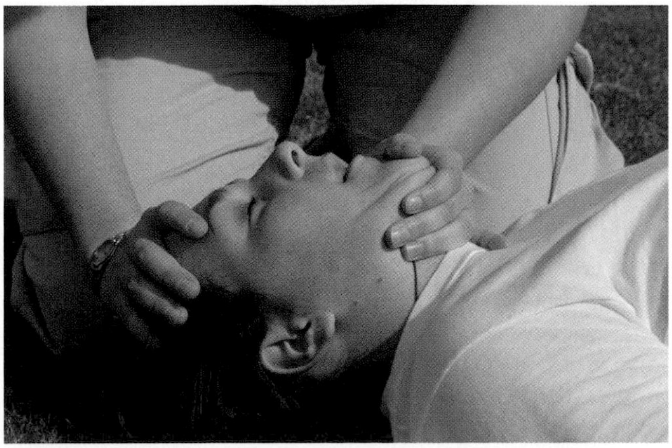

FIGURE 7-6 When an individual is unconscious, the tongue can fall back and block the airway. The head-tilt chin-lift method can be used to open an obstructed airway.

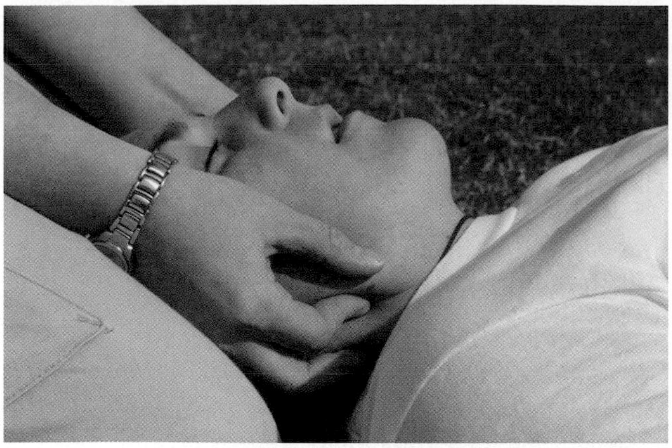

FIGURE 7-7 If the airway is obstructed and a neck injury is suspected, the athletic trainer should use the jaw-thrust method to open the airway.

As the name implies, these devices are automatic and are not difficult to use. Even untrained personnel can successfully use an AED because each unit provides both pictorial and verbal directions. Today's units deliver an electrical shock to the heart only when the machine's sensors have identified a true problem. If the heart is not in distress, the unit does not deliver a shock. The AED uses the enclosed pads to analyze the person's heart rate (Figure 7-8). If the heart is malfunctioning, the AED

automatic external defibrillator (AED) device that delivers an electrical shock to help correct the firing of the heart's internal circuits in an emergency

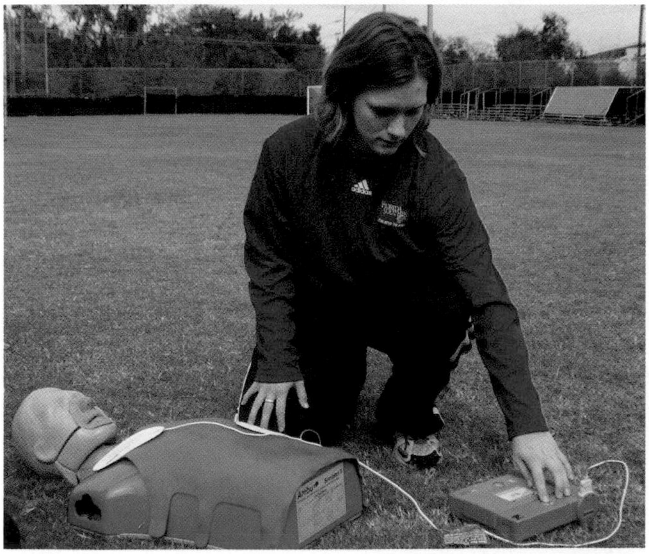

FIGURE 7-8 If an athlete experiences cardiac distress, the athletic trainer can use the automatic external defibrillator (AED) to deliver an electrical shock that can help reestablish a normal heart rhythm.

Points to Ponder
Where should you keep the only AED at a high school? Would the office, gymnasium, football practice field, or track be most practical?

fires (shocks) in an effort to return the electrical impulse of the heart back to a normal rhythm.[5] Timely use of an AED can help save someone's life.

Cervical Spine Control

Another important skill to master in emergency management is maintaining control of the cervical spine in either an unconscious athlete or an athlete with a potential injury to the cervical spine. Cervical spine control is merely the application of manual stabilization to the cervical spine until a cervical collar can be applied and the athlete can be moved as a unit onto a spine board. Athletic helmets, such as those used in football or lacrosse, must be left on the athlete during stabilization and transport to a hospital. Other helmets, such as motorcycle helmets, should be removed to protect the cervical spine during transportation to a hospital.

Establishing cervical spine control requires the athletic trainer to move to the top of the injured person's head and, if the athlete is lying supine (on his or her back), to place his or her hands on either side of the athlete's face (Figure 7-9). This hand position allows the middle, or ring, fingers to be available for a modified jaw thrust, if necessary.

If the athlete is not lying supine, he or she must be "log rolled" into that position as a unit. If the athlete must be repositioned to his or her back, it is best to log roll him or her directly onto a spine board, a procedure that is described in greater detail in the next section. This motion requires that the person at the head of the athlete be in charge of coordinating all assistance. It is imperative to move the body as a unit with minimal movement, and cervical spine and head alignment must be maintained throughout the log-roll process. Any steps taken to prevent unnecessary movement of the cervical spine help reduce the risk of further injury. If the athlete is not breathing and is wearing a helmet with a face mask, immediate removal of the face mask (not the helmet) should be performed with the use of appropriate tools, such as an electric screwdriver, trainer's angel, or other appropriate device.

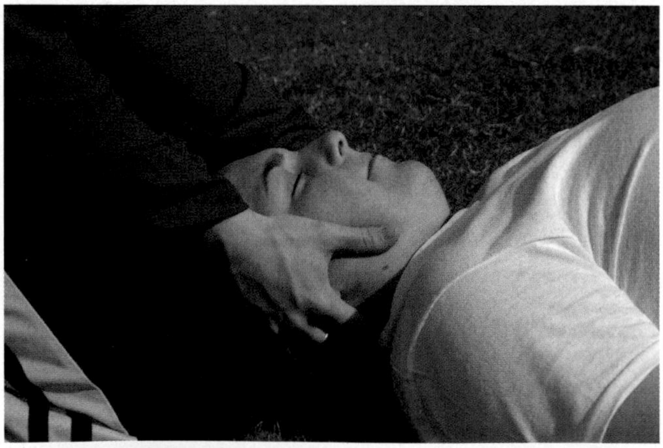

FIGURE 7-9 In an emergency situation, the establishment of cervical spine control is vital, especially when a neck injury is suspected. This process involves the application of manual stabilization—for example, with the injured person on his or her back, the athletic trainer would place a hand on either side of the face—until the person can be properly stabilized on a spine board and transported to a medical facility.

Use of a cervical collar is not a difficult skill to master, but it does require a little practice.[1] Several types of cervical collars are commercially available to meet the needs of nearly every setting and budget (Figure 7-10). The best styles of collars on the market are adjustable for both neck length and width.

Backboard or Spine Board

Frequently, patients are placed on a spine board (Figure 7-11) because a spine injury is suspected or because it is a safer way to transport someone with a serious injury.[1] Safely placing an injured person onto a backboard and securing him or her for transport is an emergency skill that the athletic trainer must master.[6] This skill requires the following equipment: spine board, strapping system, head restraint (or tape), and at least three other people to assist. If enough skilled personnel are not present or the athletic trainer does not feel comfortable performing these skills, the best option is to wait until EMS personnel arrive and let them place the athlete on the spine board. In the interim, the athletic trainer may safely stabilize the patient, maintaining the position of the injured body part, monitoring vital signs, and preventing shock while providing verbal support and encouragement.

Several methods are commonly used to position a person onto a spine board.[7] The most common technique used for transfer is the aforementioned log roll. This technique requires three to five people and consists of rolling the individual to one side as the spine board is slid underneath (Figure 7-12). The injured person's body is moved as a unit, meaning that all four extremities, the trunk, and the head are moved simultaneously onto the spine board. This movement should be performed in a smooth and gentle manner. If the position of the patient allows, the athletic trainer should attempt to place a head immobilizer or cervical collar on the patient to keep his or her head and neck in a stationary position. Straps that have been attached to the spine board can be used to hold the patient in place

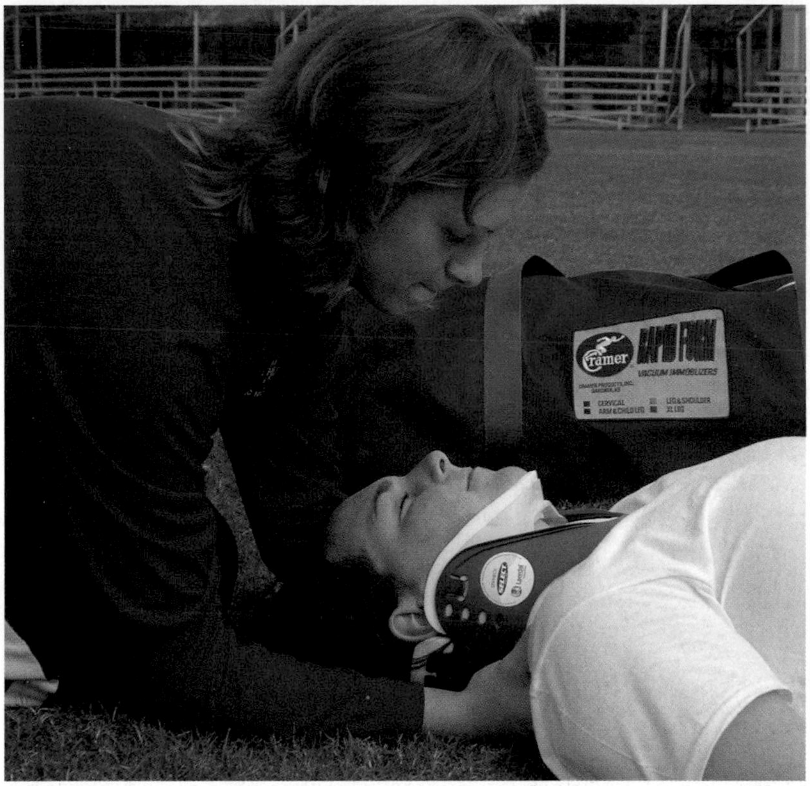

FIGURE 7-10 A cervical collar can help prevent any unnecessary movement of the cervical spine during assessment and transportation to a medical facility.

and keep the arms and legs from moving unnecessarily. Any extraneous movement of either the head and neck or arms and legs can significantly increase the severity of the injury.

Splinting

Before an injured person is moved for transport, the athletic trainer should apply the appropriate **splint** if a fracture or dislocation is suspected. When splinting any extremity, the athletic trainer checks the patient's distal pulse, motor reflexes, and sensations both before and after splinting (Figure 7-13). A list of items to note when splinting is listed in Box 7-2.

Next, the joint should be splinted above and below the injury site. Many types of splints are currently available. Rigid splints (Figure 7-14) require that the area to be splinted be held straight and in an anatomically correct position. Any material that is firm and can hold its shape, such as plastic, cardboard, magazines, or wood, may be used as a rigid splint. Rigid splints offer the most support for the injured body part, but they are not useful when the injured area is deformed. Formable splints include air splints, vacuum splints, and SAM Splints. Vacuum splints (Figure 7-15) and SAM Splints (Figure 7-16) are the most commonly used in athletic settings. They are easy to apply and do

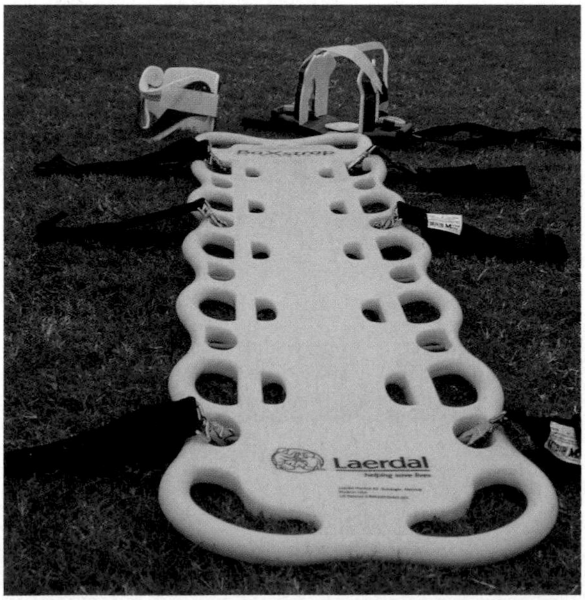

FIGURE 7-11 The backboard, or spine board, is used to prevent further injury during transport of individuals with suspected spine injuries.

splint rigid or formable device used to immobilize a body part when a fracture or dislocation is suspected

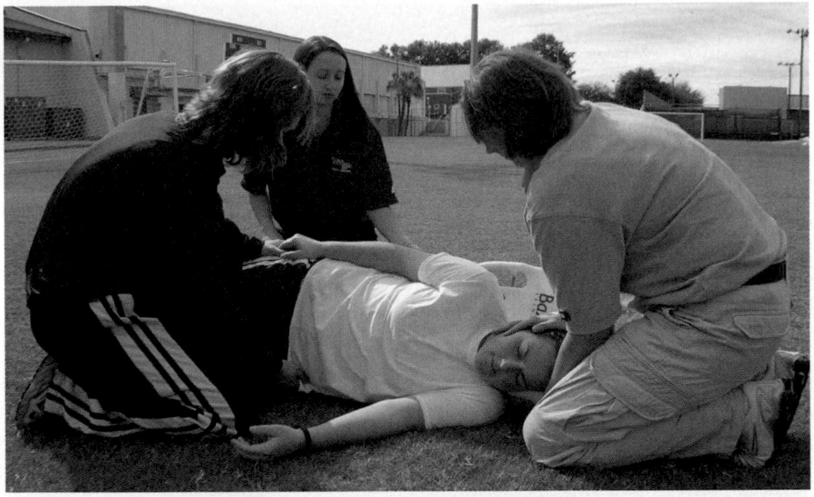

FIGURE 7-12 The log-roll method is commonly used to transfer an injured individual onto a spine board. It involves moving the individual onto his or her side in one unit (head, trunk, and extremities) while the board is slid underneath the individual's body. The log-roll method requires three to five people.

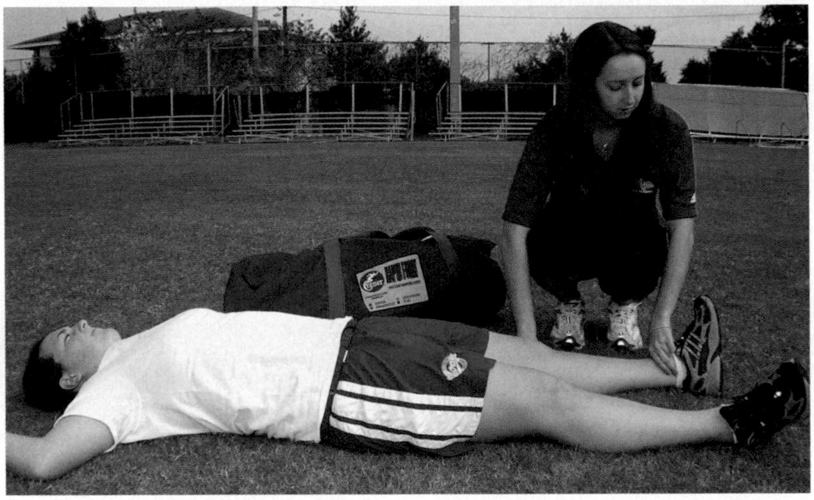

FIGURE 7-13 Before and after splinting any extremity, the athletic trainer should check the individual's distal pulse, motor reflexes, and sensations.

BOX 7-2 Splinting Checklist

- ✓ **P** Distal pulse
- ✓ **M** Monitor reflexes
- ✓ **S** Check sensations

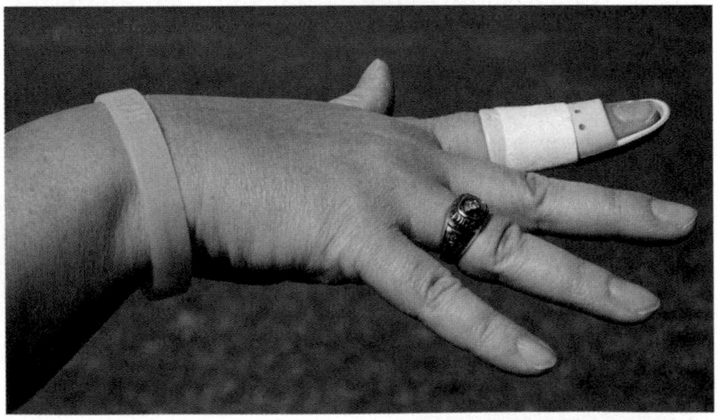

FIGURE 7-14 A rigid splint allows the athletic trainer to immobilize an extremity by holding it in an anatomically correct position.

not require any movement of the injured area, allowing the patient to be transported in the position in which he or she is found. Formable splints are most useful when a dislocation or a displaced fracture has created a deformity. The vacuum splint works by removing air from the splint, forming a rigid splint around the injured area. To decrease the risk of exacerbating the injury, practice is important with the application of any type of splint.

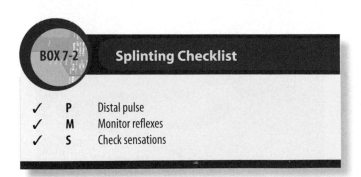

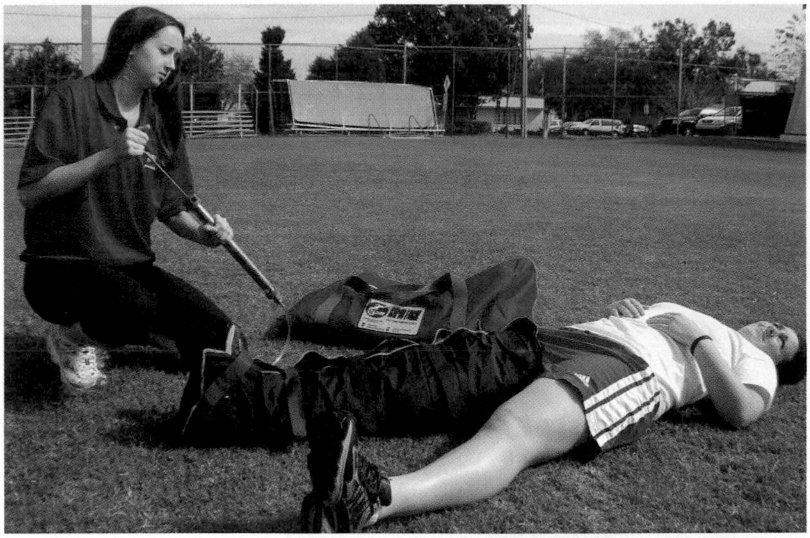

FIGURE 7-15 The vacuum splint, which is formable, removes air from the splint and forms a rigid enclosure around the injured area.

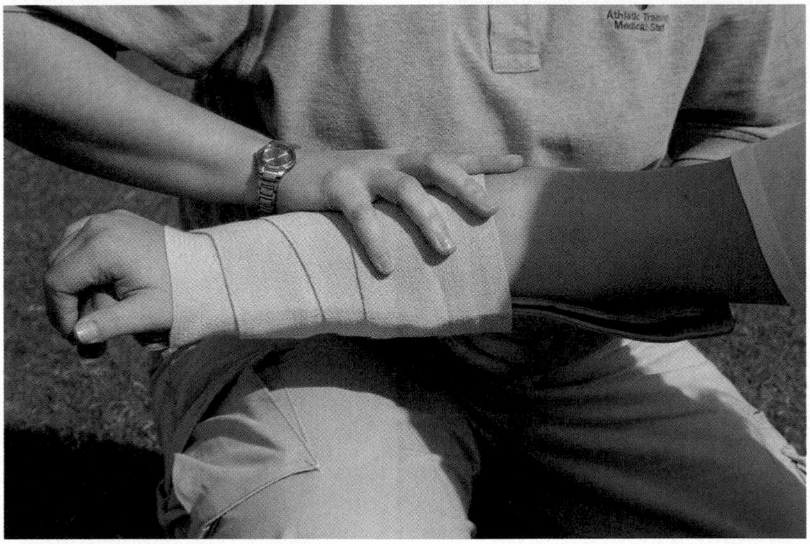

FIGURE 7-16 The SAM Splint is made of a thin core of aluminum alloy situated between two layers of foam. Composed of formable materials, it creates a strong splint when bent into one of three simple curves.

EpiPen and Inhaler

Athletic trainers should also be prepared to assist with the administration of an **EpiPen** (Figure 7-17) or the administration of an inhaler. Because these items are both prescription medications, athletic trainers may only assist the individual in administering these medications. An EpiPen is a preloaded syringe that auto-injects medicine (usually a form of epinephrine) when it is firmly pressed against the thigh. The EpiPen is used by people who have allergies to insect stings or certain foods. Epinephrine constricts the blood vessels, helping to normalize blood pressure and relax the airway passages, which often spasm with severe allergies.

A person who has asthma or another illness that makes normal breathing difficult may use a **metered-dose inhaler** for either prevention or emergency relief of an attack. The device propels medication into the respiratory system through inhalation. It is important that the athlete follow proper technique when using the inhaler to ensure that the medication reaches the bronchioles and does not just remain in the mouth. Most manufacturers recommend that patients use a spacer,

EpiPen preloaded syringe used to administer an emergency dose of epinephrine

metered-dose inhaler device used to deliver medication to the respiratory system during an asthmatic attack

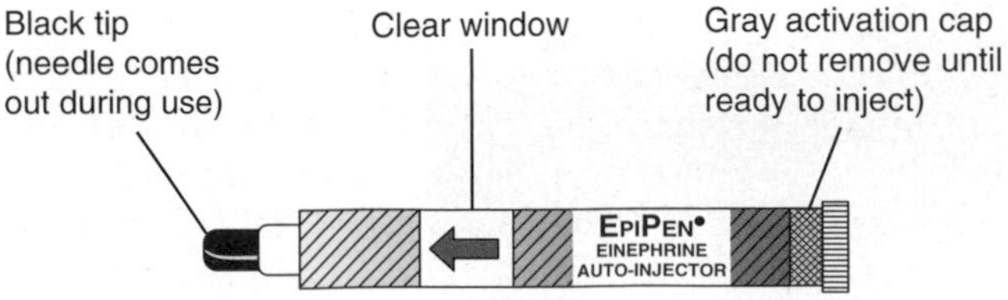

FIGURE 7-17 The EpiPen is an emergency preloaded supply of epinephrine that auto-injects the medicine when it is firmly pressed against the patient's thigh. It is commonly used to treat allergic reactions to foods and insect stings. (From Lehne RA: *Pharmacology for nursing care,* ed 6, Box 17-1, p. 156, Philadelphia, 2007, Saunders/Elsevier.)

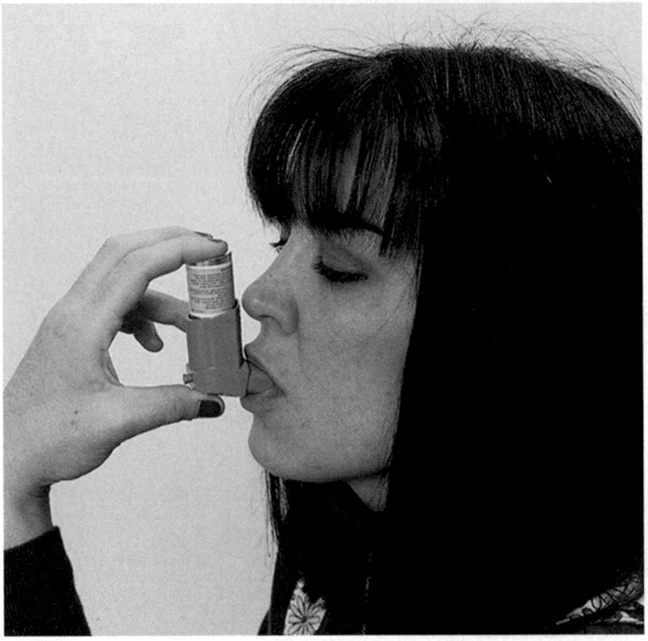

FIGURE 7-18 A metered-dose inhaler is a pocket-sized device used to administer a bronchodilator to an individual experiencing breathing difficulties during an asthmatic attack. (From Perry AG, Potter PA: *Clinical nursing skills and techniques,* ed 6, Step 4d[1], p. 672, St. Louis, 2006, Mosby/Elsevier.)

a long tube, or a holding chamber attached to the inhaler that increases the amount of medication being inhaled into the lungs with each dosage[8] (Figure 7-18).

EMERGENCY ASSESSMENT

Athletic trainers are in a unique position to observe most of the emergent injuries that occur during athletic participation. This opportunity makes it imperative that they pay close attention to the event at hand.

Mechanism of Injury or Illness

A thorough first-hand understanding of how the injury occurred is a great asset in the assessment of the injury. Actually observing the mechanism of injury, or the way in which the injury occurred, provides important clues regarding the type of injury and helps the athletic trainer make a valid emergency assessment. Was it a contact or noncontact injury? Was it a twisting or a shear injury? Was it a high-velocity injury? Was it a direct blow to the head, face, or extremity? Each of these types of mechanisms produces a specific type of injury. A noncontact twisting injury to the knee indicates a possible anterior cruciate ligament (ACL) injury. A contact injury to the back of the head may indicate a concussion or a closed head injury, such as a subdural hematoma. A high-velocity injury may be caused by a projectile, such as a batted ball traveling in excess of 120 mph when it strikes the athlete; such force can cause severe soft tissue injury or fractures (or both). Directly observing the mechanism of injury may expedite the emergency assessment and allow the athletic trainer to make a speedier assessment of the athlete's status, thus increasing the quality of care provided to the patient.

Vital Signs

Vital signs play an important role in helping the athletic trainer to complete an accurate emergency assessment. In some emergencies, no obvious mechanism of injury is apparent. In these situations, learning to take and interpret vital signs gives the athletic trainer clues about what has really happened to the injured person. Vital signs are outward signs, or indicators, of what is going on inside the body.[1] They include respiration, respiration rate, pulse, pulse quality, blood pressure, skin color, skin temperature, pupil reaction, temperatures (oral, tympanic, or rectal), and perhaps oxygen saturation.

The athletic trainer should observe both the rate and the quality of breathing when assessing respirations. The rate of breathing varies according to the age of the patient. For adults, the rate is approximately 12 to 20 respirations per minute; for school-age children, 15 to 30; for infants and toddlers, 20 to 70; and for newborns, 30 to 50. The quality of breathing is subjectively assessed by observing the patient inhale and exhale. Observation includes not only watching but also listening. Quality is graded as either normal, shallow, labored, or noisy. Box 7-3 lists the ways in which respiration is described.

The athletic trainer must consider rate and quality when checking the patient's pulse. A normal pulse rate in an adult is 60 to 100 beats per minute; for adolescents, 60 to 105; for children, 70 to 110; for toddlers,

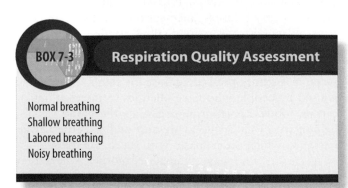

BOX 7-3 Respiration Quality Assessment

Normal breathing
Shallow breathing
Labored breathing
Noisy breathing

TABLE 7-1 Vital Signs: Normal Readings

AGE GROUP	RESPIRATIONS	PULSE
Adult	12–20	60–100
Adolescent	12–20	60–105
Child	15–30	70–110
Toddler	20–70	80–130
Infant	20–70	90–140
Newborns	30–50	90–140

80 to 130; and for infants, 90 to 140[1] (Table 7-1). A rapid pulse rate is called **tachycardia** (i.e., above 100 beats per minute), whereas a slow pulse rate is called **bradycardia** (i.e., below 60 beats per minute). Pulse quality is divided into rhythm (regularity) and force (pressure of pulse waves). A resting pulse rate in a well-conditioned person, such as a runner or swimmer, may be as low as 40. An abnormally slow pulse rate may indicate head injury, drug abuse, or certain heart problems. A high heart rate may indicate fright, fever, exertion, or shock. Anyone who complains of sickness usually has an elevated pulse rate.

Taking and reading blood pressure are skills that require frequent practice to maintain proficiency. Athletic trainers must always remember to use the correct cuff size, especially when evaluating large athletes or very small athletes. At the minimum, athletic trainers should have available a normal adult-size blood pressure cuff and an extra-large cuff for larger athletes.

Systolic blood pressure represents the force of the blood in the arteries while the ventricles of the heart are contracting, and diastolic blood pressure represents the left ventricle relaxing and refilling. The systolic pressure is represented by two consecutive beats while the cuff is being deflated, whereas the diastolic reading is the point at which the sound disappears. When a blood pressure value is recorded on the medical chart, the systolic is the top number and the diastolic is the bottom number. The normal value for systolic pressure is between 90 and 150, and the normal value for diastolic pressure is between 60 and 90. High blood pressure readings may indicate a medical condition, physical exertion, or excessive fatigue, and low blood pressure readings may indicate acute blood loss or shock. Although taking pulse or blood pressure readings in a quiet setting is easy, athletic trainers must be able to perform these emergency skills in any environment, even in a stadium surrounded by 100,000 screaming fans or on the floor of a huge industrial plant. Taking vital signs under varying conditions is a skill that should be practiced repeatedly to ensure accurate, consistent, and proficient readings.

The next vital sign to assess is the temperature and color of the patient's skin. Skin temperature, which is assessed using the back of the hand, has the following possible characteristics: cool and clammy (shock), cold and moist (losing heat), cold and dry (cold), hot and dry (high fever or serious heat illness), hot and moist (high fever or mild to moderate heat illness), and goose pimples (chills, cold, pain, fear). For Caucasian athletes, skin color is generally pink (normal). Skin color variations include the following: pale (blood loss, hypotension, emotional distress); cyanotic, or blue (lack of oxygen); flushed, or reddish (exposure to heat or emotional excitement); or yellow (liver disease) (Table 7-2).

In assessing pupil reaction, the athletic trainer must first ascertain whether both pupils are responding equally to light. When exposed to light, pupils should constrict and become smaller. The opposite should occur as the pupils respond to darkness; they should dilate, or get bigger. Pupils of unequal size may indicate a closed head injury. To obtain the ideal assessment of pupil reaction, the athletic trainer should remember the acronym PEARL: *p*upils *e*qual *a*nd *r*eactive to *l*ight.

Primary Assessment

The primary assessment, a rapid, systematic evaluation of the injured person, is designed to help the athletic trainer make quick decisions regarding the patient's status.[1,5] Using the emergency skills and equipment discussed in the previous sections, athletic trainers will be prepared to provide emergency care. Combining these

tachycardia rapid pulse rate (>100 bpm)
bradycardia slow pulse rate (<60 bpm)

TABLE 7-2 Assessment of Skin Temperature and Color

SKIN TEMPERATURE	POSSIBLE CONDITION(S)
Cool and clammy	Shock
Cold and moist	Losing heat
Cold and dry	Cold
Hot and dry	High fever or serious heat illness
Hot and moist	High fever or mild/moderate heat illness
Goose pimples	Chills, cold, pain, fever, or excitement
SKIN APPEARANCE	**POSSIBLE CONDITION(S)**
Pink	Normal
Pale	Blood loss, hypotension, or emotional stress
Blue (cyanotic)	Lack of oxygen
Flushed/reddish	Heat exposure or emotional excitement
Yellow	Liver condition or disease

skills in an orderly process allows the athletic trainer to move confidently from one step to the next, gathering all of the information necessary to make an appropriate decision.

For example, to assess a fallen worker at an industrial plant, the athletic trainer must first determine whether the scene is safe enough to enter. Another example in moving sequentially through the appropriate steps of the primary assessment is establishing an open airway before checking for circulation. On many occasions, much of the primary assessment is performed as the athletic trainer approaches the injured person. The athletic trainer should observe whether the patient is moving because mobility requires a patent airway and circulation. If the patient is not moving, the athletic trainer should look for the patient's chest to rise and fall. If the patient is unconscious, the athletic trainer should assume that he or she has sustained a cervical spine injury and act accordingly. Primary assessment involves nine steps, which are outlined in the following sections.

Step 1: Ensure Scene Safety

- Visually inspect surroundings for any objects that may compromise safety.
- Ensure that the game or practice has been stopped and that the playing area is safe to enter.
- Scan the playing area for other injured persons; if more than one is present, determine who needs your attention first.
- Ascertain whether EMS, fire rescue, or other help is needed, and make the call immediately. If other potential rescuers are nearby, have them activate the EAP by making the 911 call while you continue your primary assessment.

Step 2: Determine the Level of Consciousness and Stabilize the Cervical Spine

- Determine the patient's level of consciousness. Assess alertness, verbal abilitics, pain lcvels, and responsiveness. Consider whether the patient is alert and talking. Does the patient respond to a pinch or the pressure of your knuckles on his or her sternum? Look for any physical or verbal responses to touch. If the athlete is unconscious, assume that he or she may also have a cervical spine injury.
- Stabilize the cervical spine by maintaining the position of the head and neck as it was found.

Step 3: Determine Life Threats

- Look for any obvious situations that may immediately threaten or compromise the patient's life. These may be beyond the athletic trainer's ability to manage.
- Call 911 to activate the EAP and initiate rapid response from EMS or fire rescue if these measures have not already been taken.

Step 4: Maintain or Establish an Open Airway

Based on your findings from the previous three steps, determine whether you need to open the airway using head-tilt chin lift or a modified jaw thrust. If no cervical injury is suspected, the standard head-tilt chin lift may be used. However, an injury to the cervical spine is possible, a modified jaw thrust is the accepted method for opening the airway.[1,5]

Step 5: Look, Listen, and Feel for Signs of Breathing

- Look for the chest to rise while listening for breath sounds as you place your hand on the patient's chest to feel it rise and fall[2] (Figure 7-19). If the patient is not breathing, administer two breaths. If air does not go in, reposition and administer two more breaths.
- If you can establish an airway and the patient is not breathing, immediately begin rescue breathing.
- If the airway is obstructed, clear it. The method used to clear the airway will be determined by the person's age and condition. Typically, a blind finger sweep is used only with unconscious adult victims. If the victim is conscious and can breathe but the airway is obstructed, perform the appropriate Heimlich maneuver to forcefully expel the lodged object.

Step 6: Assess Circulation

- By placing two fingers on the carotid artery, you can determine whether the injured person has a pulse. Find the carotid pulse by sliding your fingers (not

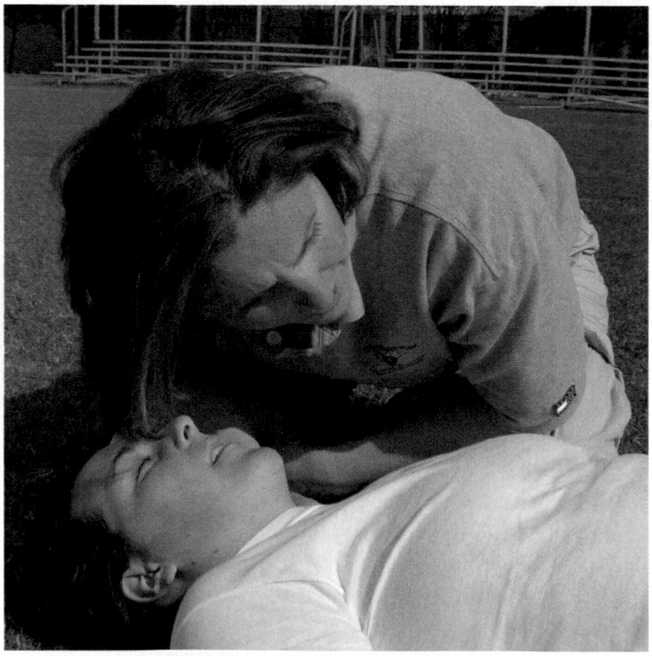

FIGURE 7-19 Breathing assessment involves looking, listening, and feeling. Look for the rise and fall of the chest while listening for breath sounds and feeling for the normal rise and fall.

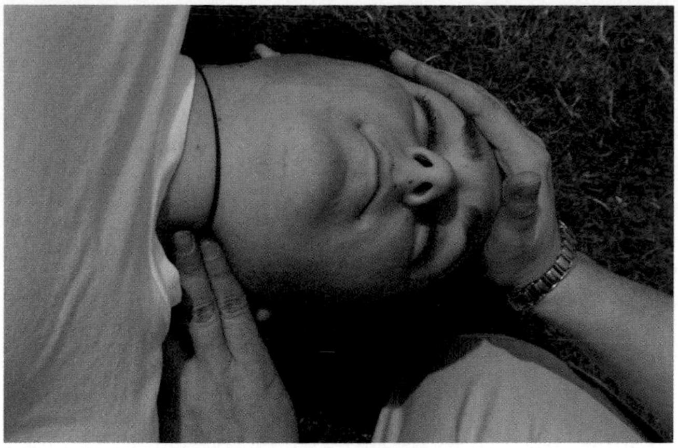

FIGURE 7-20 To assess an individual's pulse, the athletic trainer can slide the fingers (not the thumb) from the midline of the neck down until a groove is felt; this is the location of the carotid artery.

your thumb) from the midline of the neck down until you feel a groove.[5] By feeling for both the rate and strength of the pulse, you can assess the presence of blood circulation (Figure 7-20).

- If there is no pulse, begin CPR immediately. (Please note that this book is not intended to take the place of CPR training. The reader should seek more detailed information on the appropriate steps before attempting CPR.)

Step 7: Assess Skin Color and Temperature

- Assess the patient's skin temperature by touching his or her face with the back of your hand.
- Check the skin for any discolorations of the face and neck and the injured area.

Step 8: Control Bleeding

- Most major bleeding may be controlled through direct pressure. Arterial bleeding, any blood loss originating from a large or diffuse area, or any suspected internal bleeding is considered major.
- Use proper universal precautions and PPE when caring for bleeding of any kind.
- With major blood loss, elevate the feet above the heart to keep the patient from slipping into shock. If a back or neck injury or any type of lower extremity fracture is possible, do not elevate the legs and control bleeding through direct pressure.

Step 9: Transport

- Determine whether the injured person requires emergency transport to a nearby hospital emergency department or trauma unit or whether the patient should remain on-site.
- If any of the aforementioned steps resulted in your performing reactive measures, the patient should be transported immediately to a hospital. Box 7-4 outlines the criteria for making decisions regarding emergency transport.
- Under no circumstances should the athletic trainer transport a person with a life-threatening injury in his or her personal vehicle. When in doubt, call 911 so that EMS personnel can transport the patient to the nearest hospital. It is always best to allow EMS personnel to transport the patient because these professionals are equipped to handle any emergency that may arise while the patient is in transit.

BOX 7-4 Reasons to Activate Emergency Transport

Any of the following conditions is sufficient reason to activate the emergency action plan and transport the injured individual to a hospital for further evaluation:

- Loss of consciousness
- Suspected cervical injury
- Unresponsiveness
- Need to establish an airway
- Performance of rescue breathing
- Performance of cardiopulmonary resuscitation
- Major bleeding that is difficult to control
- Any obvious or suspected fracture

The athletic trainer is at a distinct disadvantage while providing care during an emergency. Unlike paramedics or emergency room staff, the athletic trainer often has a personal relationship with the patient. Because emergencies are often highly emotional situations, it is imperative that the primary assessment be so ingrained in the athletic trainer's behavior that each step is taken as part of a rehearsed script, with emotions suppressed in the interest of making rational decisions. The appropriate response to an emergency situation must be rehearsed and practiced often, and all those assisting the athletic trainer in the EAP should be familiar with the primary assessment.

Points to Ponder
Why should you never transport an injured athlete in your personal vehicle?

Secondary Assessment

A secondary assessment is performed after the primary assessment and is designed to determine nonlife-threatening injuries or injuries that are not immediately obvious that could become life threatening. The secondary assessment involves evaluating the body systematically from head to toes. A thorough history is the first step to a secondary assessment, followed by systematic inspection of the body both visually and through palpation. If the athlete is able to tell the athletic trainer the specific location of the injury, the athletic trainer can focus the secondary assessment on that body part; this process is covered in subsequent chapters. Steps in the secondary assessment are listed in the following sections.

Step 1: Obtain an Accurate History

Question the patient about type of pain, signs and symptoms, allergies, medications, other pertinent history, last oral intake, and any events preceding the injury or illness.[1] The acronym SAMPLE, as follows, is useful to remember in diagnosing injuries and illnesses:

S	Signs and symptoms
A	Allergies
M	Medications
P	Pertinent past history
L	Last oral intake (food, hydration, medications)
E	Events leading up to the injury

Step 2: Visually Inspect the Pupils

The acronym PEARL assists in remembering the way the eyes function in response to light. If any deviation is present, make an appropriate medical referral as quickly as possible. PEARL stands for the following:

P	Pupils
E	Equal
A	and
R	Reactive to
L	Light

Step 3: Visually Inspect the Mouth, Nose, and Neck

- Look for any signs of fluid coming out of the mouth, nose, or ears.
- The neck should be inspected visually to ensure that the trachea is in the midline and has not deviated to either side. A trachea that has deviated to the side is a medical emergency.
- Examine the jugular veins looking for abnormalities or distention. If distention is present, a heart problem is typically the cause. Again, even though this information is obtained in the secondary assessment phase, this situation is now a medical emergency that requires immediate transport to a hospital by ambulance.

Step 4: Palpate the Body from Head to Toe

The next step in the secondary assessment is the tactile portion. Never palpate a body part without first visually inspecting it. Begin the palpations by using the DCAP-BTLS acronym, "dee-cap beetles," to remember the palpation foci—deformities, contusions, abrasions, punctures or penetrations, burns, tenderness, laceration, and swelling:[1]

D	Deformities
C	Contusions
A	Abrasions
P	Punctures or penetrations
B	Burns
T	Tenderness
L	Lacerations
S	Swelling

Palpations progress systematically, moving down the body from the head, as follows:

Cervical spine: Look and feel for obvious deformity, swelling, or point tenderness. Point tenderness over the spinous processes is a particular cause for concern because it may indicate a cervical spine fracture. Point tenderness and any neurological complaints, as well as any restricted movements, suddenly turn this nonemergency into an emergency. Steps to maintain cervical stabilization should be taken at this time.

Chest: Look and palpate for signs of rib fractures or paradoxical motion (movement of a section of the chest that moves in an opposite direction from the rest of the chest; this implies flail chest). If flail chest is present or the athlete is in respiratory distress, activate the EAP immediately.

Abdomen: Divide the abdomen into four quadrants using the navel as the midpoint of the quadrants. Palpate each quadrant, feeling for tenderness, rigidity, or rebounding from any of the major organs in each quadrant (see Chapter 5).

Pelvis: Assess the pelvis by palpating each iliac crest. If a fracture is suspected, the patient should be transported to a hospital as directed by the EAP.

Lower extremities: Assess the lower extremities by palpating first at the trunk and moving outward. Assess for pulse, reflexes, sensory responses, deformity, swelling, and point tenderness, as previously discussed.[1]

Upper extremities: Repeat the protocol for lower extremities with the upper extremities.

Posterior aspects: Once the preceding steps are completed, begin assessment of the posterior aspects of the body. Use the DCAP-BTLS (dee-cap beetles) mnemonic to systematically move through this assessment. Move head to toe, as in the anterior assessment.

Step 5: Reassess Vital Signs as Necessary

If the vital signs warrant it, the athletic trainer may need to refer the individual to a physician or to EMS.

MANAGEMENT OF EMERGENCY SITUATIONS

Many injuries occur daily in athletic training settings, ranging from minor to limb- or life-threatening. An athletic trainer's responsibility is to manage the injury or illness as well as possible so that a nonemergency does not become an emergency. Some situations, however, result in injuries and illnesses that unexpectedly develop into emergencies. At these moments, the decisions and actions of the athletic trainer can help save a limb or a life. Understanding emergent situations and their proper management can prevent the unthinkable from happening.

The injury-response decision tree provides a sequential process to determine whether the individual may return to play or work or is referred to a medical facility, or whether the EAP must be activated (Figure 7-21). The ultimate goal with all injuries and illnesses is a complete return to activity without limitations. The reality, on the other hand, is that some injuries or illnesses prevent individuals from returning to their prior levels of activity. With that in mind, the athletic trainer must endeavor to properly manage every situation so that the lives and limbs of athletes under their care do not become compromised—or, in the event that injuries do occur, that they result in as little permanent damage as possible.

The rest of this chapter deals with injuries that the athletic trainer may see in the course of a career. Starting with the most serious and potentially life- or limb-threatening conditions, descriptions and treatment steps are provided to ensure that adequate care is provided. Other emergent injuries and conditions not mentioned in this chapter are addressed later in this book, in the context of diagnosis and management.

Cardiac Emergencies

Cardiac emergencies occur during athletic activities every year. The key to handling cardiac emergencies

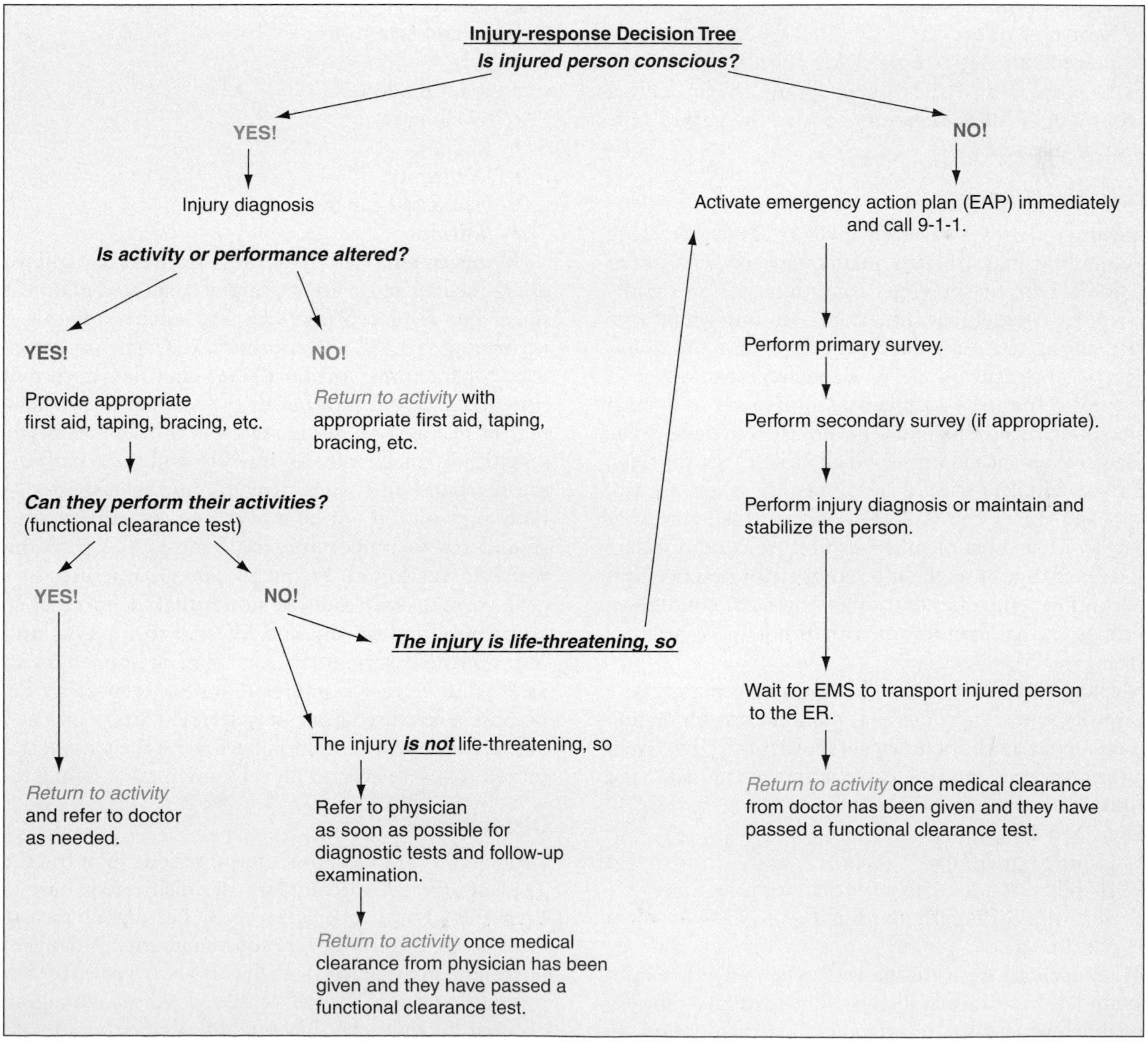

FIGURE 7-21 The injury-response decision tree provides the athletic trainer with a tool to assess whether an injured athlete may return to play, whether that individual must be referred to a physician, or whether the EAP should be activated.

is preparation: having the right equipment, knowing how to use the equipment, conducting an appropriate primary assessment, and executing the EAP. All cardiac emergencies are potentially life threatening. When a cardiac emergency arises, the EAP should be activated immediately.

Mechanism: Cardiac emergencies often have an insidious onset but can also result from severe blunt force trauma or genetic abnormalities.

Signs and symptoms: Most often, there are no symptoms until the patient goes into cardiac arrest or experiences any of the following symptoms:

- Chest pains
- Pain radiating down the arm or between the shoulder blades
- Nausea
- Profuse sweating
- Tightness of the chest
- Shortness of breath

Management: Activate the EAP, and call 911. Begin steps to employ an AED if appropriate. Begin CPR if appropriate; all steps necessary to save the person's life should be initiated.

Respiratory Distress

Respiratory distress is the term given to severe breathing difficulty that may result in inadequate oxygenation of the blood. Like the previous conditions, it can rapidly turn into an emergent situation. An important step in preventing this emergency situation is to establish which, if any, athletes or workers have asthma or a history of respiratory problems. Complaints of asthma or a respiratory illness should never be taken lightly. The athletic trainer should know which athletes use inhalers, and these inhalers should be accessible when needed, not locked up in the athlete's locker. Make sure that athletes with asthma or other respiratory conditions are able to exchange enough air to compete or practice. It is important to remember that other emergent conditions, including cardiac conditions, can result in respiratory distress.

Mechanisms: All of the following can bring about a respiratory emergency: asthma, pleural effusion, hemothorax, pneumothorax, hyperventilation, hypoventilation, apnea, airway obstructions, trauma, and pneumonia.

Signs and symptoms:

- Labored breathing
- Inability to adequately ventilate or oxygenate
- Shortness of breath (dypsnea)
- Weakness

Management: Activate the EAP when anyone exhibits complete respiratory distress. The primary concern is establishing normal oxygenation and ventilation. In cases of incomplete respiratory distress, determine the severity and potential cause. Assist the athlete with his or her inhaler if appropriate. The return to normal respiratory function will decrease the burden on the heart and prevent a worrisome cascade of events. If respiration does not quickly return to normal, activate the EAP.

Fractures

Fractures usually are the result of excessive loading. They can occur from being kicked, planting and twisting rapidly, being hit by an object, or undergoing repetitive stress over a prolonged period. Although bones are generally very durable, excessive external loading or trauma can cause them to fracture.

Mechanism: Fractures may result from external loading with any variation (e.g., twisting, bending, compression) that is greater than normal—for example, getting kicked in the lower leg while playing soccer, falling off a ladder onto an outstretched hand, or dropping a heavy load on a toe.

Signs and symptoms:

- Pain
- Point tenderness
- Swelling
- Redness
- Deformity
- Decreased range of motion
- Warmth

Management: Ice and immobilization (i.e., splinting) are immediate steps for the care of suspected minor fractures. For displaced fractures, immediate splinting and activation of EMS are appropriate. Casts are typically used for fractures; for more severe injuries, open reduction and external fixation or other surgical procedures may be necessary. The management of fractures depends specifically on the type of fracture and the condition of the surrounding tissues. If a fracture is suspected, the body part should not be moved and the athletic trainer should try to immobilize the bone in the position in which it was found. Frequently, minor fractures of fingers, toes, or scaphoids or nondisplaced fractures may be immobilized on-site and referred to a physician for X-ray; if necessary, a cast or splint is applied as soon as possible. Other fractures require transport by EMS. Because a fractured bone may sever an artery or a nerve, all fractures must be immobilized, with the patient transported to a safe area to prevent any further damage.

Dislocations

Dislocations are sometimes more serious than fractures. The soft tissues surrounding the dislocated joint may be stretched and torn so severely that drastic measures must be taken to restore the joint's integrity. A dangerous possible consequence of dislocations is nerve or blood vessel disruption. Nerve or blood vessel damage can occur at the moment of injury or during reduction of the dislocation. The athletic trainer must exercise extreme caution to keep from inflicting further damage to the joint beyond the original injury. The athletic trainer should never attempt to reduce major joints but should instead immobilize them and activate EMS. Dislocations and fractures can turn into life- and limb-threatening emergencies if the blood supply or nerves become compromised.

Mechanism: Dislocations are often caused by violent trauma that involves separation of the bones at the joint.

Signs and symptoms:
- Gross deformity at a joint
- Pain
- Swelling
- Loss of movement and function
- Decreased range of motion

Management: Immobilize the limb(s), and activate EMS if a major joint is dislocated. The potential for arterial bleeding or rupture warrants immediate transport of these individuals. Dislocations of minor joints can be managed on-site by immobilization, ice, compression, elevation, and referral to a physician as soon as possible for further diagnostic tests and reduction.

Bleeding

Bleeding is very common and can occur both internally and externally. Internal bleeding typically results after soft tissue injuries and traumatic blunt force trauma. Traumatic internal bleeding injuries are uncommon but potentially quite serious because the outward signs are not readily obvious. The athletic trainer should be prepared for these situations, which can turn into emergencies if not properly identified and managed. External bleeding is frequently associated with various tears of the skin such as lacerations (i.e., cuts), abrasions, and punctures. Arterial blood spurts out and is bright red in color. Venous blood seeps out slowly and steadily, whereas capillary blood tends to trickle out.

Mechanism: Internal bleeding results from blunt force trauma, whereas external bleeding results from any tearing or penetration of the skin.

Signs and symptoms: Internal bleeding is not always obvious, especially when it occurs in the abdomen, but it may be accompanied by the following:
- Abdominal rigidity
- Nausea
- Discomfort

Internal bleeding in the extremities results in the following:
- Swelling
- Point tenderness
- Redness or hemorrhaging
- Warmth

External bleeding results in the following:
- Swelling
- Skin deformities
- Increased skin temperature at the site of injury

Management: Minor internal bleeding (i.e., hemorrhage) in a muscle or joint is best managed by following the tenets of PRICES, an acronym that stands for *p*articipation, *r*ecovery, *i*ce, *c*ompression, *e*levation, and *s*tabilization. Internal bleeding in the abdomen must be recognized and referred for medical intervention and further diagnostic tests. Minor external bleeding is managed by cleansing the wound and covering it with a sterile bandage held in place with an adhesive tape or bandage. Excessive external bleeding is best managed by applying direct pressure over the wound with a dressing. As the blood soaks through the dressing, new dressings should be applied on top of the original one. Use of PPEs and adherence to standards developed by the Occupational Safety and Health Administration (OSHA) regarding bloodborne pathogens are of utmost importance with all bleeding injuries.

Shock

A medical emergency, shock always requires activation of the EAP. Shock is the body's reaction to a decrease in blood circulation to the vital organs. It may be caused by massive external or internal bleeding or an allergic reaction to certain stimuli. The major forms of shock that athletic trainers are most likely to encounter are **hypovolemic shock** and **anaphylactic shock**.

Mechanism: Hypovolemic shock is the result of decreased blood volume occasioned by internal or external bleeding. Usually, it is due to traumatic injuries. Anaphylactic shock is the result of a severe reaction to a stimulus, such as a bee sting, medications, and certain foods or perfumes. Cardiogenic shock is the result of ineffective pumping of the heart and is associated with damage to the heart.

Signs and symptoms:
- Very low blood pressure
- Depending on the specific type of shock, one or more of the following:
  - Anxiety or agitation
  - Rapid, weak pulse
  - Confusion
  - Rapid, shallow breathing
  - Cold, pale, clammy skin
  - Bluish lips and fingernails
  - Dizziness, light-headedness, or faintness
  - Low or nonexistent urine output
  - Profuse sweating, moist skin
  - Unconsciousness

hypovolemic shock reaction to decreased blood volume caused by internal or external bleeding

anaphylactic shock severe reaction to a stimulus (allergen) such as a bee sting, medication, or food

Management: Activate the EAP immediately. Perform a primary assessment, and act accordingly. Monitor breathing and pulse at least every 5 minutes. Perform a secondary assessment. If there are no obvious fractures or head, neck, or spine injuries, place the patient in the **shock position** by raising the legs approximately 12 inches above the heart while the patient is in a supine position. Never elevate the head. Keep the patient as warm and comfortable as possible while waiting for EMS to arrive,[1] and respond to any findings from the secondary assessment.

Abdominal Distress

Any type of pain or discomfort in the abdomen is considered abdominal distress. Careful attention must be made to the type and location of the pain because these are good indicators of the underlying conditions. Abdominal pain may be referred from other injuries or illnesses. Frequently, because of the generalized nature of the infection, a severe case of cold or flu may cause systemic pain and result in pronounced soreness or tenderness of the stomach or groin. Pain may also be indirectly proportional to the severity of the injury. It is important to rely on knowledge of the abdominal organs housed in each quadrant. Pain or distress in any region will help the athletic trainer isolate the true cause and underlying condition(s).

Mechanisms: Abdominal distress may result from splenic rupture, appendicitis, traveler's diarrhea, gastritis, pancreatitis, gallbladder or kidney stones, trauma, internal bleeding, and infection.

Signs and symptoms:

- Pain
- Point tenderness
- Rigidity over organs
- Fever
- Pain in the chest, neck, or shoulder
- Blood in vomit or stool
- Inability to defecate

Management: Severe, acute onset of abdominal pain should prompt the activation of the EAP. However, the athletic trainer should be able to distinguish between the abrupt onset of intolerance to foods and true abdominal distress that results from trauma or illness. If the onset is gradual, medical attention is still warranted but not necessarily in an emergent fashion. Perform the secondary assessment palpating the uninvolved side before palpating the involved side. Depress the abdomen to a depth of approximately 1 inch to locate the organs. A normal abdomen is soft, whereas a firm abdomen indicates an internal injury. Watch for specific areas of point tenderness.

Diabetic Emergencies

At some point during his or her career, the athletic trainer is likely to work with a diabetic individual. Diabetic emergencies are typically the result of **hypoglycemia** or **hyperglycemia**. Hypoglycemia, the most common diabetic emergency, is due to low blood sugar levels. A high blood sugar level, or hyperglycemia, is seen less frequently. As with chronic respiratory disorders, knowing which individuals have diabetes is the athletic trainer's first line of defense in managing these situations. To best respond to the emergency, the athletic trainer must determine whether the athlete is suffering from hypoglycemia or hyperglycemia. Also, knowing whether the individual takes insulin, how much, and how often he or she needs it will help the athletic trainer respond quickly and appropriately to the athlete's needs.

Mechanism: Diabetic emergencies result from inappropriate amounts of circulating blood sugars (glucose).

Signs and symptoms:

Hypoglycemia

- Confusion
- Combativeness
- Dizziness
- Sweating
- Weakness
- Incoherence
- Shaking, seizures
- Unconsciousness
- Hunger
- Headache

Hyperglycemia

- Fruity breath
- Deep and rapid breathing
- Nausea or vomiting
- Dry skin and mouth
- Flushed face
- Stomach pain

Management: For hypoglycemia, monitor the patient's vital signs. Blood glucose may be monitored with a blood glucose meter. If the athlete is conscious, offer juice, hard candy, sport gels, sugar, or oral glucose tablets and wait about 15 minutes. If the athlete is stabilizing, then merely monitor him or her and eventually allow normal food and fluid intake. If the athlete does not stabilize, administer more sugar. If the athlete does not regain normal status, activate the EAP. Oral glucose tablets or another form of nonperishable sugar should be kept in the athletic training or trauma kit. The athletic training kit should also contain a blood glucose meter if any of the athletes are known to have diabetes.

If any symptoms suggest that an individual is suffering from hyperglycemia, activate the EAP immediately.

---

hypoglycemia abnormally low circulating blood sugar (glucose)

hyperglycemia abnormally high circulating blood sugar (glucose)

Hyperglycemia is an emergent situation that could turn into a life-or-death situation.

Soft Tissue Injuries

Athletic trainers encounter a great number of soft tissue injuries. Not all soft tissue injuries are the same. Sprains (i.e., ligamentous injuries), strains (i.e., muscular or tendinous injuries), contusions (i.e., bruises), tendinitis (i.e., inflammation of musculotendinous tissue), and bursitis (i.e., inflammation of the joint bursa sacs) are the most common soft tissue injuries. Because other underlying injuries may occur simultaneously, athletic trainers must perform a thorough secondary assessment to rule out further complications.

Mechanism: Most soft tissue injuries occur because of blunt force trauma or overuse.

Signs and symptoms:

- Discomfort
- Decreased range of motion
- Swelling
- Redness
- Lumps or depressions
- Point tenderness.

Management: Acute injuries can typically be managed with PRICES:

P	Participation in activity or sport on some level
R	Recovery (rest or appropriate exercises)
I	Ice modalities
C	Compression with ace wraps, braces, or immobilizers
E	Elevation of the body part above the heart
S	Stabilization of the injured body part

Chronic injuries can typically be managed with CHEAT":

C	Compression
H	Heat modalities
E	Elevation
A	Active exercise
T	Timely return to activity

Syncope

Syncope, or fainting, occurs for several reasons, ranging from mild to serious. Typically, low blood pressure, resulting in decreased blood flow to the brain, incites a syncope episode. The most common cause of syncope in younger athletes is a vasovagal response, which may be caused by a sudden change in position (e.g., from supine to standing) or a response to a traumatic situation or pain. There are other more serious causes for syncope, but these are usually not immediately apparent to the athletic trainer at the scene. The most important thing to remember is that the person in syncope is unconscious.

Mechanism: Syncope results from a vasovagal response caused by decreased venous return or reaction to pain, from cardiac conditions, or from epilepsy.

Signs and symptoms:

- Nausea
- Blurred vision
- Sweating
- Dizziness followed by unconsciousness

Management: The athletic trainer must perform a primary assessment to understand the cause of the syncope. The patient may regain consciousness very quickly or experience respiratory distress or cardiac failure. Continue to follow the steps of the primary assessment, and activate the EAP. If the athlete regains consciousness quickly, remember that the underlying cause of the syncope episode must still be identified. Even if the syncope resolves without intervention, the patient should not return to normal activities without appropriate medical clearance.

SUMMARY

Athletic trainers respond to many situations over the course of their careers. Some of these situations begin as emergencies, and others become emergencies during the primary assessment. The athletic trainer's most important responsibility is to ensure the best possible outcome for these individuals by knowing how to respond properly and efficiently. The athletic trainer's ability to make appropriate decisions depends on the availability of appropriate emergency equipment and the presence of personnel who know how to use it. Quickly activating the EAP and contacting 911 when necessary are crucial steps in deterring a limb- or life-threatening event. Understanding the steps involved in the primary and secondary assessments will help the athletic trainer to make critical decisions during these unusually demanding circumstances. Practicing the use of the equipment and training with the assessment tools are paramount in making the right decision at the right time. After all, these situations are called emergencies because they come without warning.

syncope fainting

Revisiting the OPENING *Scenario*

An athlete has just collapsed on the track after a 15 minute warm-up, on a hot day, after making himself vomit and then standing rapidly. You approach him to begin your primary assessment. You assess his breathing and level of consciousness as you move toward him. He does not respond to verbal commands but does seem to respond to a sternal rub. You open his airway using the head-tilt chin lift because you do not suspect a cervical injury and look, listen, and feel for respirations. He is breathing, fortunately, which means that he has circulation. You check the quality of the pulse and skin color and temperature and confirm that the athlete, though unconscious, is breathing and has circulation. You activate the EAP, and call 911. You notice also in the primary survey that his skin was warm to the touch and sweaty.

While waiting for EMS, you soak him in ice towels to treat his heat illness and get out your trauma bag.[9] Your next step is to begin the secondary assessment while waiting on help to arrive. Remember that the first step in the secondary assessment is the recording of vital signs. As you begin to take his vital signs, the athlete begins to regain consciousness and attempts to stand up. The athlete is alert and oriented to his surroundings and the events preceding his collapse. You continue your secondary assessment until the athlete is transported to a local hospital, where he is evaluated and released. In your final diagnosis, you describe a bout of sudden fainting caused by a rapid change in blood pressure and stimulation of the vagal nerve after induced vomiting.

Issues & Ethics

Once again, Mary Helen is the marquee performer in the show. Her athletic abilities, flexibility, and grace have drawn people from all over the Northeast. She moves across the stage with an ease and authority that bedazzle even the most sophisticated spectator, earning standing ovations every night.

Mary Helen is the reason that most people come to see this show. Tonight, as she draws the crowd members to their feet, she lands slightly off balance on her last combination of moves with her partner. You notice that he attempts to support her and carries her through their last move. As they move closer to where you watch offstage, it becomes obvious that she cannot bear weight on her left leg. Once she's offstage, you notice that she has marked swelling starting just above the lateral malleoli and down into her toes, and she complains of a loss of sensation in her great toe.

Only 2 hours remain until the next show begins. You have already been informed by the box office that several newspaper critics will be attending the evening performance. During yesterday's practice, her understudy failed even to remember simple voice cues from the director. What are your options? Do you attempt to tape and wrap her leg in the hope that she can make it through the performance without exacerbating the injury? Do you let the director know the severity of her injury? Tonight is a once-in-a-lifetime moment for Mary Helen's career, possibly her last chance to make it to Broadway.

Web Links

American Heart Association: www.americanheart.org

American Red Cross: www.redcross.org

Minneapolis Heart Institute Foundation: "Sudden Death in Athletes": www.nata.org/employers/cu/emer_medplan.pdf

National Athletic Trainers' Association, Position Statement: "Emergency Planning": http://www.nata.org/statements/position/emergencyplanning.pdf

National Athletic Trainers' Association, Consensus Statements: "Appropriate Medical Care for Secondary School-Age Athletes": www.nata.org/statements/consensus/Consensus%20Statement_Final%20Version_Sept02.pdf

National Center for Catastrophic Sport Injury Research: www.unc.edu/depts/nccsi/

National Collegiate Athletic Association, *2006–07 NCAA Sports Medicine Handbook*: www.ncaa.org/library/sports_sciences/sports_med_handbook/2006-07/2006-07_sports_medicine_handbook.pdf

National Registry of Emergency Medical Technicians: www.nremt.org

University of Georgia Sports Medicine Emergency Plan: www.nata.org/employers/cu/emer_medplan.pdf

References

1. Limmer D, O'Keefe M, editors: *Emergency care*, ed 10, Upper Saddle River, NJ, 2005, Prentice Hall/Pearson Education.
2. National Athletic Trainers' Association: *Athletic training educational competencies*, ed 4, Dallas, 2006, Author.
3. Board of Certification: *Role delineation study*, ed 5, Omaha, Neb, 2003, Author.
4. University of Georgia: *University of Georgia sports medicine emergency plan*, Athens, Ga, 2001, Author. Retrieved June 24, 2007, from www.nata.org/employers/cu/emer_medplan.pdf.
5. The American National Red Cross: *CPR/AED for the professional rescuer*, San Bruno, Calif, 2001, StayWell.
6. Kleiner D et al: Prehospital care of the spine-injured athlete: a document from the inter-association task force for appropriate care of the spine-injured athlete, Dallas, 2001, National Athletic Trainers' Association.
7. Browner B, Lenworth J, editors, and American Academy of Orthopedic Surgeons: *Emergency care and transportation of sick and injured*, ed 7, Sudbury, Mass, 1999, Jones and Bartlett.
8. Miller MG et al: National Athletic Trainers' Association position statement: management of asthma in athletes, *J Athl Train* 40:2, 2005.
9. Binkley HM et al: National Athletic Trainers' Association position statement: exertional heat illness, *J Athl Train*, 37:3, 2002.

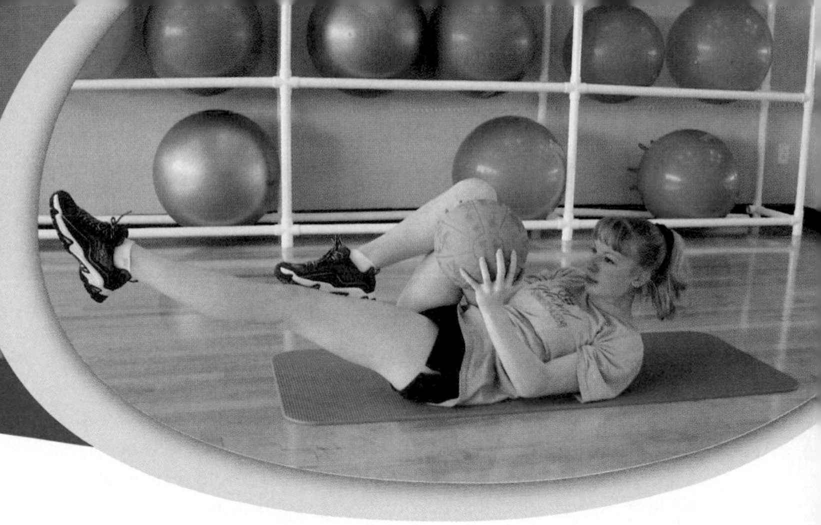

8 Therapeutic Techniques

NANCY H. CUMMINGS AND SUE STANLEY-GREEN

Learning Goals

1. Demonstrate the ability to develop rehabilitation goals for various diagnoses.
2. Identify various modalities used in the rehabilitation process to assist in the healing of acute, as opposed to chronic, injuries and illnesses.
3. Employ effective strategies in selecting appropriate therapeutic modalities.
4. Describe the importance of conditioning and rehabilitative exercises in the overall return-to-activity plan of care and in the prevention of injuries.
5. Understand various modes of exercise and the timeliness of each in returning clients to their activities.
6. Create a comprehensive return-to-activity program for various diagnoses.

One of the most rewarding aspects of being an athletic trainer is watching injured clients return to activity in a manner that exceeds their expectations and allows them to resume their daily lives. A recent study examining the work skills and responsibilities of athletic trainers revealed that their knowledge of sports injuries and rehabilitation skills were exceptional[1] (Figure 8-1). Before clients may resume their previous level of activity (i.e., be rehabilitated), several things must happen. Obtaining a correct diagnosis provides the groundwork for establishing a plan of care that will enable clients to return to their chosen activities as quickly and as safely as possible. Determining the cause of the injury or illness and understanding the client's pain and current phase of injury healing are critical. It is also necessary to know all the pertinent details about the activity to which the client wishes to return. What type of activity is it? What position does the client play, and how much playing time does the client generally get? How significant is the client's presence on the team? What are the client's activity demands, and what level of play is he or she expected to resume? Answering these questions helps the athletic trainer in developing a comprehensive rehabilitation plan specific to the individual client. Once the plan is established, the key to success lies in remaining open to making modifications when the client's circumstances change, as they inevitably will. This chapter provides readers with the information needed to demonstrate a basic level of understanding and application of therapeutic techniques or rehabilitation skills. By building on this foundational knowledge, readers will eventually develop exceptional rehabilitation skills.

THERAPEUTIC REHABILITATION PROGRAMS

The most important aspect of designing a therapeutic rehabilitation program is to start with the end in mind. Before the athletic trainer can create a successful plan of care, he or she must know what the program is supposed to be accomplishing. For example, Bob wants to be an Olympic runner; he does not go to the track every day merely to run for exercise. He knows not to go to the gym and lift weights for 5 hours every day. Finding a balanced blend of exercises that train his body to respond appropriately is critical to his success. He considers all of the factors that go into the making of an Olympic champion and creates a plan accordingly. Factors such as cardiorespiratory fitness, flexibility, proprioception, strength, explosive power, and core stability all come together to create physical success. He also must consider

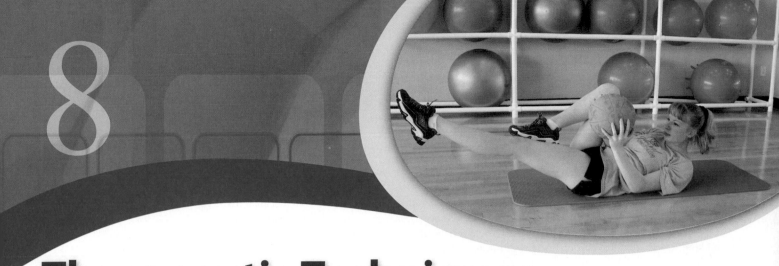

OPENING *Scenario*

Noah, a 44-year-old veteran employee at the local automobile manufacturing plant, reported that he was lifting a heavy load during his final shift at work last night. He was unable to find another co-worker to help, so he tackled the job himself. While he was lifting one of the boxes, which weighed at least 150 pounds, he pivoted on his left leg and rotated to his left side to place the box on a bench. He did not have much space to maneuver at the job site. It was near the end of his shift, and his wife had been home all day with their sick baby. He was anxious to get home to relieve his wife and to check on his daughter. After that last load was moved, he knew he could quit for the day and be home with his family.

Today Noah is complaining of diffuse pain and stiffness across his lower back, a burning sensation down the back of his left leg that stops above the knee, and a tightness that affects his left buttock and hamstring regions. Although his injury is less than 24 hours old, he needs to return to work as soon as possible so that he can continue to earn money for his family. The upcoming holidays are an unusually stressful time this year because his wife was recently laid off and is currently not working outside the home. Noah feels the pressure of being the sole source of income for the family. As the on-site athletic trainer providing acute care triage to the industrial workers at the plant, you are responsible for making a diagnosis and creating a plan of care. At your disposal are a fully equipped athletic training room and a rehabilitation room with resistance and cardiovascular equipment, exercise balls, medicine balls, and exercise tubing.

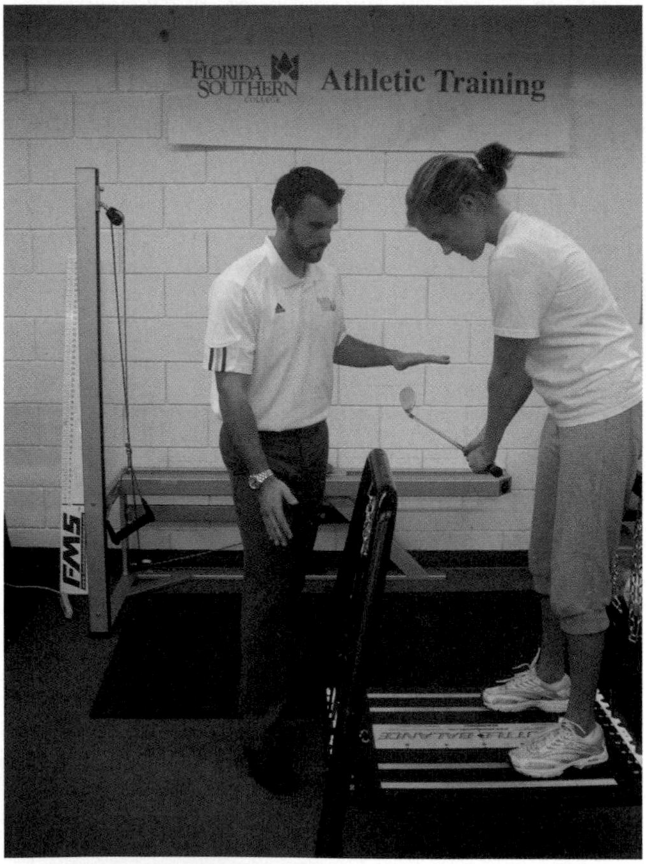

FIGURE 8-1 Facilitating a comprehensive rehabilitation program that allows return to play is a rewarding part of being an athletic trainer.

any modalities that he could use to either prevent soreness and pain or rehabilitate injuries as they occur. Mastery of all these factors is required if the human body is to perform exactly as it needs to and when it needs to. This, too, is the goal in designing a comprehensive rehabilitation program (Figure 8-2). Regardless of the type of activity that the athletic trainer is addressing, it is necessary to know, to the most detailed level possible, what the desired outcome should look like.

Combining modalities with conditioning and rehabilitative exercises is what constitutes the **therapeutic rehabilitation program. Acute injuries**, injuries that have occurred in the previous 24 to 48 hours, generally must be treated initially with modalities to relieve pain and inflammation. Then, if needed, exercises are incorporated into the treatment plan to allow for return to activity. **Chronic injuries**, injuries that have been persistent for more than 2 or 3 weeks, require a different approach. Exercise becomes the primary focus in the program. Modalities may be used as needed to complement the conditioning and rehabilitative exercises. The primary difference for program design is that acute injuries are modality intensive and chronic injuries are exercise intensive. Athletic trainers must be knowledgeable about both modalities and exercises to properly manage the injury, thus preventing re-injury and allowing for full return to activity.[2]

Diagnosing the Injury: Step One

An accurate diagnosis, based on careful attention to the client's description of his or her symptoms, is the most

therapeutic rehabilitation program plan of care combining modalities with conditioning and rehabilitative exercises

acute injuries injuries that have occurred in the last 24 to 48 hours

chronic injuries injuries that have persisted for longer than 2 or 3 weeks

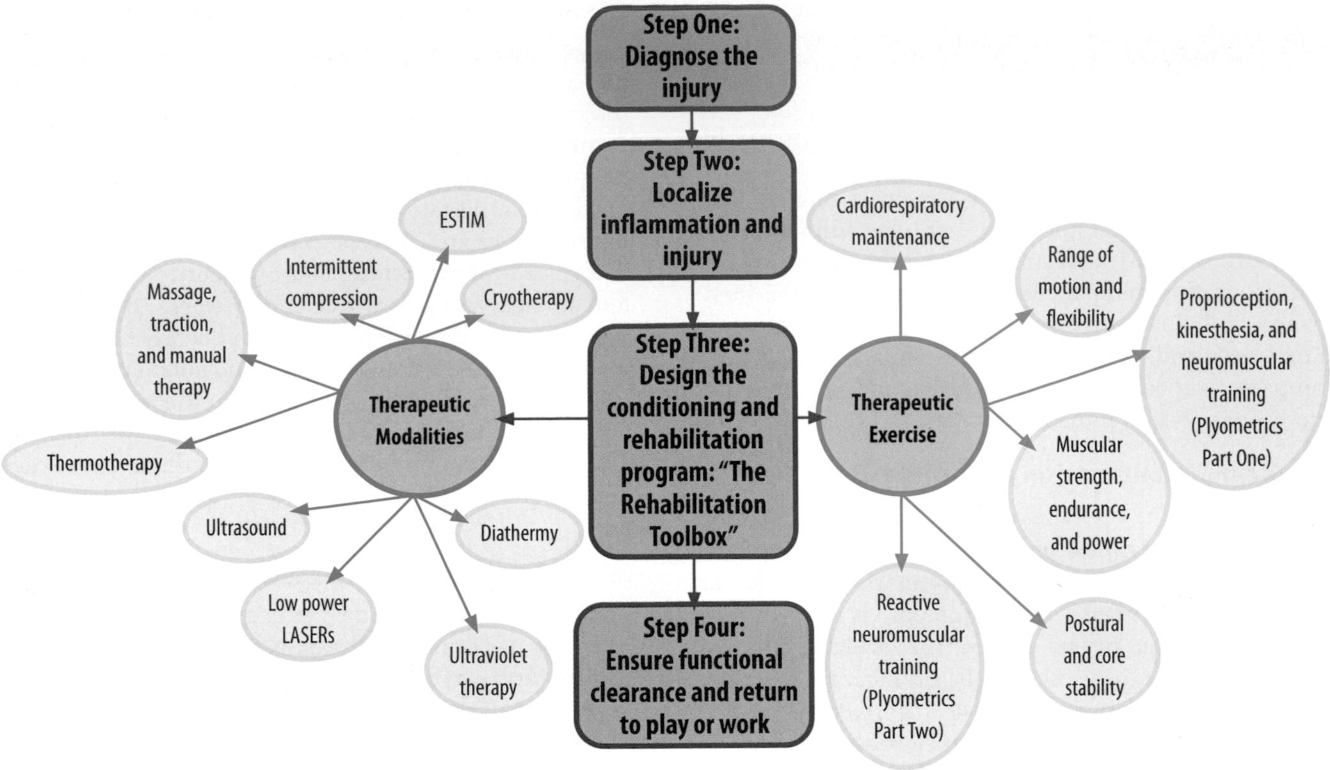

FIGURE 8-2 The major components that make up the comprehensive rehabilitation program.

important factor in guaranteeing a successful rehabilitation plan (Figure 8-3). Asking specific, relevant questions and then listening intently to the responses will lead to a more accurate diagnosis. The more detail elicited from the client, the easier the diagnostic process becomes.

Being on-site when the injury occurs is most helpful. Witnessing the injury or accident provides important information regarding the **mechanism of injury**, or why and how it occurred. These injuries are acute, or of recent onset, and are typically simple to diagnose. They respond well to immediate intervention.

Other injuries are more insidious; they do not have a definitive onset and often seem to appear from nowhere. After questioning, most people vaguely recall being annoyed by a seemingly insignificant injury. Usually, they ignore these injuries, assuming that they will eventually go away. Consequently, injuries of this type are often more challenging to diagnose because the answers to most of the athletic trainer's questions are frustratingly unclear. Clients simply cannot remember much about the mechanism of injury or even the injury itself. Injuries that emerged more than 2 weeks before the client sought treatment are considered chronic. As previously discussed, the physiological symptoms of chronic and acute injuries are markedly different. Therefore the rehabilitation programs reflect these differences in both modality and exercise selection.[2]

Knowing the mechanism of injury is an important factor in obtaining a correct diagnosis and selecting specific

mechanism of injury the "why" and "how" of an injury

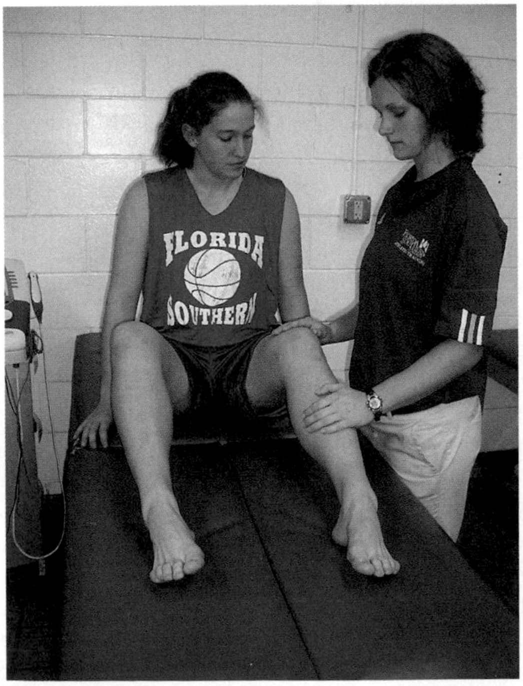

FIGURE 8-3 Proper diagnosis of the injury is the first step in the successful rehabilitation program.

exercises to include or avoid in the rehabilitation program. Clients are asked frequently, "How did the injury happen?" If the athletic trainer knows that the cross country runner tore her meniscus running on a rocky course last week, the athletic trainer can attempt to educate her on environmental awareness and stabilizing her core while running on uneven terrain, strategies that will decrease the likelihood that her knee will move into awkward or stressful positions. This athlete's rehabilitation program should focus on strengthening the hamstrings and quadriceps, developing core strength and endurance, and strengthening the ankles. All of these components combined decrease the likelihood of re-injury and prepare her to return to activity.

Localizing Inflammation and Injury: Step Two

After determining the type of injury and its mechanism, the athletic trainer must proceed with the next step. The location of the pain and inflammation should be immediately identified.[3–5] Although pain is necessary for proper diagnosis of an injury, the athletic trainer's priority after diagnosis should be eradicating the pain. Relieving pain is critical because it allows the injured person to move through the phases of healing and repair as quickly and safely as possible. The best method to eliminate pain and reduce the inflammation is to choose an appropriate modality. As addressed later in the chapter, certain modalities work best with acute injuries, and others work best with chronic injuries. Knowing the diagnosis and time frame of the injury helps in selecting the correct modality.

Designing the Conditioning and Rehabilitation Program: Step Three

Recognizing the limitations and **contraindications** of the injury or illness provides further direction in the development of the conditioning and rehabilitation program. Contraindications are modalities or exercises that should not be performed. Depending on the diagnosis, the athletic trainer might ask the following questions: What should the injured body part be doing (or not doing)? Is it more effective to involve body segments above and below the injury to enhance the rehabilitation outcome and prevent re-injury? Certain movement patterns expedite tissue repair, whereas other movement patterns impede the repair and may even create setbacks or exacerbate the injury. For example, consider the softball pitcher whose right shoulder is still very sore after a rotator cuff repair. Any range of motion above the shoulder is contraindicated in the early phases of rehabilitation because this movement could damage the surgical repair. To increase her chance of returning to play on time, the athletic trainer should work on the player's range of motion and strength within the available, pain-free range and progress as the protocol and her pain levels allow.

Conditioning and Rehabilitation Goals

Envisioning the projected outcome is only one part of the formula in designing a conditioning and rehabilitation program. Developing a system of goals with the client is another critical aspect of the process.[6] Short-term and long-term goals are necessary in establishing the direction of the rehabilitation program and in demonstrating improvement and success to the individual (Table 8-1).

Typically, **short-term goals** are designed to be met within four to eight visits or within 2 to 4 weeks, depending on your practice setting. These goals frequently focus on pain management, reduction of swelling and inflammation, range of motion, basic levels of function and activity, ambulation, and self-care skills. The time frame for **long-term goals** ranges from 4 weeks to several months and even years.

contraindications modalities or exercises that should not be performed on the basis of a particular diagnosis

short-term goals goals that are designed to be met within four to eight visits or within 2 to 4 weeks

long-term goals goals that are designed to be met at any point from 4 weeks to several months and even years

TABLE 8-1 Conditioning and Rehabilitation Program Goals

TYPE OF GOAL	TIME FRAME	REHABILITATION FOCUS
Short-term goals	4–8 visits, or 2–4 weeks	Manage pain Limit injured area Limit edema and swelling Increase cardiorespiratory fitness Improve range of motion Improve flexibility Promote proprioception Promote kinesthesia Promote neuromuscular control
Long-term goals	4 weeks to months to years	Increase muscular strength Increase muscular endurance Increase muscular power Promote postural and core stability Achieve reactive neuromuscular training Achieve functional progressions Provide necessary taping, bracing, strapping Promote psychosocial well-being Achieve functional clearance Foster education and prevention Return client to activity

These goals usually include functional strengthening, mastery of job- or sport-specific skills, return to work or play, ongoing home exercise programs, extensive education, and frequent re-assessments. The successful accomplishment of long-term goals for any individual requires a carefully planned comprehensive rehabilitation program that includes both therapeutic modalities and exercises.

Activity Requirements

The steps outlined in the previous sections deal with the specific activity performed by the client, the type of injury or illness, and the rehabilitation goals that will allow the client to return to the required or desired activity. To design an effective rehabilitation program, the athletic trainer must now incorporate the remaining part of the formula: Examine the specific requirements of the activity that the client wishes to resume.[7,8] The best way to discover what the activity imposes on the body is to study the activity from both a biomechanical and a bioenergetic point of view.

Biomechanical. **Biomechanical analyses** of human activity are an attempt to explain how and why movements occur through an observation of linear and angular motion.[6] **Linear motion** occurs when all points within a body or an object move at the same time and over the same distance. This motion may follow a straight or curved path. The paths of a runner, a baseball pitch, or a gymnast performing a triple back flip are all examples of linear motion (Figure 8-4). **Angular motion** occurs when a body segment, the entire body, or an object moves about a fixed axis. A golfer swinging a driver, the forearm moving about the axis of the elbow in a biceps curl, and a water skier performing a complex move about a fixed axis are classic examples of angular motion (Figure 8-5). All human movements involve at least one of these types of motion and are typically a combination of both. Understanding the way the body moves and its relationship to the environment is paramount to understanding how to properly design a rehabilitation program that allows the client to resume his or her chosen activity.

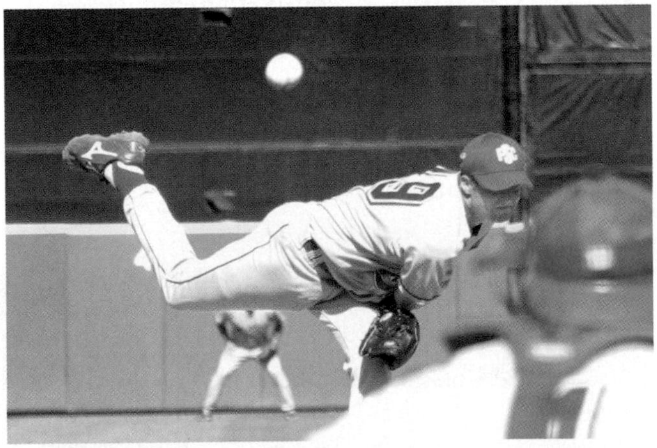
FIGURE 8-4 The path of the baseball after it is pitched is an example of linear motion.

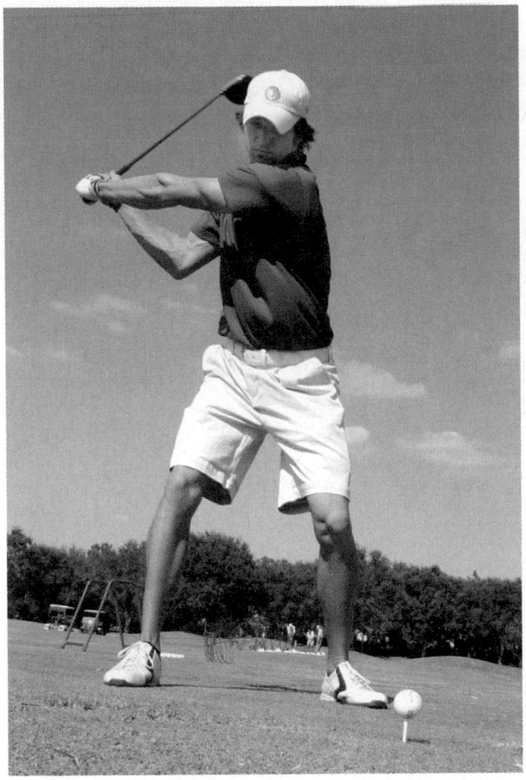
FIGURE 8-5 The path of the driver as it is swung by the golfer is an example of angular motion.

Bioenergetic. In a **bioenergetic analysis**, the activity is examined from an energy system utilization standpoint. Which energy system does the activity primarily target? Does the job require long, sustained repetitive movements? If so, it is tapping into the aerobic system (Figure 8-6). Does the job require short bursts of activity with high levels of intensity? If so, it calls on the anaerobic system

biomechanical analysis a physical analysis that determines how and why movements occur through linear and angular observations
linear motion movement that occurs when all points within a body or object move at the same time and over the same distance
angular motion movement that occurs when a body segment, the entire body, or an object moves about a fixed axis
bioenergetic analysis a physical analysis that looks at activity from an energy system utilization standpoint

(Figure 8-7). Are there moments of both activities interspersed throughout the activity or workday? The answers to these questions allow the athletic trainer to recognize the primary system of energy in use and will ultimately dictate the program design represented in sets and repetitions.[8] If an athlete does a lot of running and repetitive jumping, the program should eventually progress to multiple sets of numerous repetitions. If a worker stands around and lifts infrequently but with heavy loads, the program design should incorporate fewer sets and fewer repetitions, with an emphasis on greater resistance. It should be noted, however, that the worker's program design should challenge the worker with much more resistance (i.e., load) than the program design of the athlete in the first example (Table 8-2).

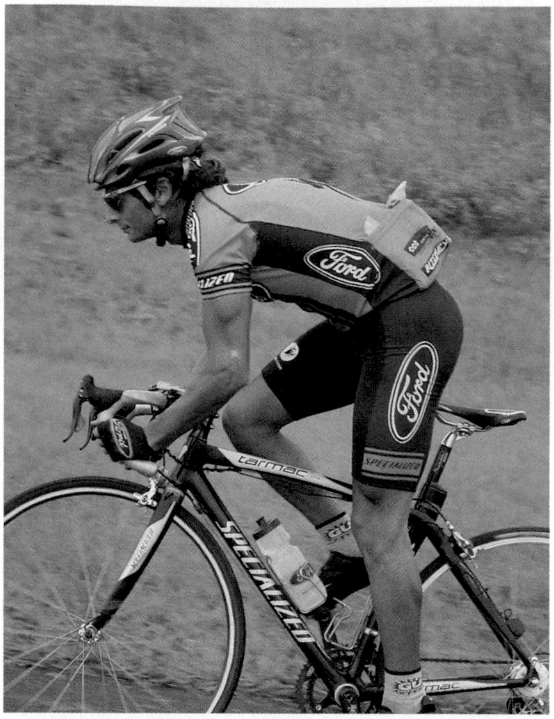

FIGURE 8-6 Long-distance cycling is an example of an aerobic activity.

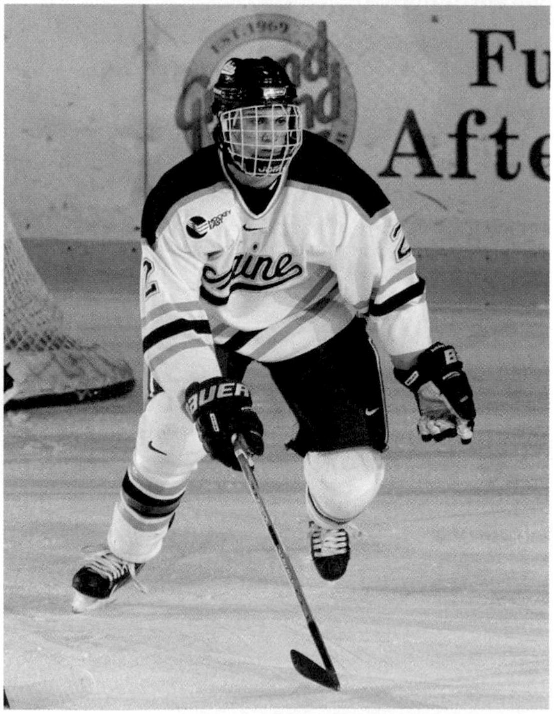

FIGURE 8-7 A hockey forward sprinting toward the goal with the puck is an example of an anaerobic activity.

Understanding the biomechanical and bioenergetic needs of the activity allows the athletic trainer to create a program based on **specificity**. *Specificity* means that the conditioning and rehabilitation program is designed in a way that is tailored to the client's chosen activity. Replicating the movement patterns to functionally train the main muscle groups (**agonists**, or prime movers) and assistors as well as the opposing muscle groups (**antagonists**) while constantly challenging the correct energy system results in an exercise program tailored to the individual. By applying the **principle of overload** throughout the exercise program, the athletic trainer continuously stimulates the body, the muscles, and soft tissues in general to become stronger. The overload is achieved by manipulating the frequency of workouts or rest intervals, the intensity of the stimulus, or the duration (i.e., time) of each workout or the number of sets and repetitions (Figure 8-8).

The **SAID principle**—an acronym that stands for *specific adaptations to imposed demands*—combines all of the aforementioned concepts and reflects the assumption that any human structure will adapt over time to the

specificity-based program a conditioning and rehabilitation program that replicates the activity in which the individual participates
agonists primary movers
antagonists muscles opposing the agonists
principle of overload fundamental law describing a stimulus that continuously overloads the muscles and soft tissues, causing them to become stronger
SAID principle fundamental law stating that any human structure will adapt accordingly over time to stressors and overloads; acronym stands for specific adaptations to imposed demands

TABLE 8-2 Sets and Repetitions for Aerobic and Anaerobic Activities

TYPE OF EXERCISE	SETS	REPETITIONS	RESISTANCE
Aerobic	2–4	10–15	Light to moderate
Anaerobic	2–3	3–8	Heavy to maximal

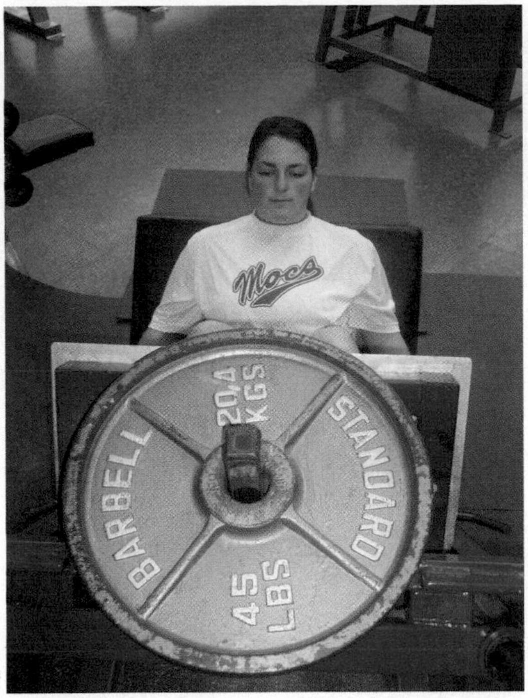

FIGURE 8-8 The principle of overload and the SAID principle are demonstrated as this athlete participates in an off-season resistance training session.

particular stressors or overloads placed on it.[9] Ideally, the client returns to activity quickly and safely. However, if the principle is not applied properly, the outcome may be deleterious, prompting re-injury or unnecessary setbacks caused by a return to activity without proper training. In light of all possible variables that the athletic trainer may manipulate to achieve performance gains, it is the actual load itself that has the potential to produce the greatest results.[10]

Implementation of the Conditioning and Rehabilitation Program

Figure 8-2 depicted the road map that is necessary to design a comprehensive rehabilitation program. Each of the four steps in this process—(1) diagnosing the injury, (2) localizing inflammation and injury while eliminating pain, (3) designing the conditioning and rehabilitation program, and (4) ensuring functional clearance with full return to activity—are important and should not be overlooked. Inclusion of these steps can all but guarantee a prompt and safe return to activity. Proper supervision of the exercises and rehabilitation program, combined with the previously stated steps, contributes to a successful program.[11] Omitting just one phase may lead to a faulty program design, resulting in partially accomplished goals. Goals that are partially accomplished or not accomplished at all increase the odds that the client will suffer a re-injury and be unable to resume the activity.[5,12] In any case, the client's life is affected and physical and mental setbacks are inevitable. Flexibility in following the rehabilitation program ensures an ever-evolving program that can meet the ongoing and dynamically changing needs of the client.

Consider once again the case of Noah in the opening scenario. Although he made great progress with his back rehabilitation program over the past 2 weeks, he sustained a setback after moving the couch so that his wife could vacuum. Clearly, continuing with the previously planned program will not help him accomplish his rehabilitation goals. At this point, the athletic trainer should perform a reassessment to obtain a new diagnosis and then redesign Noah's rehabilitation program according to the current physical findings. His long-term goals and return to activity remain the same. Flexibility is necessary when adjusting his program and short-term goals. The athletic trainer must identify and then eliminate the new acute pain and facilitate Noah's progress through the phases of injury repair and healing. Once Noah progresses through the phases of injury repair and healing, the final functional exercise program will help him make the transition to his required activities. The athletic trainer's choices in exercises and modalities allow Noah to return to activity as promptly and safely as possible so that he does not need to miss any of his scheduled work shifts.

Ensuring Functional Clearance and Return to Activity: Step Four

The functional clearance is probably the most important aspect of a client's return to activity. Obviously, the goal from the outset is to return the client to the required or desired level of activity as soon and as safely as possible. Throughout the course of the conditioning and rehabilitation program, the requisite level of function necessary to return to play has emerged. Once the athletic trainer fully understands all the components of the activity that the client is attempting to resume, the next and final step in providing high-quality care is to create a functional clearance test that will provide substantive evidence that the client is ready to return to activity without risk of re-injury.

For example, a setter in volleyball must display both aerobic and anaerobic strength and endurance. She must also demonstrate agility, speed, change of direction, explosive power, reactive neuromuscular control, core stability, and endurance, as well as all the sport-specific demands of her position in gamelike scenarios. (These are discussed later in this chapter.) Levels of achievement in these areas are typically best demonstrated throughout the conditioning and rehabilitation program, culminating in a final clearance test on the volleyball court (Figure 8-9). Creating a volleyball-specific clearance test that replicates all facets of her position and having her perform this test, followed by game simulation and then live-game play, will provide sufficient quantitative evidence that she is ready to return to play without undue risk of re-injury.

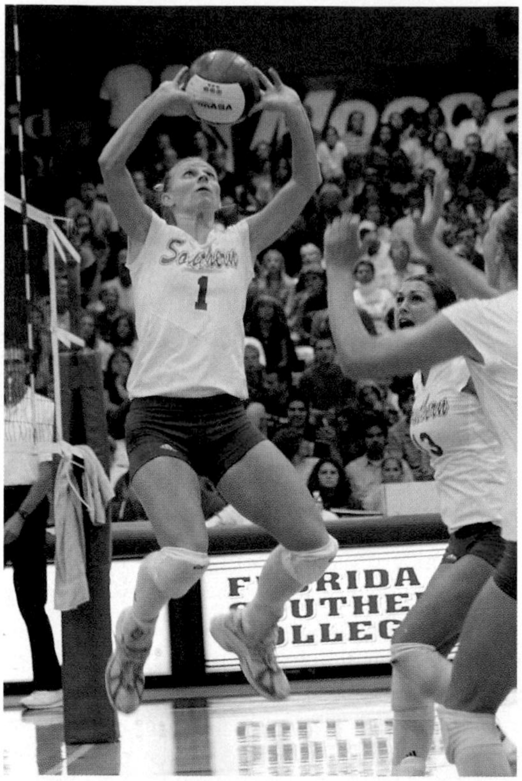

FIGURE 8-9 Before this athlete may safely resume activity, a functional clearance test must be performed to ensure that there are no deficits in her performance on or off the volleyball court.

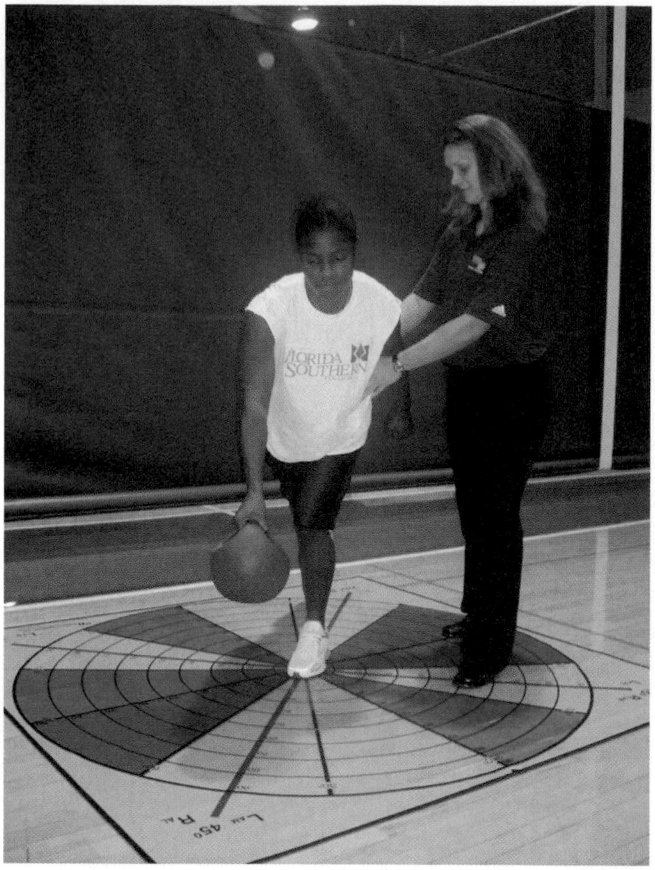

FIGURE 8-10 Becoming familiar with all of the resources at the job site will help the athletic trainer make the employee's conditioning and rehabilitation programs both creative and comprehensive.

Points to Ponder

A wrestler goes down during a match with a serious knee injury. What does it take to get him back to competition pain-free, and how should the athletic trainer implement that program?

THERAPEUTIC TECHNIQUES: THE REHABILITATION TOOLBOX

Athletic trainers have a vast amount of resources available for use in designing the conditioning and rehabilitation program (Figures 8-10 and 8-11). Experienced professionals know that they are limited only by their own levels of creativity. An effective program design represents the marriage of art and science. Often, therapeutic modalities and therapeutic exercises are skillfully woven together. The science is in knowing exactly what each modality and exercise can accomplish for the individual client. The art comes into play when the athletic trainer is innovative and daring but still operates within known confines. Pushing the envelope just a bit regarding the application of modalities and the implementation of exercises is what propels the profession forward and allows athletes to achieve seemingly impossible feats (Figure 8-12).

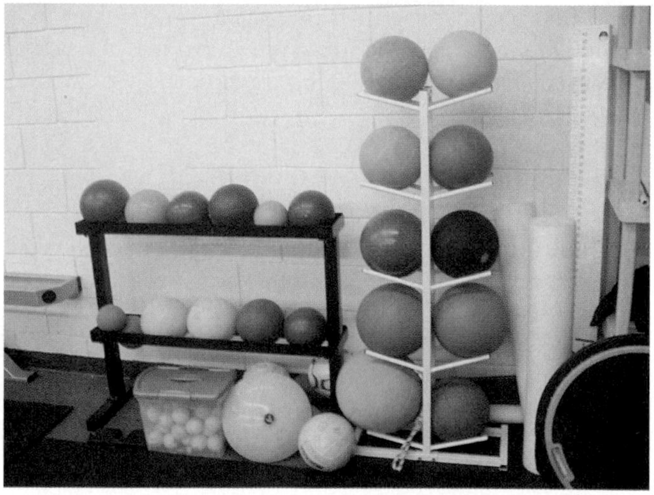

FIGURE 8-11 Common rehabilitation and conditioning equipment includes machines for resistance training as well as medicine balls, foam rolls, and dumbbells, which can be used for many forms of exercise.

Athletic trainers who are most successful in designing conditioning and rehabilitation programs usually benefited from the tutelage of a professional who was not afraid to combine modalities and exercise in a creative way. These athletic trainers have an arsenal

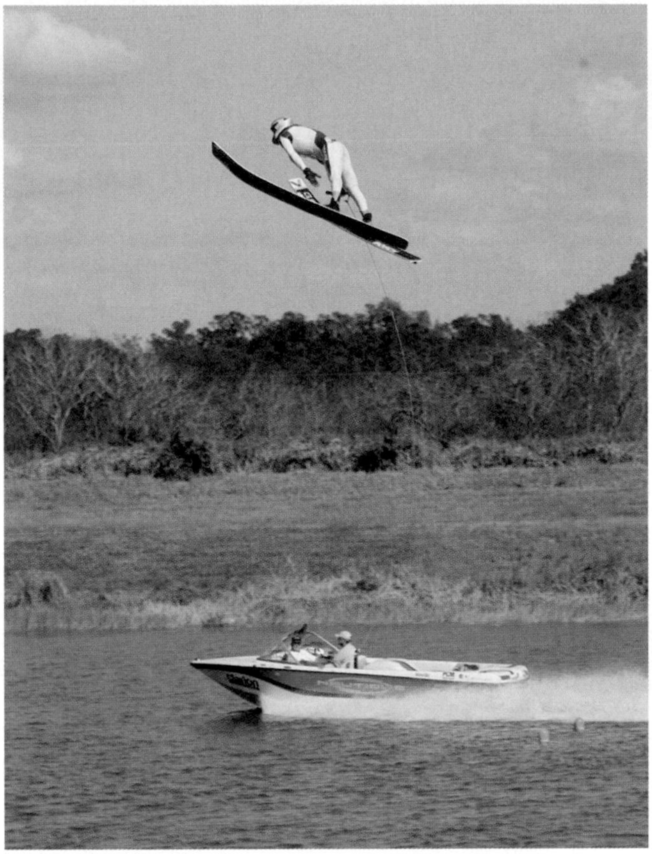

FIGURE 8-12 A carefully planned and executed combination of resources and creativity leads to a successful conditioning and rehabilitation program, one that allows clients to do amazing things.

of preferred modalities and exercises to help them accomplish specific program goals. This arsenal is sometimes called the *rehabilitation toolbox*. The more options in modalities and exercises that the athletic trainer has in the toolbox, the better equipped he or she will be in successfully designing conditioning and rehabilitation programs.

Therapeutic Modalities

Noah's description of his low back pain in the opening scenario underscores the need for pain in the initial diagnostic phase. As previously discussed, pain guides the athletic trainer in determining an accurate diagnosis, but it should be alleviated once the diagnosis is obtained. The athletic trainer uses appropriate modalities to immediately decrease the pain and inflammation caused by the injury. In consideration of the three phases of injury repair (i.e., inflammation, proliferation, and maturation), the athletic trainer selects modalities and exercises tailored to the stage of injury, the levels of reported pain, and the current rehabilitation goals. If Noah's injury is still in the inflammation phase, the athletic trainer is not likely to treat him with heat and aggressive core stabilization and strengthening exercises. Heat will counteract the goal of the inflammation stage, which is to contain the injury, and aggressive exercise will most likely exacerbate his pain. In fact, these measures would prevent the injury from moving beyond the first stage and interfere with the client's rehabilitation goals and return to activity.

Injuries and individuals heal at different rates. The athletic trainer can, however, estimate the length of time that a typical injury may persist in each phase of healing. If diagnosed and treated properly, injuries usually move through the first phase, the inflammation phase, after approximately 4 days. After that, they enter the proliferation phase, which may last as long as 6 weeks. The third and final phase may linger on for several years, depending on the client's response to the rehabilitation program and possible re-injury. Box 8-1 shows the average length for each phase of a typical injury, and Figure 8-13 demonstrates the injury cycle with healing phases and therapeutic interventions.

Points to Ponder

How do the stages of injury repair influence the selection of modalities and exercises?

Factors That Impede Healing

Not only does the improper selection of modalities and exercises impede the healing process, but other factors also drastically alter the rehabilitation program. For example, internal and external healing factors come into play at various times during the rehabilitation process. Internal factors include edema, hemorrhage, muscle spasm, poor vascular supply, the speed and effectiveness with which the injury is limited (or not), the amount of tissue separation and damage incurred, and even excessive scarring in the form of **keloids**. Humidity, infection, smoking, steroids, nutrition, and exercise habits are all

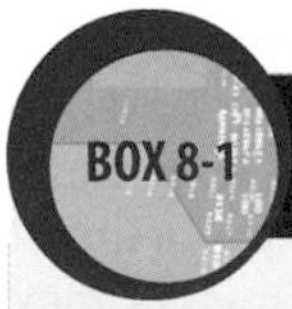

Phases and Duration of Injury Healing and Repair

Phase I: Inflammation (0 to 4 days)
Phase II: Proliferation or repair (2 days to 6 weeks)
Phase III: Maturation or remodeling (3 weeks to 2 years)

keloids raised formation of fibrous scar tissue; caused by excessive scarring

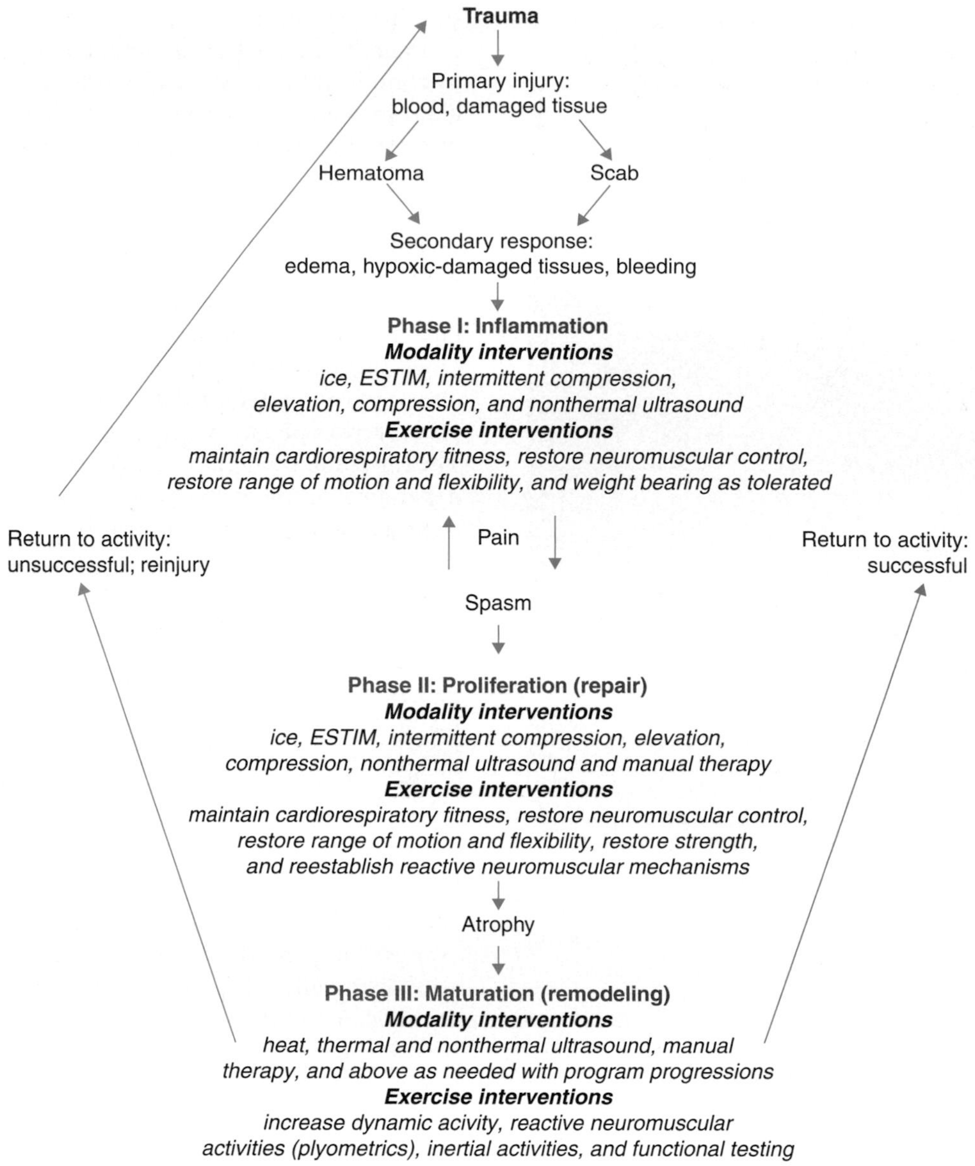

FIGURE 8-13 Phases of healing and interventions in the injury cycle.

external factors that contribute in some fashion to the overall outcome of an injury or illness. Properly managing these factors and having a flexible approach to treatment enable the athletic trainer to move successfully through the stages of injury repair and safely return the individual to his or her activity (Box 8-2). Athletic trainers may need to schedule time to educate clients about their role in assisting with their own healing process.[2]

Pain Control Theories

When selecting a modality to use for pain management and various diagnoses, the athletic trainer should make a choice that is based on an understanding of existing pain control theories. Many mental processes modulate a person's perception of pain, including previous experiences and memories of painful stimuli endured in the past. An essential element of pain control is the notion that these mental processes are not mutually exclusive but instead interdependent, acting on one another as the pain signal travels to and from the brain.

In brief, the four pain control theories discussed here involve the nociceptive pathways, gate control (or ascending afferent pathways), descending efferent pathways, and opiate production (Table 8-3). According to the nociceptive pathways theory, chemicals are released from the nociceptive neuron as the pain stimulus travels along the afferent ascending pathway. Upon release of these chemicals, the ability of the nerve to detect pain, or a noxious stimulus, is diminished. According to the gate control theory of pain, large-diameter afferent nerves regulate and stimulate the dorsal horn and inhibit pain signals from reaching smaller neurons. This action triggers a shutting or blocking mechanism within the ascending pathways to the brain; subsequently, the pain signal does not reach the brain. Release of enkephalins may also occur, providing another means by which to shut the gate. The descending efferent pathways theory states that these pathways can be desensitized by neurotransmitters released from the hypothalamus, which block the pain stimulus as it passes along the efferent descending pathway. Finally, according to the opiate theory, beta-endorphins and opioids are released after long periods of stimulation of the afferent fibers; these substances produce an analgesic effect, thus diminishing the perception of pain. This theory presumes that the analgesic effect deters the nerves from perceiving the painful stimulus. Keep in mind that the original signal occurs at the sensory receptors within the tissue and travels along the same afferent-efferent pathway as it travels back to the muscle or tissue. The athletic trainer's own beliefs as to which theory of pain control is most plausible will generally dictate the modalities he or she selects.

A hierarchical system exists within the body to address tissue sensitivity (Box 8-3). The periosteum surrounding bone and joint capsules is the tissue that is most sensitive to painful stimuli. Ligaments, tendons, and subchondral bone are somewhat less sensitive, followed by muscles and cortical bone. Finally, the least sensitive tissues are articular cartilage and joint synovium. This hierarchy explains why a contusion is less painful than an avulsion fracture and why an inflamed bursa is less painful than a dislocated shoulder. The potential for perceived pain is directly related to the type of tissue involved in the injury. Understanding this pain progression helps in designing comprehensive rehabilitation programs based on the injured body part and involved tissues.

BOX 8-2 Factors Affecting Healing

Internal Factors

Edema
Hemorrhage
Muscle spasm
Poor vascular supply
Quick response in limiting of the extent of the injury
Tissue separation and damage
Excessive scarring (keloids)
Diabetes

External Factors

Humidity
Infection
Smoking
Steroids
Nutrition
Allergens
Exercise
Certain medications

BOX 8-3 Tissue Sensitivity Within the Body*

Periosteum
Joint capsule
Ligaments
Tendons
Subchondral bone
Muscles
Cortical bone
Articular cartilage
Joint synovium

*In descending order of sensitivity.

TABLE 8-3 Pain Control Theories

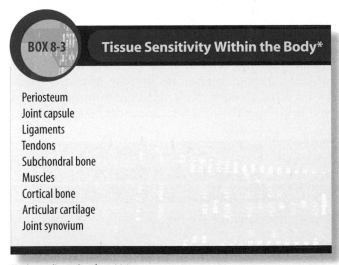

PAIN CONTROL THEORY	EXPLANATION	COMMON MODALITY APPLICATIONS
Nociceptive pathways	Chemicals are released to inhibit perception of noxious stimuli.	Ice, intermittent compression
Gate control	Large afferent nerves stimulate the dorsal horn and discourage pain signals from reaching smaller neurons; enkephalins can be released, shutting the gate as well.	ESTIM (depends on settings)
Descending efferent pathways	Neurotransmitters are released from the hypothalamus, keeping the pain signal from traveling down the descending efferent pathways.	ESTIM (depends on settings)
Opiate	An analgesic effect is produced by the release of beta-endorphins and opioids.	Heat, massage

ESTIM, Electric stimulating currents.

Therapeutic Modalities Color Spectrum

Before considering the vast array of modalities available for use, the athletic trainer should have a working knowledge of all the available options. Each modality is slightly different in its depth of penetration, indications, and contraindications. These subtle nuances will guide the athletic trainer to select appropriate modalities according to the injury diagnosis, stage of injury repair, and rehabilitation goals. After making the diagnosis, athletic trainers should bear in mind that their primary goal is to get rid of the client's pain. The selected modality will determine how quickly and effectively this and other goals are achieved.

To facilitate proper modality selection, the athletic trainer may determine the location of each modality on the color spectrum (Table 8-4). The color on the spectrum associated with each modality identifies the potential depth of penetration of the treatment within the human body. The spectrum ranges from the invisible to ultraviolet. Notice that the progression through the spectrum encompasses both movement through the standard color spectrum (Figure 8-14) and linearly increasing (or decreasing) depths of penetration. Depths that can be achieved with current modalities range from approximately 5 centimeters to approximately 1 millimeter. While studying this table, remember first to diagnose the injury and then to establish the stage of injury repair. Be mindful that acute injuries are modality intensive, whereas chronic injuries are exercise intensive. These two criteria, along with the client's past medical history, will help the athletic trainer choose the best modalities.

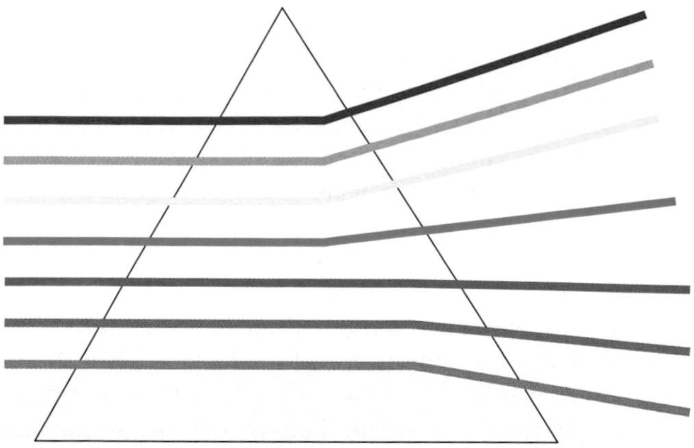

FIGURE 8-14 The standard color spectrum made up of the colors that stand for ROY G BIV: red, orange, yellow, green, blue, indigo, violet.

It should be noted that most modalities actually fall within two different spectrums—the electromagnetic spectrum and the acoustic spectrum—that have been conveniently placed in this therapeutic modalities color spectrum. The **electromagnetic spectrum** deals primarily with radiant energy produced by moving electrons that can travel through either space or a vacuum. Most modalities

electromagnetic spectrum range of radiation frequencies that primarily involves radiant energy produced by moving electrons that can travel through either space or a vacuum

TABLE 8-4 **Modality Color Spectrum**

THERAPEUTIC MODALITIES	COLOR SPECTRUM	DEPTH OF PENETRATION
Electrical stimulating currents HVPS TENS IF NMES Iontophoresis MENS	Invisible to the naked eye	Effects possible at any point between the electrodes (bigger electrodes and increased distance between electrodes increases depth of penetration)
Shortwave diathermy	Invisible to the naked eye	3 cm and 5 cm
Cryotherapy (cold packs, ice massage, cold whirlpool, ice immersion)	Infrared	1 cm
Thermotherapy (hot whirlpool, paraffin, hydrocollator, infrared lamps, fluidotherapy)	Infrared	1 cm
Low-power LASER	Red to violet	5 cm to 15 mm
Ultraviolet	Ultraviolet	1 mm
Ultrasound (T = thermal; N = non-thermal, P = phonophoresis)	Ultraviolet	>1 mm (1 MHz goes deeper than 3 MHz; slower movement of the sound head increases depth of penetration)
Intermittent compression	Ultraviolet	> 1 mm

HVPS, high-voltage pulsed stimulation; *TENS*, transcutaneous electrical nerve stimulation; *IF*, interferential stimulation; *NMES*, neuromuscular electrical stimulation; *MENS*, microcurrent electrical stimulation.

used by athletic trainers fall into this spectrum. The **acoustic spectrum**, which is traditionally referred to as *ultrasound*, involves mechanical vibrations or sound waves that can travel only through specific mediums, such as gels, lotions, water, or viscous bladders.

The following modalities listed in the color spectrum are those most frequently seen and used by athletic trainers. To enhance understanding and application, the modalities are grouped and introduced as they should be used for acute and/or chronic injuries. Acute injuries have a recent onset (e.g., within the past 24 to 48 hours). Chronic injuries have been present and symptomatic for 2 to 3 weeks. However, some modalities, such as ice and electrical stimulating currents (ESTIM), may be used throughout the entire healing process. Understanding the indications and contraindications for each modality helps the athletic trainer decide when to use the modality during the specific phases of the injury.

Points to Ponder

To ensure proper application and results, modalities should be selected on the basis of depth of penetration. How does the modality's depth of penetration affect healing?

Modalities for Acute Injuries

Acute injuries present unique issues that must be addressed immediately to ensure that the injury does not worsen unnecessarily. Elimination of pain, inflammation, and swelling is usually the primary goal when choosing modalities for acute injuries because the client wants to return to activity as soon as possible.[12] Depending on the mechanism of injury and the diagnosis, other factors to consider while selecting the best modalities for acute injuries are stopping muscle spasms, preventing loss of muscle strength or size (i.e., atrophy), and maintaining neuromuscular pathways for proper muscle recruitment and firing (i.e., muscle re-education). Modalities that work best with acute injuries include cryotherapy, ESTIM, intermittent compression, and low-power LASERs.

Cryotherapy. Cryotherapy modalities exist in the infrared portion of the color spectrum. Most forms of **cryotherapy** reach a penetration depth of approximately 1 centimeter. Cold packs, ice massage, ice immersion, cold sprays, mechanical cooling systems, and cold whirlpools are examples of the most common forms of cryotherapy (Figure 8-15). Benefits, or indications, of cryotherapy are acute injuries, analgesic effects, vasoconstriction, and decreased inflammation and muscle guarding or spasms.[2,12–15] Contraindications to cryotherapy are relatively few. This, along with its important benefits, makes cryotherapy a first choice for athletic trainers.[2,16,17] A familiar saying among athletic trainers is "Ice is nice!" Known contraindications are circulatory impairment, impaired wound healing, hypertension, and previous allergic reactions to any form of cryotherapy. Table 8-5 summarizes the specific effects of cryotherapy.

Electrical Stimulating Currents. **Electrical stimulating currents** (ESTIM) can be discussed as a group with respect to the color spectrum and depth of penetration.

acoustic spectrum range of frequencies involving mechanical vibrations or sound waves that can travel only through certain mediums

cryotherapy family of modalities that primarily induces vasodilation; examples include cold packs, ice massage, ice immersion, cold sprays, mechanical cooling systems, and cold whirlpools

electrical stimulating currents (ESTIM) group of modalities that have a physiological effect at any point between positioned electrodes; examples include high-voltage pulsed stimulation (HVPS), transcutaneous electrical nerve stimulation (TENS), interferential stimulation (IF), neuromuscular electrical stimulation (NMES), iontophoresis, and microcurrent electrical stimulation (MENS)

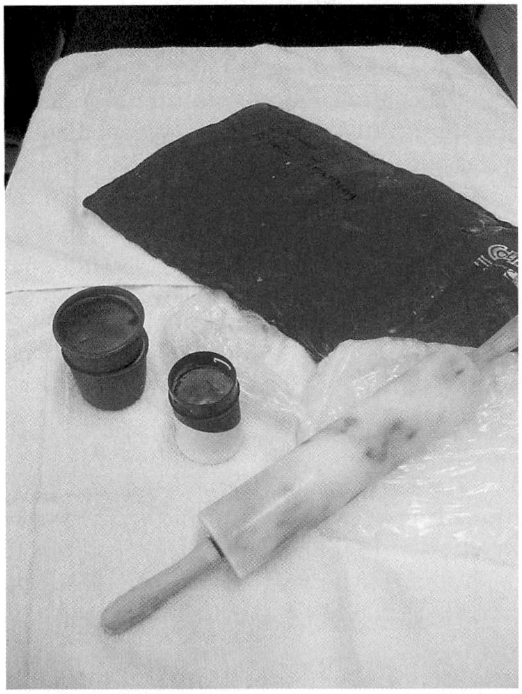

FIGURE 8-15 Examples of various cryotherapy modalities: ice cups, ice packs, ice bags, and frozen massage sticks.

TABLE 8-5 Specific Effects of Cryotherapy

	INDICATIONS	CONTRAINDICATIONS OR PRECAUTIONS
Cryotherapy: 15–20-minute treatment time, depending on modality	Acute injury or pain, vasoconstriction, analgesic, anesthetic, edema and inflammation, muscle spasm and guarding, neuralgia, delayed onset muscle soreness, small burns, chronic pain	Infection, circulatory impairments, sensitivity to cold, open wounds, hypertension, respiratory or cardiac involvement, advanced diabetes, lupus, Raynaud's disease

All modalities in this family exist in a color spectrum range that is invisible to the naked eye, and they can produce a physiological effect at any point between the positioned electrodes. Each diagnosis, each stage of injury repair, and each client presents a unique set of conditions that must be assessed for applicable ESTIM modality indications and contraindications. Consider, for example, a soccer player who has recently been diagnosed with breast cancer. This condition alone, regardless of the immediate injury that requires attention, forces the athletic trainer to rule out numerous modalities. Similarly, an athlete who has an implanted pacemaker/defibrillator in his chest may not be a good candidate for certain modalities, notwithstanding his torn rotator cuff or recent ACL repair (Figure 8-16).

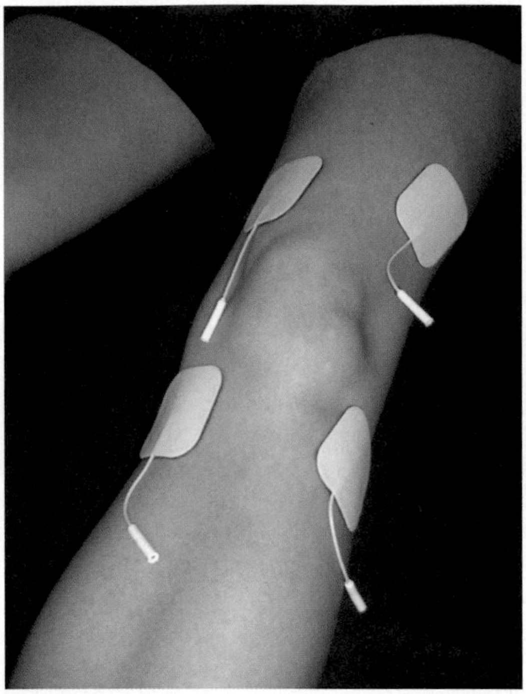

FIGURE 8-16 Electrodes attached and in position for an interferential stimulation treatment session.

Common ESTIM applications include re-educating muscles, stimulating muscle contractions, increasing strength, preventing tissue atrophy, managing pain, and increasing range of motion.[2] Other applications, governed by specific modality parameters, include pain control, analgesic effects, stimulation of sensory nerves, and promotion of wound healing. General contraindications for the various ESTIM modalities are pacemakers, malignancies, infections, skin lesions, thrombophlebitis, and any skin allergies. Typical ESTIM modality choices for the athletic trainer include high voltage pulsed stimulation (HVPS), transcutaneous electrical nerve stimulation (TENS), interferential stimulation (IF), neuromuscular electrical stimulation (NMES), iontophoresis, and microcurrent electrical stimulation (MENS). Even though the ESTIM currents have common indications and precautions, certain effects are unique to each modality (Table 8-6).

Intermittent Compression. Another widely used modality for acute injuries is intermittent compression. This modality is in the ultraviolet range of the color spectrum, with a penetration depth of approximately 1 millimeter. Intermittent compression uses a mechanical pressure to promote increased venous and lymphatic drainage. Pressure fills the boot or sleeve in a distal-to-proximal sequence to encourage the accumulated fluids to return back towards the torso, thus allowing reabsorption. Several devices are available for this application. Most important to remember is that intermittent compression appears to produce remarkable results in reducing edema in acute and subacute injuries when used with cryotherapy and elevation (Figure 8-17).[17] Indications for intermittent compression include lymphedema, acute and chronic edema, and postoperative swelling. Contraindications consist of deep vein thrombosis (blood clots in a deep vein, typically found in the legs), superficial infections, congestive heart failure, malignancies, and displaced fractures. The athletic trainer must use caution while supervising these treatments, however, because it is not possible to visually monitor the client's response to treatment until the treatment has ended. Table 8-7 lists the effects of intermittent compression.

Low-Power Lasers. Low-power lasers—the word *laser* is an acronym for *light amplification for the stimulated emission of radiation*—have been used in the medical field for a relatively short time compared with other modalities. Low-power lasers are also called *cold lasers*

TABLE 8-6 Specific Effects of Electrical Stimulating Currents and Modalities

TYPE OF ELECTRICAL STIMULATION	INDICATIONS	CONTRAINDICATIONS OR PRECAUTIONS
HVPS: 15- to 20-minute treatment time	Pain, acute injuries, edema, insufficient muscle recruitment, inadequate muscle contractions, atrophy, muscle weakness, limited ROM, fracture	Pacemakers, thrombophlebitis, superficial skin lesions, malignancy, infections
TENS: 15- to 20- minute treatment time	Pain	Pacemakers, thrombophlebitis, superficial skin lesions, malignancy, infections
IF: 15–20 minute treatment time	Pain, insufficient muscle recruitment, inadequate muscle contractions, fracture healing, limited ROM, muscle spasms	Pacemakers, thrombophlebitis, superficial skin lesions, malignancy, infections
NMES: 15- to 20-minute treatment time	Neuromuscular deficits, muscle weakness, limited ROM, atrophy, muscle spasms	Pacemakers, thrombophlebitis, superficial skin lesions, malignancy, infections, soft tissue lesions affected by contractions
Iontophoresis: varying treatment times	Inflammation, arthritis, tendonitis, chronic pain	Contraindications to the medication, unknown or phantom pain
MENS: 15- to 20-minute treatment time	Pain, ligament/tendon injuries, wounds, fracture	Malignancy, infections

HVPS, high-voltage pulsed stimulation; *TENS,* transcutaneous electrical nerve stimulation; *IF,* interferential stimulation; *NMES,* neuromuscular electrical stimulation; *MENS,* microcurrent electrical stimulation.

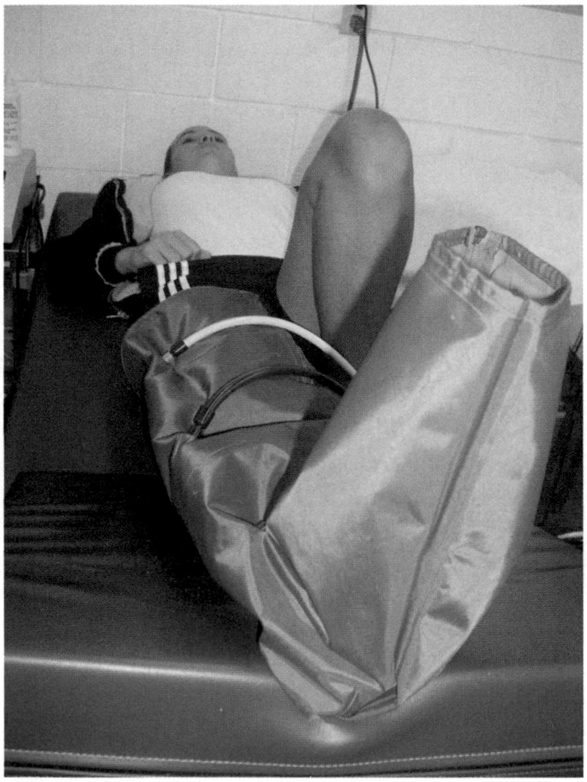

FIGURE 8-17 Intermittent compression being applied to an acute ankle injury, with the lower leg elevated to assist in reducing inflammation and edema.

because they produce photochemical effects instead of thermal effects.[18] On the color spectrum, low-power lasers are in the red-to-violet range, with a depth of penetration of approximately 1 millimeter. Indications include expediting wound healing, decreasing scar tissue and inflammation, and managing pain.[18] Contraindications are pregnancy, application over the eyes, and malignancies. Table 8-8 summarizes the effects of low-power lasers.

TABLE 8-7 Specific Effects of Intermittent Compression

	INDICATIONS	CONTRAINDICATIONS OR PRECAUTIONS
Intermittent compression: 15- to 20-minute treatment time	Acute bleeding, lymphedema, edema, postsurgical wounds	Circulatory impairment, displaced fractures, malignancy, deep vein thrombosis, congestive heart failure, cardiac dysfunction

Modalities for Chronic Injuries

Chronic injuries require a different approach during the selection of modalities. Reducing muscle guarding, spasm, pain, and chronic inflammation and promoting circulation and tissue remodeling are common goals in the treatment of chronic injuries. The focus shifts from eliminating pain, inflammation, and swelling to returning the client to an activity that has been strictly curtailed for several weeks.[2] The athletic trainer must select a modality that will assist in the client's healing process and facilitate a safe return to activity. Modalities that are best suited for chronic injuries include ESTIM, thermotherapy, ultrasound, shortwave diathermy, and ultraviolet therapy.

TABLE 8-8 Specific Effects of Low Power Lasers

	INDICATIONS	CONTRAINDICATIONS OR PRECAUTIONS
Low-power Lasers: varying treatment times	Pain, inflammation, wounds, musculoskeletal pain, fractures, arthritis	Pregnancy, malignancy, eye problems, hemorrhagic areas

Thermotherapy. Thermotherapy resides next to cryotherapy on the color spectrum. Both modalities are infrared and reach a penetration depth of approximately 1 centimeter. There is some disagreement regarding the pros and cons of heat and cold, two markedly different modalities. Thermotherapy leads to vasodilation rather than vasoconstriction. In acute injuries, this difference can be critical. Imagine an athlete who experiences an acute ankle sprain during a basketball game. During half-time, the athletic trainer has the choice to apply ice or heat and chooses heat, making a devastating error in judgment. Heat will exacerbate this acute injury by promoting vasodilation around the injured area, which in turn causes increased edema and swelling. Knowing the injury to be acute, the athletic trainer should have opted to apply ice, which encourages vasoconstriction of the injured area and restricts blood flow.

Forms of thermotherapy include hydrocollator packs, paraffin baths, warm whirlpools, infrared lamps, and fluidotherapy (Figure 8-18). Care should be taken when selecting the best thermotherapy modality because evidence suggests that during warm water immersion, considerable fluctuations occur in the blood flow during the course of treatment.[19] Thus hydrocollator packs and paraffin baths are the thermotherapy modalities of choice among most athletic trainers. Contraindications for thermotherapy include acute injuries, poor circulation, and malignancies. Despite the ongoing debate regarding cryotherapy versus thermotherapy, some people still use contrast baths, in which the injured limb is placed first in cold water and then in hot water. This alternating of cold and hot is performed for several cycles that last a specific length of time. Contrast baths should always end with a cryotherapy modality to prevent unnecessary edema and fluid accumulation. Localizing the initial injury and inflammatory response is paramount to recovery, and concluding with cryotherapy ensures this outcome. Table 8-9 outlines the effects of thermotherapy.

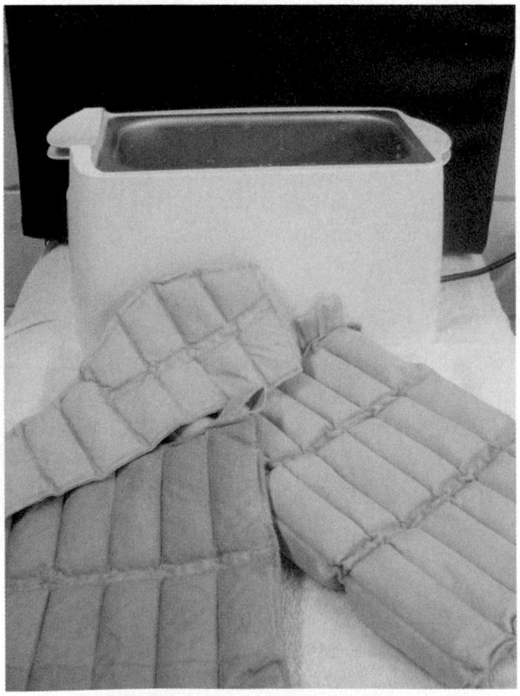

FIGURE 8-18 Examples of commonly used thermotherapy modalities: moist hot packs and paraffin bath.

Ultrasound. Ultrasound is another modality used predominantly for chronic soft tissue injuries. It is in the ultraviolet range, with a penetration depth of approximately 1 millimeter. As previously described, ultrasound is truly in the acoustic spectrum, unlike most other modalities, which are in the electromagnetic spectrum. A medium, or barrier, is required for the safe and effective use of ultrasound. These media include water, gels, lotions, and fluid-filled bladders placed directly over the area to be treated. Once the medium is applied, the ultrasound sound head is placed directly on the medium, where

TABLE 8-9 Specific Effects of Thermotherapy

	INDICATIONS	CONTRAINDICATIONS OR PRECAUTIONS
Thermotherapy: 15- to 20-minute treatment time, depending on modality	Muscle guarding and spasm, impaired nerve conductivity and decreased tissue elasticity, vasodilation, sub-acute or chronic pain, infection, decreased metabolic activity, decreased venous return and capillary permeability, wounds	Acute conditions, poor circulation, skin anesthesia, malignancy (infrared), open wounds (immersion), advanced arthritis, thrombophlebitis, cardiac and vascular concerns

thermotherapy family of modalities that primarily induces vasodilation; examples include hydrocollator packs, paraffin baths, warm whirlpools, infrared lamps, and fluidotherapy

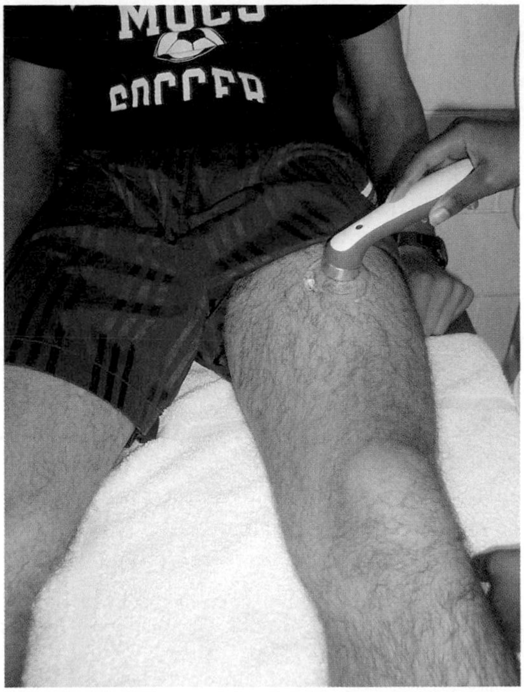

FIGURE 8-19 Ultrasound is being applied to the quadriceps to reduce acute inflammation and pain and increase circulation.

it maintains direct contact throughout the treatment session (Figure 8-19). Thermal (continuous setting) and nonthermal (pulsed setting) benefits are available. Thermal benefits include pain modulation, decreased joint stiffness and muscle spasms, increased blood flow, and collagen extensibility,[20] as well as an inflammatory response.[16] Thermal settings are typically used for chronic injuries. Nonthermal benefits include increased blood flow and protein synthesis, soft tissue healing,[21] and fracture repair.[22] Nonthermal settings can be used with acute injuries. Contraindications for the use of ultrasound are infections, acute injuries, pregnancy, malignancies, pacemakers, application over the eyes, total joint replacements, and epiphyseal injuries. The modality is also inappropriate for younger patients (Table 8-10).

Shortwave Diathermy. **Shortwave diathermy** lies in the invisible realm on the color spectrum. With this modality, however, the depth of penetration has changed. A depth of approximately 3 to 5 centimeters is possible if shortwave diathermy is properly used. A high-frequency current is introduced into the tissues and results in a deep heating of the specific area.[19] Shortwave diathermy can be used for its thermal (continuous setting) effects and for its nonthermal (pulsed setting) benefits. General thermal benefits include increased circulation and metabolic activity, decreased spasm and muscle guarding, and reduced inflammation. It promotes wound healing and often has an analgesic effect. Contraindications for diathermy thermal applications include metal implants, pacemakers, malignancies, pregnancy, application over the eyes, and the use of wet dressings; these may create excessive heat absorption by the tissues. Table 8-11 summarizes the special effects of shortwave diathermy.

shortwave diathermy modality that introduces a high-frequency current into the tissues to produce deep heating

TABLE 8-10 Specific Effects of Ultrasound

TYPE OF ULTRASOUND	INDICATIONS	CONTRAINDICATIONS OR PRECAUTIONS
Thermal ultrasound: 5- to 9-minute treatment time	Pain, muscle spasm and guarding, scar tissue, tissue dysfunction, inflammation, circulatory issues	Acute conditions, infection, epiphysis, pregnancy, malignancy, eye problems, pacemakers, reproductive organs, total joint implants, metal implants, deep vein thrombosis, pelvic area during menses
Nonthermal ultrasound: 5- to 9-minute treatment time	Scar tissue, inflammation, circulatory issues, joint contractures, acute inflammation	Infection, epiphysis, pregnancy, malignancy, eyes, pacemakers, reproductive organs, total joint implants, metal implants, deep vein thrombosis, pelvic area during menses

TABLE 8-11 Specific Effects of Shortwave Diathermy

	INDICATIONS	CONTRAINDICATIONS OR PRECAUTIONS
Shortwave diathermy: varying treatment times	Decreased circulation and metabolism, pain, muscle spasm and guarding, inflammation, vasodilation, post-acute musculoskeletal injuries, wounds, collagen deficiencies	Metal implants, pacemakers, malignancy, wet dressings, joint effusion, pregnancy, ischemia, acute injury and inflammation, areas of decreased sensitivity, areas of reduced blood flow, eye problems, fluid-filled organs, reproductive organs, IUDs

IUD, Intrauterine device.

Ultraviolet Therapy. Not surprisingly, ultraviolet therapy resides in the ultraviolet range on the color spectrum. The depth of penetration obtained is approximately 1 to 2 millimeters; therefore effective applications generally involve the superficial treatment of skin conditions. Examples, or indications, are acne, tinea capitis, septic wounds, sinusitis, pressure sores, and folliculitis. These conditions are frequently chronic. Contraindications include acute psoriasis, acute eczema, herpes simplex, renal or hepatic insufficiency, and advanced arteriosclerosis. Table 8-12 summarizes the effects of ultraviolet therapy.

Other Modalities

Several modalities exist that do not lie within the therapeutic modality color spectrum. Iontophoresis, contrast baths (previously discussed), massage, traction, and manual therapy techniques are crucial assets in any comprehensive rehabilitation program. Understanding these modalities and being able to properly combine them with the aforementioned ones will enable the athletic trainer to return clients to activity as quickly and safely as possible.

Iontophoresis. **Iontophoresis** combines a low-dose electrical current with an ionized medication to introduce the treatment into the body. Typically, the medication is applied to a special electrode pad, and the electrical current drives the medication into the affected area. The treatment time depends on factors such as the body part being treated, medication dosage, and patient tolerance to the electrical current. Iontophoresis may be used with acute and chronic injuries. The electrodes are applied in the same way as with any other electrical modality.

Massage. Massage exists in many forms and can be used for various purposes as an adjunct in the healing process. Various types are employed in the rehabilitation paradigm, particularly cross-friction massage, trigger point massage, myofascial release, and sports massage (Figure 8-20). Each of these forms of massage has specific techniques that have been developed and modified over time. Massage, generally speaking, increases circulation and range of motion, decreases pain and spasm, removes waste buildup in the venous system and the soft tissues, and facilitates the body's ability to recover from numerous soft tissue and neurological conditions.[23,24] However, its true effects on physical performance remain unclear even though it is assumed to enhance performance and decrease injury potential.[25] Massage is typically used to treat chronic soft tissue injuries.

Traction. Traction, either mechanical or manual, is a great adjunct to the previously described modalities and exercises. Traction helps to alleviate pain, neurological impairment, dysfunction, and sensitivities caused by the physical separation of the particular bony components being manipulated.[26] Mechanical traction is performed by applying an external device to the body part and is

iontophoresis modality that combines a low-dose electrical current with an ionized medication to introduce treatment

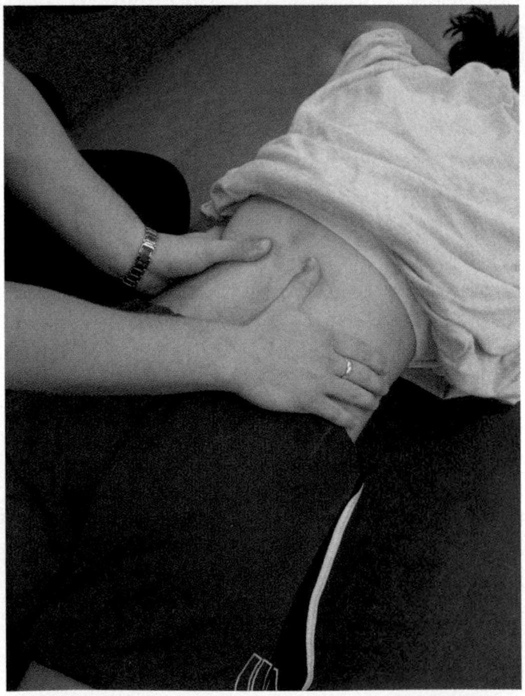

FIGURE 8-20 Massage treatments can be an added benefit in the comprehensive rehabilitation program in helping to increase range of motion and circulation while decreasing pain and spasm, both of which can severely curtail performance.

TABLE 8-12 Specific Effects of Ultraviolet Therapy

	INDICATIONS	CONTRAINDICATIONS OR PRECAUTIONS
Ultraviolet therapy: varying treatment times	Acne, aseptic wounds, pressure sores, psoriasis, sinusitis, folliculitis, exfoliation, septic wounds, pityriasis rosea, tinea capitis	Pregnancy, eye problems, malignancy

controlled electronically or by another outside force, such as a weight. Typically, mechanical traction is used in the cervical and lumbar regions (Figure 8-21). Manual traction can be applied to the cervical region as well as to most of the other joints in the body. Usually, manual traction is synonymous with long-axis distraction and is performed by gently pulling the long bone away from the involved joint[27] (Figure 8-22). This movement creates a traction akin to that performed on the spine. Mechanical and manual traction work well with acute injuries and can be used in conjunction with other modalities in the treatment of chronic injuries. Traction can also be applied through gravitational forces, as in the use of over-the-door cervical traction units.[27]

Manual Therapy. Manual therapy techniques, which are numerous and wide-ranging, are often modified by the athletic trainer to benefit the client's specific diagnosis. Joint mobilizations and glides employ the use of passive movement at the joint within normal, available ranges of motion.[2] Most athletic trainers who specialize in manual therapy techniques have studied one or two techniques and usually develop a unique method that works best for them in their settings (Figure 8-23). A number of manual therapy certifications are available, with benefits that positively affect rehabilitation outcomes. Depending on the technique being used, manual therapy is appropriate for acute and chronic injuries.

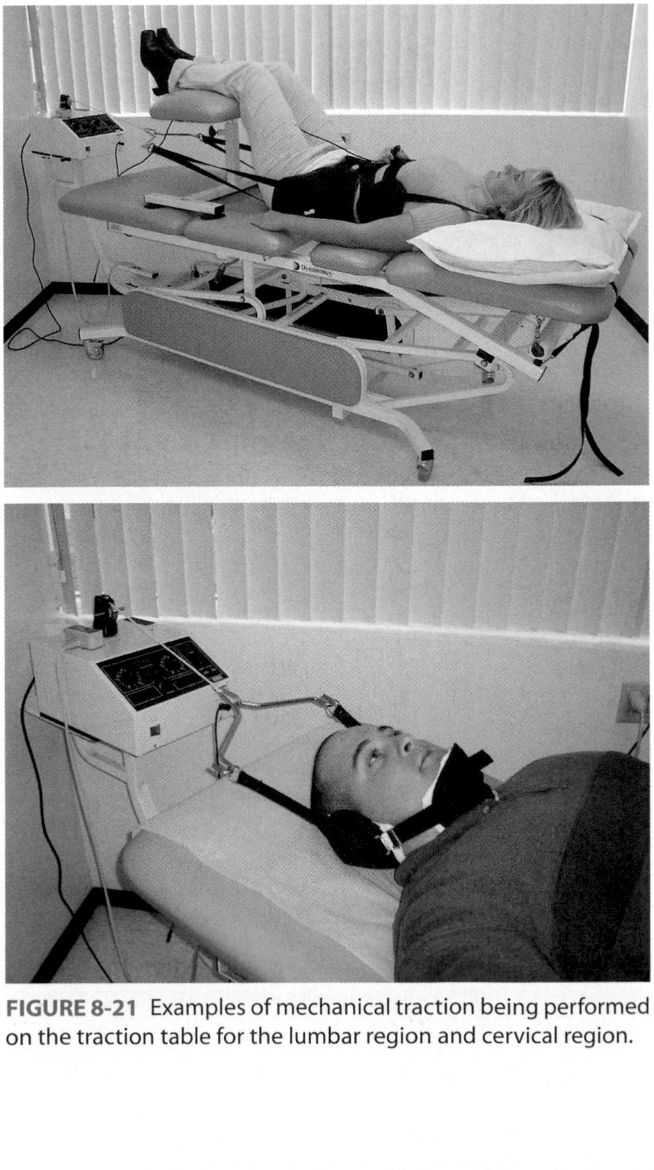

FIGURE 8-21 Examples of mechanical traction being performed on the traction table for the lumbar region and cervical region.

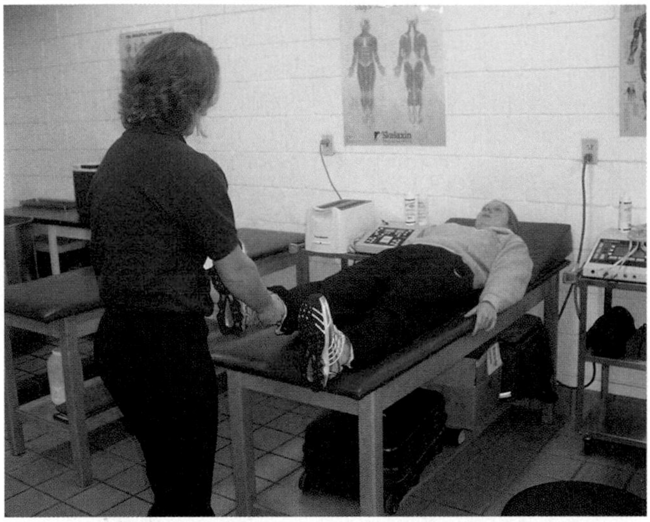

FIGURE 8-22 Long-axis distraction, a form of manual traction, helps primarily to alleviate pain and dysfunction.

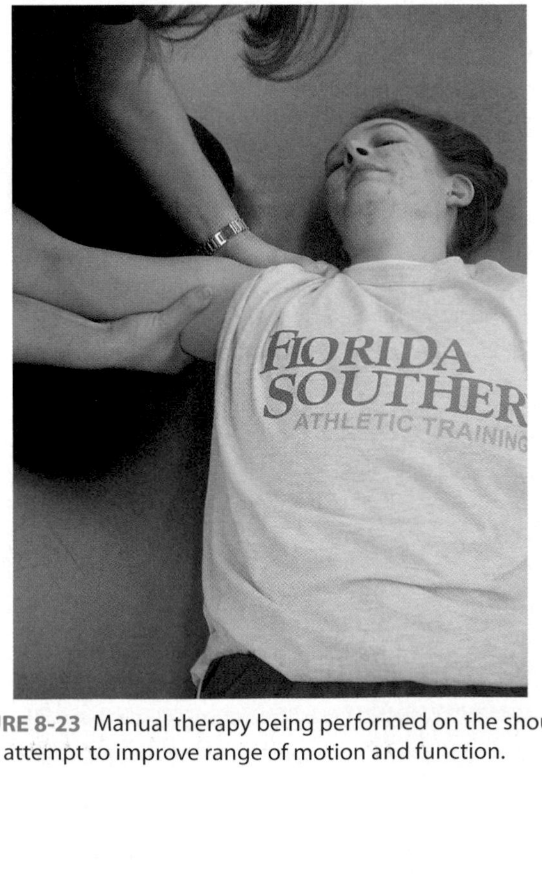

FIGURE 8-23 Manual therapy being performed on the shoulder in an attempt to improve range of motion and function.

Conditioning and Rehabilitative Exercise

Consider Noah and his back injury again. After interpreting his pain complaints to identify and diagnose the injury, the athletic trainer must create a plan of care using therapeutic modalities to manage this pain; the next step is to begin a conditioning and rehabilitation program to safely and quickly return Noah to his required activities. Exercise often begins simultaneously with the initiation of modalities. The athletic trainer's priority is to determine the specific demands of the activity that Noah would like to resume. Taking the time to analyze his job or sport requirements ensures that the athletic trainer will design a proper exercise program, one that will physically and mentally prepare Noah to return to work capable of performing his duties.

Exercise Progressions

To select the best exercises for Noah, the athletic trainer must understand the concept of progression through an exercise program. This understanding helps the athletic trainer choose the proper exercises with which to begin the conditioning and rehabilitation program. As previously mentioned, the athletic trainer must begin with the end in mind. Having a working knowledge of where Noah needs to be at the completion of the program makes it easier to create the road map to get him there. Resuming activity as quickly and as safely as possible is the ultimate goal for everyone with whom the athletic trainer will work.[12]

Most athletic trainers follow certain protocols that have pre-established progressions based on outcomes observed over time and safety precautions tailored to the specific diagnosis. Box 8-4 is an example of a general preoperative ACL reconstruction protocol illustrating specific goals and exercises to achieve the desired goals.

Extensive research studies demonstrate the effectiveness of certain protocols. Regardless of the evidence supporting a particular protocol, it is essential for the athletic trainer to remember that the protocol is a guideline, not a standard. Clients fluctuate in their responses to protocols and rehabilitation plans, with varying healing times, pain tolerance, and adherence to home exercise programs and prescribed limitations'; sometimes outcomes vary as a result of even slight differences in surgical procedures or stages of injury repair. No two individuals with the same diagnosis will respond the same way to even the best rehabilitation program ever devised. Ongoing assessments and flexibility and creativity in the rehabilitation program design allow clients under the athletic trainer's care to heal appropriately and achieve their individual goals.[8]

BOX 8-4 Preoperative ACL Reconstruction Protocol

Protocol Goals

Regain full ROM
Decrease swelling (modalities)
Control inflammatory response (modalities)
Decrease pain (modalities)
Normalize gait pattern
Restore 75% to 80% strength of uninvolved leg
Educate client regarding the HEP immediately after surgery
Prepare psychologically for surgery and rehab

ROM Exercises in Order of Progression

Heel slides
Supine wall slides
Stool hang
Prone hang
Leg stretches
Bike
Stair climber
Elliptical trainer

Strength Exercises in Order of Progression

Quad sets
Hamstring sets
Gluteal sets
Toe/heel raises (3-way: out, straight forward, and in)
Balance stance
Minisquats
Wall sits
Step ups (front and/or lateral)
Step-overs
Standing hamstring curl
Rocker board
One-leg minisquats
SLR (4-way: hip flexion, abduction, adduction, extension)
Prone hamstring curl
Gluteal strengthening
Leg press
Multi-hip strengthening
Treadmill (retro)

ACL, Anterior cruciate ligament; *HEP,* home exercise program; *ROM,* range of motion; *SLR,* straight leg raise.

Periodization

Periodization is a method to help ensure progress through conditioning and rehabilitation exercises. It is merely a means to manipulate exercise variables in order to achieve certain performance goals at certain times.[9] These performance goals can be occupational, athletic, or functional (e.g., activities of daily living). Individual clients have specific goals that they need to accomplish to be able to perform at their expected levels. True to the basic tenets of exercise, the parameters available to scientifically control (i.e., periodize) performance include the specific exercise itself, sets, repetitions, rest and/or recovery periods, intensity of exercise, frequency of exercise, and duration.

Traditionally, periodization has been applied mostly to athletes and teams. Consider, for example, a soccer team that aspires to qualify for the National Tournament this year. In order to accomplish this goal, the players must be at their peak levels of conditioning and skill execution at prime moments toward the end of the season. If they cannot perform at the apex of their abilities during certain key games, they will lose and thus not qualify for the tournament. Their chances can also be ruined by injury. A full and speedy return to activity without limitations requires the application of periodization principles to the rehabilitation program. Knowing these principles is pivotal in successfully returning injured athletes to their former activity status.

The prudent athletic trainer will study these principles and modify them to fit his or her own conditioning and rehabilitation paradigm. Following a properly periodized rehabilitation plan helps any client make progress, regardless of the diagnosis. It guarantees that the client is performing the exercises in a timely and systematic way to accomplish the intended outcomes.[9] Programs based on the principles of periodization often result in outcomes that far surpass other comparable conditioning and rehabilitation programs.[10,28,29] Full return to activity is always the goal. Table 8-13 outlines periodization cycles used in conditioning and rehabilitation programs.

Components of the Rehabilitation Program

When developing a comprehensive rehabilitation program, athletic trainers must target several key areas in order to provide the best program outcomes for the individual client. These areas often overlap and are addressed simultaneously. They are not hierarchical; the client does not pass from one to the next as if they were phases. However, athletic trainers often prefer to address them in a particular order or grouping because doing so allows for proper healing, safe progression, and full return to activity. Most rehabilitation programs include the following critical areas: cardiorespiratory maintenance; range of motion and flexibility; proprioception, kinesthesia, and neuromuscular control; muscular strength, endurance, and power; postural and core stability; and reactive neuromuscular training (Box 8-5). All of these elements, when applied and periodized appropriately, ensure that the client will eventually return to work or play.

Cardiorespiratory Maintenance. One of the basic premises of athletic training is that the client must maintain, if not improve, his or her level of cardiorespiratory fitness. Depending on the injury and the length of time that the client has been incapacitated, one of the primary goals is to ensure that cardiorespiratory function adequately supports the client's chosen activity. Based on the athletic trainer's bioenergetic analysis, the focus is typically on either aerobic or anaerobic function. Unfortunately, however, athletic trainers sometimes neglect this important assessment. Declines in cardiorespiratory fitness happen rapidly. Postoperative ACL-surgery status, an acute hip flexor strain, a cervical fracture, an Achilles tendon rupture—each of these injuries presents various challenges. Taking inventory of all available equipment and creatively and safely modifying activities help athletic trainers perform cardiorespiratory work with minimal concerns. Box 8-6 lists several ways to incorporate cardiorespiratory activities in the conditioning and rehabilitation program (Figure 8-24).

Range of Motion and Flexibility. An individual can be strong only through his or her available range of motion. The greater the distance that a joint can move safely and efficiently, the more strength and power an individual

periodization a method to facilitate progress toward conditioning and rehabilitation goals that involves manipulating exercise variables to achieve certain performance goals at certain times

BOX 8-5 Rehabilitation Program Components

- Cardiorespiratory maintenance
- Range of motion and flexibility
- Proprioception, kinesthesia, and neuromuscular control: Part A to training (or retraining) the central nervous system
- Muscular strength, endurance, and power
- Postural and core stability
- Reactive neuromuscular training: Part B to training (or retraining) the central nervous system

TABLE 8-13 **Periodization Cycles**

CYCLE	GOALS	VOLUME	WEIGHTS	CARDIO
Hypertrophy—A Strength endurance	Build muscle mass Build strength Decrease body fat Build aerobic foundation Promote mental regrouping Increase flexibility Develop recovery ability Decrease risk of injuries	High volume Low intensity	4 times per week 2–3 sets 12–15 repetitions 30- to 60-second rest RPE* 2–4	4 times per week 30–40 minutes THR† 50%–70%
Hypertrophy—B Cellular adaptations	Build muscle mass Build strength Decrease body fat Build aerobic foundation Promote mental regrouping Increase flexibility Develop recovery ability Decrease risk of injuries	High volume Low intensity	4 times per week 2–3 sets 9–12 repetitions 45- to 90-second rest RPE* 2–4	4 times per week 30–40 minutes THR 70%–75%
Strength	Increase sport-specific strength Increase power Increase speed Maintain flexibility Increase recovery ability Increase work capacity Technique and mechanics	Moderate volume High intensity	3 times per week 3–4 sets 6–8 repetitions 2- to 3-minute rest RPE 6–8	4 times per week 35–60 minutes THR 75%–80%
Cellular maintenance and refining	Maintain all fitness levels Build anaerobic capacity Train to compete Improve technique and skills	Moderate volume Moderate intensity	2 times per week 2–3 sets 9–12 repetitions 45- to 90-second rest RPE 5–7	4 times per week 25–30 minutes THR 70%–80%
Strength/power (neural adaptations)	Heighten strength Heighten power Anaerobic capacity Maintain flexibility Refine explosiveness Promote mental regrouping	Low volume Very high intensity	Every third day 4–8 sets 1–5 repetitions 3- to 5-minute rest RPE 8–10	3 times per week 25–30 minutes THR 85%–100%
Active rest	Improve cross-training Promote mental recovery Encourage playful activity Rehabilitate injuries	Very low volume Every other day		

* *RPE,* Rating of perceived exertion (0 = very easy; 10 = very difficult)
† *THR,* training heart rate (220 – Age = X; X × THR% = training heart rate)

has at his or her disposal. The ability of a joint to move through a desired range depends on several conditions. First, the joint structures (i.e., ligaments, joint capsules, cartilage, bones) must be intact and in proper alignment, allowing for specific movement at the joint itself.[30] This is referred to as **range of motion**. Second, the tissues external to the joint (i.e., muscles, tendons, fascia) must be supple, flexible, and strong enough to allow movement through the available range at a particular joint.[2] This is called **flexibility**. Combined, these two qualities provide the framework for joint movements and degrees of motion. After injury, any of these structures can become compromised, thus limiting the range of motion and flexibility of that particular body part or segment. Any limitation in available motion will predispose the affected body part to injury[2,31,32] (Figure 8-25).

range of motion the specific movement provided at a joint by the joint structures (ligaments, joint capsules, cartilage, bones)

flexibility movement through an available range allowed at a joint by the tissues external to that joint (muscles, tendons, fascia)

BOX 8-6 Cardiorespiratory Options

Upper body ergometer (UBE)
Upright bicycle
Recumbent bicycle
Treadmill
Elliptical trainer
Rower
Stair climber
Slide board
Pool (or other aquatic options)

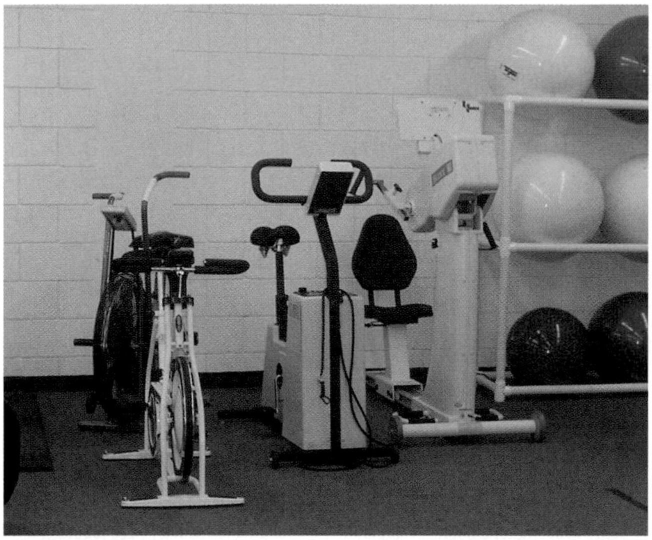

FIGURE 8-24 Options for improving cardiorespiratory fitness are plentiful and can be easily incorporated throughout the entire rehabilitation program.

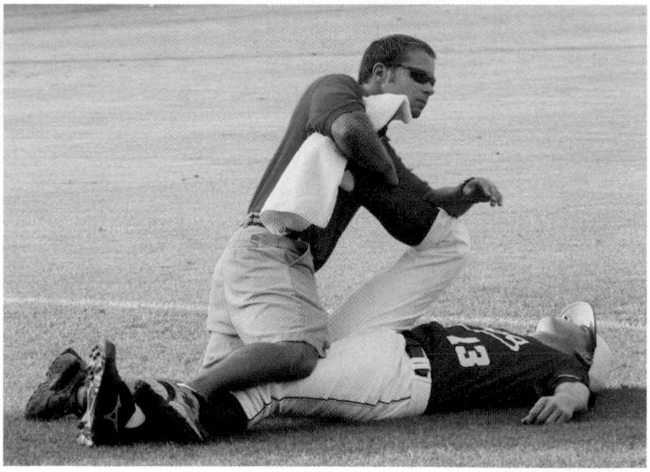

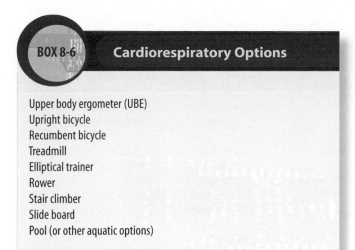

FIGURE 8-25 Addressing range of motion in all phases of the rehabilitation program will help ensure that the client achieves motion through the available range, which in turn helps to prevent re-injury.

When helping a client resume activity, the athletic trainer addresses range of motion and flexibility by way of stretching techniques. These techniques are most effective when performed in a progressive order based on the client's diagnosis and the severity of the injury.[33] Athletic trainers should always remember that joint swelling, along with any structural insult incurred secondary to the trauma or surgery, often limits the client's activity. A good rule of thumb, when determining a safe range of motion for joints, is to start with passive stretching, then progress to active stretching, and conclude with resistive stretching or proprioceptive neuromuscular facilitation (PNF). PNF is achieved by alternating muscle contractions and stretches in functional movement patterns. Each form of stretching has specific foci that must be fully understood before being incorporated in the rehabilitation program. Table 8-14 summarizes stretching techniques and their specific parameters.

Proprioception, Kinesthesia, and Neuromuscular Training: Part A to Training the Central Nervous System. Proprioception, kinesthesia, and neuromuscular control are different but equally important concepts in the early stages of physical rehabilitation. These three concepts are considered "Part A" in training (or retraining) the central nervous system (CNS). **Proprioception** is simply awareness, be it conscious or unconscious, of a joint relative to the rest of the body and the environment. **Kinesthesia** is the ability to perceive joint motion or movement by way of input that is transmitted to the spinal cord through sensory pathways. **Neuromuscular control** is the motor response to the kinesthetic (sensory) input. Exercises that fall in this category are diverse, ranging from merely standing upright and practicing full weight bearing through the injured body part (Figure 8-26) to balancing erect on an exercise ball while catching a medicine ball in one hand with the eyes closed. Exercises of this nature have been shown to help in the prevention of injuries.[34–37] Athletic trainers should always start with simple proprioceptive activities (e.g., weight bearing) to establish the base level of ability. Once this is determined, progressing safely and quickly with kinesthetic and neuromuscular training will

proprioception awareness of a joint relative to the rest of the body and the environment surrounding it
kinesthesia the ability to perceive joint motion or movement
neuromuscular control the motor response to kinesthetic (sensory) input

TABLE 8-14 Stretching Techniques

TECHNIQUE	DESCRIPTION	MOVEMENT	GRAVITY	PRECAUTIONS
Passive	You move the client's body part through a certain range of motion (*manual stretching*)	Hold for 15–30 seconds	Antigravity position	Watch for physical responses to pain and/or stretching.
Active-assistive	Something assists the client's body part through a certain range of motion (e.g., *pulleys, finger ladders*)	Hold for 15–30 seconds	Gravity-dependent position most common	Monitor for excessive stretching beyond desired range of motion.
Active-dynamic	The client moves the body part through a certain range of motion (e.g., *walking lunge, overhead rainbows*)	Smooth, continuous, active movements	Gravity-dependent position	Monitor for technique and safety.
Resistive/PNF	The client resists against a force, typically the athletic trainer (e.g., *contract-relax, resisted-active movement*)	Smooth movements, either with a 5- or 10-second hold or continuous	Antigravity position most common	Monitor for excessive stretching and resistance.
Ballistic	A rapid, bouncing stretch with a particular body part	Bouncy, rapid movements	Antigravity position	Monitor for excessive stretching, technique, and safety.

PNF, Proprioceptive neuromuscular facilitation.

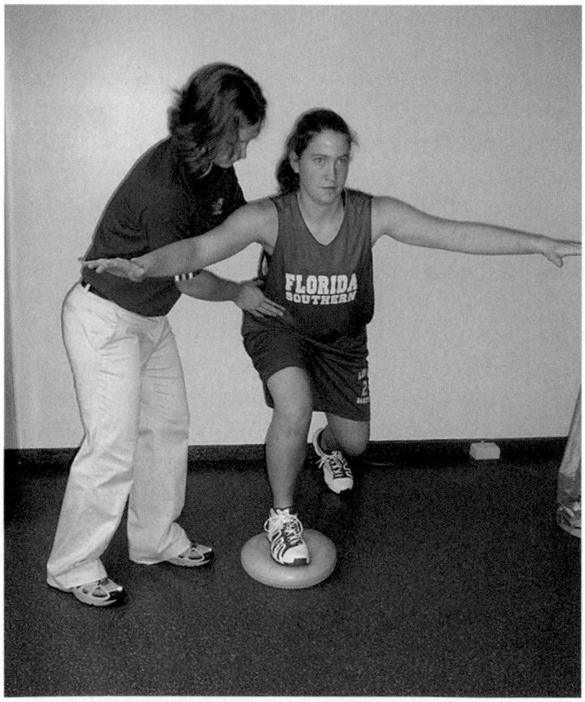

FIGURE 8-26 Performing progressive exercises that challenge proprioception, kinesthesia, and neuromuscular control will prepare the client to return to activity in the best condition possible.

create a productive environment that promotes the body's capacity to respond to internal and external stimuli, culminating, perhaps, with balancing on the exercise ball. This component of the rehabilitation program can be started at the onset of the rehabilitation program, depending on the injury and the stage of injury repair.

Muscular Strength, Endurance, and Power. Muscular strength is necessary to move any body part. The complex movements imposed on the body by athletes and working people place significant demands on the muscles. Movements range from heavy lifting to complex fine motor skills to repetitive endurance movements. Many sports and occupations require a combination of movements, tapping into various forms of strength. The basis for all movement is to establish a foundation of strength. By performing biomechanical and bioenergetic analysis, athletic trainers ascertain whether the activity requires more pure strength, power, or endurance. **Muscular strength** is the ability to generate force against a resistance (Figure 8-27). **Muscular endurance** is the ability to perform repeated muscular contractions over time. **Muscular power** is the ability to produce a large amount of force in a relatively short period (Figure 8-28). Once a good strength base is established, the athletic trainer may then focus on endurance or power, both of which require a solid foundation of strength to be truly effective.

Figure 8-29 demonstrates the strength continuum in repetitions that would be emphasized during training of that particular strength form.

muscular strength the ability to generate force against a resistance

muscular endurance the ability to perform repeated muscular contractions over a period of time

muscular power the ability to produce a large amount of force in a relatively short period of time

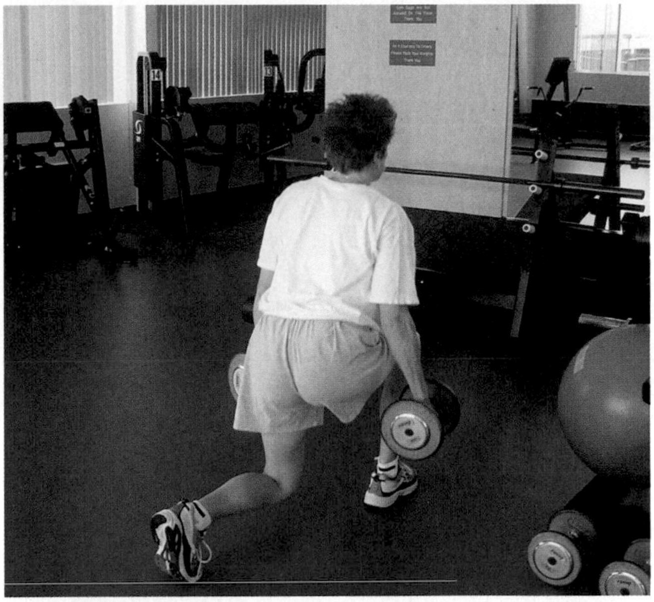

FIGURE 8-27 Muscular strength is frequently improved by performing specific movement patterns with external resistance or loads.

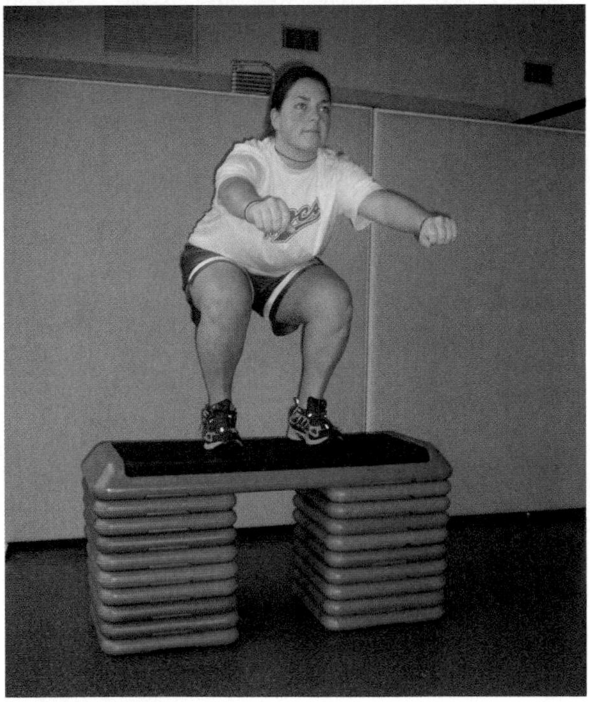

FIGURE 8-28 Muscular power can be developed in many ways and frequently accounts for the difference between a good performance and a great performance.

Modes of training strength include isometric, isotonic, and isokinetic activities. **Isometric exercise** is performed by resisting a movement pattern but without moving the body part involved. Isometrics have approximately a 15-degree carryover effect. In other words, if someone is performing an isometric biceps curl at 90 degrees, the carryover strength benefit is from 75 degrees to 105 degrees. **Isotonic exercise** is performed with a constant weight (e.g., dumbbell) while performing either concentric (i.e., muscle shortening) or eccentric (i.e., muscle lengthening) contractions. Many functional strengthening exercises—that is, exercises that require multijoint and multimuscle recruitment in all planes of motion—involve a combination of concentric and eccentric contractions, which is how the human body truly moves (Figure 8-30). Thus rehabilitation programs that train the body in this manner are most effective. **Isokinetic exercise** involves a device that has a fixed speed and allows for varying resistances through the predetermined range of motion[2,32] (Figure 8-31). Isokinetics are frequently performed as diagnostic tools to determine levels of readiness through the rehabilitation process. Usually, an isokinetic test is one of the final criteria that an individual must fulfill before resuming activity.

Postural and Core Stability. Building on the gains made in addressing the proprioception, kinesthetic, and neuromuscular components, the athletic trainer next incorporates postural and core stability techniques, which ensure that the body can respond adequately to the required internal and external stimuli. Initially, the client must be able to maintain a neutral posture in order to maneuver safely through the demands of his or her job or sport. The **postural neutral position**, sometimes called the functional

isometric exercise resistance training that does not involve moving the involved body part

isotonic exercise resistance training performed with either concentric or eccentric contractions, causing movement of the limb

isokinetic exercise resistance training that involves a device with a fixed speed and allows for varying resistances through a predetermined range of motion

postural neutral position the functional position; a neutral posture

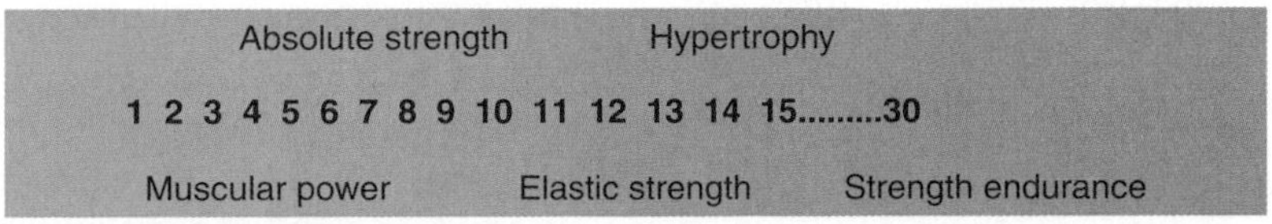

FIGURE 8-29 Strength continuum designed to help the athletic trainer determine the proper number of repetitions.

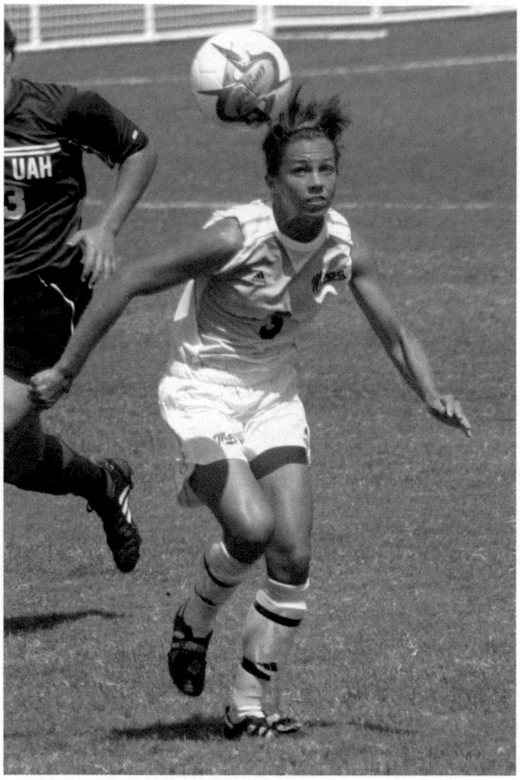

FIGURE 8-30 Isotonic exercises, the most common form of strength training, involve a consistent resistance (e.g., dumbbell, medicine ball, weighted bar) during a particular movement, much like the majority of all sport movements.

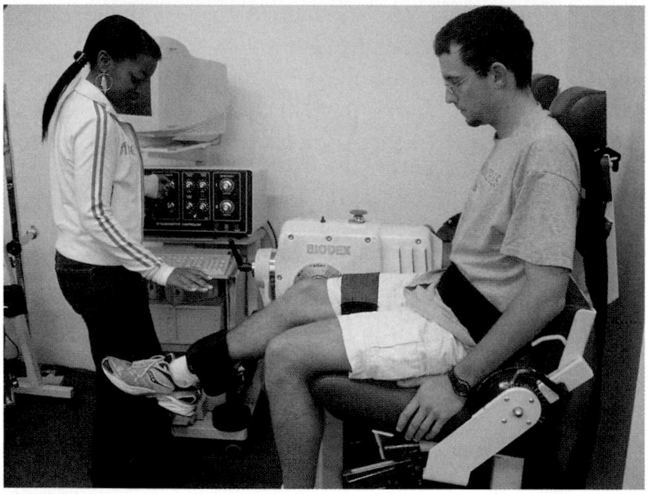

FIGURE 8-31 Isokinetic exercises involve a consistent speed, instead of resistance, that is performed through a particular range of motion; the computer program controls the speed and range of motion while the individual controls the resistance exerted.

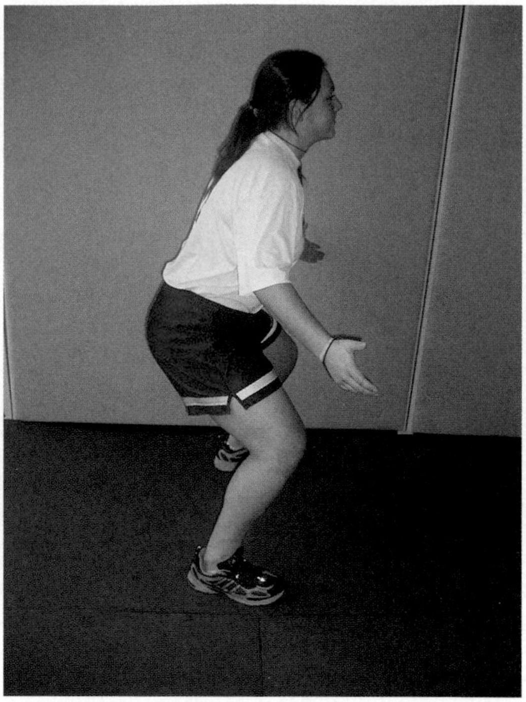

FIGURE 8-32 In the functional position (also called the *postural neutral position*), the ankles, knees, and hips are slightly flexed with the hips and buttocks placed slightly behind the center of mass and the knees positioned over the midfoot; the core is strong and tight, and the upper trunk and arms are relaxed in preparation for the next movement.

position (Figure 8-32), requires sensory input and motor control of the spine, head, and core.[38] The core consists of the lumbar, pelvis, and hip structures.

After demonstrating the ability to maintain the functional position, the client must next demonstrate the ability to move the body in various patterns while managing external loads.[2] Again, the biomechanical and bioenergetic analysis will reveal precisely what movements are needed to prepare the client for this goal. The athletic trainer should be careful to replicate the required demands in the rehabilitation program before allowing the client to return to activity. A useful rule of thumb is that most human movements begin and end with the core.[2] The importance of postural and core stability in physical rehabilitation cannot be overstated.[2,38] The key to preventing future injuries or further injury is often found in the development of a strong and stable core.

Points to Ponder

Describe three movements that negate the assumption that human movement begins and ends at the core.

Reactive Neuromuscular Training (Plyometrics): Part B to Training the Central Nervous System. **Plyometrics** are exercises of a relatively independent motor quality that condition the neuromuscular system to allow faster and more powerful changes of direction and production

plyometrics reactive training that stimulates changes in the neuromuscular system, enhancing the ability of the muscle groups to respond more quickly and powerfully to slight and rapid changes in muscle length of force. In other words, plyometrics allow an athlete to change directions running down the field more quickly and more accurately or to jump and rebound a ball, land, and turn around quickly enough to sprint down the court on a fast break. Plyometrics are also known as reactive training, elastic training, the stretch-shortening cycle, and the myotatic stretch reflex. This type of exercise stimulates changes in the neuromuscular system, enhancing the ability of the muscle groups to respond more quickly and powerfully to slight and rapid changes in muscle length. Plyometrics involves the neuromuscular system at levels beyond those generated by other types of training. An individual can be very strong but not powerful because of an inability to rapidly contract already strong muscles. Because plyometrics are rapidly executed, maximal speed is reached without the allowance of time to adjust movements during performance. Reactive neuromuscular training, or plyometrics, can help decrease the risk of injuries,[31,39] improve performance outcomes,[39–44] and increase bone mass in adolescent girls[45] (Figure 8-33).

To design a safe and effective plyometric program, the athletic trainer must begin with some basic knowledge. The following areas must be considered when determining both the potential effectiveness of plyometrics and the feasibility of performing them: chronological age; training age within the sport; body composition; postural alignment; strength, flexibility, and fitness levels; medical history; current training cycle and the specific job or sport demands. If clients do not have the required strength and flexibility to handle plyometrics, if they are in the middle of a competition cycle, or if they are just beginning to train, a plyometrics program should not be attempted. Negative training effects will occur, most likely leading to injury. Plyometrics are extremely demanding and should be performed only by individuals equipped to handle each level safely and properly. Table 8-15 describes proper plyometric progressions for the lower body.

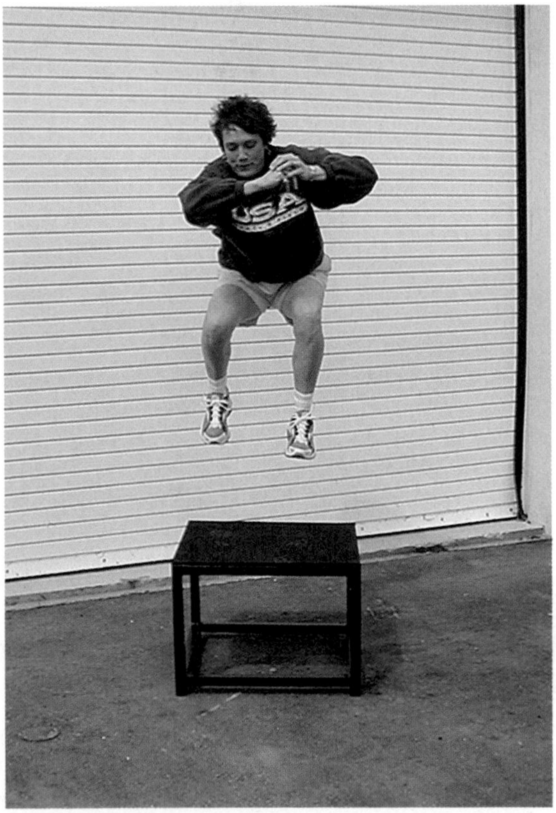

FIGURE 8-33 When plyometrics are properly taught and performed in conditioning and rehabilitation programs, increases in performances are possible as well as the reduction or prevention of certain injuries.

Return to Activity. Before returning the client to his or her previous activity, the athletic trainer must design a functional clearance test, as described earlier in this chapter. This test demonstrates the client's ability to perform the required activities.[5,12] The athletic trainer's analysis of the activity dictates the specific movements with which the client should be challenged.[13] The design of the functional clearance test should be progressive, starting with simple exercises that increase in complexity. For the client to resume activity, merely passing the test is not sufficient. The client's readiness depends on successfully meeting the rehabilitation goals established at the onset of the rehabilitation program, with continual monitoring of the client's psychosocial status. Nurturing the mind as well as the body hastens recovery, increases the client's confidence in his or her capabilities, and lessens his or her fear of reinjury. Box 8-7 provides a sample clearance test for a lower extremity injury.

Points to Ponder

Clients should move through the progressive exercises of a rehabilitation program with a good understanding of the rationale behind its components. What factors should the athletic trainer take into account when creating the conditioning and rehabilitation program?

COMBINING MODALITIES AND EXERCISE

As mentioned throughout this chapter, the best rehabilitation programs incorporate both modalities and exercises to return the client to activity as quickly and safely as possible. In the early stages of injury repair, modalities are the primary focus because the goal at this point is to limit inflammation and cellular trauma. Alleviating pain and swelling is crucial for healing to occur. As the client progresses through the stages, the focus shifts from modalities to exercise. Modalities can be used throughout the conditioning and rehabilitation program to enhance healing and deter negative physiological responses to increased training and activity loads. Also, exercise can be initiated at the beginning of some

TABLE 8-15 Lower Extremity Plyometrics Continuum

LEVEL	GOALS	PLYOMETRIC EXERCISES
Level 1: very low impact	Teach plyometric concepts	Minitrampoline marching Minitrampoline ankle bounces Lunge series Cone lunges Step-overs Minitrampoline jogging Weighted squat series Unilateral squat Squat with medicine ball pick-up Squat throws
Level 2: low impact * Do not progress to the next level until mastery has been achieved at each level	Teach landings Teach core stabilization Teach "triple extension" take-off	Ankle bounces (pogos) Squat jump series Tuck jump series Split-squat jumps Butt-kick jumps Scissors jumps
Level 3 : medium impact		
A	Horizontal displacement of center of gravity (COG)	Bilateral long jumps Bilateral hurdle jumps Hurdle strides Unilateral long jumps
B	Advanced horizontal displacement of COG	Bilateral hop series Bilateral zig-zag hop series Unilateral hop series High barrier hop series Lateral barrier hop series
C	Horizontal displacement of COG with velocity	Skip series Power skip series Retro skips Bounding series Bilateral stair bound series
Level 4: high intensity (box jumps)	Vertical displacement of COG	
A	Getting "to" the box	Unilateral push-off Alternating push-offs Lateral push-off Side-to-side push-off series
B	Getting "on" the box	Box jump-ups Box leap-overs Lateral jump-ups Jump down series Jump on to squat series
Level 5: very high intensity (depth jumps)	Develop explosive power	Depth jump series Mixed height box series Depth jump to long jump Unilateral depth jump Depth jump to lateral series

rehabilitation programs provided that it is not contraindicated. Recovery sessions must be scheduled into the program as the gains made in training actually manifest during recovery.[46] A well-planned program combines modalities with exercise and incorporates recovery periods at just the right times to properly move the individual through the stages of injury repair without prompting any setbacks.

SUMMARY

When developing a conditioning and rehabilitation program, athletic trainers must consider many issues. Obviously, the type of injury and its current stage of repair are crucial factors. A proper diagnosis is necessary for the design of a high-quality program. A thorough biomechanical and bioenergetic analysis of the activity provides the foundation of the program.

BOX 8-7 Lower Extremity Functional Clearance Test

- Toe and heel raises
- Minisquats
- Lunge series
- Two leg, 1-inch hops
- Front-to-back and side-to-side hops
- One-leg, 1-inch hops
- One-leg, front-to-back and side-to-side hops
- Broad jump series
- Lateral shuffle
- Cariocas
- Multi-angle zig-zag runs
- Stop-and-start series
- Backward running
- Jumps and hops (90- and 180-degree)
- Squat jump
- Tuck jump
- Rapid step-up series
- Sprint series
- Activity-specific balance, agilities, and plyometrics

While designing the program, the athletic trainer should remember that modalities and exercises can be employed simultaneously. Programs for acute injuries tend to be modality intensive, whereas programs for chronic injuries tend to be exercise intensive. The ultimate goal is to return the client to activity as quickly and safely as possible. The athletic trainer's selection of modalities and exercises is a crucial part of making this happen.

Revisiting the OPENING Scenario

An examination of Noah reveals that he has strained his low back, specifically his quadratus lumborum. In addition, he has pinched his sciatic nerve, which is the reason for the burning sensation radiating from his left gluteals down to his hamstring. Because circumstances compel him to return to work, a good rehabilitation program might include a comprehensive stretching and dynamic lumbar strengthening program that incorporates the simultaneous application of ESTIM and cryotherapy in the clinic. Noah should be advised to continue the clinic visits so that he can make progress with the recommended modalities, and his functional abilities should be monitored as he moves through the stages of injury repair. At every visit, Noah should be re-assessed to determine the efficacy of the modalities and exercises as well as his ability to perform his activity-specific duties.

Issues & Ethics

Brandon is a 20-year-old junior transfer on your college basketball team. He began complaining about a sore hamstring about 4 weeks ago, when preseason practices started. When his coach and other teammates are around, he walks with a limp and favors his left leg. However, several times while you have been walking across campus, you have seen Brandon walking without an altered gait; still more surprising, you even saw him run on two occasions. You know that Brandon recently transferred from a school across the state, where he was the star player. At your school, a preseason contender for the championship title, he is one of many stars vying for the same starting position. Today Brandon is complaining about increased soreness and an inability to run or jump. Listening to him, you feel conflicted. On the one hand, he may need a comprehensive rehabilitation program to address what appears to be strength and range of motion deficits. On the other hand, he also appears to be faking his injury, possibly in response to the unexpected pressure of making the team. What do you do?

Web Links

American Sorts Medicine Institute: www.asmi.org
National Athletic Trainers' Association: www.nata.org
National Strength and Conditioning Association: www.nsca-lift.org

References

1. Greene JJ: Athletic trainers in an orthopedic practice, *Athletic Therapy Today* 9(5): 56–57, 2004.
2. Stanos SP, McLean J, Rader L: Physical medicine rehabilitation approach to pain, *Medical Clinics of North America* 91: 57–95, 2007.
3. Man IOW, Morrissey MC, Cywinski JK: Effect of neuromuscular electrical stimulation on ankle swelling in the early period after ankle sprain, *Physical Therapy* 87(1): 53–65, 2007.
4. Stalzer S, Wahoff M, Scanlan M: Rehabilitation following hip arthroscopy, *Clinics in Sports Medicine* 25: 337–357, 2006.
5. Cascio BM, Culp L, Cosgarea AJ: Return to play after anterior cruciate ligament reconstruction, *Clinics in Sports Medicine* 23: 395–408, 2004.
6. Hamill J, Knutzen M: *Biomechanical analysis of human movement*, ed 2, Baltimore, 2003, Lippincott Williams & Wilkins.
7. Riemann BJ: Is there a link between chronic ankle instability and postural instability? *Journal of Athletic Training* 37(4): 386–393, 2002.
8. Nyland J, Nolan MF: Therapeutic modality: rehabilitation of the injured athlete, *Clinics in Sports Medicine* 23: 299–313, 2004.

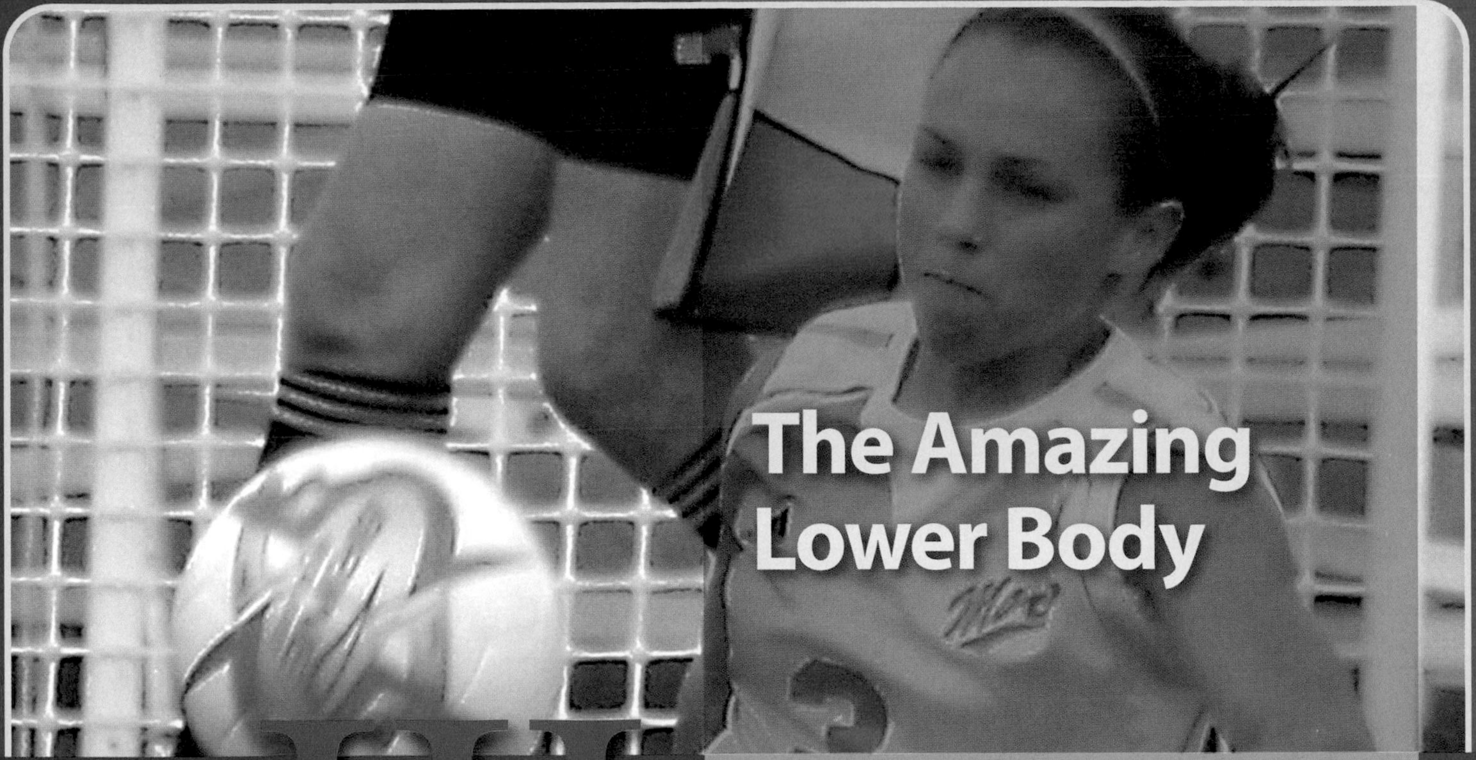

The Amazing Lower Body

III

UNIT THREE

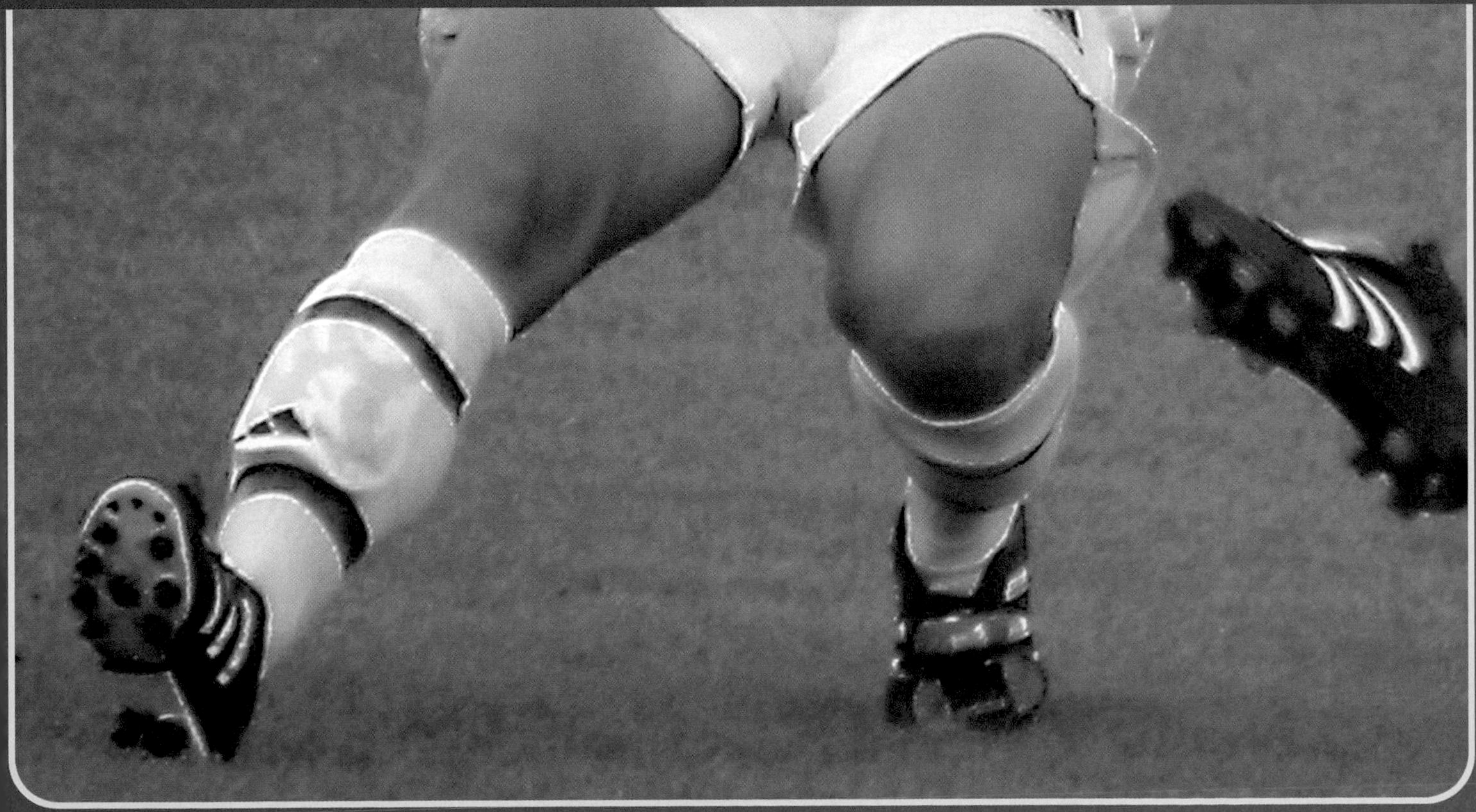

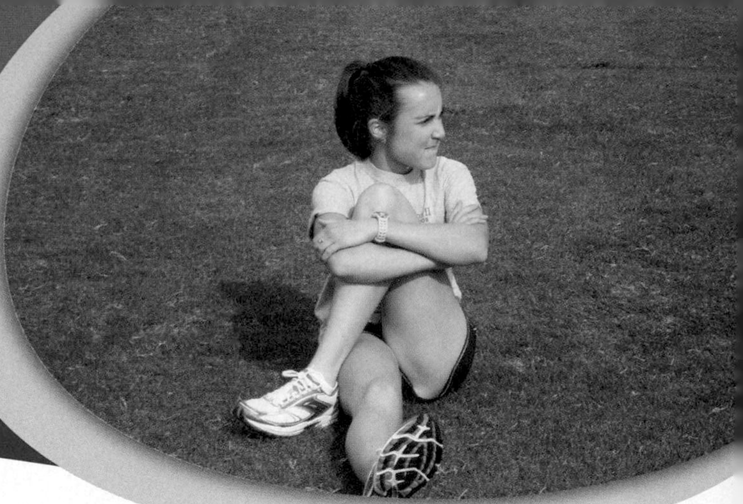

9 Anatomy of the Lower Body

ROBERT MOSS

Learning Goals

1. Name and describe the basic anatomical structures—bones, ligaments, muscles, tendons, nerves, arteries, and veins—their unique aspects, and locations relative to the lower body.
2. List the anatomical structures of the lower body using the appropriate terminology.
3. Describe the interdependent relationships of the structures of the lower body.
4. Describe the complex structures of the lower body.
5. Identify how the role or function of each of the anatomical structures may change with various movements that occur in areas above or below it.

Lower body anatomy is amazing for several reasons. The following two are probably the most important: (1) Almost every activity that the body performs relies on its lower half in some way to accomplish that activity most effectively; (2) most of the time, people are unaware of the extent to which their lower bodies are responsible for movement. Consider, for example, the act of throwing a ball. Obviously, a ball can be thrown while the thrower is sitting, but it cannot be thrown as far or as hard as when the thrower is standing and using the legs to help generate force that can be transferred up to the arm. When the foot pushes off the ground during walking, running, and jumping, the foot bones naturally lock, allowing the foot to become a rigid lever with which the body is pushed off the ground in an efficient manner. In a similar fashion, the foot bones unlock, becoming flexible so that they may better absorb forces when landing. The bones of the foot lock and unlock without the need for conscious thought. The amazing lower body allows people to run marathons, squat 600 pounds, bounce babies on their knees, dance, and so much more.

Terms that appear in boldface green type are defined in the book's glossary.

FUNCTIONS OF THE LOWER BODY

In this chapter, the lower body is defined as encompassing everything from the pelvis and hips down to the toes. The pelvis is also discussed in Chapter 13 because it serves as a central station where forces that come from below are transferred up to the spine and upper body and where forces from the upper body and spine are transferred down to the lower body. The lower body has two general functions (Box 9-1). One function is to support all the structures and weight that are above it. The second function is to produce movement. *Movement* is defined as taking a body part or the entire body from one place to another and maintaining balance along the way. Although supporting weight may seem like a relatively simple function, it becomes complicated when movement is involved or when relative weight is not predictable, such as when supporting the body on just one limb. Similarly, movement itself does not seem especially difficult until we try to imitate a professional basketball player's agile pivots and explosive changes of direction or a champion golfer's subtle lower body movements when hitting a golf ball. To facilitate an understanding of the component parts that have a role in these two general functions (i.e., support and movement), as well as other, more specific movements, this chapter presents the anatomy of the amazing lower body.

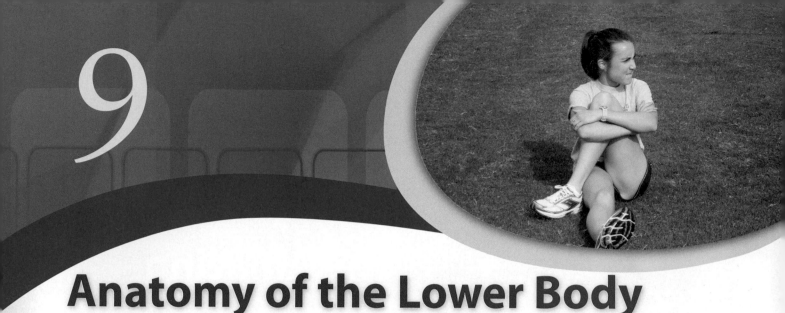

BOX 9-1 Two Main Functions of the Lower Body

1. To support all of the structures and weight above the lower body.
2. To move and balance while performing various activities.

BONES OF THE LOWER BODY

The bones of the lower body are also the foundation of almost every physical activity in which at least one foot is on the ground (Figure 9-1 and Box 9-2). With regard to these structures and those more **proximal**, consider the following factors: (1) how the individual parts work together to become compilations of structures, (2) how these structures assume a number of different functions or responsibilities depending on the activity, and (3) the uniqueness of these structures among individuals.

Bones of the Ankle and Foot Area

The normal foot has 26 bones "plus two." The 28 bones are classified in a couple of different ways according to their location in the foot. The first classification is relative to each bone's location in the rearfoot, midfoot, or forefoot (Figure 9-2) There are two bones in the rearfoot: the calcaneus and the talus. The midfoot comprises five bones: the navicular, the cuboid, and the three cuneiforms (medial, middle [or intermediate] and lateral; Figure 9-3). The forefoot contains twenty-one bones (including two sesamoid bones): five metatarsals and fourteen phalanges. All the foot bones may also be grouped according to location, relative to their original Greek or Latin derivation. For example, seven of the foot bones—the calcaneus, talus, navicular, cuboid, and three cuneiforms—are also called *tarsals* (from the Greek word *tarsus,* for ankle). The five metatarsals come from the Greek words *meta* and *tarsal,* which means "beside" or "after" the ankle, and the 14 phalanges come from the Greek and Latin word *phalanx,* which means "log" or "battle array." The "plus two" bones are two small sesamoid (from a Greek word that means "shaped like a sesame seed") bones located **inferior** to the **distal** end of the first metatarsal. Note that the shape of the foot includes three sets of arches. There are two longitudinal arches,

proximal closer to the midline or center of the body relative to another landmark
inferior under or beneath
distal farther away from the body's midline or center relative to another landmark

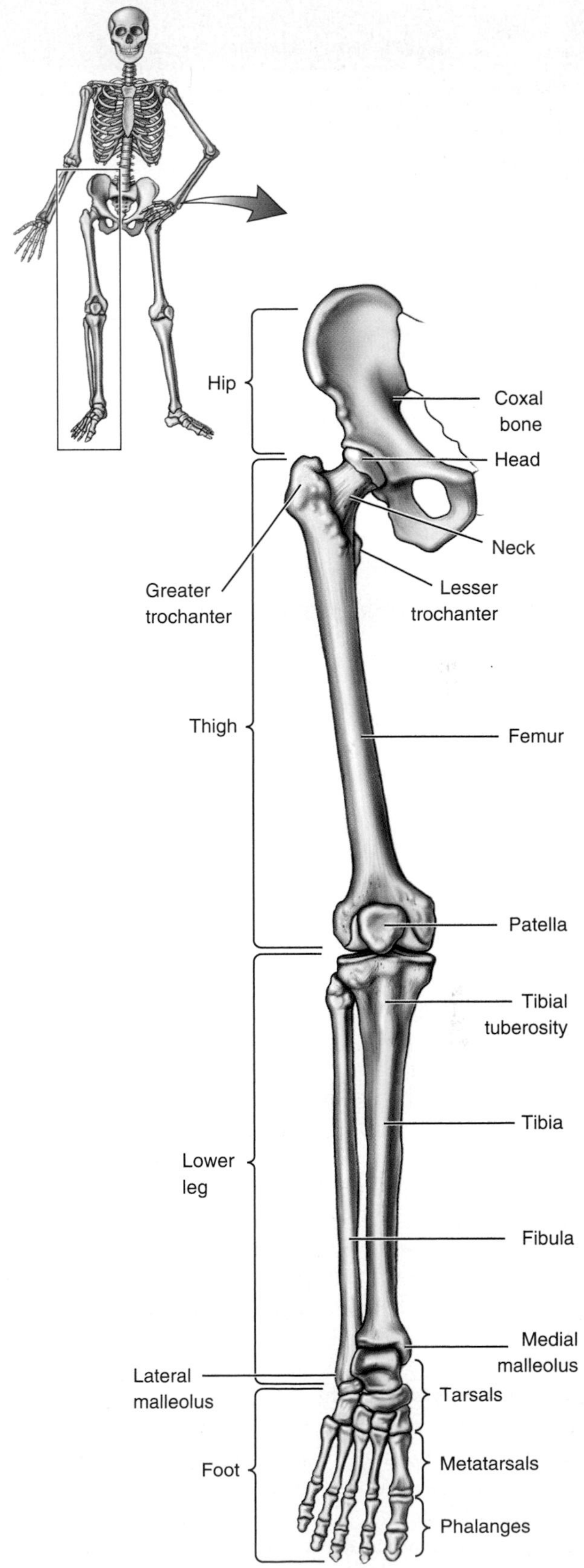

FIGURE 9-1 Bones of the lower body, anterior view. (From Herlihy B: *The human body in health and disease,* ed 3, p. 126, Philadelphia, 2007, Saunders/Elsevier.)

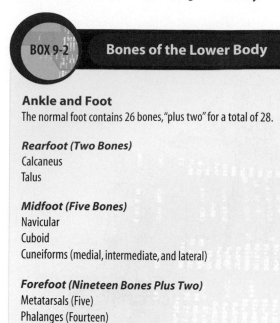

BOX 9-2 Bones of the Lower Body

Ankle and Foot

The normal foot contains 26 bones, "plus two" for a total of 28.

Rearfoot (Two Bones)

Calcaneus
Talus

Midfoot (Five Bones)

Navicular
Cuboid
Cuneiforms (medial, intermediate, and lateral)

Forefoot (Nineteen Bones Plus Two)

Metatarsals (Five)
Phalanges (Fourteen)
Sesamoids ("plus two"—medial [tibial] and lateral [fibular])

Leg

Tibia
Fibula

Thigh and Thigh Area

Femur
Patella (knee)

Pelvis

Ilium
Ischium
Pubis

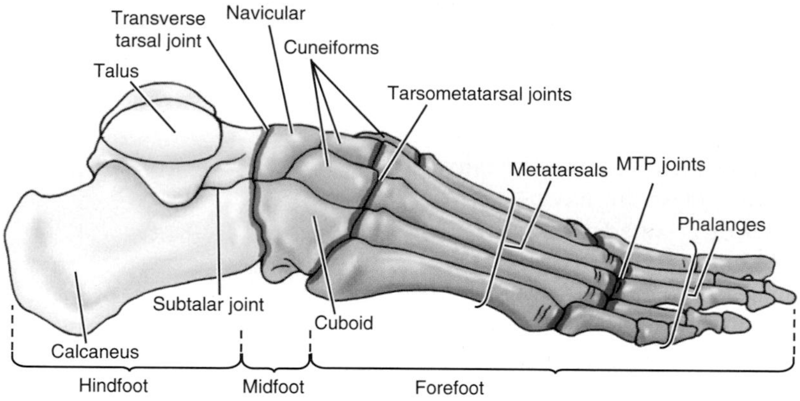

FIGURE 9-2 Foot bones, lateral view. (From Muscolino JE: *Kinesiology: the skeletal system and muscle function,* p. 331, St Louis, 2006, Mosby/Elsevier.)

one on the **medial** side and one on the **lateral** side. There is also a transverse arch spanning across the forefoot (Figure 9-4).

Calcaneus

The calcaneus serves the important purpose of being the body's first point of contact with the ground during walking or running. It is an irregular-shaped bone covered on the bottom by a specialized tissue called the *calcaneal fat pad.* This fat pad helps absorb ground reaction forces when the calcaneus makes contact with the ground. The calcaneus also serves as the attachment site for many muscles, tendons, and ligaments. It has a significant landmark in that it has a unique shelf of sorts called the *sustentaculum tali.*

Talus

The other rearfoot bone is the talus, which rests on top of the sustentaculum tali of the calcaneus in a rather precarious position. The positioning of the talus on the calcaneus is analogous to that of a saddle (the talus) on a horse (the calcaneus). The talus is an irregular-shaped bone that is unique in the human body because it has no muscular or tendinous attachments. However, it does play an extremely important and unsung role in **gait.**

medial toward the midline or center of the body (inner aspect) relative to another landmark
lateral away from the midline or center of the body (outer aspect) relative to another landmark
gait pattern or technique of walking or running

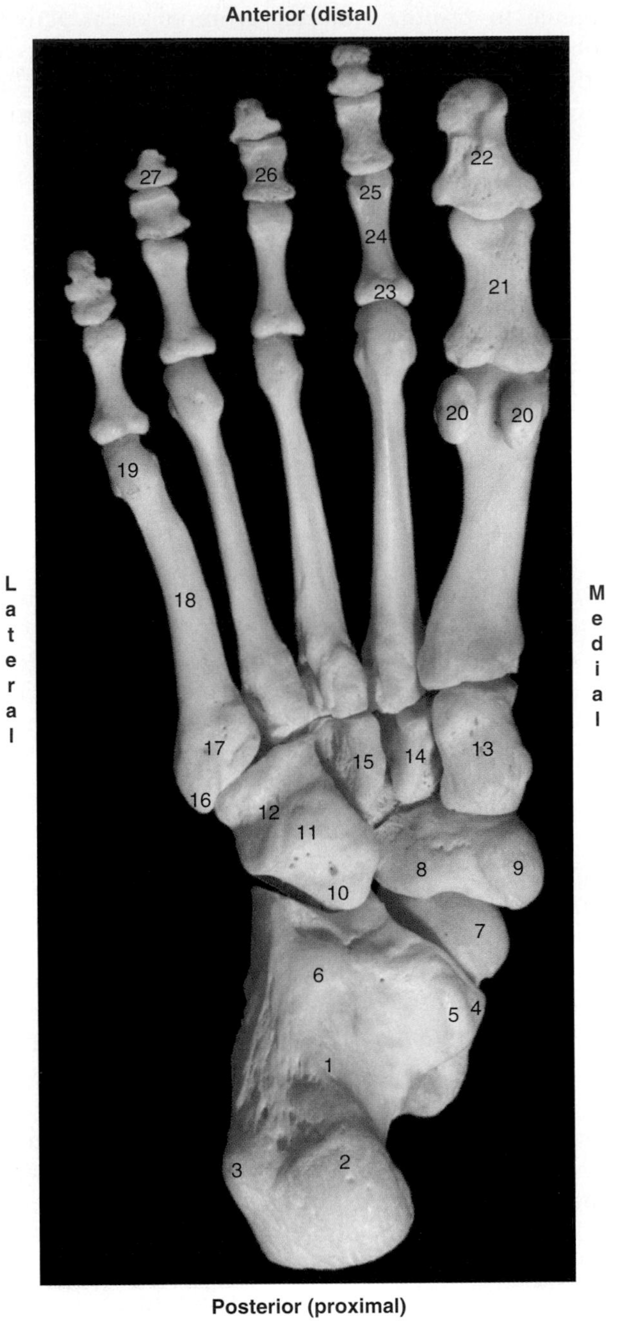

FIGURE 9-3 Foot bones, inferior view. *1,* Calcaneus; *2,* medial process of calcaneal tuberosity; *3,* lateral process of medial tuberosity; *4,* sustentaculum tali of calcaneus; *5,* groove for distal tendon of flexor hallucis longus muscle (on sustentaculum tali); *6,* anterior tubercle of calcaneus; *7,* head of talus; *8,* navicular; *9,* navicular tuberosity; *10,* cuboid; *11,* tuberosity of cuboid; *12,* groove for distal tendon of fibularis longus muscle; *13,* first cuneiform; *14,* second cuneiform; *15,* third cuneiform; *16,* tuberosity of base of fifth metatarsal; *17,* base of fifth metatarsal; *18,* body (shaft) of fifth metatarsal; *19,* head of fifth metatarsal; *20,* sesamoid bone of big toe; *21,* proximal phalanx of big toe; *22,* distal phalanx of big toe; *23,* base of proximal phalanx of second toe; *24,* body (shaft) of proximal phalanx of second toe; *25,* head of proximal phalanx of second toe; *26,* middle phalanx of third toe; *27,* distal phalanx of fourth toe. (From Muscolino JE: *Kinesiology: the skeletal system and muscle function,* p. 133, St. Louis, 2006, Mosby/Elsevier.)

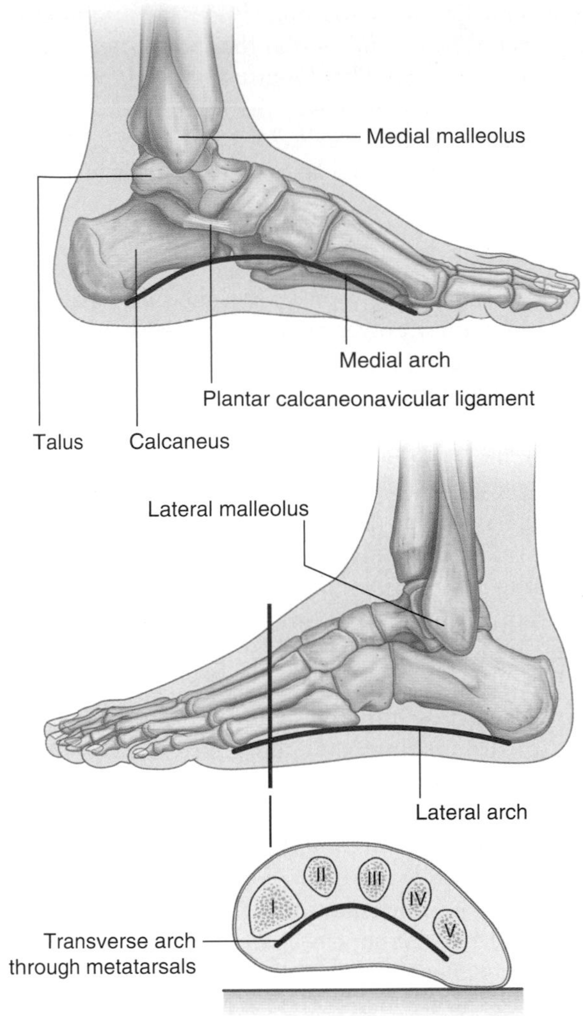

FIGURE 9-4 Arches of the foot. (From Drake RL, Vogl W, Mitchell ADM: *Gray's anatomy for students,* p. 475, Philadelphia, 2005, Elsevier/Churchill Livingstone.)

(This role is discussed in greater detail later in the chapter.) Although it has no muscle attachments, the talus is surrounded by tendons and has many ligaments that provide it with stability. The weight of the body running through the tibia, which rests **superior** to the talus, also helps hold the talus in place.

Midfoot Bones

The navicular, cuboid, and three cuneiform bones compose the structure of the midfoot. These bones work together to form the arch of the foot and serve to transmit force from the ball of the foot through the rearfoot and up into the lower leg.

superior above or on top

Navicular. The navicular bone is located just **anterior** to the talus on the medial side of the foot. Often called the "keystone" of the medial **longitudinal** arch, it is situated in such a way that makes it the bone most responsible for maintaining the concavity of the arch. The concavity of the arch provides its shock-absorbing ability. The navicular also serves as a key attachment site for muscles and ligaments.

Cuboid. Shaped like a cube, the cuboid is also a midfoot bone with a **posterior** (i.e., situated behind) aspect that lies lateral to the navicular and anterior to the calcaneus. Although the cuboid also has muscles and ligaments attached to it, one of its most important functions is to serve as a pulley for the tendon of the fibularis longus muscle, which is discussed later in the chapter. Like the navicular and the medial longitudinal arch, the cuboid is key in maintaining the integrity of the lateral longitudinal arch. The anterior aspect of the cuboid is located just lateral to the three other midfoot bones, the three cuneiforms.

Cuneiforms. The three cuneiforms (Latin for "wedge shaped") are small, rectangular bones that complete the midfoot. The medial cuneiform is also called the *first cuneiform;* the middle, or intermediate, cuneiform is also called the *second cuneiform;* and the lateral cuneiform is also called the *third cuneiform.* They all lie anterior to the navicular, and the third lies medial to the cuboid. A unique aspect of the cuneiforms is that the second cuneiform is smaller and more recessed than the first or third cuneiform; it is truly "wedged in" (see Figure 9-3).

Forefoot Bones

The forefoot comprises 21 bones: five metatarsals, fourteen phalanges, and two sesamoids. These are described in detail in the following sections.

Metatarsal Bones. The five metatarsals have similar properties—a base proximally, a head distally, and a body in between. They are miniature versions of the long bones (i.e., fibula, tibia, radius, ulna) that will be presented later. The first metatarsal is the most medial, the shortest, and the strongest of the metatarsals. It plays an important, if often overlooked, role in weight bearing of the foot. It allows a smooth transition from heel contact to toe-off during gait. The second metatarsal is long and relatively slender, and its base is wedged between the first and third cuneiforms. Its shape, size, and positioning, as well as the stresses placed on it, can make the second metatarsal susceptible to stress fractures. The bases of the first, second, and third metatarsals lie anterior to the cuneiforms and posterior to the bases of the fourth and fifth metatarsals. The third and fourth metatarsals are long, relatively slender, and generally immune to trauma resulting from physical activity. Note that this immunity does not apply to extreme situations, such as being stepped on or having a bowling ball dropped on the foot. A relatively rare condition that can occur between the bodies of the third and fourth metatarsals is the formation of a small **neuroma.** On the most lateral aspect of the foot is the fifth metatarsal, another long, relatively slender bone that is susceptible to injury. The base of this bone is in partial contact with the proximal cuboid to aid in the stability of the lateral longitudinal arch of the foot. A relatively large **tuberosity** is also present on the lateral aspect of the base of the metatarsal. This area of the base and tuberosity is susceptible to fractures, as discussed in the next chapter. All of the metatarsals have sites for the attachment of muscles, tendons, and ligaments (see Figure 9-3).

Phalanges. Distal to the metatarsals are the toes. The five toes are composed of fourteen phalanges. The first digit (known as the big toe or great toe) has two rather large and strong phalanges, the proximal phalange being larger and stronger than the distal phalange. Digits (i.e., toes) two, three, and four all have three phalanges, which decrease in size from proximal to distal relative to each phalange. The fifth digit has three tiny phalanges. Similar to the metatarsals, each phalange has a base proximally, a head distally, and a body between.

Sesamoids. The last two bones of the forefoot are the sesamoids, called the *medial* and *lateral sesamoids* or the *tibial* and *fibular sesamoids,* respectively. They both lie under the head of the first metatarsal, with the medial sesamoid being more palpable. Like the cuboid, the sesamoids serve as an important pulley for a muscle, the flexor hallucis longus. Sesamoid bones generally function to help reduce friction, modify pressure in an area, and alter or control the angle of pull on a muscle. To approximate the sensation of a bruised or fractured sesamoid of the foot, put a pea-sized pebble under the head of the first metatarsal and try to walk or run. It will change your gait and help you appreciate the proper function of a very small bone, the importance of which is often overlooked.

anterior in front of something else; toward the front
longitudinal occurring along the midline of a bone
posterior behind something else; toward the back
neuroma small area of inflammation that forms around a nerve
tuberosity a normal outgrowth or bump on a bone

Everyone in the classroom should remove their shoes and socks. Next, each student should be asked which of their toes is the longest. Generally speaking, the great toe is the longest. However, in some cases the second toe appears to be longest. These individuals have a condition known as Morton's foot (named after Dr. Dudley Morton). This foot type may predispose them to particular overuse injuries that will be discussed in Chapter 10.

Bones of the Leg

The area between the ankle and the knee is the leg. It is composed of two bones: the tibia (Latin for "shin bone") and the fibula (Latin for "pin"). In addition to being the site for many muscles, these two bones transmit the ground reaction forces from the foot and ankle up to the femur. Note that the distal part of the leg becomes part of the ankle and the proximal part of the leg becomes part of the knee (Figure 9-5).

Tibia

The larger of the two leg bones, the tibia is located on the anterior and medial side of the leg. There is a bump on the distal, medial aspect of the tibia called the medial **malleolus** (Latin for "small hammer"); this is also called the *inner ankle bone*. It is possible to feel

malleolus the distal end or knob of the tibia or fibula recognized as the ankle

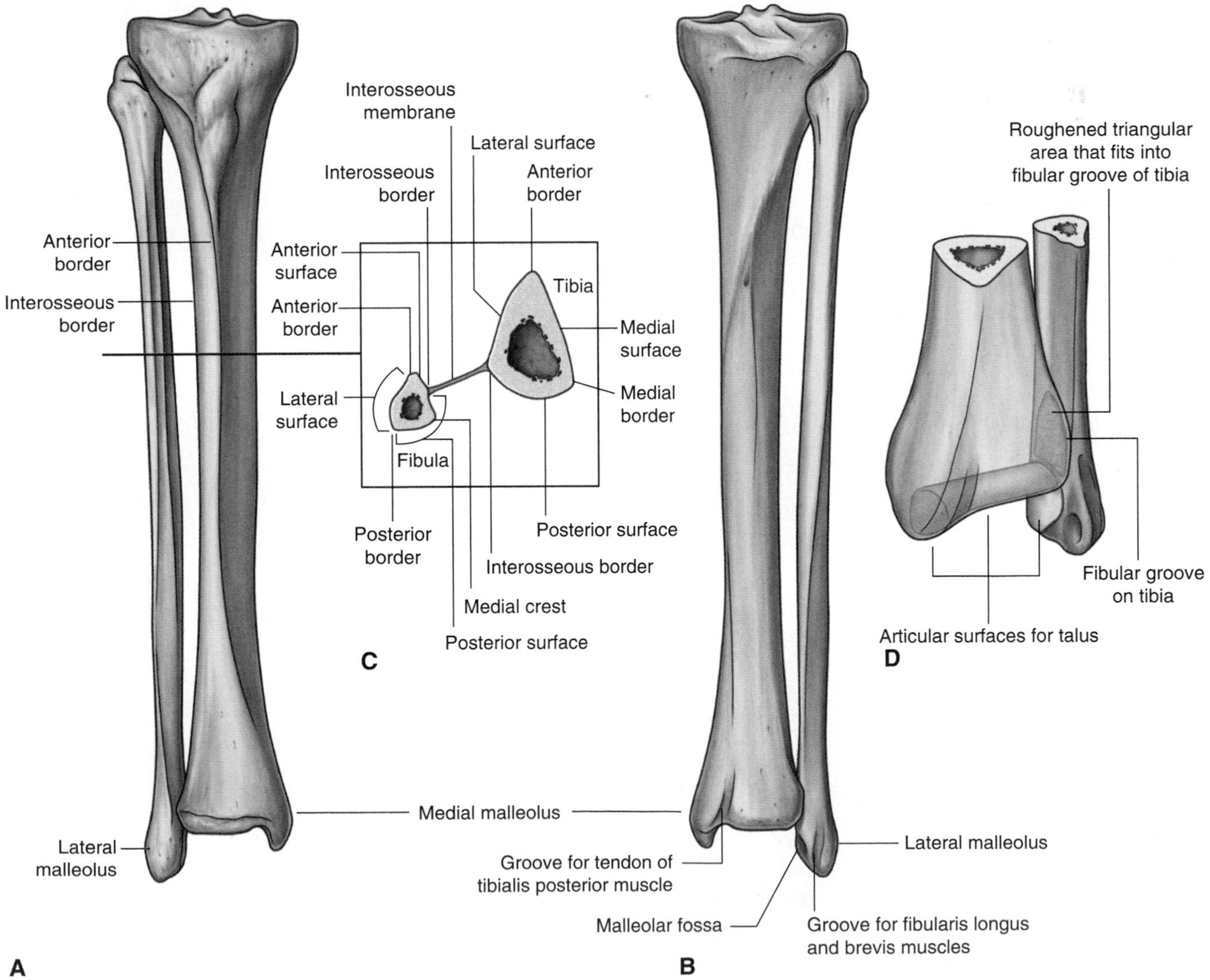

FIGURE 9-5 Leg bones, **A**, Anterior view. **B**, Posterior view. **C**, Cross-section through shafts. **D**, Posteromedial view of distal ends. (From Drake RL, Vogl W, Mitchell ADM: *Gray's anatomy for students*, p. 544, Philadelphia, 2005, Elsevier/Churchill Livingstone.)

the rather large medial malleolus by running the fingers down the inside, medial aspect of the tibia; this marks the most distal aspect of the tibia. The shaft of the tibia progresses proximally up and gradually widens to form the tibial plateau, which receives the distal femur and forms the knee joint. The shaft is almost triangular, forming a posterior surface, an anterior-medial surface, and an anterior-lateral surface. The anterior edge of the tibia is not protected very well and is often the site of pain after being kicked. These surfaces serve as the origination sites of muscle. The tibial plateau has two cushions, a medial and a lateral meniscus that will be discussed later in the chapter in reference to the knee joint. Just below the tibial plateau on the anterior aspect of the tibia is another landmark, the tibial tuberosity. The tibia has many muscle, tendon, and ligament attachments (Figure 9-6).

Fibula

The **fibula** is a long, thin bone found on the lateral aspect of the leg. Proximally is the landmark known as the head of the fibula. Distally, the fibula has a large bump called the *lateral malleolus.* Both the fibular head and lateral malleolus are palpated easily. By tracing the fibula up the side of your leg, you can feel it quickly disappear under the lateral musculature of the leg; however, as you continue, you will eventually get to the head of the fibula, which is just inferior and lateral to the knee joint. The fibula is connected to the tibia by a dense connective tissue called the *interosseous membrane.* The interosseous membrane is reinforced both proximally and distally by ligaments.

The lateral malleolus is positioned slightly posterior and distal to the medial malleolus. Athletic trainers will find this information valuable when examining an injured ankle and distinguishing abnormal from normal anatomical relationships. Both the medial and lateral malleoli (plural of malleolus) have small pointed inferior projections that are the sites of ligament attachments. These projections also serve as important pulleys for muscles and tendons. The tibia and fibula serve as sites for muscle attachments—particularly for most of the muscles that send tendons across the ankle into the foot. Most of the muscle attachments are located proximally and not down by the ankle. The tibia is responsible for transmitting most of the forces that come from the ground up to the rest of the body. The fibula makes a significant contribution to the lateral stability of the ankle. It also bears about 17% of the weight transmitted up through the leg during gait.

Bones Associated With the Thigh

The thigh is the part of the body between the hip and the knee. Unlike the lower leg, the upper leg (thigh) consists of a single bone—the femur. Another bone associated with the thigh is the patella, or kneecap.

Femur

The area of the lower extremity between the knee and the hip is the thigh (Figure 9-7). The **femur,** the longest bone in the body, is responsible for transmitting those ground reaction forces from the leg to the pelvis. Resting on top of the tibial plateau are the medial and lateral condyles (Latin for "knuckles") of the femur. The medial condyle projects slightly farther distally than the lateral condyle. The medial and lateral menisci of the tibia cup both condyles. On the outer aspects of each of these condyles are landmarks called the *epicondyles.* (*Epi* means "outer"; the epicondyle is the outermost part of the condyle.) Both the medial and lateral

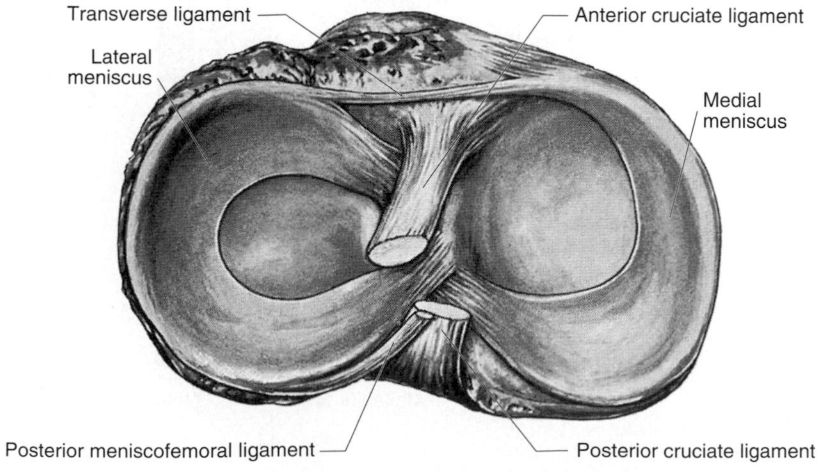

FIGURE 9-6 Menisci of the tibia, superior view. (From Standring S: *Gray's anatomy: the anatomical basis of clinical practice,* ed 39, p. 1476, Edinburgh, 2005, Elsevier/Churchill Livingstone.)

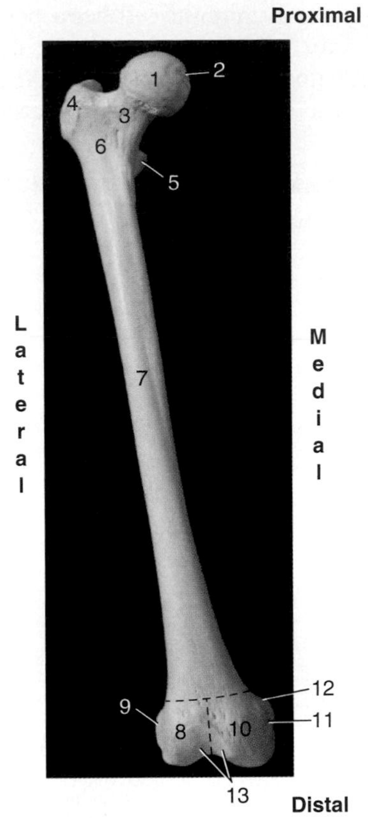

FIGURE 9-7 Femur, anterior view. *1,* Head; *2,* fovea of the head; *3,* neck; *4,* greater trochanter; *5,* lesser trochanter; *6,* intertrochanteric line; *7,* body (shaft); *8,* lateral condyle; *9,* lateral epicondyle; *10,* medial condyle; *11,* medial epicondyle; *12,* adductor tubercle; *13,* articular surface for patellofemoral joint. (From Muscolino JE: *Kinesiology: the skeletal system and muscle function,* p. 122, St Louis, 2006, Mosby/Elsevier.)

epicondyles are sites for the attachment of ligaments. Between the two condyles is the intercondylar notch, or fossa, which houses the cruciate ligaments and other important vessels. The notch is more pronounced when it is observed from the posterior aspect.

On the anterior side of the distal femur is a shallow groove in which the patella glides during knee movements. Just above the condyles, the femur narrows and forms the shaft of the femur. The shaft continues proximally until it reaches the greater and lesser tuberosities, which also serve as landmarks for the neck of the femur. The shaft of the femur, **concave** posterior, allows for some imperceptible flexing when walking, running, and jumping, thereby helping in the dissipation of forces that could otherwise result in injuries. The neck of the femur angulates medially at approximately 120 degrees in adults. At birth, the femoral neck is straighter. With increased age, the femoral neck is a common site of fracture, particularly in individuals with osteoporosis. The most proximal aspect of the femur is the head. The femur is the site of many ligament and muscle attachments. In fact, the greater and lesser tuberosities serve as the attachment site for many muscles of the hip region. Muscles cover the femur on all sides, rarely leaving any bone tissue susceptible to blunt trauma as the tibia does.

Patella

A bone that is closely associated with the femur is the patella, or kneecap (Figure 9-8). The patella, the largest sesamoid bone in the body, is irregularly shaped. Embedded in the quadriceps tendon, the patella functions to protect the distal anterior femur from direct blows and prevent the quadriceps tendon from rubbing on the femur. The posterior surface of the patella has a protective surface, which in some ways is similar to the Teflon coating of a nonstick frying pan. A **hyaline cartilage** protects the patella and the femoral groove as the patella glides in the groove during **flexion** and **extension** of the knee. Another important function of the patella is that it slightly elevates the quadriceps tendon away from the femur, which gives the quadriceps muscles a better mechanical advantage while working eccentrically and concentrically.

Bones of the Pelvis

The most proximal part of the lower body is the pelvis. The Latin definition of *pelvis* is "basin," which refers to the shape of the pelvis. Although some might say the pelvis is part of the torso, back, and abdomen, it plays a very significant role in the lower body because it transmits the forces absorbed by the lower extremities up to the spine. The pelvis also is the site of many muscle attachments, some that go up to the back and abdomen and some that go down to the lower extremities. Many

concave a type of curve rounded inward like a bowl
hyaline cartilage smooth, shiny cartilage that allows one bone to glide smoothly over another
flexion bending of a joint; decrease in the angle
extension straightening of a joint; increase in its angle

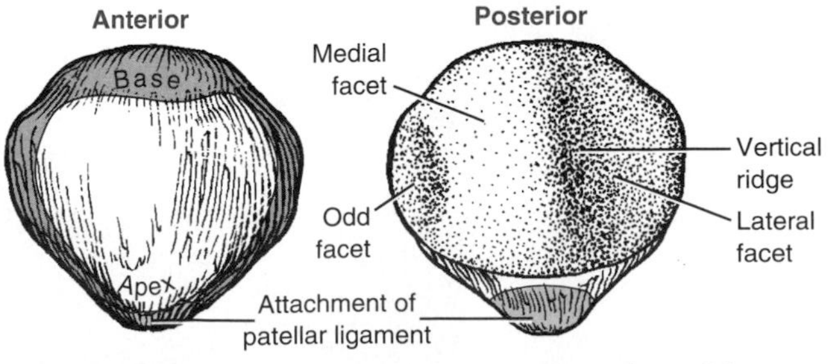

FIGURE 9-8 Patella. (From Neumann DA: *Kinesiology of the musculoskeletal system,* p. 437, St Louis, 2002, Elsevier/Mosby.)

internal organs and important nerves and vessels also are located in the pelvis, and some pass through the pelvis.

Ilium, Ischium, Pubis, and Sacrum

The pelvis comprises seven bones that most people consider fused. The following bones are paired: the ilium, ischium, and pubis (Figure 9-9). One set of each of the bones forms a right and left **hemi**-pelvis. The two hemi-pelvises are connected anteriorly by the pubic symphysis and posteriorly by the sacrum. The ilium, ischium, and pubis converge on their lateral side and

hemi indicating half of something

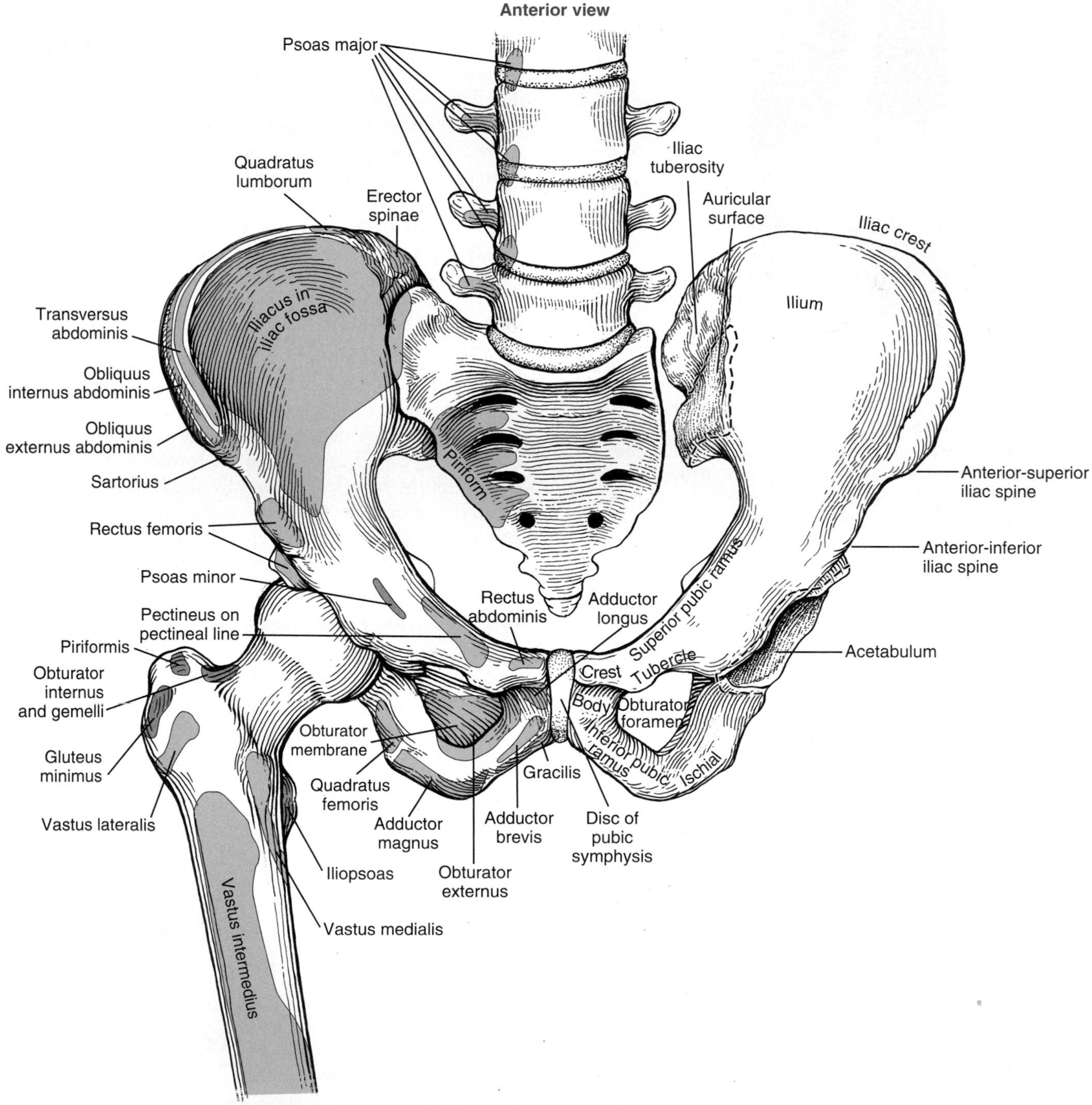

FIGURE 9-9 Anterior pelvis. (From Neumann DA: *Kinesiology of the musculoskeletal system,* p. 389, St Louis, 2002, Elsevier/Mosby.)

form a hollowed-out area called the *acetabulum* (Figure 9-10). *Acetabulum* is Latin for "vinegar cup"; it is the cup-shaped hip socket that holds the head of the femur in the hip joint.

Each ilium flares out, with the ischium posterior and inferior and the pubis anterior and inferior. Both the ischium and pubis bones are extremely irregular in shape. Because of this irregularity, there are many notches and openings, including an inferior opening, in the pelvis for muscles and vessels. Structural variations exist between men and women (Figure 9-11). The pelvis has three main functions:

1. To protect internal organs
2. To serve as an attachment site for muscles and ligaments
3. To transmit forces from the lower extremity to the spine by way of the sacroiliac joint

JOINTS AND LIGAMENTS OF THE LOWER BODY

Joints, in the most basic sense, form wherever a ligament connects two bones. Given the structure of the foot and the configuration of its 28 bones, it comes as no surprise that many joints are present. Because there are so many joints in this area, this chapter covers only those joints and ligaments relevant to a general introduction of the topic. The many joints of the foot and ankle are responsible for maintaining balance, initiating ground reaction force absorption (i.e., landing on the ground during gait and jumping), and then initiating force production (i.e., propelling off the ground during gait and jumping). The knee joint is in the middle of the lower body and probably receives more attention than other joints because it is susceptible to a variety of injuries. Its placement in the middle of the lower extremity makes it vulnerable to stressors below, at the foot and ankle, and stressors above, at the pelvis and hip. The hip joint is the strongest joint in the body because it has the largest muscles attached to it and the largest ligaments stabilizing it. This area transmits forces between the lower body and the spine and the upper body. Box 9-3 summarizes the joints and ligaments of the lower body.

Joints of the Foot

The foot has several joints in it because it has several bones. With its complex array of joints, the foot is able to make subtle shifts and movements to maintain

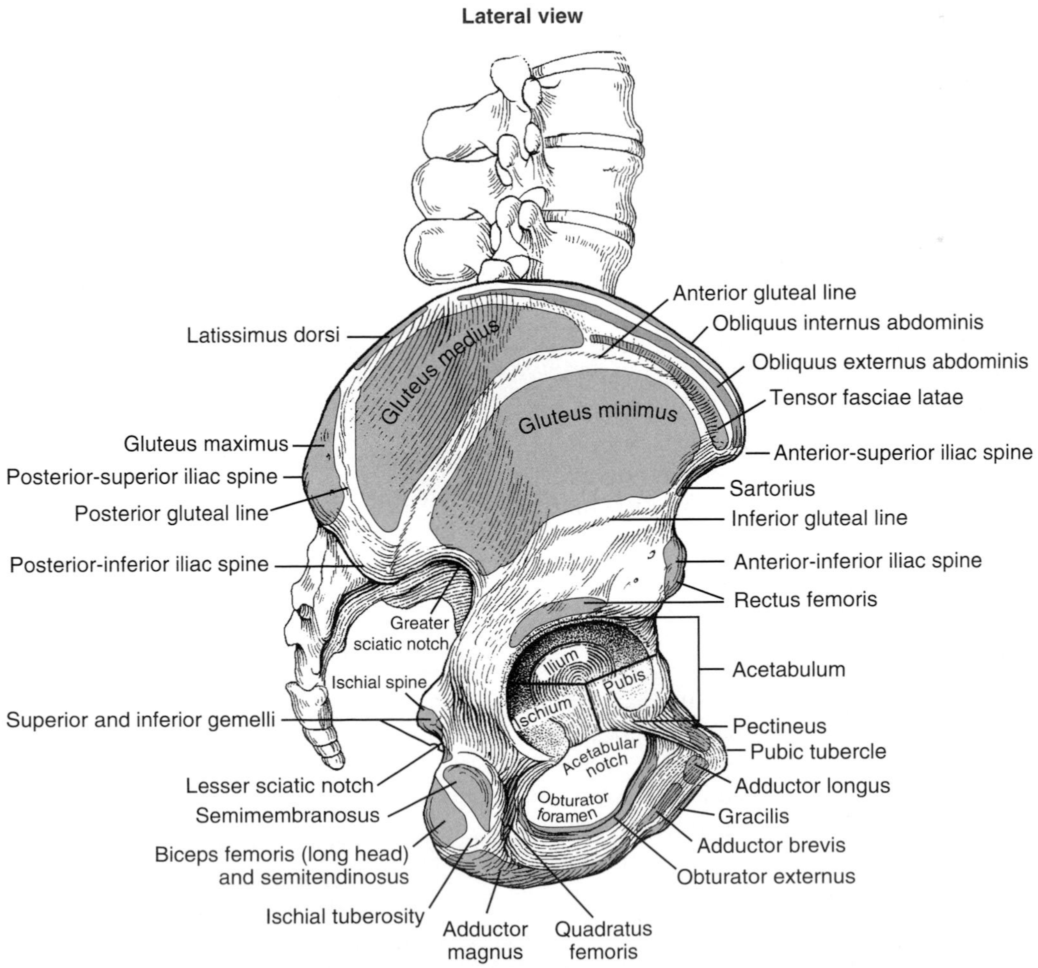

FIGURE 9-10 Lateral pelvis. (From Neumann DA: *Kinesiology of the musculoskeletal system,* p. 388, St Louis, 2002, Elsevier/Mosby.)

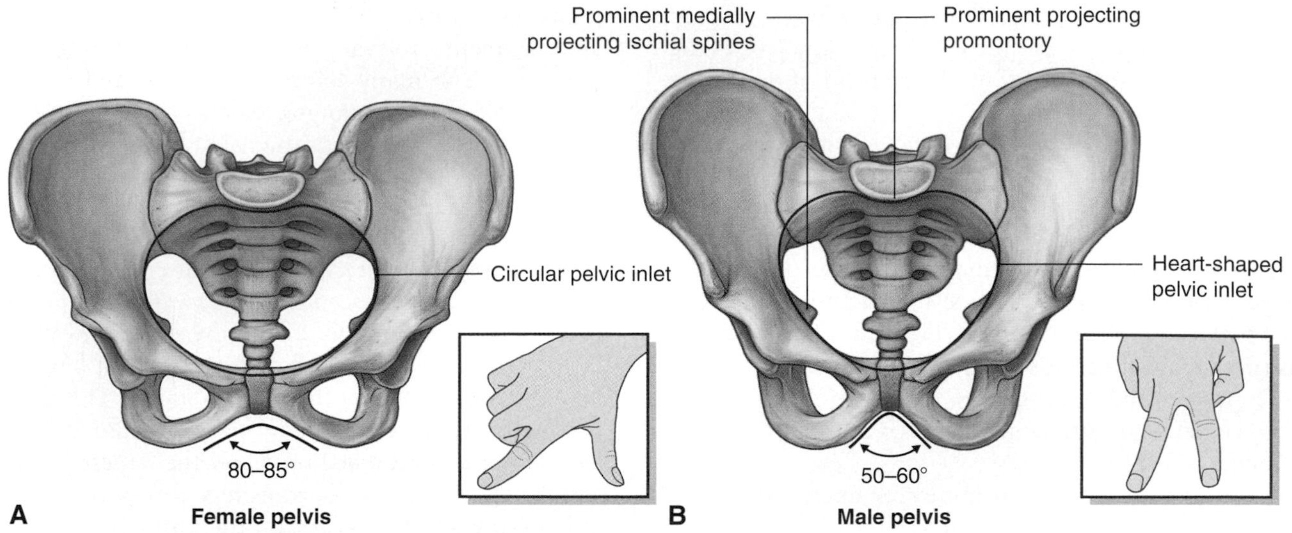

FIGURE 9-11 Female **(A)** and male **(B)** pelvis. (From Drake RL, Vogl W, Mitchell ADM: *Gray's anatomy for students,* p. 386, Philadelphia, 2005, Elsevier/Churchill Livingstone.)

balance and to generate great leverage in propelling the body during walking or running. Because the joints of the foot are so numerous, no single joint has to move far to bring motion throughout the whole foot. Each joint moves only slightly, or shifts, as needed.

Subtalar Joint

Starting posteriorly, the foot begins with the talus and calcaneus. The joint between the talus and the calcaneus is called the subtalar joint; *sub* means "below," and in this case, refers to the talus. The subtalar joint is formed by the concave undersurface of the body of the talus and the convex posterior-superior surface of the calcaneus that gives the appearance of a saddle on a horse's back. Visualize a saddle that has not been cinched tight, and the potential movements of the talus on top of the calcaneus become apparent. Most of the anatomical stability of this joint comes from interosseous ligaments that are below the talus and on top of the calcaneus. This arrangement is fairly unusual because ligaments around the joint or just outside the joint usually stabilize the joint (Figure 9-12). Because there are no muscle attachments to the talus, structural stability for the subtalar comes from ligaments and from the weight of the body. Some of the ligaments in this area simply appear as thickenings in the thin joint capsule that encompasses the talus and calcaneus.

There are also two other strong ligaments that control the integrity of the subtalar joint. Both are located in the sinus tarsi, a landmark of interest that is associated with this joint. If you palpate just anterior to your lateral malleolus with your index finger, you will feel the finger dive into a hole of sorts. This hole is the sinus tarsi (Latin for "opening in the tarsals"). Keeping your finger in the sinus tarsi, roll the sole of your foot inward as if you were spraining your ankle. You should be able to feel the superior, lateral, and anterior aspects of the talus push into your finger. This landmark is critical in the assessment of foot and ankle injuries as well as anatomical relationships. The subtalar joint, one of the unsung heroes of anatomy, allows many important movements to occur. These movements eventually allow other structures, above and below the foot, to do their jobs, thus highlighting the importance of the subtalar joint.

Inversion, eversion, and **circumduction** are the primary movements that occur at the subtalar joint. To *invert,* the verb form of the term *inversion,* means to "turn in" (Figure 9-13). In this case, the sole or bottom of the foot turns in (i.e., moves medially). *Eversion* means the opposite: The sole of the foot turns out (i.e., moves laterally: Figure 9-14). Circumduction is the movement of something in a circular direction. The subtalar joint is the joint primarily responsible for inversion, eversion, and circumduction.

inversion a turning in (turning medially)
eversion a turning out (turning laterally)
circumduction movement in a circular direction

Points to Ponder

Consider what happens when you stand on one leg and slowly rotate the body back and forth (you may want to lightly grasp something for balance). The talus moves medially as you rotate inwardly, and it moves laterally as you rotate outwardly. What keeps it from sliding all over the place or falling off the calcaneus? Imagine what happens at the subtalar joint when you are playing soccer, basketball, or golf. If the talus moves slightly off center during a twisting motion, you will either fall or be forced to catch yourself as you lose you balance.

BOX 9-3 Joints and Ligaments of the Lower Body

Foot

- Subtalar joint
  Interosseous ligaments
  Two ligaments at sinus tarsi
  Associated movements: inversion, eversion, circumduction
- Talocalcaneonavicular joint
  Plantar calcaneonavicular ligament ("spring ligament")
  Connective tissue: plantar fascia (stability)
  Associated movements: involved in walking, running, jumping
- Transverse tarsal joints
  Transverse (mid) tarsal joint: composed of talocalcaneonavicular and calcaneocuboid joints
  Small ligaments connecting adjacent bones
  Associated movements: involved in twisting, eversion, and inversion
- Tarsometatarsal joints
  Many ligaments between surfaces that connect cuneiforms and cuboid with metatarsals
  Lisfranc's ligament of specific interest
  Associated movements: many subtle movements, including limiting of dorsiflexion
- Metatarsophalangeal joints (five)
  Medial and collateral ligaments
  Plantar ligament
  Associated movements: plantar flexion, abduction, adduction, limiting of dorsiflexion; involvement in walking, running, and jumping
- Interphalangeal joints
  Proximal interphalangeal joint (PIP)
  Distal interphalangeal joint (DIP)
  Associated movements: plantar flexion and dorsiflexion

Ankle

- Talocrural joint
- Called a mortise joint
- Lateral ligaments: anterior talofibular ligament, calcaneofibular ligament, posterior talofibular ligament
- Medial ligament: deltoid ligament
- Distal tibiofibular joint (just proximal to ankle joint)
- *Associated movements:* plantar flexion and dorsiflexion

Knee

- Tibiofemoral joint
  Medial collateral ligament (MCL)
  Lateral collateral ligament (LCL)
  Anterior cruciate ligament (ACL) and posterior cruciate ligament (PCL)
  Medial and lateral menisci (stability)
  Associated movements: prevention of valgus (buckling in) and varus (buckling out) movements
- Proximal tibiofibular joint
  Anterior fibular head ligament
  Posterior fibular head ligament
  Associated movements: minimal; slight upward movement of fibula during foot eversion and downward during inversion
- Patellofemoral joint
  Medial retinaculum (stability)
  Medial and lateral femoral condyles (support)
  Associated movements: involved in stretching of quadriceps to stabilize and support knee

Hip

- Hip joint
  Iliofemoral (anterior side), pubofemoral (anterior side), and ischiofemoral (posterior side) ligaments
  Labrum (cartilaginous ring; helps in stability)
  Ligamentum teres (connective tissue not involved in stability)
  Associated movements: flexion, extension, abduction, internal (medial) and external (lateral) rotation, and circumduction

Other factors, such as stability, play a role in the function of the subtalar joint. Stability comes from the placement of the talus, which is surrounded by the mortise, a rectangular cavity formed by the distal tibia and fibula. The mortise, in tandem with the weight of the body, helps control the movements of the talus. The mortise is considered to be the ankle joint, which will be discussed later in this chapter.

Talocalcaneonavicular Joint

Distal from the subtalar joint is the talocalcaneonavicular joint. This joint is formed by the inferior talus resting on the superior, medially located sustentaculum tali portion of the calcaneus and the posterior concave navicular surface matching up with the anterior convex aspect of the talar head. A strong, relatively thick plantar calcaneonavicular ligament connects the anterior, medial sustentaculum tali of the calcaneus with the entire width of the inferior navicular. This ligament blends in with the deltoid (triangular) ligament, which will be discussed later.

Another term for the plantar calcaneonavicular ligament is the "spring ligament," thus called because of its relative fibroelastic properties, which allow it to serve as a sling for the head of the talus so that the medial longitudinal arch can collapse and then spring back. Other small ligaments in this area attempt to stabilize the bones as forces try to separate them. Another undergirding stabilizer of the medial longitudinal arch is the plantar fascia, a tough connective tissue thickening (similar to

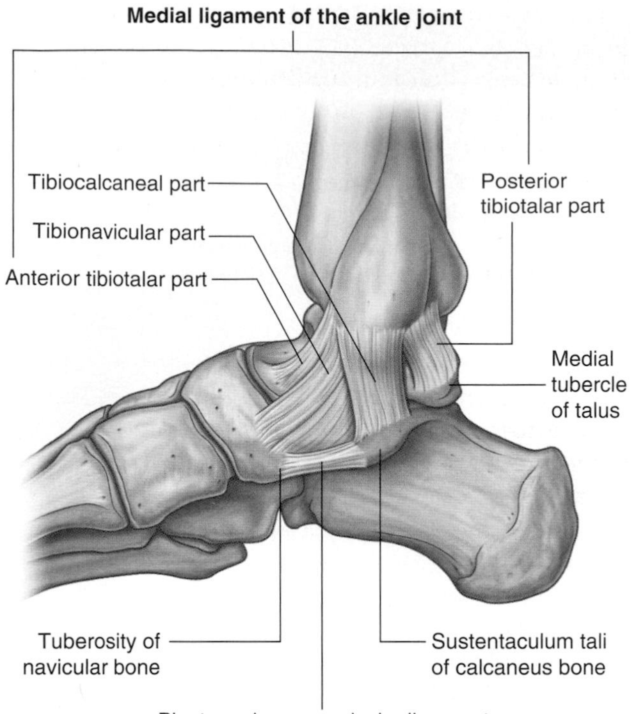

FIGURE 9-12 Medial joints of foot and ankle. (From Drake RL, Vogl W, Mitchell ADM: *Gray's anatomy for students,* p. 563, Philadelphia, 2005, Elsevier/Churchill Livingstone.)

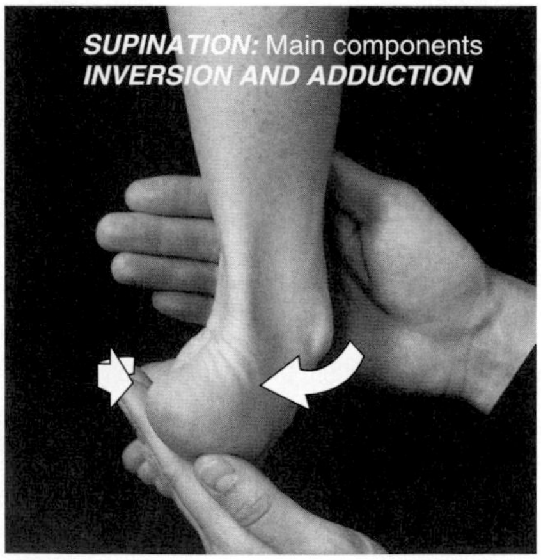

FIGURE 9-13 Inversion of the right foot. (From Neumann DA: *Kinesiology of the musculoskeletal system,* p. 490, St Louis, 2002, Elsevier/Mosby.)

a thin leather strap) that is a part of the fascial network running throughout the body. The distal inferior aspect of the calcaneus serves as an attachment site for the plantar fascia, which runs to the junction of the metatarsal heads and phalangeal bases.

Any movement that causes the medial longitudinal arch to collapse stresses this area. Muscles help stabilize this joint and the medial longitudinal arch. These structures, found in a relatively small area, play an important role in handling the weight and forces that run down through this area during walking, running, and jumping.

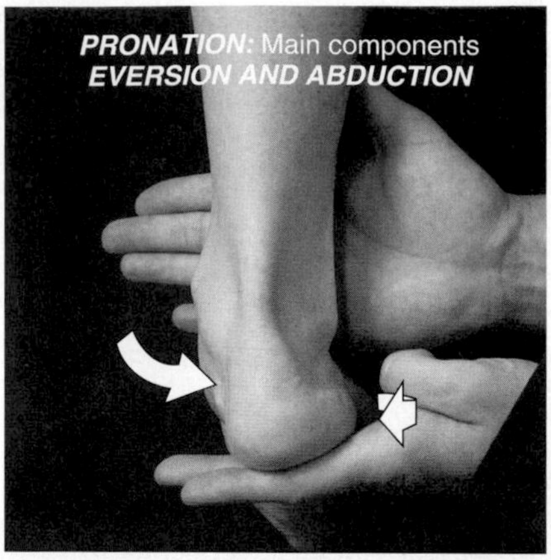

FIGURE 9-14 Eversion of the right foot. (From Neumann DA: *Kinesiology of the musculoskeletal system,* p. 490, St Louis, 2002, Elsevier/Mosby.)

Transverse Tarsal Joint

The transverse (mid) tarsal joint is composed of the talocalcaneonavicular and calcaneocuboid joints. Running almost perpendicular to the medial longitudinal arch, the transverse tarsal joint allows twisting motions. When everything is working well, the midfoot and forefoot can twist, invert, and evert on a longitudinal axis that runs roughly from the distal phalange of the second metatarsal posterior through the medial third of the calcaneus. Again, the support here is from small ligaments connecting the adjacent bones. However, because of the amount of movement that must occur in this area, the ligamentous strength is limited in a way that is relative to the amount of movement required.

Tarsometatarsal Joints

Tarsometatarsal joints are plentiful because they are formed between the three cuneiforms and the cuboid, as well as the five metatarsal bases. There are many ligaments located on both the dorsal aspect, plantar aspect, and between the surfaces that connect these bones. The three cuneiforms and the cuboid form the transverse tarsal arch. Subtle movements in many directions occur here as the foot adapts to different surfaces. Perhaps most valuable to the foot, the ligaments here limit dorsiflexion of the distal bones in the joint with their respective proximal bones. A ligament of interest is Lisfranc's ligament, which connects the distal aspect of the first cuneiform to the base of the second metatarsal (see Figure 9-3). Although an injury to this area is not typically considered serious, damage to Lisfranc's ligament or any of the ligaments in this area usually results in significant debilitation.

Metatarsophalangeal Joints

The distal aspects of the metatarsals articulate with the phalanges to form the five metatarsophalangeal (MTP) joints. These joints are capsular with strong thickenings on the medial, plantar, and lateral aspects. The medial and lateral collateral thickenings (i.e., ligaments) prevent motion in their opposite directions, the medial ligaments prevent lateral motion of the distal segments, and the lateral ligaments prevent movements in the medial direction. The plantar ligament helps limit **dorsiflexion** of the phalanges (i.e., toes). Toes two through five have tendons crossing over and under them that also help stabilize this joint. Normal motions are **plantar flexion**, dorsiflexion, **abduction** (i.e., motion away from the midline by the distal segment), **adduction** (i.e., motion toward the midline by the distal segment), and circumduction. The first metarsophalangeal (i.e., big toe) is involved in any walking, running, and jumping activities, and as a result of these ongoing stressors is quite susceptible to injury.

Interphalangeal Joints

Proximal interphalangeal (PIP) and distal interphalangeal (DIP) joints complete the joints of the foot. Toes two through five each have three phalanges, so there are two interphalangeal joints—one proximal and one distal. The first toe has only two phalanges, which means that it has only one interphalangeal joint. There are strong medial and lateral collateral ligaments for all the interphalangeal joints; consequently, the only true movements that occur here are plantar flexion and dorsiflexion. A strong plantar connective tissue helps limit dorsiflexion. A unique aspect of these joints is the fact that the DIP of the fifth toe often becomes immobile later in life because of lack of use.

Ankle Joint

The ankle, sometimes called the talocrural joint (*crural* is Latin for "leg"; the talocrural joint is the point at which the talus joins the tibia and fibula), is the joint that transmits forces from the ground and foot to the leg. Because it is a commonly injured joint, it receives a great deal of attention. The ankle is made up of the distal tibia on the medial side and above, the distal fibula on the lateral side, and the talus below. The configuration of these bones is similar to that of a mortise joint used in carpentry. Therefore the ankle joint is called a *mortise joint.* Because of the way that the talus articulates with the tibia and fibula, the only appreciable movements at this joint are plantar flexion and dorsiflexion, not inversion and eversion.

Although minimal inversion and eversion motions are possible, any significant movements of this kind occur at the subtalar joint. Bony stability from the medial malleolus of the tibia, the lateral malleolus of the fibula, and their associated ligamentous attachments help limit inversion and eversion while still allowing plantar flexion and dorsiflexion.

Anterior Talofibular Ligament, Calcaneofibular Ligament, and Posterior Talofibular Ligament

Three lateral ligaments work to prevent excessive inversion. These ligaments—the anterior talofibular ligament, the calcaneofibular ligament, and the posterior talofibular ligament—are named according to their locations. The ligaments on the medial side are considered fused as a single unit and collectively called the *deltoid ligament.* The ankle joint is especially stable when it is maximally dorsiflexed because the talus then fits quite snugly in the overhanging mortise. Dorsiflexion and plantar flexion are essential movements in many common activities, including walking, running, jumping, and getting in and out of a chair.

Distal Tibiofibular Joint

Just proximal to the ankle joint is the distal tibiofibular joint, the point at which the tibia and fibula connect to help form the mortise. There are anterior and posterior sections, and the anterior inferior tibiofibular ligament and the posterior inferior tibiofibular ligament, respectively, stabilize them. The interosseous membrane reinforces the entire tibiofibular complex.

Knee Joints

A joint very susceptible to injury is the knee. It seems commonplace that we hear of someone who "blew out their knee" while performing any variety of activities. Injuries of the knee are discussed in more detail in Chapter 11. For a proper understanding of the underlying cause of knee injuries, the anatomy of the knee must first be understood (Figure 9-15).

The main movements of the knee are flexion and extension, both of which are initiated and controlled primarily by the hamstrings and quadriceps muscles. When the leg is off the ground and the knee is flexed, the tibia can also rotate a small amount under the femur. Similarly, the femur can rotate slightly on the tibia when the foot is planted and the knee is flexed.

Tibiofemoral Joint

The true knee joint, the tibiofemoral joint, is formed by the tibial plateau of the tibia and the femoral condyles of the femur. The condyles actually rest in the concave menisci on top of the tibia. The knee is stabilized on its medial and lateral aspects by the medial and lateral collateral ligaments. The medial collateral ligament (MCL) is also called the *tibial collateral ligament* because it attaches to the medial proximal tibia distally and then runs up to the medial femoral epicondyle. The

dorsiflexion upward movement by the distal segment; used to describe motion in the toes or ankle
plantar flexion downward motion by the distal segment; used to describe motion in the toes or the ankle
abduction movement away from the midline of the body
adduction movement toward the midline of the body

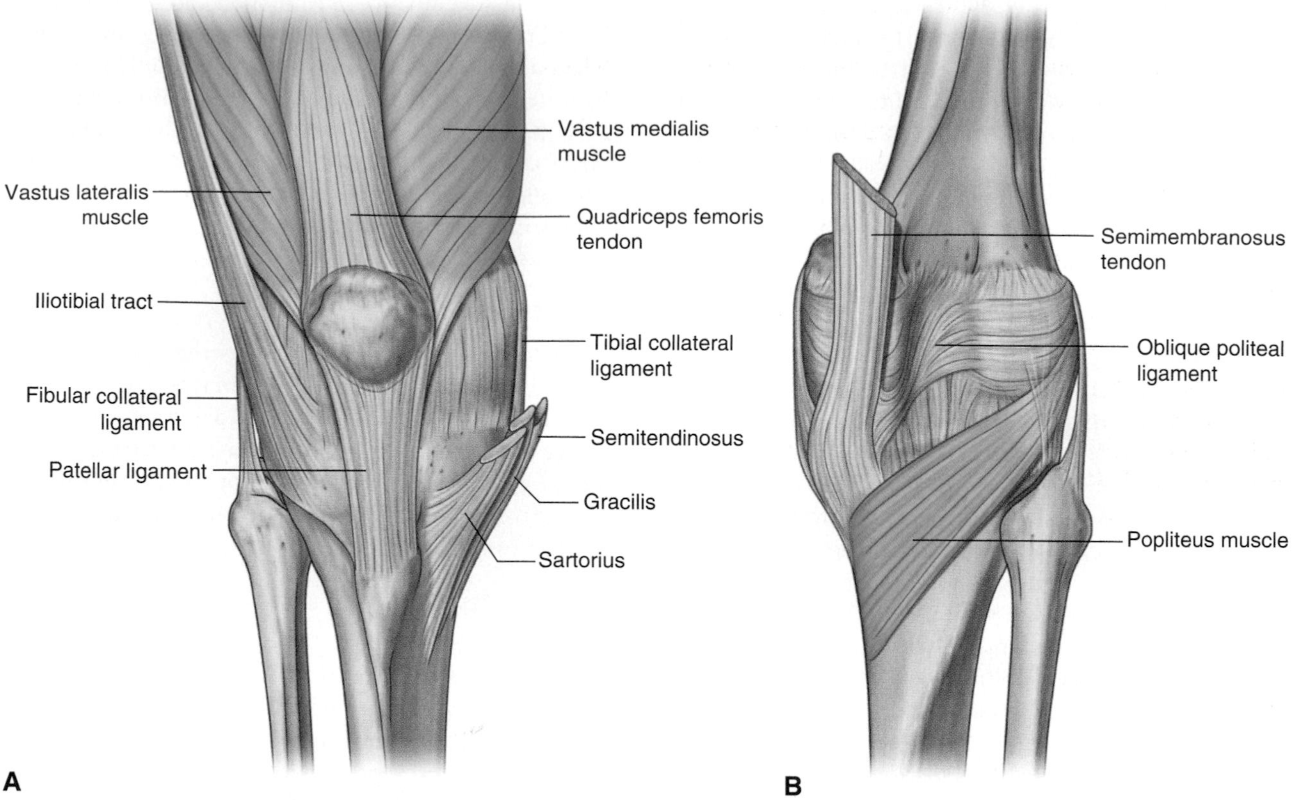

FIGURE 9-15 Anterior **(A)** and posterior **(B)** views of the knee joint. (From Drake RL, Vogl W, Mitchell ADM: *Gray's anatomy for students,* p. 536, Philadelphia, 2005, Elsevier/Churchill Livingstone.)

lateral collateral ligament (LCL) is called the *fibular collateral ligament* because it attaches on the proximal, lateral fibula and then continues up to the lateral epicondyle of the femur. The medial collateral ligament (MCL) is shorter, wider, and stronger than the lateral collateral ligament and is composed of two parts. The deep part is shorter and has attachments on the medial meniscus.

It is possible to determine the movements that these ligaments prevent by understanding what would happen if the ligaments were torn. If an MCL is torn, the knee buckles in, or moves medially. This buckling movement is also called a **valgus movement**. A valgus movement is a movement in which the distal end of the distal segment of a joint moves outward. An MCL tear usually occurs when an individual is hit on the outside of the knee, which drives the knee inward. Anything that drives the knee inward may be considered a valgus force because it causes the distal end of the distal segment of the joint to move outward. How such a force and movement could cause the MCL to be stretched beyond its breaking point and eventually torn is readily apparent. These injuries often result in what many call the "knock-kneed" look. However, do not be misled, since most individuals generally have a slight valgus deviation of their knees because the medial condyle of the femur extends distally a bit farther than the lateral femoral condyle. The LCL helps prevent the knee from buckling out in what is called a **varus movement**. A varus movement occurs when the distal aspect of the distal segment moves inward. The normal mechanism of injury to the LCL occurs when an individual is hit on the inside of the knee. This does not happen as often as being hit on the outside of the knee because the contralateral (opposite) lower extremity partially protects the knee.

Anterior and Posterior Cruciate Ligaments. Between the tibia and femur, running through the femoral notch, are the anterior and posterior cruciate ligaments. Although many associate *cruciate* with *crucial,* it actually comes from the word *crucifix;* it is so called because the two ligaments cross each other. The rest of the name, *anterior* or *posterior*, is based on the location at which each ligament attaches on the tibial plateau. The anterior

valgus movement movement in which the distal segment is forced outwardly, away from the midline of the body

varus movement movement in which the distal segment is forced inward, toward the midline of the body cruciate ligament (ACL) attaches on the anterior, middle tibial plateau and runs back to the posterior, medial aspect of the lateral femoral condyle. The posterior cruciate ligament (PCL) attaches on the posterior, middle tibial plateau and runs forward to the anterior, lateral aspect of the medial femoral condyle. One way that you can picture how these ligaments run is to use your hand, the same one that is on the side of the knee that you are evaluating. If you are considering your right knee, turn your right hand so that it is in a palm-down position. Next, cross your index finger over your middle finger. Your index finger represents the PCL as the distal end of your finger goes up and over the ACL to the anterior, medial aspect of the lateral femoral condyle, and your middle finger represents the ACL as the proximal aspect of the middle finger runs up to the posterior, lateral aspect of the medial condyle.

Medial and Lateral Menisci. The medial and lateral menisci are cartilaginous discs that play a crucial role in stabilizing this joint. The medial meniscus is a little larger than the lateral meniscus and is shaped like a semicircle as it opens toward the center of the knee joint. The lateral meniscus is smaller and more circular. The cuplike shape of the menisci helps hold the condyles on the tibia, preventing the tibial plateau from gliding back and forth under the femoral condyles and the femoral condyles from gliding back and forth over the tibial plateau.

The locations of the ACL and PCL dictate the movements that these ligaments prevent. The ACL prevents the tibia from sliding forward under the femur and the femur from sliding backward over the tibia. It also helps prevent excessive internal and external rotation of the tibia under the femur. Young women seem to be particularly susceptible to injuries of the ACL. Researchers are studying the factors that contribute to these injuries; one of the only absolutes to emerge is that these factors are numerous. Just as in other parts of the body, one structure relies on other structures. The same holds true for the ACL, wherein the menisci, the shape of the femoral condyles, and the strength and timing of the firing of the muscles all can help or hinder function.

Proximal Tibiofibular Joint

Another joint that is located in the general area of the knee is the proximal tibiofibular joint. It is different from the distal tibiofibular joint in that only the tibia articulates with the bone superior to it (the femur) and distally both the tibia and fibula articulate with the bone below it (the talus). Holding the fibula next to the tibia are the anterior and posterior fibular head ligaments, which connect the fibular head to the tibia. Although not much movement occurs here, it is possible to feel the head of the fibula move up when the foot is everted and move down when the foot is inverted.

Patellofemoral Joint

The last joint in the area of the knee is the patellofemoral joint (see Figure 9-7). This joint is intimately associated with the knee—in fact, injuries to the patellofemoral joint are often misidentified as knee injuries. In this joint, the patella glides on the distal anterior femoral surface, fittingly called the *patella groove.* The stability of this joint is unique in that it generally comes from the quadriceps muscle rather than ligaments. As the knee flexes, the quadriceps stretches and pulls the patella deeper into the femoral groove.

Sit on the floor with your legs straight out in front of you. Relax your quadriceps, and grab your patella with your thumb and middle finger as if it were a computer mouse. Notice how easy it is to slide it back and forth. Next, bend your knee to approximately a 45-degree angle, and try moving the patella again. Finally, bend your knee to approximately a 90-degree ankle, grab your patella, and try to move it around. Notice how difficult it is to move the patella when it is pulled tightly into the femoral groove.

The medial **retinaculum** stabilizes the patella on the medial side. On the lateral side, an additional retinaculum comes off the iliotibial band and keeps the patella from sliding medially. Providing further support are the medial and lateral femoral condyles., which form the borders of the patella groove.

Hip Joint

The last joint in this chapter is the hip joint, which consists of the head of a femur and the acetabulum of a hemi-pelvis (Figure 9-16). This joint is built more for stability than mobility, but it still can still perform some impressive movements. Normal movements here are flexion; extension; abduction; adduction; **internal,** or **medial, rotation** (in which the anterior surface of the distal segment moves toward the midline of the body); **external,** or **lateral, rotation** (in which the anterior surface of the distal segment moves away from the midline of the body); and circumduction. The hip joint is the largest joint in the body and its movements are protected by

retinaculum tight, tough connective tissue (keeps the patella from sliding laterally or medially)

internal (medial) rotation movement in which the anterior surface of the distal segment moves toward the midline of the body

external (lateral) rotation movement in which the anterior surface of the distal segment moves away from the midline of the body

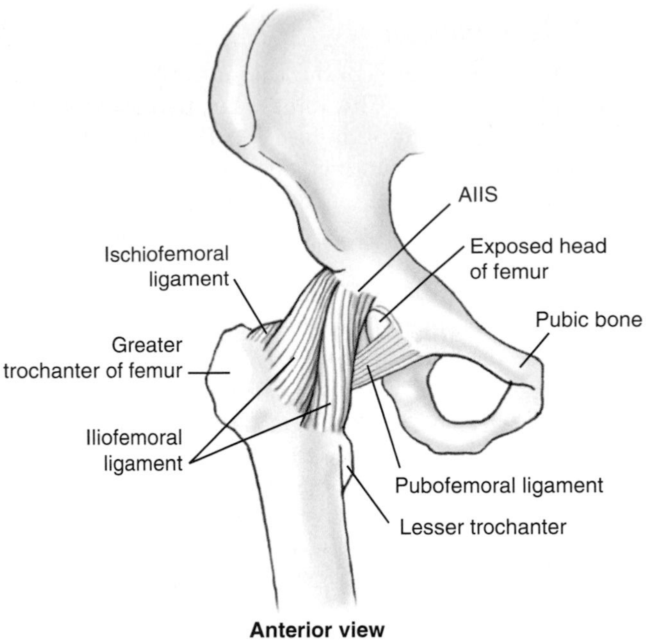

FIGURE 9-16 Anterior view of hip joint. (From Muscolino JE: *Kinesiology: the skeletal system and muscle function,* p. 311, St Louis, 2006, Mosby/Elsevier.)

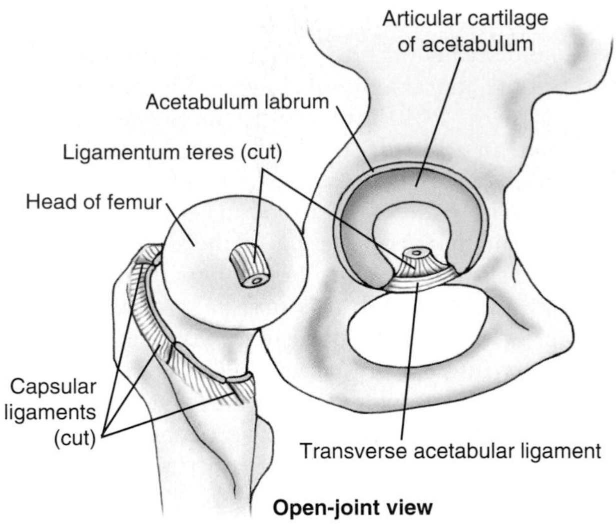

FIGURE 9-17 Internal view of hip joint. (From Muscolino JE: *Kinesiology: the skeletal system and muscle function,* p. 311, St Louis, 2006, Mosby/Elsevier.)

the three strongest ligaments in the body: the iliofemoral, pubofemoral, and ischiofemoral ligaments. Once again, their location dictates their names. The iliofemoral and pubofemoral ligaments are on the anterior side of the hip joint, generally limiting extension, abduction, and external rotation of the femur. The ischiofemoral ligament is on the posterior side, which helps limit flexion, abduction, and internal rotation.

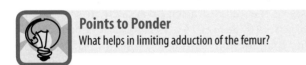

Points to Ponder
What helps in limiting adduction of the femur?

Also adding stability to the hip is the labrum, or cartilaginous ring, which serves as a small extension of the acetabulum and helps hold the head of the femur. Muscles that are in this area also stabilize this joint. When a person stands, the weight of the body helps keep the acetabulum positioned over the femoral head.

One other ligament that comes up in discussions of the hip is the ligamentum teres, a hollow connective tissue structure that encases an artery supplying blood from the pelvis to the head of the femur. Although its name suggests otherwise, it does not provide any stability to the hip (Figure 9-17).

MUSCLES, NERVES, AND ARTERIES OF THE LOWER BODY

The chapter thus far has presented the bones and major ligaments and joints of the lower body. Although these structures are important, they cannot move without muscles and their respective tendons. The names of the muscles often describe their size, shape, actions, and locations. The muscles, individually and collectively, are encased by fascia, specialized connective tissue that runs throughout the body and serves to help hold structures in place. *Fascia* is Latin for "band," as in banding or tying something together. In the leg, these bands of fascia group muscles into compartments that are named according to their location relative to the tibia.

Muscles of the Lower Body

The muscles in the lower body serve to stabilize the joints, move the leg, and control balance. They often cross more than one joint and therefore control range of motion in more than one joint.

Foot Muscles

The muscles of the foot can be categorized as intrinsic (i.e., all aspects of the muscle are within the confines of the foot) or extrinsic (i.e., some aspect originates outside of the foot). The small intrinsic muscles usually perform small movements or help stabilize an area. There are four layers of the small intrinsic muscles (Figure 9-18) located under the plantar surface of the foot.

Small **intrinsic muscles** are responsible for abduction and adduction of the toes. *Abduction* and *adduction* have slightly different meanings in reference to the toes and fingers. In abduction of the toes, the toes move away from the second toe; in adduction of the toes, the toes move toward the second toe. Although this is not the section

intrinsic muscles muscles that start and end (originate and insert) within the foot, without extending to the ankle or lower leg

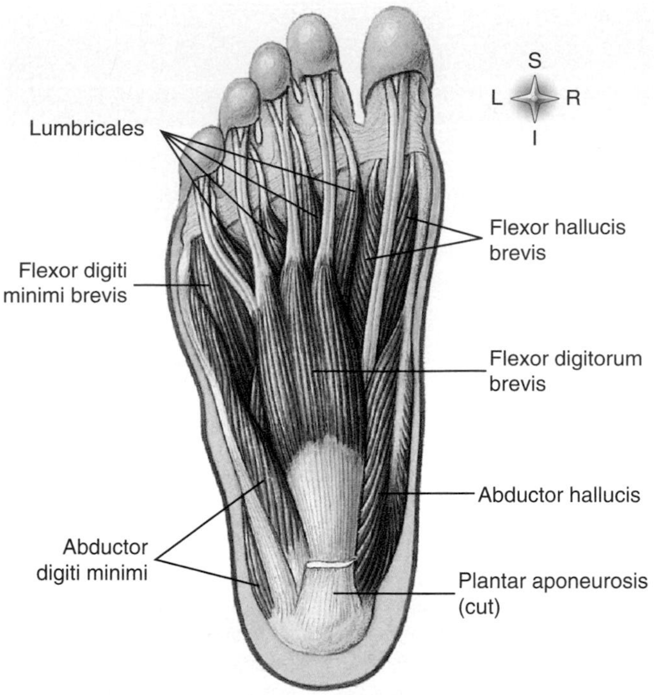

FIGURE 9-18 Intrinsic foot muscles, plantar view. (From Thibodeau GA, Patton KT: *Anatomy & physiology,* ed 6, p. 388, St Louis, 2007, Mosby/Elsevier.)

dealing with the hand and fingers, it bears mentioning that abduction and adduction of the fingers use the third finger as the point of reference. Separate small muscles control abduction and adduction of the big toe and small toe, and one group of muscles controls abduction and adduction of the middle three toes. Separate small muscles are also involved in flexion and extension of the big toe, small toe, and middle three toes. Terms for the small or short muscles of the foot typically include the word *brevis,* which is Latin for "short." It is important to remember that muscles work in three ways: They can initiate a movement (i.e., concentric contraction), they can stabilize a movement (i.e., isometric activity), and they can control a movement as it occurs (i.e., eccentric activity).

Leg and Ankle Muscles

Extrinsic muscles generally serve as the primary controllers of foot and ankle movements. The extrinsic muscles of the foot originate on the leg and proceed down to attach on some aspect of the foot. They are best considered in the context of their compartments. There are four compartments of muscles in the leg (Figure 9-19 and Table 9-1). The anterior compartment, located on the anterior, lateral aspect of the tibia, contains several muscles. Three of these muscles, listed from medial to lateral relative to their position on the top of the ankle or foot, are the tibialis anterior, extensor digitorum longus, and the extensor hallucis longus. Note that another small muscle, the fibularis tertius, considered by some to be an offshoot of the extensor digitorum longus, is also located here.

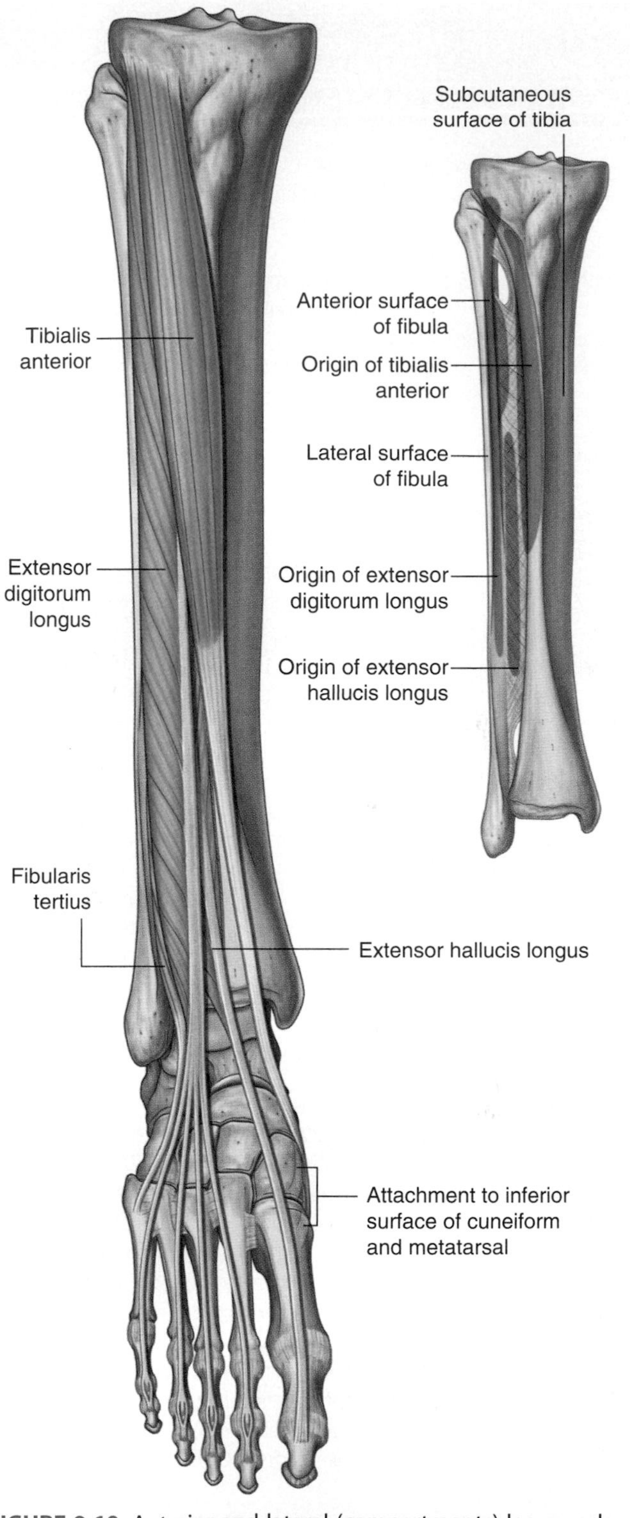

FIGURE 9-19 Anterior and lateral (compartments) leg muscles. (From Drake RL, Vogl W, Mitchell ADM: *Gray's anatomy for students,* p. 553, Philadelphia, 2005, Elsevier/Churchill Livingstone.)

extrinsic muscles muscles that originate in the leg and proceed down to attach on some aspect of the foot

TABLE 9-1 Muscles of the Leg and Ankle

MUSCLE(S)	LOCATION	FUNCTION*
Anterior Compartment (4)		
Tibialis anterior	Originating on the superior lateral tibia and interosseous membrane, it travels distally and medially to insert on the navicular.	Concentrically, it inverts and dorsiflexes the ankle. Eccentrically, it helps control pronation and the collapsing of the medial longitudinal arch.
Extensor hallucis longus	Originating on the midanterior fibula and interosseous membrane, it runs distally to insert on the distal phalanx of the big toe.	It extends the big toe and helps dorsiflex the foot.
Extensor digitorum longus	Originating on the superior lateral tibia, the proximal two thirds of the medial tibia and interosseous membrane, it runs almost straight down the front of the leg and then, while over the foot, splits into four tendons to insert onto the middle and distal phalanges of toes 2 through 5.	It extends the toes and helps dorsiflex the ankle.
Fibularis tertius	This muscle is relatively insignificant.	This muscle is relatively insignificant.
Lateral Compartment (2)		
Fibularis longus	Originating on the proximal two thirds of the fibula, it travels down posterior to and under the lateral malleolus, under the cuboid, and crosses under the foot to the base of the first metatarsal.	It uses the lateral malleolus as a lever to plantar flex the foot, and then as it goes under the cuboid, it changes its direction and becomes an evertor of the foot. Eccentrically, it helps control pronation.
Fibularis brevis	Originating on the distal two thirds of the fibula before going posterior to and under the lateral malleolus, it attaches to the base of the fifth metatarsal.	It everts and helps to plantar flex the foot. By attaching to the base of the fifth metatarsal, it helps stabilize the cuboid, which serves as a pulley for the fibularis longus.
Superficial Posterior Compartment (3)		
Gastrocnemius	Having two origins that cross the back of the knee and insert just proximal to the knee on the medial and lateral aspects of the posterior femur, it inserts distally on the back of the calcaneus, forming part of the Achilles tendon	It is a strong plantar flexor and a weak knee flexor.
Soleus	Originating on the posterior, superior aspect of the tibia and fibula, it runs deep to the gastrocnemius and inserts distally on the back of the calcaneus, forming part of the Achilles tendon.	It is a strong plantar flexor.
Plantaris	Originating between the gastrocnemius and the soleus is the plantaris muscle and tendon that originate on the posterior distal femur. It inserts distally on the back of the calcaneus, forming part of the Achilles tendon.	It is a weak plantar flexor.
Deep Posterior Compartment (4)		
Popliteus	Originating on the posterior lateral condyle of the femur, the popliteus then runs diagonally and medially to the superior, posterior, medial tibia.	It is a very weak flexor of the knee and an important internal rotator of the tibia as the knee flexes.
Tibialis posterior	Originating on the back of the midtibia and fibula, it then runs under the medial malleolus distally to attach to the navicular, cuneiforms, and cuboid and the bases of metatarsals two through four.	It works to plantar flex as it uses the medial malleolus as a pulley, and it helps the tibialis anterior invert the foot. Eccentrically, it helps control pronation.
Flexor digitorum longus	Originating on the midposterior tibia, it continues downward behind the tibialis posterior and the medial malleolus, attaching to the distal phalanges two through five.	It helps plantar flex the ankle and, as its name implies, flexes toes two through five.
Flexor hallucis longus	Originating on the inferior half of the fibula and interosseous membrane, the flexor hallucis longus continues distally under the sustentaculum tali of the calcaneus before traversing through the sesamoid bones under the first MCP joint to the distal phalanx of the big toe.	It serves as the main flexor of the big toe. Eccentrically, it helps control pronation.

*Remember that a function of all of these muscles is that they cover some anatomical structure and thereby protect it.

Tibialis Anterior. The tibialis anterior originates on the superior, lateral tibia and interosseous membrane. It traverses distally and medially to insert on the navicular. Note that when it contracts, it inverts and dorsiflexes the foot.

Extensor Hallucis Longus. The extensor hallucis longus originates on the midanterior fibula and interosseous membrane and runs distally to insert on the distal phalanx of the big toe. It extends the big toe and helps dorsiflex the foot. Notice the similarities (e.g., origins, insertions) among the tibialis anterior, the extensor hallucis longus, and the extensor digitorum longus. The tibialis anterior tendon is palpable as a tight cord just over the top of the ankle joint when the ankle is dorsiflexed. The tendons of the extensor digitorum longus and extensor hallucis longus are apparent over the top of the foot when the four most lateral toes and the great toe are extended. If you put your fingers on the anterior, lateral aspect of your leg as you perform any of the aforementioned movements, you can feel this compartment bulge.

Extensor Digitorum Longus. The extensor digitorum longus starts on the superior lateral tibia, the proximal two thirds of the medial tibia and interosseous membrane. It runs almost straight down the front of the leg and then, while over the foot, splits into four tendons to insert onto the middle and distal phalanges of toes two through five. As its name and location suggest, this muscle extends the toes and dorsiflexes the ankle. Note that a small muscle, the fibularis tertius, closely accompanies the extensor digitorum longus.

Lateral Compartment Muscles

The lateral compartment has two muscles, the fibularis longus and fibularis brevis. It is called the lateral compartment because it covers the lateral aspect of the leg (Figure 9-20).

Fibularis Longus. The fibularis longus originates on the proximal two thirds of the fibula, travels distally down under the lateral malleolus, under the cuboid, and crosses under the foot to the base of the first metatarsal. It uses the lateral malleolus as a lever to plantar flex the foot, and then, as it goes under the cuboid, it changes direction and becomes an evertor of the foot.

Fibularis Brevis. The fibularis brevis originates on the distal two thirds of the fibula before going under the lateral malleolus to attach to the base of the fifth metatarsal. This muscle everts and helps plantar flex the foot. By everting your foot, you can feel the fibularis tendons just distal to the lateral malleolus. Its attachment to the base of the fifth metatarsal helps stabilize the cuboid that serves as a pulley for the fibularis longus.

Superficial Posterior Compartment Muscles

There are two posterior compartments, superficial (i.e., closer to the skin) and deep. Both compartments are posterior to the tibia and the fibula. The superficial posterior compartment contains three muscles (Figure 9-21).

All three of the muscles outlined in the following sections come together distally to form the Achilles tendon, which inserts on the posterior distal calcaneus. Together these three muscles plantar flex the ankle and keep the

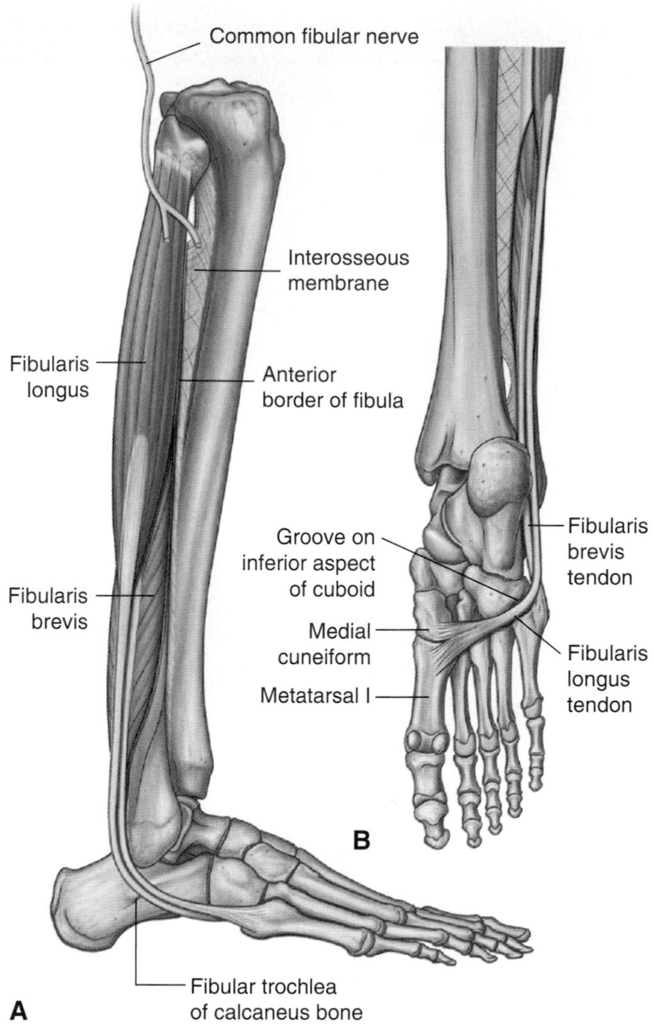

FIGURE 9-20 Lateral (compartment) leg muscles. **A**, Lateral view. **B**, Inferior view of left foot with foot plantar flexed at the ankle. (From Drake RL, Vogl W, Mitchell ADM: *Gray's anatomy for students,* p. 552, Philadelphia, 2005, Elsevier/Churchill Livingstone.)

tibia from dorsiflexing too far over the foot when the foot is planted.

Gastrocnemius. The gastrocnemius has two origins that cross the back of the knee and insert just proximal to the knee on the medial and lateral aspects of the posterior femur. It inserts distally on the back of the calcaneus, forming part of the Achilles tendon, and is a strong plantar flexor and a weak knee flexor.

Soleus. The soleus runs just under the gastrocnemius and originates on the posterior, superior aspect of the tibia and fibula. It inserts distally on the back of the calcaneus, forming part of the Achilles tendon, and is a strong plantar flexor.

Plantaris. Between the gastrocnemius and the soleus are the plantaris muscle and tendon, which originate on the

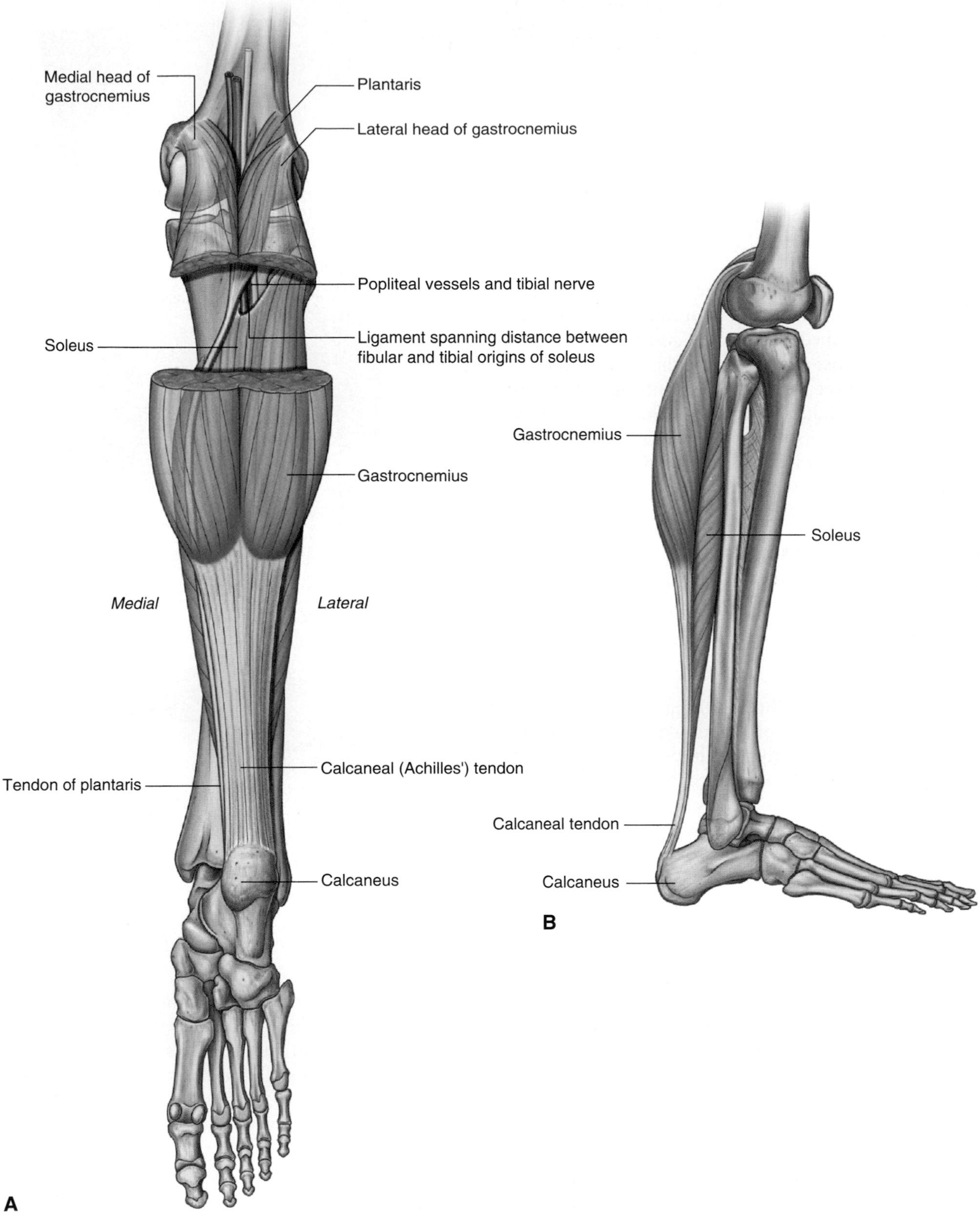

FIGURE 9-21 Posterior superficial (compartment) leg muscles. **A**, Posterior view. **B**, Medial view. (From Drake RL, Vogl W, Mitchell ADM: *Gray's anatomy for students,* p. 547, Philadelphia, 2005, Elsevier/Churchill Livingstone.)

posterior distal femur. The plantaris inserts distally on the back of the calcaneus, forming part of the Achilles tendon, and is a weak plantar flexor.

Deep Posterior Compartment Muscles

The deep posterior compartment lies underneath, or deep to, the superficial posterior compartment and comprises three muscles plus one. The plus one, the popliteus, is a deep and relatively small muscle behind the knee, and the three other muscles start about halfway down the leg and continue as tendons crossing the ankle. The three muscles by the ankle are sometimes nicknamed Tom (*t*ibialis posterior), Dick (flexor *d*igitorum longus), and Harry (flexor *h*allucis longus) according to the letters of their significant names and the order of their respective tendon locations just above and behind the medial malleolus (Figure 9-22).

Popliteus. The popliteus has an attachment on the posterior lateral condyle of the femur and then runs diagonally and medially to the superior, posterior, medial tibia. Although it is often included in the posterior deep compartment of the leg, it actually works more on the knee. It is a very weak flexor of the knee and an important internal rotator of the tibia as the knee flexes (Figure 9-23).

Tibialis Posterior. The tibialis posterior muscle (i.e., "Tom") originates on the back of the midtibia and fibula and then runs under the medial malleolus distally to attach on to the navicular, cuneiforms, and cuboid and the bases of metatarsals two through four. It works to plantar flex using the medial malleolus as a pulley, and it helps the tibialis anterior muscle invert the foot.

Flexor Digitorum Longus. The flexor digitorum longus (i.e., "Dick") originates on the midposterior tibia and continues downward behind the tibialis posterior and the medial malleolus. After it passes the medial malleolus, it continues distally to distal phalanges two through five and flexes them. Because it crosses the back of the ankle, it also helps plantar flex the ankle, and, as its name implies, it flexes toes two through five.

Flexor Hallucis Longus. The flexor hallucis longus (i.e., "Harry") originates on the inferior half of the fibula and interosseous membrane. It continues distally under the sustentaculum tali of the calcaneus before traversing through the sesamoid bones under the first metacarpophalangeal (MCP) joint to the distal phalanx of the big toe, where it serves as the main flexor of the big toe. Together, this deep posterior group helps invert and plantar flex the foot (primarily as a result of the muscles' medial insertion) and provides support to the medial longitudinal arch. Small bony

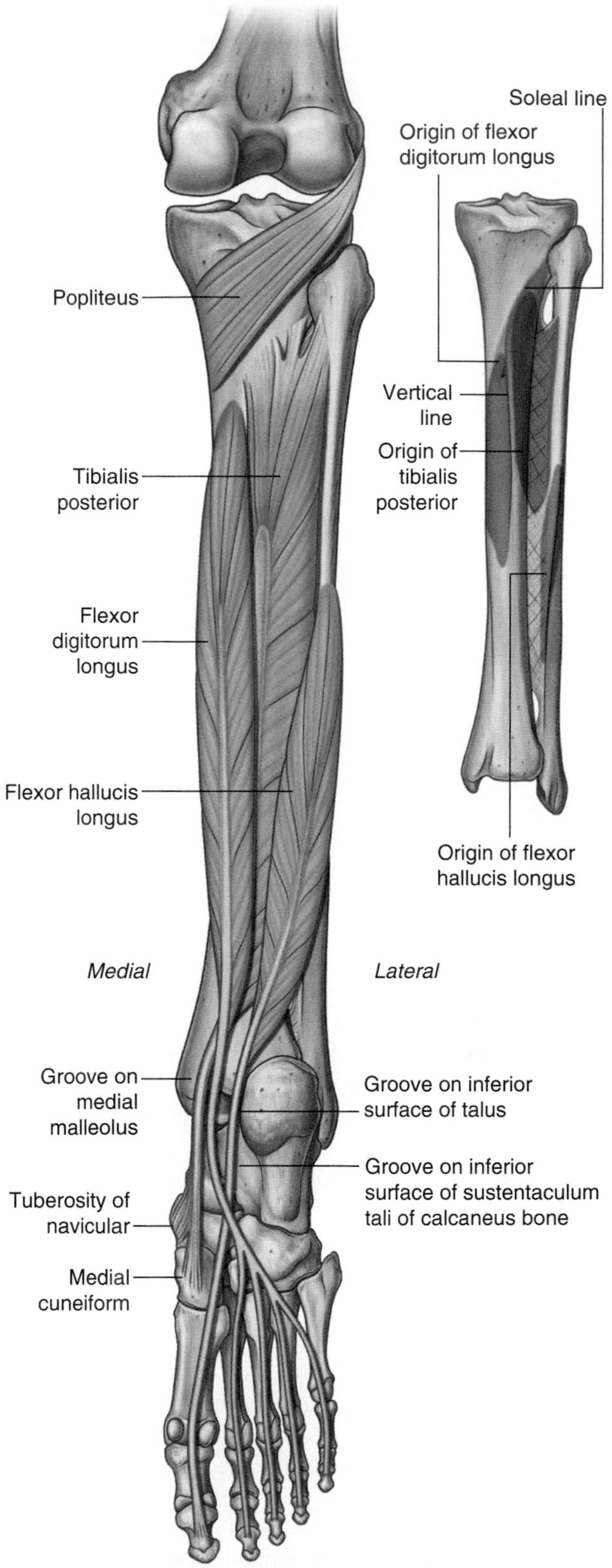

FIGURE 9-22 Posterior deep (compartment) leg muscles. (From Drake RL, Vogl W, Mitchell ADM: *Gray's anatomy for students*, p. 549, Philadelphia, 2005, Elsevier/Churchill Livingstone.)

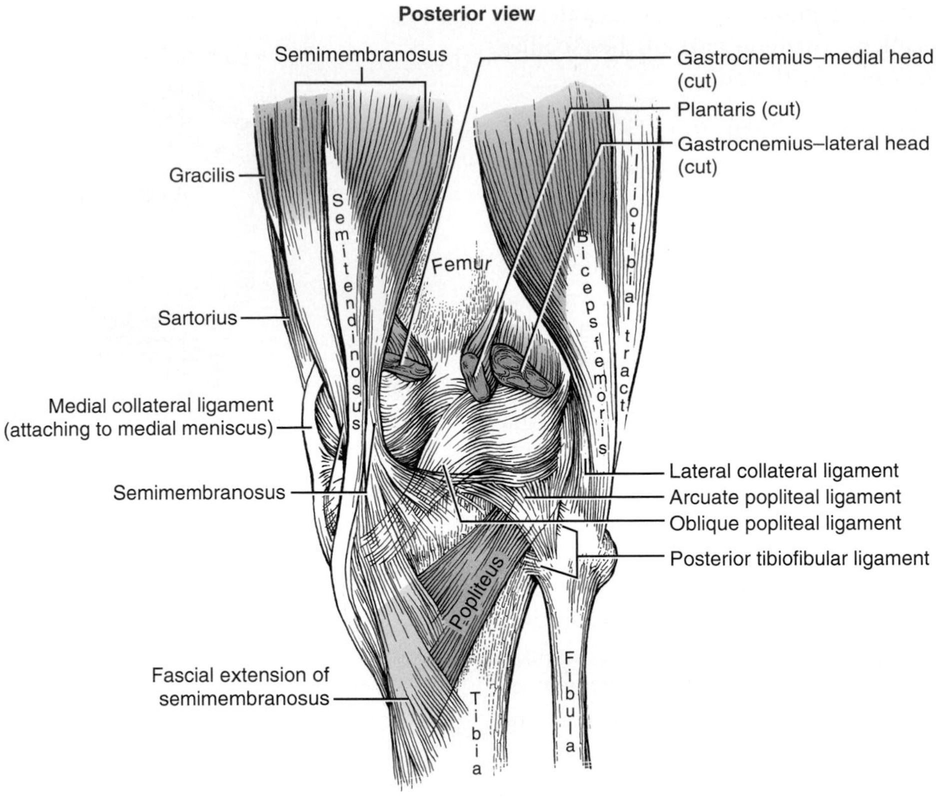

FIGURE 9-23 Popliteus and posterior knee. (From Neumann DA: *Kinesiology of the musculoskeletal system,* p. 441, St Louis, 2002, Elsevier/Mosby.)

pulleys—the medial malleolus, the sustentaculum tali, and the sesamoid bones—help these muscles function.

Retinaculum. Another unique anatomical structure that is located in the deep posterior compartment is the retinaculum. *Retinaculum* is Latin for "halter." It serves to cinch down the tendons, gently separating them from the muscle of the leg as they pass over the ankle and go to the foot. The retinaculum functions to improve the performance of the muscles and keep them from interfering with other structures.

Knee and Thigh Muscles

The muscles and tendons of the knee and thigh have a relationship that is similar to that of the muscles and tendons of the ankle and leg. In other words, the muscle bellies are generally located above the joint on which they work, and tendons from these same muscles cross over the joint to the distal segment of the joint. In the case of the knee, the muscles run from the femur down to the tibia or fibula, and in some cases the muscles run down from the pelvis and gluteal areas all the way to the leg (i.e., tibia and fibula). The muscles of the hip have a similar pattern insofar as the bellies are proximal to the joint and the tendons run to the distal segment of the joint.

Table 9-2 summarizes the thigh muscles, which are described in detail in the following sections.

Anterior Thigh Muscles

Muscles of the thigh can, like those of the foot and ankle, also be grouped according to their respective locations. The anterior aspect of the thigh includes the pectineus, iliopsoas, tensor of the fasciae latae, sartorius, and the quadriceps (Figure 9-24).

Pectineus. The pectineus is a relatively small muscle that runs from the pubic bone to the lesser trochanter of the femur. As its angle of pull suggests, it adducts the thigh and helps with flexion.

Iliopsoas. The iliopsoas is really two muscles: the iliacus, which lines the ilium, and the psoas, which comes off the lumbar vertebrae. These two muscles merge in the pelvis and then exit the pelvis as one, inserting on the lesser trochanter of the femur. This muscle is the strongest flexor of the thigh.

Tensor Fasciae Latae. The tensor fasciae latae is actually located on the anterior lateral aspect of the thigh. Although it has a bony attachment proximally on the iliac crest, its distal attachment is actually not bone but

TABLE 9-2 **Muscles of the Thigh**

MUSCLE(S)	LOCATION	FUNCTION*
Anterior		
Pectineus	The pectineus originates on the pubic bone and runs to the lesser trochanter of the femur.	It adducts the thigh and helps with flexion.
Iliopsoas	The iliopsoas is two muscles: the iliacus, which lines the ilium, and the psoas, which comes off the lumbar vertebrae. They merge in the pelvis and then exit the pelvis as one, inserting on the lesser trochanter of the femur.	This muscle is the strongest hip flexor of the thigh.
Tensor fasciae latae	Originating on the iliac crest, the tensor fascia lata runs about a third of the way down the thigh into the IT band. The IT band inserts onto the lateral, superior tibia on a small bump called Gerdy's tubercle.	It helps stabilize the lateral aspect of the thigh and can help in hip flexion, internal rotation of the thigh, and abduction. It can also be a weak extensor or flexor of the knee depending on the flexion angle of the knee.
Sartorius	Originating just medial to the IT band on the anterior superior iliac spine of the ilium, the sartorius crosses over the quadriceps, inserting on the superior medial tibia. This insertion point is called the *pes anserine*.	It flexes, abducts, and externally rotates the thigh while also flexing the knee.
Quadriceps (4 Plus 1)		
Rectus femoris	Originating off the femur, on the anterior, inferior ilium, the rectus femoris runs straight down the thigh to merge with the three other quadriceps muscle bellies to form the quadriceps/patellar tendon on the tibial tuberosity.	It flexes the hip and, with the other quadriceps muscles, extends the knee. Eccentrically it serves the important function of controlling knee flexion as the foot hits the ground during gait and jumping.
Vastus lateralis	Originating off the superior lateral femur, the vastus lateralis then merges distally with the quadriceps/patellar tendon.	It extends the knee and eccentrically helps with the important function of controlling knee flexion.
Vastus medialis	Originating off the superior medial femur, the vastus medialis then merges distally with the quadriceps/patellar tendon.	It extends the knee and eccentrically helps with the important function of controlling knee flexion.
Vastus medialis oblique	Originating off the distal vastus medialis, it has some insertion on the medial retinaculum of the patella and with the quadriceps/patellar tendon.	It helps with the medial stability of the patella and the quadriceps/patellar tendon.
Vastus intermedius	Originating off the superior middle femur, the vastus intermedius then merges distally with the quadriceps/patellar tendon.	It extends the knee and eccentrically helps with the important function of controlling knee flexion.
Medial Adductors (3)		
Adductor brevis	Originating on the pubic bone, the adductor brevis runs down to the proximal, posterior, medial aspect of the femur.	Of the three muscles that serve to adduct the femur, the magnus is the most powerful.
Adductor longus	Originating on the pubic bone, the adductor longus attaches to the middle one third of the posterior, medial femur.	
Adductor magnus	Originating on the pubic bone, the adductor magnus has two attachment sites on the distal medial femur, one proximal and one distal.	The distal attachment helps extend the thigh, and the proximal part helps flex the thigh.
Others		
Gracilis	Originating on the medial pubic bone, the gracilis runs straight down to the superior medial tibia, inserting with the sartorius and semitendinosus at the pes anserine.	It is a weak knee flexor and thigh adductor.
Obturator externus	Originating from the obturator foramen of the ilium, the obturator externus runs mostly horizontal out to the junction of the neck and shaft of the femur.	It externally rotates the femur and stabilizes the hip.
Posterior Hamstrings (3)		
All three hamstrings originate on the ischial tuberosity of the ischium.		
Semitendinosus	The semitendinosus inserts on the medial, superior tibia with the gracilis and the sartorius.	It internally rotates the tibia and flexes the knee.
Semimembranosus	The semimembranosus continues down to insert on the posterior, medial tibial condyle.	It internally rotates the tibia and flexes the knee.
Biceps femoris	The biceps femoris also has an origin on the midposterior femur. It runs distally and laterally to the head of the fibula.	It externally rotates the tibia and flexes the knee.

*Remember that a function of all of these muscles is that they cover some anatomical structure and thereby protect it.

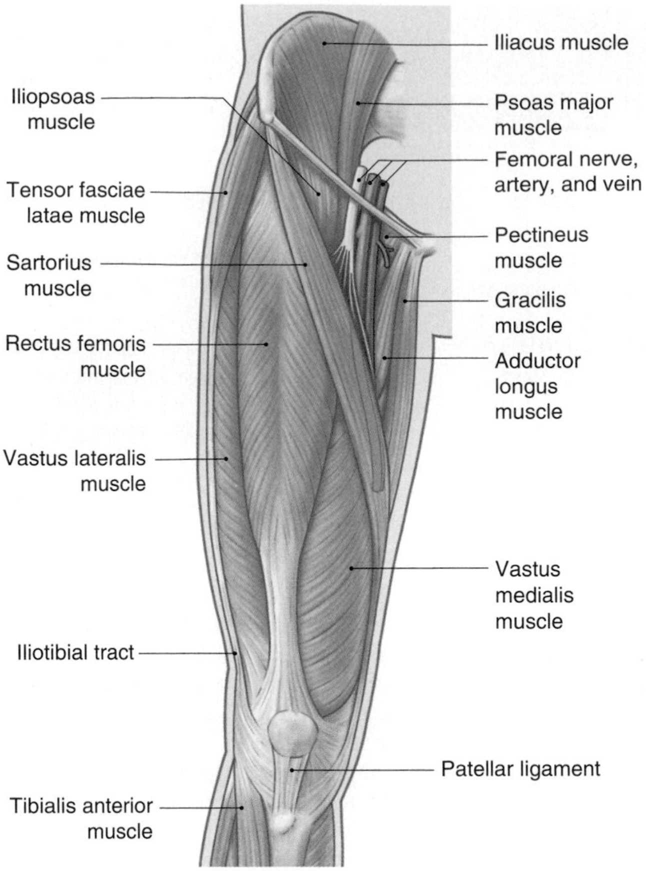

FIGURE 9-24 Anterior and medial thigh muscles. (From Moses K et al: *Atlas of clinical gross anatomy,* p. 488, St Louis, 2005, Elsevier/Mosby.)

thickened fascia, called the *iliotibial (IT) band,* about a third of the way down the thigh. The IT band consists of tough connective tissue and covers the lateral aspect of the thigh, running from the iliac crest to the lateral, superior tibia. The insertion point of the IT band on the lateral, superior tibia feels like a small bump. This bump is referred to as *Gerdy's tubercle.* The tensor fasciae latae muscle helps stabilize the lateral aspect of the thigh and can help in hip flexion, internal rotation of the thigh, and abduction. It may also be a weak extensor or flexor of the knee depending on the flexion angle of the knee. If the knee is flexed less than 20 degrees, the tensor fasciae latae acts more as an extensor of the knee; if the knee is flexed more than 20 degrees, the tensor fasciae latae acts more as a flexor of the knee.

Sartorius. The sartorius, which starts just medial to the IT band, is the longest muscle in the body. It originates on the anterior superior iliac spine of the ilium and then crosses over the quadriceps, inserting on the superior medial tibia. This insertion point is called the *pes anserine* (*anserine* is Latin for "gooselike" and *pes* is Latin for "foot") and is also the insertion point of the gracilis and the semitendinosus. In combination, the attachments of these three muscles resemble a goose's foot—hence the name. The sartorius, often called the *tailor's muscle,* flexes, abducts, and externally rotates the thigh while also flexing the knee.

Quadriceps. The quadriceps is so named because it is a four-headed muscle. The most superficial muscle, the rectus femoris, is also the only muscle that originates off the femur on the anterior, inferior ilium. It then runs straight down the thigh to merge with the distal aspects of the three other quadriceps muscle bellies on the tibial tuberosity. Whereas all the other quadriceps muscles originate on the thigh and act only on the knee, the rectus femoris can also act as a hip flexor because it crosses the front of the hip joint. The other muscle bellies and their heads are named according to their location. They all originate on the anterior superior femur and, from lateral to medial, are called the vastus lateralis, the vastus intermedius, and the vastus medialis. The vastus medialis is unique in that the distal fibers run in a more oblique direction than those of the vastus lateralis; therefore it provides more medial pull on the patella, which is embedded in the quadriceps tendon. The distal fibers of this muscle form another muscle called the vastus medialis oblique, so called because its fibers run at an oblique angle compared with those of the rest of the vastus medialis. The structure generally called the quadriceps tendon is so named because it connects the quadriceps muscle to the patella, a sesamoid bone within the tendon. The structure running from the patella down to the tibial tuberosity is called the *patella tendon.* The tendon that runs from the patella to the tibial tuberosity is also called the *patellar tendon.*

Medial Thigh Muscles

The muscles of the medial thigh assist with movement of the hip and knee. Because they tend to cross both joints at times, they move bones of both joints at times. As a group, these muscles are commonly called the *groin muscles.*

Adductor Muscles. There are five muscles on the medial aspect of the thigh. The adductor group consists of three muscles whose names reflect their respective sizes. These adductor muscles are the adductor brevis, adductor longus, and adductor magnus. All three muscles originate on the pubic bone, with the brevis traveling down the femur to attach on the proximal, posterior, medial aspect. The longus attaches to the middle third of the posterior, medial femur, and the magnus has two attachment sites on the femur. Both attachments are on the medial aspect of the femur, with one proximal and one distal, leaving a small opening through which vessels can pass. Although all three muscles serve to adduct the femur, the magnus is the most powerful.

Gracilis. The gracilis is also considered an adductor because of its location and angle of pull. Its name means *graceful*, and as one would imagine, it is not very powerful. In fact, it might be better known as the muscle or tendon often used to replace the ACL after surgical reconstruction. The gracilis is also a weak knee flexor and thigh adductor. It runs from the medial pubic bone straight down to the superior medial tibia, inserting with the sartorius and semitendinosus at the pes anserine.

Obturator Externus. The fifth muscle of this group, the obturator externus, is a short, flat muscle that lies deep to the other muscles of this area and works primarily to externally rotate the femur. It runs in a mostly horizontal direction from the obturator foramen of the ilium out to the junction of the neck and shaft of the femur.

Posterior Thigh Muscles

There are many muscles on the posterior aspect of the hip and thigh. Some are short, and some are long; some are superficial, and some are deep; some are primary movers, and some are stabilizers (Figures 9-25 and 9-26).

Hamstrings. The hamstrings represent the main posterior thigh muscles. They are long, superficial prime movers consisting of the semitendinosus and the semimembranosus on the medial posterior aspect and the biceps femoris on the lateral posterior aspect. All of these muscles originate on the ischial tuberosity, with the biceps femoris also having an origin on the midposterior femur. The two heads of this muscle account for its name (*bi* means "two," and *ceps* means "heads"). It continues distally and laterally to the head of the fibula. The semitendinosus continues distally from the ischial tuberosity and inserts on the medial, superior tibia with the gracilis and the sartorius. This common point of insertion is called the *pes anserine.* The semimembranosus continues down to insert on the posterior, medial tibial condyle. When sitting with your knees flexed, you

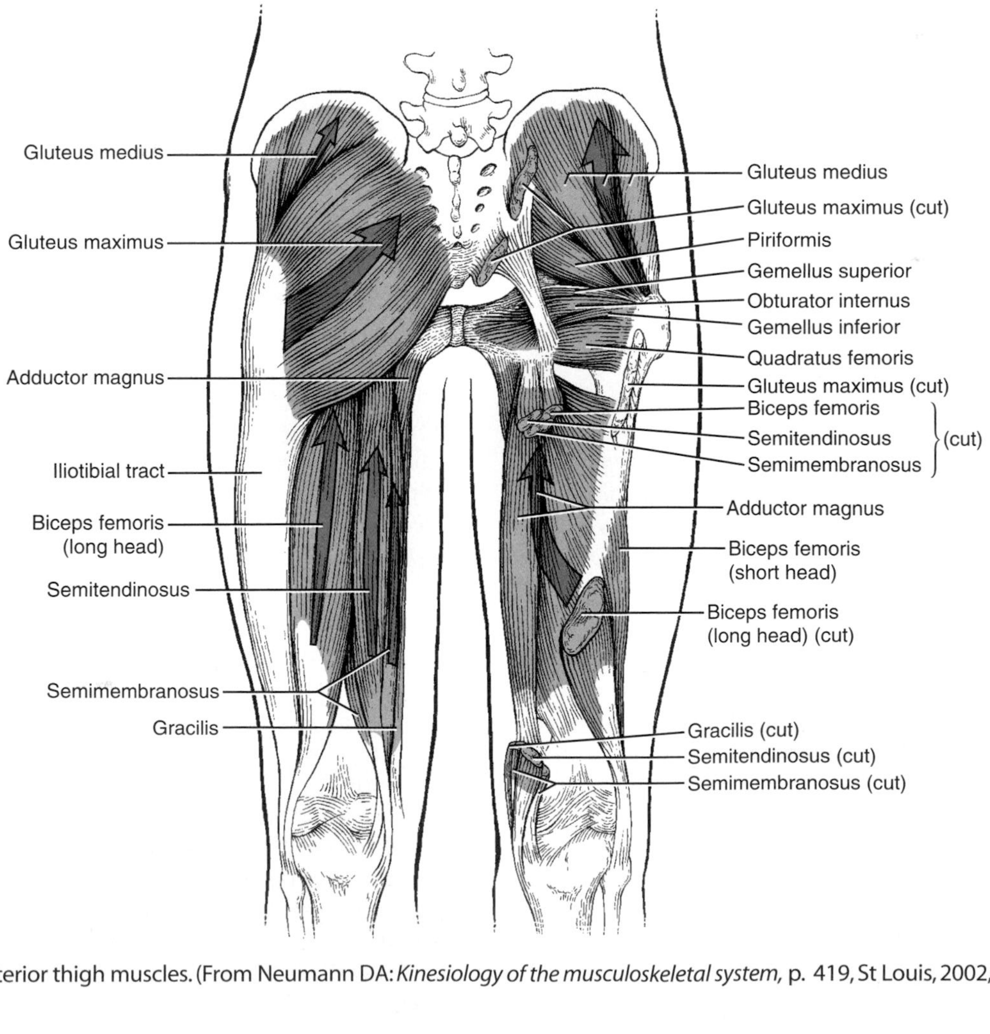

FIGURE 9-25 Posterior thigh muscles. (From Neumann DA: *Kinesiology of the musculoskeletal system,* p. 419, St Louis, 2002, Elsevier/Mosby.)

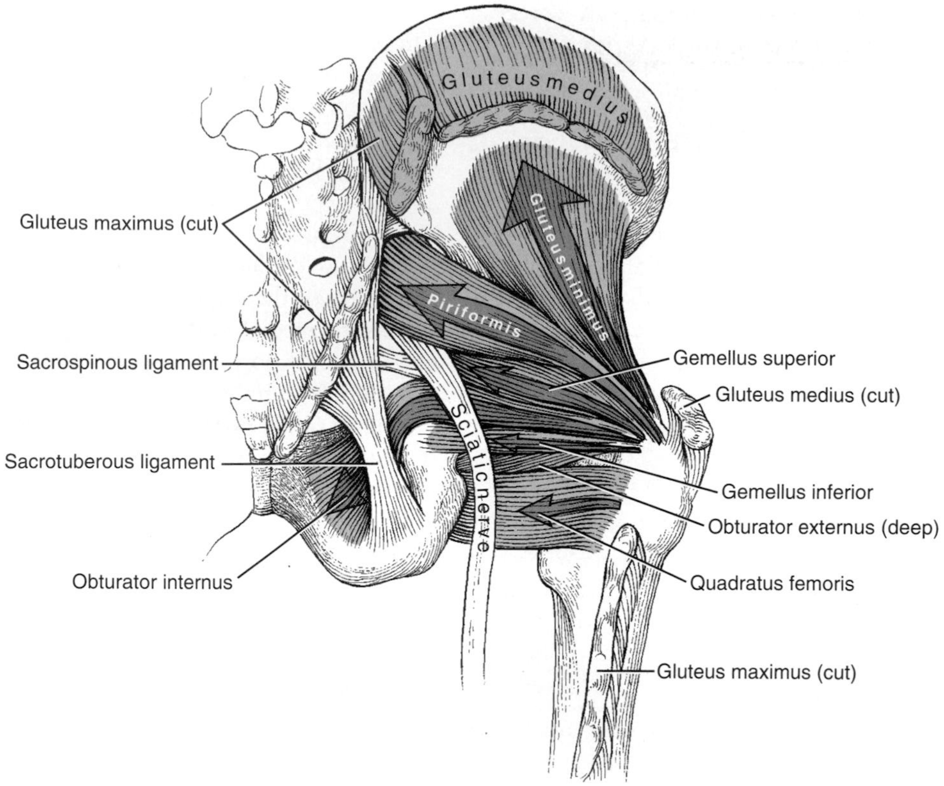

FIGURE 9-26 Deep posterior thigh muscles. (From Neumann DA: *Kinesiology of the musculoskeletal system,* p. 421, St Louis, 2002, Elsevier/Mosby.)

can feel the tendons of these three muscles by putting your index and middle fingers under your knee at the point of flexion. The soft and fleshy area behind the knee, between the tendons of the hamstrings, is called the *popliteal fossa.* Deep in this area are the popliteal artery and the tibial nerve, both of which are vital to the leg.

Gluteal Muscles

There are three gluteal muscles. The largest and most powerful muscle, as indicated by its name, is the gluteus maximus. It originates on the external ilium and inserts into the posterior, superior iliotibial band. Its main functions are to extend and externally rotate the thigh. The gluteus medius is just deep to the gluteus maximus and is about half its size. Although the gluteus medius also originates on the external ilium, it inserts on the lateral aspect of the greater trochanter of the femur in such a way that it internally rotates the femur and abducts it. Injury to the gluteus medius results in a lurching gait on the side opposite to the site of injury; this happens because the gluteus medius cannot hold the ilium up against the femur as the opposite side swings through during gait. Deep to the gluteus medius is the gluteus minimus, which runs a similar course but inserts on the anterior greater trochanter. The functions of the gluteus minimus are to help with internal rotation and abduction of the femur.

Table 9-3 summarizes the gluteal and hip area muscles, including the external rotators, which are described in detail in the following section.

Small Hip External Rotators. Inferior to the gluteus minimus are five small external rotators of the femur. They are, from proximal to distal, the piriformis, the obturator internus, the gemelli brothers, more commonly known as the superior and inferior gemellus, and the quadratus femoris. The muscle most often implicated in pathology is the piriformis; it is very close to the sciatic nerve and can put pressure on the nerve, causing radicular signs and symptoms.

Nerves and Arteries of the Lower Body

Nerves transmit information from outside the body to the brain for interpretation. They form the biological wiring that sends commands from the brain to the rest of the body about how to relate and react to that information.

Arteries are one of the components of the superhighway of vessels that bring nutrients to the tissues of the body and help transfer waste products from the tissues to the appropriate disposal and processing sites elsewhere in the body. These nutrients, primarily oxygen, are carried in the bloodstream through this intricate network of blood vessels.

TABLE 9-3 **Muscles of the Gluteal and Hip Regions**

MUSCLE(S)	LOCATION	FUNCTION*
Gluteal		
Gluteus maximus	The gluteus maximus originates on the external ilium and inserts into the posterior, superior iliotibial band.	The main functions are to extend and externally rotate the thigh.
Gluteus medius	The gluteus medius originates on the external ilium and inserts on the lateral aspect of the greater trochanter of the femur.	It internally rotates the femur and abducts it. Injury to the gluteus medius produces a lurching gait to the side opposite to the injury.
Gluteus minimus	The gluteus minimus runs a similar course to the medius but inserts on the anterior greater trochanter.	It functions to help with internal rotation and abduction of the femur.
External Rotators of Hip		
Piriformis Obturator internus Superior gemellus Inferior gemellus Quadratus femoris	These muscles originate on the anterior sacrum, ischium, and obturator foramen and then insert on the greater trochanter.	They all work to rotate the femur externally.

*Remember that a function of all of these muscles is that they cover some anatomical structure and thereby protect it.

Nerves of the Lower Body

Bones, ligaments, and muscles are the structures that get the most attention. However, they would not function properly without nerves, arteries, and veins. Nerves cause the muscles to fire, and arteries bring oxygen and nutrients to the muscles and bones so that they are viable living structures. Nerve roots exit from the spinal cord through the fourth and fifth lumbar vertebrae and the first, second, and third sacral vertebrae to form the sciatic nerve. The sciatic nerve travels through the thigh and leg all the way to the toes. Nerves of the leg, ankle, and foot all come off the sciatic nerve, which splits into the common fibularis and tibial nerves in the area just above the posterior knee. The common fibularis nerve divides again as it crosses over the head of the fibula. A deep branch extends into the anterior compartment. A **superficial** branch travels down between the two fibularis muscles in the lateral compartment. The tibial nerve continues distally into both of the posterior compartments. After passing through the posterior compartments, the tibial nerve splits and covers the foot as medial and lateral plantar nerves.

Nerves send signals to activate both the extrinsic and small intrinsic muscles so that movements and activities enhance the stability of the foot. The sensory nerves provide feedback regarding the foot to the central nervous system (e.g., Is the toe or foot being tickled, scratched, or pinched?) and thereby initiate the appropriate motor nerve function. One of the most important sensory functions of these nerves is to give **proprioceptive** feedback regarding joint position and muscle tension. Proprioception, an unconscious process, determines the amount of force that a muscle must create to achieve a desired response.

Arteries and Veins of the Lower Body

Just as the nerves of the leg, ankle, and foot come from the thorax area, so do the arteries and veins. The heart is responsible for sending out blood, the life-giving fluid of the body. The femoral artery comes down out of the thorax and pelvis into the thigh. It continues behind the knee as the popliteal artery for a short distance and then splits into the anterior and posterior tibial arteries. Both of these arteries continue down all the way into the foot. Veins return the unoxygenated blood back up to the heart. Superficial (i.e., saphenous) and deep (i.e., popliteal and femoral) veins are responsible for this function. The impressive and abundant communication between the smallest arteries and veins often goes unacknowledged.

Pronation and Supination. The foot, ankle, and their component structures serve as the foundation for movements and activities that require the individual to be upright. Bones serve as the rigid framework for this foundation. The relationships formed by each set of adjoining bones, or joints, are critical in the proper functioning of the foot. An often overlooked concept is that the responsibilities of the bones, joints, and structures of the lower body are different when the foot is in contact with the ground than when the foot is in the air, in a nonweight-bearing state. When the foot is not in contact with the ground, no ground reaction forces pass up the kinetic chain formed by the musculoskeletal structures of the body. When the foot is planted or in contact with the ground, it has a lot of influence on the structures above it. Two movements of the foot that occur naturally with every step are pronation and supination.

superficial closer to the skin's surface of the body; farther away from the layer of tissue near the bone and closer to the skin

proprioceptive describes information sent to the brain concerning body position and muscle tension; used to maintain balance and coordination

Pronation allows the foot and lower body to absorb the forces that occur during walking, running, and jumping. *Pronation,* loosely defined, is the combination of movements that begins with calcaneal eversion, forefoot abduction, and ankle dorsiflexion (Figure 9-27). Following these movements, the talus, which rides on top of the calcaneus, pulls the tibia into internal rotation. Above the tibia, the knee flexes, the femur internally rotates, and the hip flexes. All of these movements allow the lower extremity to absorb forces and are a natural biomechanical reaction to the foot landing on the ground and "rolling in," or pronating. Pronation is a natural occurrence that varies according to the individual's anatomy. The bones of the foot, in concert with the ligaments, muscles, and other interacting structures, actually assume a looser-than-normal relationship during pronation. This looseness allows the foot and the leg above it to better absorb forces. Individuals who are unable to dissipate forces properly are more likely to sustain overuse injuries.

Supination, the opposite of pronation, is the movement that allows the foot and ankle to become a rigid lever so that pushing off the ground can occur efficiently and effectively (Figure 9-28). If the foot were to stay flexible during push off, it would be like pushing off in a bowl of mashed potatoes, with all propulsive force lost. Fortunately, the foot naturally transforms from a loose structure to a rigid one when push off occurs. The calcaneus inverts, the forefoot adducts, and the ankle plantar flexes (i.e., the angle between the front of the

pronation combination of movements resulting in the rolling-in movement of the foot as it lands on the ground

supination movement of the foot and ankle that allows the food and ankle to become a rigid lever to enhance the pushing-off motion of the foot from the ground

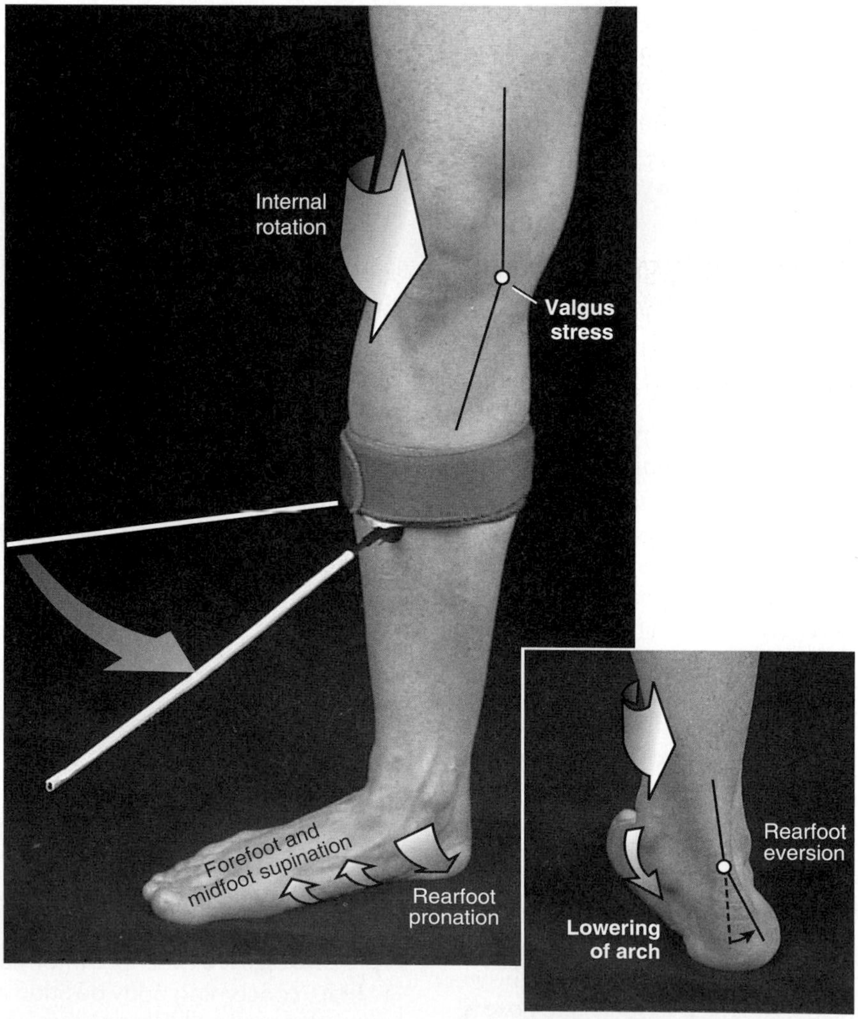

FIGURE 9-27 Rearfoot pronation. (From Neumann DA: *Kinesiology of the musculoskeletal system,* p. 500, St Louis, 2002, Elsevier/Mosby.)

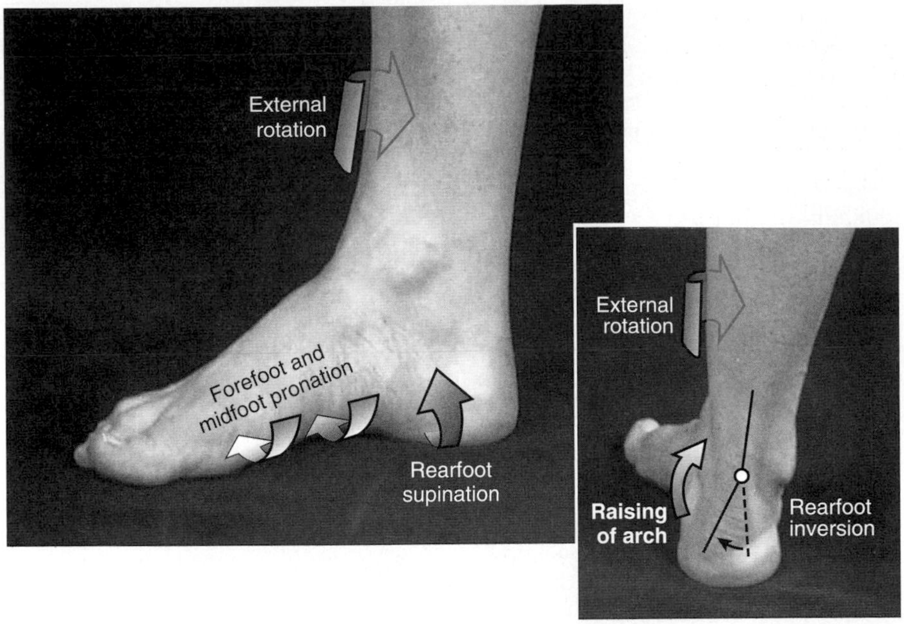

FIGURE 9-28 Rearfoot supination. (From Neumann DA: *Kinesiology of the musculoskeletal system,* p. 502, St Louis, 2002, Elsevier/Mosby.)

tibia and the foot gets larger). This series of events causes the talus to pull the tibia externally, the knee extends, the femur externally rotates, and the hip extends. These movements in turn cause the bones, muscles, tendons, and ligaments of the leg, thigh, and pelvis to propel foot and body away from the ground. When the foot becomes rigid, it allows the foot and leg to better transmit muscular forces to the ground for propulsion. During running or walking, or any forward-moving activity in which the foot pushes off the ground, the foot and ankle should supinate during the push-off phase. Supination initiates a rigid foot position that enhances push off. Sometimes the individual's anatomy does not allow supination to occur as described. Because these people do not supinate effectively, they cannot create the rigid lever that is needed to propel the body up or forward in the usual manner. Consequently, they are more vulnerable to lower extremity overuse injuries such as muscle strains and tendonitis, as discussed in Chapter 10. Pronation and supination play significant roles in absorbing force and serving as rigid levers, both functions of the lower extremity that are initiated at heel contact. If these functions are not performed, ground reaction forces are not absorbed effectively and push off is less efficient.

SUMMARY

The lower extremity has many functions, many of which are needed to allow movements to be performed in the trunk, abdomen, and upper body. The lower extremity is capable of producing both very powerful movements and very delicate, discrete movements. Each bone, ligament, muscle, tendon, nerve, and vessel is obviously an entity in its own right, but these structures are most impressive when working with other structures.

The lower extremity is capable of amazing feats: tightrope walking, championship sprinting, and tap dancing, to name a few. From the runner who competes in ultramarathons to the football player who kicks the ball 50 yards for the winning field goal, athletes depend on the lower extremity to achieve their dreams.

Web Links

Body Worlds Project: www.koerperwelten.de/en/pages/home.asp

Medical Gross Anatomy Learning Resources (University of Michigan): http://anatomy.med.umich.edu/

The Anatomy Lesson: http://mywebpages.comcast.net/wnor/homepage.htm

The Visible Human Project (National Library of Medicine, National Institutes of Health): www.nlm.nih.gov/research/visible/visible_human.html

Web Anatomy (University of Minnesota): www.msjensen.gen.umn.edu/webanatomy/

Bibliography

Applegate E: The *Anatomy and physiology learning system*, ed 3, Philadelphia, 2006, Saunders/Elsevier.

Cuppett M, Walsh KM: *General medical conditions in the athlete*, St Louis, 2005, Elsevier/Mosby.

Drake RL, Vogl W, Mitchell ADM; *Gray's anatomy for students*, Edinburgh, 2005, Elsevier/Churchill Livingstone.

Gray G: *Chain reaction: functional biomechanics* [workshop and workbook]. Adrian, Mich, 1992, Winn Publishing.

Griffin LY: *Prevention of noncontact ACL injuries*, Rosemont, Ill, 2001, American Academy of Orthopaedic Surgeons.

Herlihy B: *The human body in health and illness*, ed 3, Philadelphia, 2007, Saunders/Elsevier.
Lambert LL: The weight bearing function of the fibula: a strain gauge study, *J Bone Joint Surgery* 53: 507–513, 1971.
Moses KP et al: *Atlas of clinical gross anatomy*, St Louis, 2005, Elsevier/Mosby.
Muscolino JE: *Kinesiology: The skeletal system and muscle function*, St Louis, 2006, Elsevier/Mosby.
Neumann D: *Kinesiology of the skeletal system: foundations for physical therapy*, St Louis, 2002, Elsevier/Mosby.
Seidel HM et al: *Mosby's guide to physical examination*, ed 6, St Louis, 2006, Mosby/Elsevier.
Standring S, editor: *Gray's anatomy: The anatomical basis of clinical practice*, ed 39, Edinburgh, 2005, Elsevier/Churchill Livingstone.
Thibodeau GA, Patton KT: *Anatomy and physiology*, ed 6, St Louis, 2007, Mosby/Elsevier.

10

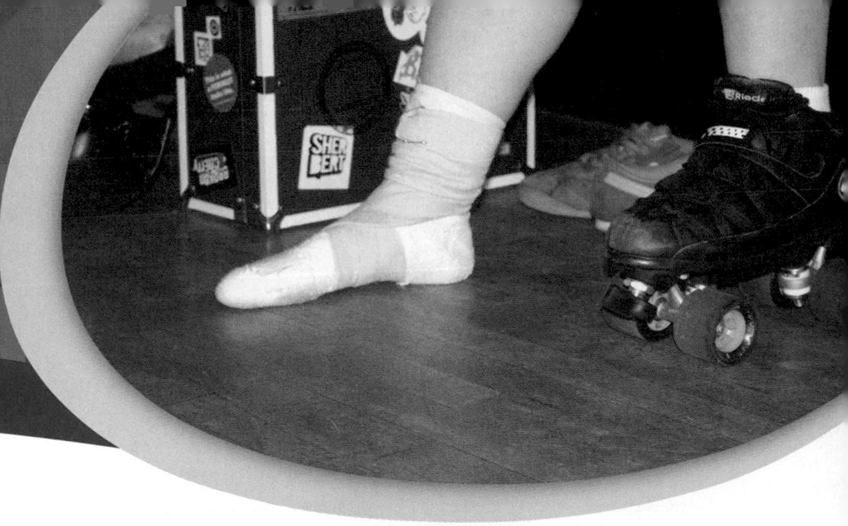

Diagnosis and Management of Lower Leg, Ankle, Foot, and Toe Injuries

GARY B. WILKERSON

Learning Goals

1. Describe appropriate procedures to evaluate and diagnose common acute and chronic injuries to the lower leg, ankle, foot, and toes.
2. Discuss the importance of a systematic assessment in the management of injuries to the lower leg, ankle, foot, and toes.
3. Identify common signs and symptoms of on-field/acute injuries to the lower leg, ankle, foot, and toes.
4. Explain the proper interventions for managing acute injuries to the lower leg, ankle, foot, and toes.
5. Identify common signs and symptoms of chronic/overuse injuries to the lower leg, ankle, foot and toes.
6. Describe the proper interventions for managing chronic/overuse injuries to the lower leg, ankle, foot, and toes.
7. Identify principles and concepts that can be applied to prevent injuries to the lower leg, ankle, foot, and toes.
8. Recognize specific age-group injuries that affect the lower leg, ankle, foot, and toes.

Terms that appear in boldface green type are defined in the book's glossary.

Injuries of the ankle and foot are extremely common in both athletic and nonathletic populations and may account for as much as 25% of all musculoskeletal injuries.[1,2] Lower leg and toe injuries are not quite as common. The complex relationships among the lower leg, ankle, foot, and toes, combined with the numerous potential combinations of dynamic human movement, make diagnosing and managing injuries in this area quite challenging. Properly diagnosing and managing these injuries can facilitate the client's prompt and safe return to activity.

A simplistic view of lower leg, ankle, foot, and toe function presents the ankle as a single joint that connects the lower leg to a relatively immobile foot segment. In reality, ankle and foot motion involves a complex system of joints (Table 10-1) that are highly integrated and interdependent. Movement occurs at the following places: the ankle, the subtalar and talocrural joints (the rearfoot), the transverse tarsal joint (the midfoot), and the tarsometatarsal and the metatarsophalangeal joints (the forefoot).

Understanding normal biomechanical function of the ankle and foot requires an awareness of the spatial orientation of each joint and its axis of motion as well as the motion that occurs simultaneously at the various joints. Injury mechanisms are often related to excessive joint motion that is induced by external forces.

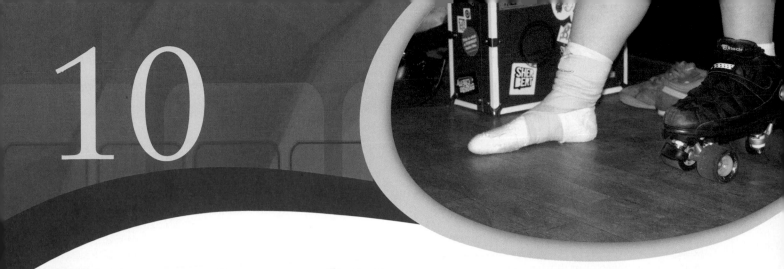

OPENING *Scenario*

Calvin, a 20-year-old starting quarterback for his college football team, went home for a visit with his family on a midseason weekend when no game was scheduled. While playing basketball in his driveway with his brothers and friends, Calvin's right foot landed on another person's foot as Calvin was coming down from a lay-up under the basket. He recounts that the sole of his foot rolled inward, causing him immediate intense pain, and the ankle quickly became swollen. Because he feared that walking on the injured ankle might cause further injury, he complied with his mother's insistence that he use a pair of crutches that had been stored in the attic. Approximately 24 hours after the traumatic episode, he comes to the athletic training room with diffuse swelling on the medial and lateral aspects of the ankle and on the dorsum of the foot. The use of a swing-through crutch gait has kept his foot in a gravity-dependent position in plantar flexion; dorsiflexion is now restricted and uncomfortable. Ecchymosis is apparent on both sides of the ankle but is considerably greater on the lateral aspect. Palpation elicits intense localized tenderness over the anterior talofibular ligament, minimal tenderness over the calcaneofibular ligament, and a moderate degree of tenderness on both the anterior and posterior tibial malleolus. Palpation does not elicit any tenderness directly over the fibular malleolus, the tibial malleolus, the navicular, or the base of the fifth metatarsal. The anterior drawer test elicits pain but does not appear to be positive for ligament laxity. The head football coach is extremely anxious to find out how long his starting quarterback will be unable to play. Since the team is in the middle of the football season, the coach needs to know when Calvin can return to a level of performance that will allow full participation in practice and games. What should be done immediately to manage Calvin's current condition, and how would you respond to the coach's desperate pleas for assurance that a high level of ankle function can be quickly restored?

TABLE 10-1 Primary Joints Providing Movement at the Ankle and Foot

JOINT(S)	LOCATION	RECIPROCAL MOTIONS
Talocrural (ankle)	Rearfoot	Dorsiflexion/plantar flexion
Subtalar	Rearfoot	Supination/pronation
Transverse tarsal	Midfoot	*OR*
Tarsometatarsal	Midfoot	Inversion/eversion
Metatarsophalangeal	Forefoot	Flexion/extension
		Abduction/adduction

The term **pathomechanics** refers to the unique combination of external forces and joint displacements that produce an injury. A working knowledge of both normal biomechanical function and pathomechanics of common injuries greatly enhances an athletic trainer's ability to determine the precise nature and severity of an injury. Information derived in this manner will guide development of a specific treatment plan that will efficiently restore optimal functional capabilities of the affected joint.[3]

CLINICAL EVALUATION AND DIAGNOSIS OF LOWER LEG, FOOT, ANKLE, AND TOE INJURIES

To evaluate, diagnose, and manage injuries of the lower leg, foot, ankle, and toe, comprehension of certain key terms is paramount. Medical literature in the United States generally uses the coupled terms *inversion-eversion* to define an injury mechanism responsible for ankle ligament damage,[4] whereas the coupled terms *supination-pronation* are generally used to describe foot position in relation to the leg during standing, walking, or running.[5] The coupled terms *adduction-abduction* generally refer to the direction of movement of the midline of the foot segment within the transverse plane (horizontal toe-in versus toe-out of the foot), whereas corresponding motion of the leg segment is universally designated as internal-external rotation. The coupled *terms plantar flexion-dorsiflexion* are universally used to designate upward and downward movement of the foot in relation to the leg.

Understanding the relationships of the involved anatomical structures and their associated movements assists in establishing a systematic evaluation and diagnosis process. Acute and chronic injuries to these areas warrant immediate attention. Preventing further injury or recurrent injuries is paramount to the active individual. Obtaining an accurate history, followed by thoroughly examining the injury, palpating the affected area, assessing range-of-motion abilities, performing special tests, and determining neurovascular status, provides the athletic trainer with the necessary information to develop a comprehensive rehabilitation program, one that will allow the client to resume activity as quickly and safely as possible.

History

The athlete with a lower leg, ankle, foot, or toe injury is usually able to relate details of the sequence of events

pathomechanics the unique combination of external forces and joint displacements that produce an injury leading up to the injury: These make up the history. The history usually includes the direction of the lower leg or foot displacement that caused the injury. Important clues about the probable pathology can be derived from careful analysis of the scenario that immediately preceded the traumatic event and the subsequent set of circumstances that existed at the moment injury occurred.[6] The likelihood of extensive damage to multiple joint structures is substantially increased by a history of high-force impact of the foot against the ground or another object, such as an improper jump landing or a sudden deceleration from running.[7] Important broad categories of history questions to ask, which will lead to a decisive mechanism of injury (MOI), include how, what, when, where, and why.

Observation/Inspection

The athletic trainer often has the opportunity to gain insight into functional limitations by observing the injured person's mode of ambulation before the actual evaluation. If the client is using a swing-through crutch gait or displays great difficulty while ambulating, a relatively severe injury may be suspected; however, the ability to ambulate without the use of an assistive device should not be interpreted as an indication of a relatively mild injury. Full weight bearing on the injured extremity may be demonstrated by individuals who are later found to have a complete ligament rupture. Furthermore, functional capabilities may dramatically improve or worsen from one day to next or even within a few hours. Observation should be performed in both nonweight-bearing and weight-bearing positions.

> **Points to Ponder**
>
> What aspects can change when viewing the foot in a weight-bearing position instead of in a nonweight-bearing position?

In terms of the purely physiological response to acute injury, the location, amount, and characteristics of swelling are key indicators of the nature and extent of pathology. The immediate appearance of localized swelling, sometimes referred to as a *goose egg,* is probably due to acute trauma-induced arterial disruption that causes hemorrhage within the tissues. The volume of blood and edema that accumulates in the injured area is generally proportional to the extent of tissue damage.

Blood within a joint is referred to as a **hemarthrosis**, whereas excessive fluid is referred to as a *joint effusion,* and blood pooled within the tissues outside a joint is referred to as a *hematoma*. The viscosity of joint fluid containing blood is much greater than that of a joint effusion. A hemarthrosis is associated with high intracapsular pressure that restricts joint motion to a much greater extent than either a joint effusion or an extracapsular edema formation, and it causes the distended skin and subcutaneous tissues to display a much firmer consistency than normal. Swelling is generally localized to the area with less severe injuries, whereas more severe injuries are associated with diffuse swelling.

Palpation

Localization of tenderness in the lower leg, ankle, foot, or toes should initially be focused on determining the likelihood of a fracture. Because of the frequent and violent nature of injuries to this area, the risk of fracture is relatively high. Also of note are the numerous bony and soft tissue landmarks that require palpation. A thorough understanding of the anatomy of this region is paramount in determining an accurate diagnosis. Palpation during an on-field evaluation should be performed only on relevant structures and should begin away from the injured area. Once the client has been taken from the activity area, a more in-depth evaluation may be initiated. Palpation aids in determining possible deformities, tenderness, swelling or effusion, increased skin temperature, crepitus, and any other abnormal findings that are unlike the uninvolved side.

Range of Motion Testing

A given body part's range of motion is often a good indicator of compromised functional abilities. The athletic trainer should have the athlete attempt active range of motion to tolerance in all planes at every possible joint. Motion displayed actively provides key information about the extent of injury and the structures involved. If the client experiences increased pain with movement, further assessments for range of motion should be stopped until further diagnostic testing is performed to rule out the possibility of fracture. Passive range of motion should be assessed after active range of motion. When appropriate, resisted range of motion can be assessed after passive range of motion. The type of end-feel noted with passive range of motion assists in determining the extent of injury. With the anatomical complexity of this region of the body and the dynamic relationship of each joint to the other, goniometric measures are exceedingly difficult to obtain except for plantarflexion and dorsiflexion.

Special Tests

Several special tests are used in evaluating and diagnosing injuries to the lower leg, ankle, foot, and toes. For the most part, special tests in this region are performed to rule out fractures and assess the severity of ligament sprains. If the athletic trainer suspects that a client needs further medical intervention, he or she should make a referral as soon as possible. Common special tests are discussed in this section and then listed with the injuries that they are used to diagnose. Other diagnosis-specific tests will be introduced in the context of the relevant injuries.

---

hemarthrosis condition in which blood is within the joint

Compression Test

For the compression test, the client is seated with the lower leg, ankle, or foot in a nonweight-bearing position, typically in a long-sitting position on the table or off the edge of a table or chair. One hand is placed on each side of the injured body part (e.g., lower leg, ankle, foot). A compressive force is applied along the length of the injured area starting distal to the injury and working in a proximal direction, if possible. Start with gentle pressure, and gradually apply more pressure. Pinpoint pain in the injured area or crepitus may indicate a fracture. If findings are positive, the client should be referred to a physician for further evaluation and X-rays.

Tap or Percussion Test

For the tap or percussion test, the individual is in the same position as for the compression test. Using the index finger, the athletic trainer should tap the bone and soft tissue surrounding the injury, beginning with the area that is most tender and then slowly working toward the involved area. A positive test produces pinpoint or radiating pain or crepitus from associated vibrations. Positive findings may indicate a fracture. The client should be referred to a physician for further evaluation and X-rays if a fracture is suspected.

Anterior Drawer Test

The anterior drawer test is widely used to assess the status of the anterior talofibular ligament (ATFL). The anterior drawer test is most effective when performed with the foot plantar flexed at 10 to 20 degrees and the calcaneus pulled forward while the lower leg is stabilized (Figure 10-1).[8–11] Performing the test with the client's foot resting on the athletic trainer's forearm may enhance relaxation of muscle tension, thereby facilitating the perception of unusual motion.[12] The anterior drawer test sometimes creates a **skin sulcus**, or dimple, on the anterolateral aspect of the talocrural joint. Interpretation of the test result is based on the athletic trainer's subjective interpretation of the amount of ligament laxity observed in response to manual force, which is generally based on comparison with the uninjured extremity. Pain-related reflexive muscle tension or swollen soft tissues may prevent joint displacement, thereby causing a high rate of false-negative test results. Some athletic trainers consider either laxity or a pain response to manual ligament stress testing to be a positive test result.[8,9]

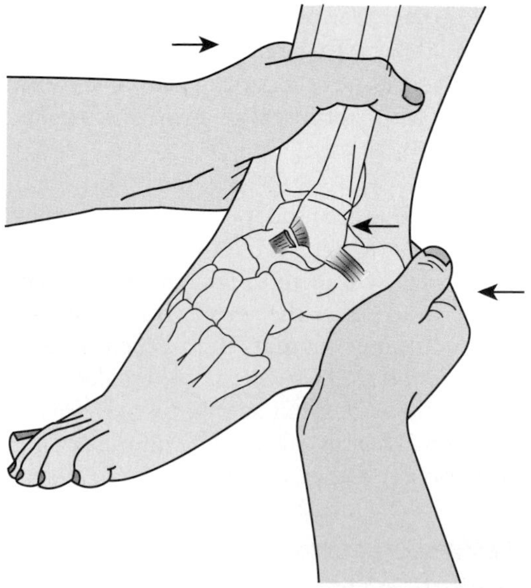

FIGURE 10-1 Anterior drawer test. (Redrawn from Eustace S et al: *Sports injuries: examination, imaging, and management*, Figure 7.18b, Philadelphia, 2007, Churchill Livingstone/Elsevier)

Points to Ponder

Why is it important that the lower leg and foot muscles be relaxed when performing the anterior drawer test?

Talar Tilt Test

The talar tilt test is used primarily to assess the status of the calcaneofibular ligament (CFL). When used as a clinical test, the foot should be positioned in either a neutral position or 10 degrees of dorsiflexion. Next, manually induce inversion of the calcaneus (Figure 10-2).[6,10,13] The amount of abnormal talocrural joint displacement produced by the talar tilt test may be very difficult to perceive, but it sometimes produces a palpable click that is distinctly different from the test response of the opposite uninjured extremity.

Interpretation of the talar tilt test result is similar to that of the anterior drawer; the test should be performed on both the involved and the uninvolved sides, with

skin sulcus a dimpling of the skin indicating a gap in the integrity of the soft tissue being tested

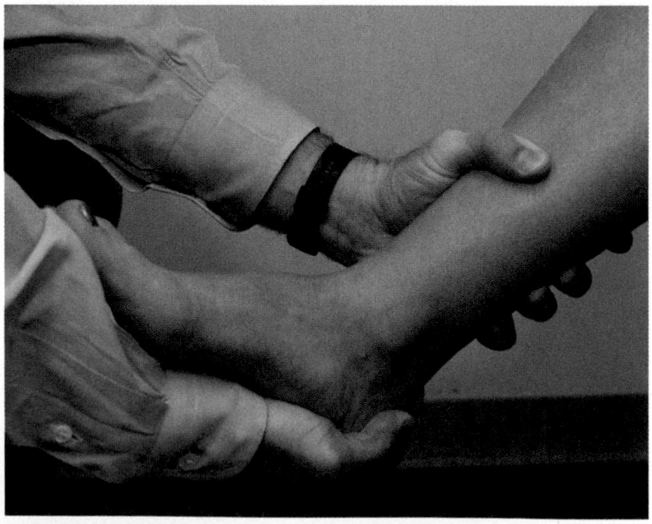

FIGURE 10-2 Performance of the anterior drawer test with the patient's foot resting on the examiner's forearm to minimize muscle guarding.

either laxity or a pain response to the tests considered to be a positive test result.[8,9]

Neurovascular Tests

A thorough evaluation of the neurovascular status of injuries to the lower leg, ankle, foot, and toes should include the testing of myotomes (i.e., a nerve's innervation of a muscle) and dermatomes (i.e., a nerve's innervation of the skin), circulation or pulse, and reflexes. A bilateral evaluation is necessary to properly determine the level of involvement. A quick and easy way to test the neurovascular status of any lower extremity injury is to have the client attempt to wiggle his or her toes and feet. This technique helps determine any loss of strength or sensation to the area. For less serious injuries, standing or gait activities are convenient methods to assess neurovascular status. If necessary, a more thorough neurovascular exam may be conducted once the client is removed from the activity. Marked loss of strength unilaterally or bilaterally constitutes an emergency because it may indicate loss of neurological abilities; as with other emergencies, it warrants an immediate referral for further diagnostic testing.

Myotomes are tested by manually resisting a muscle or group of muscles that a particular nerve innervates. In essence, it is akin to conducting isolated manual muscle tests. Dermatomes are assessed by running a finger or another object over the client's lower leg, ankle, foot, or toes while the client's eyes are closed. Any difference in sensation between one side and the other should be noted. If no loss or difference in sensation is apparent, the response is considered normal. If a difference in strength or sensation is detected, the response is considered abnormal and referral to a physician should occur as soon as possible.

Next, vascular status should be evaluated by checking the dorsal pedis pulse and performing a capillary refill test. A normal capillary refill test should demonstrate nail bed refill within 2 to 3 seconds (Box 10-1).The nail should appear white when pinched and then refill, turning a pinkish-red color.

Reflexes are evaluated by striking the distal tendon of a specific muscle with a neurological hammer or other solid object. Normal reflexes result in the involuntary contraction of the muscle after the tendon is struck. If the neurovascular exam shows any bilateral loss of strength, sensation, circulation, or reflexes, immediate referral to the emergency room is warranted.

BOX 10-1 Capillary Refill Test

1. The capillary refill test is easily performed by squeezing an unaffected nail bed for several seconds.
2. Upon release, the nail bed should refill or "pink up" within 2 seconds.
3. Capillary refill that takes more than 3 seconds may indicate compromised blood flow and the possible presence of a severe injury.

Referrals and Diagnostic Tests

Because most injuries to the lower leg, ankle, foot, and toes are fractures or soft tissue injuries, referrals are usually preferred so that radiographs (X-rays) can be used to rule out common injuries to this area. Fractures are estimated to be present in approximately 15% of individuals who seek care in an emergency room after having experienced a traumatic injury to the ankle.[14] With rare exceptions, the remainder of injuries that produce ankle pain and swelling are associated with either partial tearing or complete rupture of one or more ligaments. To help with the diagnosis and subsequent management of ankle fractures, the **Ottawa ankle rules** state that if any of the following are present, X-rays should be taken: tenderness to palpation anywhere in the area between the midline and the posterior margin of the most distal 6 cm of either the tibial malleolus or the fibular malleolus (Figure 10-3), tenderness elicited directly over the navicular bone or the base of the fifth metatarsal, or an inability to bear weight on the injured extremity for four steps. A modification of the Ottawa ankle rules limits the area of malleolus palpation to only the midline of the distal 6 cm of the tibial malleolus and the fibular malleolus (Figure 10-4).[15] Because palpation-elicited pain along the posteroinferior margin of either the tibial malleolus or the fibular malleolus could be attributable to ligament damage, this modification is believed to result in fewer false-positive clinical predictions.

MANAGEMENT OF ON-FIELD OR ACUTE LOWER LEG, ANKLE, FOOT, AND TOE INJURIES

Injuries to the lower leg, ankle, foot, and toes that are acute tend to be relatively serious (Figure 10-5). Proper diagnosis helps ensure that the client is able to return to activity in a timely and appropriate manner. Also, proper diagnosis allows the athletic trainer to determine when and how the individual should return, thus lessening the risk that injuries will develop into more debilitating conditions.

Lower Leg Injuries

Acute lower leg injuries include fractures, musculotendinous strains, **compartment syndromes**, and peroneal nerve contusions. The tibia and fibula articulate with the foot and

Ottawa ankle rules a clinical model designed to assist with the diagnosis and management of suspected ankle fractures

compartment syndrome condition characterized by increased pressure generally within the anterior compartment, restricting blood supply to nearby muscles and potentially compromising the nerve

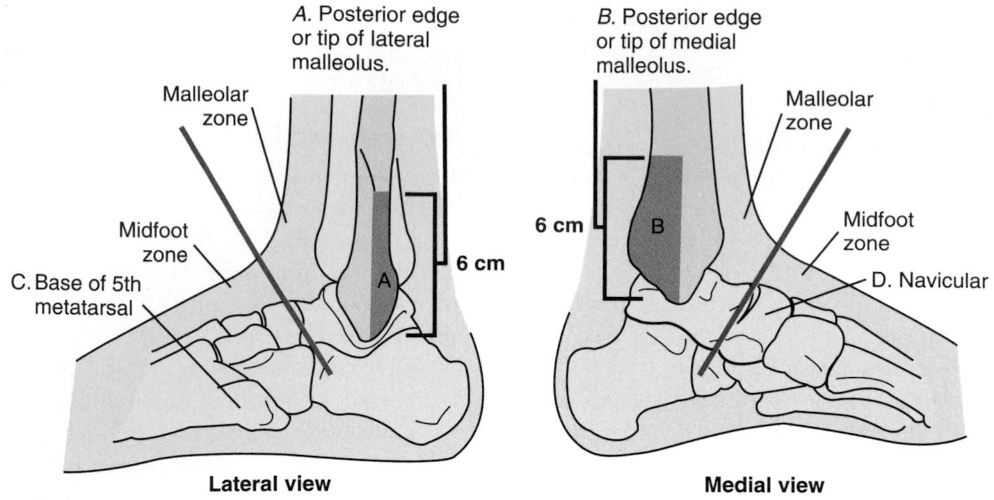

FIGURE 10-3 Areas of palpation to assess the likelihood of fracture according to the original Ottawa ankle rules. (Redrawn from Leddy JJ et al: Prospective evaluation of the Ottawa ankle rules in a university sports medicine center: with a modification to increase specificity for identifying malleolar fractures, *Am J Sports Med* 26: 158–165, 1998.)

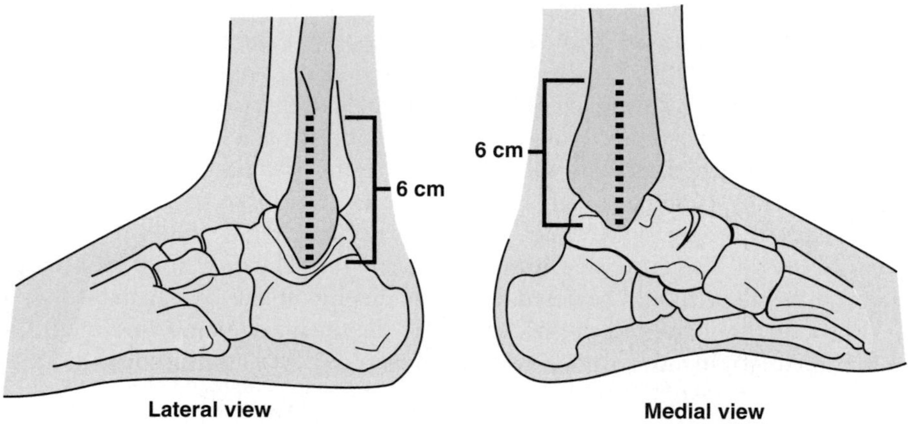

FIGURE 10-4 Areas of palpation for assessment of fracture likelihood according to the "modified" Ottawa ankle rules. (Redrawn from Leddy JJ et al: Prospective evaluation of the Ottawa ankle rules in a university sports medicine center: with a modification to increase specificity for identifying malleolar fractures, *Am J Sports Med* 26: 158–165, 1998.)

form the ankle, and the four compartments of the lower leg house not just muscles and tendons but also arteries, veins, and nerves. With a lack of surrounding girth from soft tissue to protect the lower leg, acute injuries to this area may be debilitating.

Tibial and Fibular Fractures

Fractures in the lower leg are common in certain activities and necessitate activation of an emergency action plan for immediate physician follow-up and diagnostic testing. Fractures (spiral, comminuted, oblique) affect the tibia, whereas avulsion fractures are common at the distal head of the fibula.

Mechanism: Regardless of the type of fracture, direct, forceful contact with an object or another person usually causes the injury. An abrupt ankle sprain, either lateral or medial, is another possible mechanism of injury.

Signs and symptoms:

- Pain
- Deformity
- Swelling
- Ecchymosis
- Loss of motion
- Possible loss of pulse and sensation (depending on the severity of the fracture)

Special tests: Tap or percussion tests can be used. In general, the deformity is so significant and obvious that no special tests are warranted to diagnose a tibial fracture. However, in many cases, fibular fractures are not detected until diagnostic tests are performed.

Immediate management: Immediate management of these fractures includes immobilization with referral to a physician for diagnostic tests. PRICES, as discussed previously, can be applied for immediate relief until transport is initiated.

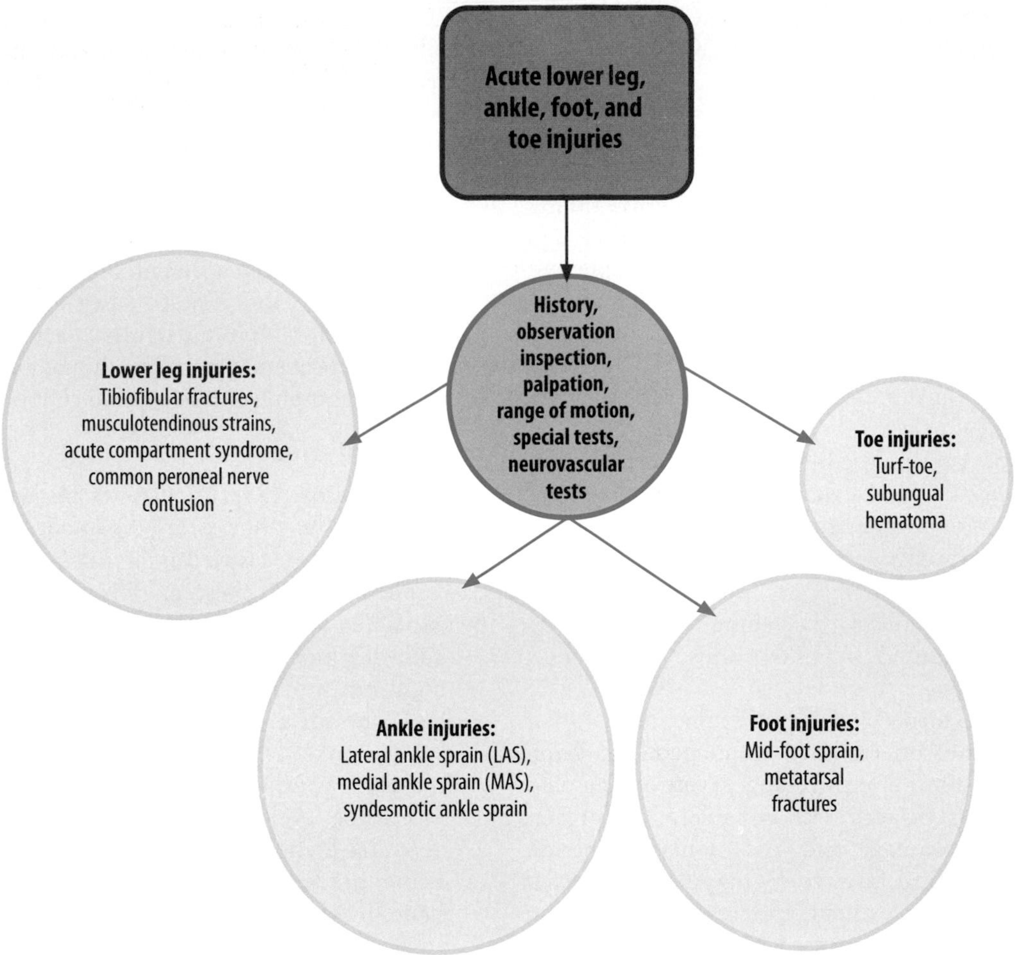

FIGURE 10-5 Concept map overview of acute injuries to the lower leg, ankle, foot, and toes.

> **Points to Ponder**
> Ice, compression, and elevation are commonly used to treat many musculoskeletal injuries. Why would compression not be used in treating anterior compartment syndrome?

Intermediate management: Simple fractures can usually be managed with immobilization, whereas displaced or comminuted fractures usually require surgical stabilization procedures.

Musculotendinous Strains

Muscle strains are common at the musculotendinous junction of the gastrocsoleus complex and within the specific muscle bellies. Tendon disruption is most likely to occur in an area of poor vascularity. Tendon disruption is usually associated with explosive activities, such as jumping, landing, cutting, and abruptly starting and stopping.

Mechanism: The connective tissue surrounding the soft tissue or the muscle itself can be either **attenuated** (stretched) or torn at any point from its origin to insertion. This mechanism can be instigated by either repetitive low-level loads or a single load of great magnitude and force.

Signs and symptoms:

- Pain
- Swelling
- Ecchymosis
- Limited range of motion, especially with dorsiflexion and plantar flexion
- Difficulty with ambulation because of painful or nonexistent gastrocsoleus or anterior tibialis contractions
- Tender to palpation

Special tests: No special tests are applicable.

Immediate management: Immediate management includes PRICES, with an emphasis on cold compression applied circumferentially to the injured area. While performing cold compression, the athletic trainer should place the client's lower leg in a position that promotes venous return; elevating it above the heart usually encourages this response. Heat is contraindicated because it will increase hemorrhage and bleeding, which causes further swelling that could compromise

attenuated tissue elongation or stretching

the involved compartment. If pain is severe, the client may require crutches until his or her gait is sufficiently restored.

Acute Compartment Syndrome

Lower leg acute compartment syndrome usually involves the anterior compartment. Here, the anterior tibialis, extensor digitorum longus, and extensor hallucis longus are housed within a fascia covering that prevents expansion as fluid begins to accumulate. Hemorrhage and edema associated with a severe contusion or fracture may cause intracompartmental pressure to increase to a level that compromises circulation to the muscles and the deep peroneal nerve.

Mechanism: A traumatic blow to the anterior shin or an unusual stress caused by inappropriate training loads may cause anterior compartment syndrome.

Signs and Symptoms:

- Severe, aching pain
- Rapid anterior lower leg swelling
- Foot drop caused by compromise of the deep peroneal nerve

Special tests: No special tests are applicable.

Immediate and intermediate management: Rapid development of anterior leg swelling, severe aching pain, and foot drop must be addressed immediately to prevent permanent tissue damage and loss of nerve function. An emergency **surgical fasciotomy** may be necessary to decompress the compartment and restore circulation. Therefore anterior compartment syndromes should be treated as a medical emergency, with prompt activation of the emergency medical plan.

Intermediate management: After medical intervention, a conservative rehabilitation plan addressing gentle range of motion, strength, tissue extensibility, and functional activities should be designed. The athletic trainer should be careful to prevent undue fluid accumulation in the compartment and attempt to balance the training and rehabilitation activities.

Common Peroneal Nerve Contusions

A direct blow to the lateral aspect of the proximal leg may lead to a contusion of the common peroneal nerve where it lies against the fibula, which in turn can cause a transient foot drop.

Mechanism: Typically, direct trauma resulting from a kick or blow by a hard object to the lateral side of the lower leg can create the nerve contusion.

Signs and symptoms:

- Immediate pain, sometimes radiating down the anterior aspect of the lower leg to the dorsum of the foot
- Ecchymosis
- Possible numbness and paresthesia
- Possible drop foot resulting from muscle weakness

Special tests: No special tests are applicable.

Immediate management: Because there is very little soft tissue between the skin and the common peroneal nerve at this location, cryotherapy application directly to the skin is contraindicated. The potential for cold-induced nerve injury should be considered whenever cryotherapy is applied to the lateral aspect of the leg and knee. Rest, compression, elevation, and protective padding may help alleviate the acute symptoms.

Intermediate management: In most cases, symptoms dissipate within 2 to 3 days of onset. Provided that the client is clear of all symptoms, return to activity can be granted. However, protective padding should be worn for several weeks to continue to lessen the likelihood of repeat injury.

Ankle Injuries

An estimated 75% to 90% of all acute ankle injuries sustained by athletes are ligament sprains.[16–18] Ankle sprains can be classified as lateral, medial, or syndesmotic (Table 10-2). Of these ankle sprains, 75% to 80% are associated with an inversion injury in which the lateral ankle ligaments are damaged.[16,17] However, pathology might not be limited to ankle ligament disruption, and ankle sprains are also sometimes associated with some types of ankle or midfoot fractures.

Ligament injuries at any joint are generally classified on a three-level scale of severity: **grade I** when a ligament is stretched and disruption in its structure is microscopic, **grade II** when a ligament is partially torn, and **grade III** when a ligament is completely torn.

surgical fasciotomy surgery to cut away the fascia to remove tension or pressure
grade I ankle sprain stretching or disruption in the integrity of the ligament
grade II ankle sprain partial tearing of the ligament
grade III ankle sprain complete tearing of the ligament

TABLE 10-2 Ankle Sprain Descriptions and Mechanisms of Injury

SPRAIN	LOCATION OF INJURY	COMMON MECHANISM OF INJURY
Inversion ankle	Lateral ankle	Outside of the forefoot making ground contact while in slight plantar flexion
Eversion ankle	Medial ankle	Internal rotation of the lower leg on a planted foot, or abrupt ankle eversion
Syndesmotic ankle	High ankle, lateral aspect	Traumatic blow to the leg with the foot in external rotation, either planted or lying on the ground

Lateral Ankle Sprain

The term **lateral ankle sprain** (LAS) is widely used to designate a lateral ankle ligament injury that has been produced by an inversion mechanism. Because severe LAS frequently involves some degree of damage to both the ATFL and the CFL, some experts advocate classification on the basis of a single ligament tear or a double ligament tear.[18] Most clinical researchers have classified an isolated rupture of the ATFL as a grade II LAS. Grade III LAS has been defined by many clinical researchers as a complete disruption of both the ATFL and CFL.[19–26] Severe LAS may involve multiple talocrural and subtalar joint structures without injury to the CFL. External clinical indicators that reflect the severity of internal ligament pathology include functional limitations, ligament laxity, localization of tenderness to palpation, amount of swelling, extent of ecchymosis, and restriction of joint motion (Table 10-3).[16,27–33]

Mechanism: The most common mechanism of LAS involves ground contact of the lateral border of the forefoot with the ankle in a plantar flexed position, which often results from landing on an uneven support surface. The lateral edge of the shoe sole acts as a fulcrum, around which inward rotation of the sole is induced by the ground reaction force. The series of joints interlock as they each reach the limit of normal motion, which causes the foot to become a rigid segment that tends to continue its inward rotation around the functional axis of the subtalar joint (Figures 10-6 and 10-7). Until the subtalar joint reaches the limit of its inversion range of motion, the calcaneus and the talus are rotating in opposite directions from each other. The articular surfaces of the talocrural joint transfer subtalar inversion torque to the tibia and fibula in a manner that produces external rotation of the leg. When the subtalar joint becomes locked at the limit of its normal range of inversion, the talus is pulled into an internally rotated position relative to the externally rotating leg, which produces a high tensile load on the ATFL (Figure 10-8).

Because the ATFL almost always tears before the CFL and the CFL is not taut in a plantar flexed position, a two-phase injury mechanism seems likely for combined ATFL and CFL ruptures. The LAS is most commonly associated with a plantar flexed position,

lateral ankle sprain injury to the lateral ankle region induced through inversion forces

TABLE 10-3 Ankle Sprain Classifications

CRITERION	GRADE I	GRADE II	GRADE III	GRADE III+ OR GRADE IV
Swelling	Minimal amount located on anterior margin of fibular malleolus	Diffuse loss of normal contours on lateral aspect of ankle and midfoot	Substantial enlargement of entire ankle and foot, including medial side	Extremely large volume in ankle, foot, and toes; joint motion restricted
Ecchymosis	None or minimal	Primarily limited to lateral aspect of ankle	Broad area on lateral side and some on medial side	Extensive areas on both sides of the ankle and dorsum of the foot
Function*	Minimal or no loss; capable of unilateral vertical hops	Unable to perform ≥ 3 unilateral vertical hops	Incapable of unilateral heel rise	Completely disabled
Gait*	Minimal limp or no limp evident	Capable of unassisted ambulation, but limp clearly evident	Unassisted ambulation extremely difficult or impossible to tolerate	Incapable of unassisted ambulation
Tenderness	Mild to moderate over ATFL	Moderate to intense over ATFL; possible over LTCL, CFL, or DTTL	Intense over ATFL and at least one other ligament: LTCL, CFL, or DTTL	Diffuse and intense over multiple ligaments
Anterior drawer	No laxity apparent; no discomfort elicited	No laxity or mild laxity apparent; pain elicited in response to manual stress	Laxity and sulcus sign apparent (unless pain and reflex splinting interfere)	Substantial laxity evident (pain and reflex splinting likely to preclude testing)
Click test or talar tilt	Negative	Negative or possibly mildly positive	Possibly positive, depending on degree of CFL injury	Positive (hemarthrosis may interfere with motion, preventing click)
Pathology	Microscopic tears within ATFL; other ligaments unaffected	Partial ATFL tear; possible partial tear of LTCL, CFL, or DTTL	Rupture of ATFL with some damage to LTCL, CFL, DTTL, or ITCL	Rupture of ATFL + CFL; with probable damage to LTCL, DTTL, or ITCL

*Function and gait assessed without ankle support by brace or tape.

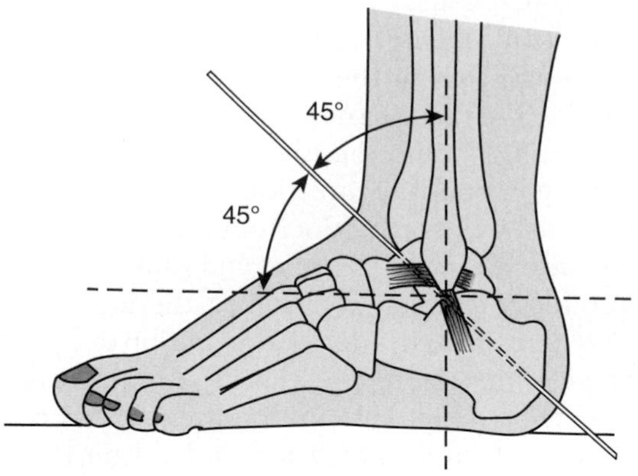

FIGURE 10-6 Approximate orientation of the functional axis of the subtalar joint in the sagittal plane. (Redrawn from Wilkerson GB: Biomechanical and neuromuscular effects of ankle taping and bracing, *J Athl Train* 37:439 [Fig. 1], 2002.)

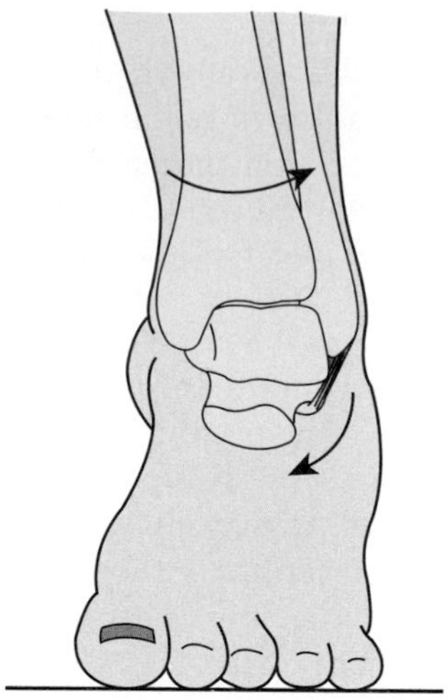

FIGURE 10-8 Development of tension within the ATFL as the leg externally rotates in relation to the foot, which resists subluxation of the anterolateral portion of the talus. (Redrawn from Wilkerson GB: Biomechanical and neuromuscular effects of ankle taping and bracing, *J Athl Train* 37:439 [Fig. 2], 2002.)

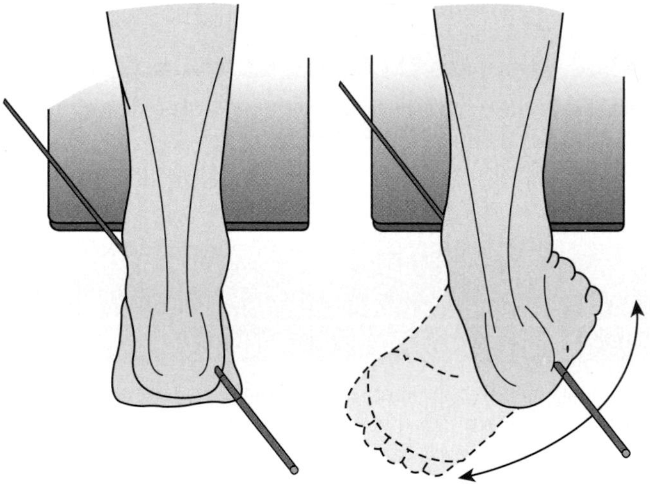

FIGURE 10-7 Approximate orientation of the functional axis of the subtalar joint in the frontal plane. (Redrawn from Hertel J: Functional anatomy, pathomechanics, and pathophysiology of lateral ankle instability, *J Athl Train* 37:364–375, 2002.)

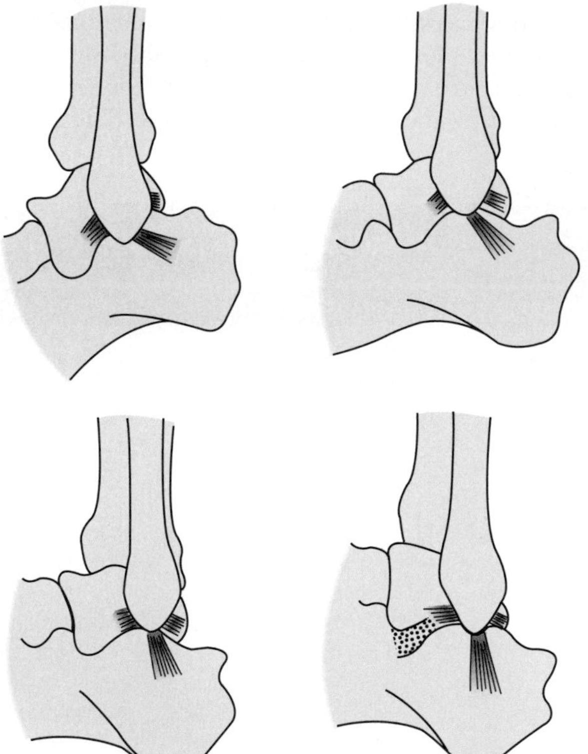

FIGURE 10-9 Change in the orientation of the ATFL and CFL with change in position of the talocrural joint. (Redrawn from Robichon J et al: Functional anatomy of the ankle joint and its relationship to ankle injuries, *Can J Surg* 15:147 [Fig. 4, *A-D*], 1972.)

whereas CFL strain is greatest in a dorsiflexed position[34,35] (Figure 10-9). The primary cause of ATFL disruption is believed to be internal rotation of the talus, induced by subtalar inversion in a plantar flexed talocrural position, which does not produce any strain in the CFL. Immediately following rupture of the ATFL in a plantar flexed position, a sudden hip and knee flexion postural reaction rapidly moves the talocrural joint into a dorsiflexed position, which may induce strain in the CFL (Figure 10-10).[20,36–38] An isolated ATFL rupture may be the result of a single-phase injury mechanism that does not involve talar tilt. Because the lateral talocalcaneal ligament (LTCL) clearly plays a role in lateral ankle stability, and its fibers sometimes blend with those of the ATFL and CFL, any injury mechanism that damages the CFL probably damages the LTCL.[39] The posterior talofibular ligament (PTFL) is the strongest and least vulnerable component of the lateral ankle ligament complex and is subjected to tensile loading only in extreme dorsiflexion.[4,39]

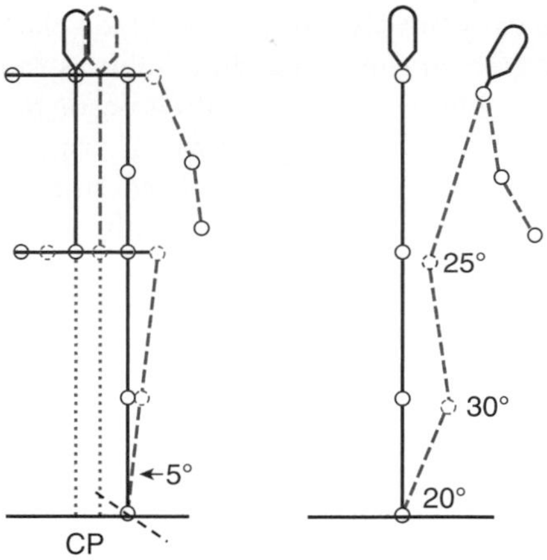

FIGURE 10-10 Postural reaction to sudden inversion of 30 degrees: anterior view and lateral view (values represent median degrees of joint displacement). (Redrawn from Konradsen L, Ravn JB: Ankle instability caused by prolonged peroneal reaction time, *Acta Orthop Scand* 6: 389 [Fig. 1], 1990. Copyright Taylor & Francis Ltd. [www.informaworld.com].)

Signs and symptoms:

- Swelling, possibly distending the joint capsule
- Immediate localized point tenderness over involved structures
- Lateral ankle pain
- Ecchymosis
- Ligament laxity

Special tests: The anterior drawer test and the talar tilt test can be performed bilaterally and used to diagnose an LAS. The combined effects of pain and swelling on test responses may vary substantially from one day to the next. If ecchymosis is present and palpation of the ATFL elicits pain, the estimated likelihood of ATFL rupture is 90%.[2] An important consideration when evaluating an inversion ankle injury in a skeletally immature athlete is the possibility that lateral ankle ligament tension may have imposed a traction force on the fibular growth plate.[40] Any degree of disruption in the growth plate is diagnosed as a Salter-Harris Type I fracture.

Immediate management: Treatment of an acute LAS is typically guided by a categorization of its severity based on the clinical signs and symptoms found during the evaluation.[41] The primary focus of acute management of LAS is control of swelling.[42–46] PRICES can help to effectively control immediate post-injury pain and swelling as well as quickly restore functional capabilities. Protection against further damage is critical. Individuals who have previously sustained LAS are about five times more likely to be injured than those who do not have such a history.[47]

The single most effective therapeutic procedure for facilitation of optimal ATFL healing and rapid restoration of normal ankle function is probably the use of a U-shaped pad or brace incorporating the pad to provide focal compression on the periphery of the fibular malleolus (Figures 10-11 and 10-12).[33,44,46] Effective control of pain and swelling during the acute and subacute phases, combined with protection of ligaments from excessive loading, can merge the treatment phases and dramatically accelerate restoration of functional capabilities.[29,33,46,48] Because dorsiflexion approximates the torn ends of the ATFL, maintenance of a dorsiflexed position enhances the quality of ligament healing during the early stage of the process.[43,49]

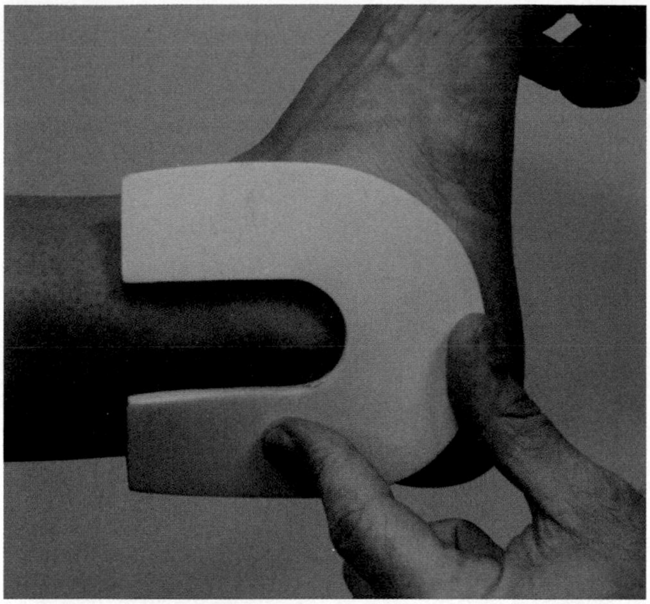

FIGURE 10-11 U-pad application to soft tissues on the periphery of the fibular malleolus.

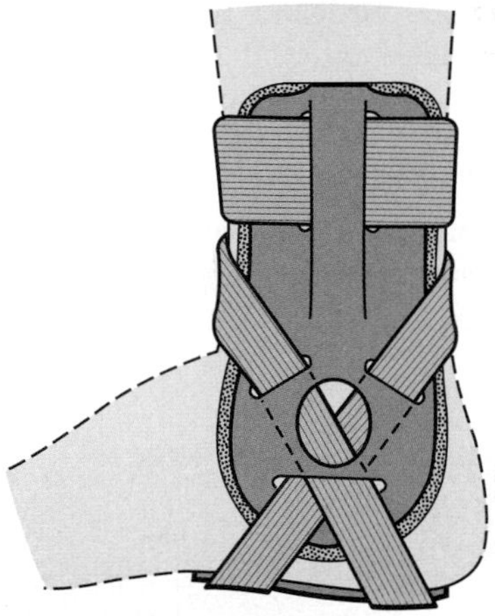

FIGURE 10-12 Stirrup-type ankle brace that incorporates a U-pad, or horseshoe pad, and molded drainage channel for application of adjustable focal compression.

Intermediate management: Weight bearing should be encouraged as soon as possible to the greatest extent that is tolerable. A heel-to-toe contact walk-through crutch gait simultaneously facilitates maintenance of dorsiflexion, promotes lymphatic drainage of ankle and foot swelling, and decreases perception of pain.[50] The client can move on to full weight bearing after demonstrating the ability to walk with a symmetrical gait. The presence of a brace on the injured ankle often provides a sense of security that accelerates restoration of a normal gait pattern. If accelerated functional progression is feasible, rehabilitative exercises for restoration of optimal strength, fatigue-resistance, and neuromuscular control should be incorporated.

Restriction of anterior translation and internal rotary displacement of the talus during ATFL healing is believed to be an extremely important factor for prevention of subsequent ankle disability, which no functional ankle brace has been shown to provide.[51]

However, an ankle taping procedure referred to as the **subtalar sling** has been shown to effectively provide such restriction.[52,53] A lateral subtalar sling consists of one or more strips of high-strength semi-elastic tape that spans all of the joints between the forefoot and leg; it is anchored on the plantar aspect of the forefoot, wrapped around the lateral border of the foot, and wrapped around the leg above the malleoli (Figure 10-13). External rotation of the leg increases tension within the tape fibers that form the lateral subtalar sling, which tends to lift the lateral border of the foot, thereby reversing the normal effect of external leg rotation on the forefoot and protecting the ATFL from tensile loading.[54]

Medial Ankle Sprain

Isolated medial ligament injuries, or **medial ankle sprains** (MASs), represent only about 5% of all ankle sprains.[16,17] Because medial ankle ligament injury and syndesmotic injury typically involve similar joint displacements of varying degree, and because these injuries to structures on opposite sides of the ankle often occur together, the evaluation is the same as that for a suspected medial ankle sprain or a suspected syndesmotic sprain.[49] Deltoid ligament injury can occur without injury to the syndesmosis and vice versa.

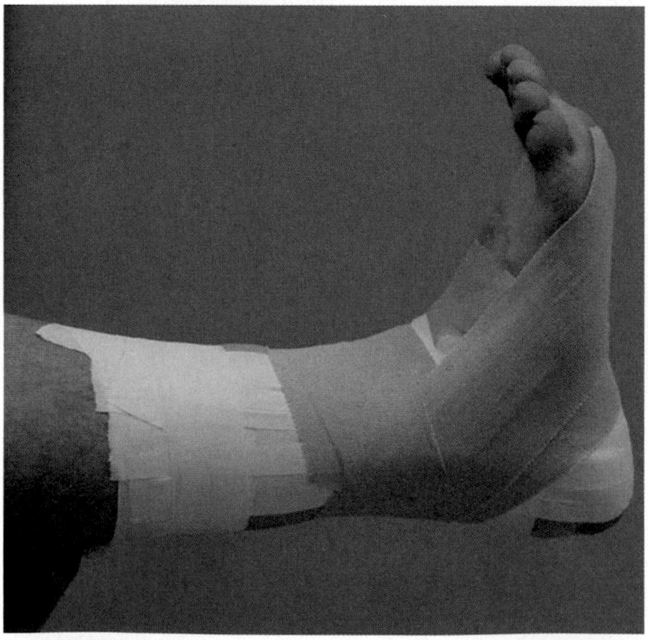

FIGURE 10-13 Subtalar stabilization ankle taping procedure: lateral subtalar sling. (From Wilkerson GB et al: Effects of the subtalar sling ankle taping technique on combined talocrural-subtalar joint motions, *Foot Ankle Int* 26:241 [Fig. 2, *A*], 2005)

Mechanism: Sprains affecting the inferior tibiofibular syndesmosis are primarily due to a mechanism involving forceful internal rotation of the leg on a fixed foot (i.e., relative external rotation of the foot), which is usually associated with eversion of the ankle that may produce a complete tear of the deltoid ligament.[49] An eversion injury mechanism produces simultaneous medial distraction and lateral compression of joint articular surfaces.

Signs and symptoms:

- Prolonged post-injury pain
- Prolonged recovery of full functional abilities
- Medial ankle pain
- Localized point tenderness over involved structures
- Ecchymosis
- Ligament laxity

Special tests: The talar tilt test may be performed bilaterally and used to diagnose MAS. As with the LAS, combined effects of pain and swelling on test responses may vary substantially from one day to the next. Due to this variability, repeated assessments should be performed to obtain an accurate ongoing diagnosis of the extent of healing.

Kleiger Test: A Kleiger test is used to determine the extent of medial deltoid injury (Figure 10-14). With the client in a seated position, the athletic trainer holds the client's lower leg down with one hand while the other hand holds the client's foot medially and rotates it laterally. Pain over the deltoid ligament suggests injury to this structure.

Immediate management: PRICES is used to manage the MAS just as it is the LAS. Complete avoidance of weight bearing for the first 4 days post-injury, followed by progressive partial weight bearing and restoration of full weight bearing beyond 6 days post-injury, is recommended.[55] Alternatively, some experts advise progressive pain-free weight-bearing crutch ambulation with up to 50% of body weight applied to the injured extremity during the acute phase of treatment. Orthotics or inserts may be used. The use of a removable lower extremity walker-boot may decrease stress during healing. Although fracture of the navicular is rare, a radiograph of the foot should be obtained if palpation elicits tenderness.

subtalar sling ankle taping procedure that helps restrict ankle movement
medial ankle sprain injury to the medial ankle region induced through eversion forces

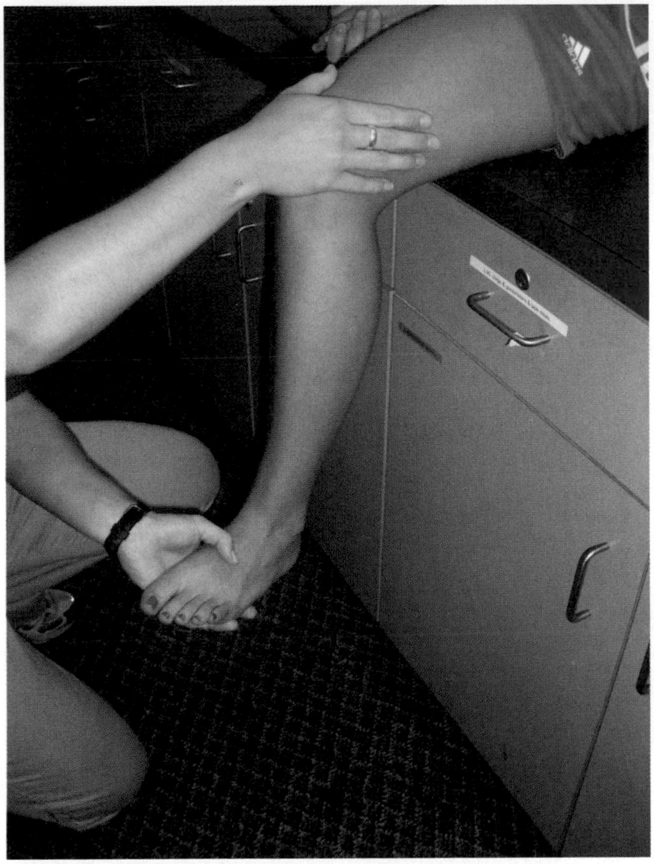

FIGURE 10-14 Performance of the standard Kleiger test for assessment of medial ankle sprain.

Intermediate management: Rehabilitative exercises are the same as those used for LAS. Lack of tolerance for weight-bearing activities with the MAS may require greater reliance on open-chain exercises until the client progresses to a later phase of the rehabilitation program. Return to activity may be facilitated by ankle taping that restricts dorsiflexion[56] or ankle taping that incorporates a medial subtalar sling.[54] Gradual restoration of a full weight-bearing walking gait during the period of 4 to 14 days post-injury may follow.[57]

Syndesmotic Ankle Sprain

Approximately 10% to 15% of all ankle sprains involve the syndesmosis, with the percentage being higher among athletes who participate in activities that may subject the ankle to an extremely high level of force.[16,17] **Syndesmotic ankle sprains,** or high ankle sprains, may occur at a rate as high as 30% for collision sports such as football and as low as 5% for noncontact sports.[16] Among athletes diagnosed with syndesmotic sprain, approximately 40% have been reported to have an associated medial ligament injury.[55] Because the severity of LAS is related to swelling, the severity of ligament pathology associated with syndesmotic injuries may be underestimated. Keep in mind that relatively severe syndesmotic injury is often accompanied by a minimal amount of visible swelling.[16,49,56–58]

Mechanism: The syndesmotic sprain almost always involves a direct blow to the lateral aspect of the leg with the foot planted in external rotation or a direct blow to the leg of an athlete lying on the ground with the foot in an externally rotated position[58] (Figure 10-15). The exact mechanism of injury varies, but some degree of dorsiflexion and eversion of the ankle is generally associated with the traumatic event.[56,57]

syndesmotic ankle sprain injury to the high, lateral ankle region induced through direct contact and external rotation of the foot

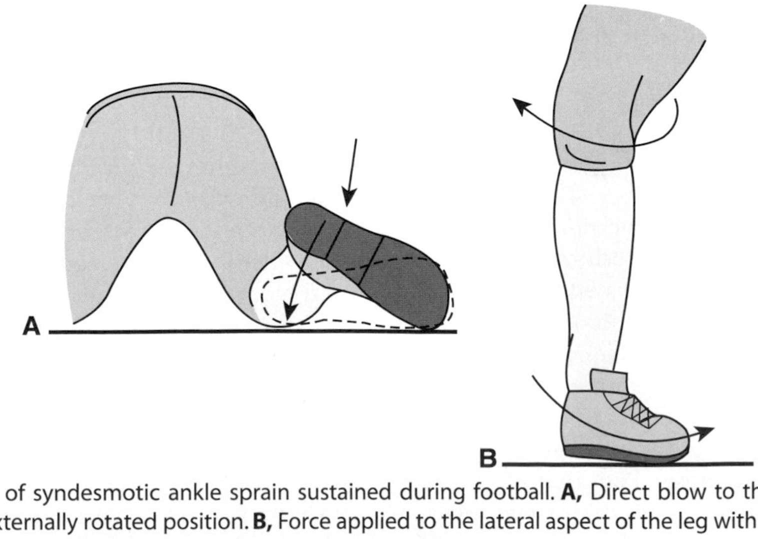

FIGURE 10-15 Mechanisms of syndesmotic ankle sprain sustained during football. **A,** Direct blow to the leg of a player lying on the ground with the foot in an externally rotated position. **B,** Force applied to the lateral aspect of the leg with the foot fixed to the ground in external rotation. (Redrawn from Boytim MJ, Fischer DA, Neumann L: Syndesmotic ankle sprains, *Am J Sports Med* 19: 297 [Fig. 5], 1991.)

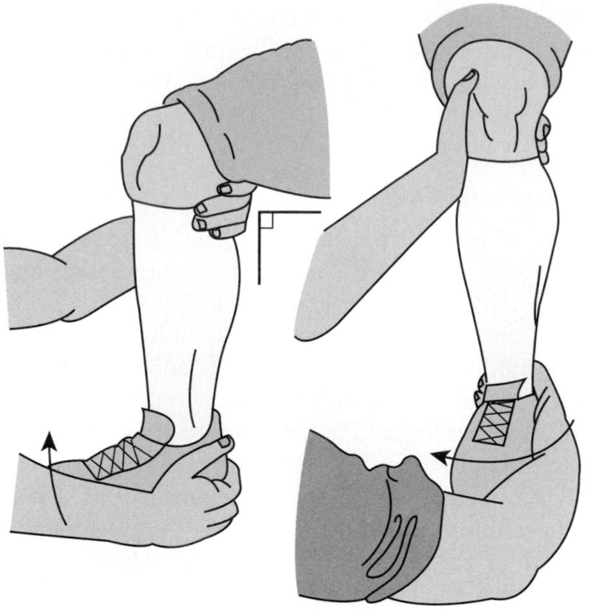

FIGURE 10-16 Performance of the external rotation (Kleiger) test for assessment of syndesmotic injury. (Redrawn from Boytim MJ, Fischer DA, Neumann L: Syndesmotic ankle sprains, *Am J Sports Med* 19: 295 [Fig. 1], 1991.)

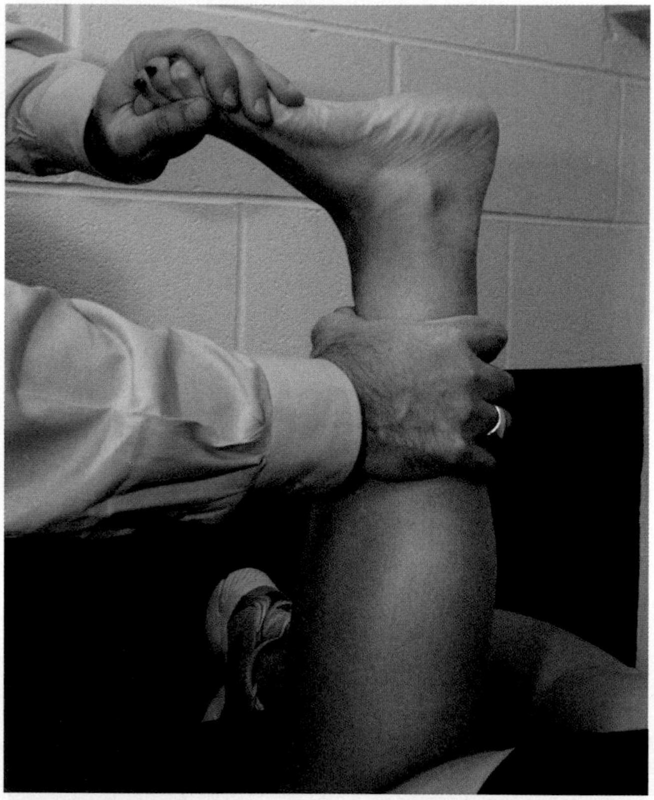

FIGURE 10-17 Performance of the external rotation test for assessment of syndesmotic injury with the patient lying prone on a table.

Signs and symptoms:
- Minimal lateral ankle swelling
- Possible medial ankle swelling
- Pain in the anterolateral lower leg
- Point tenderness over the deltoid ligament with less severe injury
- Point tenderness over the anterior syndesmotic (tibiofibular) ligament (ASL), the interosseus membrane, the posterior syndesmotic (tibiofibular) ligament (PSL) , and the posterior talofibular ligament (PTFL) with more severe injuries
- Point tenderness over the superior tibiofibular syndesmosis, adjacent to the knee joint, with a relatively severe injury
- Discomfort with active range of motion (AROM) dorsiflexion
- Possible loss of ankle function

Special tests:

Kleiger test: The external rotation (Kleiger) test is performed with the client seated on a table with the knee at 90 degrees of flexion and the talocrural joint in neutral position[58] (Figure 10-16). Performance of the external rotation test with the patient lying prone on a table may increase the sensitivity of the test by providing the athletic trainer with a greater mechanical advantage for manual production of external rotation torque on the client's foot (Figure 10-17). The test is considered positive when forced passive external rotation of the foot elicits pain at the syndesmosis. Pain that is elicited proximal to the syndesmosis in the interosseus membrane is interpreted as evidence of a more severe injury than pain that is limited to the syndesmosis. This test appears to be superior to the squeeze test for identification of syndesmotic injury and prediction of disability duration.[6,55]

Squeeze test: The first special test reported in the literature for evaluation of syndesmotic injury was the squeeze test. This test involves manual compression of the fibula toward the tibia at the midpoint of the calf (Figure 10-18). The squeeze test is considered positive when distal lower leg pain is elicited.

Immediate and intermediate management: Management of syndesmotic sprains is similar to that of LAS and MAS. It should be noted, however, that syndesmotic sprains require a period of immobilization. Immobilization for 6 weeks has been recommended for syndesmotic injuries that demonstrate more than 1 mm of ankle mortise widening on a stress radiograph.[59] Therefore the total recovery time tends to be lengthened. Syndesmotic sprains without this complication do not appear to cause chronic dysfunction and are not associated with long-term susceptibility to recurrent injury.[60]

Foot Injuries

In light of the complexity of the anatomical structure of the foot and the intimate relationship of the foot to human movement, the opportunity for injury to this

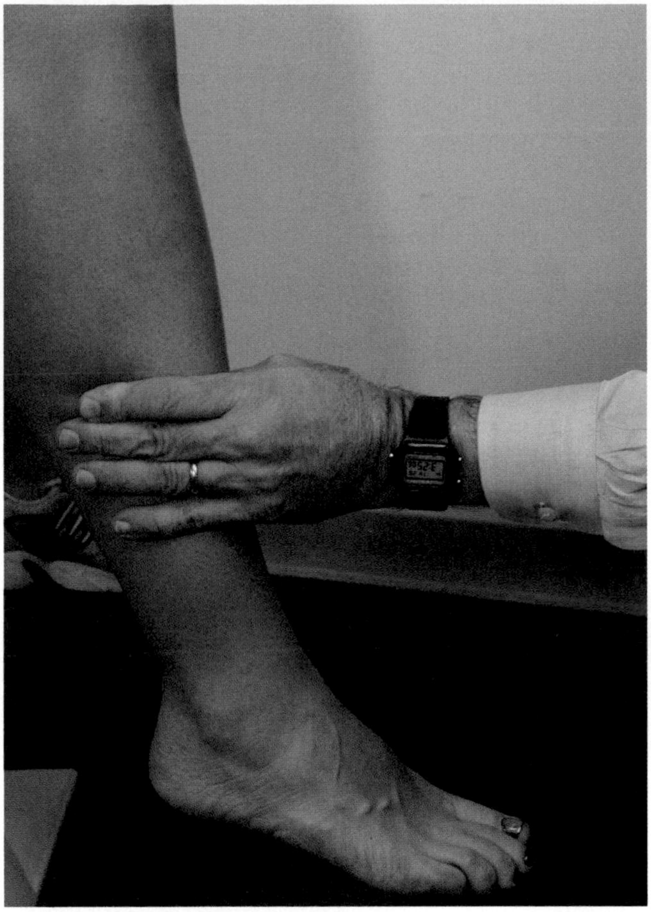

FIGURE 10-18 Performance of the squeeze test for assessment of syndesmotic injury.

area is great. Any miscue in landing, jumping, gait, or change of direction, or even a different playing surface, has the potential to induce foot injury. External forces can cause fracture, sprain, contusion, or a combination of injuries to the various anatomical structures of the foot. Common types of acute injuries experienced by active individuals include midfoot sprain and metatarsal fractures.

Midfoot Sprain

The set of articulations between the five metatarsal bases and the adjacent tarsal bones are sometimes collectively referred to as *Lisfranc's joint.* The same term is also used as a specific designation for the second tarsometatarsal joint.[40]

Mechanism: Axial loading of the metatarsals with the foot in a plantar flexed position may disrupt the ligament between the medial cuneiform and second metatarsal. This results in **diastasis** of the first and second metatarsal bases with weight bearing. This ligament disruption is widely referred to as a *Lisfranc's sprain,* or *midfoot sprain.* Concomitant fracture may occur, producing a fracture dislocation of the midfoot.

Signs and symptoms:
- Localized pain and tenderness to palpation
- Localized swelling
- Inability to bear weight
- Prolonged pain

Special tests: Tap and percussion tests may be attempted to rule out possible midfoot fractures.

Immediate and intermediate management: Referral to a physician for diagnostic testing allows for a more systematic return to functional activity. Use of orthotics, taping procedures, and heel lifts may help decrease the stressful forces transmitted through the injured area. Severe diastasis may require surgical intervention to reduce or stabilize the excessive movement noted with weight bearing.

Metatarsal Fracture

An acute fracture of the proximal portion of the shaft of the fifth metatarsal is commonly referred to as a *Jones' fracture,* although any metatarsal may be acutely fractured.

Mechanism: Jones' fractures typically result from a forceful ground impact. Often, the acute fracture is preceded by a chronic stress reaction to excessive loading that is associated with microfractures, possibly the consequence of mistakes in training. High external force may cause fracture, but most metatarsal fractures result from chronic overuse situations.

Signs and symptoms:
- Localized pain
- Immediate swelling
- Possible difficulty bearing weight and ambulating

Special tests: Tap and percussion tests may be used to diagnose metatarsal fractures.

Immediate and intermediate management: Nonunion is often a problem with Jones' fracture; it may require surgical internal fixation and a bone graft.[49] If surgery is not warranted, ambulation with crutches starting with partial weight bearing and progressing to full weight bearing as soon as possible is indicated. Full weight bearing should be attempted only if pain is eliminated. Functional return to activity may begin as soon as the client can tolerate the rehabilitation program.

Toe Injuries

Injuries to the toes are common among active people. Jumping, kicking, and stopping and starting mechanics can cause various injuries to the toes, as can dropping heavy objects on them.

diastasis a disunion between two adjoining bones or a complete disarticulation of a nonmobile joint

Turf-Toe

The term **turf toe** came about because of the prevalence of first metatarsophalangeal (MTP) joint sprains among football players who play on artificial turf.[49] Hyperdorsiflexion of the first MTP joint can damage the cartilaginous plantar plate that spans the joint and to which the flexor hallucis brevis muscle and the sesamoid ligaments attach.

Mechanism: Excessive dorsiflexion of the great toe results in turf toe. It can result from a single incident or repetitive microtrauma, most often caused by shoes that are either too small in the toe box or too flexible for the ground surface.

Signs and symptoms:

- Intense localized pain
- Localized swelling
- Increased pain with functional activities, especially running and jumping
- Difficulty bearing weight and ambulating

Special tests: No special tests are applicable.

Immediate and intermediate management: PRICES can be used to manage pain and swelling. Persistence of discomfort during activity and recurrent injury is not uncommon. Beyond standard treatments for acute joint sprain symptoms, extreme dorsiflexion should be restricted by use of either tape or a stiff inner sole within the athletic shoe.

Subungual Hematoma

Hemorrhage beneath the toenail, or subungual hematoma, looks more debilitating than it actually is. In most cases, affected persons can continue to participate in their daily activities without limitations.

Mechanism: A compressive force concentrated on the toenail can cause a painful high-pressure hematoma to develop beneath the nail. Hematomas may result from a heavy object being dropped on the toe or an opponent stepping on it.

Signs and symptoms:

- Ecchymosis
- Possible localized discomfort

Special tests: No special tests are applicable.

Immediate and intermediate management: The condition can be effectively managed by drilling a hole in the nail, which frees the blood from beneath it. Maintain a sterile environment by keeping the nail bed clean and covered with a bandage dressing.

Box 10-2 summarizes acute injuries to the lower leg, ankle, foot, and toe and the appropriate special tests used to help diagnose each condition.

Prevention of Acute Injuries

Because most acute injuries to the lower leg, ankle, foot, and toes are traumatic in origin, prevention is multifaceted. Equipment, uniforms, playing surfaces, technique, and conditioning all play major roles. Prevention is challenging because it requires the cooperation of other parties to refrain from causing injury (e.g., by kicking another player's lower leg), stepping on his or her toes, dropping a weight. Even reliance on

turf toe sprain of the first metatarsophalangeal joint; common in football athletes playing on artificial turf

BOX 10-2 Acute Lower Leg, Ankle, Foot, and Toe Injuries and Appropriate Special Tests

Lower Leg Injuries
- Tibial and fibular fractures
  - Tap or percussion tests
- Musculotendinous strains
  - No appropriate special tests
- Acute compartment syndrome
  - No appropriate special tests
- Common peroneal nerve contusions
  - No appropriate special tests

Ankle Injuries
- Lateral ankle sprains
  - Anterior drawer test
  - Talar tilt test
- Medial ankle sprains
  - Talar tilt test
  - Kleiger's test
- Syndesmotic ankle sprain
  - Kleiger's test
  - Squeeze test

Foot Injuries
- Midfoot sprains
  - Tap and percussion tests
- Metatarsal fractures
  - Tap and percussion tests

Toe Injuries
- Turf toe
  - No appropriate special tests
- Subungual hematomas
  - No appropriate special tests

the physical environment presents challenges; holes in the field, slippery court surfaces, and tree roots on the running path all have the potential for causing injury. By prescribing conditioning and warm-up activities that include all the fitness components—such as power, speed, agility, reaction time, muscular strength, endurance, and flexibility—the athletic trainer can reduce the possibility of injury. Exercises that incorporate neuromuscular control, balance, and proprioception best prepare the lower leg, ankle, foot, and toes to withstand excessive forces. The more fit the individual is, the less likely he or she is to sustain an injury while participating in an activity.

MANAGEMENT OF CHRONIC AND OVERUSE LOWER LEG, ANKLE, FOOT, AND TOE INJURIES

Chronic and overuse injuries to the lower leg, ankle, foot, and toes involve repetitive microtrauma (Figure 10-19), which results from the demands that are placed on these structures in most activities. The more an individual participates, both in frequency and in intensity, the greater the stresses that are placed on these body parts and the greater the likelihood of subsequent injury.

Lower Leg Injuries

Chronic or overuse injuries to the lower leg are relatively common. The demands placed on this part of the body during activity are intense. Typically, repetitive trauma prompts the onset of injury, as do gross training errors and poor mechanics.

Achilles Tenosynovitis, Tendinosis, and Tendinitis

The term *tenosynovitis* designates an inflammatory reaction in a tendon that is surrounded by a synovial sheath. *Tendinosis* is the progressive structural degeneration of a tendon, which may ultimately weaken the tendon to the point that sudden loading produces a tendon rupture. *Tendinitis* refers to a combination of peritendinitis and tendinosis. Because the Achilles tendon is not surrounded by a synovial sheath but is covered by a layer of highly vascularized tissue (called a *paratenon*), it is susceptible to peritendinitis, or inflammation of the paratenon.

Mechanism: Increased training volume or intensity may overload musculotendinous units, resulting in microscopic structural damage. A resulting inflammatory reaction follows in the outermost layer of tissue that surrounds the tendon.

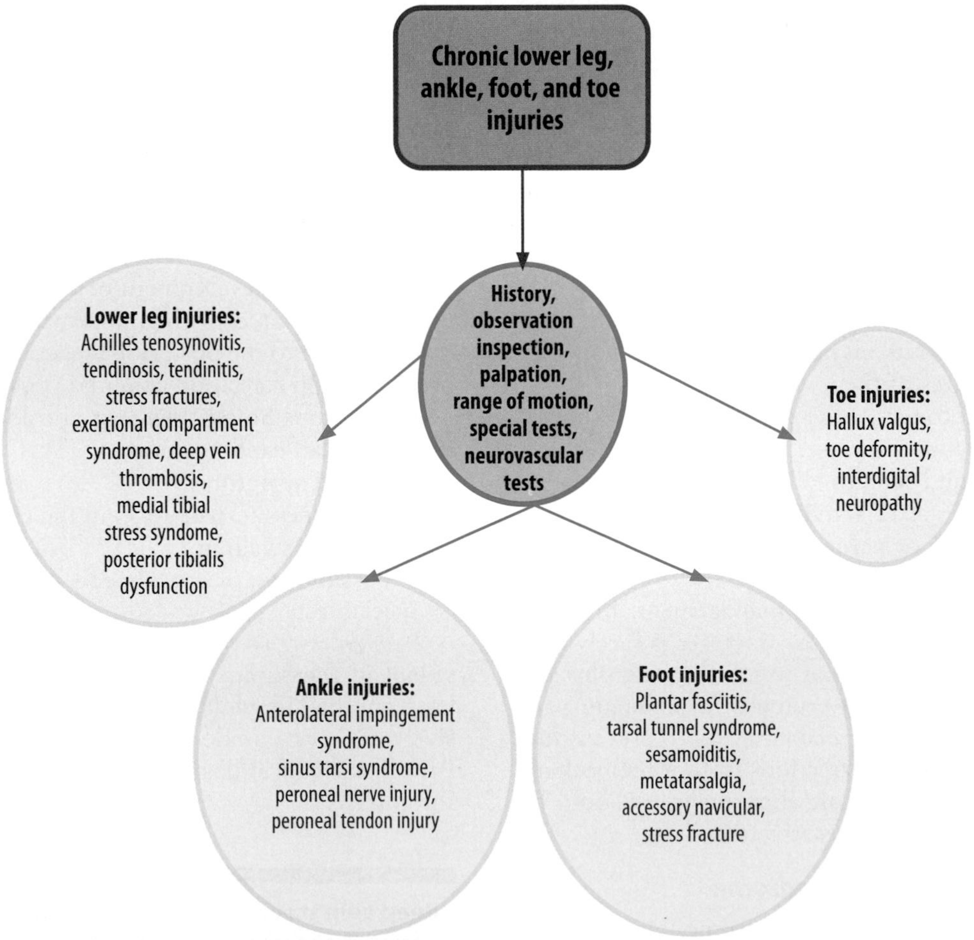

FIGURE 10-19 Concept map overview of chronic injuries to the lower leg, ankle, foot, and toes.

Signs and symptoms:
- Pain
- Tendon stiffness
- Possible decreased plantar flexion
- Possible decreased flexibility in the gastrocnemius and soleus muscles
- Increased pain with hill running
- Difficulty standing on toes and walking or running

Special tests: No special tests are applicable.

Immediate management: PRICES may be used for early management. As the injury progresses, reducing stress to the tendon is the key to recovery and return to activity.

Intermediate management: A comprehensive rehabilitation program focusing on strength, flexibility, and proper mechanics helps alleviate further complications. The athletic trainer should be careful not to overload the tendon by recommending exercise in excess of the tendon's current capabilities. This mistake may exacerbate the injury and delay return to activity. Ultrasound and manual therapy techniques may be employed to promote healing.

Tibial and Fibular Stress Fractures

Long-distance runners and triathletes are the athletes who most commonly report stress fractures. Athletes who are out of training or not properly conditioned succumb to stress fractures caused by attempting loads that are greater than what they can handle. Individuals with structural defects of the foot or imperfections in their gait mechanics are particularly susceptible to lower leg stress fractures. A stress fracture on the anterior aspect of the tibia presents the greatest risk for development of a complete fracture and is associated with the greatest incidence of nonunion.

Mechanism: Errors in training (i.e., too much too soon, unfamiliar terrain, inappropriate shoes) frequently cause stress fractures of the lower leg.

Signs and symptoms:
- Immediate pain is diffuse.
- Ongoing pain becomes localized.
- Pain increases after activity.

Special tests: Tap or percussion tests may be used to diagnose lower leg stress fractures.

Immediate and intermediate management: Immobilization of tibia and fibula stress fractures is rarely necessary, but initial restriction of weight-bearing physical activity is essential. Use of crutches to eliminate pain with weight bearing can be encouraged. To prevent further or recurrent injury, corrections to foot biomechanics, technique issues, and gait abnormalities should be addressed before the client returns to activity.

Exertional Compartment Syndrome

As with acute compartment syndrome, the anterior compartment is most often involved with exertional compartment syndrome. The deep posterior compartment may become compromised as well. The condition is often bilateral and may be associated with the appearance of a fascia herniation on the anterolateral aspect of the lower one third of the leg while intracompartmental pressure is elevated.

Mechanism: An increase in the tissue fluid pressure within the compartment is normal with activity. However, a repetitive increase that does not abate over time causes the syndrome to occur. Either the pressure increases too much with exercise or remains too high after exercise.

Signs and symptoms:
- Pressure
- Cramping
- Pain during activity; onset becoming predictable over time
- Achy sensation
- Ischemia
- Prompt subsidence of symptoms after activity stops

Special tests: No special tests are applicable.

Immediate and intermediate management: PRICES often helps alleviate symptoms. If symptoms continue, surgical intervention to release the pressure and prevent neurological damage may be warranted.

Deep Vein Thrombosis

Aching pain on the posterior aspect of the leg should always be carefully evaluated to rule out formation of a life-threatening blood clot known as **deep vein thrombosis**. Clots can move through the vascular system to a location where they lodge and occlude circulation to a vital organ. Immediate medical referral is mandatory for these individuals.

Mechanism: Development of a clot in a deep leg vein may be associated with a recent surgical procedure, direct trauma to the posterior aspect of the leg, a genetic predisposition for blood coagulation, or interruption of normal venous blood flow (e.g., prolonged sitting with the knee in a flexed position).

Signs and symptoms:
- Tenderness to palpation in the calf complex
- Possible swelling
- Possible loss of dorsal pedis pulse

Special tests:

Homan test: To perform **Homan's test**, place the individual in the supine position on a plinth. Elevate the leg from the hip while the knee is in full extension. Passively move the ankle into dorsiflexion (Figure 10-20). Pain in the calf indicates a positive result for deep vein thrombosis.

---

deep vein thrombosis blood clot in a major vein, often in the leg; life-threatening condition

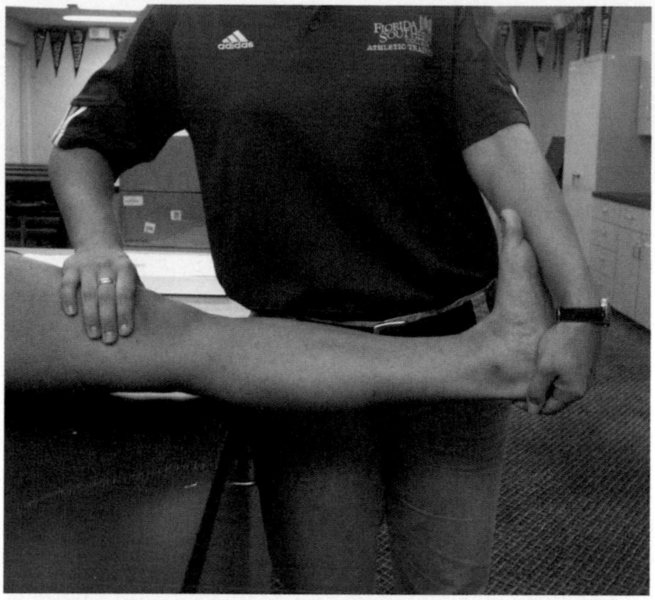

FIGURE 10-20 Performance of Homan test for assessment of deep vein thrombosis.

Immediate and intermediate management: Referral to a physician, with subsequent diagnostic testing, should ensue as soon as a deep vein thrombosis is suspected.

Medial Tibial Stress Syndrome

Formerly known as shin splints, medial tibial stress syndrome (MTSS) is more defined in scope. MTSS is either a tibial stress fracture or a soft tissue overuse syndrome.

Mechanism: Microscopic tears in the muscle attachment site on the posteromedial aspect of the lower one third of the tibia may produce a painful inflammatory response. MTSS is typically due to repetitive microtrauma resulting from inappropriate training techniques, improper equipment, soft tissue tightness, and muscle weakness or imbalances.

Signs and symptoms:

- Pain (grade I: after activity; grade II: during and after activity without altering participation; grade III: before, during, and after and altering participation; grade IV: making participation impossible)
- Possible loss of function
- Possible loss of motion

Special tests: No special tests are applicable.

Immediate management: The client should be referred immediately to a physician for further diagnostic testing. The need to rule out stress fractures is paramount. PRICES may be performed to promote healing in the acute phase.

Intermediate management: As with other chronic and overuse lower leg injuries, the athletic trainer should attempt to determine the root cause of MTSS. Mechanics with activity, technique, equipment, training and conditioning programs, and soft tissue flexibility should all be assessed. The appropriate corrections should be made so that the injury does not worsen or recur.

Posterior Tibialis Dysfunction

The posterior tibialis (PT) muscle plays a critical role in maintaining dynamic stability of the medial longitudinal arch[61] (Figure 10-21). The PT contracts eccentrically to control the rate of pronation during the transition from heel strike to the midstance phase of gait. It also contracts concentrically to produce supination during the transition from midstance to push off.[62]

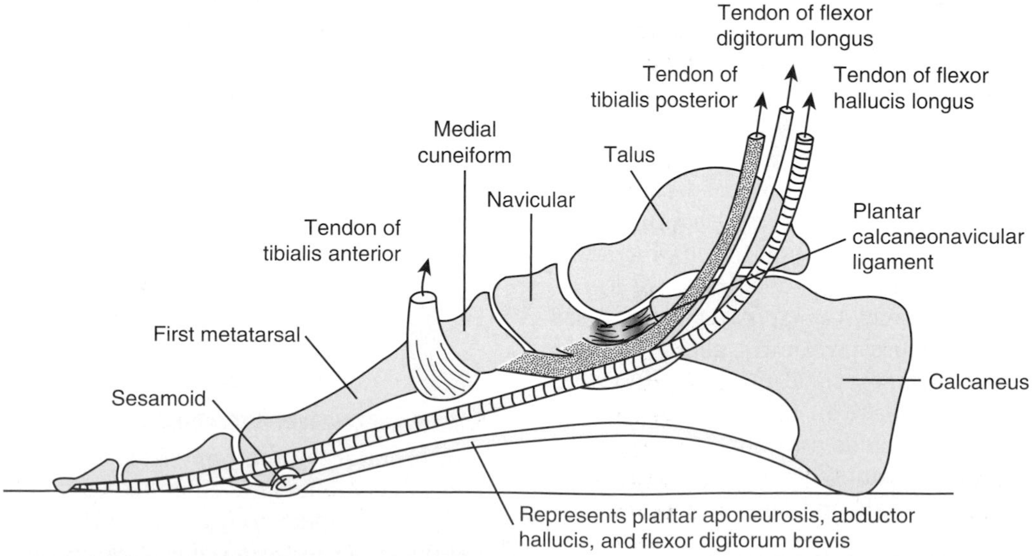

FIGURE 10-21 Anatomical structures of the medial longitudinal arch of the foot. (Redrawn from Hamilton JJ, Ziemer LK: Functional anatomy of the human ankle and foot. In Kiene RH, Johnson KA, eds: *American Academy of Orthopaedic Surgeons symposium on the foot and ankle,* Figure 1-5, St Louis, 1983, Mosby.)

Mechanism: PT dysfunction is commonly seen in runners, jumpers, and individuals who perform lateral agilities. These motions cause repetitive microtrauma. Loss of static support for the medial longitudinal arch imposes an increased load on the PT muscle. PT tenosynovitis and PT weakness may lead to the development of other pronation-related overuse syndromes. Loss of PT function decreases the stability of the talonavicular joint, which is essential for transmission of force from the rearfoot to the forefoot for effective push off.

Signs and symptoms:

- Localized pain along the tibial malleolus
- Localized swelling
- Tenderness to palpation in the posterior tibial malleolus
- Possible localized edema
- Pain with resisted inversion and plantar flexion

Special tests: No special tests are applicable.

Immediate and intermediate management: PRICES may be used to manage the pain and edema associated with this condition. Taping and orthotics may be used to help with foot biomechanics and weight transfers during attempts to return to activity.

Ankle Injuries

In the context of ankle injury, the term *chronic* describes an injury in which symptoms last longer than 3 months.[63] The severity of chronic symptoms, such as pain during activity, recurrent swelling, and giving-way sensations, does not appear to be related to the severity of the initial injury.[16,27,64,65] The likelihood of LAS recurrence is 70% to 80%,[66] with a 20% to 40% prevalence of chronic symptoms among individuals who have a history of LAS.[16, 27, 64,65,67–69] Only about 40% of individuals who have symptoms of chronic ankle instability demonstrate ligament laxity on stress radiographs.

Inadequate restraint of ankle motion may be due to ankle ligament laxity, a deficiency in neuromuscular control, or a combination of the two factors.[3,70–72] Impaired neuromuscular control of ankle motion is almost certainly a contributing factor in most cases of chronic ankle instability, but the presence of ligament pathology that is not readily identifiable by conventional diagnostic tests may be an equally important consideration. Biomechanical abnormalities may also influence neuromuscular function, which may be manifested as decreased muscle responsiveness, muscle weakness, alteration in the strength relationship of antagonistic muscles, or impaired postural stability. Evaluation of an individual with chronic ankle instability should include a through assessment of postural balance, joint position sense, reflex responses, cutaneous sensation, strength, and range of motion.[71]

Anterolateral Impingement Syndrome

Synovial hypertrophy and development of fibrotic scar tissue in the anterolateral gutter between the fibular malleolus and the lateral articular facet of the talus after LAS are possible sources of chronic lateral ankle pain during activity.[73–76] This condition is known as **anterolateral impingement syndrome.**

Mechanism: Some experts believe that the synovial absorption of hemarthrosis associated with LAS induces chronic synovitis and extensive formation of adhesions.[74] Fibrotic tissue may develop in the anterolateral portion of the talocrural joint, which impinges on the articular surface of the dome of the talus and can ultimately cause chondromalacia.[73]

Signs and symptoms:

- Pain with activity
- Tenderness to palpation around the lateral fibular malleolus with activity
- Swelling
- Absence of ankle instability

Special tests: A combination of assessments is used to diagnose anterolateral impingement syndrome. If at least five of the following six clinical indicators present as positive, it is highly likely that the individual has anterolateral impingement syndrome: (1) anterolateral ankle joint tenderness, (2) anterolateral ankle joint swelling, (3) pain with forced eversion and dorsiflexion of the affected ankle, (4) pain with single-leg squat on the affected ankle, (5) pain with activity, and (6) absence of ankle instability.[76]

Immediate and intermediate management: Arthroscopic debridement of fibrotic scar tissue is indicated for resolution of the condition.

Sinus Tarsi Syndrome

The sinus tarsi separates the anterior and posterior articulations of the subtalar joint and contains the interosseus talocalcaneal ligament (ITCL), the cervical ligament (CL), and the ligament-like roots of the inferior extensor retinaculum. The roots of the retinaculum contribute to the restriction of subtalar inversion. Inflamed fibrotic tissue within the sinus tarsi, combined with symptoms of persistent lateral foot pain and perceived instability, is a common complication following LAS.[77,78] This condition is known as **sinus tarsi syndrome.**

Mechanism: Hemarthrosis associated with subtalar ligament damage is believed to play a role in the development of this chronic inflammatory condition.

anterolateral impingement syndrome soft tissue impingement of the anterolateral gutter as a result of synovial hypertrophy and fibrotic scar tissue

sinus tarsi syndrome clinical syndrome of the opening on the outside of the foot between the ankle and heel; causes pain and restricts movement

Signs and symptoms:
- Pain
- Localized tenderness to palpation
- Pain relieved with localized antiinflammatory injections or anesthetics

Special tests: No special tests are applicable.

Immediate and intermediate management: PRICES may be attempted to control immediate pain and swelling. Referral to a physician is necessary for further diagnostic testing and medicinal intervention.

Peroneal Nerve Injury

Decreased conduction velocity of the superficial and deep peroneal nerves following LAS may contribute to a delay in reflexive activation of the evertor muscles in response to sudden inversion.[79–81]

Mechanism: Overstretching of the superficial peroneal nerve is most likely to be induced by inversion, whereas the deep peroneal nerve is most likely to be stretched by extreme plantar flexion.[79] Compression to the deep peroneal nerve secondary to anterior compartment syndrome, ill-fitting shoes, trauma, or improper technique and mechanics can also cause injury.

Signs and symptoms:
- Inability to distinguish sensations (mostly with superficial peroneal nerve injury)
- Possible drop foot
- Possible loss of ankle stability

Special tests:

Slump test: During the slump test, the client starts by sitting on the edge of the table with thighs supported, hands behind the back, and hips positioned in neutral. The test is performed in the following seven-part sequence (Figure 10-22): (1) While maintaining the client's chin in neutral position, have the client slump forward by curving the thoracic and lumbar spine; (2) apply downward overpressure with one arm across the shoulders; (3) have the client flex the neck and head as far as possible; (4) carefully apply overpressure to the back of the head, maintaining flexion throughout the spine; (5) with the opposite hand, dorsiflex the foot; (6) have the client extend the knee; and finally (7) have the client extend the neck and head. If pain results or symptoms increase at any point, testing should be stopped and a positive result should be noted.

Immediate and intermediate management: Management of peroneal nerve injury is similar to that of common peroneal nerve contusions.

Peroneal Tendon Injury

The peroneus longus (PL) and peroneus brevis (PB) tendons are held within a shallow groove on the posterior margin of the fibular malleolus by retinacular ligaments, which are essentially thickenings of the sheath that covers the tendons.[49] Rupture of the CFL is usually accompanied by a tear of the medial portion of the common peroneal tendon sheath.[4]

Mechanism: Hemorrhagic tenosynovitis can result from direct tendon damage,[77] or **extravasation** of blood into the common peroneal sheath from a hemarthrosis

extravasation the movement of fluid from a physiological space (e.g., a blood vessel or intracapsular joint space) into surrounding tissues

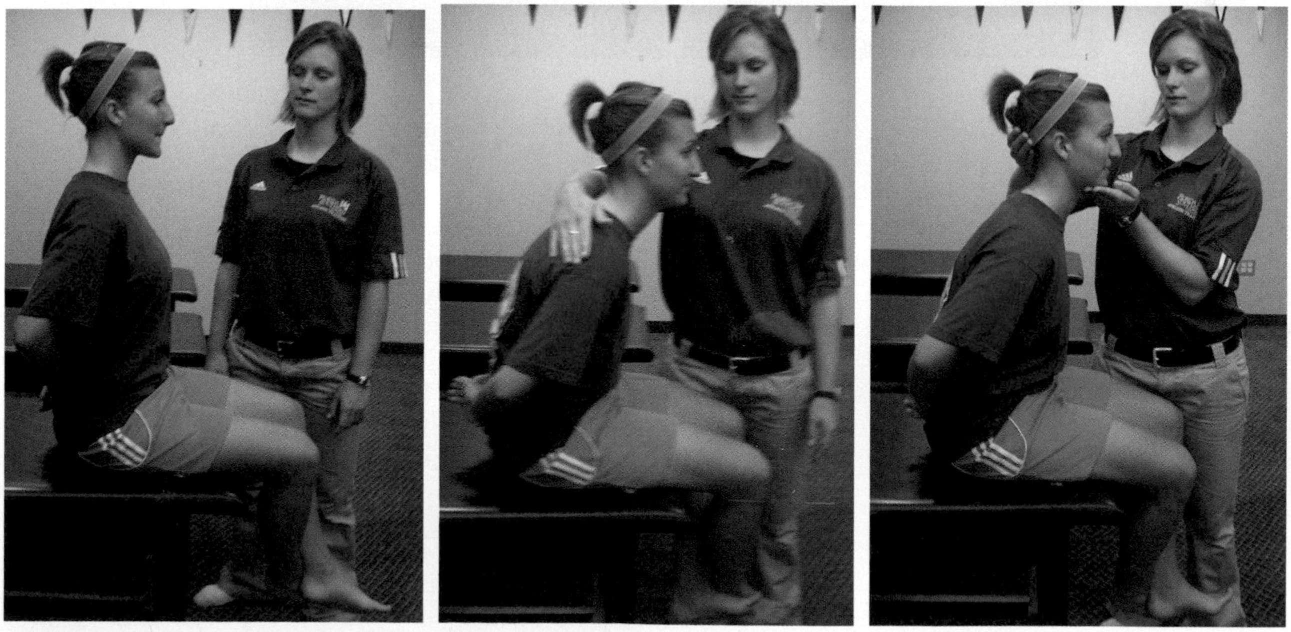

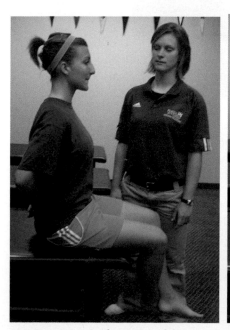

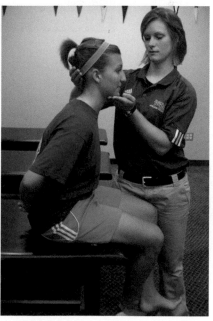

FIGURE 10-22 Performance of the seven-part slump test for assessment of peroneal nerve injury. See the text above for detailed descriptions of the steps involved.

Continued

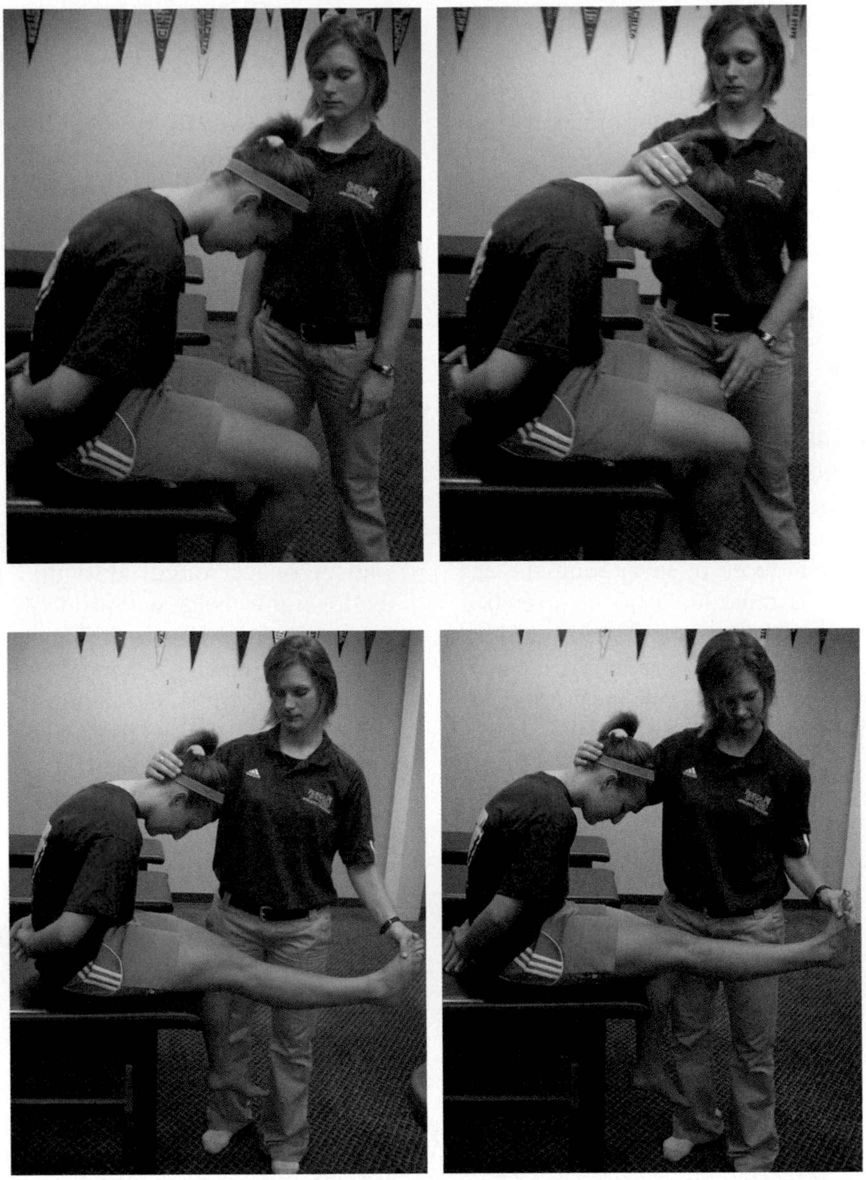

FIGURE 10-22, Cont'd

of either the talocrural or subtalar joints. Longitudinal tendon tearing or fraying is referred to as *tendinosis.* Powerful contraction of the peroneal muscles can tear the superior peroneal retinaculum on the posterior margin of the fibular malleolus, which may result in repetitive anterior subluxation of the peroneal tendons.[82]

Signs and symptoms:

- Localized pain
- Tenderness to palpation
- Swelling
- Possible loss of function
- Possible loss of motion

Special tests: No special tests are applicable.

Immediate management: PRICES may be used to manage peroneal tendon injuries. As with LAS, focal compression with pads or braces with pads should be used in conjunction with the modalities to optimize their ability to reduce swelling.

Intermediate management: Once swelling and pain have subsided, a conservative comprehensive rehabilitation program may be implemented that focuses on range of motion, flexibility, strength, neuromuscular control, and balance.

Foot Injuries

Immediately after heel strike of the foot in a slightly supinated position, the subtalar joint and adjacent joints dissipate ground reaction forces by moving into a maximally pronated position during transition to the midstance phase of gait. From the maximally pronated position at midstance, the foot moves into a supinated position that increases its rigidity as the heel rises and body weight is shifted to the forefoot. Thus foot pronation is a normal characteristic of gait that is essential for proper dampening of forces created by weight-bearing activities. Excessive or prolonged pronation is associated with an altered distribution of forces on foot, ankle, or leg structures that can lead to degenerative changes and chronic inflammation, which often occurs in both extremities.

Plantar Fasciitis

The plantar fascia provides stability to the dorsum of the foot and maintains the integrity of the longitudinal arch. Weight bearing in daily activities, as well as athletic endeavors, creates significant force on the fascia. Simple changes in routine, such as wearing different footwear, running, jumping, and shifting weight toward your toes while standing, may produce an unusual tension that eventually begins to damage the plantar fascia and contribute to the development of a condition known as **plantar fasciitis,** which involves microscopic tears and painful inflammation.

Mechanism: Flattening of the medial longitudinal arch increases the distance between the posterior and anterior attachments of the plantar fascia. This forced lengthening produces microscopic tears at the calcaneal origin of the plantar fascia that initiate a painful and persistent inflammatory response.[77] Plantar fasciitis is often precipitated by shoes that lack proper support, errors in training, poor technique and mechanics, and gait abnormalities.

Signs and symptoms:

- Pain upon initial weight bearing in the morning
- Pain at the plantar fascial attachment on the calcaneus
- Pain after prolonged sitting
- Pain that dissipates after several weight-bearing steps are taken

Special tests: No special tests are applicable.

Immediate management: Short-term relief of symptoms may be achieved with medication and therapeutic modalities (e.g., PRICES, ultrasound, manual therapy), but correction of the underlying biomechanical cause is necessary to minimize recurrent problems and prevent the development of progressively greater dysfunction.

Intermediate management: Dramatic relief of symptoms caused by excessive pronation is sometimes realized through the use of custom-fabricated orthotics that provide support beneath the talonavicular joint and extend to the metatarsal heads in the forefoot. Orthotics constructed from a relatively stiff material resist medial longitudinal arch flattening that the superincumbent body weight tends to induce during the midstance phase of gait and enhance the rigidity of the foot during push off by splinting the joints that lie between the Achilles tendon insertion on the calcaneus and the toes.

Tarsal Tunnel Syndrome

The *tarsal tunnel* refers to the concavity adjacent to the posterior margin of the tibial malleolus, which contains the PT, flexor digitorum longus (FDL), and flexor hallucis longus (FHL) tendons, along with the posterior tibial artery, vein, and nerve. These structures are collectively encased by fascia and a fibrous roof that is formed by the flexor retinaculum. Trauma or overuse can constrict the structures within the tunnel and cause pain, burning, or numbness during activity, a condition known as **tarsal tunnel syndrome.**

Mechanism: Trauma or overuse can produce fibrotic thickening of the encasing tissues, which constricts the structures within the tunnel.

Signs and Symptoms:

- Diffuse pain
- Localized burning
- Numbness along the medial and plantar aspects of the foot with activity

Special tests: Tinel's sign.

Immediate and intermediate management: Because excessive pronation increases traction stress on the posterior tibial nerve, an orthotic device may relieve the symptoms. Surgical release of the constrictive tissue is sometimes necessary. Conservative medications and modalities may help lessen the symptoms.

Sesamoiditis

The medial and lateral sesamoid bones lie beneath the first MTP joint. Acute fracture is possible, but a stress fracture is the most common cause of sesamoiditis and sesamoid pain.

Mechanism: Repetitive loading and impact often make the sesamoid bones susceptible to injury.

Signs and symptoms:

- Localized pain under the great toe
- Tenderness to palpation
- Pain increased with passive dorsiflexion
- Possible pain and difficulty with gait

Special tests: No special tests are applicable.

Immediate and intermediate management: Custom fabricated orthotics may help alleviate pain associated with sesamoiditis. To promote tissue healing and decrease inflammation, it may be necessary to curtail activity for

plantar fasciitis painful condition caused by excessive wear and strain on the plantar fascia of the foot

tarsal tunnel syndrome condition in which the posterior tibial nerve is compressed within the tarsal canal, causing pain and burning several weeks. Surgical resection of a fractured sesamoid or a bipartite sesamoid is sometimes necessary for resolution of the condition.

Metatarsalgia

Pain that is localized beneath the metatarsal heads typically is called **metatarsalgia.** In many cases, metatarsalgia is exacerbated by calluses that develop beneath the affected metatarsal heads.

Mechanism: Metatarsalgia may be a secondary condition following plantar fasciitis or other foot injuries. It can also be brought on by repetitive trauma caused by a tight gastrocnemius and soleus complex that alter gait mechanics.

Signs and symptoms:
- Localized pain
- Flattened appearance of the metatarsal heads
- Swelling
- Stiffness
- Possible loss of motion

Special tests: No special tests are applicable.

Immediate and intermediate management: Periodic callus shaving, use of a metatarsal pad, and a nonsteroidal antiinflammatory drug (NSAID; see Chapter 23) may provide some degree of symptom relief. Surgical debridement, synovectomy, or osteotomy is often necessary for severe cases that do not improve in response to conservative treatment. To prevent further or recurrent injury, mechanical and technique issues that incite metatarsalgia should be addressed before return to activity is granted.

Accessory Navicular

A relatively small percentage of athletes have a small accessory bone on the inferomedial aspect of the navicular bone, in the area of the PT tendon insertion. When present, it usually appears bilaterally.

Mechanism: The small accessory navicular bone is subjected to tensile stress as a result of the pull of the PT muscle during activity.

Signs and symptoms:
- Localized pain
- Tenderness to palpation
- Localized swelling

Special tests: No special tests are applicable.

Immediate and intermediate management: Conservative treatment, consisting of modified activity, NSAIDs, and orthotics, may help alleviate symptoms.

Stress Fracture

The term *stress fracture* is used to designate a broad range of pathological conditions of the bone. The prevalence of stress fractures is greatest for long-distance runners, and female athletes exhibit greater susceptibility than do male athletes. The second and third metatarsals are the foot bones most commonly affected, but a stress fracture may develop in any of the metatarsals, the sesamoid bones, the talus, the calcaneus, or the navicular.

Mechanism: Overuse, a traumatic event, or a combination of both types of tissue loading may be responsible for symptom onset. Stress fractures may occur either suddenly or gradually.

Signs and Symptoms:
- Insidious onset of vague pain
- Tenderness to palpation
- Possible loss of function

Special tests: No special tests are applicable.

Immediate and intermediate management: Bone scan images will identify the existence of a pathological condition before radiographic evidence appears. When the volume of weight-bearing physical activity is reduced, the pain associated with a metatarsal stress fracture rapidly diminishes, and the condition typically resolves without complications. If this conservative treatment fails, surgical fixation and bone grafting will probably be necessary. Because the incidence of navicular fracture nonunion is high, typical initial treatment for a navicular stress fracture is nonweight-bearing immobilization for 6 to 8 weeks, with full return to participation often not allowed until 16 to 20 weeks after the injury.

Toe Injuries

Abnormalities in the alignment of the bones of the toes may be congenital or acquired. Regardless of how and when they occur, these injuries may become bothersome and sometimes prevent affected individuals from performing their usual activities.

Hallux Valgus

Hallux valgus is a deformity of the first metatarsophalangeal (MTP) joint that involves lateral angulation of the great toe (i.e., the hallux). This angulation causes the medial aspect of the first metatarsal head to protrude on the medial border of the forefoot. The protrusion is referred to as a *bunion*, and it becomes more prominent as shoe pressure causes the development of a callus. Pressure against the medial aspect of the first metatarsal head may lead to chronic bursitis, eventual fibrotic thickening of the bursa, and formation of osteophytes.

Mechanism: A genetic predisposition and tight shoes with tapered toes are believed to cause the angulated position of the first MTP joint, which progressively worsens as the direction of pull of the EHL and FHL tendons on the hallux is altered.[40]

metatarsalgia tenderness and burning within the metatarsal region

hallux valgus deformity of the first metatarsophalangeal joint involving lateral angulation of the great toe

Signs and symptoms:
- Localized tenderness
- Localized swelling
- Enlargement of the first metatarsal joint
- Possible loss of function
- Possible pain with gait

Special tests: No special tests are applicable.

Immediate and intermediate management: Alignment of the first MTP joint may be improved by the use of a toe spacer between the first and second toes; this device discourages lateral displacement of the hallux. Uncomfortable bunion pressure may be alleviated by use of a silicone pad. Properly fitting shoes and orthotics may also help diminish symptoms. If conservative management does not help, surgical intervention may be required.

Toe Deformity

Claw toes and hammer toes are both characterized by hyperextension of the MTP joint and flexion of the proximal interphalangeal (PIP) joint in one or more toes. Secondarily, the skin on the dorsal aspect of the PIP joint highly becomes susceptible to shoe pressure and friction.

Mechanism: A claw toe is characterized by flexion of the distal interphalangeal (DIP) joint, whereas a hammer toe exhibits a neutral or extended DIP joint (resembling a finger boutonnière deformity).

Signs and symptoms:
- Localized swelling
- Localized pain
- Possible blistering over the affected joint
- Possible loss of function
- Possible pain with gait

Special tests: No special tests are applicable.

Immediate and intermediate management: Either condition may be associated with neuropathy, dysfunction of the foot's intrinsic muscles, or metatarsalgia, which may be idiopathic or secondary to foot trauma. Therefore the best form of management is to relieve the pressure causing the pain and dysfunction by applying and using orthotics or pads, wearing appropriate footwear, or regularly shaving the callus surrounding the affected area.

Interdigital Neuropathy

Mechanical compression of an interdigital nerve may cause demyelination and fibrotic scarring. This condition, often called *Morton's neuroma,* frequently occurs where the nerve splits to innervate adjoining toes. The term *neuroma* is a misnomer in this context because a true nerve tumor does not exist. The third interdigital nerve, which lies between the third and fourth metatarsal heads, is usually involved.

Mechanism: Compression on the nerve caused by irritation from improper foot mechanics, ill-fitting shoes, or inappropriate training increases may result in the formation of the neuropathy.

Signs and symptoms:
- Localized burning
- Severe pain that diminishes when weight-bearing activity ceases
- Tingling sensations
- Numbness of affected toes

Special tests: No special tests are applicable.

Immediate and intermediate management: Padding, NSAIDs, and reduction in activity volume are usually effective for relief of symptoms. In some cases, injection of a corticosteroid or surgical excision of the nerve is necessary. Before the athlete returns to activity, mechanics, technique, and footwear must be assessed to prevent recurrence.

Box 10-3 summarizes the chronic injuries to the lower leg, ankle, foot, and toe and the appropriate special tests used in diagnosis.

Prevention of Chronic Injuries

During participation in high-demand physical activities, the lower leg, ankle, foot, and toes are subjected to very high forces and stressors. To allow the body to meet these demands, preventive measures should be taken to thwart injury. Protective padding and properly fitting equipment (e.g., shoes) are priorities. Maintaining a high level of fitness emphasizing strength, flexibility, neuromuscular control, and balance is equally important to prevent many chronic and overuse injuries. By being attentive to training programs and progressions, athletes can improve their performance without suffering undue setbacks. Also, an unstable ankle should be protected by ankle taping or an ankle brace; this measure may dramatically improve sports performance capabilities and decrease activity-related ankle discomfort.

TAPING, BRACING, AND RETURN TO PLAY

Taping and bracing are common techniques in the management of injuries to the lower leg, ankle, foot, and toes. Taping and bracing methods are diverse and plentiful, but all are intended to protect the injury and promote healing, as well as to prevent further injury. Given this variety, specific techniques will not be addressed here. However, it is important to remember that taping and bracing may help alleviate some of the symptoms associated with these injuries, allowing a safe and speedy return to activity. As always, before returning a client to activity, athletic trainers should perform a comprehensive evaluation and functional clearance test to ensure that the client can execute the required skills.

Orthotics are another adjunct that can be used to promote healing and return to activity. Inexpensive and

orthotics a pair of semi-rigid supportive devices for both feet that facilitate maintenance of normal alignment

BOX 10-3 Chronic Lower Leg, Ankle, Foot, and Toe Injuries and Appropriate Special Tests

Lower Leg Injuries

Achilles tenosynovitis, tendinosis, tendinitis
- No appropriate special tests

Tibial and fibular stress fractures
- Tap or percussions tests

Exertional compartment syndrome
- No appropriate special tests

Deep vein thrombosis
- Homan's test

Medial tibial stress syndrome
- No appropriate special tests

Posterior tibialis dysfunction
- No appropriate special tests

Articular cartilage lesions
- No appropriate special tests

Ankle Injuries

Anterolateral impingement syndrome
- Combination of assessments

Sinus tarsi syndrome
- No appropriate special tests

Peroneal nerve injury
- Slump test

Peroneal tendon injury
- No appropriate special tests

Foot Injuries

Plantar fasciitis
- No appropriate special tests

Tarsal tunnel syndrome
- Tinel's sign

Sesamoiditis
- No appropriate special tests

Metatarsalgia
- No appropriate special tests

Accessory navicular
- No appropriate special tests

Stress fractures
- No appropriate special tests

Calcaneal apophysitis
- No appropriate special tests

Toe Injuries

Hallux valgus
- No appropriate special tests

Toe deformity
- No appropriate special tests

Interdigital neuropathy
- No appropriate special tests

effective orthotics are easily fabricated from thermoplastic material that is molded directly to the contours of the foot. Prone positioning of the patient, with the knee at 90 degrees of flexion and the ankle in a neutral position, facilitates maintenance of both the rearfoot and forefoot in a neutral horizontal alignment (i.e., absence of rearfoot-forefoot twist) and allows for gravity-assisted formation of the thermoplastic material while it is in its heat-malleable condition. After the material has cooled and the contours are set, comfort may be enhanced by gluing a thin high-density foam rubber cushioning material to the upper surface of the orthotic and grinding its edges to minimize material bulk in locations that can cause uncomfortable pressure against the foot. If the client is large, an area of high-density material (e.g., ethyl vinyl acetate, which is used to construct athletic shoe midsoles) should be glued to the undersurface of the orthotic beneath the medial longitudinal arch to resist deformation of the orthotic under high loading conditions. Ideally, the orthotics should have sufficient width to fit snugly against the sides of the shoes.

THE AGE GROUP ATHLETE

Several injuries to the lower leg, ankle, and foot are specific to certain populations of active people. Articular cartilage lesions and calcaneal apophysitis are fairly common in the adolescent and pediatric populations. Conversely, Achilles tendon ruptures are most common in males over the age of 30. Proper early diagnosis and management are important to ensure that these injuries do not worsen and that involvement in future activities and sports will be possible.

Pediatric Athletes

The delay in growth plate closure during youth makes young athletes particularly susceptible to injury. The immaturity of the bones and musculotendinous attachments is a factor in most injuries to this area.

Articular Cartilage Lesions

Chondral lesions, also called *articular cartilage lesions*, that do not involve a fracture of the subchondral bone are often associated with LAS.[7,83,84] Osteochondritis dissecans, a detachment of the cartilage from the talus, is usually associated with insidious onset of ankle pain in young athletes.[40]

Mechanism: A single traumatic event or repetitive microtrauma caused by shear forces from recurrent ankle sprains may cause these cartilage lesions.

Signs and symptoms:
- Pain
- Possible catching or locking in the ankle

- Localized effusion
- Possible loss of function
- Possible pain with gait

Special tests: No special tests are applicable.

Immediate and intermediate management: Because chondral lesions found in chronically unstable ankles are more severe than those associated with acute injuries, prevention of recurrent sprains has been suggested as the best treatment.[84] Although the ankle is not generally regarded as susceptible to development of arthritis, an association between severe ligament trauma and arthritic degeneration has been documented.[85] Arthroscopic removal of an osteochondral fragment may be necessary for relief of chronic symptoms.[49]

Calcaneal Apophysitis

Skeletally immature athletes, typically between the ages of 8 and 13 years old, sometimes experience aching pain in the heel region.[40] The secondary center of ossification of the calcaneus is subjected to traction forces by the attachments of the Achilles tendon and plantar fascia, which create an inflammatory condition of the apophysis designated by some as *Sever's disease* but generally known as **calcaneal apophysitis.**

Mechanism: Achilles tendon tightness is a predisposing factor, and bilateral occurrence is common.

Signs and symptoms:

- Localized pain
- Diminished pain after activity

Special tests: No special tests are applicable.

Immediate and intermediate management: The condition is self-limiting and typically resolves with PRICES, reduced training volume, heel padding, and Achilles tendon stretching.

Aging Athletes

Proper conditioning and use of protective equipment reduce the mature athlete's risk of incurring injury. However, Achilles tendon rupture is common in men over the age of 30 who are involved in ballistic or jumping activities.

Achilles Tendon Rupture

Achilles tendon rupture is a very painful and traumatic injury. Even worse, most affected individuals will not be able to return to their previous levels of activity after experiencing this injury.

Mechanism: Abrupt movements such as those required for jumping, landing, and quickly changing directions are common causes of Achilles tendon rupture.

Signs and symptoms:

- Sudden sharp pain that coincides with injury
- Pain that quickly diminishes after injury occurs
- Swelling
- Ecchymosis
- Point tenderness
- Deformity with complete ruptures
- Loss of function
- Loss of ability to ambulate

Special tests:

Thompson test: For the Thompson test, the client assumes a prone position, with legs extended and the feet off the edge of the table, while the athletic trainer squeezes the calf at midbelly (Figure 10-23). If no plantar flexion is noted or plantar flexion is reduced compared with that of the other leg, a positive result is noted for an Achilles tendon rupture.

Immediate and intermediate management: A conservative approach is recommended to promote optimal healing. In most cases, a period of immobilization with no weight-bearing activity will be prescribed while PRICES is implemented as an adjunct therapy. Surgical intervention may be necessary. A comprehensive rehabilitation program focusing on stretching, strengthening, and neuromuscular control will facilitate a return to activity.

SUMMARY

The severity of injuries to the lower leg, ankle, foot, and toes does not necessarily correspond directly to the extent of activity limitation that is imposed. Understanding the intimate and dynamic relationships of the involved anatomical structures in this area makes evaluation and diagnosis of injuries less difficult.

calcaneal apophysitis inflammatory condition of the apophysis in which the heel bone (calcaneus) is subjected to traction forces; most common in athletes between ages 8 and 13.

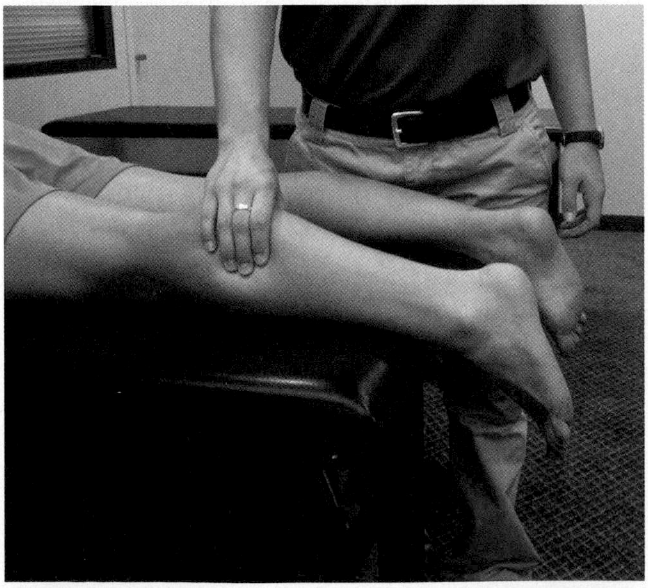

FIGURE 10-23 Performance of Thompson test for assessment of Achilles tendon rupture.

The best way for the athletic trainer to ensure a return to activity is to obtain a thorough history, which is required for a proper diagnosis of the injury. Management and intervention strategies rely heavily on assessing biomechanical issues, footwear, training programs, and the use of orthotics and taping or wrapping with a U-pad. Prevention, the ideal method of reducing the risk of injury, includes comprehensive conditioning focusing on strength, flexibility, neuromuscular control, balance, and proper technique.

Revisiting the OPENING *Scenario*

Because the athlete's acutely swollen and plantar flexed ankle precludes immediate assessment of his or her ability to walk on the injured extremity, the presence of a fracture cannot be authoritatively excluded on the basis of the Ottawa ankle rules. Immediate referral for radiographic evaluation would not be inappropriate, but the referral decision could be delayed if the ankle is carefully protected until the ability to bear weight on the injured extremity can be better assessed.

Cryotherapy generally decreases the perception of ankle pain, which facilitates restoration of dorsiflexion to the extent that a neutral position of the ankle may be maintained. The forefoot should be wrapped with a cohesive elastic material to facilitate resolution of edema on the dorsum of the foot, and a U-shaped pad should be applied to the periphery of the fibular malleolus to simultaneously compress underlying soft tissues and redirect lateral ankle swelling in a proximal direction up the leg. A rocker-sole walking boot may be used to maintain the ankle in a neutral position for a period of 12 to 24 hours. Alternatively, an ankle stirrup brace or ankle taping may be used to protect the ankle ligaments. Either of the latter options should be combined with the application of an athletic shoe that can be fitted over the ankle support (preferably a running shoe or cross-training shoe with a padded nylon tongue), which will facilitate use of a walk-through crutch gait to the extent that weight bearing on the injured extremity is tolerated. The coach should be advised that the extent of the injury cannot be precisely determined on the basis of a single acute phase assessment and that the athlete's response to treatment over the next 24-hour period will provide a great deal of additional information about the severity of the ankle ligament disruption.

Approximately 48 hours after the traumatic event and 5 days before the next game, the athlete's functional status is dramatically improved. He now demonstrates the ability to walk unassisted with a minimally perceptible limp, his dorsiflexion range of motion is nearly normal, and the surface contours of his foot and ankle demonstrate that swelling is substantially decreased. Ecchymosis is considerably greater on the lateral aspect of the ankle, particularly within the channel area created by the U-pad. Palpation elicits intense pain directly over the anterior talofibular ligament, no tenderness is elicited over the calcaneofibular ligament, and considerably diminished tenderness is evident on the medial aspect of the ankle joint compared with the prior assessment. The anterior drawer test elicits a lesser degree of discomfort than it did before, but a mild degree of anterior translation of the talus is clearly evident. The athlete is capable of performing a unilateral heel raise using the injured extremity, but he experiences some discomfort and has difficulty maintaining postural balance as his heel rises. On the basis of the Ottawa ankle rules, the existence of a fracture is highly improbable. The overall clinical presentation is consistent with diagnostic criteria for classification as a grade II lateral ankle sprain.

The coach should be advised that full restoration of normal functional capabilities is likely within 2 weeks. Near-normal function may be regained sooner, depending on the athlete's tolerance for progressively more demanding physical activities that will be attempted with protective ankle support. If the athlete clearly demonstrates tolerance for normal sport-specific functional demands while wearing a protective support, the timing of return to full participation mostly depends on the coach's assessment of his performance in relation to that of other candidates for the starting quarterback position. Symptoms should be carefully monitored throughout the ensuing weeks and months to ensure that any previously unrecognized pathological condition associated with the injury does not contribute to the development of chronic ankle dysfunction.

Issues & Ethics

Shawn is a 17-year-old forward recently selected for the U.S. ice hockey team. He has played hockey since he was 5 years old and has always dreamed of making the national team. He has 12 school and state scoring records. Before joining the team, he underwent two surgeries to repair damage to his left ankle caused by chronic lateral ankle sprains. He trains hard and does all the right things. Understandably, he seems frustrated at times by his limitations and ongoing pain. During practice yesterday, he was making a break to the goal with no defenders in sight. As he approached the goal, his feet became tangled with the goalie's feet. Shawn went down to the ice grimacing in pain and grabbing his left ankle. Upon evaluation, he was diagnosed with a rupture of his recently repaired ATFL and CFL. It also was noted that he had sustained a distal fibular head fracture. Because the fibula is technically a nonweight-bearing bone, Shawn requests that the injury be treated with PRICES and heavy taping and strapping. Logic tells you that this approach is merely temporary and that further injury is inevitable. What do you do?

Web Links

American Academy of Orthotists and Prosthetics: www.oandp.org
American College of Foot & Ankle Surgeons: www.acfas.org
American Orthopedic Foot & Ankle Society: www.aofas.org
American Podiatric Medical Association: www.apma.org
Ankle Sprain, Brigham & Women's Hospital: http://healthgate.partners.org/browsing/browseContent.asp?fileName=12051.xml&title=Ankle%20Sprain
Ankle Sprain, Massachusetts's General Hospital: http://healthgate.partners.org/browsing/LearningCenter.asp?fileName=12051.xml&title=Ankle%20Sprain
Foot and Ankle Problems, Cleveland Clinic: http://cms.clevelandclinic.org/ortho/body.cfm?id=20&oTopID=9
Foot Injuries & Disorders: www.nlm.nih.gov/medlineplus/footinjuriesanddisorders.html
Nail Disease: www.nlm.nih.gov/medlineplus/naildiseases.html

References

1. Pijnenburg ACM et al: Treatment of ruptures of the lateral ankle ligaments: a meta-analysis, *J Bone Joint Surg Am* 82: 761–773, 2000.
2. van Dijk CN: Management of the sprained ankle, *Br J Sports Med* 36: 83–84, 2002.
3. Hertel J: Functional anatomy, pathomechanics, and pathophysiology of lateral ankle instability, *J Athl Train* 37: 364–375, 2002.
4. Kelikian H, Kelikian AS: *Disorders of the ankle*, Philadelphia, 1985, Saunders.
5. Hamilton JJ, Ziemer LK: Functional anatomy of the human ankle and foot. In Kiene RH, Johnson KA, editors: *American Academy of Orthopaedic Surgeons Symposium on the foot and ankle*, St Louis, 1983, Mosby.
6. Eustace S et al: *Sports injuries: examination, imaging, and management*, Edinburgh, 2007, Churchill Livingstone Elsevier.
7. van Dijk CN, Bossuyt PM, Marti RK: Medial ankle pain after lateral ligament rupture, *J Bone Joint Surg Br* 78: 562–567, 1996.
8. Becker H-P et al: Stress diagnostics of the sprained ankle: evaluation of the anterior drawer test with and without anesthesia, *Foot Ankle* 14: 459–464, 1993.
9. van Dijk CN et al: Physical examination is sufficient for the diagnosis of sprained ankles, *Bone Joint Surg Br* 78: 958–962, 1996.
10. Bahr R et al: Mechanics of the anterior drawer and talar tilt tests: a cadaveric study of lateral ligament injuries of the ankle, *Acta Orthop Scand* 68: 435–441, 1997.
11. Tohyama H et al: Biomechanical analysis of the ankle anterior drawer test for anterior talofibular ligament injuries, *J Orthop Res* 13: 609–614, 1995.
12. van Dijk CN et al: Correspondence: physical examination is sufficient for the diagnosis of sprained ankles, *Bone Joint Surg Br* 79: 1039–1040, 1997.
13. Magee DJ: *Orthopedic physical assessment*, ed 2, Philadelphia, 1992, Saunders.
14. Steill IG et al: Interobserver agreement in the examination of the acute ankle injury, *Am J Emerg Med* 10: 14–17, 1992.
15. Leddy JJ et al: Prospective evaluation of the Ottawa ankle rules in a university sports medicine center: with a modification to increase specificity for identifying malleolar fractures, *Am J Sports Med* 26: 158–165, 1998.
16. Gerber JP et al: Persistent disability associated with ankle sprains: a prospective examination of an athletic population, *Foot Ankle Int* 19: 653–660, 1998.
17. Garrick JG, Requa RK. The epidemiology of foot and ankle injuries in sports, *Clin Sports Med* 7: 29–36, 1988.
18. Black HM, Brand RL, Eichelberger MR: An improved technique for the evaluation of ligamentous injury in severe ankle sprains, *Am J Sports Med* 6: 276–282, 1978.
19. Ferran NA, Maffulli N: Epidemiology of sprains of the lateral ankle ligament complex, *Foot Ankle Clin N Am* 11: 659–662, 2006.
20. Robichon J et al: Functional anatomy of the ankle joint and its relationship to ankle injuries, *Can J Surg* 15: 145–150, 1972.
21. Cass JR, Settles H: Ankle instability: in vitro kinematics in response to axial load, *Foot Ankle* 15: 134–140, 1994.
22. Boruta PM et al: Acute lateral ankle ligament injuries: a literature review, *Foot Ankle* 11: 107–113, 1990.
23. Ardevol J et al: Treatment of complete rupture of the lateral ligaments of the ankle: a randomized clinical trial comparing cast immobilization with functional treatment, *Knee Surg Sports Traumatol Arthrosc* 10: 371–377, 2002.
24. Bergfeld J et al: Symposium: management of acute ankle sprains, *Contemp Ortho* 13: 83–116, 1986.
25. Dias LS: The lateral ankle sprain: an experimental study, *J Trauma* 19: 266–269, 1979.
26. Frey C et al: A comparison of MRI and clinical examination of acute lateral ankle sprains, *Foot Ankle Int* 17: 533–537, 1996.
27. Kannus P, Renstrom P: Treatment for acute tears of the lateral ligaments of the ankle operation, cast, or early controlled mobilization, *J Bone Joint Surg Am* 73: 305–312, 1991.
28. Beynnon BD et al: A prospective, randomized clinical investigation of the treatment of first-time ankle sprains, *Am J Sports Med* 34: 1401–142, 2006.
29. Jackson DW, Ashley RL, Powell JW: Ankle sprains in young athletes: relation of severity and disability, *Clin Orthop* 101: 210–215, 1974.
30. Kaikkonen A, Kannus P, Jarvinen M: A performance test protocol and scoring scale for the evaluation of ankle injuries, *Am J Sports Med* 22: 462–469, 1994.
31. Lassiter TE Jr, Malone TR, Garrett WE Jr: Injury to the lateral ligaments of the ankle, *Orthop Clin North Am* 20: 629–640, 1989.
32. Milgrom C et al: Risk factors for lateral ankle sprain: a prospective study among military recruits, *Foot Ankle* 12: 26–30, 1991.
33. Wilkerson GB, Horn-Kingery HM: Treatment of the inversion ankle sprain: comparison of different modes of compression and cryotherapy, *J Orthop Sports Phys Ther* 17: 240–246, 1993.
34. Stephens MM, Sammarco GJ: The stabilizing role of the lateral ligament complex around the ankle and subtalar joints, *Foot Ankle* 13: 130–136, 1992.

35. Colville MR et al: Strain measurements in lateral ankle ligaments, *Am J Sports Med* 18: 196–200, 1990.
36. Konradsen L, Ravn JB: Ankle instability caused by prolonged peroneal reaction time, *Acta Orthop Scand* 6: 388–390, 1990.
37. Konradsen L, Voigt M, Hojsgaard C: Ankle inversion injuries: the role of the dynamic defense mechanism, *Am J Sports Med* 25: 54–58, 1997.
38. Uys HD, Rijke AM: Clinical association of acute lateral ankle sprain with syndesmotic involvement: a stress radiography and magnetic resonance imaging study, *Am J Sports Med* 30: 816–822, 2002.
39. Safran MR et al: Lateral ankle sprains: a comprehensive review. Part 1: Etiology, pathoanatomy, histopathogenesis, and diagnosis, *Med Sci Sports Exerc* 31: S429–S437, 1999.
40. Omey ML, Micheli LJ: Foot and ankle problems in the young athlete, *Med Sci Sports Exerc* 31: S470–S486, 1999.
41. DeSimoni C et al: Clinical examination and magnetic resonance imaging in the assessment of ankle sprains treated with an orthosis, *Foot Ankle Int* 17: 177–182, 1996.
42. Hutton PAN: Ankle lesions. In Jenkins DHR, editor: *Ligament injuries and their treatment*, Rockville, Md, 1985, Aspen Systems.
43. Smith RW, Reischl SF: Treatment of ankle sprains in young athletes, *Am J Sports Med* 14: 465–471, 1986.
44. Weiker GG: Ankle injuries in the athlete, *Prim Care* 11: 101–108, 1984.
45. Safran MR et al: Lateral ankle sprains: a comprehensive review. Part 2: Treatment and rehabilitation with an emphasis on the athlete, *Med Sci Sports Exerc* 31: S438–S447, 1999.
46. Wilkerson GB: Treatment of the inversion ankle sprain through synchronous application of focal compression and cold, *Athl Train* 26: 220–237, 1991.
47. McKay GD et al: Ankle injuries in basketball: injury rate and risk factors, *Br J Sports Med* 35: 103–108, 2001.
48. Hettinga DL: Inflammatory response of synovial joint structures. In Gould JA, editor: *Orthopedic and sports physical therapy*, St Louis, 1990, Mosby.
49. Black HM Jr, Brand RL: Injuries of the foot and ankle. In Scott WN, Nisonson B, Nicholas JA, editors: *Principles of sports medicine*, Baltimore, 1984, Williams and Wilkins.
50. Gardner AMN et al: Reduction of post-traumatic swelling and compartment pressure by impulse compression of the foot, *J Bone Joint Surg Br* 72: 810–815, 1990.
51. Hintermann B, Valderranbano V: The effectiveness of rotational stabilization in the conservative treatment of severe ankle sprains: a long-term investigation, *Foot Ankle Surg* 7: 235–239, 2001.
52. Wilkerson GB: Comparative biomechanical effects of the standard method of ankle taping and a taping method designed to enhance subtalar stability, *Am J Sports Med* 19: 588–595, 1991.
53. Wilkerson GB et al: Effects of the subtalar sling ankle taping technique on combined talocrural-subtalar joint motions, *Foot Ankle Int* 26: 239–246, 2005.
54. Wilkerson GB: Biomechanical and neuromuscular effects of ankle taping and bracing, *J Athl Train* 37: 436–445, 2002.
55. Nussbaum ED et al: Prospective evaluation of syndesmotic ankle sprains without diastasis, *Am J Sports Med* 29: 31–35, 2001.
56. Briner WW Jr, Carr DE, Lavery KM: Anteroinferior tibiofibular ligament injury: not just another ankle sprain, *Physician Sportsmed* 17: 63–69, 1989.
57. Brosky R et al: The ankle ligaments: consideration of syndesmotic injury and implications for rehabilitation, *J Orthop Sports Phys Ther* 21: 197–205, 1995.
58. Boytim MJ, Fischer DA, Neumann L: Syndesmotic ankle sprains, *Am J Sports Med* 19: 294–298, 1991.
59. Edwards GS Jr, DeLee JC: Ankle diastasis without fracture, *Foot Ankle* 4: 305–312, 1984.
60. Hopkinson WJ et al: Syndesmosis sprains of the ankle, *Foot Ankle* 10: 325–330, 1990.
61. Conti SF: Posterior tibial tendon problems in athletes, *Orthop Clin North Am* 25: 109–121, 1994.
62. Hintermann B: Tibialis posterior dysfunction: a review of the problem and personal experience, *Foot Ankle Surg* 3: 61–70, 1997.
63. Vaes P, Gheluwe BV, Duquet W: Control of acceleration during sudden ankle supination in people with unstable ankles, *J Orthop Sports Phys Ther* 31: 741–752, 2001.
64. Peters JW, Trevino SG, Renstrom PR: Chronic lateral ankle instability, *Foot Ankle* 12: 182–191, 1991.
65. Dettori JR: Early ankle mobilization. Part II: A one-year follow-up of acute, lateral ankle sprains, *Milit Med* 159: 20–24, 1994.
66. Hertel J et al: Talocrural and subtalar joint instability after lateral ankle sprain, *Med Sci Sports Exerc* 31: 1501–1508, 1999.
67. Freeman MAR, Dean MRE, Hanham IWF: The etiology and prevention of functional instability of the foot, *J Bone Joint Surg Br* 47: 678–685, 1965.
68. Itay S et al: Clinical and functional status following lateral ankle sprains, *Orthop Rev* 11: 73–76, 1982.
69. Verhagen RA, de Keizer G, van Dijk CN: Long-term follow-up of inversion trauma of the ankle, *Acta Orthop Trauma Surg* 114: 92–96, 1995.
70. Hubbard TJ, Hertel J: Mechanical contributions to chronic lateral ankle instability, *Sports Med* 36: 263–277, 2006.
71. Hertel J: Functional instability following lateral ankle sprain, *Sports Med* 29: 361–371, 2000.
72. Wilkerson GB, Nitz AJ: Dynamic ankle stability: mechanical and neuromuscular interrelationships, *J Sport Rehabil* 3: 43–57, 1994.
73. Ferkel RD et al: Arthroscopic treatment of anterolateral impingement of the ankle, *Am J Sports Med* 19: 440–446, 1991.
74. Guhl JF: Soft tissue (synovial) pathology. In Guhl JF, editor: *Ankle arthroscopy, pathology, and surgical techniques*, Thorofare, NJ, 1988, Slack, Inc.
75. Kim S-H, Ha K-I: Arthroscopic treatment for impingement of the anterolateral soft tissues of the ankle, *J Bone Joint Surg Br* 82: 1019–1021, 2000.
76. Liu SH, Nuccion SL, Finerman G: Diagnosis of anterolateral impingement: comparison between magnetic resonance imaging and clinical examination, *Am J Sports Med* 25: 389–393, 1997.
77. Duddy RK et al: Diagnosis, treatment, and rehabilitation of injuries to the lower leg and foot, *Clin Sports Med* 8: 861–876, 1989.
78. Lektrakul N et al: Tarsal sinus: arthrographic, MR imaging, and pathologic findings in cadavers and retrospective

study data in patients with sinus tarsi syndrome, *Radiology* 219: 802–810, 2001.
79. Kleinrensink GJ et al: Lowered motor conduction velocity of the peroneal nerve after inversion trauma, *Med Sci Sports Exerc* 26: 877–883, 1994.
80. Nitz AJ, Dobner JJ, Kersey D: Nerve injury and grades II and III ankle sprains, *Am J Sports Med* 13: 177–182, 1985.
81. van Cingel REH et al: Repeated ankle sprains and delayed neuromuscular response: acceleration time parameters, *J Orthop Sports Phys Ther* 36: 72–79, 2006.
82. Safran MR, O'Malley D, Fu FH: Peroneal tendon subluxation in athletes: new exam technique, case reports, and review, *Med Sci Sports Exerc* 31: S487–S492, 1999.
83. Hintermann B, Boss A, Schafer D: Arthroscopic findings in patients with chronic ankle instability, *Am J Sports Med* 30: 402–409, 2002.
84. Taga I et al: Articular cartilage lesions in ankles with lateral ligament injury: an arthroscopic study, *Am J Sports Med* 21: 120–127, 1993.
85. Valderrabano V et al: Ligamentous posttraumatic ankle osteoarthritis, *Am J Sports Med* 34: 612–620, 2006.

11

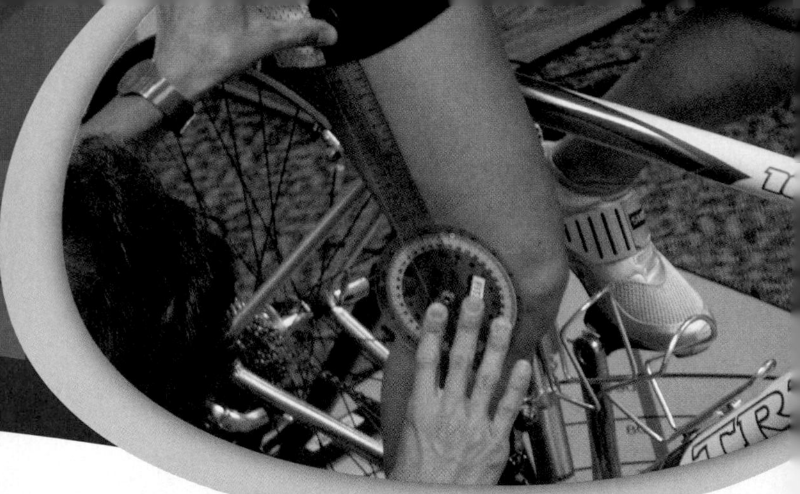

Diagnosis and Management of Knee and Thigh Injuries

ROBERT C. MANSKE AND JAMES W. MATHESON

Learning Goals

1. Describe assessment and diagnostic procedures for evaluation of common acute injuries to the knee and thigh.
2. Identify common signs and symptoms of acute athletic injuries that affect the knee and thigh.
3. Describe assessment and diagnostic procedures for evaluation of common chronic injuries to the knee and thigh.
4. Identify common signs and symptoms of chronic athletic injuries that affect the knee and thigh.
5. Develop a differential diagnosis system to identify the injury and provide proper care and management for acute and chronic injuries to the knee and thigh.
6. Identify risk factors for knee and thigh injuries associated with athletic participation.
7. Develop methods to identify and employ injury prevention procedures for athletic injuries to the knee and thigh.
8. Identify precautions and risks associated with athletic participation by athletes of various age groups and how these factors influence injuries to the knee and thigh.

The knee and thigh are frequently injured in sports and activities of daily living. These injuries are both acute and chronic and range from short-term setbacks with minimal impact to long-term and possibly career-ending injuries. Acute injuries to this area generally are quite simple to diagnose and manage. They usually are the result of traumatic direct-contact situations. It is the chronic or overuse injury that presents the greatest challenge to the athletic trainer. Most often, these injuries have such an innocuous onset that the athlete has difficulty describing the symptoms.

Because most people today are active in their younger years, knee and thigh injuries are common in the pediatric and adolescent populations. Most of these injuries are due to repetitive trauma during growth spurts or just excessive loading that the body part cannot handle. Regardless of age or injury symptoms, athletic trainers must have a thorough understanding of the involved anatomy, mechanisms of injury, and possible pathological conditions for proper evaluation and diagnosis. Management of these injuries is necessary to prevent recurring symptoms and allow a safe and timely return to activity. The goal of this chapter is to provide a systematic process that allows appropriate diagnosis and management of acute and chronic/overuse knee and thigh injuries.

CLINICAL EVALUATION AND DIAGNOSIS OF KNEE AND THIGH INJURIES

Knee injuries can be serious or emergency situations or they can be mere nuisances. An awareness of potential emergencies is always beneficial. Knee and thigh injuries

Terms that appear in boldface green type are defined in the book's glossary.

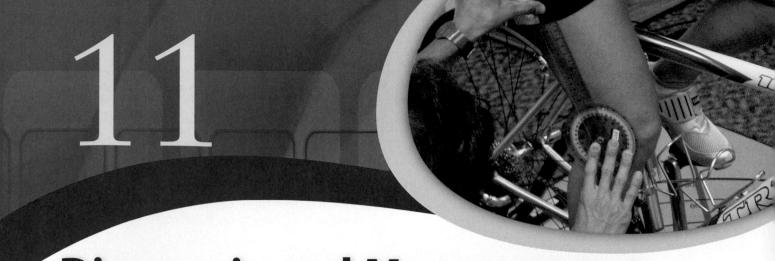

OPENING Scenario

A 22-year-old senior on the varsity college basketball team comes to the athletic training room. The team has been practicing for 1 week. On the day that he first noticed his knee symptoms, a few days after practice began, the team had performed multiple cutting and pivoting drills following a timed 2-mile run. He complains today of medial knee pain with weight-bearing activities such as cutting, pivoting, and landing with his knee in a flexed position. Furthermore, he complains of an occasional painful popping and catching sensation. Positions that elicit pain include jumping, squatting, and stooping. Minimal knee effusion can be detected visually, and some tenderness is noted along the medial joint line of the knee. His active and passive knee range of motion appears to be full, although overpressure with passive knee flexion causes some discomfort. Ligament stress testing reveals normal and intact collateral and cruciate ligaments. He is also neurovascularly intact. McMurray and Apley's tests appear positive; each test causes substantial pain and popping when performed. After a consultation with the team orthopedic surgeon, a magnetic resonance imaging examination is ordered; the film suggests a minor knee effusion but no other clear evidence of pathology. The athletic training staff attempts conservative therapy for 6 weeks, but these efforts do not relieve the athlete's pain. The orthopedic surgeon and the athlete both decide that a diagnostic arthroscopy is the best treatment option.

fall into two very broad categories: those in which the athlete comes to the athletic trainer with a recent onset of injury (i.e., acute) and those in which the athlete informs the athletic trainer of the injury a long time after the symptoms first appeared (i.e., chronic). Both types of injuries have the potential to be serious.

During the evaluation of either acute or chronic knee and thigh injuries, a thorough history and meticulous physical examination process should be used to establish an appropriate diagnosis. This systematic examination process should be practiced often to ensure efficiency and accuracy. In an emergency, time is of the essence. Whether the athlete is able to leave the playing area by his or her own volition or not, the initial portion of any acute examination begins with a triage assessment or the assignment of treatment priorities.[1] If the athlete is moving normally or rolling on the ground in pain, the athletic trainer knows that the athlete is conscious and has an intact central nervous system. A primary survey is performed to discover any immediate life-threatening problems, including loss of consciousness, cardiovascular or pulmonary complications, profuse bleeding, and obvious deformity resulting from fracture or dislocation. After the primary survey, the athletic trainer may perform a more thorough secondary evaluation that will assess for less serious injuries, such as contusions, hematomas, bleeding, or minor deformities. Generally speaking, the athlete may be transferred from the field of play, if necessary, at this time.

History

By obtaining a detailed history, the athletic trainer gains insight into the specific knee and thigh structures that might be injured. One of the first history questions that the athletic trainer should ask involves the mechanism of injury (MOI). The MOI in a knee or thigh injury can provide critical clues regarding which structures are at fault. The relationship of the MOI to the knee and subsequent injuries is presented in Table 11-1. The athletic trainer should consider whether the leg was in a weight-bearing position when the foot was planted during the injury. Especially with knee injuries, the athletic trainer should always ascertain whether the client felt or heard a pop or experienced a tearing sensation. Often, when the anterior cruciate ligament is disrupted, a pop is felt, whereas a tearing sensation often accompanies damage to the medial collateral ligament.

Inspection and Observation

The inspection should begin as soon as the athletic trainer enters the area and begins observing the client. The inspection of a knee injury may require removal of clothing such as pants, shorts, protective equipment, and

TABLE 11-1 Mechanisms of Injury for Knee Injuries and Affected Structures

MECHANISM OF INJURY	AFFECTED STRUCTURES
Knee flexion with posterior directed force to tibia	PCL
Knee hyperextension	ACL, PCL, ACL/PCL combination
Valgus force	MCL
Valgus force with external rotation	MCL, ACL and meniscus
Varus force	LCL
Varus force with internal rotation	LCL and ACL
Anterior blow (tibia driven forward)	PCL
Posterior blow (tibia driven backward)	ACL
Femoral rotation with weight bearing	Meniscus, patellar dislocation
Flexed knee valgus with tibial	Patellar dislocation

PCL, Posterior cruciate ligament; *ACL*, anterior cruciate ligament; *MCL*, medial collateral ligament; *LCL*, lateral collateral ligament.

padding. During the initial visual assessment, the athletic trainer should look for obvious deformity, open fractures, swelling, or discoloration (e.g., ecchymosis). Because some deformities may be subtle, the athletic trainer may need to refer to the other extremity for comparison.

Observation of lower extremity alignment (in both injured and noninjured legs), resting posture, and gait pattern provides the athletic trainer with information about possible biomechanical causes of injury.

Standing Postural Examination

A key function of the knee is to transmit and dissipate forces from the long bones of the tibia and femur. Akin to the automatic transmission of an automobile, the knee may also be characterized as a "complex set of asymmetrical moving parts acting together as a living biologic transmission."[2] The knee is required to accept the **asymmetrical** forces created by the contact of the foot, ankle, and tibia and the ground, forces that are then transmitted up the shaft of the femur. Likewise, the knee must transmit the weight and forces generated by the upper limbs, torso, pelvis, and hips to the tibia and foot. Thus an examination of the knee would be incomplete if biomechanical asymmetries of the proximal and distal lower extremity are not evaluated. Box 11-1 highlights key aspects of a standing lower extremity postural examination.

asymmetrical irregular or uneven

BOX 11-1 Standing Postural Examination of the Lower Extremities

	Anterior View	Lateral View	Posterior View
Hip and Pelvis	• Does the athlete demonstrate any abnormalities of the bony and soft tissue contours at the waist and thighs? • Does the athlete rotate one hip in or out to a greater degree than the other? • Is bruising or skin discoloration apparent?	• Does the athlete exhibit any signs of gluteal muscle atrophy? • Does the athlete have an increased or decreased lumbar lordosis? An increased lordosis may be a result of decreased length of the hip flexors, whereas a decreased lordosis may be secondary to decreased length of the hamstring muscles.	• Does the athlete demonstrate any abnormalities of the bony and soft tissue contours at the waist and thighs? • Does the athlete exhibit any signs of buttock or posterior thigh muscle atrophy? • Observe lumbar spine for scoliosis and/or unilateral paraspinal muscle hypertrophy.
Knee	• Does the patient demonstrate either a genu valgum (knock-knee) or genu varum (bowleg) deformity? • What are the positions of the patella? Do they face straight ahead or tilt inward (squinting) or outward (grasshopper eyes)? • Does the patient have any signs (scars) of a previous knee surgery? • Do the inferior poles of the right and left patella appear level with each other?	• When the athlete extends his or her knees, is genu recurvatum (hyperextension) present? • Are one or both patellae lower (patella baja) or higher (patella alta) than normal? A "camel sign" may be present in an athlete with a high-riding patella. From a lateral view, it will appear as two "humps" present at the knee • Does the inferior pole of the patella appear to tilt inward toward the infrapatellar fat pads?	• Is any swelling present in the athlete's right or left popliteal spaces?
Leg	• Does the athlete's proximal tibia demonstrate a bowleg deformity (tibia varum)? • Is the tibial tuberosity rotated outward (lateral tibial torsion) or inward (medial tibial torsion)?	• Does the athlete exhibit any signs of gastrocnemius muscle atrophy?	• Does the athlete exhibit any signs of gastrocnemius muscle atrophy?
Foot and Ankle	• Examine the athlete from both an anterior and an anterosuperior view. • Do the feet turn inward (pigeon toes) or outward? If yes, does this relate to either a medial or a lateral tibial torsion? • Does the athlete exhibit excessive supination or pronation of the foot? • Does the patient demonstrate a bunion (hallux valgus) or bunionette deformity?	• Examine the longitudinal arches of the foot. Compare and contrast the heights of the medial and lateral longitudinal arches.	• Does the athlete's Achilles tendon(s) curve out or in? • Does the athlete have a buildup of bone on the calcaneus (pump bump)? • What is the athlete's rearfoot angle?

Gait Analysis

Gait assessment or analysis is a skill that requires a great deal of practice and sound knowledge of the gait cycle. To investigate the complexity of gait, researchers at universities and large hospitals have developed elaborate biomechanical laboratories employing **electromyography**, force platforms, and high-speed video motion analysis systems. Significant technical skill is required in these settings; in many cases, teams of clinicians are needed to run the gait laboratory alone. Although many athletic training settings do not have this wealth of equipment and technical support, a standard digital video camera and relatively inexpensive video analysis and editing software are excellent tools, well within the range of the average athletic department's budget. Armed with camera and laptop, the athletic trainer can examine the client's biomechanics during his or her daily functional activities. By reviewing these activities in slow motion, the athletic trainer can identify any deficits. The athletic trainer can also use these tools to assess the effectiveness of interventions such as knee braces and foot orthotics. Consideration of environmental factors (e.g., training surface), lower extremity alignment and training equipment (e.g., footwear) on the kinematics of the individual's gait is often necessary to determine the cause of the injury.

Palpation

Numerous bony and soft tissue structures can be palpated in or around the thigh and knee. When performing an on-field examination, the athletic trainer should assess only those structures immediately pertinent to the injury. A more thorough assessment may be performed once the athlete has been taken off the field. Box 11-2 is a complete list of bony and soft tissue structures to be palpated.

Palpation should begin in an area near the suspected problem but not directly over the injured tissue, at least initially. This approach will inspire the client's confidence and trust; ideally, the client will be able to relax during the examination of the actual injury site. The athletic trainer should palpate gently and attempt to identify any point tenderness or palpatory deformities, both of which are good indicators of underlying fractures or dislocations.

Range of Motion Testing

After asking the client to move the knee through the available range of motion (ROM), the athletic trainer should watch carefully to see how far the client is able to move the injured knee. Beginning with active range of motion (AROM) and progressing to passive range of motion (PROM) then resisted range of motion (RROM), allow the athlete to stop any ROM exercise when it becomes painful. Because an injured knee and thigh may be fractured or dislocated, the leg should not be forced past the client's limits of pain through passive ROM exercises. If the athlete is unconscious, passive ROM should not be performed until fracture and dislocation have been definitively ruled out as a cause of injury.

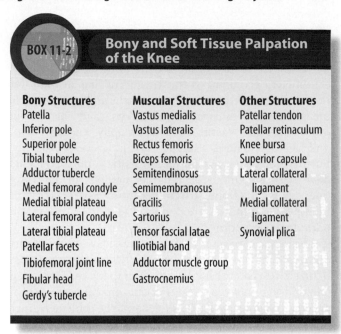

BOX 11-2 Bony and Soft Tissue Palpation of the Knee

Bony Structures	Muscular Structures	Other Structures
Patella	Vastus medialis	Patellar tendon
Inferior pole	Vastus lateralis	Patellar retinaculum
Superior pole	Rectus femoris	Knee bursa
Tibial tubercle	Biceps femoris	Superior capsule
Adductor tubercle	Semitendinosus	Lateral collateral ligament
Medial femoral condyle	Semimembranosus	Medial collateral ligament
Medial tibial plateau	Gracilis	Synovial plica
Lateral femoral condyle	Sartorius	
Lateral tibial plateau	Tensor fascial latae	
Patellar facets	Iliotibial band	
Tibiofemoral joint line	Adductor muscle group	
Fibular head	Gastrocnemius	
Gerdy's tubercle		

Special Tests

Special tests are used to help confirm a suspected diagnosis of an injury to the knee and thigh. These tests assess girth and leg length, manual muscle strength, muscle length (flexibility), and injury-specific factors. In the presence of an obvious or suspected joint dislocation or fracture, the athletic trainer should perform only the special tests necessary to determine the best way to immobilize and move the injured person to safety. Any other special tests should be deferred at this time.

Injury-specific special tests will be discussed with the relevant diagnoses later in this chapter. Special tests reproduce the injury mechanism to stress specific structures in an attempt to evaluate the integrity of contractile and noncontractile tissues. By stressing these structures, the athletic trainer can establish laxity, tightness, instability, or fractures within them. There is a specific special test unique to each body part or joint. Only the applicable special tests should be performed with each diagnosis, and these should be performed bilaterally. The athletic trainer must be careful when performing any special test because it could exacerbate the injury.

electromyography in patient care, a test used to determine whether a person's muscle weakness is caused by a disease within the muscle or by a problem in the nerve supplying the muscle

Girth and Leg Length Measurement

Circumferential measurements should be taken 20 centimeters proximal to the knee joint line, 10 centimeters proximal to the knee joint line, at the joint line, and 15 centimeters distal to the joint line. These measurements illustrate quadriceps and hamstring muscle atrophy, vastus medialis atrophy, knee effusion, and gastrocnemius soleus atrophy, respectively.[3,4] Furthermore, similar circumferential measurements have been shown to be reliable methods of assessing knee joint effusion.[5] Circumferential asymmetries in the lower extremities are common and do not suggest a pathological condition.[6]

Leg length measurements are taken in both supine and standing positions. The athletic trainer must recognize two types of leg length discrepancies. A true leg length discrepancy is a result of anatomical or structural anomaly. To measure true leg length, the athletic trainer must first square the athlete's pelvis and lower extremities on the examination table. The legs are positioned 15 to 20 centimeters apart in neutral rotation. Any asymmetry in limb placement (e.g., hip adduction, abduction, rotation) may result in a false measurement.[7] After carefully positioning the client, the athletic trainer completes the leg length measurement by noting the distance from the inferior portion of the most prominent point of the anterior superior iliac spine (ASIS) to the inferior portion of the medial malleolus.[8] In contrast to an anatomical leg length difference, a functional leg length discrepancy may be the result of unilateral genu recurvatum, unilateral pronation, or spinal scoliosis. Functional leg length discrepancy may be assessed with a tape measure while the client is standing, using the same landmarks as described for the supine method.

Assessment of Lower Extremity Muscle Strength

Comprehensive strength testing of all major muscle groups surrounding the hip, knee, and ankle provides the athletic trainer with important information when examining a knee injury. Weakness at any point along the lower extremity kinetic chain may place increased force on the tibiofemoral or patellofemoral joints and contribute to injury.[9–11] By determining the athlete's specific muscle weakness, the athletic trainer is better prepared to prescribe specific strengthening exercises and develop an appropriate exercise program. To improve the validity and reliability of muscle testing, the use of a digital or analog hand-held digital **dynamometer** is recommended[11–13] (Figures 11-1 and 11-2). In addition, instrumented strength testing allows the athletic trainer to assess antagonist-to-agonist muscle ratios.

Assessment of Lower Extremity Muscle Length

After observing the client's gait and posture, the athletic trainer performs a thorough assessment of lower extremity flexibility for all knee and thigh injuries. The assessment

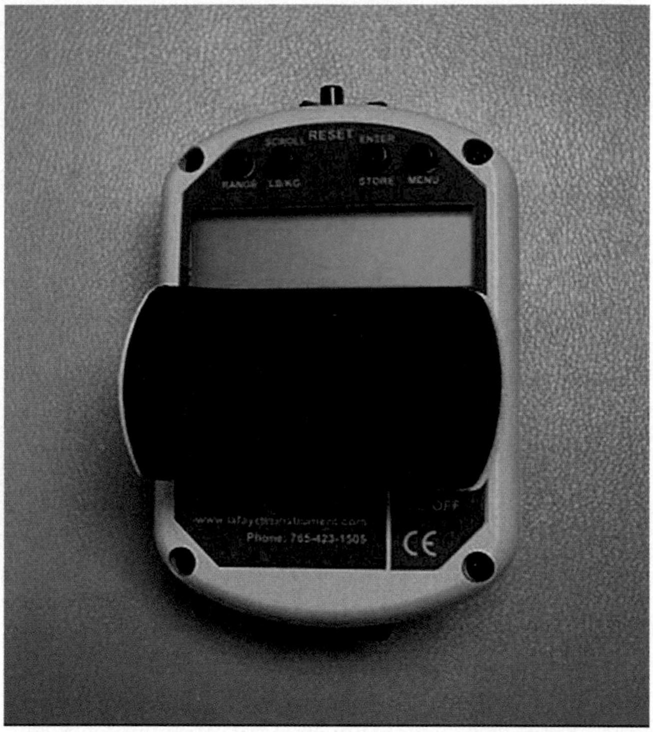

FIGURE 11-1 Lafayette hand-held dynamometer.

of muscle iliopsoas, hamstring, quadriceps, and the iliotibial band/tensor fasciae latae (ITB/TFL) length helps the athletic trainer in determining structural asymmetry in the lower extremities that may be placing increased stress on the tissues of the knee and thigh. When testing muscle length, the athletic trainer should carry out the following tests on both the injured and uninjured extremities for the purpose of a bilateral comparison.

Iliopsoas Length. The Thomas test is a common method to assess fixed flexion deformities of the hip. The athlete lies supine while the athletic trainer checks for excessive lumbar lordosis. The examiner then passively flexes the extremity not being tested, bringing the athlete's knee to his or her chest to flatten the lumbar spine. The athlete is instructed to hold his or her knee against the chest. The hip being tested, the straight leg will remain on the examination table if no flexion deformity exists. If a deformity exists, the extended extremity will remain off the table in a slightly flexed position. The examiner then measures the angle between the table and the hip.

Hamstring Length. Hamstring muscle length may be assessed by two different methods. The **passive straight leg raise test** is performed by having the athlete

dynamometer device for measuring muscle strength

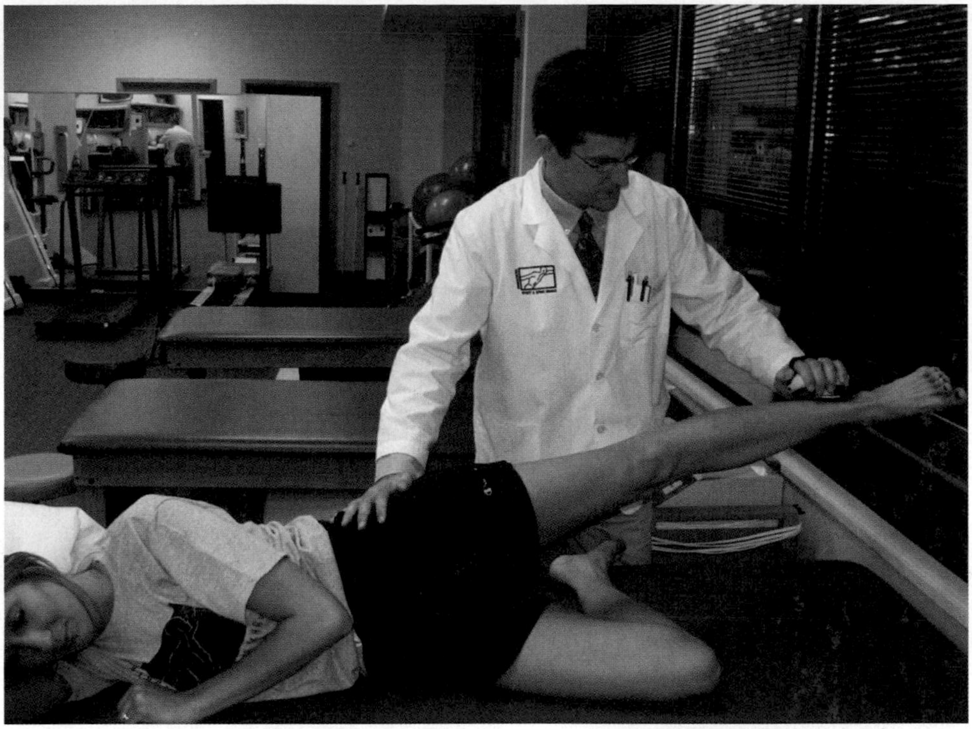

FIGURE 11-2 Use of hand-held dynamometer to assess hip abduction strength.

positioned supine on the table with the opposite leg extended and flat on the table to minimize posterior pelvic tilt. An inclinometer may be placed on the anterior border of the distal tibia of the leg to be tested. The test leg is passively raised to end range or until firm resistance is felt.[14] A second method to measure hamstring length is the 90/90 straight leg raise.[15,16] Similar to the passive straight leg raise test, the 90/90 straight leg raise test is performed by having the athlete assume a supine position on the table with the opposite leg extended and flat against the surface of the table to minimize posterior pelvic tilt. The hip of the lower extremity to be tested is flexed to 90 degrees. The knee is then passively extended to end range or until a firm resistance is felt. The **popliteal angle** is recorded. Both of these methods have been shown to be reliable. However, athletic trainers are cautioned not to use them interchangeably when repeating measures on the same athlete. Also, the passive straight leg raise is recommended for athletes with generalized joint hypermobility, who may "zero out" before reaching their physiological end range when being assessed with the 90/90 straight leg raise test.[14,15]

Quadriceps Length. Quadriceps muscle length is assessed by use of the Ely test.[7] The Ely test is performed by positioning the athlete in the prone position and measuring passive knee flexion with an inclinometer or **goniometer**. An alternative to using a goniometer is to measure the distance between the athlete's heel and buttock with a tape measure. Substitution patterns to avoid are those involving ipsilateral hip flexion and anterior tilting of the pelvis or lumbar spine extension.[7,14]

Iliotibial Band/Tensor Fasciae Latae Length. The Ober test is primarily used to assess the length and mobility of the iliotibial band/tensor fasciae latae (ITB/TFL) complex in individuals with lower extremity complaints. To assess the length of the ITB/TFL complex, the athletic trainer asks the client to assume a side-lying position with the upper or test leg above and the lower hip flexed enough to remove any lumbar lordosis. The knee of the upper leg is flexed to 90 degrees and cradled by the athletic trainer. The athletic trainer's other hand is used to press firmly down on the athlete's ilium to stabilize the pelvis during testing. Holding the knee at a right angle, the test leg is flexed, abducted, and extended until the hip is in line with the trunk. The examiner then allows gravity to adduct the test leg. If the test leg remains above the horizontal plane, the test indicates a shortened ITB/TFL complex. An inclinometer or goniometer may be used to quantify the degree of hip abduction above the horizontal plane.[14,17,18]

popliteal angle widely used means of assessing hamstring length

goniometer an apparatus to measure joint movements and angles

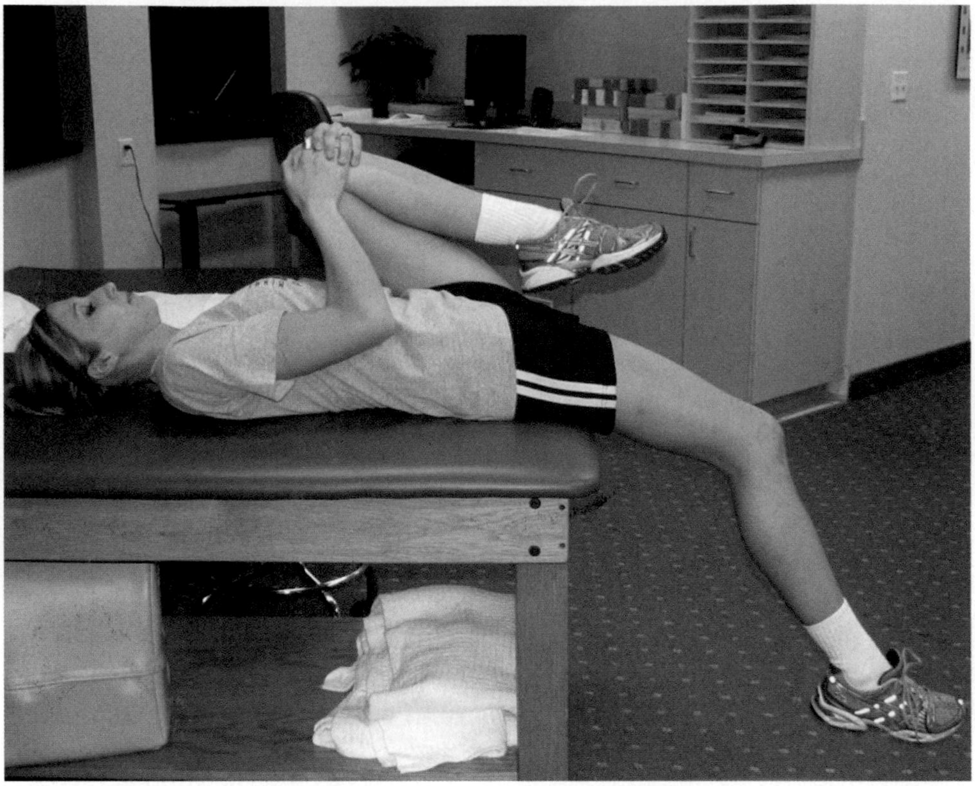

FIGURE 11-3 Modified Thomas test.

The Modified Thomas Test. The modified Thomas test assesses iliopsoas, quadriceps, and ITB length. The athlete sits on the edge of the treatment table and then rolls back onto the table, holding both knees to the chest. These steps ensure that the lumbar spine is flat on the plinth and a posterior tilt of the pelvis is obtained. The athlete then firmly holds the **contralateral** knee to the chest as the examiner passively lowers the extremity to be tested toward the floor (Figure 11-3). The athletic trainer records hip flexion, knee flexion, and hip abduction angles, making note of any asymmetries between the involved and uninvolved limbs.

Neurovascular Tests

Evaluation of neurovascular function in an injured knee or thigh is paramount because many nerves and vessels that are crucial to the lower extremity are in close proximity to the knee. These structures may be easily injured in tandem with knee or thigh fractures, dislocations, or contusions. As long as the client is present, the athletic trainer should perform a thorough neurovascular evaluation at a minimum of every 30 minutes.[1]

Pulse

The athlete's pulse should be assessed distally from the site of injury. With most knee or thigh injuries, the location of choice for pulse assessment is either the posterior tibial artery or the dorsalis pedis artery (Figure 11-4). Athletic trainers must always remember that a pulseless limb is dying until circulation is restored. Therefore a lack of pulse is a medical emergency requiring emergency care.[1]

Capillary Filling Time

Capillary filling time may be assessed with firm pressure on either the nail bed or the skin near a nail bed (Figure 11-5). Pressure to the nail or skin in this area will cause the nail to blanch, or turn white. Once pressure is released, a quick return to a normal pink should occur within approximately 2 to 3 seconds. Capillary refill that takes longer than 2 to 3 seconds indicates impaired circulation. Depending on the level of impairment, poor capillary refill may also represent a medical emergency.[1]

Sensation

An athlete's ability to perceive light touch in the limb distal to the site of injury is a good indication that the nerve supply is intact. All dermatomes in the leg distal to the site of injury should be assessed for light touch sensation.

contralateral opposite

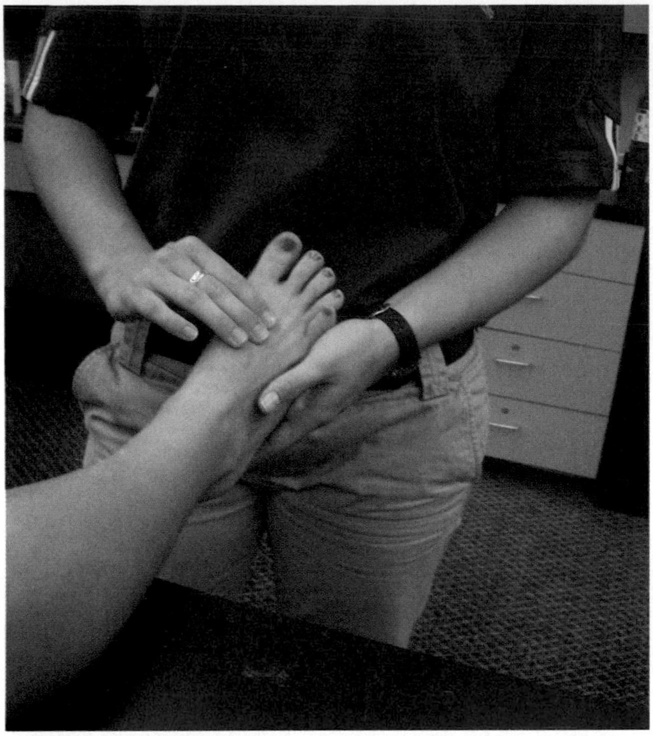

FIGURE 11-4 Dorsalis pedis artery palpation.

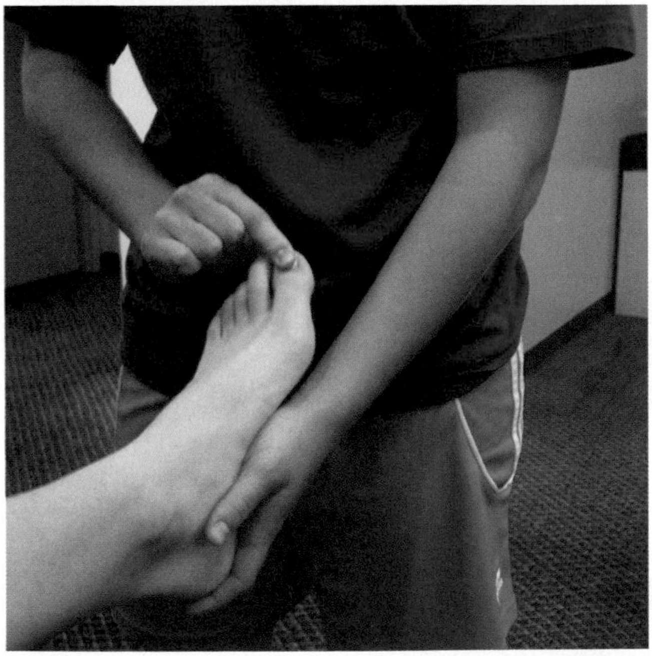

FIGURE 11-5 Capillary refill assessment.

Motor Function

The athlete's ability to actively move the limb using muscles or groups of muscles indicates the level of motor function. However, a better indicator involves the use of manual muscle testing (Table 11-2). If strength testing reveals full strength with no discomfort, the injury is probably minimal. If the strength testing is significantly

TABLE 11-2 Manual Muscle Test Grading

MMT GRADE	RESPONSE FELT DURING TESTING
5/5	The athlete is able to perform the break test, against gravity, with full resistance.
4/5	The athlete is able to perform the break test, against gravity, with some resistance.
3/5	The athlete is able to perform the break test, against gravity, with no resistance. The athlete can get the body part into position but is not able to provide any resistance.
2/5	The athlete is able to get into position, without gravity resistance, but cannot provide any resistive strength.
1/5	The athlete is not able to move the body part into position, even after gravity resistance is removed. The muscle is contracting but not strongly enough to move the body part.
0/5	No muscle contraction is occurring visibly or through palpations.

MMT, Manual muscle testing.

weak and/or painful, further injury-specific special testing will be necessary.

Referrals and Diagnostic Tests

Many knee and thigh injuries cause long-term disability if not properly managed. If, however, they are treated in a timely manner, most of the injuries can be managed without permanent loss of function. Typically, radiographs are used as the first line of diagnostic tools to detect abnormalities in bones and rule out any bony injuries. They may also be used to rule out potential avulsion or epiphyseal fractures in youth. When radiographs are negative but symptoms persist, magnetic resonance imaging (MRI) may be used to diagnose most soft tissue injuries. Keep in mind that any injury accompanied by severe pain or loss of pulse, sensation, or function requires immediate referral to a physician.

MANAGEMENT OF ON-FIELD AND ACUTE KNEE AND THIGH INJURIES

Acute on-field knee and thigh injuries usually involve significant trauma. These injuries include ligament injuries, muscle and tendon ruptures, fractures, and dislocations. If the injury occurs to structures near major arteries or nerves, proper emergent care necessitates activation of your emergency action plan. Figure 11-6 is an overview of the issues surrounding the evaluation, diagnosis, and management of chronic injuries to the knee and thigh.

Ligament Injuries

Of all the acute injuries to the knee, ligamentous injuries provoke the most discussion. Because of the dynamic

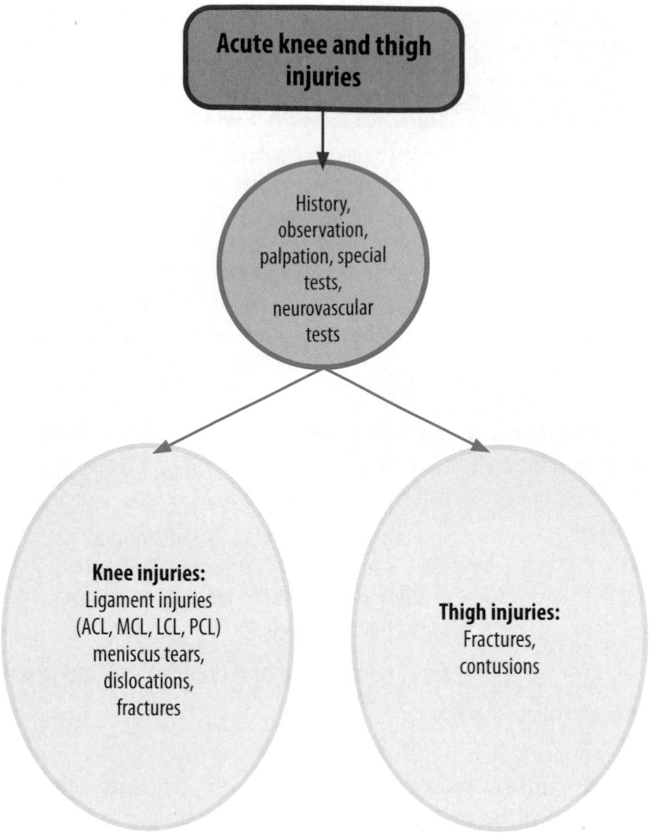

FIGURE 11-6 Concept map overview of acute injuries to the knee and thigh.

nature of sport and most physical occupations, trauma to the knee is a common occurrence. The most frequently injured ligaments in the knee include the anterior cruciate and the medial collateral ligaments.

Ligament Stress Testing

General orthopedic and sports ligament stress testing continues to be the preferred method for evaluation of knee ligament injuries. Although subjective descriptions of mild, moderate, and severe instability are common, objective descriptions are more reliable because they produce more consistent results among examiners. Table 11-3 shows a description of common grades of ligament injury.

Anterior Cruciate Ligament Injury

The anterior cruciate ligament (ACL) provides restraint to anterior translation of the tibia on the femur while in 30 degrees of knee flexion.[19] Additionally, the ACL also assists in controlling varus and valgus stresses on the knee[20] and control of hyperextension stresses.[21–23]

Mechanism: The mechanism of injury for the ACL involves noncontact, plant, and cutting maneuvers in which the foot is firmly on the ground while the knee twists. Additionally, a jump-stop or landing from a jump is another common cause of ACL rupture.

Signs and symptoms:

- Pain
- Instability
- Palpable or audible pop
- Large hemarthrosis that forms with rapid onset
- Decreased ROM and function

Special tests:

Lachman's test: One of the more accurate tests for single-plane ACL integrity is **Lachman's test**. This test accurately assesses the integrity of both the anterior medial band and the posterolateral band of the ACL. To perform Lachman's test, the athletic trainer asks the client to lie supine in a relaxed position holding his or her knee in approximately 20 degrees of knee flexion. To test the right knee, the athletic trainer uses his or her left hand to stabilize the athlete's thigh by grasping firmly just above the knee. The athletic trainer firmly grasps just below the medial side of the right knee on the medial tibia with his or her right hand. While the outer hand maintains (i.e., stabilizes) the thigh, the inner hand draws the tibia anteriorly on the femur (Figure 11-7). A clinical pearl when performing Lachman's test: The athletic trainer places the elbow of his or her outside

TABLE 11-3 Common Grades of Ligament Injury

	FIRST-DEGREE SPRAIN	SECOND-DEGREE SPRAIN	THIRD-DEGREE SPRAIN
Adjunct term	Mild sprain	Moderate sprain	Severe sprain
Symptoms			
Pain	Mild	Moderate	Severe
Swelling	Minimal to none	Minimal to moderate	Severe
ROM	Normal	Minimal to moderate	Moderate to severe
Disability	Mild	Moderate	Severe
Tenderness	Mild	Moderate	Severe
Pathology	Minor tearing	Partial tearing	Complete rupture
Joint opening	<5.0 mm	5.0–10.0 mm	>10.0 mm

ROM, Range of motion.

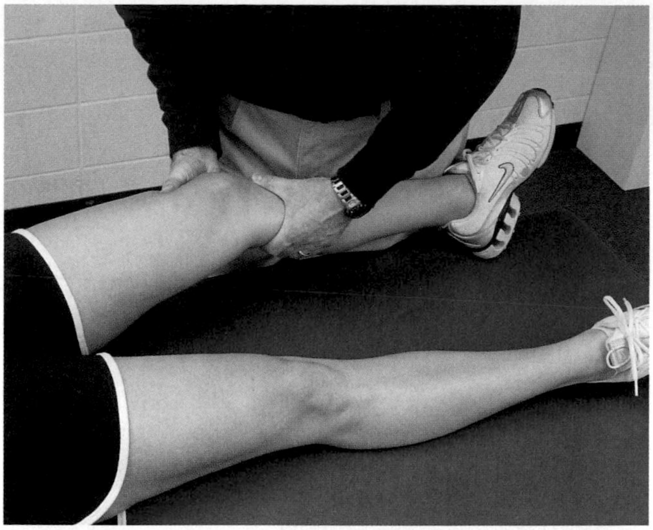

FIGURE 11-7 Lachman's test.

arm on their own iliac crest to assist in stabilization of the femur.[24] In performing this test, the athletic trainer assesses both the quantity (i.e., amount) and the quality (i.e., end-feel) of the anterior translation and compares them to those of the uninjured knee. Testing athletes with large or heavy thighs may be difficult, especially if the athletic trainer has small hands.

Points to Ponder

How could you modify Lachman's test in order to properly assess a suspected rotational knee ligament injury versus a straight ACL injury?

Anterior drawer test: To perform the anterior drawer test, the athletic trainer places the client's knee in 80 to 90 degrees of flexion, with the client's hip flexed at 45 degrees. Some evidence suggests that performance of the anterior drawer examination procedure more accurately tests the anteromedial bundle of the ACL.[25–27] The athletic trainer usually sits on the athlete's outer foot to stabilize the leg in the 80- to 90-degree flexed position. The athletic trainer's hands and fingers are wrapped around the client's proximal tibia. By pulling the tibia in an anterior direction, the athletic trainer can assess the function of the ACL. Just as with the Lachman's test, the athletic trainer assesses for both quality and quantity of the end-feel. Keep in mind that three situations may lead to false readings. First, the hamstrings in this position are antagonistic to the anterior pull of the tibia. Also, a large, tense hemarthrosis of the knee will not generally allow the tibiofemoral joint to achieve the range of 80 to 90 degrees of knee flexion needed to ensure the accuracy of this test. Finally, the shape of the tibiofemoral joint and the intra-articular meniscus may block anterior movement of the tibia on the femur, giving the false impression of an intact ligament.

Immediate management: Immediate management of the ACL injury includes PRICES (protection, rest, ice, compression, elevation, and stabilization). Protection at this juncture includes some form of bracing until it has been determined that the ACL is torn. Because most ACL injuries result in dramatic swelling within approximately 12 hours, cold therapy and compression are almost always indicated. Elevation of the limb promotes proximal drainage of swelling and, even more important, prevention or reduction of edema in the lower leg. If the client is unable to ambulate with a normal gait pattern, use of an assistive device may be warranted until normal gait is achieved.

Intermediate management: An athlete with recurrent instability should be referred to an orthopedic surgeon, because continuing activity with an unstable knee also creates risk of injury to the articular cartilage at the ends of the femur and tibia. Most orthopedic surgeons recommend ACL reconstruction because a functioning ACL is needed for high-level activities and the ACL-deficient knee usually leads to progressive deterioration.[28–33] The ACL is presently repaired with several forms of graft sources, the most common being the bone-patellar tendon-bone repair followed closely by the semitendinosus-gracilis hamstring reconstruction.

Medial Collateral Ligament Injury

The medial collateral ligament (MCL) is often injured as a result of a valgus or combined valgus and external rotation force that exceeds the tensile strength of the ligament.[34] The MCL is primarily responsible for protecting the knee from valgus stress–related mechanisms of injury.

Mechanism: The most common mechanism of injury for the MCL is a clipping force applied to the lateral side of the knee. Other mechanisms for an MCL injury resemble those for an ACL injury. In many cases, both the ACL and the MCL are injured concomitantly. Therefore if one is suspected, the other should also be tested and ruled out.

Signs and symptoms:

- Medial knee pain
- Swelling
- Medial joint laxity (valgus)

Special tests:

Valgus stress test: To perform the valgus stress test of the knee, the athletic trainer asks the client to lie supine with the knee in either full extension or 30 degrees of flexion. Performing the valgus stress test in 30 degrees of flexion isolates the MCL, whereas the same test in full extension stresses multiple structures, including the MCL, ACL, and posterior oblique and the medial portions of the posterior capsule. With the athlete's hip in relative extension and the knee in full extension, the athletic trainer applies a gentle valgus stress by grasping the medial side of the foot with the distal hand, while a

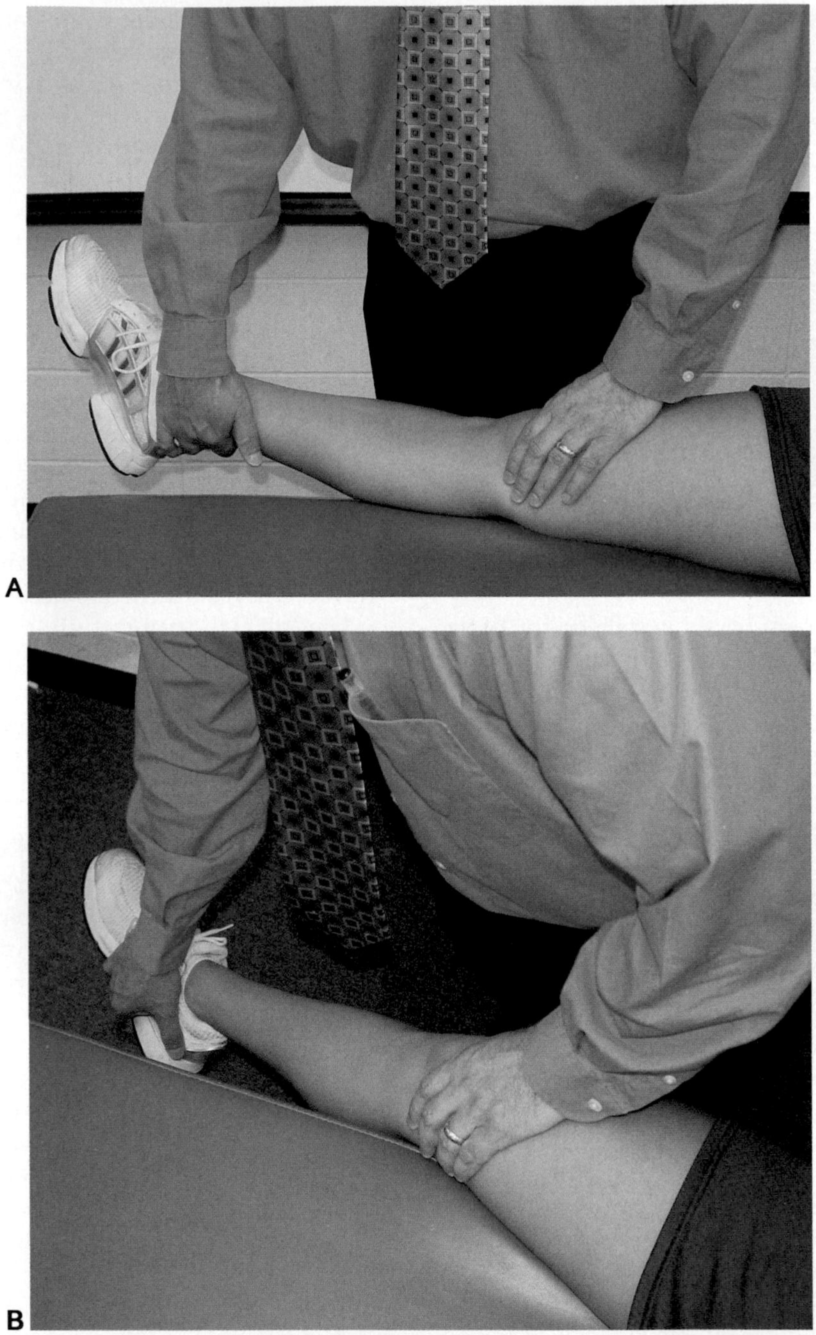

FIGURE 11-8 **A,** Valgus stress test at full knee extension. **B,** Valgus stress test at 30 degrees of knee flexion.

fulcrum is placed at the lateral side of the athlete's knee by the athletic trainer's thigh (Figure 11-8, *A*). A clinical pearl: The athletic trainer first closes the joint into varus to enable palpation of the true joint opening, a method that allows the athletic trainer to feel the medial joint opening. A medial joint opening that is larger than the uninvolved side with a soft end-feel indicates MCL instability. The same description is used when testing at 30 degrees of knee flexion (Figure 11-8, *B*). When the test is positive at 30 degrees of knee flexion, an isolated tear of the MCL is the diagnosis.

Immediate management: Immediate management of the MCL injury is almost identical to that of the ACL. When acute, the MCL injury should be treated in accordance with the PRICES principle. The knee will likely require a double upright hinged knee brace for stability. If the knee can reach full extension without causing pain, the brace should be locked in this position. If terminal extension is painful, the brace can be locked in 20 to 30 degrees of knee flexion until swelling begins to decrease and full extension is possible. If ambulation is painful, crutches should be used until the pain dissipates.

Intermediate management: A nonsurgical approach to treatment of MCL injuries, with early mobilization for even grade III MCL ligament sprains, has become acceptable.[35–37] Most studies have shown excellent healing of the MCL tear without surgical intervention.[38] Grades I and II MCL injuries are treated with early ROM and a short stint in an upright brace until clients achieve full functional ROM without pain or discomfort. Once full ROM is achieved, a progression of resistive exercises, balance drills, and functional exercises may be implemented.

Lateral Collateral Ligament Injury

Lateral collateral ligament (LCL) injuries are rare compared with other ligamentous injuries in the knee. Isolated injuries of the LCL account for only approximately 2% of all knee injuries.[39]

Mechanism: The mechanism of injury for isolated LCL injuries is a varus force applied to the knee, such as would occur if a laterally directed force was applied to the medial knee. LCL sprains and ruptures, which are relatively rare, are responsible for several problems or sequelae (i.e., a disease or disorder that is caused by a preceding disease or injury). If sufficient force is generated, a concomitant injury to the peroneal nerve may occur.

Signs and symptoms:

- Lateral knee pain
- Localized lateral knee edema
- Ecchymosis
- Lateral joint laxity (varus)

Special tests:

Varus stress test: The test of choice for an LCL injury is the varus stress test. As with the valgus stress test, the athletic trainer asks the client to lie supine with his or her knee in either full extension or 30 degrees of flexion. Performing the varus stress test of the knee in 30 degrees of flexion isolates the LCL, whereas the same test in full extension stresses multiple structures, including the LCL, posterolateral capsule, arcuate-popliteus complex, iliotibial band, biceps femoris tendon, ACL, posterior cruciate ligament, and the lateral head of the gastrocnemius muscle.[40] With the individual's hip in relative extension and the knee in full extension, the athletic trainer applies a gentle varus stress by grasping the lateral side of the foot with the distal hand as a fulcrum is placed at the medial side of the individual's knee by the athletic trainer's thigh. A clinical pearl: The athletic trainer first closes the joint into valgus to enable palpation of the true joint opening, a method that allows the athletic trainer to feel the lateral joint opening. A lateral joint opening that is larger than the uninvolved side with a soft end-feel indicates LCL instability. The same applies when testing at 30 degrees of knee flexion.

Immediate management: Immediate management of the torn LCL is identical to that of the MCL: PRICES.

Points to Ponder

After performing a varus or valgus stress test, you determine that the individual has a positive finding in full extension. Knowing that the ACL can also be compromised, you perform Lachman's test, with positive findings. What could be the possible mechanisms of injury (MOI) that resulted in a combined anteromedial and anterolateral instability?

Special care should be taken to assess peroneal nerve function because peroneal nerves may be injured concomitantly. A double upright hinged brace used soon after the injury occurs may help control varus forces on the knee. Weight bearing should progress as tolerated; the client may start out with crutches if ambulation is painful.

Intermediate management: Depending on the severity of injury, a regimen of progressive resistive exercises can usually be initiated between 4 and 6 weeks after injury. Crutches may be discontinued when the client can achieve full passive knee extension and control his or her body weight while performing a single-leg mini-squat through 30 degrees of knee flexion on the involved side.[38] Sometimes, the orthopedic surgeon and the client decide that surgery is the best option.

Posterior Cruciate Ligament Injury

The posterior cruciate ligament (PCL) spans the posterior intercondylar region of the tibia to the medial condyle of the femur. It prevents the tibia from moving posterior relative to the femur. The PCL is not commonly injured.

Mechanism: Several mechanisms can cause rupture of the PCL. Probably the most common is a direct blow to the anterior tibia, which drives it in a posterior direction.[41] This injury, sometimes called a "dashboard injury," usually occurs as the result of a motor vehicle accident in which the passenger is moving in a forward (anterior) direction while his or her tibia hits the dashboard, driving it in a posterior direction. This injury also may occur when an athlete falls and lands directly on the anterior tibia. Other causes include hyperflexion and hyperextension maneuvers, which often injure the ACL concomitantly.

Signs and symptoms:

- Large, tense knee effusion
- Little discomfort in 30 degrees of flexion
- Discomfort attempting to flex the knee beyond 90 degrees

Special tests:

Tibial sag test: A tibial sag test, by which the examiner may evaluate a potential PCL rupture, can be performed in several ways. The client may be placed in a supine position with both knees flexed at approximately 80 degrees, with the hips flexed at 45. With the quadriceps and the hamstrings relaxed in this position, the

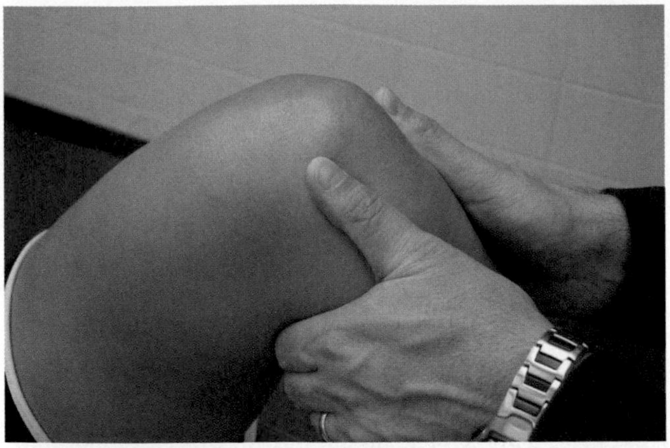

FIGURE 11-9 Step-up test.

tibia on the involved side should sag posteriorly compared with that of the uninvolved side.

Step-up test: The step-up test uses the same position as that used for the tibial sag test. The athletic trainer places his or her thumb pads on the distal femoral condyles and the interphalangeal joints of the same thumbs on the tibial plateau. In a normal stable knee, the tibial plateau should be about 1 centimeter anterior to the distal condyles of the femur (Figure 11-9). An absence of this step-up appearance indicates PCL rupture.[24]

Posterior drawer test: The posterior drawer test somewhat resembles the anterior drawer used to test the ACL. With the athlete supine, the hip flexed 45 degrees, and the knee flexed 80 degrees, the athletic trainer wraps his or her fingers around the proximal tibia. The athletic trainer gives a posteriorly directed force to the proximal tibia with his or her thumbs. The test is positive when the examiner determines that the translation was increased or detects a soft end-feel during the testing.

Immediate management: Immediate management is to that of the other knee ligament injuries discussed: PRICES. Neurovascular assessment helps the athletic trainer rule out any neurovascular injuries as a potential cause of symptoms. The client will need to apply cold and compressive dressings to the knee.

Intermediate management: Protected weight bearing should be instituted until a physician rules out other potential conditions. In the past, these injuries were generally treated conservatively, although reconstruction for PCL injuries has recently become more commonplace.

Meniscus Tears

The medial and lateral **menisci** are cartilaginous structures that lie between the femur and the tibia and fibula. They provide shock absorption during weight bearing and structural integrity to the knee and also disperse friction with movement. Concave on the top so that the femur can glide smoothly, the menisci are relatively stable on the tibia as a result of their flat underside. Both menisci are attached to the tibia.

Mechanism: The meniscus may be injured in several ways, and most incidents appear at first to be relatively insignificant. These injuries usually occur with some form of planting and twisting, possibly the result of landing in an awkward manner. Meniscus injuries may also be caused by severe trauma that injures other ligaments and structures in the knee. It is not uncommon for the meniscus to be injured along with the ACL.

Signs and symptoms:

- Catching
- Locking
- Pain
- Swelling
- Possible effusion (vascular tears have increased swelling)

Special tests:

McMurray test: The classic meniscus test, the McMurray test,[42] is performed while the subject assumes a supine position. The athletic trainer grasps the client's knee with the proximal hand while the distal hand grasps the athlete's foot and ankle. The tibia is internally rotated on the femur with a force applied at the athlete's foot. The more proximal hand at the knee palpates the joint line to assess for clicking or popping sensations. The proximal hand also imparts a varus stress to the medial knee as it is moved into and then out of a flexed position. A second flexion movement is then performed with a valgus stress to the lateral portion of the knee while the foot is externally rotated, again moving from an extended to a flexed position (Figure 11-10). Several symptoms may indicate a meniscus tear, including clicking, snapping, popping, locking, pseudolocking, and pain in the lateral or medial joint line.

The recurvatum test: In most cases, a positive recurvatum test indicates a radial tear that extends into the anterior portion of the medial or lateral meniscus.[24] While the client lies in a relaxed supine position, the athletic trainer passively extends the client's knee with overpressure at the end range of motion. Medial or lateral joint line pain that replicates the client's symptoms is considered a positive response.

Immediate management: Immediate diagnosis and management of this injury is sometimes difficult, especially when the tear is small. Much easier to diagnose is the large bucket handle tear, which causes a substantial block to knee flexion or extension (or both). Treatment obviously depends on symptoms and the degree of tear. Absolute surgical indications are reserved for those with a bucket handle tear that causes the knee to lock. Otherwise, conservative treatment to relieve pain,

menisci cartilaginous structures that lie between the femur and the tibia and fibula; provide shock absorption and stability to the knee

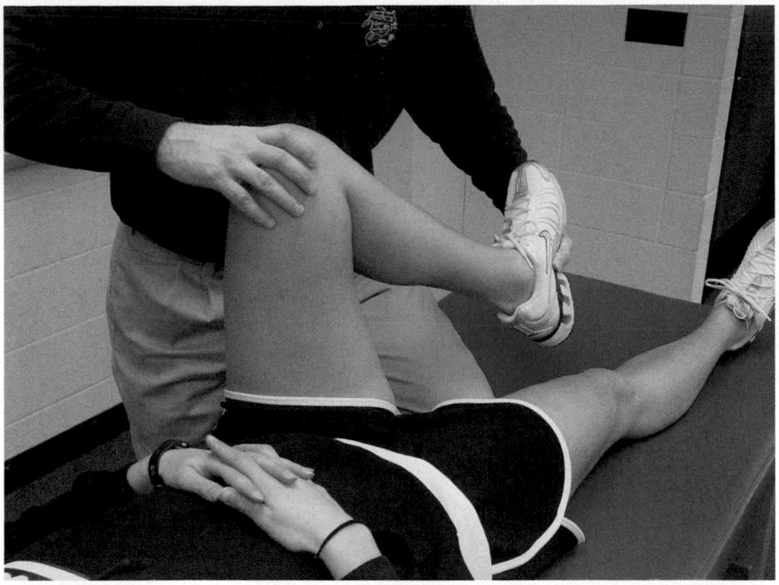

FIGURE 11-10 McMurray test.

swelling, and intermittent catching and locking should commence (i.e., PRICES).

Intermediate management: If symptoms are not relieved after 6 to 12 weeks, surgery may be indicated.[43] Surgical procedures for a torn meniscus depend on the type of tear. If the tear is in the inner portion of the meniscus where there is less blood supply, the edges are simply smoothed down. If the tear is in a portion of the meniscus that has a good blood supply, it will be repaired by use of fixation devices such as sutures, tacks, or darts.

Knee Dislocations

Dislocations of the knee involve either the tibiofemoral joint or the patellofemoral joint. Because of the size of the joint and the structures located in the popliteal fossa, the tibiofemoral dislocation is typically a medical emergency. Patellofemoral joint dislocation is much less serious, albeit a very painful injury that requires adequate emergent treatment.

Tibiofemoral Dislocations

Of all the injuries discussed to this point, tibiofemoral knee dislocation is the injury that presents the greatest risk for loss of the leg. Because of the location of vasculature in the posterior knee, a tibiofemoral dislocation carries an extremely high risk for resultant vascular insult. Therefore a suspected tibiofemoral dislocation always should be considered an extreme medical emergency until proven otherwise, one that requires activation of the emergency action plan.

Mechanism: Tibiofemoral dislocations are the result of violent impact to the knee. They can be caused by direct impact from another object or a fall onto an object or the ground. Knee dislocations are generally classified in terms of the tibial displacement with respect to the femur[44] (Figure 11-11).

Signs and symptoms:

- Deformity (obvious or slight)
- Pain
- Effusion
- Loss of, or altered, function
- Possible affected pulse distal to the injury
- Possible affected neurological findings distal to the injury

Special tests: No special tests are applicable.

Immediate management: Immediate management of this condition involves immobilization and referral to the emergency room for evaluation and monitoring of neurovascular structures. Of potential concern is that devastating insult may occur to the popliteal artery after a dislocation despite the fact that pulses may still exist on clinical examination.[45] Additionally, careful attention should be paid to the peroneal and tibial nerves, which are commonly injured with this type of dislocation. Because these injuries are usually the result of high-energy trauma, possible fracture should always be suspected. If it appears as though the knee has been dislocated, the athletic trainer should not attempt to move the limb or realign it. If no evidence of deformity exists, the knee may be placed in an immobilizer. Assessment of both circulation and nerve function should be done serially every several minutes until the client is in the care of emergency medical personnel. Definite reasons for immediate transfer to a medical facility include loss of pulse distal to the injured site, loss of superficial sensation, discoloration, and coldness.[46]

Intermediate management: Depending on the clinical findings at the hospital, conservative treatment and rehabilitation may begin once all neurovascular and

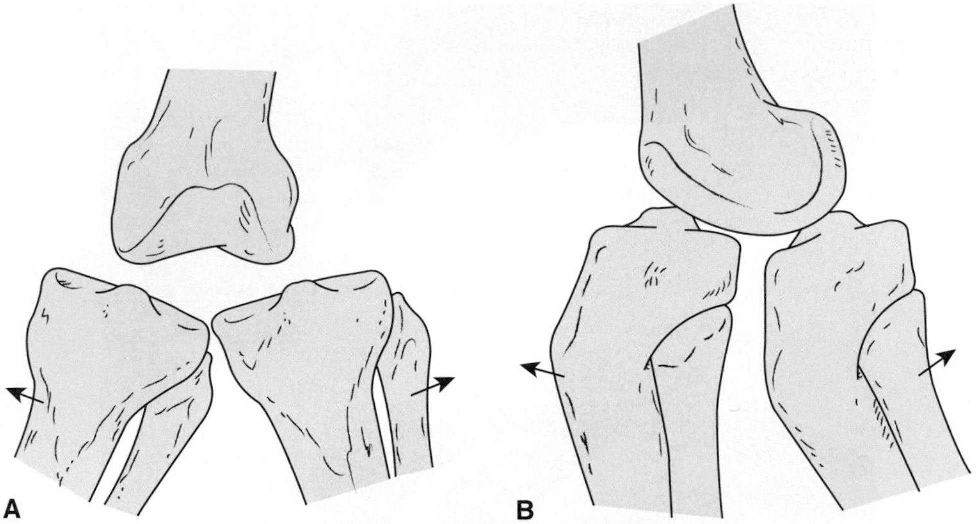

FIGURE 11-11 Tibiofemoral dislocation. **A,** Medial–lateral. **B,** Anterior–posterior.

fracture concerns are addressed. Because other structures may be involved in this injury, management is frequently tailored to each specific case.

Patellofemoral Dislocations

The patella may be either subluxed or dislocated. Most subluxations or dislocations occur in the lateral direction. Patellar subluxation occurs when the patella is partially displaced from the trochlea of the anterior distal femur. A patellar dislocation occurs when the patella, a sesamoid bone, is completely displaced out of the knee joint.

Mechanism: Patellofemoral dislocations usually result from one of two insults. First, internal rotation of the thigh during weight bearing while the foot is planted may cause an unusual load or pull of the quadriceps. The rapid change of direction forces the quadriceps to contract in an abnormal alignment, thus allowing the patella to be pulled laterally. Second, blunt force trauma may cause the patella to dislocate. Note that most patella dislocations occur in women, who have wider pelvises and resulting Q-angles.

Signs and symptoms:
- Giving-way sensation
- Deformity (lateral displacement)
- Sensation of knee shifting medially
- Effusion
- Hemarthrosis
- Severe ecchymosis (mostly medial)
- Tenderness (typically medial)

Special tests:

Fairbank test: The Fairbank test of patellar apprehension is performed with the knee in full extension.[47] For assessment of a patellar dislocation or patellar instability, a straight lateral glide is imparted onto the patella. In an individual with patellar instability, an urge to maintain knee stability will ensue after a contraction of the quadriceps muscle to prevent the patella from subluxing or dislocating when mobilized by the athletic trainer. An important clinical pearl: This test may elicit apprehension rather than outright pain.

Points to Ponder

One individual reacts to the Fairbank test by constantly contracting the quadriceps each time you attempt to perform the lateral patellar glide. Another individual complains of intense pain each time you attempt to perform the lateral patellar glide. Do both test positive for patellar instability? How can you determine which individual may have a more recent patellar dislocation?

Immediate management: If still dislocated, the knee will probably be in a flexed position in which the femoral condyles are very prominent. Reduction may occur as the client extends the knee. Although this reduction may significantly reduce the level of the individual's pain, other potential injuries, such as a fracture or an osteochondral defect, may be present. Therefore immediate management includes immobilization and transportation to an appropriate medical facility for radiographic evaluation.[48]

Intermediate management: As with tibiofemoral dislocation, conservative treatment of patellofemoral dislocation may begin once all possibilities of neurovascular involvement and fractures are ruled out.

Knee Fractures

Knee fractures result from a very violent blow to the leg, possibly from coming into contact with another person or object or stopping and planting with the foot and leg in an awkward position. Various fractures may occur in this region. However, patellar fractures are the most common sports-related knee fracture. Fractures of any kind are a medical emergency; therefore the emergency action plan should be activated immediately.

Regardless of the type of fracture, decisions must be made to justify the need to obtain a radiograph. To prevent unnecessary exposure, two clinical rules have been established to help in this decision-making process: The first rule, the **Pittsburgh knee rule**, recommends obtaining a radiograph for patients with a recent history of a fall or blunt trauma, those who are younger than 12 years of age or older than 50 years, and those who are unable to take at least four weight-bearing steps in the emergency department. The second rule, the **Ottawa knee rule**, is more sensitive. It specifies that a radiograph should be obtained if the individual exhibits any of the following five conditions: The patient is age 55 years or older, experiences tenderness at the head of the fibula, experiences isolated tenderness of the patella, is unable to flex the knee to 90 degrees, and is unable to bear weight for four steps immediately and in the examination room regardless of limping.[49]

Patellar Fractures

Patellar fractures are divided into several categories: transverse, vertical, upper pole, lower pole, comminuted, and osteochondral. Each of these fractures can be displaced or nondisplaced. Often, the mechanism of injury determines whether the fracture is displaced or not.

Mechanism: Fractures of the patella in active individuals may be caused by direct or indirect forces. A direct force occurs when some form of blunt trauma affects the knee, such as when two opposing players make patella-to-patella contact during a soccer match or a marathon runner trips and lands with full body weight directly onto the anterior knee. Indirect forces involve a forceful contraction of the quadriceps muscle in a patella that has lost full strength. This indirect mechanism has been known to happen among athletes returning from an ACL repair in which a portion of the tibia was removed for the reconstructed graft, a procedure that weakens the existing patella.[50,51]

Signs and symptoms:
- Inability to flex or extend the knee because of severe pain
- Pronounced, immediate swelling
- Deformity
- Possible gapping at the injury site

Special tests:

Tap or percussion test: The tap or percussion test may be used to identify a patellar fracture. Gently tapping on an area of the patella that does not appear to be involved should elicit a pain that radiates directly to the fractured site. Because the patella is not a long bone, as typically prescribed for the tap or percussion test, this should not be used as a primary means of diagnosis.

Immediate management: Immediate management of a patellar fracture includes immobilization with referral to a physician for diagnostic tests.

Intermediate management: Simple fractures are usually managed with immobilization, whereas displaced or comminuted fractures generally require surgical repair.

Thigh Injuries

Acute thigh injuries often include fractures and contusions. Not only is the thigh composed of the largest bone in the human body, the femur; it is also surrounded by several of the largest muscles in the body, including the quadriceps and hamstring groups. Acute injury to this area often leads to the development of a debilitating condition.

Femur Fractures

Femur fractures are common in sporting activities and require activation of the emergency action plan for immediate physician follow-up and diagnostic testing. Common forms of fractures found in the active population include distal femoral and supracondylar fractures.

Mechanism: Direct, forceful contact with an object or another person can cause fractures. Falling onto a hard surface is another mechanism of injury.

Signs and symptoms:
- Pain
- Deformity
- Swelling
- Ecchymosis
- Loss of motion
- Possible loss of pulse and sensation (depending on the severity of the fracture)

Special tests: Tap or percussion tests may be used. In most cases, the deformity is so significant and obvious that no special tests are warranted to diagnose a thigh fracture.

Pittsburgh knee rule recommends obtaining a radiograph for patients with a recent fall or blunt trauma, those who are younger than 12 years of age or older than 50 years, and those who are unable to take at least four weight-bearing steps in the emergency department

Ottawa knee rule specifies that if the individual exhibits any of the following five conditions, a radiograph should be obtained: age 55 years or older; tenderness at the head of the fibula; isolated tenderness of the patella; inability to flex the knee to 90 degrees; and an inability to bear weight for four steps immediately and in the examination room regardless of limping

Immediate management: Immediate management of a thigh fractures includes immobilization with referral to a physician for diagnostic tests.

Intermediate management: Simple fractures are usually managed with immobilization, whereas displaced or comminuted fractures generally require surgical stabilization procedures.

Quadriceps Contusion

Sports-related quadriceps contusions are common. Depending on the specific activity, athletes may sustain contusions regularly. The management of these contusions, which can become quite a nuisance, is what ultimately determines the athlete's outcome.

Mechanism: Quadriceps contusions are particularly likely to occur in contact sports such as football, soccer, hockey, rugby, and basketball, as a result of blunt force trauma from an object or contact with the opposing player's body.

Signs and symptoms:

- Pain
- Swelling
- Ecchymosis
- Limited range of motion, especially with knee flexion
- Difficulty with ambulation caused by painful or nonexistent quadriceps contractions
- Tenderness during palpation

Special tests: No special tests are applicable.

Immediate management: Immediate management includes PRICES, with the focus on cold compression to the anterior knee. While cold compression is being applied, the knee should be placed in as much flexion as the client can tolerate. Heat is strongly discouraged because it will increase bleeding and cause further swelling. Additionally, soft tissue massage is discouraged because it may disrupt the normal clotting process and restart the active bleeding process in the anterior knee. As pain decreases, knee flexion ROM should be continually increased to tolerance.[52] If pain is severe, the athlete may require crutches for assistance with ambulation until sufficient quadriceps firing has returned.

Intermediate management: Decreasing bleeding in the thigh after a contusion may lessen the risk of **myositis ossificans.** This complication is common when severe contusions continue to receive traumatic blows. Essentially, bone begins to develop in the midst of all the red blood cells that have accumulated as a result of hemorrhage. Monitoring the healing rate of the contusion as well as providing ample padding to prevent repeated blows can also decrease the likelihood that myositis ossificans will develop. Pain-free activities should begin as soon as possible, as should activities to increase ROM.

Box 11-3 summarizes the acute injuries of the knee and thigh and the appropriate special tests associated with each.

BOX 11-3 Acute Knee and Thigh Injuries and Appropriate Special Tests

Ligament Injuries

Anterior Cruciate Ligament Injury
Lachman's test
Anterior drawer test

Medial Collateral Ligament Injury
Valgus stress test of the knee

Lateral Collateral Ligament Injury
Varus stress test of the knee

Posterior Collateral Ligament Injury
Tibial sag test
Step-up test
Posterior drawer test

Meniscus Tears

McMurray test
Recurvatum test

Knee Dislocations

Tibiofemoral Dislocations
No special tests applicable

Patellofemoral Dislocations
Fairbank test

Knee Fractures

Patellar Fractures
Tap or percussion test

Thigh Injuries

Femur Fractures
Tap or percussion test

Epiphyseal Fractures
Tap or percussion test

Quadriceps Contusion
No special tests applicable

Prevention of Acute Injuries

Prevention of acute injuries relies on adequate conditioning and warm-up activities as well as protective equipment. Conditioning and warm-up activities should address muscular strength, muscular endurance, and muscle tendon unit flexibility as well as other fitness components, such as power, speed, agilities, and reaction

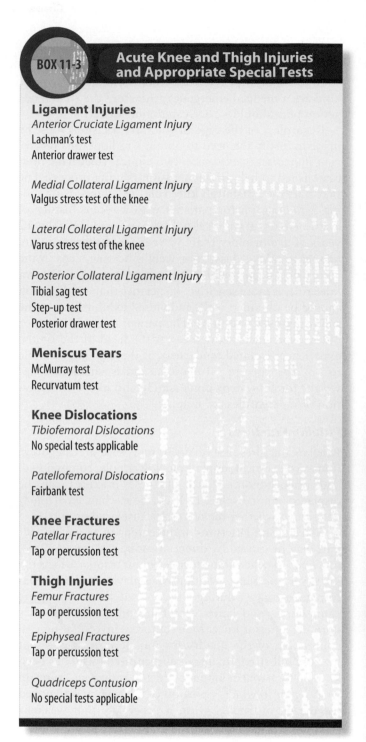

myositis ossificans inflammation of muscle tissue marked by ossification of the intramuscular fascia time. The more fit an individual is, the less likely he or she is to sustain an injury. Some people believe that prophylactic knee bracing may be beneficial for some knee injuries. As with most sports injuries, however, complete prevention of injury is impossible to achieve and should not be expected.

MANAGEMENT OF CHRONIC AND OVERUSE KNEE AND THIGH INJURIES

Knee and thigh overuse injuries are often caused by repetitive microtrauma related to specific activity that overloads the various connective tissues, tendons, muscles, and bones surrounding the affected area. Clients with overuse injuries often complain of localized knee or thigh pain and do not have a history of acute injury or macrotrauma.

More than 100 years ago, anatomists recognized that biological tissue adapts to the level of stress placed on it.[53,54] A **stress-strain curve** illustrates the way in which connective tissue adapts to physical stress (Figure 11-12). If the stress-strain load on the connective tissue exceeds the tensile strength of the collagen fibers, fiber failure occurs, resulting in injury. Similarly, when the combination of stress and strain exceeds the elastic characteristics of the connective tissue, permanent tissue elongation (i.e., lengthening or flexibility) occurs. This adaptation may be a desirable result of the activity. Several clinicians have applied this concept to musculoskeletal overuse injuries,[2,55,56] with the premise being that all biological tissues accommodate their structure and composition to meet the mechanical demands placed on them.

After injury, the tissues can no longer tolerate stresses to the same degree. The stress thresholds have been lowered, and athletes are less equipped to tolerate activities that they could easily perform before the injury (Figure 11-13). Stress levels that did not cause pain before the injury may now result in pain and further tissue damage. It is up to the athletic trainer to assist clients in reducing the stresses applied to the area until they have achieved a certain level of tissue homeostasis. Once inflammation has subsided, clients may begin to load the joint under supervision, which promotes tissue adaptation and resumption of their prior level of activity. Applying this tissue-stress model helps the athletic trainer in treating overuse injuries of the knee and thigh in a consistent and logical manner, even when the exact mechanism of the overuse injury is unknown. A five-step process summarizing the use of a tissue-stress model in the diagnosis and management of overuse injuries is shown in Table 11-4.

Figure 11-14 is a concept map overview of the issues surrounding evaluation, diagnosis, and management of chronic injuries to the knee and thigh.

stress-strain curve concept illustrating how connective tissue adapts to physical stress

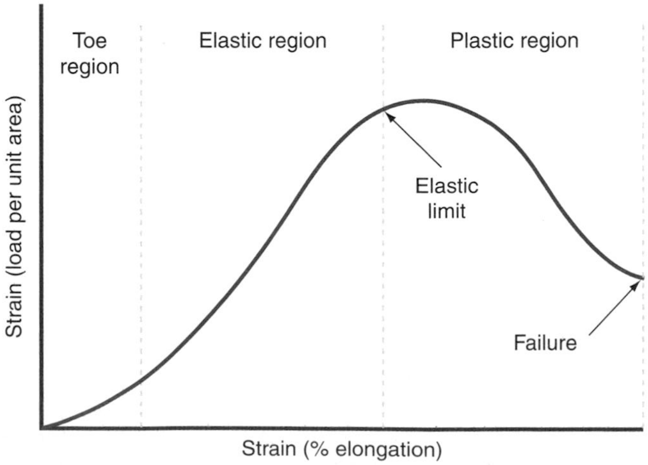

FIGURE 11-12 Stress-strain curve for connective tissue. Elastic region is that portion of the curve in which tissue returns to its original length when the stress is removed. Plastic region is that portion of the curve that results in permanent elongation when the stress is removed. (Modified from Kisner C, Colby, LA: *Therapeutic exercise: foundations and techniques*, ed 3, Philadelphia, 1996, FA Davis.)

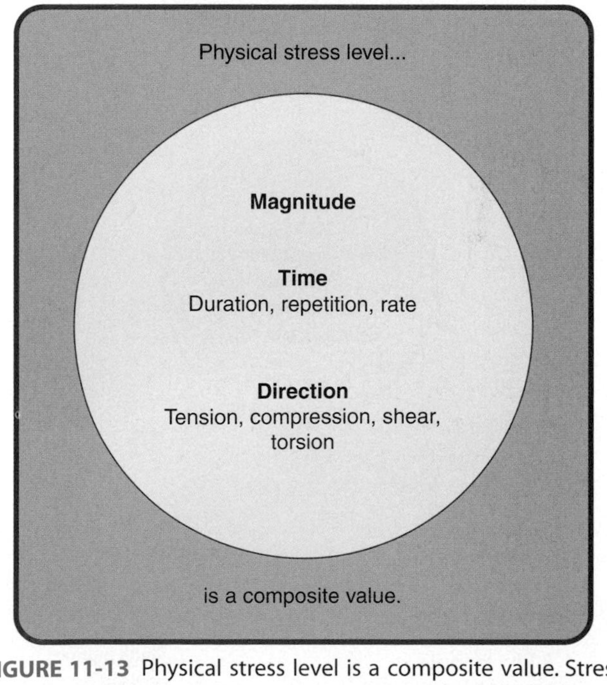

FIGURE 11-13 Physical stress level is a composite value. Stress magnitude refers to the amount of stress (force per unit area) on a tissue. Time factors include the duration, number of repetitions, and the rate at which stress is applied to tissues of the body. Stress will have a different effect depending on whether it is applied in tension, compression, shear, or torsion. (Redrawn from Mueller MJ, Maluf KS: Tissue adaptation to physical stress: a proposed "Physical Stress Theory" to guide physical therapist practice, education, and research, *Phys Ther* 82[4]:383–403, 2002.)

TABLE 11-4 Diagnosis and Management of Overuse Injuries Using a Tissue Stress Model

STEP	DESCRIPTION
Step 1: History	Identify biological tissue being stressed. This is accomplished by careful questioning of the athlete regarding their current symptoms, training habits, and current sport demands.
Step 2: Examination	Careful examination of the patient using selected tests and measures to reproduce the stresses described in step 1. The goal is to load the tissues in a controlled manner and thereby reproduce the athlete's symptoms.
Step 3: Evaluation	Using the results of the testing in step 3, determine whether the athlete's complaints are a result of excess tissue loading. Consider the factors of force magnitude, time application of force, and force direction.
Step 4: Interventions	Develop a treatment protocol that will reduce tissue stress, promote healing, and allow the tissues to return to a level of homeostasis.
Step 5: Re-evaluation	Repeat tests used in step 2, and assess effectiveness of interventions used in step 4. Reduce or increase tissue stress in order to return athlete's knee to an envelope of function that includes all desired athletic activities.

Modified from McPoil TG, Hunt GC: Evaluation and management of foot and ankle disorders: present problems and future directions, *J Orthop Sports Phys Ther* 21(6):381–388, 1995.

Stress Fractures of the Femoral Shaft

Stress fractures are fatigue-failure injuries of bone common among endurance and repetitive motion athletes such as runners, dancers, jumpers, and skaters.[57,58] They constitute 10% of all sports-related injuries, with the most common site being the tibia.[58] Femoral stress fractures are not as common as tibial stress fractures, constituting approximately 5% of all sports-related stress fractures.[57,59] Use of the tissue-stress model facilitates the appropriate diagnosis and management of these overuse injuries.

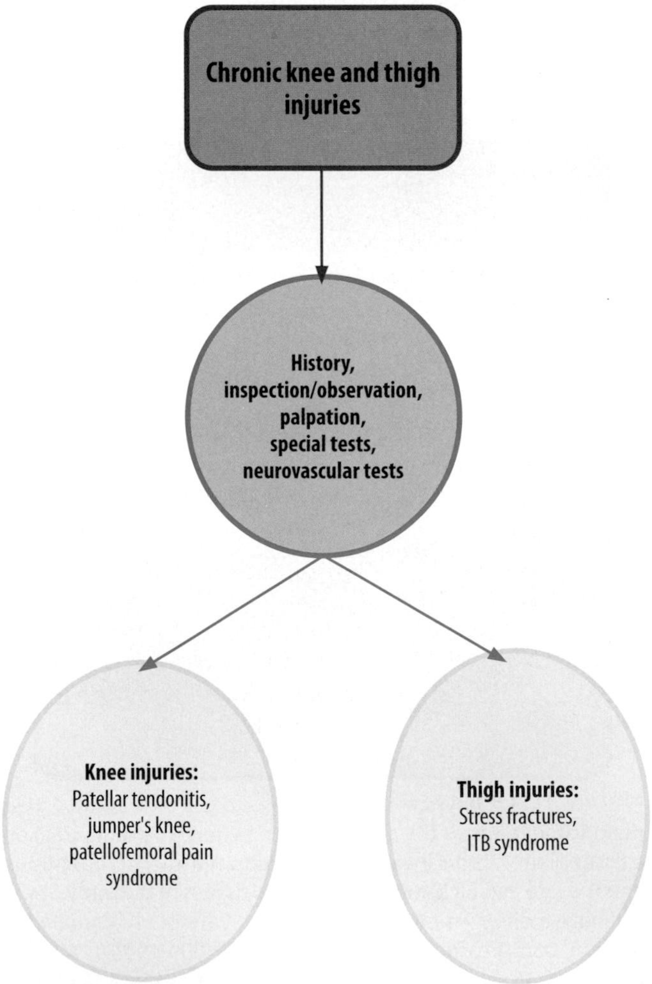

FIGURE 11-14 Concept map overview of chronic injuries to the knee and thigh.

Mechanism: A stress fracture is the result of an injury causing an initial stress reaction to the point of bony microfailure but without true disruption in the integrity of the bone.[60] Femoral stress fractures, or overuse injuries, represent a failure of the bone that results from an accumulation of repetitive microtrauma. This excessive loading creates an imbalance between bone formation and reabsorption. The athlete's threshold of injury, or "envelope of function," has been breached, preventing continued activity at the previous level.

Signs and symptoms:

- A history of repetitive impact exercise
- A nondescript history reflecting no specific mechanism of injury
- Insidious onset
- Pain with weight bearing that is relieved with rest
- Recent change in the intensity or volume of the training regimen

Special tests:

Hop test: The **hop test** is performed by asking the client to hop on the injured leg.[57] If the client's symptoms are reproduced, the test is considered positive.

Fulcrum test: The **fulcrum test** is performed by having the client sit on the examination table while one of the athletic trainer's arms is placed under the client's thigh.[61] This arm is used as a fulcrum under the thigh while gentle pressure is applied to the ventral side of the knee with the opposite hand (Figure 11-15). The test is repeated several times as the fulcrum arm is moved proximally under the thigh.

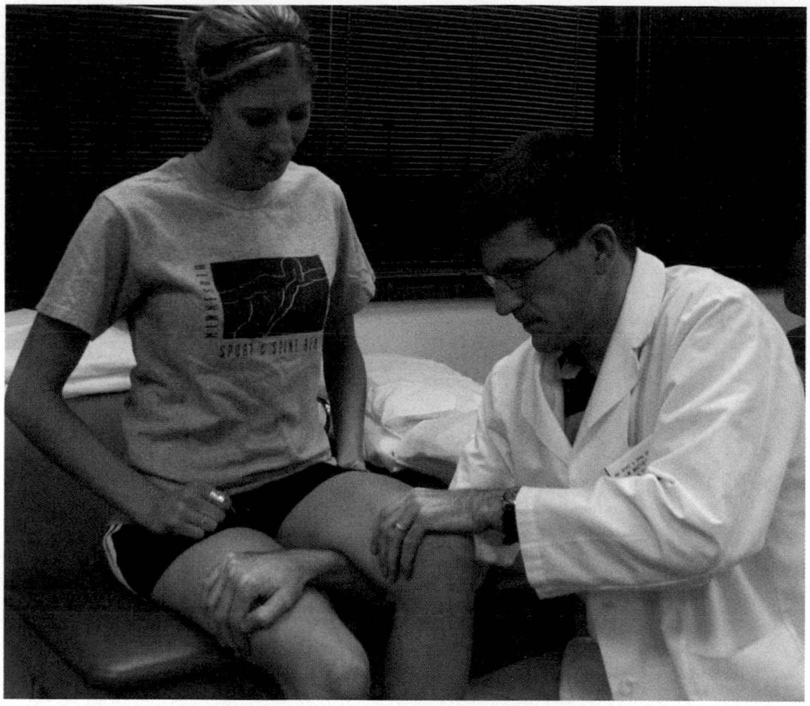

FIGURE 11-15 Fulcrum test for femoral shaft stress fracture.

Immediate management: With early accurate diagnosis, an initial period of nonweight bearing and modification of the client's activities is quite successful. Radiographs are always obtained to rule out serious bony abnormalities. Diagnosis of stress fractures is typically confirmed by either nuclear bone scan or magnetic resonance imaging. A four-phase treatment algorithm for the management of femoral shaft stress fractures[62] is shown in Figure 11-16.

Intermediate management: A delayed diagnosis may lead to progression to a complete fracture, which requires surgical stabilization and intense rehabilitation before previous activities may be resumed.

Iliotibial Band Syndrome

Iliotibial band (ITB) syndrome is one of the most common causes of chronic lateral knee pain in triathletes, cyclists, and distance runners.[63] Often, when the athlete is experiencing symptoms only during activity, the results of the physical examination are normal and no tenderness over the ITB is present. Runners with ITB syndrome have been found to have weak hip abductors and rotators, weak knee flexors and extensors, and a tight ITB/TFL complex.[10,64]

Mechanism: Frequently, overuse or the inappropriate timing of a training session initiates or aggravates the client's knee symptoms. Moreover, overuse, fatigue, breakdown of technique, and poor timing all can exacerbate an ITB injury. Running downhill, sprint training on a track or bike, frequent running on the same side of crowned surfaces (paved roads), a sharp increase in mileage, and prolonged sitting with the knees higher than the hips also cause ITB syndrome.

Signs and symptoms:

- Sharp pain or burning occurs in the lateral knee.
- Activity does not cause pain at first; symptoms arise after a certain distance or time.
- Pain subsides after activities stop but returns as soon as activity is resumed.
- Activities of daily living, especially ascending or descending stairs, are adversely affected.

Special tests:

Compression test: For the compression test, the client assumes a supine position with the knee flexed to 90 degrees (the hip flexes as well). The athletic trainer then applies pressure with the thumb at the lateral femoral epicondyle while the client slowly extends the knee. The test is positive if the client complains of pain and the symptoms are reproduced at 30 degrees over the lateral femoral epicondyle.[7,63]

Immediate management: Initially, a brief period of rest from the repetitive activities of running or cycling is recommended. The athlete may use an upper body ergometer or swim with a pool buoy between the legs to maintain cardiovascular fitness. ROM and muscle length issues may be addressed with daily stretching and foam roll mobilization routines.

iliotibial band (ITB) syndrome chronic syndrome responsible for lateral knee pain in triathletes, cyclists, and distance runners characterized by weak hip abductors and knee flexors and extensors and a tight ITB/tensor fasciae latae (TFL) complex

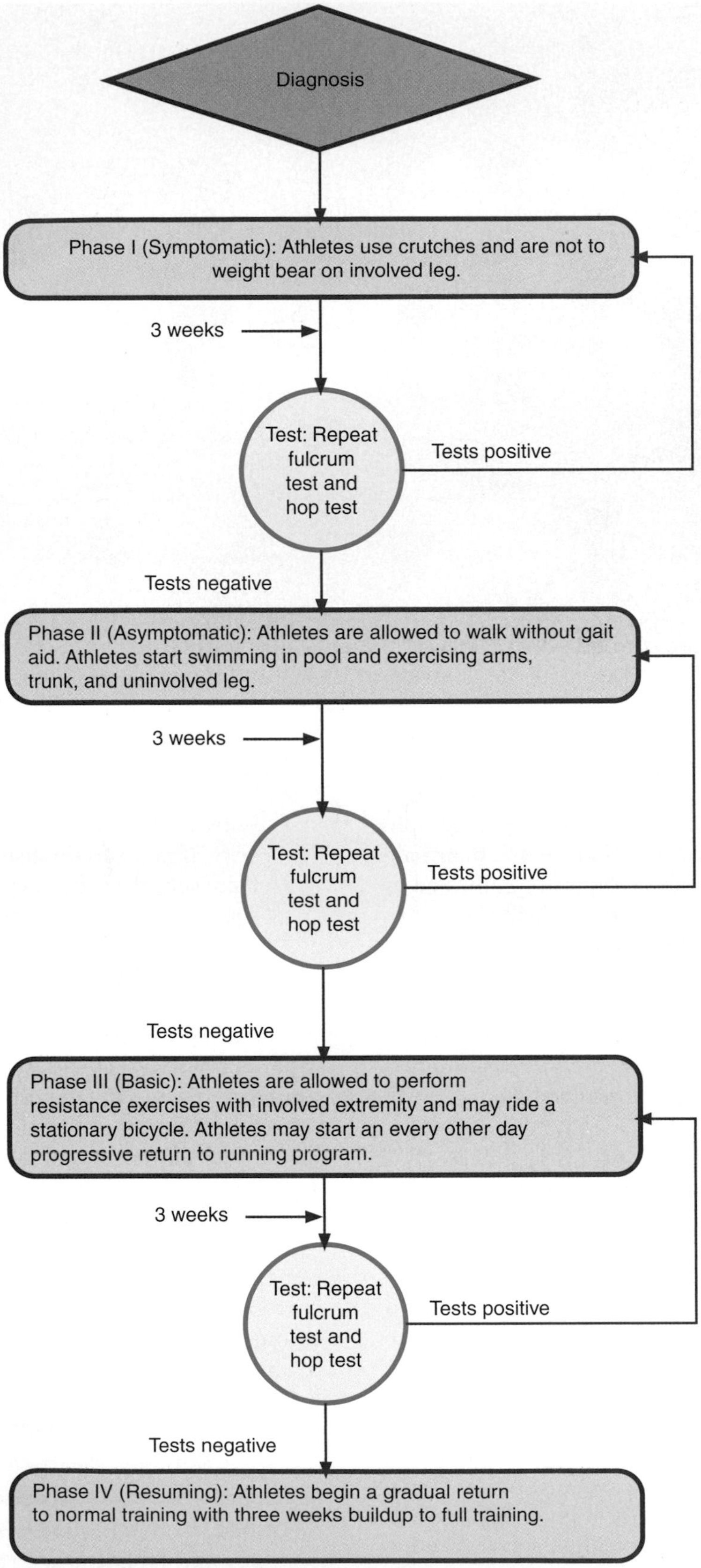

FIGURE 11-16 Femoral shaft stress fracture treatment algorithm. (Redrawn from Ivkovic A, Bojanic I, Pecina M: Stress fractures of the femoral shaft in athletes: a new treatment algorithm, *Br J Sports Med* 40[6]: 518–520, 2006.)

Intermediate management: Strengthening exercises may be initiated once ROM and myofascial restrictions are normalized. Strengthening exercises should focus on functional strengthening of the lumbopelvic and lower extremity muscle groups. First, a program of concentric side-lying hip abduction, single leg step-downs, and pelvic drop exercises is implemented.[64] Once the athlete has mastered these exercises, these single plane exercises may be increased to multiple plane exercises with integrated functional movement patterns. As exercises are advanced, eccentric loading of the gluteus minimus, gluteus medius, and TFL in a single-leg stance is emphasized.[11]

Patellar Tendonitis/Tendinopathy (Jumper's Knee)

A common misconception is that symptomatic tendon injuries represent an inflammatory process. Consequently, **patellar tendinopathy** (jumper's knee) is often mislabeled as patellar tendonitis.[65,66] Acute inflammatory tendon injuries do exist. However, many athletes arrive for evaluation with chronic knee symptoms suggesting a degenerative, disorganized condition in the patellar tendon that should be labeled correctly as patellar tendinosis or tendinopathy. The clinical differentiation between tendonitis and tendinosis is based on the chronicity of the knee pain and presence, or lack thereof, of inflammation. If the condition has been present for more than 2 to 3 weeks, patellar tendinosis should be suspected. Patellar tendonitis, the acute response, is accompanied by inflammation.

Mechanism: Patellar tendinopathy is common in individuals who jump a lot during their daily activities (e.g., basketball and volleyball players, high jumpers, dock loaders, and shipping/delivery workers).

Signs and symptoms:

- Pain at the proximal patellar tendon that increases with activity
- Pain with the onset of activity that may be described as severe or sharp; may or may not decrease as activity progresses
- Pain that remains constant with activity in severe or more chronic conditions

Special tests:

Patellar tendon palpation: Palpate the patellar tendon at its insertion on the inferior pole of the patella. This will elicit pain in the individual with tendinopathy.

Resisted knee extension: Ask the client to perform resisted knee extension with the knee in full extension. Reproduction of symptoms indicates possible patellar tendinopathy.

Immediate management: Tendonitis resolves quickly (1 to 2 weeks), and the treatment of choice is active rest and antiinflammatory modalities. In contrast, tendinosis is often recalcitrant to treatment, takes months to resolve, and does not respond to antiinflammatory modalities. The clinical diagnosis is confirmed with either ultrasonography or magnetic resonance imaging.

For patellar tendinopathy, relative rest is an important component of treatment, given that structural damage to the tendon has occurred. Affected individuals should refrain from engaging in impact activities (e.g., running, jumping, hiking) until they are pain free during normal activities of daily living.

Deep transverse friction massage to the proximal portion of the patellar tendon is also recommended to reduce pain in athletes with patellar tendinopathy.[66] Cryotherapy may be a useful modality for short-term pain relief.[67]

Intermediate management: Once the client can engage in activities of daily living without pain, he or she may begin a strengthening program. Clinical research has demonstrated the effectiveness of eccentric exercise in the management of athletes with tendinopathies.[66,68–72] The premise is that the mechanical loading of the eccentric exercises accelerates metabolic activity within the tendon and may speed tendon repair.[65,73] In addition to eccentric loading of the patellar tendon, a strengthening program must also address biomechanical faults or muscle weaknesses identified in the trunk, hip, or ankle. Isolated strengthening of hip and knee muscle groups, as well as functional total leg and core strengthening, should be implemented. Concentric quadriceps activity of the involved knee should be avoided as much as possible.

Patellofemoral Pain Syndrome

Patellofemoral pain syndrome is one of the most common disorders of the knee and affects athletes and nonathletes alike. It is especially common in runners and has been reported to account for 30% of all sports injuries. Approximately 50% of athletes report bilateral symptoms.[74,75] Patellofemoral pain is seen in 9% of all young athletes, with a 10% incidence in young female athletes and a 7% incidence in young male athletes.[74,76]

Mechanism: No single biomechanical factor (e.g., patellar tracking, muscle weakness, muscle length, proximal and distal biomechanical forces) has provided an adequate explanation for patellofemoral pain. However, consideration of the biological factors involved (e.g., synovial lining, fat pads, metabolic activity) allows athletic trainers to improve both their understanding and their effectiveness in treating the enigma of patellofemoral pain.

patellar tendinopathy overuse injury commonly called "jumper's knee" in which the patellar tendon becomes inflamed and may tear or degenerate; common cause of pain in the inferior knee region

Signs and symptoms:
- Anterior knee pain before and after activity
- Pain after prolonged sitting with the knee in flexion ("movie theater sign")
- Dull and achy pain
- Stiffness
- Crepitus
- Diffuse pain that cannot be pinpointed

Special tests: Until better examination and treatment algorithms (e.g., clinical decision rules) are developed, tests that produce a specific cluster of signs and symptoms can help the athletic trainer place the client with anterior knee pain into a subgrouping.[76]

Immediate and intermediate management: Treatment should address all factors, both intrinsic and extrinsic, that have caused the client to cross his or her injury threshold. To better address these intrinsic and extrinsic factors, the athletic trainer may find it helpful to classify the patellofemoral disorders (Table 11-5). Management protocols based on this classification are shown in Table 11-6.

Box 11-4 summarizes chronic injuries of the knee and thigh and the appropriate special tests used with each.

Prevention of Chronic/Overuse Injuries

As with the prevention of acute injuries, adequate conditioning and warm-ups, as well as attentive detail to technique and mechanics, are crucial in preventing chronic and overuse injuries to the knee and thigh. Changes in training programs must be planned with scrupulous care. What appears to be a simple, modest change in the program could result in an ongoing injury that prevents the client from performing his or her regular activities for a prolonged periods.

TAPING, BRACING, AND RETURN TO PLAY

During rehabilitation of knee and thigh injuries, the goal is to improve muscle strength, muscle endurance, and muscle flexibility. This focus allows the client to return safely and as quickly as possible to his or her previous activities. Along with a comprehensive rehabilitation program, knee bracing has become a significant adjunctive treatment choice.[77,78] Knee bracing is most commonly broken into several categories: prophylactic, functional, and rehabilitative. **Prophylactic bracing** is intended to prevent or reduce the severity of injuries. **Functional bracing** is designed to provide stability for an unstable joint. **Rehabilitative bracing** allows protected controlled motion during exercises and rehabilitation. The use of bracing also depends on physician preference and the activity to which the individual is returning.

Returning the client to activity should include not just clinical findings and observations but also functional testing. Frequently, reproducing the client's activity is sufficient to determine his or her abilities. With the knee and thigh, several other components of functional abilities must be addressed, including quality of movement and balance.

Functional Testing

Functional testing safely challenges the injured body part. Functional testing offers an excellent means to assess long-term and ongoing progress during the course

prophylactic bracing type of bracing intended to prevent or reduce the severity of injuries

functional bracing bracing designed to provide stability for an unstable joint

rehabilitative bracing a type of bracing that allows protected controlled motion during exercises and rehabilitation

TABLE 11-5 Proposed Classification of Patellofemoral Disorders

CLASSIFICATION	PATELLOFEMORAL CONDITIONS FOUND WITHIN SPECIFIC CLASSIFICATION
Patellar compression syndrome	Excessive lateral pressure syndrome Global patellar pressure syndrome
Patellar instability	Acute patellar dislocation Recurrent patellar dislocation Chronic patellar subluxation
Biomechanical dysfunction	Miserable malalignment syndrome Muscle length and strength asymmetries
Direct patellar trauma	Isolated articular cartilage lesion Fracture/dislocation Articular cartilage lesion with associated malalignment
Soft tissue lesions	Acute Medial retinaculum / medial patellofemoral ligament pain Iliotibial band friction syndrome Bursitis Acute or chronic Symptomatic plica Fat pad syndrome
Overuse syndromes	Adults Patellar tendinopathy Quadriceps tendinopathy Pediatric athletes with open growth plates Osgood-Schlatter syndrome (tibial osteochondrosis) Sinding-Larsen-Johanssen syndrome (patellar osteochondrosis)
Osteochondritis dissecans (OCD)	Osteochondritis dissecans (OCD)
Neurological disorders	Complex regional pain syndromes I and II

Modified from Wilk KE et al: Patellofemoral disorders: a classification system and clinical guidelines for nonoperative rehabilitation, *J Orthop Sports Phys Ther* 28(5): 307–322, 1998.

TABLE 11-6 Classification and Management of Patellofemoral Pain Disorders

CLASSIFICATION/SUBTYPE	POSSIBLE EXAMINATION FINDINGS	POSSIBLE TREATMENT OPTIONS
Classification: Patellar compression syndrome **Subtype:** Excessive lateral patellar pressure syndrome	Tight hamstrings	Stretching program
	Tight hip flexors and/or quadriceps	Stretching program
	Tight ITB/TFL complex	Stretching program, cross friction massage
	Decreased patellar medial glide and medial tilt (lateral hypomobility)	Patellar mobilization, stretching program, taping patella into a position of a medial glide and tilt as a means to gain a long duration low-load stretch to the superficial patellar retinaculum
	Quadriceps weakness	Strengthening program avoiding painful ROM and patellofemoral joint shear
	Suspected inflammation of the synovium	Active rest and antiinflammatory modalities
Classification: Patellar compression syndrome **Subtype:** Global patellar pressure syndrome	Tight hamstrings	Stretching program
	Tight hip flexors and/or quadriceps	Stretching program
	Tight ITB/TFL complex	Stretching program, cross friction massage
	Decreased patellar medial and lateral glides and tilts (global hypomobility)	No tape; may increase compression Emphasis on patellar mobilizations, frequent knee AROM without resistance; possible to nourish cartilage through cycling with a high seat, at a high rpm level without resistance
	Quadriceps weakness	Strengthening program avoiding painful ROM and patellofemoral joint shear Multi-angle isometrics progressing to protected ROM on the leg press machine and eccentric step-downs
	Suspected inflammation of the synovium	Active rest and antiinflammatory modalities
Classification: Soft tissue lesion **Subtype:** Infrapatellar fat pad syndrome	Inflammation of the infrapatellar fat pads (Hoffa's sign) in terminal extension	Active rest and antiinflammatory modalities such as cryotherapy and iontophoresis
	Abnormal biomechanics and lower extremity malalignment	Complete foot evaluation and possibly orthotics Temporary heel lifts for 1 to 2 weeks to unload fat pad tissue Running video analysis to examine biomechanics
	Soft tissue stress	Counter force bracing or taping
Classification: Patellar instability **Subtype:** Chronic patellar subluxation	Generalized hypermobility	Taping and bracing
	Excessive patellar glides and tilts	Strengthening program avoiding painful ROM and patellofemoral joint shear
	Quadriceps weakness	Foot orthotics
	Abnormal biomechanics and lower extremity malalignment	Running video analysis to examine biomechanics
Classification: Overuse syndrome **Subtype:** Tendinopathy	Chronic/recalcitrant (>4 weeks)	Possible tendinopathy; should not be treated as tendinitis
	Painful palpation of patellar tendon	
	Quadriceps weakness	Eccentric strengthening program (decline squat, leg press)
	Abnormal biomechanics and lower extremity malalignment	Dynamic stabilization program for hip and trunk (core) musculature; possible that improved hip and lumbopelvic strength will help prevent fatigue-related kinematic changes that stress patellofemoral joint Possibly foot orthotics Running video analysis to examine biomechanics

Modified from Wilk KE et al: Patellofemoral disorders: a classification system and clinical guidelines for nonoperative rehabilitation, *J Orthop Sports Phys Ther* 28(5):307–322, 1998.

of treatment. Repeated functional tests can provide a global assessment of the client's progress and ability to perform specific and required activities.

Quality of Movement During the Lateral Step-Down Test

For the lateral step-down test, the client is asked to stand on the involved limb on a step that is 20 centimeters high. The client places his or her hands on the waist while weight bearing in full knee extension with the toes near the edge of the step. The contralateral leg is held hanging down toward the floor adjacent to the step in knee extension. The client then squats until the nonweight-bearing limb touches the floor and then returns to the start position[14] (Figure 11-17). The client attempts to complete five repetitions in a slow and deliberate manner. The athletic trainer faces the client and scores the test as described in Table 11-7.

Star-Excursion Balance Test

Dynamic balance is a key requirement of any activity. Thus quantification of balance or postural control is a necessary part of the comprehensive physical examination of the athlete or client returning to play.

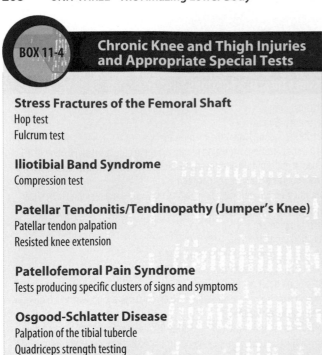

BOX 11-4 Chronic Knee and Thigh Injuries and Appropriate Special Tests

Stress Fractures of the Femoral Shaft
Hop test
Fulcrum test

Iliotibial Band Syndrome
Compression test

Patellar Tendonitis/Tendinopathy (Jumper's Knee)
Patellar tendon palpation
Resisted knee extension

Patellofemoral Pain Syndrome
Tests producing specific clusters of signs and symptoms

Osgood-Schlatter Disease
Palpation of the tibial tubercle
Quadriceps strength testing

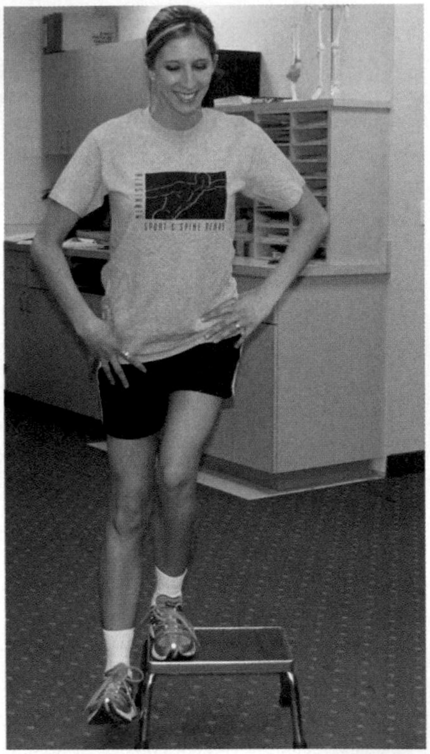

FIGURE 11-17 Lateral step-down test. If scored according to the criteria described in Table 11-7, this athlete would score a "medium quality of movement" or score of three because of her medial knee position and unlevel pelvis.

The star-excursion balance test (SEBT) offers a reliable[79–81] clinical method to examine dynamic balance.[79,82] The SEBT consists of a series of lower extremity reaching tasks in eight directions to challenge postural control, strength, ROM, and balance abilities. The farther the client can reach on one leg while balancing on the other leg, the greater his or her level of function.

The SEBT is performed with the client standing barefoot at the center of a grid (either purchased or laid on the floor with athletic tape). There should be eight lines extending at 45-degree increments from the center of the grid. The geometric center of the weight-bearing foot is aligned with the center of the grid. The client is asked to reach and gently touch the farthest point possible on the desired line with the most distal part of the reaching foot. The athletic trainer records this distance in centimeters. The client then returns to a bilateral stance in the center of the grid. The process is repeated for each of the SEBT lines (Figure 11-18).

TABLE 11-7 Scoring of the Quality of Movement During the Lateral Step-Down Test

CRITERION	SCORE CRITERIA	SCORE
Arm strategy	Any arm movement or arm positioning used in attempt to maintain balance	+1
Trunk movement	If any trunk lean to either the right or left is observed	+1
Pelvis plane	If the pelvis is observed as being rotated or elevated to one side	+1
Knee position	If the knee deviated medially and the tibial tuberosity crossed an imaginary vertical line over the second toe, add one point. If the knee deviated medially and the tibial tuberosity crossed an imaginary vertical line over the medial border of the foot, add two points.	+1 or +2
Maintenance of steady unilateral stance	If the stance limb became unsteady or the subject placed more than toe-touch weight on the contralateral limb.	+1

A total score of quality of movement between 0 and 5 is possible.
A total score of 0 to 1 is classified as good quality of movement
A total score of 2 or 3 is classified as medium quality of movement
A total score of 4 or 5 is classified as poor quality of movement

From Piva SR et al: Reliability of measures of impairments associated with patellofemoral pain syndrome, *BMC Musculoskelet Disord* 7:33, 2006.

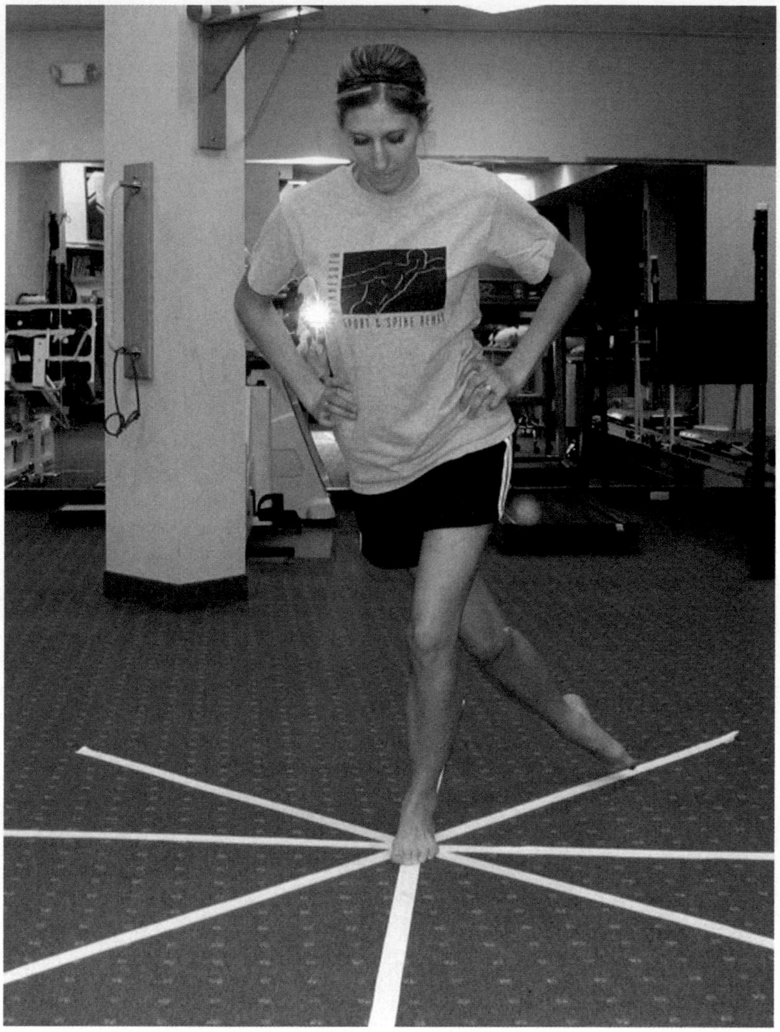

FIGURE 11-18 Star-excursion balance test (SEBT).

Balance and Reach Test for Time

The balance and reach test is used to assess patellofemoral pain.[83,84] To begin, the client stands with the toes just behind a taped line on the floor. The client reaches forward with one leg so that the heel touches the floor, with most of the body weight placed through the weight-bearing (test) leg. Distance is recorded from the start line to the heel of the reaching leg. The athlete performs three trials, and the maximum distance reached with the heel is recorded. The athletic trainer calculates 80% of this maximum value and marks it on the line. Then, the number of touches that the athlete can reach beyond the 80% mark in 30 seconds is recorded. The test is repeated on the opposite limb, preferably with the involved leg being tested first.

THE AGE GROUP ATHLETE

Several knee and thigh injuries are specific to young active people. Epiphyseal fractures, Osgood-Schlatter disease, and Sinding-Larssen-Johansson syndrome are fairly common in the adolescent and pediatric populations. Because of the nature of these injuries, early diagnosis and management are critical to ensure that involvement in future activities and sports will not be compromised or prevented.

Epiphyseal Fractures

Distal femoral epiphyseal fractures are potentially serious because they may damage the growth plate. In most cases, these injuries affect adolescents between the ages of 10 and 14 years old. Special care must be taken to ensure appropriate and timely treatment. Approximately 70% of the growth of the femur occurs at the physes.[85]

Mechanism: The mechanism of injury is similar to that of other fractures in this area: violent direct contact or extremely strong contractions of the quadriceps or hamstring muscles.

Signs and symptoms:

- Pain at the site of injury
- Inability to bear weight

Immediate management: Immediate treatment, as with most fractures, is application of an immobilizer and immediate referral to a physician for diagnostic testing.

Intermediate management: Surgical intervention may be required as a procedure to repair the fracture, depending on the severity of the injury. A comprehensive and progressive rehabilitation program allows a safe return to activity.

Osgood-Schlatter Disease

Osgood-Schlatter disease is a common cause of knee pain in the pediatric athletic population. Also known as tibial osteochondrosis, this condition develops from repetitive microtrauma to the tibial tubercle apophysis.

Mechanism: Repetitive trauma from jumping and impact activities during the beginning of a growth spurt may lead to Osgood-Schlatter disease. Most often, it is noticed in boys between the ages of 10 to 15 years, with most cases reported in subjects who are between 13 and 14 years of age. In girls, the age of onset is between 8 and 13 years, with most cases reported in subjects who are between 10 and 11 years of age. Bilateral complaints are reported in approximately 20% to 30% of all cases.[86]

Signs and symptoms:

- Pain at the tibial tubercle
- Swelling at the tibial tubercle
- Bony or cartilaginous prominence present at the tibial tubercle

Special tests: Palpation of the tibial tubercle is used as the primary means to diagnose Osgood-Schlatter disease. Tenderness to palpation signifies a positive finding. Also, pain that is reproduced with quadriceps strength testing (especially in >90 degrees flexion) indicates a positive finding. Sometimes, the athlete has tight quadriceps and hamstring muscles as well when thoroughly examined.

Immediate management: The treatment of Osgood-Schlatter disease is based on the severity of symptoms and individual tolerance. It begins with resting or performing activities that do not cause knee pain. Application of ice and other antiinflammatory modalities may be recommended. Activity limitations and relative rest for several weeks eventually alleviate the symptoms.

Intermediate management: A change in activity or sport position (e.g., catcher to outfielder) may alleviate symptoms and allow continued participation. Individuals with severe Osgood-Schlatter disease may need to avoid sports that require significant running, jumping, or kneeling for several months to a year. The athlete and family members must be reassured that the condition, which is usually self-limiting, gradually improves over time. Occasionally, bracing and padding are advised. Stretching of any tight muscle groups in the knee is an important part of treatment. Conservative treatment of Osgood-Schlatter disease is successful in all but the most recalcitrant cases. If surgery is required, ossicle excision or tibial tubercle prominence resection is an option.[87,88]

Sinding-Larsen-Johansson Syndrome

Sinding-Larsen-Johansson syndrome, or patellar osteochondrosis, is an overuse traction apophysitis of the inferior pole of the patella that results from repetitive microtrauma to the area. Although the pathology is the same as for Osgood-Schlatter disease, Sinding-Larsen-Johansson syndrome differs in that the apophysitis occurs at the insertion point of the patellar tendon on the patella rather than on the tibial tubercle.

Mechanism: This condition is seen in adolescents between 10 and 14 years of age who participate in jumping sports such as basketball or volleyball.[89,90]

Signs and symptoms:

- Pain and palpable tenderness at the inferior pole of the patella
- Swelling at the inferior pole of the patella
- Bony or cartilaginous prominence present at the inferior pole of the patella
- Pain with running, jumping, and stair climbing

Immediate and intermediate management: Treatment is the same as for Osgood-Schlatter disease.

SUMMARY

Proper management of acute and chronic knee and thigh injuries requires careful evaluation to ensure proper diagnosis. Once a proper diagnosis is determined, every attempt should be made to use appropriate intervention strategies that will allow the client to return to activity safely and quickly. Numerous knee and thigh injuries afflict the active population and present myriad diagnosis and management opportunities. At times, no clear evidence dictates a definitive treatment approach. Clinical intuition and experience working with specific diagnoses will help the athletic trainer establish an effective and comprehensive rehabilitation program. The ultimate goal of rehabilitation is to safely return the client to the highest level of function in the shortest amount of time possible.

Osgood-Schlatter disease a common cause of knee pain in young athletes that causes swelling, pain, and tenderness just below the knee, over the shin bone; occurs mostly in boys who are having a growth spurt during their preteen or teenage years

Sinding-Larsen-Johansson syndrome inflammation of the knee cap

Revisiting the OPENING *Scenario*

Diagnostic arthroscopy revealed that the athlete had a very irritated medial synovial fold that was rubbing along the medial femoral condyle with every cycle of motion involving knee flexion and extension. This fold, or pleat, is a very common cause of pathology and is sometimes lumped into the patellofemoral pain category. When thickened and irritated, this fold may rub against the condyle, producing painful popping and snapping sensations in the medial knee. The athlete's menisci and cartilage surfaces were perfect, with no sign of articular cartilage defects. After 4 weeks of a comprehensive rehabilitation program, the athlete was back on the basketball court with no remaining symptoms.

OPENING *Scenario Differential Diagnosis*

EVALUATION TECHNIQUE	DIFFERENTIAL DIAGNOSIS: MENISCUS TEAR	DIFFERENTIAL DIAGNOSIS: SYNOVIAL FOLD
History	Acute or chronic	Acute or chronic
Inspection	Swelling: depends on severity	Swelling: generally mild
Palpation	Point tenderness	Point tenderness
AROM	Depends on severity; can be locked	May be decreased but generally no limitation
PROM	Depends on severity; can be locked	Generally full
RROM	Depends on severity	Depends on severity
Neurological	Normal	Normal
Special tests	McMurray test (+)	McMurray test may appear (+)
Diagnostic test	Radiographs (−) MRI (+)	Radiographs (−) MRI (−)

AROM, Active range of motion; PROM, passive range of motion; RROM, resisted range of motion.

Issues & Ethics

Justin, a college senior point guard, is a top pick for the upcoming NBA draft. While playing in his last collegiate basketball game, he was running a fast-break when an opponent fouled him during a lay-up. Justin fell to the floor, landing on his left knee. The on-site medical team evaluated him and diagnosed a possible meniscal tear and bone bruise of the knee. He was allowed to re-enter and finish his final collegiate game. Weeks passed as he aggressively performed his rehabilitation program, but he did not make the hoped-for progress. Because he is both rehabilitating his injury and attempting to train for the upcoming NBA camp, his improvement is of utmost importance to many people. He still cannot perform sprints or lift heavy weights. Further and repeat diagnostic tests are ordered. The findings indicate that he was originally misdiagnosed; a tibial epiphyseal fracture and a ruptured bursa are found. How do you explain the misdiagnosis? Do you allow him to train through the pain and injury so he can go, as scheduled, to the NBA camp? Do you brace him up and slow down his rehabilitation and training even if it prevents him from entering the draft as a top pick this year?

Web Links

American Orthopaedic Society for Sports Medicine: www.aossm.org
Journal of Athletic Training:www.nata.org/jat
Evidence in Motion: www.evidenceinmotion.com
Wheeless' Textbook of Orthopaedics: www.wheelessonline.com/
Comprehensive medical textbook for all clinical fields: www.emedicine.com/
Integrated medical information and educational tools: www.medscape.com/home
Healthcare information: www.orthosupersite.com/

References

1. *Athletic training and sports medicine*, ed 2, Rosemont, Ill, 1991, American Academy of Orthopedic Surgeons.
2. Dye SF: The knee as a biologic transmission with an envelope of function: a theory, *Clin Orthop Relat Res* 325: 10–18, 1996.
3. Davies GJ, Larsen R: Examining the knee, *Phys Sportsmed* 7: 48–73, 1978.
4. Manske RC, Davies GJ: A nonsurgical approach to examination and treatment of the patellofemoral joint. Part I. Examination of the patellofemoral joint, *Crit Rev Phys Rehabil Med*, 15(2): 141–166, 2003.
5. Soderberg GL, Ballantyne BT, Kestel LL: Reliability of lower extremity girth measurements after anterior cruciate ligament reconstruction, *Physiother Res Int*, 1: 7–16, 1996.
6. Johnson LL, et al: Clinical assessment of asymptomatic knees: comparison of men and women, *Arthroscopy*, 14(4): 347–359, 1998.
7. Magee DJ: *Orthopaedic physical assessment*, ed 4, Philadelphia, 2002, Saunders/Elsevier.
8. Woerman A, Binder-MacLeod S: Leg length discrepancy assessment: accuracy and precision in five clinical methods of evaluation, *J Orthop Sports Phys Ther* 5: 230–239, 1984.
9. Nicholas JA, Marino M: The relationship of injuries of the leg, foot, and ankle to proximal thigh strength in athletes, *Foot Ankle*, 7(4): 218–228, 1987.
10. Devan MR, et al: A prospective study of overuse knee injuries among female athletes with muscle imbalances and structural abnormalities, *J Athl Train* 39(3): 263–267, 2004.
11. Niemuth PE, et al: Hip muscle weakness and overuse injuries in recreational runners, *Clin J Sport Med* 15(1): 14–21, 2005.
12. Andrews AW, Thomas MW, Bohannon RW: Normative values for isometric muscle force measurements obtained with hand-held dynamometers, *Phys Ther* 76(3): 248–259, 1996.
13. Bohannon RW: Test-retest reliability of hand-held dynamometry during a single session of strength assessment, *Phys Ther* 66(2): 206–209, 1986.
14. Piva SR, et al: Reliability of measures of impairments associated with patellofemoral pain syndrome, *BMC Musculoskelet Disord* 7: 33, 2006.
15. Gajdosik RL, et al: Comparison of four clinical tests for assessing hamstring muscle length, *J Orthop Sports Phys Ther* 18(5): 614–618, 1993.

16. Youdas JW, et al: The influence of gender and age on hamstring muscle length in healthy adults, *J Orthop Sports Phys Ther* 35(4): 246–252, 2005.
17. Gajdosik RL, Sandler MM, Marr HL: Influence of knee positions and gender on the Ober test for length of the iliotibial band, *Clin Biomech (Bristol, Avon)* 18(1): 77–79, 2003.
18. Reese NB, Bandy WD: Use of an inclinometer to measure flexibility of the iliotibial band using the Ober test and the modified Ober test: differences in magnitude and reliability of measurements, *J Orthop Sports Phys Ther* 33(6): 326–330, 2003.
19. Grood ES, et al: Ligamentous and capsular restraints preventing straight medial and lateral laxity in intact human cadaver knees, *J Bone Joint Surg* 63A: 1257–1269, 1981.
20. Takeda Y, et al: Biomechanical function of the human anterior cruciate ligament, *Arthroscopy* 10: 140–147, 1994.
21. Fiebert I, et al: Comparative measurements of anterior tibial translation using a KT-1000 knee arthrometer with the leg in neutral, internal rotation, and external rotation, *J Orthop Sports Phys Ther* 19: 331–334, 1994.
22. King S, Butterwick DJ, Ceurrier JP: The anterior cruciate ligament: a review of recent concepts, *J Orthop Sports Phys Ther* 8: 110–122, 1986.
23. Norkin CC, Levange PK: The knee complex. In: *Joint structure and function: A comprehensive analysis*, ed 2, pp. 337–377, Philadelphia, 2005, FA Davis.
24. Manske RC, Stovak M: Preoperative and postsurgical musculoskeletal examination of the knee, In Manske RC, editors: *Postsurgical orthopedic sports rehabilitation: Knee and shoulder*, St Louis, 2006, Mosby/Elsevier.
25. Johnson BC, Cullun MJ: The anterior cruciate ligament: injuries and functions in anterolateral rotary instability, *Athl Train* 17: 79–83, 1982.
26. DiStefano VJ: The enigmatic anterior cruciate ligament, *Athl Train* 16: 244–249, 1981.
27. Girgis FG, Marshall JL, Al Monajem ARS: The cruciate ligaments of the knee joint: anatomical, functional, and experimental analysis, *Clin Orthop* 106: 216–231, 1975.
28. Clancy WG, Ray JM, Zoltan DJ: Acute tears of the anterior cruciate ligament, *J Bone Joint Surg* 70A: 1483–1488, 1988.
29. Fetto JF, Marshall JL: The natural history and diagnosis of anterior cruciate ligament insufficiency, *Clin Orthop* 147: 29–38, 1980.
30. Levy M, Torzilli PA, Warren FR: The effect of medial meniscectomy on anterior-posterior motion of the knee, *J Bone Joint Surg* 64A: 883–888, 1982.
31. Marshall JL, Olsson SE: Instability of the knee: a long term experimental study in dogs, *J Bone Joint Surg* 53A: 1561–1570, 1971.
32. McDaniel WJ, Dameron TB: The untreated anterior cruciate ligament rupture, *Clin Orthop*, 172: 158–163, 1983.
33. McDaniel WJ, Dameron TB: Untreated ruptures of the anterior cruciate ligament: a follow-up study, *J Bone Joint Surg* 62A: 696–705, 1980.
34. Wilk KE et al: Assessment and treatment of medial capsular injuries, In Ellenbecker TS, editors: *Knee ligament rehabilitation*, Philadelphia, 2000, Churchill Livingstone.
35. Indelicato PA: Non-operative treatment of complete tears of the medial collateral ligament of the knee, *J Bone Joint Surg* 65A: 323–329, 1983.
36. Ellsasser JC, Reynolds FC, Omohundro JR: The nonoperative treatment of collateral ligament injuries of the knee in professional football players, *J Bone Joint Surg* 56A: 1185–1190, 1974.
37. Derscheid GL, Garrick JG: Medial collateral ligament injuries in football: nonoperative management of grade I and grade II sprains, *Am J Sports Med* 9(6): 365–368, 1981.
38. Sutton G, Smith JP: Treatment of collateral ligament injuries of the knee. In Manske RC, editor: *Postsurgical orthopedic sports rehabilitation: knee and shoulder*, St Louis, 2006, Mosby.
39. Miyasaka KC et al: The incidence of knee injuries in the general population, *Am J Knee Surg* 4: 3–8, 1991.
40. Irrgang JJ, Safran MR, Fu FH: The knee ligamentous and meniscal injuries, In Zachazewski JE, Magee DJ, Quillen WS, editors: *Athletic injuries and rehabilitation*, Philadelphia, 1996, WB Saunders.
41. Parolie JM, Bergfeld JA: Long-term results of nonoperative treatment of isolated posterior cruciate ligament injuries in the athlete, *Am J Sports Med* 14: 35–38, 1986.
42. McMurray TP: The similunar cartilages, *Brit J Surg* 29: 407–414, 1941.
43. Stone KR: Current and future directions for meniscus repair and replacement, *Clin Orthop* 367(suppl): S273–S280, 1999.
44. Bucholz RW, editors: *Orthopedic decision making*, ed 2, St. Louis, 1996, Mosby.
45. Wolin PM: Limb-threatening emergencies, In Cantu RC, Micheli LJ, editors: *ACSM's guidelines for the team physician*, Philadelphia, 1991, Lea and Febiger.
46. Grant HD, Murray RH, Bergeron D: *Emergency care*, ed 5, Englewood Cliffs, NJ, 1990, Prentice Hall.
47. Fairbank KA: Internal derangement of the knee in children, *Proc R Soc London*, 3: 11, 1937.
48. Dick BH, Anderson JM: Emergency care of the injured athlete, In Zachazewski JE, Magee DJ, Quillen WS, editors: *Athletic injuries and rehabilitation*, Philadelphia, 1996, WB Saunders.
49. Bachmann LM, Haberzeth S, Steurer J, ter Riet G: The accuracy of the Ottawa knee rule to rule out knee fractures: a systematic review, *Ann Intern Med* 140: 121–124, 2004.
50. Viola R, Vianello R: Three cases of patella fracture in 1,320 anterior cruciate ligament reconstruction with bone-patellar tendon-bone autograft, *Arthroscopy* 15: 93–97, 1999.
51. Simonian PT, Mann FA, Mandt PR: Indirect forces and patellar fracture after anterior cruciate ligament reconstruction with the patellar ligament: case report, *Am J Knee Surg* 8: 60–64, 1995.
52. Starkey C, Ryan J: The pelvis and thigh, In Starkey C, Ryan J, editors : *Evaluation of orthopedic and athletic injuries*, ed 2, Philadelphia, 2002, FA Davis.
53. Huiskes R: If bone is the answer, then what is the question? *J Anat*, 197: 145–156, 2000.
54. Lee TC, Taylor D: Bone remodelling: should we cry Wolff? *Ir J Med Sci* 168: 102–105, 1999.

55. McPoil TG, Hunt GC: Evaluation and management of foot and ankle disorders: present problems and future directions, *J Orthop Sports Phys Ther* 21(6): 381–388, 1995.
56. Mueller MJ, Maluf KS: Tissue adaptation to physical stress: a proposed "Physical Stress Theory" to guide physical therapist practice, education, and research, *Phys Ther* 82(4): 383–403, 2002.
57. Matheson GO et al: Stress fractures in athletes: a study of 320 cases, *Am J Sports Med* 15(1): 46–58, 1987.
58. Brukner P et al: Stress fractures: a review of 180 cases, *Clin J Sport Med* 6(2): 85–89, 1996.
59. Bennell KL, Brukner PD: Epidemiology and site specificity of stress fractures, *Clin Sports Med* 16(2): 179–196, 1997.
60. Diehl JJ, Best TM, Kaeding CC: Classification and return-to-play considerations for stress fractures, *Clin Sports Med* 25(1): 17–28, vii, 2006.
61. Johnson AW, Weiss CB, Wheeler DL: Stress fractures of the femoral shaft in athletes: more common than expected: a new clinical test, *Am J Sports Med* 22: 248–256, 1994.
62. Ivkovic A, Bojanic I, Pecina M: Stress fractures of the femoral shaft in athletes: a new treatment algorithm, *Br J Sports Med* 40(6): 518–520, discussion 520, 2006.
63. Noble CA: The treatment of iliotibial band friction syndrome, *Br J Sports Med* 13(2): 51–54, 1979.
64. Fredericson M et al: Hip abductor weakness in distance runners with iliotibial band syndrome, *Clin J Sport Med* 10(3): 169–175, 2000.
65. Khan K, Cook J: The painful nonruptured tendon: clinical aspects, *Clin Sports Med* 22(4): 711–725, 2003.
66. Wilson JJ, Best TM: Common overuse tendon problems: a review and recommendations for treatment, *Am Fam Physician* 72(5): 811–818, 2005.
67. Bleakley C, McDonough S, MacAuley D: The use of ice in the treatment of acute soft-tissue injury: a systematic review of randomized controlled trials, *Am J Sports Med* 32(1): 251–261, 2004.
68. Sayana MK, Maffulli N: Eccentric calf muscle training in non-athletic patients with Achilles tendinopathy, *J Sci Med Sport* 10(1): 52–58, 2007.
69. Peers KH, Lysens RJ: Patellar tendinopathy in athletes: current diagnostic and therapeutic recommendations, *Sports Med* 35(1): 71–87, 2005.
70. Alfredson H, Lorentzon R: Chronic Achilles tendinosis: recommendations for treatment and prevention, *Sports Med* 29(2): 135–146, 2000.
71. Jonsson P, Alfredson H: Superior results with eccentric compared to concentric quadriceps training in patients with jumper's knee: a prospective randomised study, *Br J Sports Med* 39(11): 847–850, 2005.
72. Purdam CR et al: A pilot study of the eccentric decline squat in the management of painful chronic patellar tendinopathy, *Br J Sports Med* 38(4): 395–397, 2004.
73. Kannus P et al: Effects of training, immobilization and remobilization on tendons, *Scand J Med Sci Sports* 7(2): 67–71, 1997.
74. Witvrouw E et al: Intrinsic risk factors for the development of anterior knee pain in an athletic population: a two-year prospective study, *Am J Sports Med* 28(4): 480–489, 2000.
75. Sandow MJ, Goodfellow JW: The natural history of anterior knee pain in adolescents, *J Bone Joint Surg Br* 67(1): 36–38, 1985.
76. Wilk KE et al: Patellofemoral disorders: a classification system and clinical guidelines for nonoperative rehabilitation, *J Orthop Sports Phys Ther* 28(5): 307–322, 1998.
77. Ott JW, Clancy WG: Functional knee braces, *Orthopedics* 16: 171–175, 1993.
78. American Academy of Pediatrics Committee on Sports Medicine: Knee brace use by athletes, *Pediatrics* 85: 228, 1990.
79. Kinzey SJ, Armstrong CW: The reliability of the star-excursion test in assessing dynamic balance, *J Orthop Sports Phys Ther* 27(5): 356–360, 1998.
80. Hertel J, Miller SJ, Denegar CR, Intratester and intertester reliability during the star excursions balance tests, *J Sport Rehabil* 9: 104–116, 2000.
81. Manske RC, Andersen J: Test retest reliability of the lower extremity functional reach test, *J Orthop Sports Phys Ther (Abst)* 34: A52, 2004.
82. Hertel J et al: Simplifying the star excursion balance test: analyses of subjects with and without chronic ankle instability, *J Orthop Sports Phys Ther* 36(3): 131–137, 2006.
83. Loudon JK, Gajewski B, Goist-Foley HL, Loudon KL: The effectiveness of exercise in treating patellofemoral pain syndrome, *J Sport Rehabil* 13: 323–342, 2004.
84. Loudon JK et al: Intrarater reliability of functional performance tests for subjects with patellofemoral pain syndrome, *J Athl Train* 37(3): 256–261, 2002.
85. Strizak AM: Knee injuries. In Nicholas JA, Hershman EB, editors: *The lower extremity and spine in sports medicine*, ed 2, St Louis, 1995, Mosby.
86. Stanitski CL: Management of sports injuries in children and adolescents, *Orthop Clin North Am* 19: 689–698, 1993.
87. Hogh J, Lund B: The sequelae of Osgood-Schlatter's disease in adults, *Int Orthop* 12(3): 213–215, 1988.
88. Mital MA, Matza RA, Cohen J: The so-called unresolved Osgood-Schlatter lesion: a concept based on fifteen surgically treated lesions, *J Bone Joint Surg Am* 62(5): 732–739, 1980.
89. Duri ZA, Patel DV, Aichroth PM: The immature athlete, *Clin Sports Med* 21(3): 461–482, ix, 2002.
90. Medlar RC, Lyne ED: Sinding-Larsen-Johansson disease: its etiology and natural history, *J Bone Joint Surg Am* 60(8): 1113–1116, 1978.

12

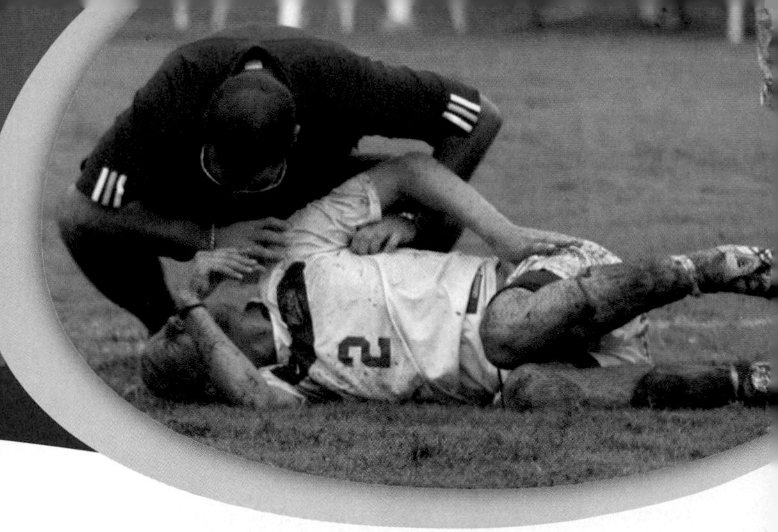

Diagnosis and Management of Hip and Pelvis Injuries

PAT GRAMAN

Learning Goals

1. Describe appropriate procedures for evaluation and diagnosis of common acute and chronic injuries to the hip and pelvis.
2. Explain the importance of a systematic assessment in the management of injuries of the hip and pelvis.
3. List common acute injuries to the hip and pelvis regions.
4. Describe the proper management of common acute injuries occurring to the hip and pelvis.
5. List common chronic injuries that are found with the hip and pelvis.
6. Describe the proper management of common chronic injuries involving the hip and pelvis.
7. Identify principles and concepts that can be applied to prevent athletic injuries to the hip and pelvis.
8. Identify precautions and risks associated with athletic participation by the age group athlete to the hip and pelvis.

Injuries to the hip and pelvis occur less often than injuries to the knee, ankle, and foot. Because the hip joint is an anatomical ball-and-socket joint, it is very well protected by the musculature of the hip and pelvis and is also structurally maintained by strong bony anatomy. Owing to this amount of protection around the hip, the incidence of injury is relatively low in this area compared with other parts of the body. In high school athletes, injuries to the hip region comprise approximately 5% to 9% of sports-related injuries.[1] Hip and pelvic injuries are more common in older active people and in military recruits.[2,3] Stress fractures of the femoral neck are the most common injury, largely because of the great number of runners across all age groups. In the general population of physically active people, hip injuries account for only 1% of total injuries; in runners, however, injuries may be as high as 15%.[2] There are occasional reports of stress fractures of the pelvis, but they are very rarely diagnosed because of the scarcity of documented cases.[3] The anatomical and biomechanical complexity of the hip and pelvis makes management of these injuries quite challenging. The hip joint handles loads of eight times the body's weight during jogging.[1] The greater the load, the higher the risk for injury and even subsequent bone failure during athletic competition.

Points to Ponder
What is unique to these populations that increases their risk of hip and pelvis injuries?

To perform a thorough evaluation, all athletic trainers must understand the anatomy and biomechanics of the hip. Obtaining an accurate diagnosis leads to a comprehensive plan for rehabilitation and return to activity. This chapter provides an overview of common hip and pelvis injuries and their proper evaluation and diagnosis.

Terms that appear in boldface green type are defined in the book's glossary.

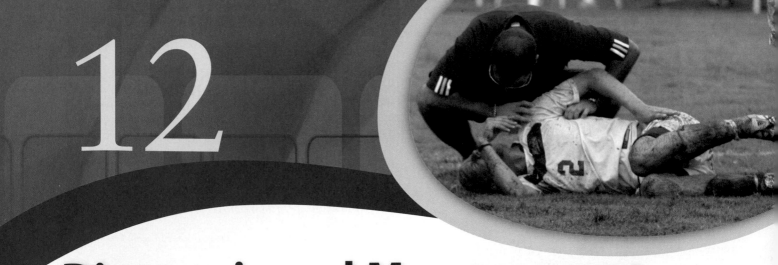

OPENING *Scenario*

John, a 19-year-old college sophomore cross-country runner, reports to the athletic trainer complaining of right hip and groin pain. He states that the pain started about a week ago and has gradually increased, occurring only when he runs. He experiences no pain or discomfort during activities of daily living. The initial evaluation demonstrates no tenderness or inflammation to palpation, and his active range of motion of the right hip is equal to the left hip. After evaluating John's passive range of motion, the athletic trainer notes that his right side has minimal deficiency and discomfort with end range hip flexion. John has normal strength in all ranges of hip motion with minimal discomfort reported in external and internal rotation. He is placed on a hip strengthening and flexibility program and cuts back on his running by 25%. One week later, he returns with complaints of increased pain with running and activities of daily living. The athletic trainer recommends X-rays and further diagnostic testing. The athletic trainer also tells John to discontinue all running activities and begin partial weight bearing with two crutches. Several possibilities could be plaguing John. What are they?

CLINICAL EVALUATION AND DIAGNOSIS OF HIP AND PELVIS INJURIES

The hip and pelvis are very well protected by soft tissue attachments, musculature, and strong bony anatomy. Therefore few acute injuries affect this area. However, despite the relative rareness of sports-related hip dislocations and fractures, they do occur. When confronted by an acute hip or pelvis injury, the athletic trainer must be familiar with the evaluation process for hip dislocations, femoral fractures, pelvic fractures, and contusions. The goal of an on-field hip and pelvic evaluation is to rule out any limb-threatening injury and minimize further trauma to the hip and pelvis through proper injury management. Many chronic hip and pelvis injuries are due to anatomical abnormalities, which result in a lack of flexibility or strength imbalances (or both). These problems typically affect the lower extremity as a whole and ultimately harm the athlete's overall performance. Although chronic hip and pelvis injuries are evaluated much the same way as acute injuries are, the evaluation is more thorough and detailed. The athletic trainer must also assess the lower back, hip, knee, and ankle. Moreover, the athletic trainer evaluating the hip and pelvis must know when the injury should be referred to a physician.

History

When performing evaluations on acute hip and pelvic injuries, the athletic trainer must ask specific and concise questions to promptly make an accurate decision on injury management, as well as to prevent an extended delay of the game or event. The questions should be phrased in an open-ended format to allow the athlete to convey the relevant information from his or her own perspective. History questions should include how the injury happened (mechanism of injury—MOI); whether any sounds were heard; and the magnitude, type, and distribution of the pain. With this type of questioning, the athletic trainer solicits feedback as to whether the athlete suffered a direct or indirect contact injury. When inquiring about pain, the examiner must keep in mind that pain may be referred to the hip from the sacroiliac joint or the lumbar spine.[4] The athletic trainer should ask whether someone hit or landed on the injured athlete and whether he or she heard a pop or crack, which may indicate a broken bone or hip dislocation. The absence or presence of pain should also be noted. The athlete's responses to these questions will indicate the severity of the pain as well as the presence of pain extending into the lower back or the leg. Numbness in the area may also extend into the lower extremity.

As previously mentioned, the athletic trainer can elicit the best information from the client by asking open-ended questions. Responses to these questions identify the nature of the injury, its duration, and its precipitating factors, as well as alleviating factors and prior injury.[5] Other factors to be considered when obtaining a history for a chronic injury is the client's specific activity, duration of participation in the activity, competitive level, cross training and nonsports-related activities, frequency of the activity per week, and training schedule; the client should also be asked about any recent changes in his or her routine and the duration of the recovery period.[5] Information regarding current treatment for the condition will guide the athletic trainer in selecting an approach for healing.

Additional information should be obtained from the female athlete with regard to **amenorrhea**, or absence of menstruation; **oligomenorrhea**, infrequent menstruation; disordered eating; weight loss; **osteoporosis**, or loss of bone mass; and a previous history of stress fractures.

amenorrhea an absence of the menstrual cycle
oligomenorrhea irregular or very light menstrual cycles
osteoporosis a disorder that causes a reduction in bone mineral density

These conditions are highly pertinent factors in the determination of stress fracture pathology.

Inspection and Observation

While attending to an injured athlete on the field, inspection and observation allow the athletic trainer to observe abnormal findings. This inspection starts immediately, as soon as the athletic trainer approaches the athlete. With a hip or pelvic injury, it is important to note the position of the individual on the ground. Anatomical structures as well as certain types of uniform and protective padding make it difficult to observe a hip dislocation. The hip will be in a position of adduction and internal rotation. For nonacute injuries, the inspection/observation phase of the evaluation process begins from the moment the patient enters the room. The athletic trainer must make a bilateral comparison of the injured and noninjured sides. Observation should include any type of abnormal gait, including a limp caused by an injury to the foot, ankle, knee, hip, or lower back. The athletic trainer should observe the way that the client ambulates and whether he or she has difficulty following instructions to go up steps, sit, lie down, or move in a consistent fluid motion. The athletic trainer should watch the client closely to assess whether the client exhibits any apprehension or hesitation about moving.

Palpation

Palpation of the injured area is an important step in the evaluation process, one that supplements the history and inspection/observation components. A systematic approach to palpating the bony anatomy and soft tissue structures of the hip and pelvis confirms the injury location, swelling, pain, muscular atrophy, and deformity that may not be readily apparent. Palpation determines the exact location of the pain and any referred pain. Pain felt in the hip may stem from the injured site or from another area away from the hip.[4] Referred pain is located at a site other than where it originates, and determining the exact location is important. There are two techniques in palpation. The first technique is to palpate the unaffected side and then the affected side, which fosters trust and allows the athlete to feel more comfortable during the examination process. The second technique is to palpate the affected side first. If the client is already experiencing a great deal of pain, he or she may already feel apprehensive about allowing the athletic trainer to examine the injured area; palpating the unaffected side first may ease the apprehension and allow the athlete to relax. When palpating the affected side, the athletic trainer should always start farther away from the injury and gradually move toward the site of injury.

Range of Motion Testing

A thorough assessment of history, inspection, and palpation must be completed before range of motion can be assessed. If the previous steps do not suggest a fracture or dislocation, the hip's range of motion can be evaluated. The three components of range of motion consist of active range of motion, passive range of motion, and resistive range of motion. They should be tested in sequential order. In the evaluation process, active range of motion, or the amount of motion in a joint that the subject can generate independently, should always be assessed first. In demonstrating active range of motion, the subject performs flexion, extension, abduction, adduction, internal rotation, and external rotation of the injured hip (Box 12-1).

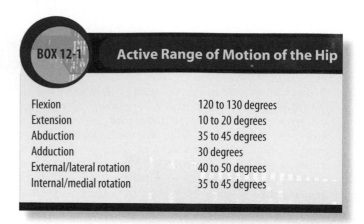

BOX 12-1 Active Range of Motion of the Hip

Flexion	120 to 130 degrees
Extension	10 to 20 degrees
Abduction	35 to 45 degrees
Adduction	30 degrees
External/lateral rotation	40 to 50 degrees
Internal/medial rotation	35 to 45 degrees

If the client is unable to perform full active range of motion, the athletic trainer should determine whether to assess passive range of motion. Assessing passive range of motion allows the examiner to evaluate anatomical restrictions of the hip or pelvis. Assessing passive range of motion allows the examiner to evaluate the amount of motion that occurs when he or she moves the client's body part through its available range of motion. At the beginning and end ranges of motion, an end-feel is determined. Assessing resistive range of motion allows the examiner to evaluate the amount of strength in the muscles involved at the joint being examined.

The athletic trainer must properly position the client before evaluating range of motion. Failure to do so may lead to inaccurate results. As with palpation techniques, bilateral comparison of all ranges must be tested in the same manner. The unaffected side may be tested before the affected side, but if the athlete is experiencing a great amount of pain, his or her apprehension will prevent the effective evaluation of range of motion. If at any time the athletic trainer suspects a fracture or dislocation, range of motion testing should be discontinued or not performed at all.

Special Tests

Implementing special tests as a component of the injury evaluation process helps the athletic trainer confirm the assessment of the injury.[4,6] The hip and pelvis special tests should be performed last, after all other components of the evaluation have been completed. If there are obvious signs of a fracture, dislocation, or loss of sensation and

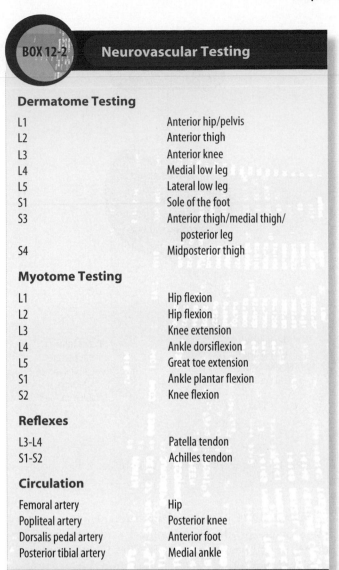

BOX 12-2 Neurovascular Testing

Dermatome Testing

L1	Anterior hip/pelvis
L2	Anterior thigh
L3	Anterior knee
L4	Medial low leg
L5	Lateral low leg
S1	Sole of the foot
S3	Anterior thigh/medial thigh/ posterior leg
S4	Midposterior thigh

Myotome Testing

L1	Hip flexion
L2	Hip flexion
L3	Knee extension
L4	Ankle dorsiflexion
L5	Great toe extension
S1	Ankle plantar flexion
S2	Knee flexion

Reflexes

L3-L4	Patella tendon
S1-S2	Achilles tendon

Circulation

Femoral artery	Hip
Popliteal artery	Posterior knee
Dorsalis pedal artery	Anterior foot
Posterior tibial artery	Medial ankle

movement, the special tests should not be performed. The client should be immobilized and referred to a physician immediately, and the emergency action plan should be implemented.

Neurovascular Tests

To evaluate the client's neurovascular status, the athletic trainer must assess dermatomes, myotomes, reflexes, and pulses. Neurovascular testing must be completed bilaterally to determine a loss of sensation, movement, reflex, and circulation in the lower quadrant (Box 12-2). By completing these tests, the athletic trainer can determine whether there is a disruption in blood flow or some form of abnormality in the hip or lower extremity region. Acute injuries to the hip, such as dislocations and fractures, may adversely affect these neurovascular structures. **Dermatomes** are assessed to identify skin sensation from a nerve root, **myotomes** are assessed to identify the motor function of the muscle from a nerve root, **reflexes** are assessed to test the state of the nerve root that supplies the reflex, and the pulse is assessed to determine the blood flow to the respective area. All results of neurological testing must be within normal limits. Any discrepancies between the unaffected and affected side must be immediately reported to a physician, who can complete further diagnostic testing.

Referrals and Diagnostic Tests

Referring the athlete to a physician or medical specialist for acute or chronic hip and pelvis injuries is imperative. Underlying secondary conditions, such as torn cartilage in the hip joint caused by a hip dislocation, may warrant a delay in advanced treatment. Improper management of hip and pelvis injuries sometimes leads to long-term disability or chronic conditions.

General Guidelines for Referral to Physicians

Athletic trainers should follow certain general guidelines in determining whether hip and pelvis injuries warrant referral to a physician. If a single trauma has occurred to the hip and the client has trouble walking or bearing weight, the client should be referred to a physician immediately to rule out fracture or dislocation.

If the client has had ongoing pain for several weeks and the condition is not improving, referral to a physician is warranted. Ongoing pain may be classified as pain that lasts for 1 week, 2 weeks, or even several months. The athletic trainer should determine the duration of the pain and seek proper medical advice.

Diagnostic Tests and Imaging

Early diagnosis and treatment of hip and pelvis injuries prevent long-term injury. Early intervention means that less time is lost from activity. Depending on the type of injury sustained, different diagnostic tools may be used in the evaluation process.

Film Radiography. Plain film radiography (X-ray) is used extensively in the diagnosis of hip and pelvic injuries in adults and children. Radiography facilitates the identification of bony abnormalities and joint injuries. The obvious difference between the skeletons of children and adults is the degree of maturity. Because the growing skeleton is more elastic than the adult skeleton, pediatric fractures often do not extend completely through the bone.[7,8] Computed tomography (CT) is considered to be superior to plain film in both

dermatomes structures that identify skin sensations from the nerve root
myotomes structures that identify the motor function of the muscle from a nerve root
reflexes predictable responses to external stimuli that test the state of the nerve root supplying the reflex

populations because it provides a three-dimensional image as opposed to the two-dimensional image produced by film radiography.

Magnetic Resonance Imaging. Magnetic resonance imaging (MRI) of the hip joint is extremely useful in the diagnosis of hip injuries and **avascular necrosis** of the hip (i.e., bone tissue death caused by diminished or interrupted blood supply to the area). Conventional MRI used for acute hip injuries and hip pain is often regarded as the standard protocol, especially if results of the plain film radiography are negative. The MRI provides a higher-quality image of the body than an X-ray does and is a preferred diagnostic tool for testing of young children because it does not involve radiation exposure.[8,9]

MANAGEMENT OF ON-FIELD AND ACUTE HIP AND PELVIS INJURIES

Proper management of acute hip and pelvis injuries is important in achieving a positive outcome. Stabilizing the injured area is of utmost importance. Most of the acute injuries to the hip and pelvis discussed in this chapter, such as dislocations and fractures, are considered medical emergencies (Figure 12-1). Individuals with these injuries should always be transported to the emergency room for physician referral and diagnostic testing. The athletic trainer's emergency action plan should always be current and reviewed periodically. Another commonly occurring acute injury, **hip pointer,** usually requires the medical attention of a physician within a 24-hour period. The athletic trainer must be aware that individuals with acute hip and pelvis injuries may go into shock as a result of the physical and emotional factors related to these injuries.

Hip Injuries

Traumatic or acute injuries of the hip usually result from collisions and violent contact. The physical demands in sports such as football, hockey, soccer, and water skiing provide the opportunity for these injuries to occur. To properly assess the severity and extent of the injury, the athletic trainer must perform the initial assessment quickly and efficiently. As discussed previously, a brief history, inspection, and palpation will determine whether the injury warrants emergency transportation. The immediate management of hip injuries is vital to prevent long-term disability.

Hip Pointer

A hip pointer is a contusion of the muscles that insert at the iliac crest. This injury occurs when the soft tissue is compressed between a hard object and the iliac crest and is seen in sports such as volleyball, gymnastics, and football in which the hip is not typically protected or padded.

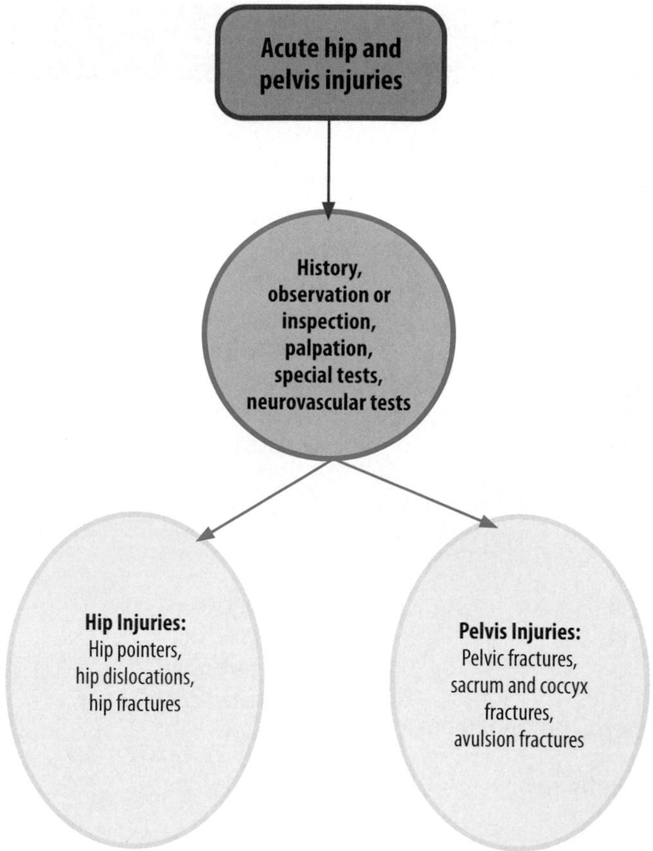

FIGURE 12-1 Concept map overview of acute hip and pelvis injuries.

Mechanism: Falling on an unprotected hip causes most hip pointers. Collision or contact with objects, teammates, or equipment may also result in a hip pointer.

Signs/symptoms:

- Localized pain at the iliac crest
- Inability to abduct or flex the leg at the hip joint
- Bruising of the area

Special tests:

Hip scouring test: The **hip scouring test** is used to determine the extent and severity of hip joint pathology. It can be used in conjunction with other tests to confirm diagnoses. The athlete is in a supine position with the hip and knee flexed to 90 degrees. The athletic trainer applies a downward pressure on the knee while rotating the hip into the internal and external position with hand placement on the anterior tibia. If the test is positive, the client experiences increased pain when the hip is moved through the ranges of internal and external rotation[6] (Figure 12-2). If positive, the athlete should be referred to a physician for further evaluation of hip joint pathology.

avascular necrosis loss of blood supply to the bone
hip pointer a bruise to the soft tissue overlying the iliac crest

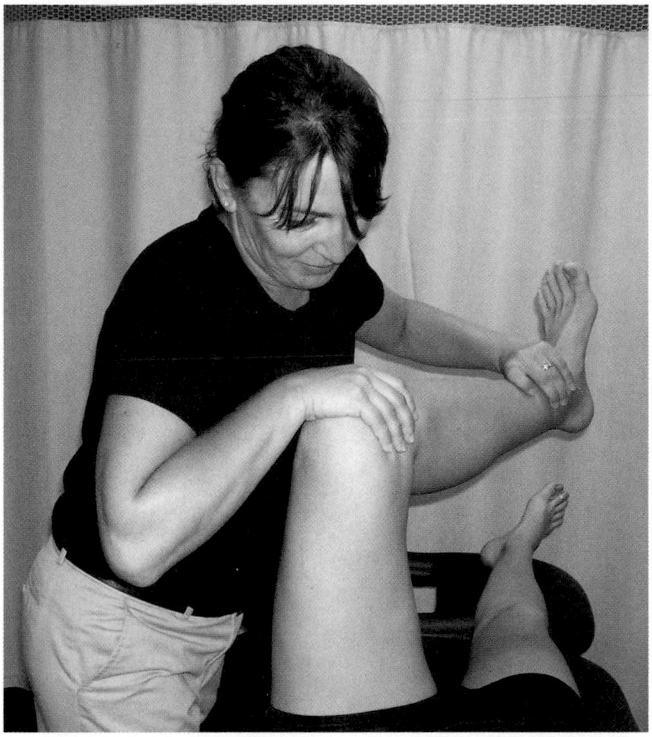

FIGURE 12-2 Hip scouring test assesses hip joint pathology.

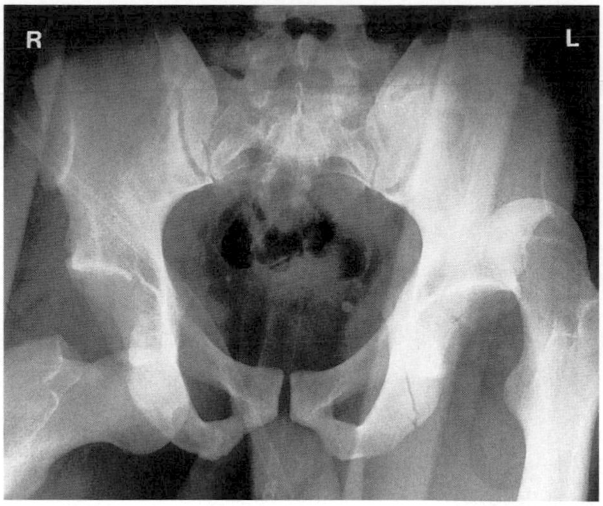

FIGURE 12-3 Hip dislocation in a patient who was in a motor vehicle accident and suffered both an anterior and a posterior dislocation of the hips. Posterior dislocation occurs 90% of the time and is seen here on the left, with the femoral head displaced superior and lateral to the acetabulum. On the right, an anterior dislocation appears, with the femoral head displaced inferiorly and medially. (From Mettler FA: *Essentials of radiology,* ed 2, Figure 8-103, Philadelphia, 2005, Saunders/Elsevier.)

Immediate management: Immediate treatment includes ice, nonsteroidal antiinflammatory medications, and rest for up to 72 hours after the injury. Crutches may be used if ambulation is difficult.

Intermediate management: The client should avoid activities that cause pain, participate in a comprehensive rehabilitation program to increase the strength and flexibility of the affected muscles, and ensure that equipment adequately protects the iliac crest. If pain persists, the client should be referred to a physician for further diagnostic testing and to rule out the possibility of fracture.

Hip Dislocations

Approximately 85% of traumatic hip dislocations occur with the hip positioned in adduction and internal rotation, which results in a posterior hip dislocation. Sports-related hip dislocations are extremely painful and primarily result from collisions during contact sports and skiing.[10] The dislocation is a result of the force placed along the femur when the hip is flexed.[1,10] The major complication of a hip dislocation is damage to the femoral head and loss of blood supply to the joint, which may lead to avascular necrosis of the femoral head. If this happens, the person will have chronic pain and instability and may eventually require a total hip replacement. Avascular necrosis also sometimes occurs when the hip subluxes. Immediate recognition, management, and treatment is important (Figure 12-3).

Mechanism: External force placed on the femur while the hip is in an adducted and flexed position causes most hip dislocations. Other mechanisms, such as a traumatic collision or fall, may also cause hip dislocations.

Signs/symptoms:

- The hip is in a position of adduction and internal rotation.
- The client is unable to perform active range of motion of the joint.
- The greater trochanter of the hip is prominent and easily palpated.
- The client experiences severe pain.

Special tests:

Hip log roll test: The purpose of the **hip log roll** is to test for pathological conditions of the hip joint (Figure 12-4). A positive sign of pain and the inability of the femoral head to roll and glide at the joint indicate a fracture or a hip dislocation. For this test, the athlete lies in a supine position and the athletic trainer places his or her hand on the distal femur to stabilize the pelvis at the anterior iliac crest. The athletic trainer then rolls the femur to the internal and external positions. The athlete should be immobilized and immediately referred to a physician if the test is positive.[6]

Immediate management: A traumatic dislocation is an orthopedic emergency. The athlete should be stabilized in the position in which he or she was found. The athletic trainer should monitor the vital signs of

Points to Ponder

How is this dislocation different from the others, and why is it a medical emergency?

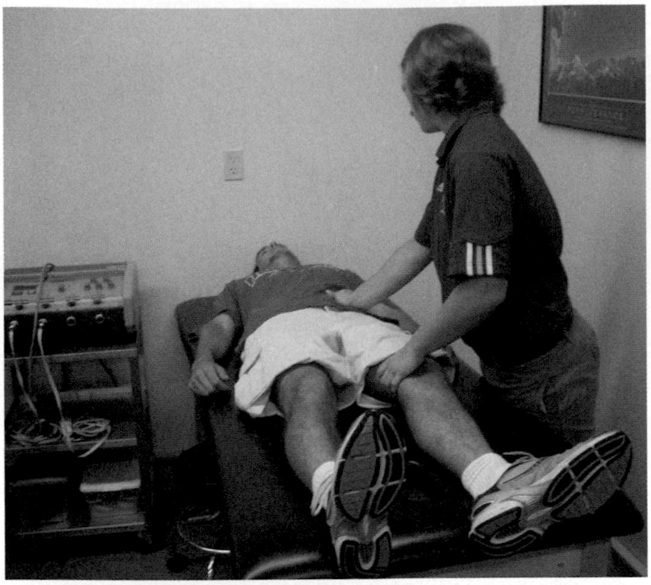

FIGURE 12-4 The hip log-roll test assesses hip joint pathology.

the lower extremity until emergency medical personnel arrive. The emergency action plan should be activated for immediate transport.

Intermediate management: Surgery is usually warranted to reduce the dislocated joint, and hardware such as metal may be needed to protect the joint from future dislocation.

Hip Fractures

Most hip fractures are the result of traumatic impact to the hip and femur. These fractures frequently occur at the neck shaft or head of the femur. Fractures of the femoral neck or shaft are considered low risk insofar as they typically do not lead to complications and respond well to individualized rehabilitation programs. On the other hand, fractures at the head of the femur are high risk because they fail to heal properly and often recur.[11] Because of the proximity of these fractures to arteries, nerves, and veins, suspected hip fractures are a medical emergency. Proper immediate injury management is of utmost importance to prevent unnecessary damage from being inflicted on these neighboring tissues.

Mechanism: High impact typically causes a hip fracture. Falls, especially in the elderly, may also cause hip fractures. People with osteoporosis are particularly susceptible to hip fractures because their bones are already weakened.

Signs and symptoms:

- Awkward position
- Severe pain
- Inability to move the leg independently
- Loss of function and possibly altered neurovascular status
- Point tenderness
- Possible bruising

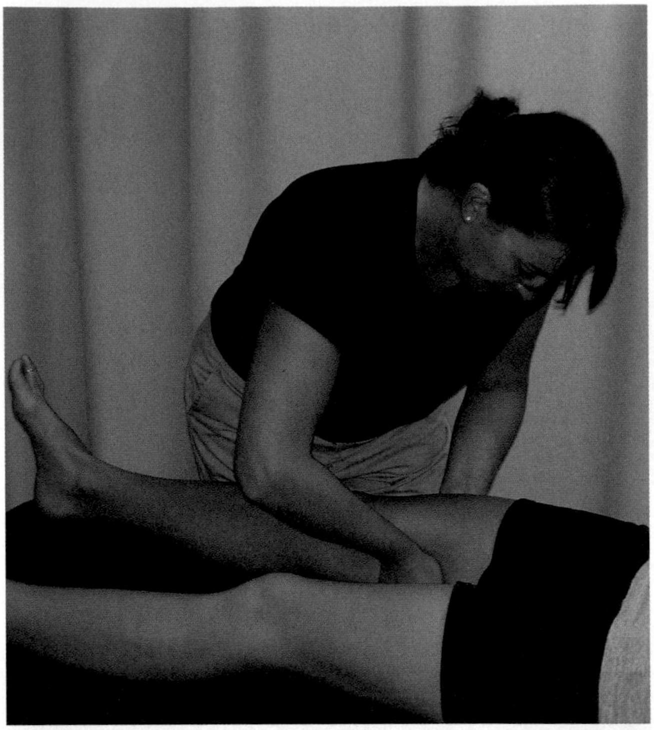

FIGURE 12-5 The long bone compression test assesses femur fractures.

Special tests:

Hip log roll test: See Figure 12-4.

Long Bone Compression Test: The long bone compression test is used to assess fractures of the femur. For this test, the athlete assumes a supine position. The athletic trainer places one hand on the client's medial thigh and one hand on the lateral thigh. Starting at the distal femur, the athletic trainer applies compression over the length of the femur. While applying pressure, the athletic trainer should gradually increase the amount of force (Figure 12-5). A positive test will produce localized or radiating pain either at the femoral neck or through the length of the femur. In this case, the athlete should be referred immediately to a physician by activating the emergency action plan and notifying emergency medical service personnel.[4,6]

Fulcrum test: The fulcrum test is used to assess femoral shaft stress fractures. For this test, the athlete is in a seated position with the knees bent at 90 degrees. The athletic trainer places one of the client's arms under the middle part of the leg. The athletic trainer places his or her opposite hand on the anterior distal femur, applying slight pressure to the anterior distal femur (Figure 12-6). If the client complains of sharp pain and exhibits apprehension when pressure is applied, the test is positive and the client should be referred to a physician for further evaluation.[4,6]

Box 12-3 summarizes acute hip injuries and the appropriate special tests used in diagnosis. A thorough evaluation consisting of the history, observation/inspection, and

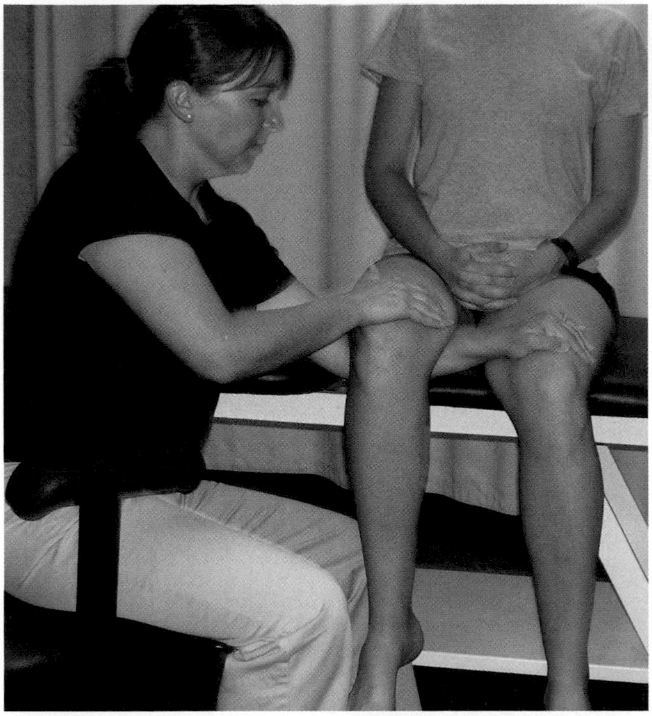

FIGURE 12-6 The fulcrum test assesses femoral shaft fractures.

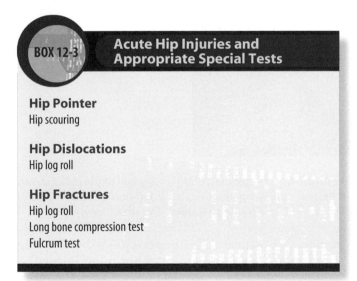

BOX 12-3 Acute Hip Injuries and Appropriate Special Tests

Hip Pointer
Hip scouring

Hip Dislocations
Hip log roll

Hip Fractures
Hip log roll
Long bone compression test
Fulcrum test

palpation helps determine which special tests are relevant to the client's condition.

Pelvis Injuries

The pelvis provides stability to the hip, abdomen, and lower back. This region is referred to as the *core of the body.* An acute disruption in the pelvis, such as a fracture or contusion, affects the function of the trunk and the entire lower extremity.

Pelvic Fractures

There is a low incidence of pelvic fractures related to athletic participation. Most pelvic fractures are caused by a direct force (Figure 12-7). Direct forces sometimes result from a high fall or major trauma. Because of the risk of internal bleeding, this injury is a medical emergency. Activation of the emergency action plan should follow any suspicion of a pelvic fracture.

Mechanism: Fractures of the pelvis occur from a traumatic force.

Signs/symptoms:

- Pain in the groin area
- Inability to ambulate
- Point tenderness
- Internal bleeding

Special tests: No specific special tests are applicable to this injury.

Immediate management: A pelvic fracture is a medical emergency. The patient should be taken to an emergency room.

Intermediate management: Surgery may be required before the client can return to activity. Any restrictions or limitations following surgery and rehabilitation should be strictly observed.

Sacrum and Coccyx Fractures

The sacrum and coccyx combine to form the distal portion of the spine. The coccyx is referred to as the *tailbone.* A fracture of the coccyx is referred to as a *break of the tailbone.* Although sacrum and coccyx fractures are relatively rare among athletes, they are common in activities such as roller skating, roller blading, motorcycle riding, and rock climbing—basically, any activity in which the participant is likely to fall on the tailbone. Sacrum and coccyx injuries are medical emergencies and warrant activation of the emergency action plan for immediate transport. Diagnostic testing and treatment will take place at the hospital.

Avulsion Fractures

Avulsion fractures are not common in adults, who usually experience a muscular strain instead. Avulsion fractures primarily occur in adolescents, whose skeletons are not yet mature. The injury mechanism for an avulsion fracture is a sudden violent muscular contraction or an excessive amount of muscle stretch over an open apophysis. They may occur at major muscle attachments in the pelvis.[1,10,12] These sites include muscular attachments at the anterior superior iliac spine, the anterior inferior iliac spine, the ischium, and the lesser trochanter of the femur.[13]

Mechanism: The most common way that athletes sustain an avulsion fracture in the pelvic region is from a sudden violent contraction. This overstretching and production of force cause the muscular attachment to rip off a small bony fragment instead of merely tearing the soft tissue.

Signs/symptoms:

- Sharp sudden pain in the pelvic or groin region
- Pain with palpation
- Swelling will be evident with palpation

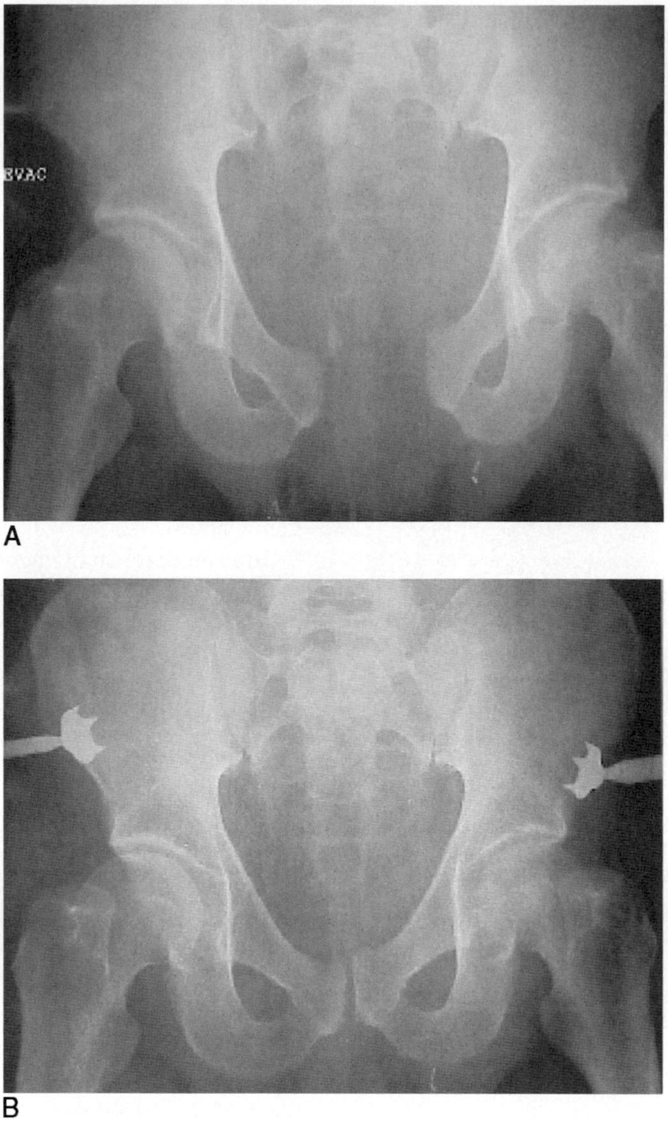

FIGURE 12-7 Pelvic fracture. Pelvic ring disruption with massive hemorrhage. **A,** Anteroposterior (AP) radiograph of the pelvis shows disruption of the symphysis pubis and the sacroiliac joint. **B,** AP view of the pelvis following reduction by application of the pelvic stabilizer. (From Townsend CM et al: *Sabiston textbook of surgery,* ed 17, Figure 21-13, *A & B,* Philadelphia, 2004, Saunders/Elsevier.)

Special tests:

Partial sit-up test: The partial sit-up test is used to determine the presence of an avulsion fracture at the pelvis. For this test, the athlete is in a supine position with the knees flexed at 90 degrees. The hands are placed behind the athlete's head, and the athlete is instructed to contract the lower abdomen and partially sit up (Figure 12-8). If the athlete experiences pain with abdominal contraction or is unable perform a partial sit-up, the test is positive and an avulsion fracture must be suspected. The client should be referred to the physician for follow-up evaluation.[4,6] A modified partial sit-up may be performed with the hands across the chest instead of behind the neck.

Immediate management: Initial treatment consists of ice and rest.

Intermediate management: The athlete should be referred to a physician for further evaluation, diagnostic testing, and treatment. The special tests used to diagnose acute pelvis injuries are shown in Box 12-4. Because of the low incidence of injuries to this area, there are fewer special tests. Also, because most injuries to the pelvis are medical emergencies, field assessments are not often performed.

MANAGEMENT OF CHRONIC/OVERUSE HIP AND PELVIS INJURIES

Chronic injuries are more common to the hip and pelvis region than acute injuries (Figure 12-9). This is primarily due to the frequency and amount of running most sports require. Of the 24% to 68% of injuries reported by runners, 2% to 11% involve the hip.[5] Chronic injuries are often a result of overtraining, poor biomechanics, and congenital and anatomical abnormalities.

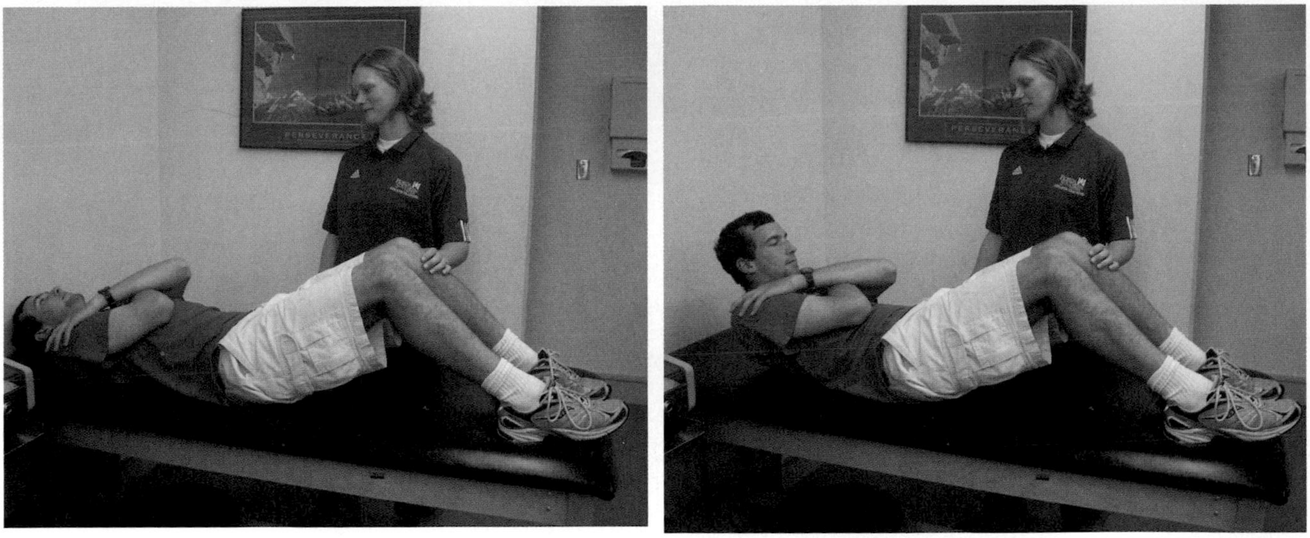

FIGURE 12-8 The partial sit-up test assesses avulsion fractures at the pelvis.

Hip Injuries

Athletes whose hip joints are subjected to a great deal of repetitive stress are susceptible to overuse injuries of the hip and pelvis. Activities such as running and jumping put the athlete at a higher risk for these types of injuries. The heavy lifting and repetitive activities associated with certain jobs predispose the hip to chronic injuries as well.

Stress Fractures

Most stress fractures are reported as overuse injuries by endurance athletes or recreational runners (Figure 12-10). Stress fractures can occur in the hip, pelvis, or thigh.[5] With the hip, stress fractures occur at the femoral neck, which is particularly susceptible because of the tendency of a tension side stress fracture to completely fracture.[2,3] A diagnosis may be delayed because the lesion is mistaken for another condition, such as a muscle strain. If not recognized, stress fractures may lead to a disabling condition such as bursitis or lower back pain.[2]

Mechanism: Repetitive overload, or stress with possible incorrect biomechanics, causes stress fractures.

Signs/symptoms:

- Onset of groin pain with a new activity
- Pain with activity that resolves with rest
- Palpable tenderness
- Possible palpable swelling

Special tests: There are no specific special tests applicable to this injury.

Immediate management: Once a stress fracture of the hip is suspected, the athlete should be referred to a physician for further evaluation and diagnostic testing. X-rays, bone scans, and computed tomography scans are used to diagnose stress fractures. Magnetic resonance imaging is frequently used to detect femoral neck stress fractures.[14] When diagnosed early and managed properly, stress fractures are likely to heal properly.

Intermediate management: After an accurate diagnosis of this injury has been made, the athlete will be required to rest. The need for crutches to immobilize the joint depends on the severity of the stress fracture. Typically, immobilization is prescribed for approximately 4 to 6 weeks. During this period, a light comprehensive rehabilitation program may be implemented.

BOX 12-4 Acute Pelvis Injuries and Appropriate Special Tests

Pelvic Fractures
No special tests

Sacrum and Coccyx Fractures
No special tests

Avulsion Fractures
Partial sit-up

Apophyseal Avulsion Fracture
No special tests

Trochanteric Bursitis

Trochanteric bursitis, which occurs in the area superficial to the greater trochanter of the femur, is an inflammatory condition that manifests as an aching pain over the lateral

trochanteric bursitis inflammatory condition that manifests as an aching pain over the lateral aspect of the hip

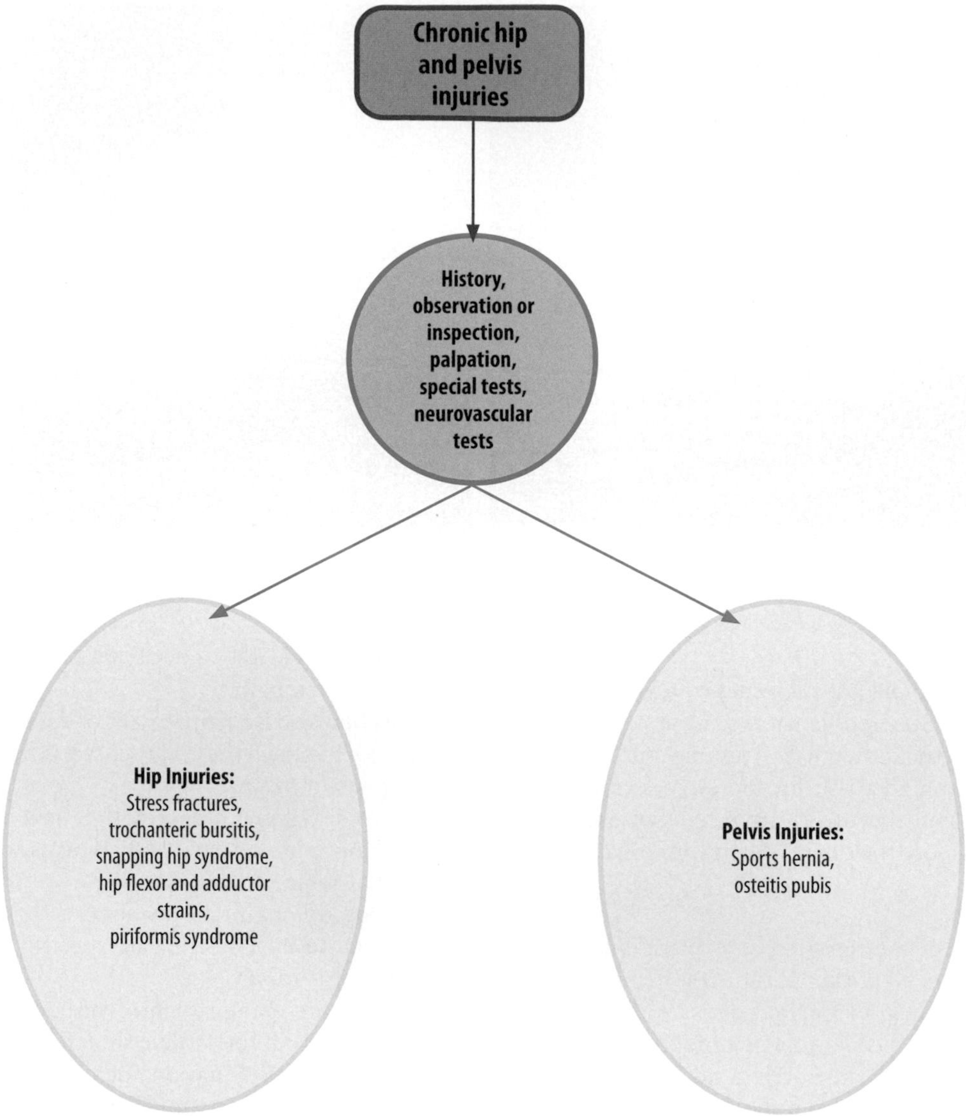

FIGURE 12-9 Concept map overview of chronic hip and pelvis injuries.

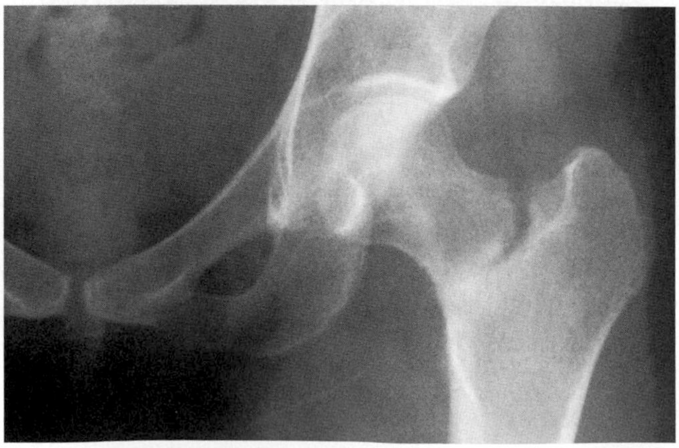

FIGURE 12-10 Stress fracture. (From Magee DJ: *Orthopedic physical assessment*, ed 4 [enhanced], Figure 11-63, Philadelphia, 2006, Saunders/Elsevier.)

aspect of the hip. This injury is caused by the friction of the gluteus medius or the iliotibial (IT) band against the greater trochanter. This condition can result from repetitive running, standing for an extended period of time, stair climbing, or direct traumatic contact to the lateral hip.[5] It is most commonly a consequence of running.

Mechanism: Repetitive forces caused by running or prolonged standing create undue stress and strain on the trochanteric bursa. This force, or friction, is related to the rubbing of the soft tissue as it moves over the greater trochanter.

Signs/symptoms:

- Lateral hip pain
- Point tenderness over greater trochanter
- Possible referred pain into the hip and groin
- Pain is produced with hip external rotation and abduction and resisted abduction

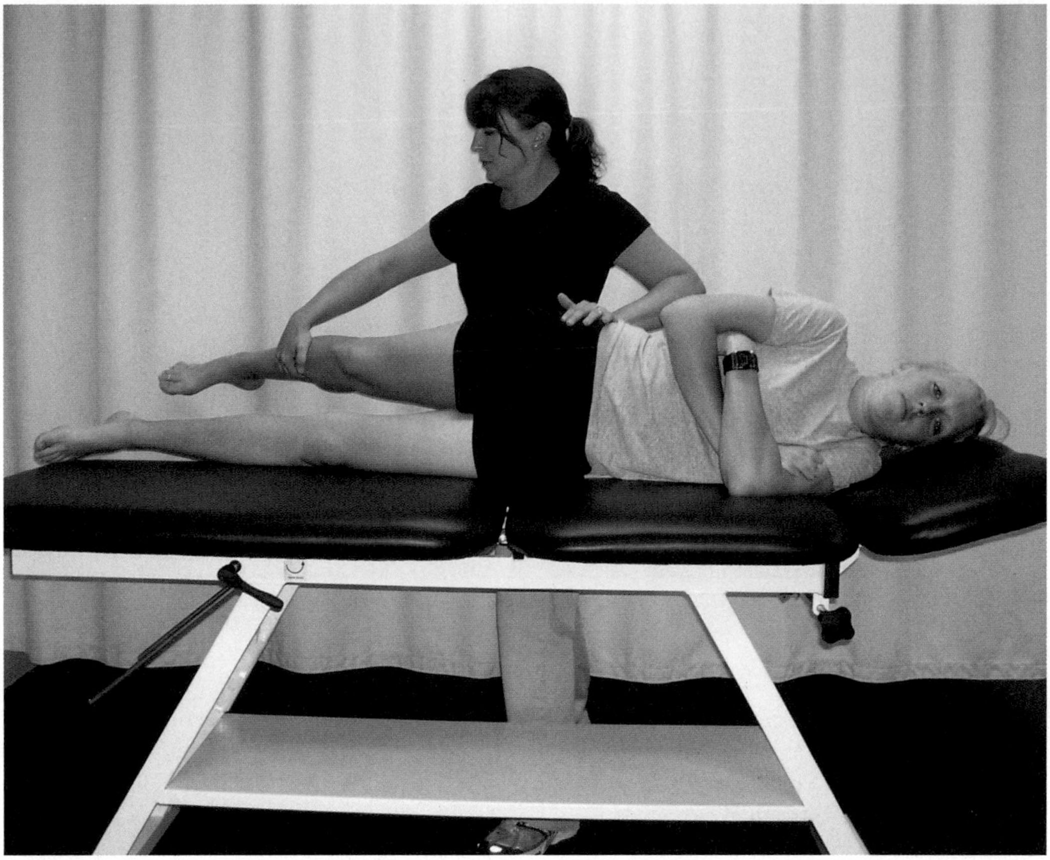

FIGURE 12-11 Ober's test assesses iliotibial band tightness.

Special tests: There are no specific special tests applicable to this injury.

Immediate management: This condition is best treated by ice, rest, and a comprehensive stretching and strengthening program focusing on the hip flexors, hamstrings, quadriceps, and IT band. Nonsteroidal antiinflammatory medications are sometimes used to control inflammation.

Intermediate management: If this condition persists, the athlete should be referred to a physician for further evaluation and treatment. Trochanteric bursitis may be relieved by aspiration of the bursa or a corticosteroid injection. Careful attention should be paid to the specific exercises being performed in the comprehensive rehabilitation program so as not to reproduce the mechanism of injury.

Snapping Hip Syndrome (Coxa Saltans)

Snapping hip syndrome, **coxa saltans,** is an audible pop or a snap heard in the hip region. The snap or pop occur during normal hip range of motion. It can be classified as either an internal or an external snapping hip. An internal snapping hip is the most common form of the condition. It is characterized by a painful sensation in the hip as the IT band snaps over the greater trochanter of the femur. It is associated with the iliopsoas muscle moving over the iliopectineal eminence, a prominence of the pelvic bone.[1,15,16] The onset of this condition is caused by rigorous activity and exercises.

Mechanism: Repetitive or strenuous activity that causes the IT band to ride over the greater trochanter is the most frequent cause of snapping hip syndrome.

Signs/symptoms:

- Dull pain
- Deep "catching" in the groin during flexion and extension of the hip
- Symptoms that may increase with activity
- Symptoms that may be intermittent because of the way that the hip changes position during activity

Special tests:

Ober's test: Ober's test is used to determine the extent of IT band tightness. The athlete lies on his or her side at the edge of the examination table with the lower hip and knee flexed. The upper leg is passively abducted and extended, allowing the IT band to cross over the greater trochanter. The leg is then passively lowered (Figure 12-11). If the test is positive, the leg will not lower to the table when the muscles are relaxed.[4,6]

coxa saltans snapping hip syndrome

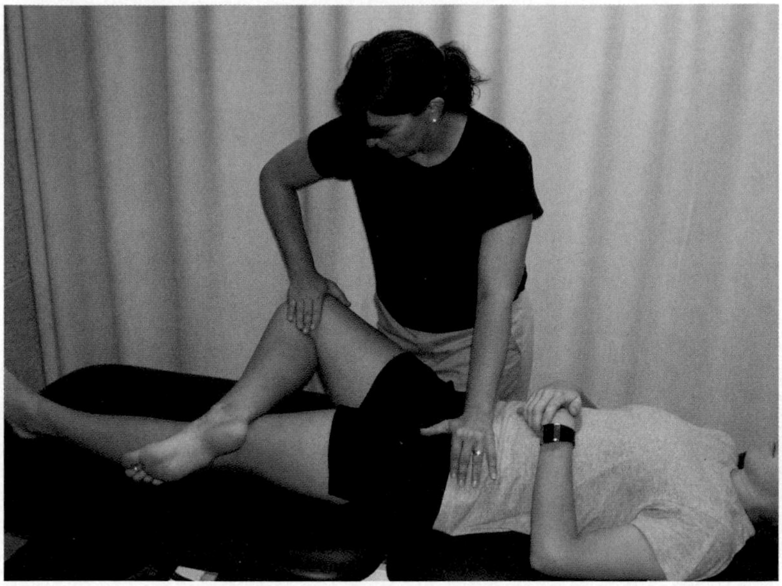

FIGURE 12-12 Patrick or Faber's test assesses iliopsoas spasm or sacroiliac involvement.

Patrick's or Faber's Test: To determine whether the athlete is suffering from an iliopsoas spasm or a sciatic joint condition, the athletic trainer should perform Patrick's or Faber's test. To perform this test, which involves flexion, abduction, and external rotation, the athletic trainer places the client in a supine position with the foot of the affected leg lying across the opposite knee (Figure 12-12). If the affected leg falls to the table or is parallel with the unaffected leg, the test is negative. A positive test indicates possible hip joint pathology in the affected leg, which is resting on across the opposite leg.[4,6]

Immediate management: This condition is treated with rest, ice, electrical modalities, nonsteroidal antiinflammatory medication, and hip flexibility exercises.

Intermediate management: If the condition is resistant to the previously described regimen, steroidal injections have been known to decrease the symptoms and allow the client to resume activity.

Hip Flexor and Adductor Strains

Hip flexor and adductor strains are common in the areas surrounding the hip and groin. These muscular strains are commonly seen in off-season and preseason training and conditioning periods. They are caused by a dynamic exertional tension force on the muscle, which is common in activities that involve sudden side-to-side motions. Hip flexor and adductor strains also sometimes result from repetitive stresses caused by a lack of strength or a muscle imbalance. People suffering from this type of injury experience a loss of strength and a significant strain.[1,5,13]

Mechanism: In many cases, individuals who attempt training or occupational loads beyond their current capacities eventually strain a muscle. Depending on the activity, the hip flexors and adductors may not be able to handle the loads being placed on them. The result is likely to be a strain to the involved muscles.

Signs/symptoms:

- Pain with palpation in the groin or medial thigh
- Palpable defect or deformity in the strained muscle
- Pain with active range of motion of hip flexion and adduction
- Loss of strength in hip flexion and adduction

Special tests:

Ely's test: Ely's test is designed to assess the tightness of the rectus femoris. The athlete is placed in a prone position as the examiner passively flexes the knee (Figure 12-13). Rectus femoris tightness is indicated

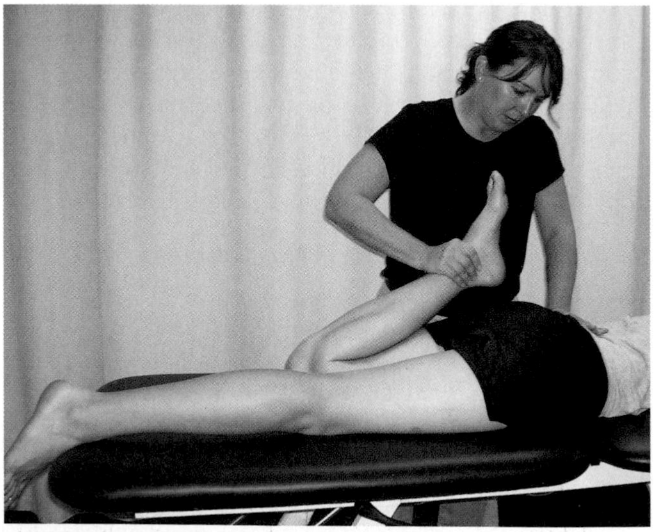

FIGURE 12-13 Ely's test assesses recurrent femoris tightness.

if the athlete's hip on the same side of the flexed knee flexes up and off the table. Both sides should be tested and compared with each other during this test.[4,6]

Thomas test: The **Thomas test** assesses hip flexor contractions (Figure 12-14). The athlete is in a supine position. Excessive lordosis in the supine position indicates the presence of tight hip flexors. Next, the athlete flexes one knee and pulls it to the chest. If the opposite leg remains flat on the table, there is no reason to suspect hip flexor tightness. However, if the opposite leg rises off the table when the involved knee is pulled to the chest, the test is positive. If the opposite leg does not rise off the table but abducts, the IT band is tight.[4,6]

Immediate management: This condition can be treated with rest, ice, electrical modalities, nonsteroidal antiinflammatory medication, and exercises that increase hip flexibility and strength.

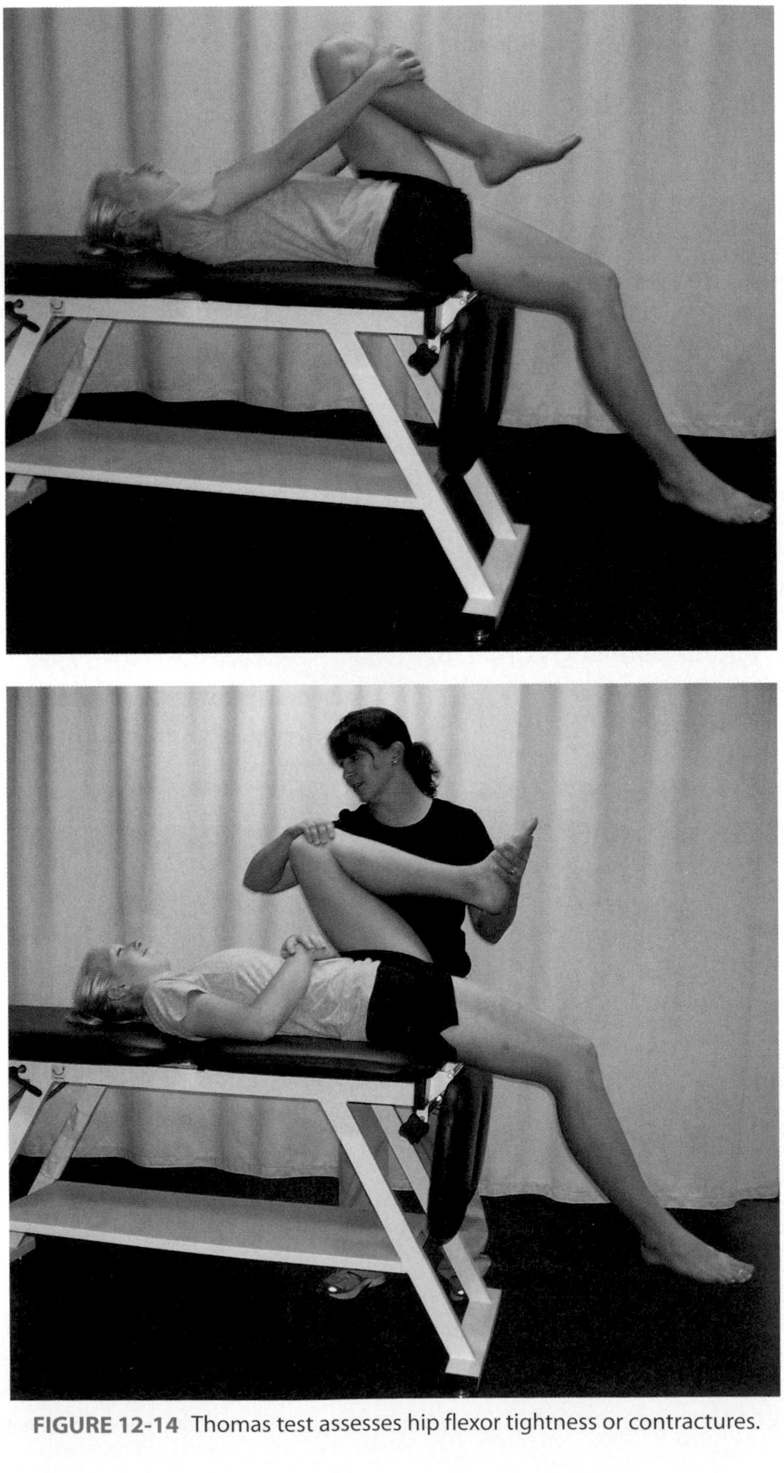

FIGURE 12-14 Thomas test assesses hip flexor tightness or contractures.

Intermediate management: Flexibility and strength exercises should be performed in all planes of motion at the hip. If the condition is resistant to this approach, the athlete should be referred to a physician for further evaluation. Magnetic resonance imaging may yield further diagnostic evidence to assist with the treatment plan.

Piriformis Syndrome

Piriformis syndrome relates to the piriformis muscle and possible compression or irritation of the sciatic nerve. The piriformis muscle attaches to the spine and to the head of the femur. It assists in rotation of the hip. Piriformis syndrome is common in runners and women, who have relatively tight hip flexors, as well as in people who sit a lot. If the irritation is sufficiently severe, pain radiates down the posterior leg and into the low back.[10]

Points to Ponder

Can you think of any other factors that may make these individuals more susceptible to this problem?

Mechanism: Structural variations of the relationship between the piriformis and the sciatic nerve and overuse or excessive strain may cause piriformis syndrome. The combination of tight hip flexors and weak gluteals may also lead to the development of this syndrome.

Signs/symptoms:

- Tightness or spasm of the piriformis muscle
- Pressure on the sciatic nerve
- Pain or point tenderness deep in the buttocks
- Burning or numbness in the buttocks, sacrum, or sciatic nerve distribution
- Pain with passive internal (medial) rotation
- Loss of strength in hip abduction and external (lateral) rotation

Special tests:

Piriformis test: For the piriformis test, the athlete is placed in a side-lying position with the unaffected side on the table. The athlete's hip should be flexed to 60 degrees with the knee also flexed. The hip is stabilized, and pressure is applied to force the affected side into internal rotation (Figure 12-15). If pain results when pressure is applied, the test is positive. Pain will be elicited in the muscle or the buttocks if the piriformis muscle is tight or if the sciatic nerve is being pinched.[4,6]

Trendelenburg test: The Trendelenburg test is used to assess the strength of the gluteus medius muscle and hip stability. The athlete starts in a standing position. The athletic trainer should be positioned behind the athlete, who should stand on one leg. The athletic trainer should observe the athlete to see whether his or her posterior iliac crests rise. If the opposite hip rises, the standing leg has normal strength. If the opposite hip drops when the athlete is standing on the affected leg, then the strength of the gluteus medius on the standing leg is decreased (Figure 12-16). This test should be performed on the unaffected side first so that the athlete can better understand the implementation of the test.[4,6]

Immediate and intermediate management: Treatment for this condition consists of a comprehensive rehabilitation plan, with special emphasis on stretching the piriformis muscle. The rehabilitation plan should involve progressive strengthening exercises of the hip in external rotation, extension, and abduction; flexibility exercises;

piriformis syndrome irritation or compression of the piriformis muscle or the sciatic nerve

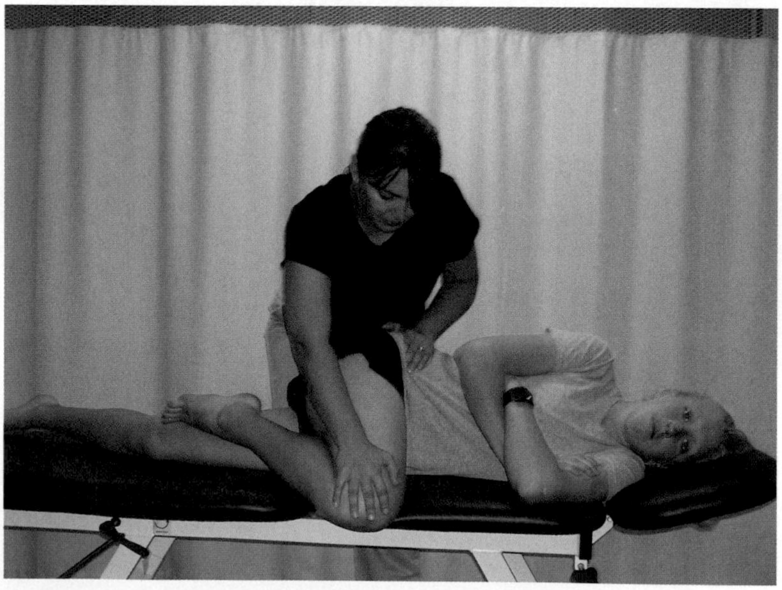

FIGURE 12-15 Piriformis test assesses piriformis tightness or sciatic nerve involvement.

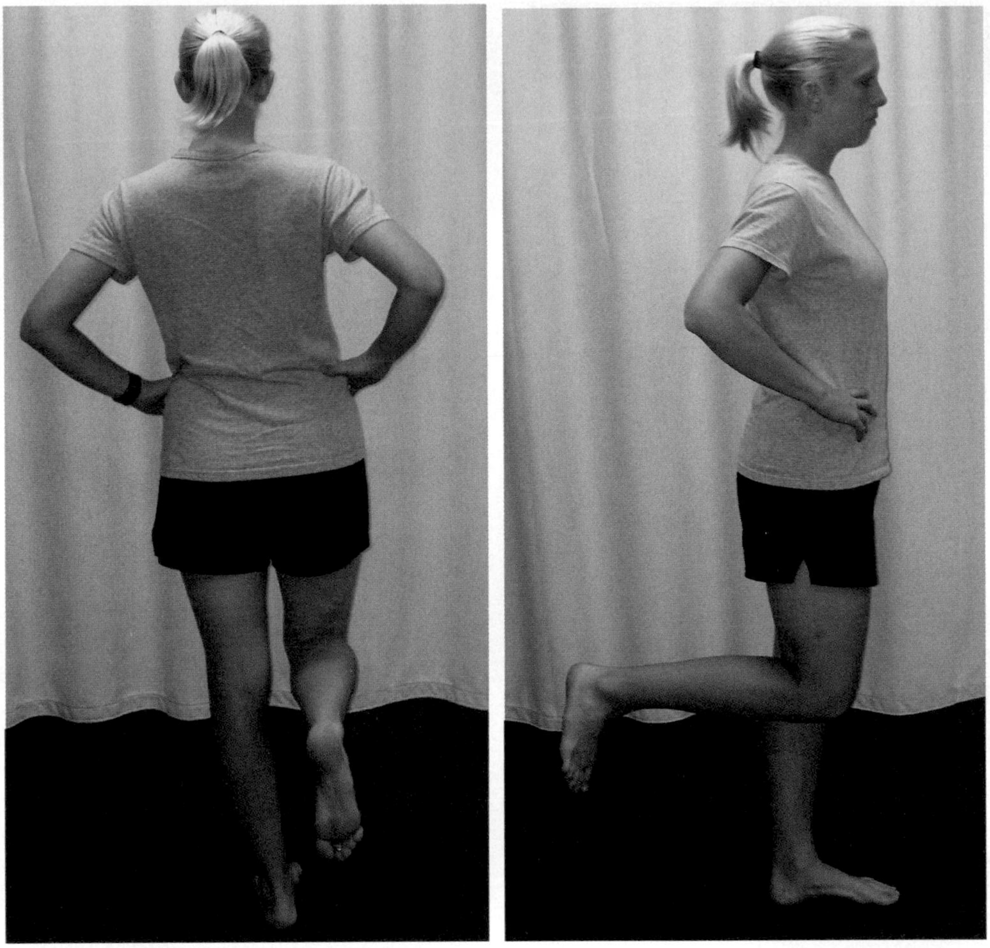

FIGURE 12-16 Trendelenburg test assesses gluteus medius strength and stability.

and combined exercises to develop neuromuscular control of the abdomen, low back, and hips.

The soft tissue involvement and movement demands of the hip region increase the risk of chronic and overuse injuries. Typically, muscle imbalances and soft tissue inflexibility are causative factors. Box 12-5 lists chronic hip injuries and the appropriate special tests used in diagnosis.

Pelvis Injuries

Chronic injuries of the pelvic region are relatively rare in the active population. Groin pain represents 5% of all athletic injuries, with sports hernias and osteitis pubis somewhat more common.[17] Sports hernias result from probable weakening of the musculature that allows other tissues or organs to protrude through the defect. Osteitis pubis often affects individuals who frequently participate in running, jumping, and kicking movements. These repetitive activities can lead to instability of the pubic symphysis, causing inflammation and irritation.[17]

Sports Hernia

Sports hernias result when the muscles or tendons of the lower abdominal wall are weakened. **Inguinal hernias** occur in the inguinal canal. When an inguinal hernia occurs, weakening of the abdominal wall can create a palpable pouch, the hernia. In the case of a sports hernia, the hernia is not palpable even though it too results from a weakening in the same abdominal wall muscles.[1,17]

Mechanism: A weakening of the abdominal musculature allows other tissues or organs to protrude through the abdominal wall. Activities involving rotation of the trunk frequently lead to sports hernias.[18]

Signs/symptoms:

- Localized pain and tenderness
- Ongoing or chronic groin pain with exercise
- Insidious presentation of pain
- Similar to groin or hip adductor strains

Special tests: There are no specific special tests applicable to this injury.

Immediate and intermediate management: The athlete should be referred to a physician for further evaluation. If the symptoms persist or worsen, surgery may be necessary.

sports hernia weakening of the muscles or tendons of the lower abdominal wall

inguinal hernia weakening of the abdominal wall

BOX 12-5 Chronic Hip Injuries and Appropriate Special Tests

Stress Fracture
No special tests

Trochanteric Bursitis
No special tests

Snapping Hip Syndrome
Ober's test
Patrick's or Faber's test

Hip Flexor and Adductor Strains
Ely's test
Thomas test

Piriformis Syndrome
Piriformis test
Trendelenburg test

Legg-Calve-Perthes Disease
No special tests

Slipped Capital Femoral Epiphysis
No special tests

Osteitis Pubis

Osteitis pubis, a painful condition in the pelvis, is an inflammation of the pubic symphysis and surrounding muscle insertions (Figure 12-17). This condition is caused by unusual stress to the pelvis with activities such as running, jumping, twisting, and weight lifting.[19]

Mechanism: Overexertion of the muscles surrounding and attaching to the pelvis causes this painful condition.

Signs/symptoms:
- Lower abdominal pain and midline anterior pelvic pain
- Insidious development of pain that progressively worsens with activity
- Difficulty walking with the increase of pain

Special tests: There are no specific special tests applicable to this diagnosis.

Immediate and intermediate management: A rehabilitation program will decrease the symptoms of this condition. This program consists of rest until the pain decreases; nonsteroidal antiinflammatory medication; exercises that increase the flexibility of the hip, abdomen, and lower back; core strengthening exercises; and strengthening exercises for the hip.

Pelvis injuries occur less frequently than hip injuries. Box 12-6 lists chronic injuries to the pelvis. It should be

osteitis pubis inflammation of the pubic symphysis and surrounding muscle insertions

BOX 12-6 Chronic Pelvis Injuries and Appropriate Special Tests

Sports Hernia
No special tests

Osteitis Pubis
No special tests

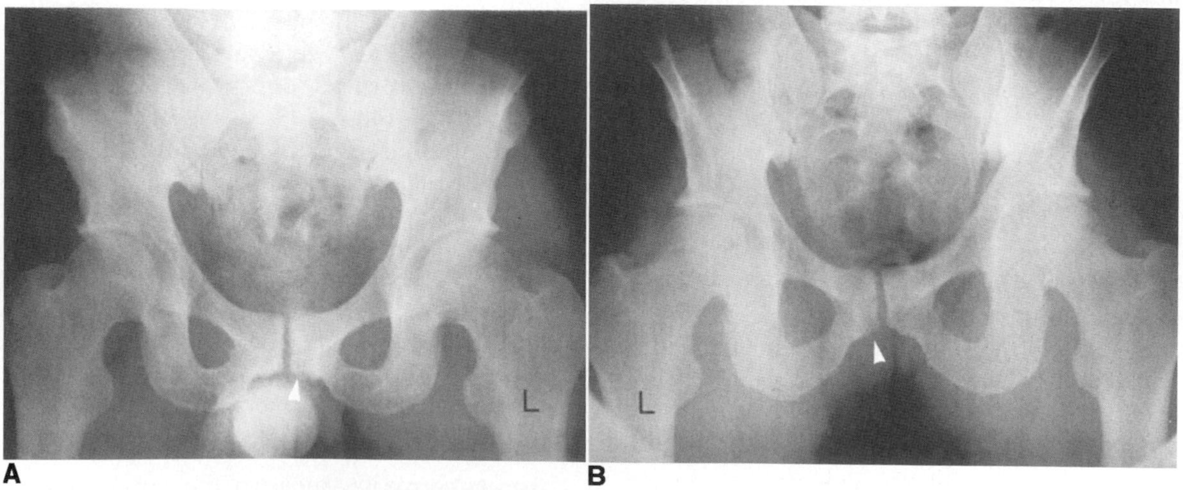

FIGURE 12-17 **A,** Anteroposterior view of pelvis showing a well-concealed bony lesion at the inferior corner of the left pubis at the symphysis *(arrowhead)*. **B,** Posterior view of the same pelvis. The bony fragment is well delineated. (From Wiley JJ: Traumatic osteitis pubis: the gracilis syndrome, *Am J Sports Med*, 11:361, 1983.)

noted that there are no special tests for these injuries. The complexity of this area makes it difficult to perform special tests.

TAPING, BRACING, AND RETURN TO PLAY

When preparing an athlete to return to play, the athletic trainer must not take shortcuts in the rehabilitation plan. Because of the biomechanical nature of the related structures of the hip and pelvis and their importance in overall function, a full rehabilitation plan must be implemented. This program should include flexibility exercises to increase joint range of motion in hip abduction, adduction, flexion, extension, and internal and external rotation. Strength training is another important aspect of rehabilitation and, like flexibility, it must be implemented in all ranges of hip motion. Make sure that the exercises focus on internal and external rotation of the hip, an area that is often overlooked in rehabilitation plans.

The rehabilitation plan must also include progressive functional activities to prepare and adapt the hip and the lower extremity to the inherent movements of the client's sport. These targeted activities will ultimately enhance the athlete's performance. The inclusion of strength and flexibility exercises, along with balance and proprioception activities[20] and neuromuscular training,[21,22] can help both to heal the existing injury and to prevent future injury in the lower extremity. Keep in mind that an athlete with a hip or pelvis injury must have full range of motion as well as full muscular strength and endurance equal to the opposite hip before returning to play.

Unlike other areas that may become injured, there is not a taping or bracing application that is strong enough to adequately support the hip and pelvic area, although use of compression shorts or a hip spica wrap can be helpful sometimes. Because of the lack of devices to assist the hip and pelvis biomechanically, injuries to these structures must be fully healed before an athlete is cleared to return to play.

THE AGE-GROUP ATHLETE

Injuries to the hip and pelvis are possible at any age. The majority of injuries that younger athletes incur result from traumatic insult or unusual responses to the growth and maturation of their bodies. Fractures, Legg-Calve-Perthes disease, and slipped capital femoral epiphysis will be discussed here. In the mature athlete, injuries frequently occur because of degenerative changes taking place over time or as a result of repetitive overuse movements executed with improper technique and mechanics. Total hip replacements are indicated in some cases.

Adolescent and Pediatric Athletes

In the adolescent and pediatric populations, athletic injuries to the hip and pelvis cover an entire spectrum of possible causes, from a single traumatic event to repetitive trauma. Most hip and pelvic injuries in adolescent and pediatric athletes are soft tissue injuries, apophyseal injuries, or underlying hip disorders.[23] Bony injuries may involve fractures, acute dislocations, and avulsion fractures. Hip dislocations account for 2% to 5% of all joint dislocations, but only 5% occur in children younger than 14 years of age.[23,24] Hip disorders include conditions such as Legg-Calve Perthes disease and slipped capital femoral epiphysis. The exact nature of any given injury depends on the age of the athlete, the nature of the trauma, the training and conditioning regimen, and the particular sport.

Apophyseal Avulsion Fractures

Apophyseal avulsion fractures of the pelvis are considered rare in the athletic population as a whole. These injuries are, however, seen in adolescent athletes between 14 and 17 years old because of the weakness of the open apophysis[9] (Figure 12-18). This weakness is due to the immaturity of the adolescent skeleton and the open growth plates. Growth plates are growing tissue at the end of the long bones in children and adolescents. As a person physically matures, the bone becomes more solid and stronger. Apophyseal avulsion fractures result from a sudden forceful contraction of the musculotendinous unit while the athlete is engaged in kicking a ball, running, or jumping. This action causes the tendon to pull a fragment of bone from the pelvis. Pain increases with palpation and passive stretching of the involved muscle.[9] This injury occurs primarily in explosive sports such as soccer, rugby, ice hockey, gymnastics, and sprinting.[9,25]

Mechanism: An abrupt contraction of the muscles causes the partially closed apophyseal plate to avulse and pull off intact with the muscle attachment.

Signs/symptoms:

- Acute onset of localized pain
- Localized swelling
- Possible referred pain to the involved tuberosity of the muscle attachment
- Loss of muscular function preventing partial sit-ups or active hip flexion

Special tests: There are no specific special tests applicable to this diagnosis.

Immediate management: Immediate treatment is ice and immobilization. The immobilization consists of being fitted for crutches to decrease weight bearing.

Intermediate management: The athlete should be referred to a physician for further evaluation and diagnostic testing.

apophyseal avulsion fracture fracture in which a forceful muscle contraction causes the tendon to pull off a fragment of the pelvis; associated with adolescent athletes

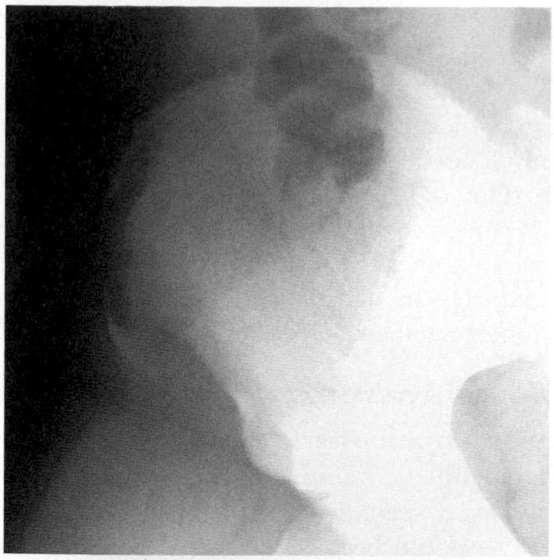

A

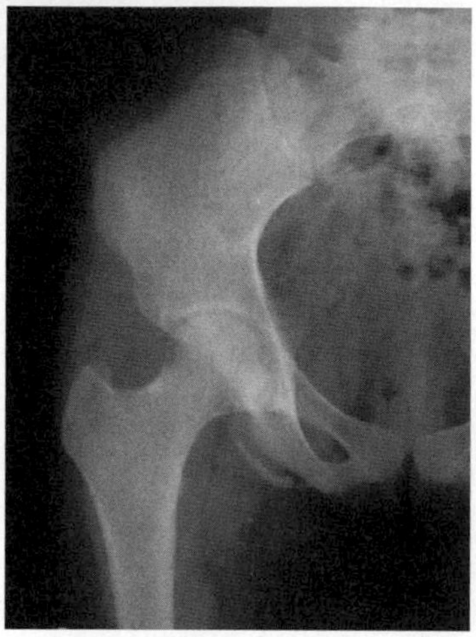

B

FIGURE 12-18 Apophyseal injuries. **A,** Anterior superior iliac spine (ASIS) avulsion fracture in an adolescent athlete. **B,** Ischial tuberosity avulsion fracture in an adolescent athlete. (From Kocher M, Tucker R: Pediatric athlete hip disorders, *Clin Sports Med* 25: 242, 2006 [Figures 1 and 2].)

Legg-Calve-Perthes Disease

Legg-Calve-Perthes disease is usually seen in children between 2 and 12 years of age and is five times more common in boys than girls.[9] This condition is characterized by a loss of blood supply to the femoral epiphysis, which causes decreased bone mass and avascular necrosis (Figure 12-19). The primary factor is that the head of the femur does not stay in the socket of the joint. Avascular necrosis occurs when the blood supply to the bone is disrupted, resulting in the death of the bone tissue of the femoral head. It is described as a form of arthritis in the hips of young children. Legg-Calve-Perthes disease is diagnosed by X-ray examination.

Mechanism: Deformity within the hip joint leads to slippage of the femoral head, causing bone loss and eventual tissue death.

Signs/symptoms:

- Onset of mild pain
- Slight limping with gait

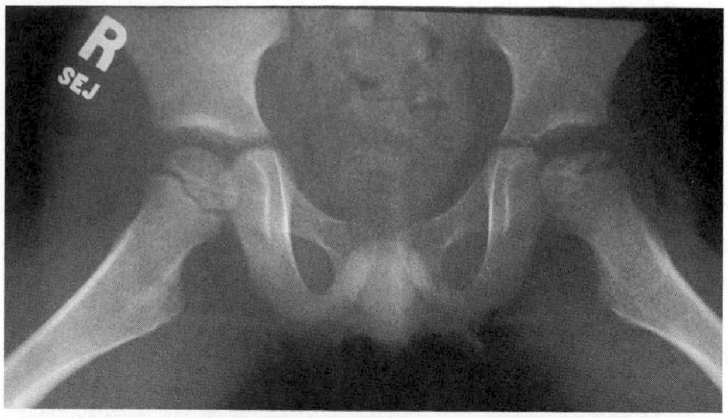

FIGURE 12-19 Legg-Calve-Perthes disease of the left hip. (From Kocher M, Tucker R: Pediatric athlete hip disorders, *Clin Sports Med* 25: 245, 2006 [Figure 5].)

- Symptoms that may be present for an extended period of time
- Pain that may mimic muscle spasms of the hip and groin

Special tests: There are no specific special tests applicable to this diagnosis.

Immediate management: Treatment consists of reducing the swelling of the hip joint, restoring the range of motion of the hip joint, and using X-ray film to ensure that the head of the femur stays within the socket while it heals.[1,9]

Intermediate management: If the hip does not maintain its position in the socket, surgery is the alternative treatment option to stabilize the hip joint.

Slipped Capital Femoral Epiphysis

Slipped capital femoral epiphysis is a condition affecting the adolescent population. It occurs more often in boys and young men than in girls and young women and usually occurs when the subject is between the ages of 10 and 16. It usually strikes after a growth spurt and the onset of puberty. The head of the femur slides out of the socket as a result of shearing forces related to extension and external rotation of the femoral neck and shaft[9] (Figure 12-20). A slipped capital femoral epiphysis may be due to a weakness in the growth plate and repetitive slippage, or it may be associated with a minor trauma or fall.

Mechanism: Extensive running, jumping, twisting, and turning or trauma causes the femoral head to repeatedly slip out of the joint socket.

Legg-Calve-Perthes disease a loss of blood supply to the femoral epiphysis causing loss of bone mass and avascular necrosis

slipped capital femoral epiphysis condition in which the head of the femur slides out of its socket; associated mainly with adolescent boys

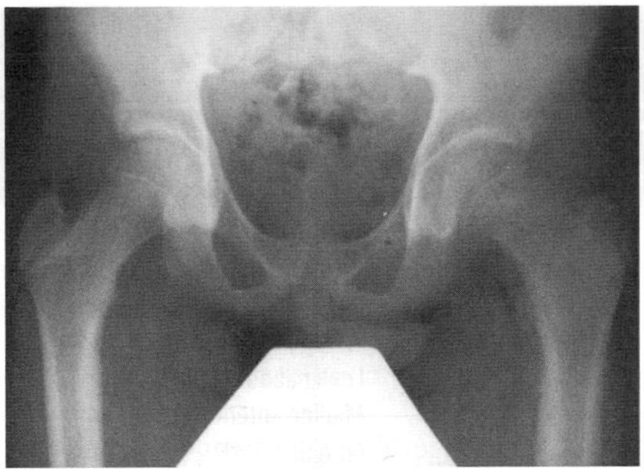

FIGURE 12-20 Anteroposterior pelvis radiograph demonstrating a left mild slipped capital femoral epiphysis. (From Kocher M, Tucker R: Pediatric athlete hip disorders, *Clin Sports Med* 25: 244, 2006 [Figure 4].)

Signs/symptoms:

- Possible history of hip, leg, or knee pain
- Noticeable limp with ambulation
- Inability to bear weight
- Possible outward-turned appearance of affected leg

Special tests: There are no specific special tests applicable to this diagnosis.

Immediate and intermediate management: Clients with a history of hip, leg, or knee pain should be referred to a physician for further evaluation and diagnostic testing.

Mature Athletes

According to some estimates, one quarter of the U.S. population will be older than age 55 by the year 2010. Older athletes are more susceptible to chronic and overuse injuries than are children, adolescents, and younger adults. As muscle ages, it begins to shrink and lose mass. The number and size of the muscle fibers decrease. With age, bones become less adaptable to the stress of physical activity because of changes in the balance between bone formation and bone absorption. Joints become more restricted, and flexibility decreases because of the breakdown of the cartilage in the joints that results from a lifetime of physical activity.[26,27]

Chronic and overuse injuries account for 70% of injuries in athletes older than 60 years of age. Only 41% of young adults are affected by such injuries. Athletic trainers should encourage older adults to adopt a consistent exercise plan emphasizing low-impact exercise to prevent chronic and overuse injuries.[26] Low impact exercises reduce the stress placed on the bones and joints.

Total Hip Replacements

Total hip replacement is a common solution for degenerating hip joints in the older adult (Figure 12-21). Recently, however, this procedure is being performed on younger patients. Athletes involved in activities that require jumping, planted hip rotation, and abrupt bracing of blocking moments are susceptible to these degenerative changes.[28] Loss of bone mass can also contribute to joint degeneration.[29] With appropriate rehabilitation, the active older adult can return to activity after a total hip replacement. Older adults who have undergone hip replacement surgery should expect not only pain relief but also the opportunity to return to their previous activities.[30,31]

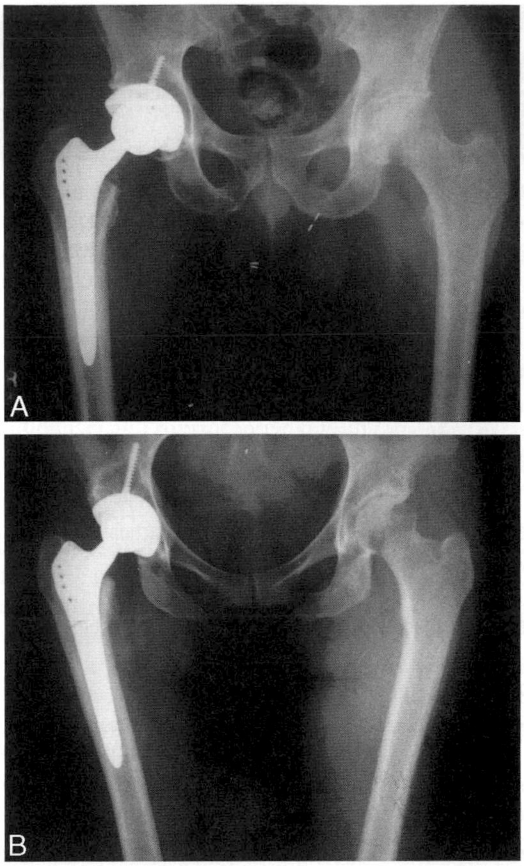

FIGURE 12-21 Total hip replacement. **A,** A 48-year-old patient, who was able to return to tournament-level beach volleyball. **B,** A 43-year old patient, who returned to work as a Pilates instructor. (From Yun A: Sports after total hip replacement, *Clin Sports Med* 25:360–361, 2006 [Figures 1 and 2].)

SUMMARY

Lower extremity injuries result from the physical demands of certain activities. Because the hip and pelvis connect the lower extremity to the trunk, they are susceptible to myriad injuries. Athletic trainers must quickly recognize the signs and symptoms of the injury and provide the appropriate management and treatment. If the athlete is not making progressive improvement during the rehabilitation process, the athletic trainer should consider referring him or her to a physician for further evaluation and diagnostic testing. If treatment of hip and pelvis injuries is delayed, long-term and possibly debilitating conditions may result.

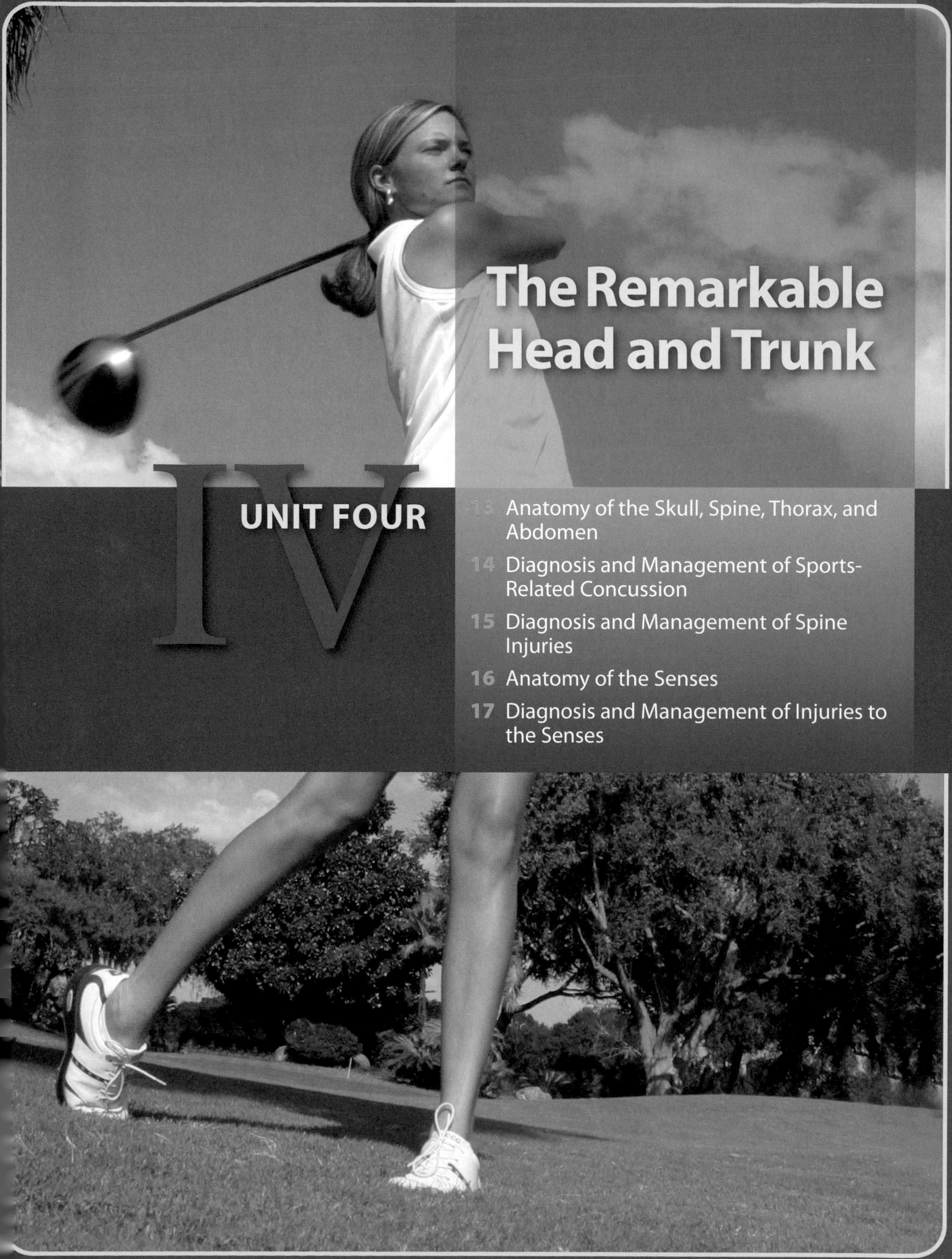

The Remarkable Head and Trunk

IV UNIT FOUR

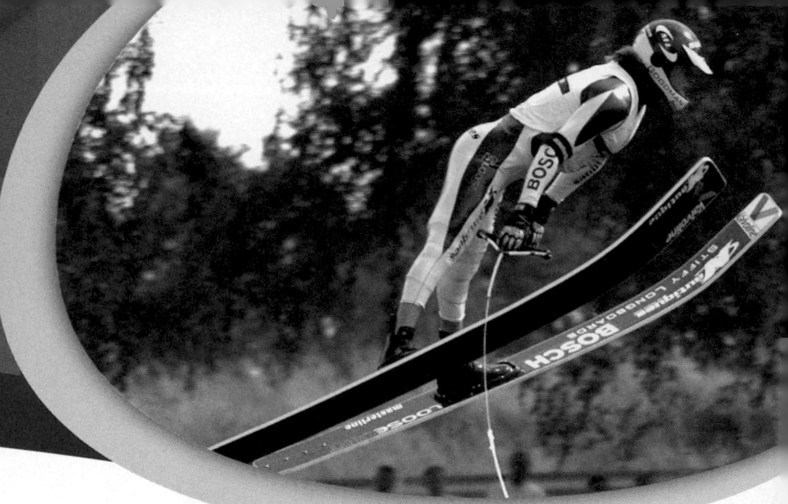

13

Anatomy of the Skull, Spine, Thorax, and Abdomen

ROBERT MOSS

Learning Goals

1. Name and describe the basic anatomical structures (bones, ligaments, muscles, tendons, nerves, arteries, veins), their unique aspects, and their locations relative to the spine, thorax, and abdomen.
2. Use appropriate terminology when describing anatomical structures of the spine, thorax, and abdomen.
3. Understand the interdependence of the structures of the spine, thorax, and abdomen.
4. Recognize the complexity of the structures of the spine, thorax, and abdomen.
5. Identify the ways in which the role or function of each of the anatomical structures may change with various movements that occur above or below them.

The spine may be described as the workhorse of the body. Like a workhorse, it gets very little attention until it is injured, at which point its importance becomes obvious. The body is rotated, flexed, extended, compressed, distracted, and laterally bent from the bottom up as the force of lower body movements is transmitted up through the pelvis to the lower spine (Figure 13-1). Likewise, the spine is rotated, flexed, extended, compressed, distracted, and laterally bent from the top down as upper body (i.e., head, trunk, and arm) movements result in forces being transmitted down through the upper spine. Often, forces are transmitted up and down the spine at the same time, and the spine is expected to handle all of them. For this reason, the spine may be compared to a mediator of sorts—caught in the middle, trying to appease the rest of the body by synchronizing forces not of its own making while attempting to carry out other important functions. The spine works hard while we are moving, and it works hard when we are just standing or sitting. About the only time the spine gets rest is when we are lying down, and even then certain positions, supine or prone, can exert problematic stress on this region.

Research suggests that more than 80% of the population may experience back pain at some point in their lives; moreover, back pain affects people of all ages. Heavy backpacks and poor posture are often blamed for back pain among children and adolescents. A sedentary lifestyle is thought to cause back pain in the middle-age population. An accumulation of factors, including obesity, are suspected to contribute to back pain in the older population.

Back injuries are a major issue for athletes. A study of injury incidence in athletes from 150 high schools and covering 10 different sports was conducted over a 3-year period. The researchers discovered that 13% of the injuries in football involved the back. A different study found that 15% of the injuries in gymnastics affected the spine. However, it is widely believed that spine injuries are underreported, because many of them result from overuse and develop gradually. The same

Terms that appear in boldface green type are defined in the book's glossary.

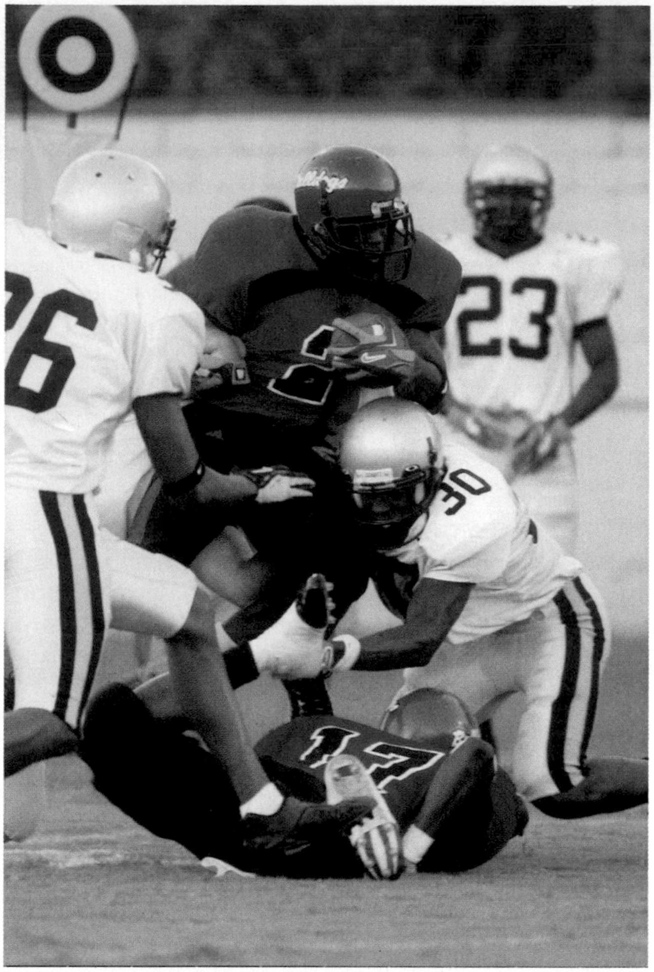

FIGURE 13-1 During physical activity the spine is often placed in compromising positions. (Courtesy Skyhawk Sports Photography, Athens, Ga.)

assumption holds true for back injuries; only a few have an acute, or a sudden, onset. Instead, they are often dismissed as an unpleasant but inevitable fact of life.

Although the focus of this chapter is the spine, other areas of the body directly related to the spine, including the skull, thorax, and abdomen, are also discussed. The skull, spine, and sternum and ribs of the thorax comprise the **axial skeleton**. The upper and lower extremities with their shoulders and hips, respectively, form the **appendicular skeleton**.

FUNCTIONS OF THE SKULL, SPINE, THORAX, AND ABDOMEN

The skull serves the obvious and critical function of protecting the brain. It also has other important responsibilities that are often taken for granted. It provides passageways throughout the body so that our senses function properly and various structures are able to take in oxygen and nutrients. The eyes, ears, nose, and mouth all serve as passageways in the skull that allow us to see, hear, smell, taste, breathe, and eat. These senses and other aspects of the face are presented

BOX 13-1 Functions of the Skull

1. The skull protects the brain from injury.
2. The skull provides passageways for oxygen, nutrients, and the organs of the senses.

in more detail in Chapters 16 and 17. At the base of the skull, there is another passageway that allows the brain to communicate with the rest of the body as the spinal cord enters the skull to unite with the brain. Box 13-1 summarizes the skull's functions.

The spine has four general functions. First, it protects the spinal cord and spinal nerves. The spinal cord serves as the main hub between the brain and the peripheral nerves in the transmission of information to the muscles, organs, and structures of the body while it also receives information from the muscles, organs and structures of the body. By sending and receiving information, the spinal cord allows the body to interact with its environment. The protective function of the vertebrae is essential to allow the spinal cord and nervous system to work as it should because so much of these structures lies within the vertebral and intervertebral **foramina**.

The second function of the spine is to support the weight of the upper body when walking, running, jumping, or performing any activity in which one foot or both feet are in contact with the ground. The spine also supports the weight of the lower body if the person is performing a movement such as a handstand, in which the hand or hands are in contact with the ground. In fact, a unique aspect of the spine is that it is made up of 26 bony segments (i.e., vertebrae) instead of being a single entity, such as a femur or tibia. This arrangement makes the weight-supporting mechanism, whether involving the upper or lower body, more precarious than if the spine were a single-structure column; however, the spine's unique composition also enhances its ability to absorb forces.

A third function of the spine is to alternate between being a rigid axis and a flexible axis for the body and for the head. Think of what the spine has to do during

axial skeleton all the bones that form the trunk and serve as an axis for the attachment of extremities

appendicular skeleton all the bones that form the upper and lower extremities (arms and legs); referring to an appendage or limb

foramina anatomical holes or openings formed by adjacent bones or within a bone; usually used as passageways for nerves or blood vessels walking or running. It has to be quite rigid so that the body can move through space. If the spine were limp like a wet noodle, the body would collapse during walking and running. The spine also has to be rigidly flexible during certain activities. Javelin throwing, ballroom dancing, and gymnastics all require strength and flexibility of the spine.

Fourth and lastly, the spine is a critical component of **posture** and movement. As most people know, poor posture is responsible for a variety of problems, including back pain. Proper posture requires the ability to maintain a stable spine and is important whether a person is standing, sitting, or moving about. Proper posture and positioning of the spine is integral in almost any movement of the human body.

Box 13-2 summarizes the functions of the spine.

The general functions of the thorax and abdomen are similar to those of the spine (Box 13-3). The thorax—which comprises the thoracic spine, ribs, and sternum—protects the lungs, heart, trachea, esophagus, and aorta. Movements of the thorax, although not of the same magnitude as those of the knee, hip, and most other joints in the body, may actually be more important because they allow proper respiration to occur. The thorax, by way of the ribs and sternum, adds stability to the thoracic spine, whereas the cervical and lumbar areas do not have these ancillary structures to provide strength. Of all the nonfused vertebral areas of the spine (i.e., cervical, thoracic, and lumbar), the articulations between the vertebrae of the thoracic spine are the least mobile.

The abdominal muscles and lumbar spine, with some help from the lower ribs, serve to protect the organs of the abdomen and add stability to the posture of the thorax and vertebral column. Abdominal organs include the stomach, spleen, liver, pancreas, gallbladder, abdominal aorta, inferior vena cava, and the intestines. Lying outside the abdomen are the kidneys, which are located in a similar transverse plane but posterior to the area generally described as the abdomen.

BOX 13-2 Functions of the Spine

1. The spine protects the spinal cord and spinal nerves, structures that lie within the vertebral and intervertebral foramina.
2. The spine supports the weight of the upper body when walking, running, jumping, or doing any type of activity in which a foot or the feet are in contact with the ground. This same function, weight-bearing by the spine, can be applied to the lower body if an individual is performing a movement in which one or both hands are in contact with the ground, such as a handstand.
3. The spine provides a rigid or flexible axis, as necessary, for the body and the head.
4. The spine serves as a critical component of posture and movement.

BOX 13-3 Functions of the Thorax

1. The thorax protects the lungs, heart, trachea, esophagus, major blood vessels, stomach, spleen, liver, pancreas, gallbladder, intestines, and kidneys.
2. The thorax supports the spine, turning it into a cylindrical axis, by simple engineering principles, making it much stronger and providing more support than the spine would provide as a simple axis.
3. The thorax allows the spine to be alternately rigid and flexible by serving as an axis for the body and for the head.
4. The thorax helps the spine maintain good posture and provide stability during movement of the entire body.

The pelvis functions to protect the organs it contains—the bladder, reproductive organs, vessels, and nerves. It also provides the spine with a strong base of support. Refer to Chapter 9, which describes the function of the pelvis in transmitting and dampening forces from the lower extremity up to the spine.

ANATOMY OF THE SKULL

This chapter confines its discussion of the anatomy of the skull to the bones, ligaments, joints, muscles, and nerves. The organs of sense are presented later, in Chapter 16. Although the skull is often conceptualized as two functional bony structures, the "skull" bone and the "jaw" bone, there are actually 28 bones that fit together almost like a jigsaw puzzle.

Bones of the Skull

The bones of the skull may be divided into three areas: (1) the cranium, (2) the face, and (3) the ear bones. The cranium, or brain case, is composed of eight bones. There are two pairs of parietal and temporal bones and one each of the frontal, occipital, sphenoid, and ethmoid bones. Paired parietal and temporal bones make up most of the **lateral** aspects of the skull. The frontal bone, as its name implies, makes up the front of the skull. The back of the skull is occupied by the occipital bone. Ethmoid and sphenoid bones are very irregular in shape and comprise most of the floor of the cranium, with the ethmoid being anterior to the sphenoid. *Sphenoid* means "wedge shaped," and it is sometimes called the "keystone" between the frontal, parietal, and occipital bones. It has also been compared

posture the means of supporting one's own body weight while sitting, standing, or walking

lateral away from the midline or center of the body (outer aspect) relative to another landmark to a "butterfly" because it appears to have wings and a body like a butterfly's. The location of the ethmoid allows it to serve as part of the posterior aspects of the eye orbits and the nasal area.

The face has 14 bones—six paired bones and one each of the vomer and mandible (Figure 13-2). Paired bones are the nasal, maxillary, zygomatic, lacrimal, palatine, and inferior nasal conchae. The two maxillae are the centerpieces of the face insofar as all the other facial bones articulate with it, except the mandible. The maxillae also hold the upper teeth. The left and right maxillae connect below the nose. Just above the nose two nasal bones serve as a bridge between the maxillae. On the upper, lateral aspects of the face the two zygomatic bones, or cheekbones, connect the maxillae to their respective temporal bones (Figure 13-3).

The very small, fingernail-sized and -shaped lacrimal bones are located just lateral and posterior to the nasal bones. The palatine bones form the posterior roof of the mouth, and the inferior nasal conchae resemble ledges in the nasal cavity. The vomer is deep to the nasal cavity and articulates with the sphenoid and ethmoid as well (Figure 13-4).

The remaining facial bone is the mandible, which might be thought of as the lower jaw (see Figure 13-3). It articulates with the temporal bone of the cranium to form the only movable joint of the skull.

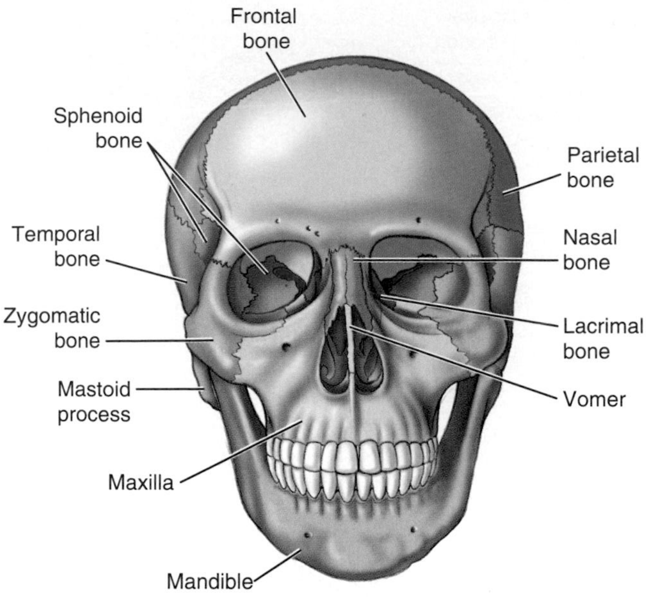

FIGURE 13-2 The anterior skull. (From Herlihy B: *The human body in health and illness,* ed 3, p. 115, Philadelphia, 2007, Saunders/Elsevier.)

Three pairs of ear bones—the auditory ossicles (Figure 13-5)— are located in what is known as the *middle ear.* They are the malleus, incus, and stapes, which resemble a miniature hammer, an anvil, and a stirrup, respectively.

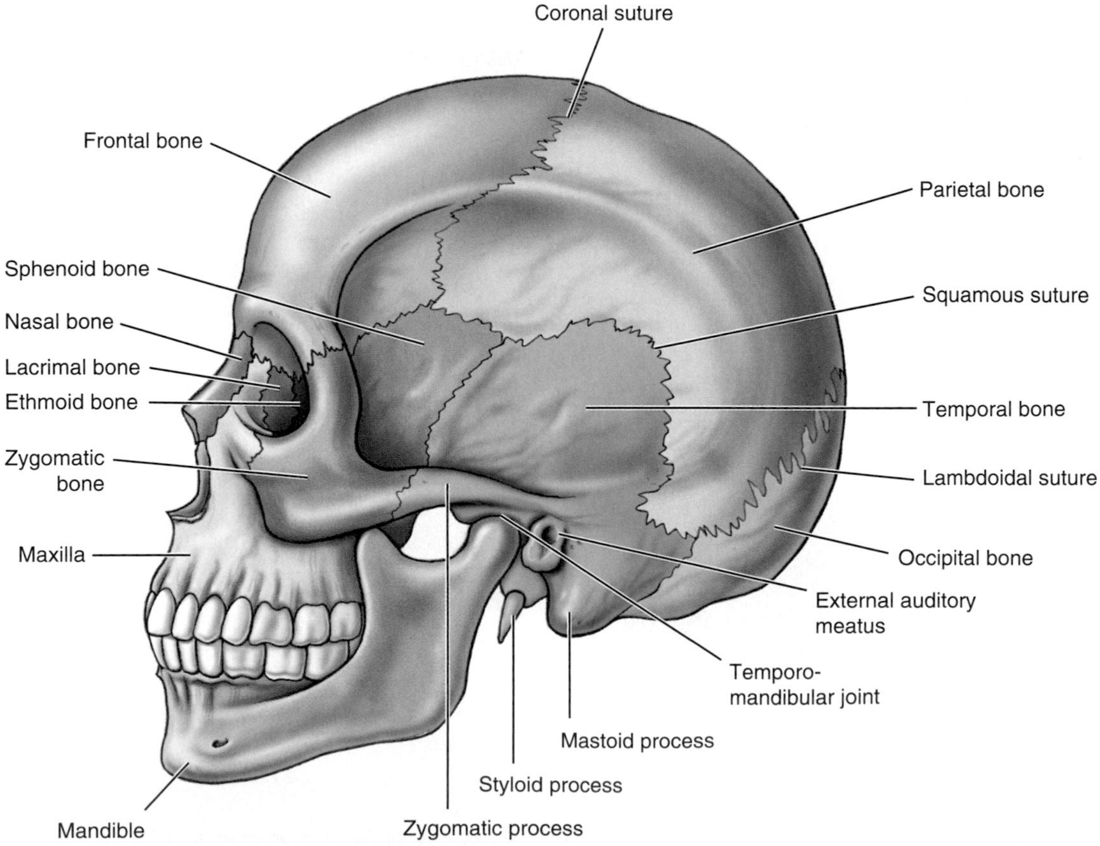

FIGURE 13-3 The left side of the skull. (From Herlihy B: *The human body in health and illness,* ed 3, p. 115, Philadelphia, 2007, Saunders/Elsevier.)

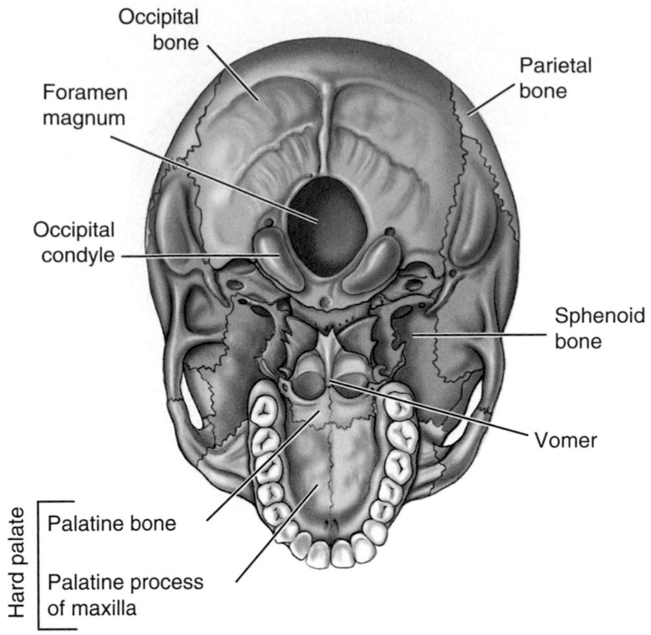

FIGURE 13-4 The cranial cavity and floor. (From Herlihy B: *The human body in health and illness,* ed 3, p. 115, Philadelphia, 2007, Saunders/Elsevier.)

Various articulations of the cranium bones and facial bones form important structures of the skull. For example, the frontal, ethmoid, lacrimal, sphenoid, zygomatic, maxillary, and palatine bones form the eye sockets. The nose and ear have passageways that allow their special senses to occur. Cavities, or spaces, in some of these bones are also known as sinuses. The frontal, sphenoid, ethmoid, and maxillary bones all have sinuses. Foramina, or small holes, are located in many of the skull bones for the passage of nerves, arteries, and veins. More details of the senses, sinuses, and facial features are discussed in Chapter 16.

Lastly, the hyoid bone, which is part of the axial skeleton, is located just below the mandible and above the larynx in the upper neck. Essentially suspended by muscles, it has the distinction of being the only bone in the body that does not articulate with any other bones.

Note that all of the bones of the skull are unique. They vary in shape, thickness, and articulation with adjacent bones. They also vary dramatically in bony landmarks. Further study of these bones will confer a sense of how remarkable they are. Their names, like those of the other bones of the body, are Greek or Latin in derivation and suggest their shape or purpose.

Box 13-4 summarizes the bones of the skull as well as the major joint of interest, which is detailed in the following section.

Joints and Ligaments of the Skull

Although it is true that joints are formed whenever two bones articulate, the types of joints that are formed vary throughout the body. Joints are often conceptualized as areas where two bones move against each other. This is generally true in the appendicular skeleton, the arms and legs. In the skull, however, only one joint functions in a fashion similar to that of the common joints of the

sinuses air cavities found in the bones of the head

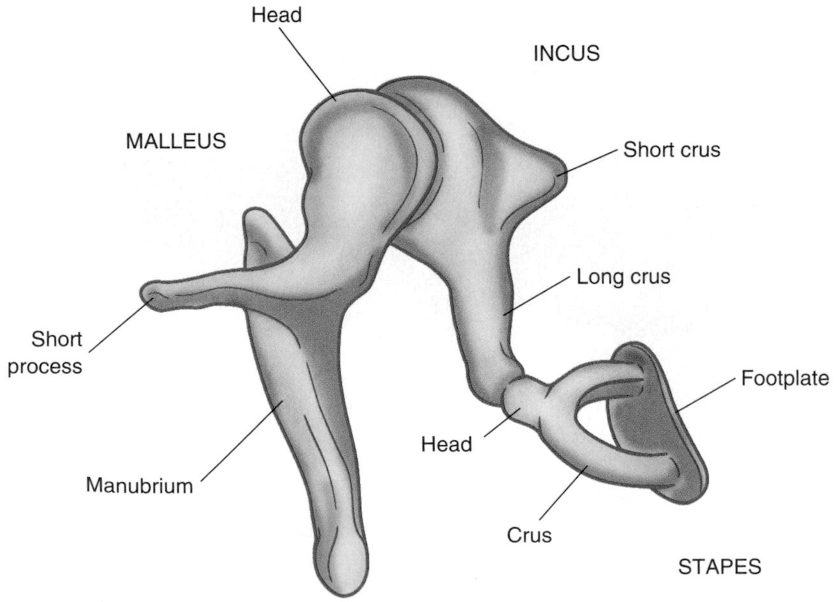

FIGURE 13-5 The auditory ossicles. (From Seidel HM et al: *Mosby's guide to physical examination,* ed 6, p. 319, St Louis, 2006, Mosby/Elsevier.)

BOX 13-4 Bones and Joints of the Skull

Bones

Cranium (8 Bones)

- Two pairs of parietal bones (lateral)
- Two pairs of temporal bones (lateral)
- Frontal bone (front of skull)
- Occipital bone (back of skull)
- Ethmoid bone (cranial floor; anterior to sphenoid)
- Sphenoid bone (wedge shaped; cranial floor)

Face (14 Bones)

- Maxillae (paired; center pieces of face)
- Nasal bones (paired; just above nose)
- Zygomatic bones (paired; cheekbones)
- Lacrimal bones (paired, small, fingernail-sized; lateral and posterior to nasal bones)
- Palatine bones (paired; form posterior roof of mouth)
- Inferior nasal conchae (paired; ledges in nasal cavity)
- Vomer (single bone; deep to nasal cavity)
- Mandible (single bone; lower jaw)

Ear (6 Bones)

- Auditory ossicles located in middle ear
- Malleus (paired; resembles miniature hammer)
- Incus (paired; resembles anvil)
- Stapes (paired; resembles stirrup)

Axial Skeleton Bone

- Hyoid (located below mandible and above larynx)

Joints

- Synovial joint: temporomandibular joint (TMJ)
- Fibrous joints: suture joints

arms and legs. That joint is the temporomandibular joint (TMJ), and it is classified as a **synovial joint**. The two words *temporal* and *mandible* distinguish the two bones that comprise the joint, and the articulation occurs just in front of the inferior ear. The TMJ is employed whenever a person opens and closes the mouth. It is often the site of pain and dysfunction.

The skull has many other articulations that are not as mobile as the TMJ; these joints are classified as **fibrous joints**, and within the classification of fibrous joints they are further classified as suture joints. Suture joints are not considered to be mobile as the TMJ, shoulder, and knee are. Suture joints are unique in that they are soft and somewhat pliable in infants, a characteristic that allows the skull to grow and accommodate to the growth of brain. These joints later become more solid so that the brain is better protected. However, some allied health practitioners believe that subtle movements of the bones of the skull occur throughout life. Currently, however, this belief is not widespread.

Muscles of the Skull

The cranium and the face contain many muscles, too many to cover within the scope of this text. The muscles discussed in this chapter are classified as the muscles of facial expression and the muscles of mastication, or chewing. These are summarized in Table 13-1.

Muscles of Facial Expression

Surprise, fear, amusement, and anger are just a few of the expressions represented by the various combinations of muscle contractions that occur about the skull (Figure 13-6). Unique to each individual are expressions of unbridled joy and extreme frustration. The occipitofrontalis is really two muscles, with the occipitalis covering the occipital bone in the back of the skull and the frontalis muscle covering the frontal bone, or forehead. These muscles are connected by a tough connective tissue called an aponeurosis. The occipitalis attaches to the occipital bone, and the frontalis attaches to the tissue of the eyebrows. Between them are the muscles that attach to the aponeurosis. Contracting these muscles allows a person to raise the eyebrows and wrinkle the forehead horizontally. The corrugator (imagine corrugated cardboard) supercilii muscle, which runs from the inferior frontal bone to the skin of the **medial** eyebrow, causes vertical wrinkles of the forehead, such as those that appear when a person frowns. Around each eye are the orbicularis (as in "orbits around") oculi, which encircle the eye and allow closing of the eye. Together, the corrugator supercilii and the orbicularis oculi allow squinting to occur. No specific muscle opens the eye.

Laughing occurs primarily because of the zygomaticus major that raises the angles of the mouth. This muscle runs from the zygomatic bone down to the

synovial joint a type of joint allowing some degree of free movement

fibrous joint a type of joint allowing little or no motion

medial toward the midline or center of the body (inner aspect) relative to another landmark

TABLE 13-1 Muscles of the Skull

MUSCLE(S)	LOCATION	FUNCTION*
	FACIAL EXPRESSION MUSCLES	
Occipitofrontalis	The occipitalis part attaches to the occipital bone, and the frontalis part attaches to the tissue of the eyebrows. Each connect by way of the aponeurosis.	This muscle allows a person to raise the eyebrows and wrinkle the forehead horizontally.
Corrugator supercilii	It runs from the inferior frontal bone to the skin of the medial eyebrow.	It causes vertical wrinkles of the forehead (frowning).
Orbicularis oculi	It encircles the eye.	It allows a person to close the eye. With the corrugator supercilii, it allows squinting to occur.
Zygomaticus major	It runs from the zygomatic bone down to the angle of the mouth.	It raises the angles of the mouth.
Buccinator muscles	They run from the side of the maxilla to the skin on either side of the mouth.	They permit smiling and blowing.
Orbicularis oris	It encircles the mouth.	It draws the lips together.
	MUSCLES OF MASTICATION	
Masseter	It runs from the zygomatic arch to the mandible.	It is the strongest muscle that closes the mouth.
Temporalis	It runs from the temporal bone to the mandible.	It helps close the mouth.
Lateral pterygoids Medial pterygoid	They attach on the undersurface of the skull and attach to the inner surface of the mandible.	They allow grating of the teeth.

*Remember that a function of all these muscles is that they cover some anatomical structure and by doing so are protecting that underlying structure.

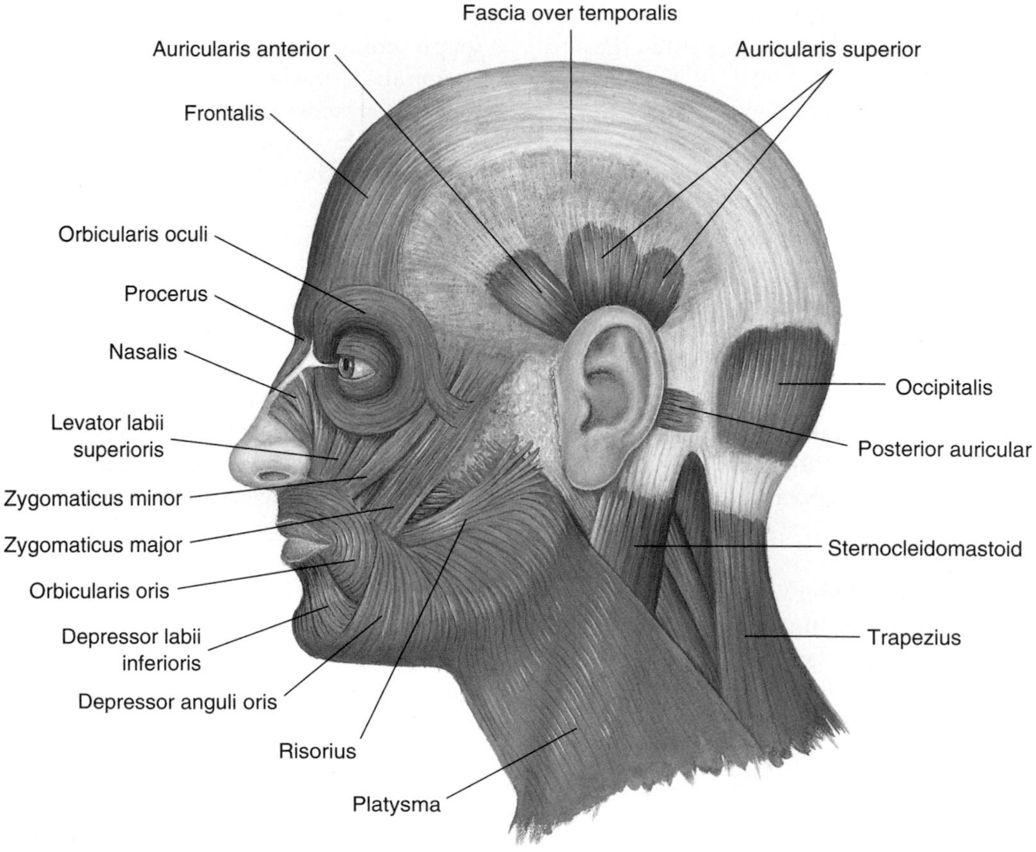

FIGURE 13-6 Muscles of facial expression. (From Seidel HM et al: *Mosby's guide to physical examination,* ed 6, p. 695, St Louis, 2006, Mosby/Elsevier.)

angle of the mouth. Helping the zygomaticus major in expressions of joy are the buccinator muscles that run from the sides of the maxilla to skin on either side of the mouth. These muscles permit smiling and blowing. The orbicularis oris encircles the mouth and draws the lips together, similar to the way in which the orbicularis oculi muscle closes the eyes. Together, the buccinator and orbicularis oris muscles pucker the mouth. Other muscles are found in the face and cranium, but the aforementioned ones are primarily responsible for facial expression.

Muscles of Mastication

Eating is one of the pleasures in life most taken for granted. It occurs primarily through the use of three muscles: (1) the masseter, (2) the temporalis, and (3) the pterygoid muscles. The masseter runs from the zygomatic arch to the mandible and is the strongest muscle that closes the mouth. It is assisted by the temporalis, which runs from the temporal bone to the mandible. The lateral and medial pterygoid muscles attach on the undersurface of the skull and the inner surface of the mandible; these allow grating of the teeth.

Neurological Considerations

Probably the most important function of the skull is to protect the brain so that it may perform all of its remarkable functions, both those that are well understood and those that remain a mystery. Starting with the outermost levels of protection, some of the attributes of the skull that help protect the brain are the skin and hair. When there is a blow to the head, the hair encourages the forces to disperse and merely glance the surface rather than be focused directly toward the underlying brain. The skin and occipitofrontalis muscle (with the aponeurosis) over the skull work in a similar way. Under the hair, skin, and muscle are the skull bones, the configuration of which is relatively unique: cortical bone on the outermost and innermost aspects with cancellous bone inside. Cortical bone is very hard, whereas cancellous bone is softer, allowing a certain degree of compression that cushions an external force to the skull. Under the skull, the brain is protected by three layers of covering called meninges (Figure 13-7). The meninges are protective coverings of the brain, spinal cord, and spinal nerves. The covering closest to the brain, spinal cord, and spinal nerves is called the pia mater. *Pia* means "delicate," and *mater* is Latin for "mother." Just outside the pia mater is the arachnoid covering. As its name suggests, the arachnoid is a spiderweb-like connective tissue. The outermost and toughest covering is called the dura mater. *Dura* is Latin for "tough." The dura mater might also have some projections into the inner aspect of the skull. It is within these coverings, the meninges, that spinal meningitis, an infection of the meninges, can take hold.

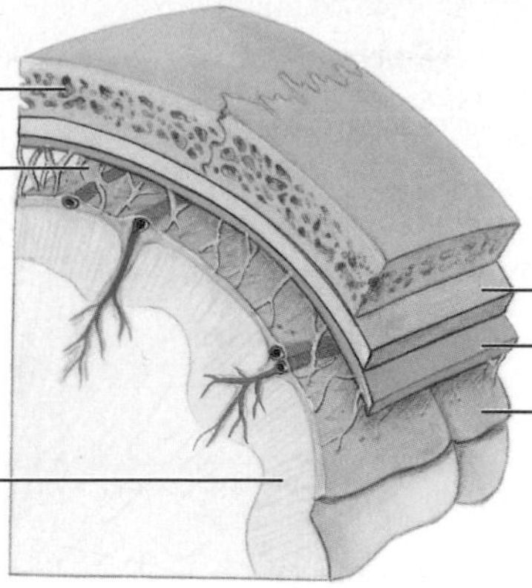

FIGURE 13-7 Brain and meninges. (From Applegate E: *The anatomy and physiology learning system,* ed 3, p. 152, Philadelphia, 2006, Saunders/Elsevier.)

The Brain

Finally, underneath all these protective coverings lies the brain. The brain, the central processing unit of the central nervous system (CNS), contains approximately 100 billion neurons, the functional cells of the nervous system. It weighs about 3 pounds. Other major components of the CNS are the spinal cord and spinal nerves (Figure 13-8). The brain is more complex than any computer. As Thibodeau and Patton memorably put it, "... [R]esearch scientists in various fields—neurophysiology, neurosurgery, neuropsychiatry, and others—have added mountains of information to our knowledge about the brain. However, questions come faster than answers, and a clear, complete understanding of the brain's mechanisms still eludes us." In other words, the more we know, the more we don't know. The brain will be briefly discussed in the following paragraphs.

There are six major divisions of the brain (Box 13-5). From the top of the skull downward are the cerebrum, diencephalon, cerebellum, midbrain, pons, and medulla oblongata. The medulla oblongata continues out of the skull as the spinal cord. The spinal cord and spinal nerves will be discussed later in this chapter.

The cerebrum is the largest division of the brain, and its surface is called the *cerebral cortex*. The cerebral cortex is responsible for the senses and plays an important role in voluntary movements, language, emotions, and short-term and long-term memory. This surface averages about 1/8-inch in thickness and consists of gray matter. The cerebrum is composed of right and left halves: the right and left hemispheres. Specialized functions have been attributed to each hemisphere. For example, it has been established that the right hemisphere is responsible for movements of the left side of the body, vision, abstract concepts, emotions, and shapes and patterns. It is sometimes thought of as the emotional, artistic, and creative

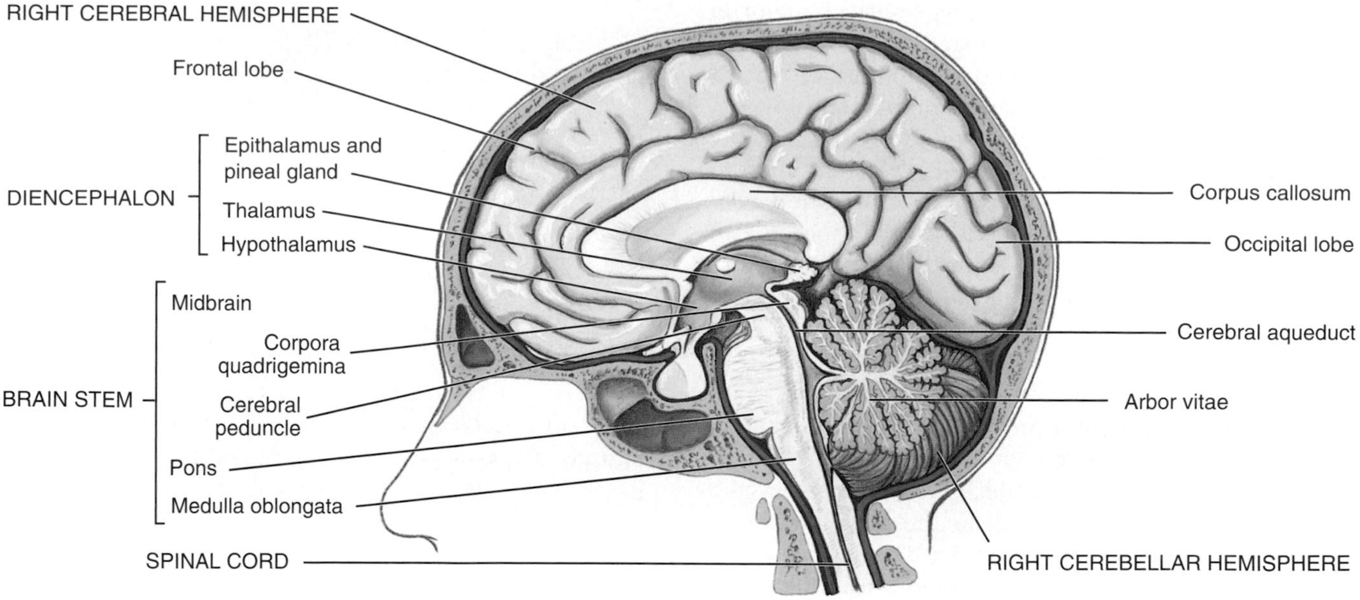

FIGURE 13-8 Central nervous system. (From Applegate E: *The anatomy and physiology learning system,* ed 3, p. 156, Philadelphia, 2006, Saunders/Elsevier.)

BOX 13-5 Major Divisions of the Brain

Cerebrum
- Largest division
- Surface known as *cerebral cortex*
- Responsible for senses and important roles in voluntary movement, language, emotions, and memory retrieval
- Right and left hemispheres

Diencephalon
- Lies below cerebrum and above midbrain
- Important role in neural impulses

Cerebellum
- Means "little brain"
- Located below posterior cerebrum and behind brainstem
- Functions to complement and assist cerebrum

Midbrain
- Together with pons and medulla oblongata, known as *brainstem*
- Located inferior to cerebrum and above pons
- Contains auditory, visual, and muscle control centers

Pons
- Located below midbrain and above medulla oblongata
- Contains centers for certain cranial nerve reflexes

Medulla Oblongata
- Most inferior part of brain
- Connects to spinal cord
- Controls vital cardiac and respiratory centers

side. The left hemisphere is responsible for movements of the right side of the body, language, details, and the establishment of a practical and orderly sequence. It is sometimes thought of as the logical, deductive, intellectual side. Even though the hemispheres have specific functions, each has been known to compensate for any deficits on the other side if an injury makes this necessary. Each hemisphere communicates with the other by way of the corpus callosum.

The **diencephalon,** which literally means "between brain," lies just below the cerebrum and above the midbrain. As its location suggests, this division plays an important role in conveying neural impulses from the divisions and spinal cord up to the cerebrum and then back down the divisions and spinal cord.

The **cerebellum,** which literally means "little brain," is located just below the posterior cerebrum and just behind the brainstem. It is believed that most of the functions of the cerebellum serve to complement and assist the cerebrum. One major function of the cerebellum is to discern incoming nerve signals and then send out nerve signals to muscles that result in coordinated movement.

The midbrain, pons, and medulla oblongata are collectively known as the **brainstem**. The **midbrain** lies just inferior to the cerebrum and above the pons. It has auditory, ocular, and muscle-control centers. The **pons** is located below the midbrain and above the medulla oblongata. It contains centers for reflexes for the fifth, sixth, seventh, and eighth cranial nerves. The most inferior part of the brain is the **medulla oblongata**, which connects to the spinal cord. The medulla oblongata is often considered the most vital part of the brain because it controls the vital centers for survival, the cardiac and respiratory centers.

Cranial nerves are summarized in Table 13-2. There are 12 pairs of cranial nerves, and they are so named because they come directly off of the brain in the cranium. The cranial nerves emerge from the inferior surface of the brain, mostly from the brainstem, and continue to their destinations. They are identified by Roman numerals and by name. The Roman numerals identify their location on the brain, moving from anterior to posterior.

ANATOMY OF THE SPINE

The anatomy of the spine consists of bones, ligaments, joints, muscles, and nerves. This chapter presents a basic overview of the anatomy of the spine so that athletic trainers will know what to expect when evaluating the spine and related structures. Although students are often intimidated by its apparent complexity, the spine is made up of the same basic elements found in every other part of the body: bones, ligaments, joints, muscles, and nerves.

TABLE 13-2 Cranial Nerves

NERVE	NAME	FUNCTION
I	Olfactory	Sense of smell
II	Optic	Vision
III	Oculomotor	Side-to-side eye movement; pupil accommodation/size
IV	Trochlear	"Looking down and in" eye movement
V	Trigeminal	Chewing movements
VI	Abducens	Lateral eye movement Head and face sensation
VII	Facial	Facial expressions Taste
VIII	Vestibulocochlear	Vestibular part: balance Cochlear part: hearing
IX	Glossopharyngeal	Swallowing Tongue sensation
X	Vagus	Gag reflex
XI	Accessory	Shrugging shoulders
XII	Hypoglossal	Tongue movements

Bones of the Spine

The spine, also often called the *vertebral column*, is composed of 33 vertebrae in children and normally 26 vertebrae in adults (Figure 13-9). This discrepancy occurs because the sacral and coccygeal vertebrae fuse later in life—usually by about 20 years of age. There are five distinct areas of the spine. They are, from superior to inferior, the cervical spine with seven vertebrae, the thoracic spine with twelve vertebrae, the lumbar spine with five vertebrae, the sacrum with five sacral vertebrae fusing to become one sacrum, and four coccygeal vertebrae fusing to become one coccyx. Particular vertebrae within each of the five areas are generally named or labeled by using the capitalized first letter of the area in question followed by the number of the vertebrae proceeding numerically in ascending order from the base of the skull downward. For example, the fourth cervical vertebra below the skull is written as C4.

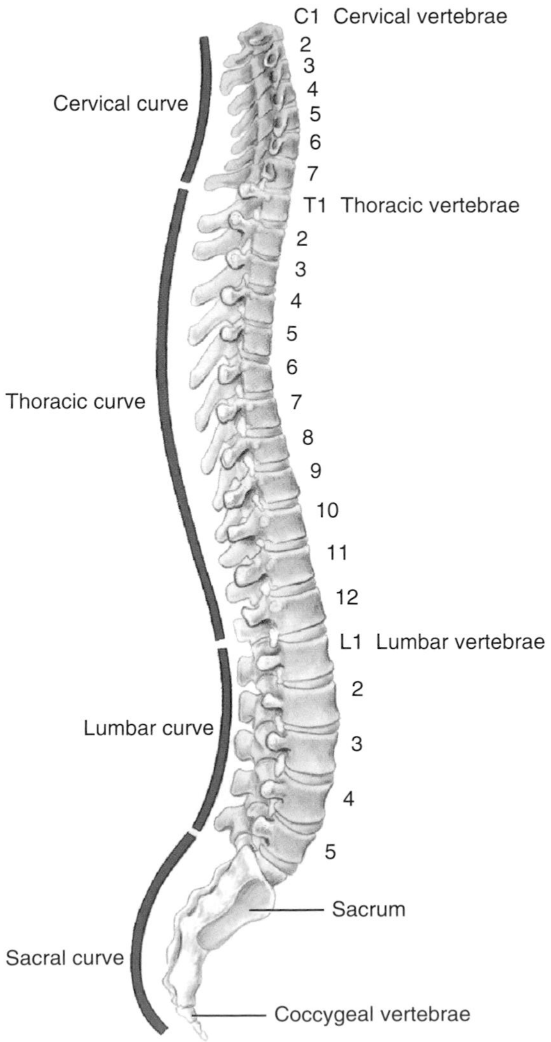

FIGURE 13-9 The vertebral column. (From Applegate E: *The anatomy and physiology learning system*, ed 3, p. 99, Philadelphia, 2006, Saunders/Elsevier.)

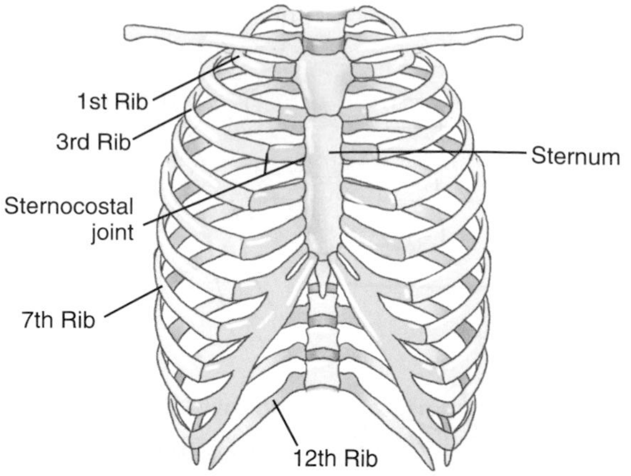

FIGURE 13-14 The thoracic cage. (From Muscolino JE: *Kinesiology: the skeletal system and muscle function,* p. 264, St Louis, 2006, Mosby/Elsevier.)

backward. If the annulus fibrosus is weakened, the nucleus pulposus may be allowed to move backward too far. When this occurs, a **herniated** disk ensues (see Figure 13-11). Pain often results when the disk pushes the spinal nerve up against the side of the intervertebral foramen.

Box 13-6 summarizes the bones of the spine and the unique aspects of the various segmental vertebrae.

Distal to the lumbar vertebrae is the sacrum. The sacrum was previously discussed in Chapter 9 within the context of the lower body. Discussing its role relative to the spine highlights some of its other important functions. The **sacrum** is a triangular bone locked between the two ilia in such a way that it serves as a strong foundation for the vertebral column. Just distal to the sacrum is the **coccyx**, or tailbone. Both the sacrum and the coccyx begin as five and four bones, respectively, but fuse later in life into one solid section of bone (Figure 13-15, *F*).

Joints and Ligaments of the Spine

The vertebral column contains a number of joints. One of them is the **intervertebral joint**, which is found between two vertebral bodies. The intervertebral disks play an important role in the stability of this joint because the annulus fibrosus is attached to each of the vertebral bodies that it separates. The annulus fibrosus is the outer concentric portion of the disk. Because of its attachments to each of the vertebrae above and below it, the disk also helps limit spine motion in all directions. For example, as the spine flexes and the vertebrae put pressure on the anterior aspect of the disk, the disk

herniated bulging, usually due to excessive pressure or force on one side

distal farther away from the body's midline or center relative to another landmark

BOX 13-6 Bones of the Spine and Unique Segmental Aspects

Cervical Vertebrae
- Seven vertebrae
- Unique aspects include the following:
  - C1 (atlas) that holds the skull
  - C1 that rotates on top of C2 (axis)
  - No disk between C1 and C2
  - Foramen in transverse process
  - Large spinous process of C7
  - Bifid spinous process
  - Large range of motion in three planes

Thoracic Vertebrae
- 12 vertebrae
- Unique aspects include the following:
  - Demifacets on bodies of thoracic vertebrae
  - Costal facets on transverse processes of thoracic vertebrae
  - Spinous processes angling down over adjacent spinous processes
  - Ribs anchored into the demifacets and transverse facets
  - Not much movement of these vertebrae because of the ribs and sternum

Lumbar Vertebrae
- Five vertebrae
- Unique aspects include the following:
  - Largest vertebral bodies
  - Short, strong spinous processes
  - Common site of herniated disks

Sacrum
- Five vertebrae in infancy that eventually fuse
- Distal to lumbar vertebrae

Coccyx
- Four vertebrae in infancy that eventually fuse
- Distal to sacrum; known as *tailbone*

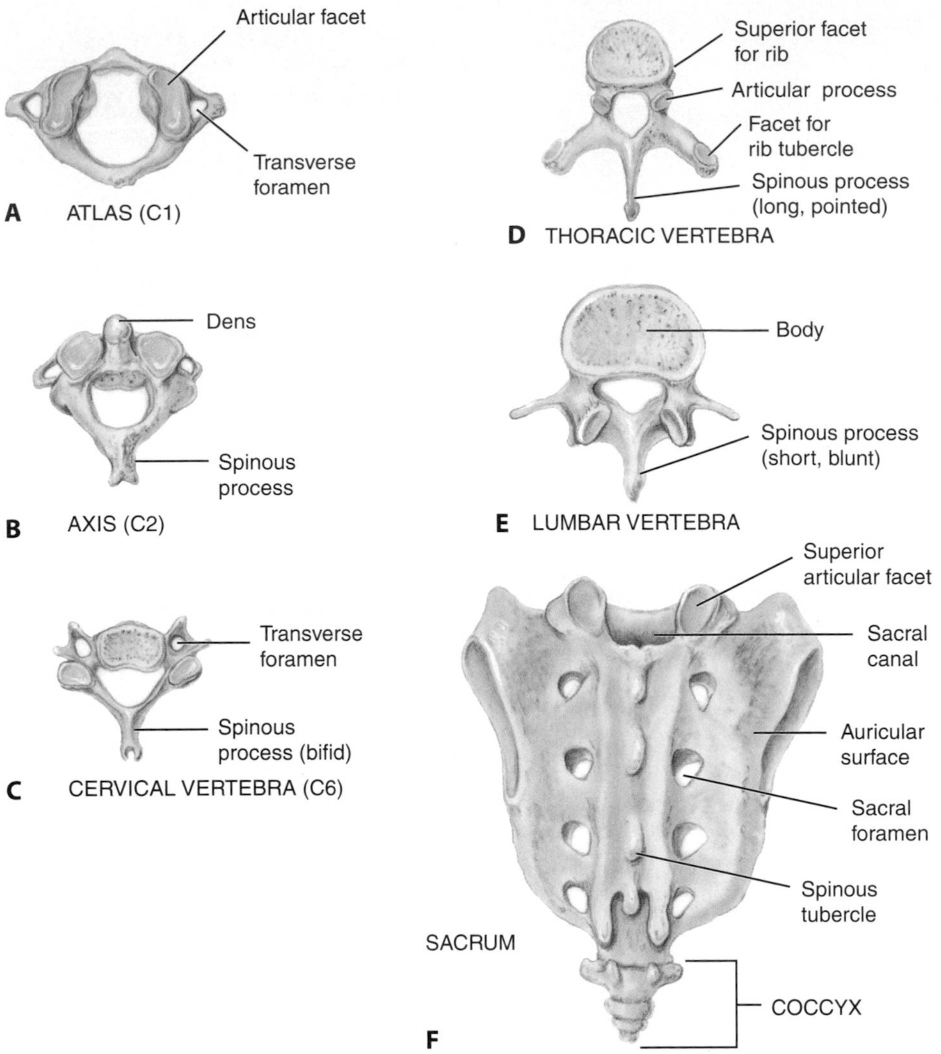

FIGURE 13-15 Structure of bones of the cervical **(C)**, thoracic **(D)**, and lumbar **(E)**, vertebrae, along with the atlas **(A)**, axis **(B)**, and sacrum and coccyx **(F)**. (From Applegate E: *The anatomy and physiology learning system,* ed 3, p. 100, Philadelphia, 2006, Saunders/Elsevier.)

attachments at the back of the vertebrae prevent them from moving apart any farther, and flexion stops. This principle works with any bending of the spine because the disk provides cushioning and stability all around the vertebral body.

Additionally, a number of ligaments help support the spine (Figure 13-16). The anterior longitudinal ligament runs the entire length of the spine in front of the vertebral bodies and helps limit extension (back bending) of the spine, whereas the posterior longitudinal ligament runs along the back of the vertebral bodies in the anterior portion of the spinal canal and helps limit flexion (forward bending). The interspinous and supraspinous ligaments connect the spine of one vertebra to the respective spines of the adjacent vertebrae and help limit forward flexion. Other ligaments that help stabilize these joints are the intertransverse ligaments, which run between the transverse processes to help limit lateral flexion. Because the ligamentum flavum connects adjacent lamina of the vertebrae, there are two ligamenta flava, just as there are two intertransverse ligaments between each pair of vertebrae. The ligamentum flavum is the only truly elastic ligament in the body, and it helps limit flexion along with the interspinous and supraspinous ligaments. In short, the movements allowed between the vertebrae are forward bending (flexion), backward bending (extension), and rotation. Often, combinations of these movements occur simultaneously as when swinging a golf club, throwing a ball, or reaching up into a cupboard. In most cases, only minimal movements take place at each intervertebral joint and the disk. The small motion from each joint adds up to allow the total motion that occurs along the spine. Most of the movement of the spine comes from the cervical and the lumbar areas because the thoracic area is relatively stable owing to the ribs' connection to the sternum.

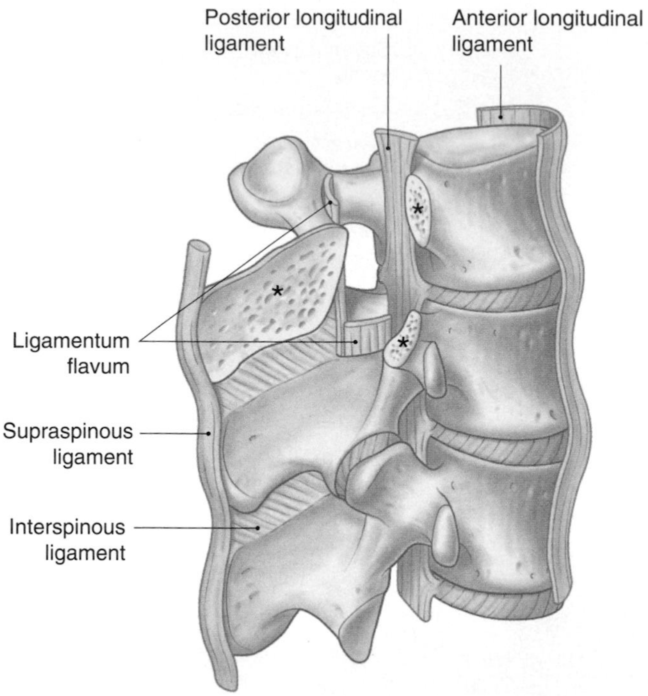

FIGURE 13-16 Vertebrae and their ligaments. (From Moses KP et al: *Atlas of clinical gross anatomy,* p. 296, St Louis, 2005, Elsevier/Mosby.)

Another set of joints that are formed between adjacent vertebrae are the facet joints (Figure 13-17). Located at the point where a superior facet of an inferior vertebra encounters the inferior facet of the superior vertebra, these joints help limit the slipping of one vertebra over another and the rotation of one vertebra over another. The facet joints are small synovial joints like the synovial joints in most of the lower and upper body.

Two other joints found in the thoracic spine are the costovertebral and the costotransverse joints. The term

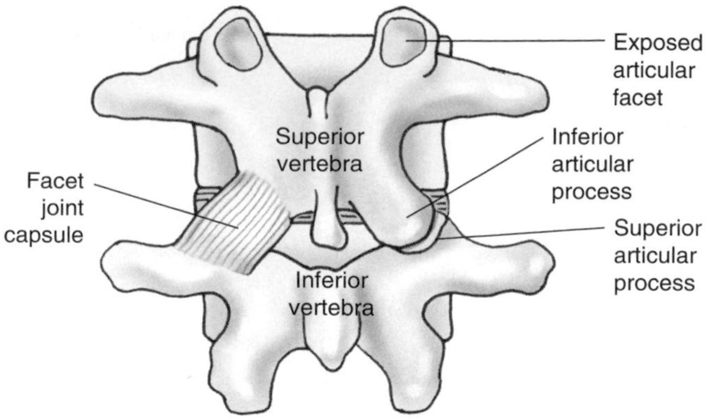

FIGURE 13-17 Facet joint. (From Muscolino JE: *Kinesiology: the skeletal system and muscle function,* p. 243, St Louis, 2006, Mosby/Elsevier.)

costo refers to the ribs. These joints represent the areas where the ribs attach to the vertebrae at two locations. One connection is made with the vertebral bodies, and the other connection is made with the transverse processes. These joints have thin, loose fibrous capsules, allowing movement during breathing and when moving the upper body and arms.

Specialized joints exist between the skull and atlas, as well as between the atlas and the axis, where nodding and rotation occur, respectively. In addition, a unique union between the sacrum and coccyx prevents any significant movement.

Box 13-7 summarizes the major joints and ligaments within the spine.

Muscles of the Spine

Muscles of the spine, thorax, and abdomen are different from those seen in the lower body and upper body. Muscles in the lower and upper body are responsible

BOX 13-7 Joints and Ligaments of the Spine

Intervertebral Joint

- Located between two vertebral bodies
- Stabilized by intervertebral disks, which limit spine motion in all directions
- Supported by the following ligaments:
  - Anterior longitudinal ligament
  - Posterior longitudinal ligament
  - Intertransverse ligaments
  - Interspinous ligament
  - Supraspinous ligaments
  - Ligamentum flavum
- *Associated movements:* forward bending (flexion), backward bending (extension), and rotation

Facet Joints

- Set of small synovial joints formed between adjacent vertebrae
- *Associated movements:* limiting of slipping or rotation of one vertebra over another

Costovertebral and Costotransverse Joints

- Located at point where ribs attach to vertebrae
- Connect with vertebral bodies and transverse process
- *Associated movements:* allowance of movement for breathing or moving upper body and arms

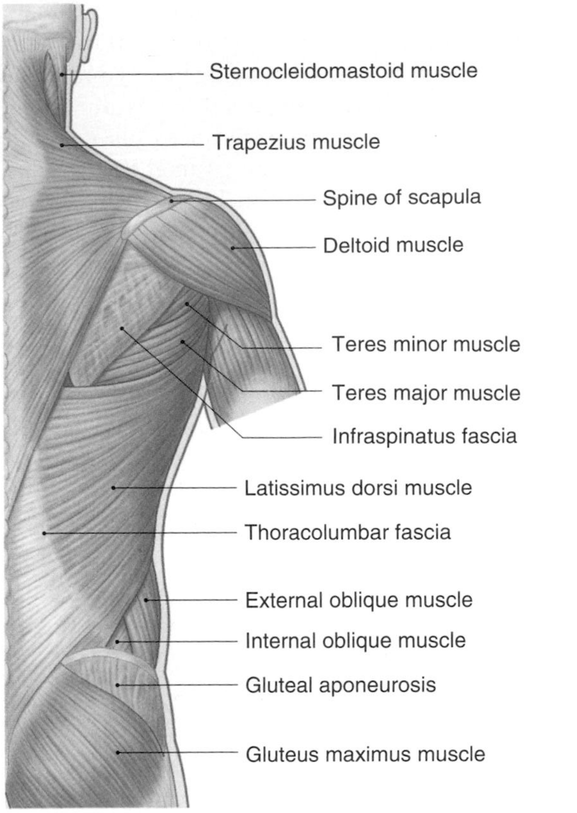

FIGURE 13-18 Superficial muscles of the back. (From Moses KP et al: *Atlas of clinical gross anatomy,* p. 322, St Louis, 2005, Elsevier/Mosby.)

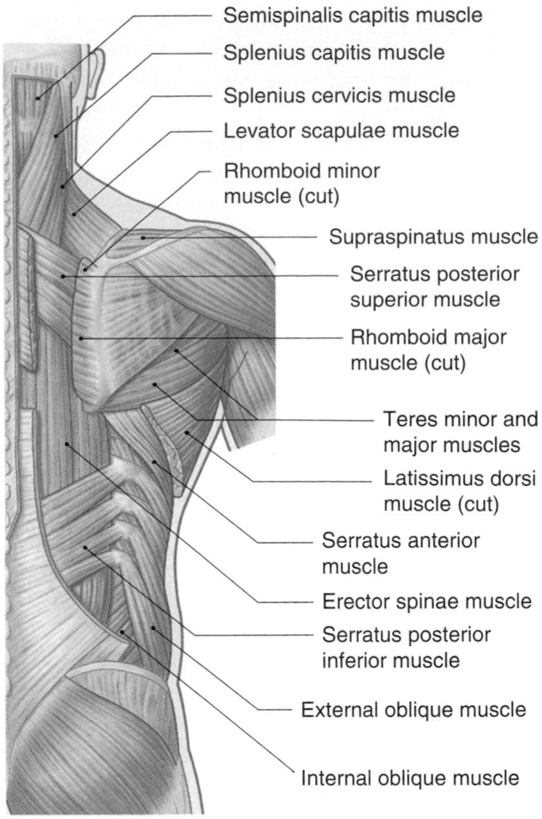

FIGURE 13-19 Deep muscles of the back. (From Moses KP et al: *Atlas of clinical gross anatomy,* p. 322, St Louis, 2005, Elsevier/Mosby.)

for major movements within those areas, whereas the primary function of the muscles of the spine, thorax, and abdomen is to stabilize and control. Some movements are initiated by these muscles but not of the same magnitude as those seen in the extremities.

Muscles of the upper back are the **trapezius, latissimus dorsi, levator scapulae, rhomboid major**, and **rhomboid minor** (Figure 13-18). Although some experts do not consider the latissimus dorsi muscles part of the upper back muscles, they cover the lateral aspect of the back and are therefore included in this discussion. The trapezius laterally flexes the neck to the same side as the contracting trapezius. When both of the trapezius muscles contract, they extend the cervical spine and head. The trapezius is a large triangular muscle, and the upper fibers are important to the upper back because they attach to the cervical spine and help control movements of the head. Attachments of the upper trapezius are on the base of the skull and the cervical and thoracic spinous processes. The attachments continue down the spinous processes to T12, flaring out to the scapula on either side. This portion of the trapezius works on the shoulder and serves as an important stabilizer of the head and neck.

Inferior and deep to the trapezius muscles are the group of muscles known collectively as the **erector spinae muscles** (Figure 13-19). There are two sets of erector spinae muscles running parallel to each other on each side of the spine. Beginning closest to the spine is the spinalis. The **spinalis muscles**, as the name implies, run along the spinous processes of the vertebrae. Just lateral to the spinalis is the **longissimus muscle**, which begins on the medial posterior iliac crest and runs up along the transverse processes of the vertebrae. The most lateral group of erector spinae muscles are the **iliocostalis muscles**, which run from the ilium up along the angles of the ribs with the cervical part of the muscle running along the transverse processes of the cervical spine. When working together, the erector spinae muscles extend the spine and, perhaps even more important, help control flexion of the spine, especially during heavy lifting and carrying. If the erector spinae muscles on just one side are activated, they cause rotation and lateral flexion to that side. The erector spinae muscles are innervated by nerves coming off the back of the spinal cord.

Another pair of deep muscles of the low back are the **quadratus lumborums**. They arise off the posterior iliac crests on their side and run up to the twelfth rib with attachments on the transverse processes of the lumbar vertebrae. The quadratus lumborum muscle, when acting on only one side, causes lateral bending to the same side and serves the important function of not allowing the pelvis to drop down to the opposite side when a person stands on one leg. When both muscles contract simultaneously, the lumbar spine extends. The nerve roots exiting the posterior spine also innervate the quadratus lumborum.

Deep to the erector spinae muscles are smaller muscles that run from one vertebra to an adjacent vertebra. Primarily stabilizing muscles (Figure 13-20), they are not big enough to provide sufficient leverage for movement. The main muscles in this group are the multifidus and rotators.

Table 13-3 summarizes and describes the muscles of the spine.

Anatomical Abnormalities

Some people are born with misshapen bones or joints of the spine. The normal curves of the spine then become exaggerated or deformed. Two of the most common spinal abnormalities are excessive kyphosis of the thoracic spine and excessive lordosis of the lumbar spine (Figure 13-21). Both of these curves are in the sagittal plane of the spine (the plane that cuts the body into symmetrical right and left halves). **Kyphosis** manifests as an exaggerated forward-angled head, an appearance caused by excessive forward flexion of the thoracic spine. Kyphosis is often seen in individuals with slouching postures. Excessive **lordosis** manifests as an exaggerated lumbar curve, or an arched back. The other abnormal curve is **scoliosis**, which occurs in the frontal plane (the plane that cuts the body into a front and back). Severe spinal abnormalities can compromise functioning of the heart and lungs.

Points to Ponder

How would abnormal spinal alignments, such as scoliosis, affect an individual's participation in athletics?

kyphosis spinal abnormality characterized by an exaggerated forward head appearance and an excessively forward-flexed thoracic spine

lordosis spinal abnormality characterized by an exaggerated lumbar curve, or arched back

scoliosis an abnormal lateral curvature of the spine

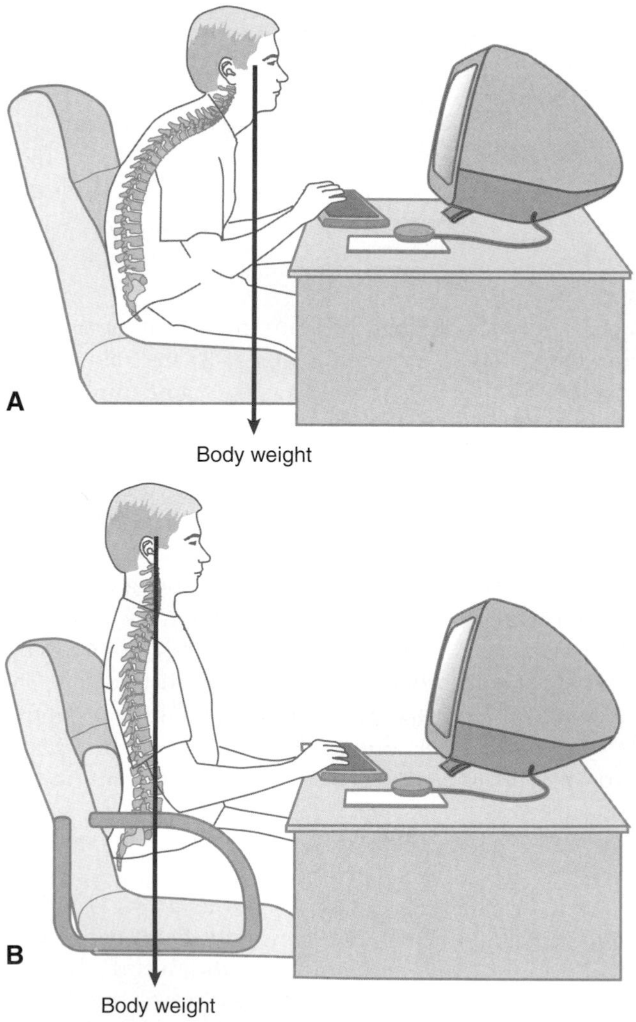

FIGURE 13-20 Posture. **A**, A slouched sitting position flexes the lumbar spine, and the head assumes a "forward" position. **B**, Proper posture facilitates a more desirable "chin-in" head position. (From Neumann D: *Kinesiology of the musculoskeletal system,* p. 302, St Louis, 2002, Mosby.)

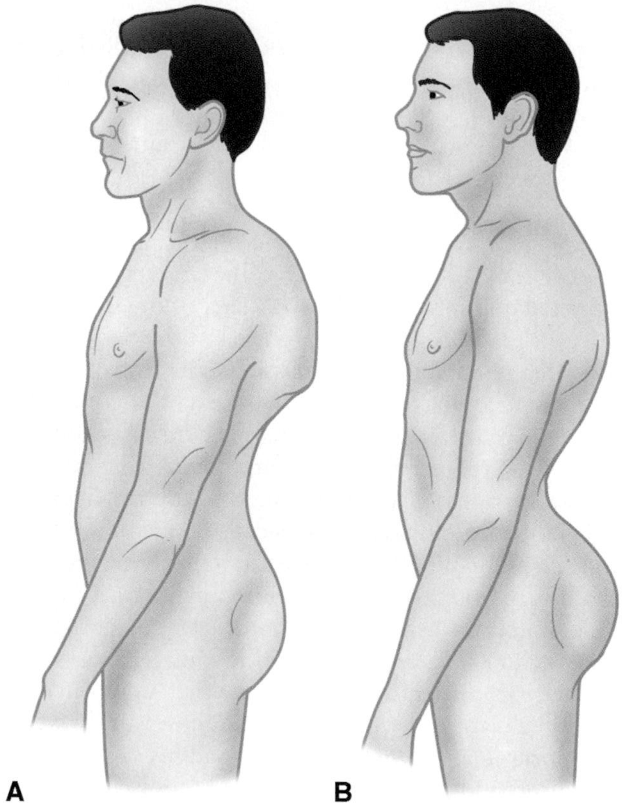

FIGURE 13-21 Abnormal spine curvatures. **A,** Kyphosis. **B,** Lordosis. (From Seidel HM et al: *Mosby's guide to physical examination,* ed 6, p. 710, St Louis, 2006, Mosby/Elsevier.)

TABLE 13-3 **Muscles of the Spine**

MUSCLE(S)	LOCATION	FUNCTION*
Trapezius	There are two trapezius muscles. Each runs from the lower back of the skull and cervical and thoracic spine out to the upper lateral back, where it attaches to the scapula.	Acting alone, each laterally flexes the head and neck to the same side as the muscle. Acting together, they extend the head and neck and control flexion of head and neck.
Latissimus dorsi	There are two latissimus dorsi muscles. Each runs from the lateral scapula to the thoracic and lumbar spine below the trapezius out and under the axilla, where it attaches to the front of the upper humerus.	Acting alone, each adducts, or pulls, the arm down such as that which occurs while swimming. Acting together, they allow such movements as pull-ups.
Levator scapulae	There are two levator scapula muscles. Each runs from the first four cervical vertebrae to the upper medial aspect of the scapula.	Acting alone, each can bend the head and neck to the same side as the muscle; however, as the name indicates, they primarily are used to elevate the scapula.
Rhomboid major	There are two rhomboid major muscles. Each runs from the first four thoracic vertebrae to the middle medial scapula. These muscles are deep to the trapezius.	Acting alone, each can retract, or pull back, the scapula closer to the spine.
Rhomboid minor	There are two rhomboid minor muscles. Each runs from the last two cervical vertebrae to the upper medial scapula. These muscles are deep to the trapezius.	Acting alone, each can retract, or pull back, the scapula closer to the spine.
Erector spinae: Spinalis Longissimus Iliocostalis	Two groups of erector spinae are deep to the trapezius and latissimus dorsi. Three muscles running parallel to each other make up a group. The spinalis runs along the spinous processes of the vertebrae, the longissimus runs along the transverse processes, and the iliocostalis runs from the posterior ilium up along the posterior ribs.	Acting alone, each bends the spine to the same side as the muscle. Acting together, they extend the spine and help control flexion of the spine.
Quadratus lumborum	There are two quadratus lumborum muscles. They are deep to the erector spinae. Each runs from the posterior iliac crest up to the twelfth rib with attachments on the transverse processes of the lumbar vertebrae.	Acting alone, each bends the lower back to the same side as the muscle and serves the important function of not allowing the pelvis to drop down on the opposite side when a person stands on one leg. Acting together, they extend the lower back and help control flexion.
Multifidus and rotators	There are a number of multifidus and rotator muscles on both sides of the spine that run diagonally from one vertebra to an adjacent vertebra or the vertebra two bones away.	Primarily stabilizing muscles, they are not big enough to provide sufficient leverage for movement. They help control flexion and rotation of the vertebra to which they attach.

*Remember that a function of all these muscles is that they cover some anatomical structure and by doing so are protecting that underlying structure.

Other relatively common abnormalities of the spine are stenosis, sacralization, lumbarization, and spina bifida occulta. These conditions are congenital, meaning that they are present at birth. Even so, certain injuries result in conditions similar to these.

Stenosis simply means "narrowing." This term is most often applied to the cervical and lumbar vertebral foramina and the intervertebral foramina in the cervical and lumbar areas. When stenosis is present, the spinal cord and spinal nerves are more likely to be injured by contact with the surrounding bony aspects.

Sacralization occurs when the last lumbar vertebra, L5, is fused with the sacrum; the term is derived from the fact that the fifth lumbar vertebra assumes the characteristics of the sacrum. Sacralization happens rarely, but when it does, it decreases the mobility of the spine. Lumbarization, recognized on X-ray examination, occurs when the first sacral vertebra is not fused with the rest of the sacrum and acts as if it were a sixth lumbar vertebrae. A slight increase in movement occurs in the lumbar area when there is a lumbarization.

Persons afflicted with **spina bifida occulta** generally experience persistent low back pain that is often exacerbated by exercise. The anomaly usually is not discovered until an X-ray examination is performed. Although spina bifida results in significant neurological problems, spina bifida occulta usually limits only certain physical activities. It is distinguished by the failure of the laminae to develop at L5 or S1, leaving the posterior portion of the spinal cord exposed.

stenosis a narrowing of a passageway, often the vertebral or intervertebral foramina in the cervical and lumbar areas

sacralization an abnormality in which the last lumbar vertebra, L5, is fused with the sacrum

spina bifida occulta congenital defect in which the laminae at L5 or S1 fail to develop, resulting in an exposed posterior spinal cord

Neurological Considerations

Probably the most important function of the vertebral column is to protect the spinal cord and the spinal nerves coming off the cord (Figure 13-22). The spinal cord is the neurological column that communicates impulses from the brain to nerves all over the body and, conversely, from the nerves all over the body back up to the brain. Sensory nerves from the skin, muscles, and joints send information to the spinal cord, which in turn sends the information up to the brain. The brain then sorts through all the information and sends signals back down the spinal cord to the motor nerves, which initiate muscle activity and movement in response to the signals from the sensory nerves. Reflexive actions of muscle can also occur. Movements such as the patellar reflex are also the responsibility of the spinal cord but do not require the intervention of the brain. For example, when the patella tendon is tapped, the knee is reflexively extended.

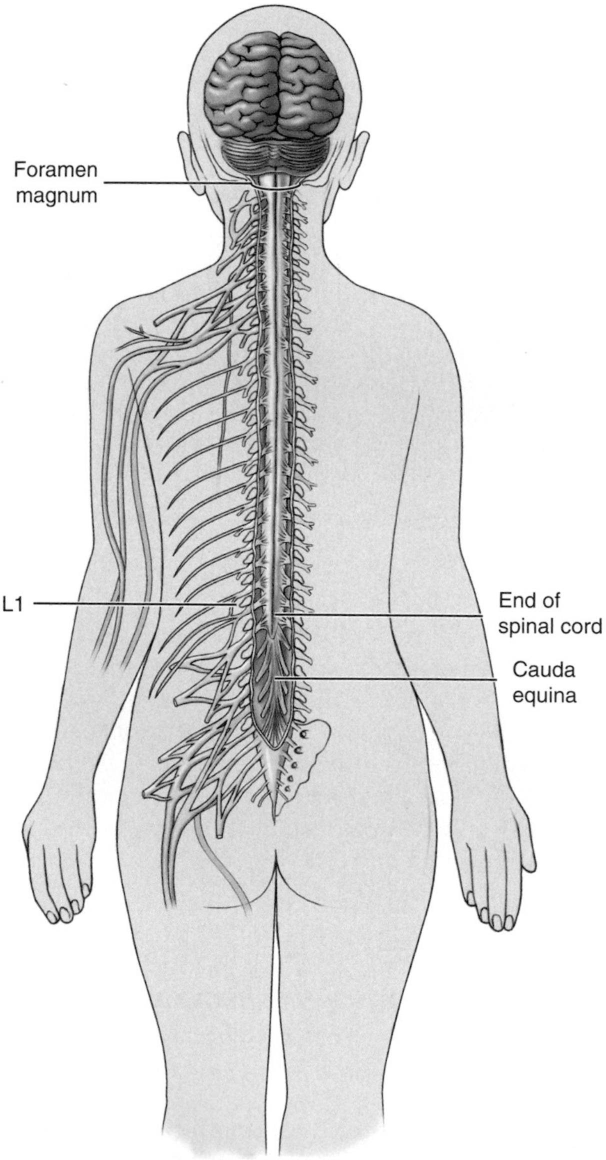

FIGURE 13-22 Spinal cord. (From Herlihy B: *The human body in health and illness,* ed 3, p. 188, Philadelphia, 2007, Saunders/Elsevier.)

The spinal cord extends from the brain down through the **foramen magnum** of the skull down to the first lumbar vertebra. At the first lumbar vertebra, the cord tapers to become the conus medullaris. Many nerve roots extend from the conus medullaris. The area where all the nerve roots of the conus medullaris are located is called the cauda equina, which is Latin for "horse's tail." All along the spinal cord, at each articulation of two vertebrae, a pair of spinal nerves extends off the cord to the right and left. These spinal nerves divide into sensory and motor nerves that continue out to various parts of the body to obtain information (sensory nerves) and send information (motor nerves). Without properly functioning nerves, the body would not be able to perform as it was created to.

Several anatomical features function to protect the cord. The bony vertebrae protect all the neural structures that run within their framework. Connecting intimately with the cord are the meningeal layers. The three layers from outside in are the dura mater, the arachnoid, and the pia mater.

ANATOMY OF THE THORAX AND ABDOMEN

The anatomy of the thorax and abdomen is a bit different from that of other areas heretofore discussed. The thoracic area moves very little, yet the muscles of the region are, to varying degrees, in nearly constant tension. This muscle action results in stability, rather than motion—a stability that serves to protect the vital organs of the thorax, such as the heart and lungs. When the thoracic region does move, it moves primarily as one large structure rather than individual segments or units.

Bones of the Thorax and Abdomen

The vertebral column, particularly the thoracic spine, provides a framework for the thorax. Twelve ribs attach to the thoracic spine, come around to the front of the thorax, and attach to the sternum to complete the part of the chest called the thorax. The superior seven ribs are called true ribs because they wrap around to the anterior thorax and connect directly to the sternum. The connection between the true ribs and sternum is by way of a costal cartilage connection. Just inferior to the true ribs are five false ribs—ribs 8 through 12—which do not directly attach to the sternum (hence the term *false ribs*). Ribs 11 and 12 are called floating ribs because they have no attachments to the sternum.

foramen magnum large opening at the bottom of the skull where the spinal cord exits

The sternum serves as a center post to the ribs on the anterior thorax. It has three parts from superior to inferior: (1) the manubrium, (2) the body, and (3) the xiphoid process. The clavicles attach to the manubrium. Ribs attach to the manubrium and the body. The thorax helps protect the contents of the thorax and provide an attachment for the upper extremity.

The abdomen is the area below the lower border of the ribs and xiphoid process. It is separated from the thorax by the diaphragm muscle. The main bony protection of the abdomen comprises the lumbar vertebrae posteriorly and the **ilia** of the hips laterally. The anterior protection is from muscle.

The primary synovial joint of the anterior thorax is the sternoclavicular joint, which is usually presented with the shoulder complex. It will be discussed further in Chapter 18.

Box 13-8 summarizes the bones of the thorax and abdomen.

Muscles of the Thorax

Many muscles of the thorax, like the muscles of the back, affect the shoulder. Within the context of the general functions of muscle throughout the body, the muscles of the thorax protect the underlying structures by deflecting and absorbing forces to the area.

The particular muscles of interest are the pectoralis minor, serratus anterior, intercostals, pectoralis major, and latissimus dorsi. As with many muscles, these are found on both the left and right sides of the thorax (Figures 13-23 and 13-24). Many of these muscles will be discussed from a functional movement and neural innervation standpoint with the shoulder.

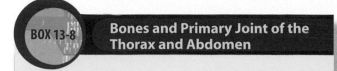

BOX 13-8 **Bones and Primary Joint of the Thorax and Abdomen**

Thorax
- Thoracic vertebrae
- Sternum
  - Manubrium
  - Body
  - Xiphoid process
- Clavicles
- Ribs (12 total)
  - True ribs (superior 7): wrap around anterior thorax and connect directly to sternum
  - False ribs (8–12): do not directly attach to sternum
  - Floating ribs (11–12): no attachments to sternum

Abdomen
- Lumbar vertebrae (posterior)
- Ilia of hips (lateral)

Main Joint
- Sternoclavicular joint

The pectoralis minor lies deep to the pectoralis major and, as its name suggests, is smaller. It connects ribs three, four, and five to the coracoid process of the scapula. Although the scapula is generally studied in

ilia plural of ilium

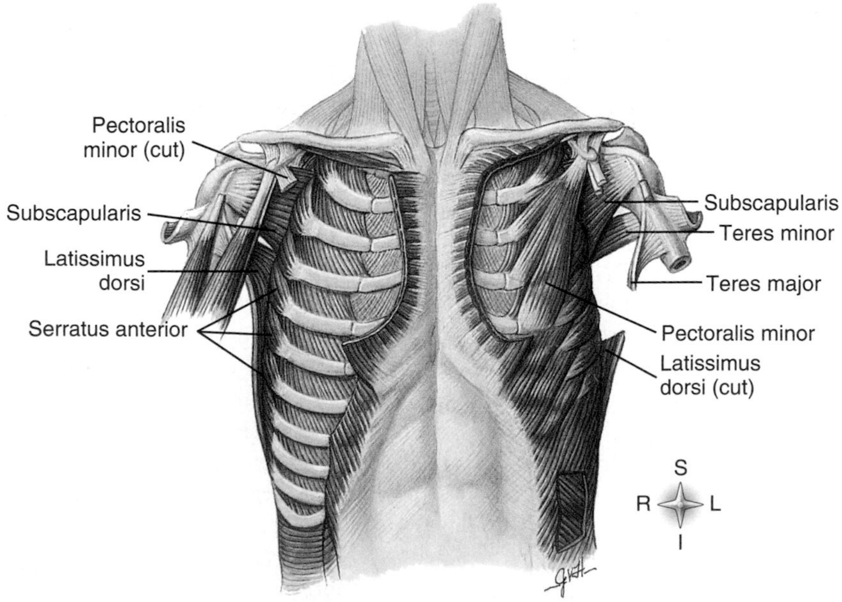

FIGURE 13-23 Deep anterior thorax muscles. (From Thibodeau GA, Patton KT: *Anatomy & physiology,* ed 6, p. 371, St Louis, 2007, Mosby/Elsevier.)

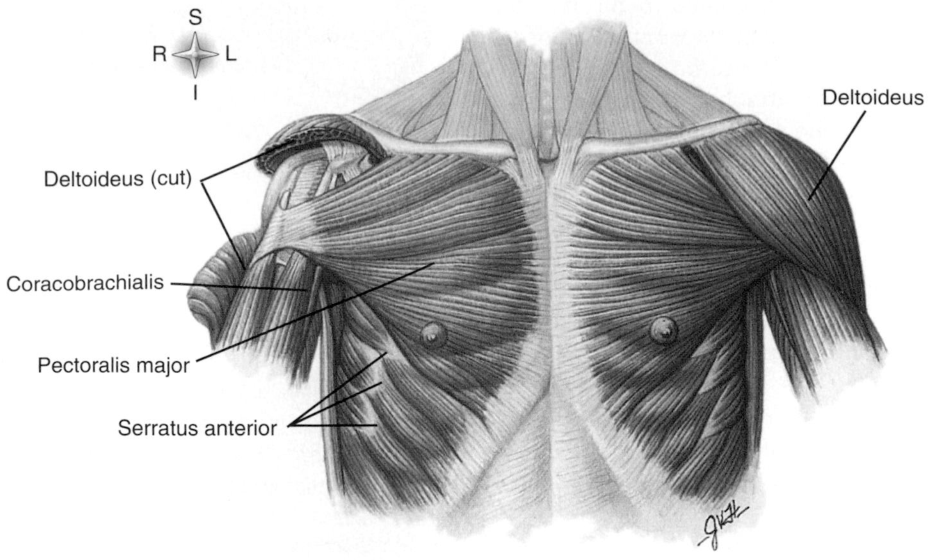

FIGURE 13-24 Superficial anterior thorax muscles. (From Thibodeau GA, Patton KT: *Anatomy & physiology,* ed 6, p. 373, St Louis, 2007, Mosby/Elsevier.)

relation to the upper body, it plays an important role in the thorax because of muscle attachments. Such interactions are seen throughout the body; therefore it is almost impossible to separate the body into totally independent areas. Observation of the lines of pull of the pectoralis minor reveal that it tends to pull the coracoid process inferiorly and medially. If the scapula is retracted, the pectoralis minor pulls the ribs out and up. The first action might be considered a stabilizing effect on the scapula, whereas the second action might be considered a means to help the breathing process by elevating the ribs.

The serratus anterior is also a relatively flat muscle that has attachments on ribs one through eight, although in some individuals it may extend to the ninth rib. The muscle then continues posteriorly to insert along the length of the anterior medial edge of the scapula. This configuration is unique in that the attachment on the scapula is hidden in most views and the resultant movements that occur are often not immediately grasped. The attachment scheme may require extra time to understand. The serratus anterior is sometimes called the "punching muscle" because it pulls or slides the scapula anteriorly around the ribs, which in turn allows the person to make a punching motion while thrusting the arm forward. *Serratus* is Latin for "sawtooth."

The intercostals, as their name implies, run between adjacent ribs. There are actually two or three layers of intercostals (depending on the interpretation), and their primary purpose is to help stabilize the chest wall of the thorax. The external intercostals also help with inspiration during breathing by elevating the lower ribs

Covering most of the pectoralis minor, serratus anterior, and intercostals are the much larger and more powerful latissimus dorsi and the pectoralis major muscles. The latissimus dorsi covers the posterior and lateral thorax with a long attachment down the spinous processes of the midthoracic, lumbar, and sacral vertebrae. The latissimus triangulates laterally and superiorly under the armpit, crossing over the medial and anterior part of the upper humerus and eventually attaching on the upper lateral humerus. As with the serratus anterior, tracing its attachment sites requires a bit of work. The actions of the muscle become evident as it is examined from end to end, whereupon it becomes clear that the primary actions are to extend the flexed humerus and to adduct and internally rotate it.

The pectoralis major has two parts, clavicular and sternal (see Figure 13-24). The clavicular and sternal parts merge before crossing laterally across the chest and attaching on the lateral aspect of the upper humerus. Hence the action of the pectoralis major is to adduct and internally rotate the humerus.

Table 13-4 summarizes the muscles of the thorax.

Muscles of the Abdomen

Consistent with all the other muscles of this area, the abdominal muscles serve the important function of protecting the abdominal contents; however, like the erector spinae group of the back, they also play a role in movement and the control of movement. The functions of these muscles include all the following and are discussed in more detail within this section:

- *Protect* the contents of the abdomen when activated isometrically
- *Support* the spine and back musculature by creating a cylinder of sorts from the spine, which otherwise serves only as an axis

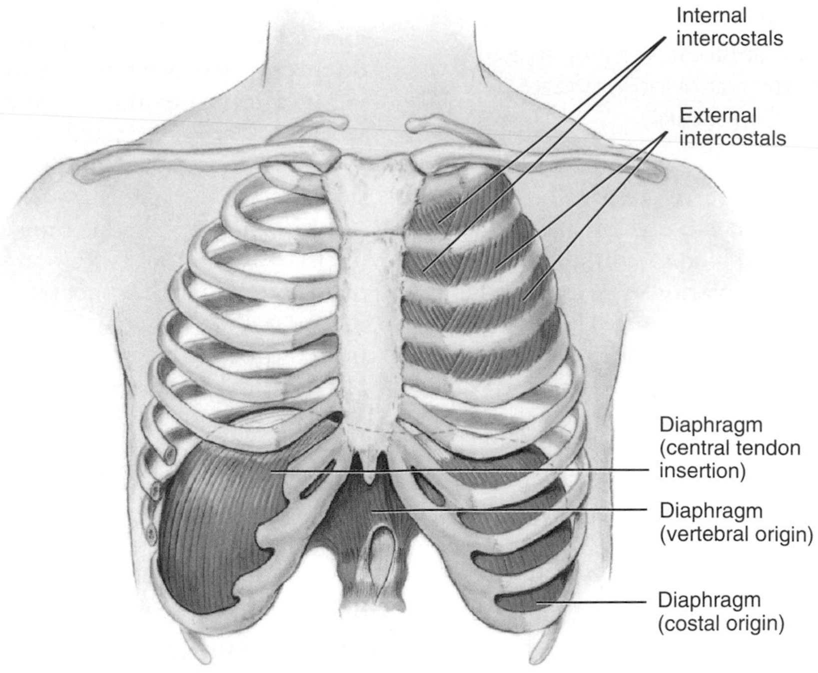

FIGURE 13-25 Diaphragm. (From Applegate E: *The anatomy and physiology learning system,* ed 3, p. 131, Philadelphia, 2006, Saunders/Elsevier.)

TABLE 13-4 Muscles of the Thorax

MUSCLE(S)	LOCATION	FUNCTION*
Pectoralis major	There are two pectoralis major muscles, and each has two parts, the clavicular and the sternal. The clavicular and sternal parts merge and form a triangular muscle that runs laterally across the chest to the upper lateral humerus.	Acting alone, each muscle adducts and internally rotates the humerus. Acting together, they are used in performing push-ups and the bench press. When they contract concentrically, they push the body or weight up; when contracting eccentrically, they control the body or weight as it is lowered.
Pectoralis minor	There are two pectoralis minor muscles. Each runs from ribs two through five up to the coracoid process of the scapula.	Acting alone, each muscle protracts, or pulls forward, the scapula.
Serratus anterior	There are two serratus anterior muscles. Each runs from ribs one through eight or nine around the ribs to the medial anterior border of the scapula.	Acting alone, each muscle protracts, or pulls forward, the scapula. This is the muscle that allows a person to thrust the arm forward when performing a punching motion.
Latissimus dorsi	See Table 13-3.	
Intercostals	There are intercostal muscles found between each adjacent pair of ribs.	The external intercostals elevate the ribs, and the internal intercostals depress the ribs.

*Remember that a function of all these muscles is that they cover some anatomical structure and by doing so are protecting that underlying structure.

- *Create* intraabdominal pressure, which helps to stabilize the entire trunk
- *Initiate and control* movements of the trunk

The **diaphragm** is a flat circular muscle that essentially forms a floor for the thorax and at the same time is a domed roof for the abdomen (Figure 13-25). Notice how it umbrellas out to the surrounding ribs. It can be thought of as connecting to the T12/L1 junction and then following around the twelfth ribs to the xiphoid process at the base of the sternum. This muscle separates the thorax from the abdomen and has the important role of influencing intrathoracic pressure and intraabdominal pressure. The diaphragm helps with breathing; it is the major muscle of inspiration. Contraction of the diaphragm causes it to bulge downward, pushing the abdominal contents down and thereby increasing the intrathoracic space so that inspiration can take place.

Points to Ponder

Would an increase in intraabdominal pressure help to increase core strength by adding stability to the abdominal muscles and low back musculature?

The diaphragm contains three holes: one for the esophagus going to the stomach, one for the descending aorta sending oxygenated blood to the abdomen and lower body, and one for the inferior vena cava bringing deoxygenated blood back up to the heart. The diaphragm is innervated by the phrenic nerve, which comes off of cervical nerves three, four, and five. When this nerve is compromised in a neck injury, the individual cannot breathe independently and will need emergent medical attention.

The other four abdominal muscles are more external, directional, and layered. They connect the ribs to the pelvis by way of the inguinal ligament. There is one abdominal muscle in the middle portion of the abdomen that runs vertically, the rectus abdominis. Activation of the rectus abdominis causes flexion of the thorax-abdomen junction and, consequently, the spine. It runs from the anterior surfaces of ribs five, six, and seven to the pubic symphysis and is relatively thick compared with the other abdominal muscles. The three other pairs of abdominal muscles tie into the right and left lateral aspects of the rectus abdominis. The deepest lateral abdominal muscle is the transverse abdominis. It attaches to the lower six ribs and the iliac crest and runs to the pubic bone and linea alba. The word *transverse* indicates the direction of the fibers as they run horizontally. The muscle's purpose is primarily to stabilize the area and hold the contents of the abdomen in place. Acting together, the abdominal muscles are important in providing core strength. They do this by increasing intraabdominal pressure and helping transform the abdominal area into a rigid cylinder when they are contracted. This entire area then serves as a core for movements that occur above and below this area.

Lying on top of the transverse abdominis are the internal oblique and external oblique muscles. Immediately covering the transverse abdominis muscles are the internal oblique muscles, which run down and away from the lower three ribs and linea alba to the iliac crest and inguinal ligament. Their function is to rotate the torso to the same side that they are located as the muscle fibers pull the rectus sheath toward the inguinal ligament. For example, the right internal oblique rotates the trunk and thorax to the right side. The outermost layer of the lateral abdominal muscles comprises the external oblique muscles. They run perpendicular to the internal obliques and up and away from the rectus abdominis and its sheath to the outer aspect of the lower eight ribs. When they are activated, they rotate the torso to the side opposite to their location as the fibers pull the ribs toward the rectus sheath. For instance, the right external obliques rotate the trunk and thorax to the left side. Therefore when the torso rotates to the left, the left internal obliques and the right external obliques work together. When all the obliques (from both the right and the left sides) are activated at the same time, they serve to help the rectus abdominis flex the trunk. Lastly, when these muscles are isometrically activated, they protect the internal organs and serve as an anterior support for the low back (Figure 13-26).

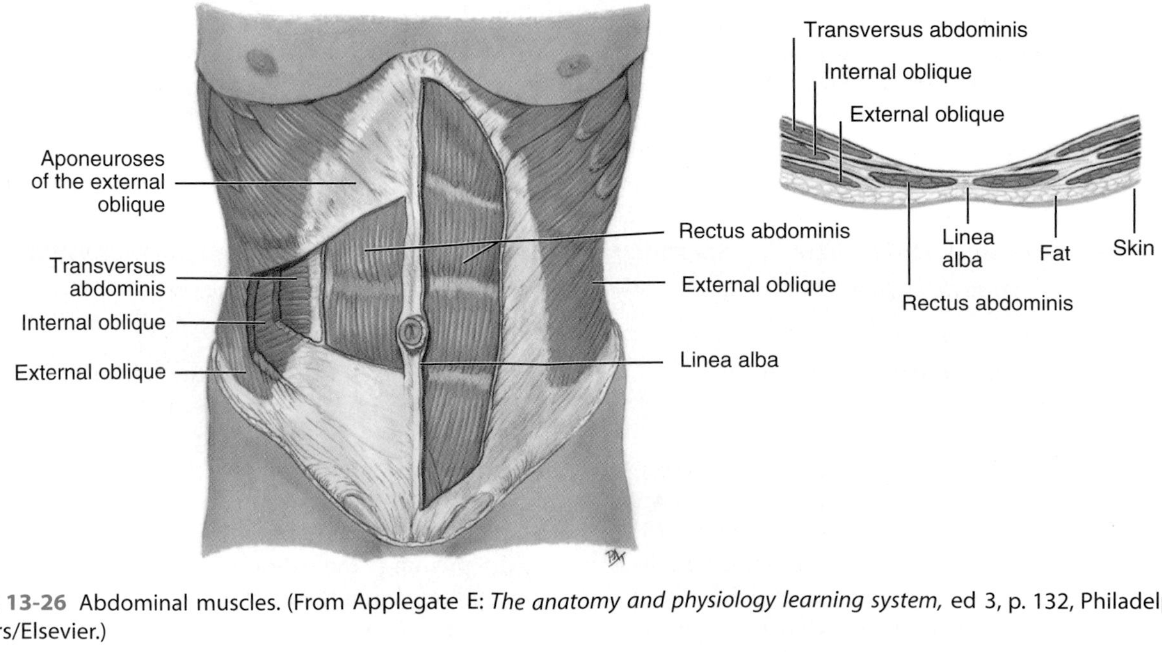

FIGURE 13-26 Abdominal muscles. (From Applegate E: *The anatomy and physiology learning system,* ed 3, p. 132, Philadelphia, 2006, Saunders/Elsevier.)

TABLE 13-5 Muscles of the Abdomen

MUSCLE(S)	LOCATION	FUNCTION*
Diaphragm	There is one diaphragm muscle. It is a flat, pancake-like muscle that attaches at the T12/L1 junction and follows the twelfth ribs around to the xiphoid process at the base of the sternum.	It is the major muscle of inspiration. Contraction of the diaphragm causes it to bulge downward, pushing the abdominal contents down and thereby increasing the intrathoracic space so that inspiration can take place.
Rectus abdominis	There is one rectus abdominis. It runs from the anterior surfaces of ribs five, six, and seven down to the pubic symphysis.	This muscle causes flexion of the thorax-abdomen junction and, consequently, the spine. It is used when doing abdominal crunches.
Transverse abdominis	There are two transverse abdominis muscles. Each attaches to the lower six ribs and iliac crest and runs to the pubic bone and linea alba.	The muscle's primary purpose is to stabilize the area and hold the contents of the abdomen in place while acting as the front wall of the abdomen.
Internal oblique	There are two internal oblique muscles. Each attaches to the lower three ribs and linea alba and runs down to the iliac crest and inguinal ligament.	Their function is to rotate the torso to the same side on which they are located.
External oblique	There are two external oblique muscles. They run perpendicular to the internal obliques and up and away from the rectus abdominis and its sheath to the outer aspect of the lower eight ribs.	Their function is to rotate the torso to the opposite side on which they are located.

*Remember that a function of all of these muscles is that they cover some anatomical structure and by doing so are protecting that underlying structure.

Table 13-5 summarizes and describes the muscles of the abdomen.

Other Organs

Several major organs are located inside the bony cage of the thorax. These organs include the heart, lungs, and major blood vessels that pass through the area. Without adequate protection from the bones of the thorax, these organs would be injured easily, with potentially catastrophic results. Chapter 5 provides more details about these essential components of the body.

SUMMARY

This chapter contains basic information about the spine, thorax, and abdomen, a foundation for subsequent chapters that cover evaluation of the structures of the spine, thorax, and the abdomen. Athletic trainers must remember, however, that every individual is unique; thus anatomical aberrations abound, both those that are readily apparent and those that require sophisticated diagnostic techniques for detection.

Web Links

Body Worlds Project: www.koerperwelten.de/en/pages/home.asp

The Anatomy Lesson: http://mywebpages.comcast.net/wnor/homepage.htm

Web Anatomy (University of Minnesota): www.msjensen.gen.umn.edu/webanatomy/

Medical Gross Anatomy Learning Resources (University of Michigan): http://anatomy.med.umich.edu/

The Visible Human Project (National Library of Medicine, National Institutes of Health): www.nlm.nih.gov/research/visible/visible_human.html

Bibliography

Applegate E: *The Anatomy and physiology learning system*, ed 3, Philadelphia, 2006, Saunders/Elsevier.

Caine CG, Caine DJ, Lindner KJ: *Epidemiology of sports injuries*, Champaign, Ill, 1996, Human Kinetics.

Cassidy JD, Carroll LJ, Cote P: The Saskatchewan health and back pain survey: The prevalence of low back pain and related disability in Saskatchewan adults, *Spine* 23(17): 1860–1866, 1998.

Cuppett M: The anatomy and pathomechanics of the sacroiliac joint, *Athletic Therapy Today* 6(4): 6, 2001.

Cuppett M, Walsh K, (eds.), *General medical conditions in the athlete*. St Louis, 2005, Elsevier/Mosby.

Drake RL, Vogl W, Mitchell ADM: *Gray's anatomy for students*, Edinburgh, 2005, Elsevier/Churchill Livingstone.

Hartman SE, Norton JM: Craniosacral therapy is not medicine, *Phys Ther* 82(11): 1146–1147, 2002.

Herlihy B: *The human body in health and illness*, ed 3, Philadelphia, 2007, Saunders/Elsevier.

Middleditch A, Oliver J: *Functional anatomy of the spine*, ed 2, Edinburgh, 2006, Churchill Livingstone/Elsevier.

Moses KP et al: *Atlas of clinical gross anatomy*, St Louis, 2005, Elsevier/Mosby.

Muscolino JE: *Kinesiology: the skeletal system and muscle function*, St Louis, 2006, Mosby/Elsevier.

Neumann D: *Kinesiology of the skeletal system: foundations for physical therapy*, St Louis, 2002, Elsevier/Mosby.

Powell JW, Barber-Foss KD: Injury patterns in selected high school sports: a review of the 1995–1997 seasons, *Journal of Athletic Training* 34(3): 277–284, 1999.

Seidel HM, et al: *Mosby's guide to physical examination*, ed 6, St Louis, 2006, Mosby/Elsevier.

Standring S., ed., *Gray's anatomy: the anatomical basis of clinical practice*, ed 39, Edinburgh, 2005, Elsevier/Churchill Livingstone.

Szanjnuk TL: Low back pain in athletes: flexion or extension?, *Athletic Therapy Today* 1(3): 47, 1996.

Thibodeau GA, Patton KT: *Anatomy & physiology*, ed 6, St Louis, 2007, Mosby/Elsevier.

14

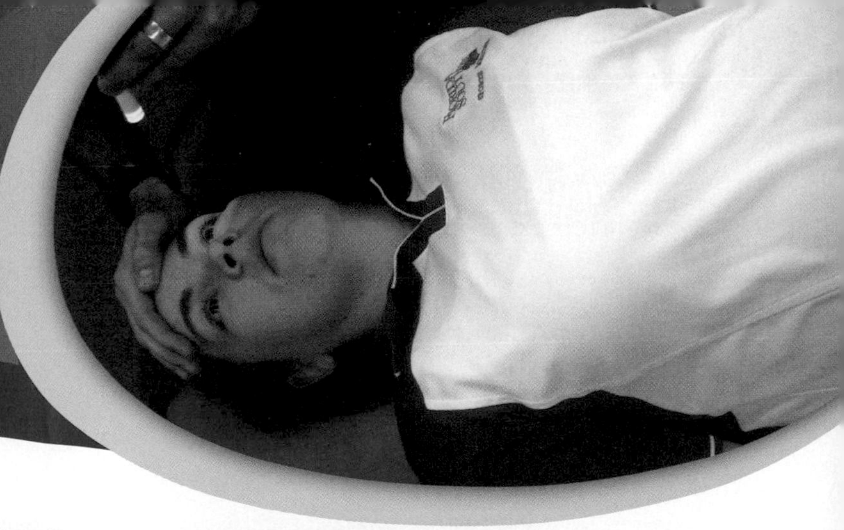

Diagnosis and Management of Sports-Related Concussion

MICHAEL S. FERRARA

Learning Goals

1. Define concussion.
2. Describe the common mechanisms that cause sports-related concussion.
3. Differentiate between the types of cerebral bleeding and the resulting signs and symptoms.
4. Explain and apply common methods used to evaluate a concussion on the sideline and in the athletic training room.
5. Develop and implement an objective management plan for sports-related concussion.
6. Describe criteria for return to play after sports-related concussion.

According to Centers for Disease Control and Prevention estimates, more than 300,000 concussions occur annually in all sports throughout the United States.[1] Most head injuries, or **concussions**—usually defined as any injury to the brain that results from an impact to the head—occur in contact sports such as football, ice hockey, wrestling, boxing, or lacrosse. Sports equipment, such as balls, bats, pucks, goal posts, or even hard surfaces, may contribute to a concussion when contact is made with them. The signs and symptoms related to concussion are often subtle, a fact that places a huge responsibility on the athletic trainer, who must be able to perform a complete and accurate evaluation. It is important to recognize the signs and symptoms of concussions, as well as those that could indicate a more significant injury or trauma to the brain.

The *Journal of Athletic Training* published the National Athletic Trainers Association (NATA) Position Statement on the Management of Sport-Related Concussion.[2] This position statement provides practical suggestions divided into eight main content areas (Box 14-1). The document serves as the standard of care and management for such injuries. All athletic trainers and health care practitioners who may provide care to athletes at risk of concussion must be familiar with these guidelines and recommendations. This chapter provides an overview of concussions: how to evaluate and manage concussions and return to play and age-related concerns regarding concussions. Suggestions from the NATA position statement are interspersed throughout the chapter.

WHAT IS A CONCUSSION?

Although the general definition of concussion is any injury to the brain that results from impact, the technical definition was first created by the Congress of Neurological Surgeons in 1966. The Congress of Neurological Surgeons defines a concussion as "a clinical syndrome characterized by immediate and transient post-traumatic impairment of neural function, such as alteration of consciousness, disturbance of vision, equilibrium due to brainstem involvement."[2] This definition was thought to be too limiting and not

concussion injury sustained from either a direct blow or an indirect force

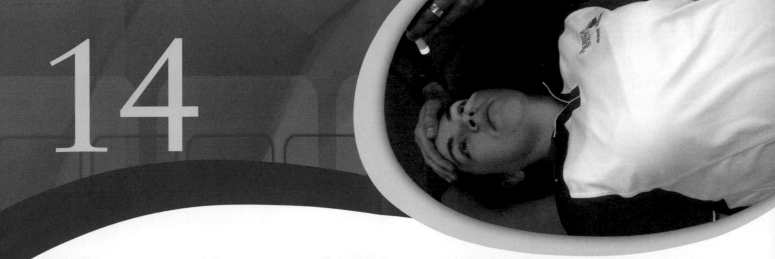

OPENING *Scenario*

A 16-year-old high school wide receiver is running a crossing pattern through the middle of the defense during a conference football game. As the ball reaches his hands, the strong safety also comes through the middle from the other direction and hits him with his shoulder pads. Direct contact appears to have been made to the side of the helmet, knocking the receiver down. After being struck, he immediately falls to the ground, hitting his head on the turf, and appears to be unconscious. The wide receiver never saw the defensive player approaching and thus the blow was completely unexpected. The crowd is quiet as medical staff employees rush to the aid of the unconscious athlete. Your supposition that this is a serious injury is accurate. But what is the exact diagnosis, and how do you know when it is safe to allow him to return to play?

BOX 14-1 NATA Position Statement on the Management of Sports-Related Concussion

1. Defining and recognizing concussion
2. Evaluating and making return to play decisions
3. Concussion assessment tools
4. When to refer an athlete to a physician after a concussion
5. When to disqualify
6. Special considerations for the young athlete
7. Home care
8. Equipment issues

Data from National Athletic Trainers' Association: NATA position statement: Management of sports-related concussions, *J Athl Train* 39(3): 280–297, 2004.

inclusive of the less severe nature of concussion typically seen in sports. In today's sports environment, where a concussion may range from minor to significant, a more comprehensive definition is needed. Therefore, at the 2001 International Symposium on Concussion in Sport, a new definition was published to fill this void and reflect a better understanding of concussive injuries. *Concussion* is now defined as a complex pathophysiological process affecting the brain induced by traumatic biomechanical forces.[3] This definition satisfies the broad range of concussion injuries, defines the common mechanism of injury, describes the typical resolution of symptoms and cognitive function, and states that imaging studies are typically normal. Several common features that incorporate clinical, pathological, and biomechanical injury constructs that may be used in defining a concussive head injury include the following[2]:

1. Concussion may be caused by a direct blow to the head, face, neck, or elsewhere on the body with any force transmitted to the head.
2. Concussion typically results in the rapid onset of short-lived impairment of neurological function that resolves spontaneously.
3. Concussion may result in neuropathological changes, but the acute clinical symptoms largely reflect a functional disturbance rather than structural injury.
4. Concussion results in a graded set of clinical syndromes that may or may not involve loss of consciousness. Resolution of the clinical and cognitive symptoms typically follows a sequential course.
5. Concussion is typically associated with grossly normal structural neuroimaging studies.

Figure 14-1 is a concept map that summarizes the issues surrounding a sports-related concussion: its type, evaluation, diagnosis, and management, as well as considerations involved in the athlete's return to play.

Hematoma of the Brain

One of the more serious consequences of a concussion is a hematoma, or bleeding, within the brain. Common types of hematomas resulting from a head injury are epidural and subdural hematomas as discussed in this chapter (Figure 14-2). Injuries that result in these kinds of hematomas are rare in sports but can certainly occur, depending on the location and force of the blow to the head. Contact sports are the most likely to produce these hematomas.

Points to Ponder
Aside from contact sports what other activities can cause this type of hematoma?

For either type of hematoma, the athletic trainer must quickly recognize the signs and symptoms to render appropriate immediate first aid and care. As the hematoma develops, the pressure inside the skull will increase and the neurological function will deteriorate rapidly. These types of injuries usually require activation of the emergency action plan and transportation by ambulance to the hospital.

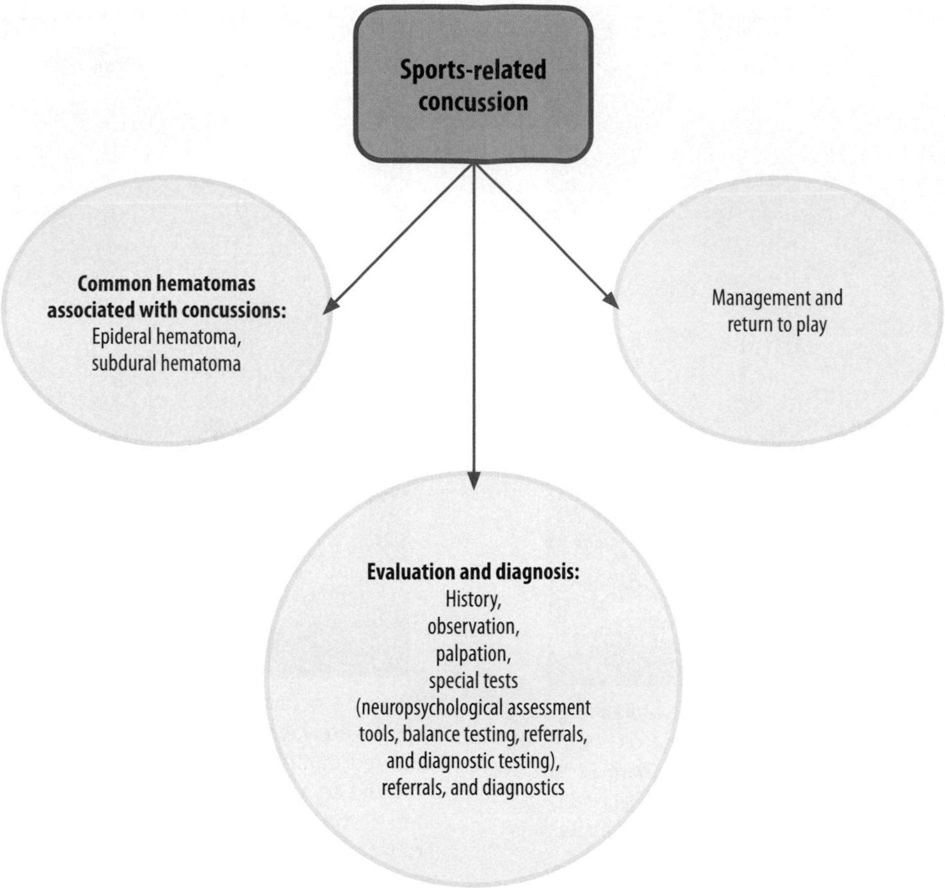

FIGURE 14-1 Concept map summarizing the issues surrounding sports-related concussion.

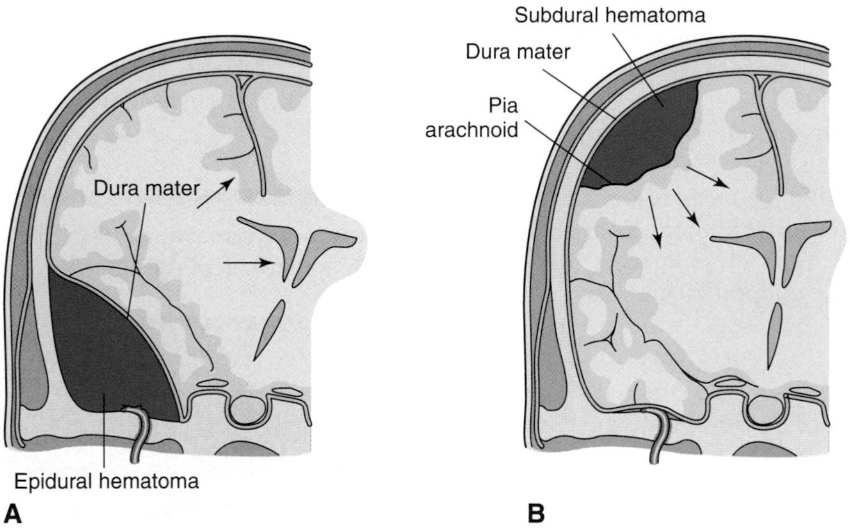

FIGURE 14-2 Common types of hematomas. **A,** Epidural hematoma. **B,** Subdural hematoma. (From Phipps W et al: *Medical-surgical nursing: health and illness perspectives,* ed 7, Figure 42-15, St Louis, 2003, Mosby/Elsevier.)

Epidural Hematoma

An **epidural hematoma** is usually an arterial bleed into the epidural space of the brain. The blood emerges from the middle meningeal artery (Figure 14-3). Those suffering from this injury experience rapid decline that results in a loss of consciousness or altered level of

epidural hematoma usually an arterial bleed into the epidural space of the brain

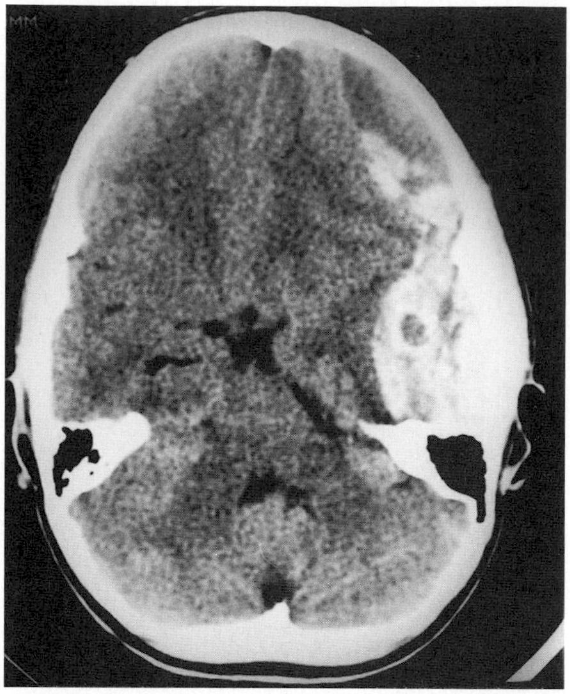

FIGURE 14-3 Computed tomographic scan showing a large left frontotemporal epidural hematoma in a 14-year-old boy. Note the different densities of blood within the lesion, characteristic of an ongoing hemorrhage. (From DeLee JC, Drez D: *DeLee & Drez's orthopaedic sports medicine,* ed 2, Figure 19B-2, Philadelphia, 2003, Saunders/Elsevier.)

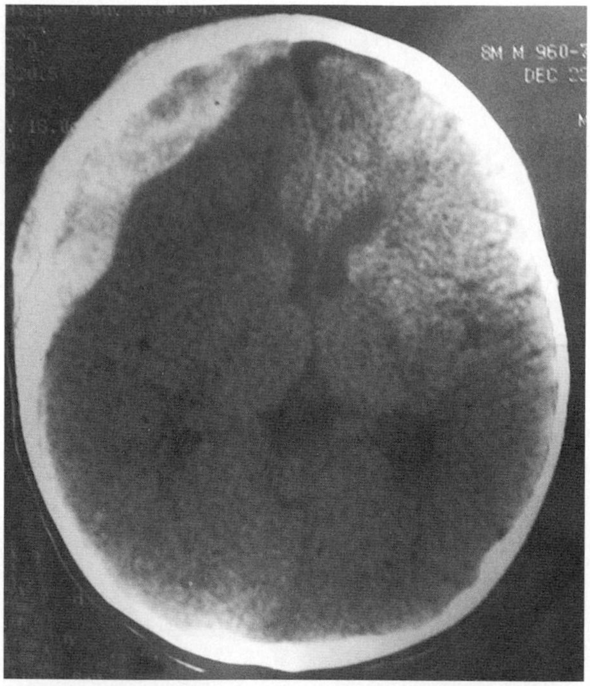

FIGURE 14-4 Large right frontotemporal subdural hematoma in a child who was tackled during a football game. The athlete was rendered immediately unconscious and rapidly transported to a trauma center. Despite emergent craniotomy, the athlete suffered a significant brain injury with a poor functional outcome. (From DeLee JC, Drez D: *DeLee & Drez's orthopaedic sports medicine,* ed 2, Figure 19B-1, Philadelphia, 2003, Saunders/Elsevier.)

consciousness. They may go in and out of consciousness. Other symptoms of this serious head injury may include increasing headache, blurred vision, speech changes, mental confusion, and dizziness. The accumulation of blood in the epidural space places pressure on the brain, which compresses the tissue and impairs its ability to function properly. Imaging techniques such as a computed tomography (CT) scan and magnetic resonance imaging (MRI) may be used to diagnose both the location and the severity of the bleeding. Typically, surgery is required to allow for drainage of the epidural hematoma.

Subdural Hematoma

A **subdural hematoma** occurs when a cerebral blood vessel tears, causing a slow bleed within the subdural space of the brain (Figure 14-4). The onset of symptoms may be more gradual than with an epidural hematoma. In some cases, symptoms may not become apparent until 24 to 72 hours after the injury. With a subdural hematoma, the collection of blood forms more slowly than it does with an epidural bleed, which accounts for the delayed onset of symptoms. The patient with a subdural hematoma will be conscious, with no obvious signs or symptoms. However, he or she will progressively get worse with the onset of myriad symptoms such as headache, nausea, dizziness, and altered mental status. The athletic trainer should always suspect bleeding or a hematoma within the brain and take a conservative approach to head injury management until these conditions are ruled out by a physician and diagnostic imaging.

Table 14-1 shows the differences between epidural and subdural hematomas. Prompt determination of the

subdural hematoma injury that occurs when a cerebral blood vessel tears

TABLE 14-1 Hematoma Comparison

TYPE OF HEMATOMA	LOCATION	ONSET	SYMPTOMS
Epidural	Arterial (bleed into epidural space)	Immediate	Altered level of consciousness, headache, blurred vision, slurred speech, sensitivity to light, mental confusion, dizziness
Subdural	Venous (bleed into subdural space)	Gradually, up to 24 to 72 hours	None initially; progress gradually to headache, nausea, dizziness, altered mental status

type of hematoma allows a timely objective decision regarding medical care and return to play.

Mechanism of Injury

The brain is a well-protected organ, enclosed by the **cranium,** or skull. Within the cranium is the cerebral spinal fluid (CSF), which acts as a cushion and allows the brain to move within the skull. However, when the brain is violently moved by a contact blow or an indirect force, the CSF is pushed away. This displacement of the CSF exposes the inner surface of the skull, providing an opportunity for the brain to collide with it.

As previously stated, concussion usually results from a direct blow with another person, equipment such as a goalpost, or the ground (Figure 14-5). This type of direct contact is called a **coup injury.** Concussion may also result from a blow to another body part in which a whiplashlike mechanism occurs to the head and neck. The brain collides with the cranium, and the injury occurs on the opposite side of the blow. This is called a **contrecoup injury.** No evidence suggests that either the coup injury or the contrecoup injury is more serious.

Mechanisms that involve a violent rotation of the head, such as a blow to the jaw or temple region that causes the head to be forcefully rotated to the side, can result in a **torsional brain injury** of the brain. This mechanism of injury causes the brain to rotate within the skull, creating a shearing mechanism that results in the tearing of vessels. A typical example of a torsion injury mechanism that results in shearing would be a boxer getting hit in the jaw from an uppercut or a football player getting hit in the side of the head. This type of blow causes an upward and lateral rotation of the head, which causes the brain to rotate within the skull, thus tearing the involved vessels.

Epidemiology of Sports-Related Concussion

Several studies have examined the injury rates and trends of concussions in sports. Thus far, football has been the most frequently studied sport. Concussion accounts for about 5% of the total injuries during a football season.[4,5] The injury rate appears to range between 0.06 and 0.55 concussions per 1000 **athlete-exposures,** or opportunities that the athlete has to either practice or compete. In an epidemiology project involving high school athletes,[5] the overall concussion injury rate was 5.5%. Of those reported concussions, almost 90% suffered from one concussion and 10% had two or more concussions during the same season. This incidence has been further confirmed, with a concussion re-injury rate of 15% within the same season.[4] Apparently, football players who handle offensive positions, positions that are subjected to high velocity collisions, tend to suffer concussions more often than other players (Figure 14-6). The top three football positions on all levels of play associated with the most concussions are quarterback, wide receiver, and tight end.[6,7] A study examining collegiate football players found that the quarterback, running back, and wide receiver are at greatest risk of concussion.[4] Another study involving high school football players found that linebackers, running backs,

cranium the skull

coup injury a direct blow that causes the brain to shift from its normal position in the skull and cerebrospinal fluid toward the point at which contact was made

contrecoup injury a severe blow that creates a whiplashlike mechanism in the brain wherein the brain shifts and collides with the cranium, a rebound effect from the coup impact, affecting the side of the head opposite to the side on which the impact was made

torsional brain injury injury that results from a severe blow to the head that causes the head to rotate on impact

athlete-exposures the number of times every athlete on a team has the opportunity to either practice or compete

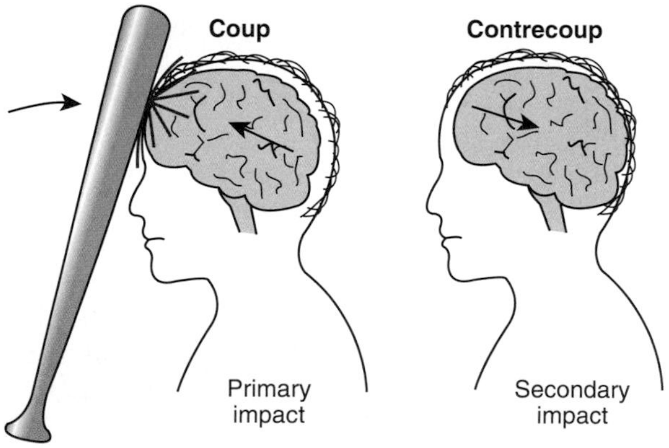

FIGURE 14-5 Coup and contrecoup injury mechanisms. (Redrawn from BrainInjury.com: *How can the brain be injured?* Waterloo, Ontario, Canada, 2001–2007, Author/Montana Publishing.)

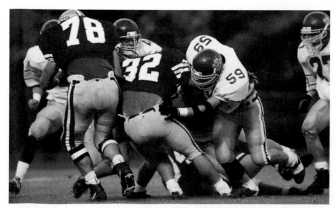

FIGURE 14-6 A high-velocity contact between football players. (Courtesy PhotoDisc.)

and offensive linemen are most likely to sustain a concussion.[5] These findings make it imperative that the athletic trainer understand the likelihood for head trauma and concussion in athletes involved with open field, high-velocity tackling.

CLINICAL EVALUATION AND DIAGNOSIS OF SPORTS-RELATED CONCUSSION

The athletic trainer must develop a thorough and systematic method for evaluating and diagnosing concussions. When evaluating a musculoskeletal injury, the athletic trainer relies on a number of physical signs and symptoms, including swelling, range of motion, and strength. When evaluating a sports-related concussion, the athletic trainer does not have as many objective measures to use as he or she does when performing a physical examination for a musculoskeletal injury. Therefore a comprehensive assessment tool should be developed and used. This tool should include a thorough history that takes into account any self-reported symptoms (SRS); a physical examination consisting of observation/inspection and palpation; and special tests related to neuropsychological functioning, balance, and exertional testing. Additionally, a number of diagnostic imaging tests may be warranted. These tests may include X-rays, CT scans, and functional MRI scans to evaluate bony and structural changes in the tissues of the brain.[8]

When first evaluating for concussion, the athletic trainer should immediately assess the athlete's vital signs to rule out life-threatening conditions. This assessment should include a check of consciousness, pulse rate, blood pressure, and respirations. Most patients with concussions demonstrate normal values for these vital signs. Any abnormal findings may indicate a more serious head injury, such as an epidural or subdural hematoma. These injuries, as previously discussed, require further medical evaluation and intervention by a physician. The athletic trainer must be quick to recognize any changes in the client's status that might indicate a more serious injury. After ruling out life-threatening conditions, the athletic trainer should be able to begin the evaluation process. The goal now is to identify other symptoms, such as amnesia, memory loss, and the potential for additional concussion-related symptoms (e.g., headache; nausea; and **tinnitus**, or ringing in the ears).

Before moving on to the evaluation process, the athletic trainer must be aware of the fact that no two concussions are the same. The signs and symptoms may be entirely different for each concussive injury. Depending on the findings of the history, the physical examination, and all the available assessment tools, the next most important area to address is whether the athletic trainer is confident that enough information is available to make a return to activity decision. Having a systematic assessment tool will help ensure a complete and thorough evaluation, making the decision more objective and reliable.

History

The athletic trainer should obtain a detailed and thorough history of the current injury and any previous concussions or head injuries. Understanding the scope and magnitude of the current injury is critical to successfully managing it and ultimately returning the athlete to activity. Knowledge of any previous head injuries becomes an integral factor in deciding how to best evaluate and treat the athlete. Guskiewicz[4] reported that an athlete may have a threefold increased risk of concussion after suffering the first concussion. Many experts believe that the most vulnerable period for re-injury is within the first 10 to 14 days after concussion.[9,10] During this time, the brain is more susceptible to injury because of the numerous chemical and glycolytic changes that are occurring after the initial (and subsequent) concussion. Any athlete with concussion-related symptoms should not be allowed to return to participation until medically cleared by a physician.

Self-reported symptoms are among the most important aspects of the history portion of the concussion evaluation. Some common symptoms include headache, nausea, trouble falling asleep, fatigue, drowsiness, irritability, vision abnormalities, balance difficulties, lethargy, and memory problems.

> **Points to Ponder**
> If you suspect a concussion injury in an individual who is not self-reporting symptoms that match his/her behavior, what could you do to corroborate your findings? Who could you talk to for more accurate information?

These symptoms should be assessed during the initial portion of the evaluation and at each subsequent re-evaluation until the injury is completely resolved. Potential concussion-related symptoms are listed in Box 14-2. The athletic trainer should assess for level of consciousness or loss of consciousness, post-traumatic amnesia (retrograde or anterograde), and any deterioration in the athlete's condition. Another important aspect of the injury evaluation is the monitoring of concussion-related symptoms such as headache, dizziness, and nausea. The diligent assessment of these concussion characteristics allows the athletic trainer

tinnitus ringing in the ears

BOX 14-2 Potential Concussion-Related Signs and Symptoms

Headache	Feeling lethargic
Nausea	Feeling in a "fog"
Difficulty falling asleep	Difficulty remembering things
Sleeping more than usual	Dizziness
Fatigue	Neck pain
Drowsiness	Vomiting
Irritability	Sensitivity to light and noise
Vision issues	Difficulty concentrating
Balance difficulties	Numbness

to document any improvement or deterioration in the status of the athlete throughout the recovery period and facilitates appropriate injury management decisions.

Observation and Inspection

As with any other injury, observation of the concussed athlete begins as soon as the athletic trainer sees the client. The observation and inspection process continues throughout the entire evaluation. During the history portion, immediate life-threatening situations are ruled out. The identification of underlying symptoms that can help establish the extent of the concussion are explored at this juncture; these are described in Box 14-3. The athletic trainer should observe the way that the athlete responds to the questions, remembers certain events, ambulates and carries himself or herself, and reacts to changes in visual stimuli. Assessment of pupil response, as discussed in Chapter 7, is also important at this point. Cranial nerves should be evaluated to definitively diagnose the type and extent of injury.

BOX 14-3 Observation/Inspection of a Concussed Athlete

- Verbal responses to questioning
- Disorientation
- Memory (retrograde amnesia or anterograde amnesia)
- Ability to focus
- Emotional responses
- Ambulation and balance
- Posture
- Coordination
- PEARL assessment
- Visual responses to various stimuli
- Cranial nerve assessment
- Level of consciousness

Initial attempts should be made to determine the athlete's level of consciousness. A common misconception is that a person must be unconscious if he or she has sustained a concussion. In fact, fewer than 10% of concussions involve any loss of consciousness[2]. However, if a loss of consciousness does occur, the athletic trainer should initially suspect both a head and a neck injury. A physical examination of the head and neck should be performed immediately. In keeping with appropriate injury management protocols, the head should be stabilized until the suspicion of fracture, dislocation, or other potentially catastrophic cervical spine injury is eliminated.

Post-traumatic amnesia (PTA) is a much more common consequence of a concussive blow. Approximately 30% of athletes have reported PTA after concussion.[2] Amnesia, either retrograde or anterograde, may be present in concussed athletes. **Retrograde amnesia** is when the athlete does not remember events preceding the injury. **Anterograde amnesia** is when the athlete does not remember events that occur after the injury.

To assess retrograde amnesia, the athletic trainer should ask questions starting from the time of injury and working backward. For example, the athletic trainer may ask questions about the score of the game, the period or quarter of the game, the score of the previous period, events from the pregame warm-up, or even transportation to the venue. The athletic trainer should assess for accuracy, speed, and clarity of the responses. Confusion and disorientation are common among athletes who suffer from retrograde amnesia.

Anterograde amnesia is more difficult to assess. A common method is to give the athlete a list of five unrelated words, such as *wagon, green, beef, diamond,* and *door.* After a period of 5 or 10 minutes, the athlete should be asked to remember and recite the words. Mistakes may indicate short-term memory impairments. Also, the athletic trainer may ask questions about the chronology of events following the concussion. Again, the athletic trainer assesses the athlete's confusion, disorientation, speed, and clarity.

post-traumatic amnesia amnesia suffered after any concussive injury in which the ability to remember is altered

retrograde amnesia amnesia in which events preceding the injury are not remembered

anterograde amnesia amnesia in which events after the injury are not remembered

TABLE 14-2 Cranial Nerves

NERVE	FUNCTION AND ASSESSMENT	TYPE
I. Olfactory	Sense of smell	Sensory
II. Optic	Visual acuity	Sensory
III. Oculomotor	Eye movement, regulation of pupil size	Motor
IV. Trochlear	Eye movement and proprioception	Motor
V. Trigeminal	Sensation of head and face, chewing	Mixed
VI. Abducens	Abduction of the eye	Motor
VII. Facial	Facial expressions, secretion of saliva, taste	Mixed
VIII. Vestibulocochlear	Balance, equilibrium, hearing	Sensory
IX. Glossopharyngeal	Taste and other sensations, swallowing, secretion of saliva	Mixed
X. Vagus	Sensation of movement of organs, regulation of heartbeat, peristalsis, contraction of muscles for voice production	Mixed
XI. Spinal Accessory	Shoulder movements, turning of head, voice production	Motor
XII. Hypoglossal	Tongue movements	Motor

Evaluation of the eyes may provide important information about the injury. The athletic trainer should perform a PEARL evaluation, as discussed in Chapter 7. Any deviation from normal may indicate a serious injury. Abnormal findings should result in immediate referral and transport to a hospital or medical facility for further evaluation.

A cranial nerve assessment should be performed to ensure proper functioning of these nerves after the injury. This assessment may help determine whether a serious injury such as a hematoma is present and also whether the brain is functioning normally. It should be done in a sequential fashion, moving logically from cranial nerve I to cranial nerve XII. Table 14-2 lists the cranial nerves and the assessment techniques relevant to each specific nerve.

Palpation

Palpation of concussed athletes is primarily performed to rule out any deformities, fractures, or neurovascular compromise to the head and neck regions (Figure 14-7). Point tenderness, swelling, muscle spasms, and loss of sensation can also be evaluated by palpating the area.

Special Tests

Several types of special tests are used to evaluate athletes who may have a sports-related concussion. These tests, or tools, help the athletic trainer accurately determine whether a concussion was sustained and ultimately provide information that assists in injury management and return to activity decisions. The tests discussed here are neuropsychological assessment tools, balance testing, and diagnostic testing.

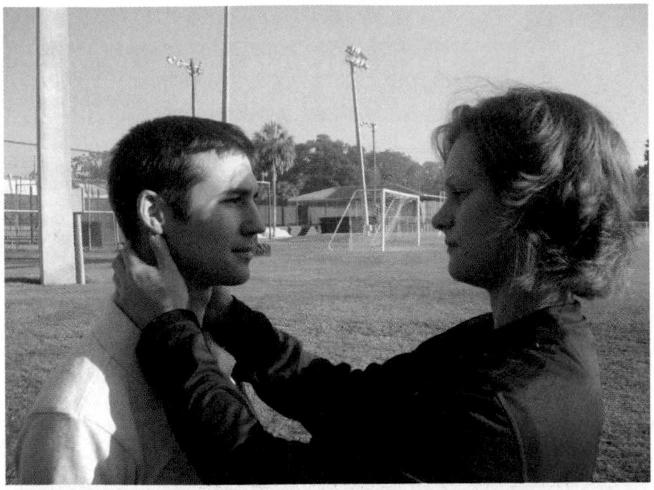

FIGURE 14-7 Palpation of the head and neck in a concussed athlete.

Neuropsychological Assessment Tools

A brief mental status examination should be performed immediately after injury. Regardless of which objective assessment tool is selected, the same examination should be repeated every 5 to 10 minutes. The purpose is to assess the athlete's current status, any possible deterioration in specific symptoms, and overall condition. This examination should include components of memory, orientation, learning, concentration, and information processing.

Head Injury Scale. The head injury scale (HIS) is a common tool used to assess concussion symptoms[11] (Table 14-3). This self-reported symptoms scale should be administered daily until the athlete no longer reports concussion-related symptoms. Typically, the time frame ranges from several days to several weeks or more, depending on the severity of the injury. Factors such as a history of previous concussion and motivation to return to play may also influence the time needed for an adequate recovery. The athletic trainer must be careful to ensure that the athlete is honest in reporting all concussion-related symptoms. Many athletes may downplay or deny their symptoms in order to return to play. Use of the HIS or other tools may reduce this risk.

Standardized Assessment of Concussion. The Standardized Assessment of Concussion (SAC) is an excellent tool to use in establishing neuropsychological functioning[12–14] (Figure 14-8). When administered preseason or pre-injury, the SAC has been found to be a reliable and valid tool for the first 48 hours after a concussion. Its setup allows the athletic trainer to compare the athlete's nonconcussed score with his or her concussed score and

TABLE 14-3 Head Injury Scale Self-Report Concussion Symptom Scale

16-ITEM HEAD INJURY SCALE							
SYMPTOM	NEVER			SOMETIMES	ALWAYS		
Headache	0	1	2	3	4	5	6
Nausea	0	1	2	3	4	5	6
Vomiting	0	1	2	3	4	5	6
Balance difficulty/dizziness	0	1	2	3	4	5	6
Fatigue	0	1	2	3	4	5	6
Trouble falling asleep	0	1	2	3	4	5	6
Sleeping more than usual	0	1	2	3	4	5	6
Drowsiness	0	1	2	3	4	5	6
Sensitivity to light and noise	0	1	2	3	4	5	6
Sadness	0	1	2	3	4	5	6
Nervousness	0	1	2	3	4	5	6
Numbness	0	1	2	3	4	5	6
Feeling "slowed down"	0	1	2	3	4	5	6
Feeling "in a fog"	0	1	2	3	4	5	6
Difficulty concentrating	0	1	2	3	4	5	6
Difficulty remembering	0	1	2	3	4	5	6

From Piland SG et al: Evidence for the factorial and construct validity of a self-report concussion symptoms scale, *J Athl Train* 38: 104–112, 2003.

document any changes in mental status. A one-point change in score from the baseline score, or a score below 25 when a baseline score is not available, indicates mental status changes caused by concussion. Another advantage of the SAC is that it is easily administered by the athletic trainer on-site or in the athletic training room.

Balance Testing

In addition to the SAC tool, a measure of balance or proprioception should be included in the physical examination. One of the easiest is the Romberg test, or stork stand (Figure 14-9). For this test, the athlete stands on one foot with hands on hips. The athlete is asked to close his or her eyes and maintain balance. The evaluator looks for the athlete to lose his or her balance or move out of an erect posture. However, even though this test provides important information about the athlete's ability to maintain balance, it lacks a normative scoring system (e.g., how much movement corresponds to a positive sign) and is therefore not objective.

The balance error scoring system (BESS) was developed to provide objective scoring to balance testing[15] (Box 14-4). The BESS uses two different surfaces (i.e., a firm surface and a foam surface) and three conditions or stances. The athlete stands in a double-leg stance, single-leg stance, and tandem-stance, first on the firm surface and then on the foam surface (Figure 14-10). The starting position for each test is hands on hips and eyes closed. The athlete is required to hold each position for 20 seconds, and the athletic trainer measures and records the number of times an athlete moves out of the starting position. It is strongly suggested that each athlete receive a baseline test before any sports-related concussion occurs to assess balance in a normal condition; this score is then compared with the post-injury score.

Referrals and Diagnostic Testing

Most sports-related concussions are considered minor. However, one must always be prepared for the worst because the potential for a concussion to become a serious and life-threatening injury is ever-present. Significant declines in alertness, mental status, or motor skills may indicate a more serious injury. For any concussion, the emergency action plan must be activated and the athlete transported for further medical evaluation. Any changes in the athlete's status may occur rapidly or over the course of several days. Because of this variability, the athletic trainer should monitor athletes with acute concussions for level of consciousness and vital signs every 5 to 10 minutes, looking for any degradation in level of consciousness and health care status. Box 14-5 contains parameters indicating when further medical attention is warranted.

MANAGEMENT OF SPORTS-RELATED CONCUSSION

The management of concussion calls for a cautious and conservative approach. In general, the athlete should not be allowed to participate in sports, and several evaluations should be performed to determine any changes in self-reported symptoms, mental status, cognitive abilities, and level of consciousness. Any athlete who loses consciousness for any amount of time (from a brief moment to a prolonged period) should be sent for a medical evaluation by a team physician, neurosurgeon, or neurologist if available. A concussion involving periods of unconsciousness necessitates immediate transport by an ambulance for further medical evaluation and diagnostic testing in the emergency room.

Home care instructions should be provided to the athlete after injury. Figure 14-11 provides suggested guidelines for home care of the athlete who has experienced a concussion. This form may be given to the athlete and a parent, guardian, spouse, or roommate. It emphasizes the need for ongoing observation of symptoms and cognitive status. It also stipulates when the athlete or caregiver should seek further medical attention. During the recovery period (i.e., while the athlete still has symptoms), rest is the recommended method of treatment. The athlete should resume going to class and participating in activities of daily living as long as the self-reported symptoms are not exacerbated by these activities. When experiencing symptoms, the athlete should exercise caution before deciding to drive a car or other type of vehicle, especially in the acute stages. As previously stated, no athlete should be returned to play if he or she exhibits any concussion symptoms.

Standardized Assessment of Concussion (SAC) Tool

1. Orientation:

Month: ______	0	1
Date: ______	0	1
Day of Week: ______	0	1
Year: ______	0	1
Time (within 1 hr): ______	0	1
Orientation Total Score ______	/	5

2. Immediate Memory: (all 3 trials are completed regardless of score on trials 1 & 2; total score equals sum across all 3 trials)

List	Trial 1		Trial 2		Trial 3	
Word 1	0	1	0	1	0	1
Word 2	0	1	0	1	0	1
Word 3	0	1	0	1	0	1
Word 4	0	1	0	1	0	1
Word 5	0	1	0	1	0	1
Total						

Immediate Memory Total Score ______ / 15

(Note: Subject is not informed of delayed recall testing of memory)

Neurologic Screening:

Loss of consciousness: (occurrence, duration)

Retrograde & Posttraumatic Amnesia:

(recollection of events pre- and postainjury)

Strength:

Sensation:

Coordination:

3. Concentration:

Digits Backward: (If correct, go to next string length. If incorrect, read trial 2. Stop after incorrect on both trials.)

4-9-3	6-2-9	______	0	1
3-8-1-4	3-2-7-9	______	0	1
6-2-9-7-1	1-4-5-2-8-6	______	0	1
7-1-8-6-4-2	5-3-9-1-4-8	______	0	1

Months in Reverse Order: (entire sequence correct for 1 point)

Dec-Nov-Oct-Sep-Aug-Jul	______	0	1
Jun-May-Apr-Mar-Feb-Jan	______	/	5

Exertional Maneuvers

(when appropriate)

5 jumping jacks
5 push-ups
5 sit-ups
5 knee bends

4. Delayed Recall:

Word 1	0	1
Word 2	0	1
Word 3	0	1
Word 4	0	1
Word 5	0	1
Delayed Recall Total Score ______	/	5

Summary of Total Scores:

Orientation	______ /	5
Immediate Memory	______ /	15
Concentration	______ /	5
Delayed Recall	______ /	5
Overall Total Score	______ /	30

FIGURE 14-8 Standardized assessment of concussion (SAC). (From McCrea M: Standardized mental status testing on the sideline after sport-related concussion, *J Athl Train* 36[3]: 274–279, 2001.)

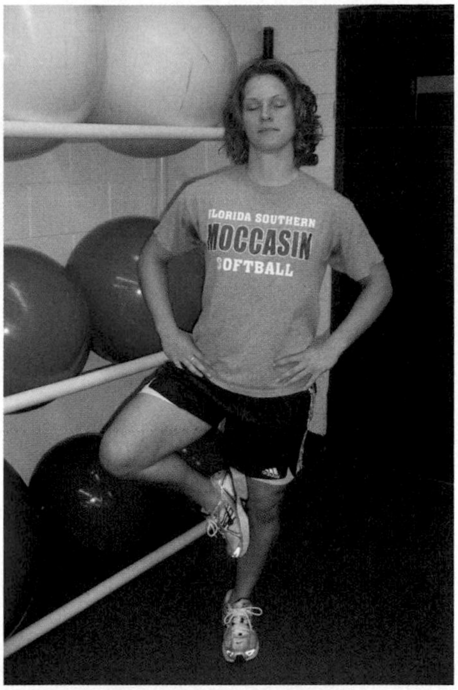

FIGURE 14-9 Athlete performing Romberg test.

RETURN TO PLAY GUIDELINES

Determining when an athlete may return to play after experiencing a sports-related concussion might be one of the most difficult decisions an athletic trainer routinely makes. Because of the lack of obvious physical signs, concussions are very challenging to diagnose and manage. With an orthopedic injury, the athletic trainer can assess swelling, joint laxity, and strength before making this decision. However, with concussion there are fewer measures by which a decision may be rendered. According to standard guidelines, the athlete should be symptom free at rest and during exertion for at least 7 days before resuming participation.[16] This is an excellent guide if there are no other putative measures to track recovery, such as postural stability or neuropsychological tests. However, these tests are considered adjuncts to the physical examination and neurological assessment. Athletes who are returned to participation too early, before recovery is complete, are more susceptible to re-injury and potentially catastrophic consequences. It is strongly recommended that any athlete who has a repeat concussion in the same season be kept from participation for at least 7 days after the athlete reports being symptom free.

When making a decision regarding a concussed athlete's ability to return to play, the athletic trainer should consistently use a graded progression method. Typically, the athletic trainer assesses the athlete's self-reported symptoms daily. A typical concussion recovery consists of a gradual reduction in the duration and severity of self-reported symptoms. This reduction will occur over the course of several days to weeks.[17] While the athlete has symptoms, complete rest should be prescribed and no exercise or participation in sport activities should be permitted in order to allow the brain recovery time following the injury. Only after the athlete reports an absence of symptoms can a graded exertional testing program begin. Figure 14-12 provides a model that can be used to allow the athlete to gradually increase activity while constantly monitoring for changes in concussion-related signs and symptoms. This exertional testing program should take several days to complete. If the athlete develops any symptoms during any phase of the exertional testing, he or she should be removed from participation until symptoms clear, and the 7-day waiting period restarts. Exertional testing can be started

BOX 14-4 Balance Error Scoring System

Test Procedure

- Test three different stances (both feet, nondominant foot, tandem), two times each (once on foam surface, once on medium-density foam 45 cm^2 × 13 cm thick, density 60 kg/m^3, load deflection 80 to 90 kg).
- Place subject's hands on iliac crests, and ask the subject to close his or her eyes.
- Once the subject's eyes are closed, test for 20 seconds.
- While the subject stands on one foot, his or her elevated leg should be maintained at 20 to 30 degrees of hip flexion and 40 to 50 degrees of knee flexion.
- Ask the subject to stand quietly in position.
- If subject loses his or her balance, make any necessary adjustments to return the subject to position.
- Add one error point for each error committed.
- The test is incomplete if subject is unable to maintain stance for more than 5 seconds.
- The maximum score is 10.

Scoring System

- Errors
- Hands lifted off iliac crest
- Opening eyes
- Step, stumble, or fall
- Moving hip into more than 30 degrees of flexion or abduction
- Lifting forefoot or heel
- Remaining out of testing position for more than 5 seconds
- One point for each error during a 20-second trial

From Guskiewicz KM: Postural stability assessment following concussion: one piece of the puzzle, *Clin J Sport Med* 11:186–187, 2001.

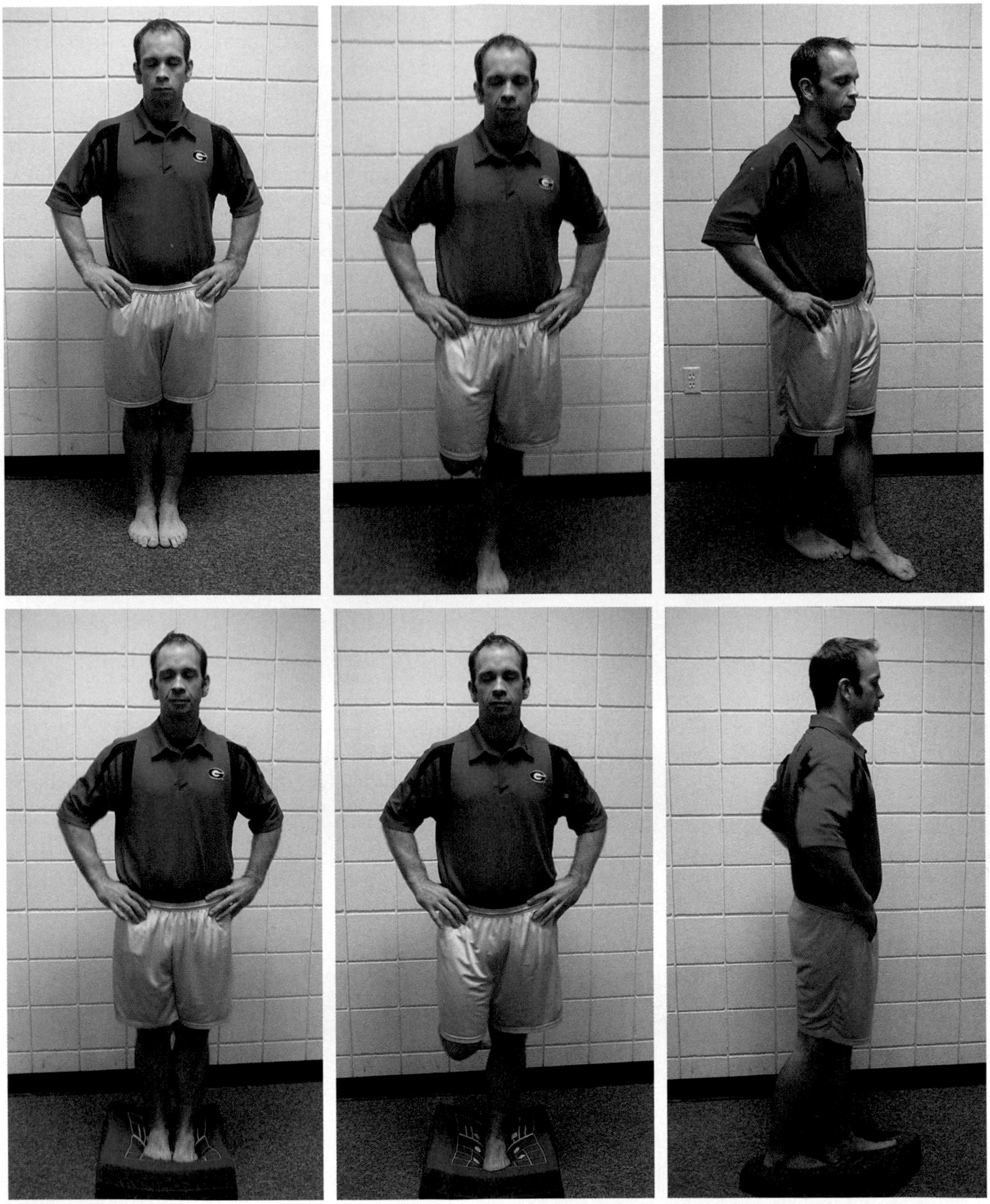

FIGURE 14-10 Athlete performing six-part balance error scoring system.

from the beginning when the athlete is symptom-free. It is strongly recommended that the athlete be evaluated by a doctor before return to participation.

THE AGE GROUP ATHLETE

Younger athletes, especially those in elementary school, are more susceptible to concussion than other athletes.[2] Because of the ongoing maturation of the brain, any injury has potentially devastating results. Therefore a more cautious approach is recommended when returning the younger athlete to play after concussion.

Points to Ponder

Why do you think younger athletes are more susceptible to concussions than older athletes? What is different that makes them sustain more concussions?

BOX 14-5 Physician Referral Checklist

Day-of-Injury Referral

1. Loss of consciousness on the field
2. Amnesia lasting longer than 15 minutes
3. Deterioration of neurological function*
4. Decreasing level of consciousness*
5. Decrease or irregularity in respirations*
6. Decrease or irregularity in pulse*
7. Increase in blood pressure
8. Unequal, dilated, or nonreactive pupils*
9. Cranial nerve deficits
10. Any signs or symptoms of associated injuries, spine or skull fracture, or bleeding*
11. Mental status changes: lethargy, difficulty maintaining alertness, confusion, or agitation*
12. Seizure activity*
13. Vomiting
14. Motor deficits subsequent to initial on-field assessment
15. Sensory deficits subsequent to initial on-field assessment
16. Balance deficits subsequent to initial on-field assessment
17. Cranial nerve deficits subsequent to initial on-field assessment
18. Postconcussion symptoms that worsen
19. Additional postconcussion symptoms as compared with those on the field
20. Athlete is still symptomatic at the end of the game (especially athletes at high school level)

Delayed Referral (After the Day of Injury)

1. Any of the findings in the day-injury category
2. Postconcussion symptoms that worsen or do not improve
3. Increase in the number of postconcussion symptoms reported
4. Postconcussion symptoms that interfere with the athlete's daily activities (e.g., sleep disturbances or cognitive difficulties)

From Guskiewicz KM et al: National Athletic Trainers' Association position statement: Management of sports-related concussion, *J Athl Train* 39(3): 297, 2004.
* Requires that the athlete be transported immediately to the nearest emergency room.

SUMMARY

The rate of concussion is approximately 5% in football, with a slightly higher or lower rate in other sports. The athletic trainer must develop a thorough and consistent method to assess concussions similar to that used for orthopedic injuries. Athletic trainers must be aware of the potential for catastrophic injury and cerebral bleeding (hematoma). These severe injuries must be considered until they are ruled out by a physician. If the athletic trainer is in doubt about the seriousness of a concussion, the athlete should be referred to the team physician for further testing. The return to play decision should be made cautiously so as not to put the athlete at further risk of injury. With respect to return to play after concussion, current standards indicate that the athlete should be symptom free for 7 days, both at rest and during exertional activities. Most concussions resolve in an orderly and predictable manner. They generally follow a normal pattern of recovery with satisfactory outcomes. The athletic trainer must be alert for any injury that does not resolve normally and make the appropriate referral for further evaluation and diagnostic tests.

Revisiting the OPENING *Scenario*

Once you reach the wide receiver's side, he regains consciousness. Subjecting him to a systematic evaluation will help determine his injury. His loss of consciousness is not enough to determine the precise diagnosis tournament. However, because it was immediate and

Issues & Ethics

Your college's softball team is on its way to winning a national title this season. Next week, the team will leave to play in the tournament after they play their last conference home game. It is the bottom of the seventh inning; there are two outs with runners on second and third base. Your team is on defense and is up by two runs. The runners on base are given the green light to go with the pitch because it is a full count and the team's best hitter is up at the plate. She smacks a triple down the left field line. One runner is in; now your left fielder fires home to stop the tying run from scoring from second base. Your catcher braces herself after quickly and cleanly fielding the ball. She gets ready to take a hard hit from the incoming runner. BAM! She is out like a light. Waking up seconds later, she is in a daze. She does not know what is going on but hears loud cheering as her teammates crowd around her. Looking at her glove, she realizes that she has saved the game by holding onto the ball and preventing the runner from scoring. However, she has suffered a concussion in doing so.

As the athletic trainer, you evaluate and diagnose your catcher. She has fewer than 7 days to prepare and play in the national tournament. Unfortunately, she has a past medical history of three previous concussions. According to school policy, three concussions could rule out an athlete from further participation. This is her third concussion, but she swears that she is okay. Her team needs her to play in the championship series next week, but from a medical perspective she is at high risk. What would you do?

Concussion Injury Information

Name ______________________ Date ____________

ID# ______________________ Date of Birth ____________

You have had a head injury or concussion and need to be watched closely for the next 24-48 hours.

It is OK to:	There is no need to:	DO NOT:
Use Tylenol (acetaminophen) Use an ice pack to head/neck for comfort Eat a light meal Go to sleep	Check eyes with a light Wake up every hour Stay in bed	**Drink alcohol** **Eat spicy foods** **Drive a car** **Use aspirin, Alleve, Advil, or other NSAID products**

Special Recommendations:

____

____

WATCH FOR ANY OF THE FOLLOWING PROBLEMS:

Worsening headache
Vomiting
Decreased level of consciousness
Dilated pupils
Increased confusion
Stumbling/loss of balance
Weakness in one arm/leg
Blurred vision
Increased irritability

If any of these problems develop, call your athletic trainer or physician immediately.

Athletic Trainer ______________________ Phone ____________

Physician ______________________ Phone ____________

You need to be seen for a follow-up examination at ________ AM/PM in the ____________ Athletic Training Room.

Recommendations provided to ______________________

Recommendation provided by ______________________

FIGURE 14-11 Concussion home care information form. *NSAID,* Nonsteroidal antiinflammatory medications.

he is also complaining of headache, confusion, and dizziness, the differential diagnosis would be that he is suffering from an epidural hematoma. Decisions regarding return to play are standard. As long as he has symptoms, he cannot return. After his symptoms have subsided and he is symptom free for 7 days, even with exertion, he may then be considered for return to play. Use of a thorough neuropsychological testing battery will help in objectively determining his status. The ability to compare test findings to the athlete's baseline score (i.e., his score before the concussion) gives the athletic trainer an advantage in recognizing the athlete's true mental and cognitive abilities.

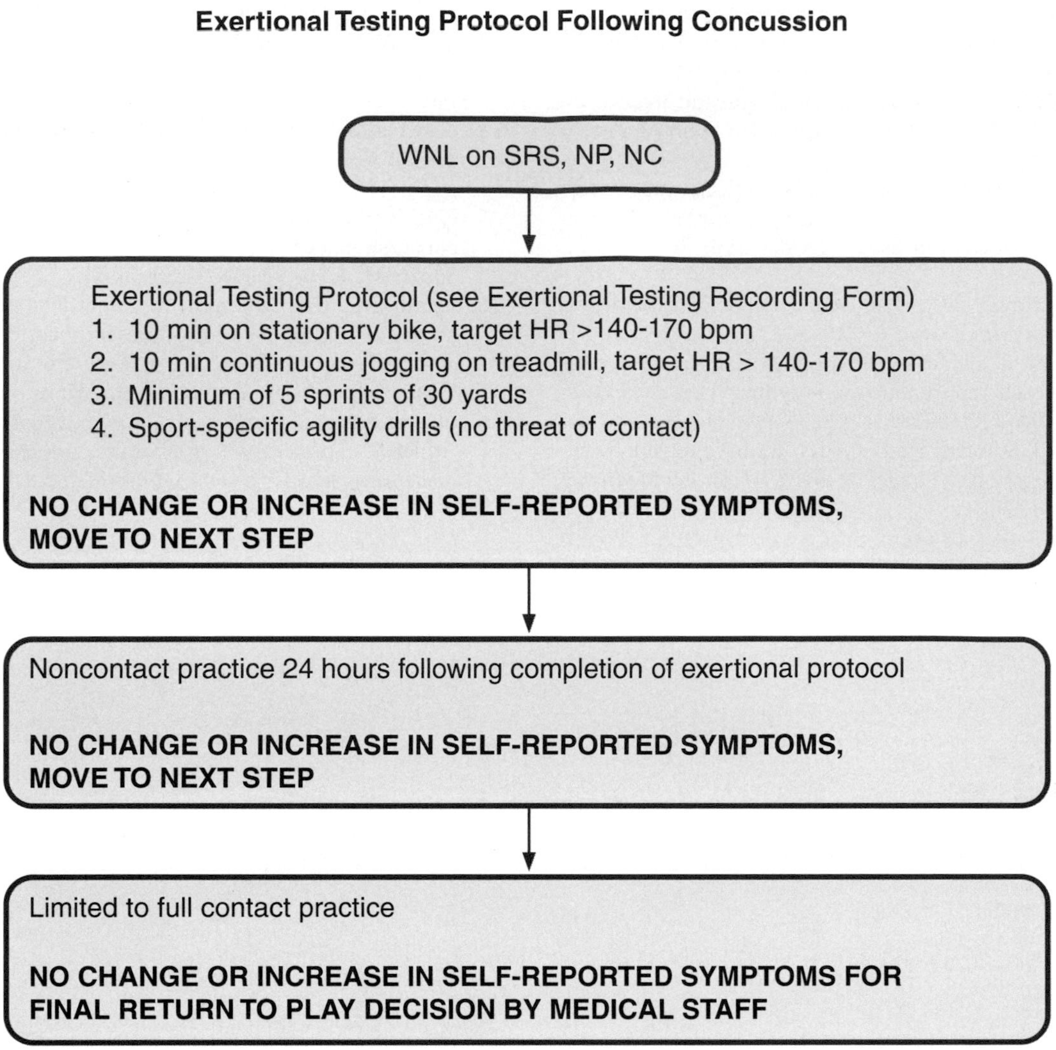

FIGURE 14-12 Exertional testing protocol after concussion. *WNL,* Within normal Limits; *SRS,* Self-reported symptoms; *NP,* neuropsychological; *NC,* neurocognitive; *HR,* heart rate; *bpm,* beats per minute.

Web Links

CDC Tool Kit on Concussion for High School Coaches: www.cdc.gov/ncipc/tbi/Coaches_Tool_Kit.htm

Concussions: http://kidshealth.org/kid/health_problems/brain/concussion.html

Concussions: http://health.howstuffworks.com/adam-200049.htm

First Aid for Concussions in Teens: http://kidshealth.org/teen/safety/first_aid/concussions.html

NATA Position Statement: Head-Down Contact and Spearing in Tackle Football: www.nata.org/statements/position/spearingps.pdf

NATA Position Statement: Management of Sport-Related Concussion: www.nata.org/statements/position/concussion.pdf

Sports-Related Concussions: Background and Significance: www.neurosurgery.pitt.edu/trauma/concussion.html

Traumatic Brain Injury: www.paems.org/eWebquiz/tbi/case_study.htm

References

1. Thurman DJ, Alverson C, Browne D: *Traumatic brain injury in the United States: a report to Congress*, Atlanta, 1999, Centers for Disease Control and Prevention.
2. Guskiewicz KM et al: National Athletic Trainers' Association Position Statement: management of sport-related concussion, *J Athl Train* 39: 280–297, 2004.
3. Aubry M et al: Summary and agreement statement of the 1st International Symposium on Concussion in Sport, Vienna 2001, *Clinical Journal of Sport Medicine* 12: 6–11, 2002.
4. Guskiewicz KM et al: Epidemiology of concussion in collegiate and high school football players, *Am J Sports Med* 28: 643–650, 2000.
5. Powell JW, Barber-Foss KD: Traumatic brain injury in high school athletes, *JAMA* 282: 958–963, 1999.
6. Pellman EJ et al: Concussion in professional football: location and direction of helmet impacts. Part 2, *Neurosurgery* 53: 1328–1340, 2003.

7. Pellman EJ et al: Concussion in professional football: epidemiological features of game injuries and review of the literature. Part 3, *Neurosurgery* 54: 81–96, 2004.
8. Johnston KM et al: New frontiers in diagnostic imaging in concussion head injury, *Clinical Journal of Sport Medicine* 11: 166–175, 2001.
9. Guskiewicz KM et al: Cumulative effects associated with recurrent concussion in collegiate football players: the NCAA Concussion Study, *JAMA* 290: 2549–2555, 2003.
10. Giza CC, Hovda DA: The neurometabolic cascade of concussion, *J Athl Train* 36: 228–235, 2001.
11. Piland SG et al: Evidence for the factorial and construct validity of a self-report concussion symptoms scale, *J Athl Train* 38: 104–112, 2003.
12. McCrea M: Standardized mental status assessment of sports concussion, *Clinical Journal of Sport Medicine* 11: 176–181, 2001.
13. McCrea M, Randolph C, Kelly JP: The Standardized Assessment of Concussion (SAC): Manual for Administration, Scoring and Interpretation, Waukesha, Wisc, 1997, CNC, Inc.
14. McCrea M, et al: Standardized Assessment of Concussion (SAC): on-site mental status evaluation of the athlete, *J Head Trauma Rehabil* 13: 27–35, 1998.
15. Guskiewicz KM: Postural stability assessment following concussion: one piece of the puzzle, *Clinical Journal of Sports Medicine* 11: 182–189, 2001.
16. Cantu RC: Posttraumatic retrograde and anterograde amnesia: pathophysiology and implications in grading and safe return to play, *J Athl Train* 36: 244–248, 2001.
17. Guskiewicz KM et al: Recommendations on management of sport-related concussion: summary of the National Athletic Trainers' Association position statement, *Neurosurgery* 55: 891–895, 2004.

15

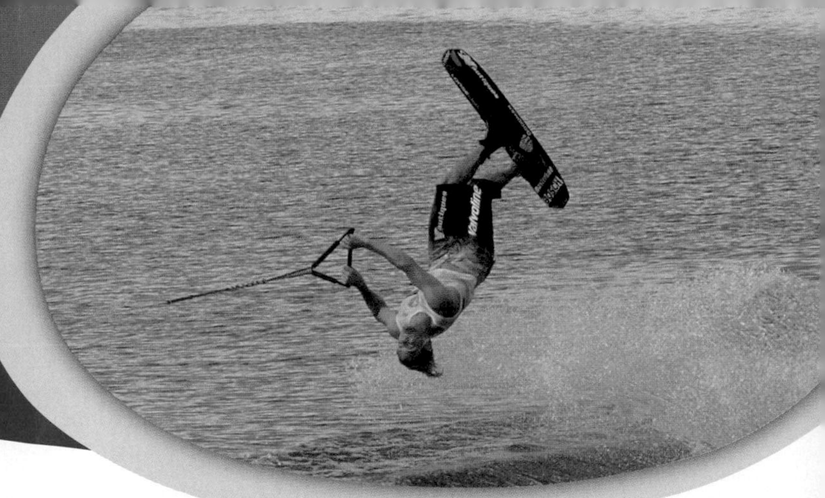

Diagnosis and Management of Spine Injuries

KATHLEEN M. LAQUALE

Learning Goals

1. Describe assessment/diagnostic procedures for evaluation of common acute and chronic injuries to the spine.
2. List the most common acute and chronic injuries occurring to the spine.
3. Define proper first aid/immediate care for managing common and acute injuries to the spine.
4. Identify principles and concepts to prevent athletic injuries to the spine.
5. Identify precautions and risks to the spine associated with athletic participation by various age groups.

Among athletes in all age groups, spinal injuries are very common, encompassing 20% to 25% of all athletic injuries.[1] Spinal injuries can be **catastrophic injuries** and are usually considered emergency situations.[2] The majority of spinal injuries are more chronic than acute, with lumbar spine pain occurring more frequently. In certain sports, such as amateur golf, low thoracic pain is the most common injury.[3] It is usually considered the second or third most common injury in basketball; 50% to 60% of football linemen have low thoracic pain.[4,5]

There are many reasons that lower thoracic injuries are so prevalent in certain sports. For example, in football, the "set" position of the offensive lineman requires the player to keep one arm extended with the fingertips on the ground. The other arm is usually resting on the player's thigh. At the same time, the offensive lineman must keep the hips and knees flexed, with body weight balanced on the ball of each foot. This position is referred to as a *three-point stance.* At the snap of the ball, the lineman must fire out from the three-point stance, driving into the defensive line. Thus the player collides with an oncoming lineman, who is performing the same mechanics (Figure 15-1). The lineman must push or lift the opposing player, which puts great stress on the lower back. At times, this repeated stress on the lower back leads to chronic low back pain. It is important to remember that low back pain is generally chronic (i.e., occurring repeatedly over time) owing to overuse or the athlete's improper technique. Acute injuries occur suddenly, as when a football player attempts a tackle using the shoulder and collides with another player's back. The tackler causes an acute injury, possibly a contusion or bruise, to the opponent's back.

Another example of a sport in which athletes experience a great deal of chronic lumbar spine pain is gymnastics. The gymnast's posture during landing and the

Terms that appear in boldface green type are defined in the book's glossary.

catastrophic injury career-ending type of injury that usually requires advanced medical care for the rest of the individual's life; not a life-threatening, but rather a life-altering, event

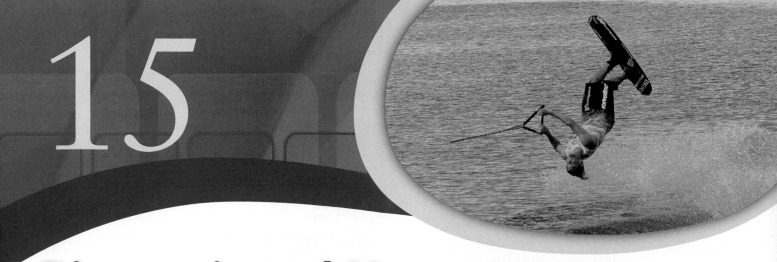

OPENING *Scenario*

A discus thrower finishes her last practice throw. As she releases the discus, she feels a slight twinge along the middle of her lower thoracic spine, approximately 2 to 3 inches away from the spine on her throwing arm. She dismisses the pain as inconsequential; does not tell you, the athletic trainer, about it; and goes home. The next morning, she feels severe pain in the same area of her thoracic spine. When she is in a seated position with her legs hanging off the edge of the bed, she experiences no pain; however, the pain returns as soon as she stands up. She goes to school and experiences the same pain during her classes. Before practice, she visits you and reports what happened at practice yesterday. She tells you that she now has pain in her back but no pain radiating down her legs.

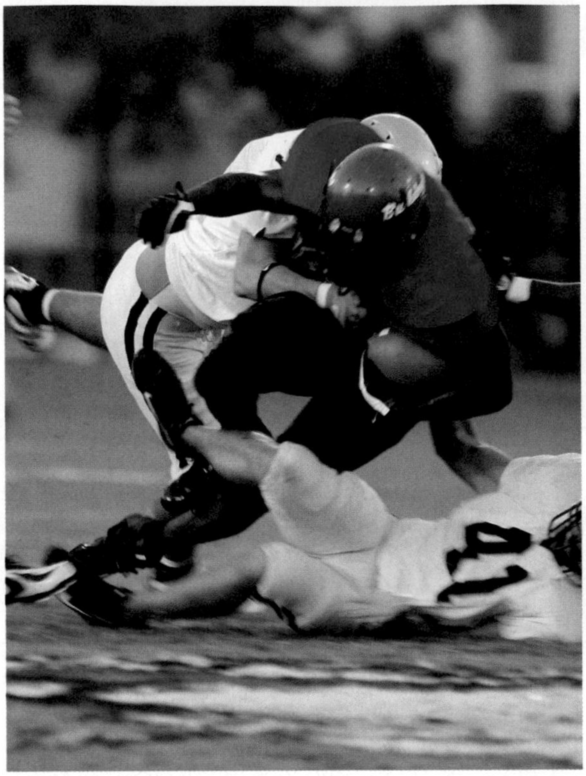

FIGURE 15-1 Proper technique and skills can lead to back pain. Improper technique can further lead to catastrophic injury. (Courtesy Skyhawk Sports Photography.)

sometimes awkward position of the back during the maneuver (on the floor, bars, beam, or vault) places strain on the low back area. The lineman's and the gymnast's low back pain is similar because of the **lordotic position**, which their very different sports both demand.

Points to Ponder

Why is it so important to understand the mechanism of injury and how it relates to an athlete's skill and technique?

Although the pain initially resolves in most individuals, frequent recurrence indicates that complete healing has not been restored. Acute trauma to both the spine and the cervical spine regions must be evaluated with extreme care using a systematic approach, with close attention paid to signs and symptoms, which may include any of the following: partial or full paralysis (inability to move), pain, and numbness (athlete states that he or she can't feel anything or is unable to discern a light touch or pin prick on the extremities). These signs and symptoms suggest that the athlete could have a serious cervical spine injury. An unconscious person should *never* be moved. What appears to be a stable situation with no compromise of the spinal cord could change in seconds if the person is improperly moved. The spinal cord and all function of the extremities could be permanently affected; the person could even become paralyzed. Whether the trauma affects the lumbar, thoracic, or cervical vertebrae, an unconscious person must always be considered as someone who may have suffered a head and cervical injury and treated as if a fracture or dislocation of the cervical spine is present. Paralysis, partial paralysis, or even death is a potential consequence of improperly treated spine and cervical injuries. This chapter covers the diagnosis and management of common spine injuries, providing a foundation that will allow the athletic trainer to make good decisions about treatment decisions and techniques.

CLINICAL EVALUATION AND DIAGNOSIS OF SPINE INJURIES

Although spinal cord injuries are not especially common in athletics, on-site medical staff members must be prepared to act in an organized fashion when this type of injury occurs. Effective on-site care of the athlete improves the outcomes of these catastrophic cervical injuries.[6] The athletic trainer is the first professional in the line of care when evaluating and treating the injured athlete. Every member of the medical team should know their individual responsibilities in the treatment plan ahead of time and act accordingly. With spinal injuries,

lordotic position position in which the spine is naturally aligned and the vertebrae form a curve anteriorly, or toward the front of the body; term "sway-back" usually describing an excessive spinal curve in this direction treatment may include the use of equipment such as a spine board, bolt cutters, or Trainer's Angel for face mask removal, rigid cervical collar, and **automatic external defibrillator** (AED). In addition, placement (by use of log roll onto a spine board) of the injured athlete onto a spine board for transportation to the emergency room *must be practiced repeatedly*. Such practice should include rehearsing the procedure in various scenarios, such as with an athlete who is conscious or unconscious, who is lying in a prone or supine position, who is breathing or not breathing, who has a mechanical (e.g., mouthpiece, gum) obstruction or anatomical (e.g., tongue) obstruction with respect to airway management, who has a pulse or no pulse (requiring the use of the AED), and who requires face mask or helmet removal (e.g., as in lacrosse).

Whether evaluating or assessing an injured athlete on the field, off the field, or in the athletic training room, the athletic trainer should follow a sequential format.[7] If a life-threatening injury is suspected, the primary and secondary survey is completed first, followed by the HIPS (history, inspection, palpation, and special tests) formula. If the athletic trainer is assessing an injury in the playing area and it is not a life-threatening injury, in many cases just the HIPS sequence or protocol is completed.

Figure 15-2 outlines the steps in the evaluation and diagnosis of spine injuries. These steps are outlined in detail in the following sections.

Primary Survey

Once the athletic trainer assesses the athlete's level of consciousness, the primary and secondary survey should be performed. Special note must be made of the following areas when conducting a primary survey involving a spine injury:

In-line stabilization: **In-line stabilization** is a method to ensure that no movement occurs at the head, cervical area, and shoulders of an athlete with a suspected head and cervical injury. The athletic trainer must always remember the Hippocratic oath: First do no harm. Several methods may be used to provide in-line stabilization. One technique is to kneel at the head of the injured athlete, place your hands on the injured athlete's shoulders, and use your forearms to cradle or stabilize the athlete's head and cervical spine. As in-line stabilization is initiated, the athletic trainer may continue the primary survey (Figure 15-3).

Cardiac/respiratory distress: If the athlete is in cardiac/respiratory distress, the primary objective is to quickly identify the cause of the distress and intercede to provide ventilation. Face mask removal is completed at this time.

automatic external defibrillator (AED) a device that uses a controlled and externally applied electrical current to restart a heart that has stopped beating or to regulate a suddenly irregular heartbeat

in-line stabilization method used to ensure that no movement occurs at the head, cervical spine, and shoulder in an athlete with suspected head and cervical injury

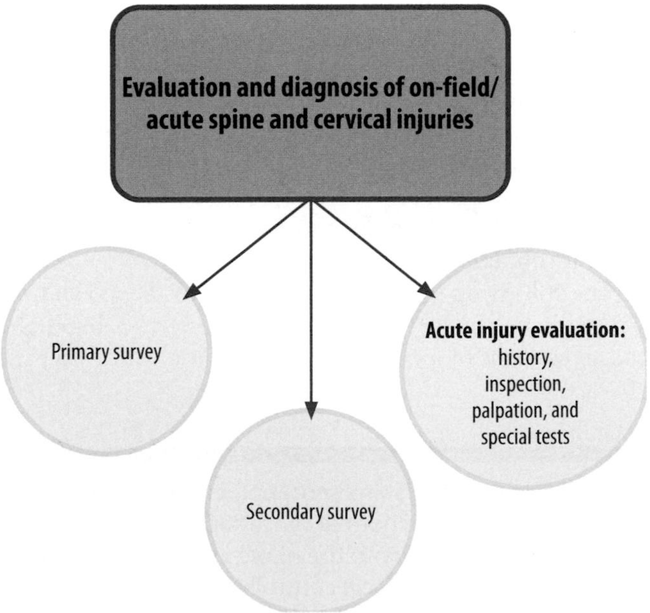

FIGURE 15-2 Concept map illustrating the evaluation and diagnosis of spine and neck injuries.

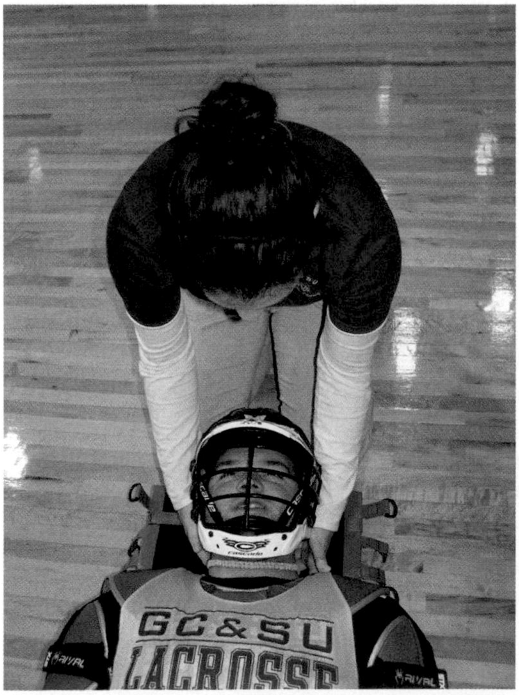

FIGURE 15-3 An athletic trainer performs in-line stabilization of an athlete lying in the supine position.

Prone position: If the athlete is prone, the top priority is always to protect the spine when performing a log roll; then the jaw-thrust maneuver must be performed to preserve axial alignment.

Dermatomes/myotomes: The athlete's **dermatomes** and **myotomes** should also be assessed at this time to determine if a nerve root from the spinal cord is injured. The athletic trainer should always remember that an unconscious athlete must always be treated as if he or she has a cervical spine injury; therefore some testing must be deferred or postponed to prevent any further damage to the spinal cord. A conscious athlete can provide feedback about sensation and help the athletic trainer identify the segment of the spine that is injured.

Points to Ponder

Students often overlook dermatomes when evaluating an injury. With consideration of the complexity of the nerve roots and the areas they innervate, describe why dermatome assessment should be a part of the evaluation protocol of a thoracic vertebrae sprain/strain.

Finally, if the athlete has a normal mental status and no respiratory or cardiac symptoms, the focus of the evaluation should be determination of the spinal cord problem.[7] Any client with a suspected cervical spine injury must be properly immobilized and prepared for transport as the emergency action plan is activated (Figure 15-4). As with any other primary survey scenario, the airway, breathing, and circulation of the injured athlete should be the primary focus. Once these areas prove satisfactory, the athletic trainer should continue the evaluation in the secondary survey.

Secondary Survey

During the secondary survey, the athletic trainer observes areas other than the spine and cervical regions for additional injuries (e.g., fractures or external bleeding in the extremities). Even if the athletic trainer has provided in-line stabilization, it is still inadvisable to release the client's head and cervical spine.

While the athletic trainer is maintaining stabilization of the head, a second person must perform the secondary survey under the athletic trainer's direction. For potential spine and neck injuries, the survey should include the following:

- *History:* to determine the position of the head and body and the type of force (mechanism of injury)
- *Inspection:* to rule out deformity of the bones of the skull and vertebrae
- *Palpation:* to rule out gross trauma and deformity
- *Functional/injury-specific special tests:* to assess dermatomes and myotomes

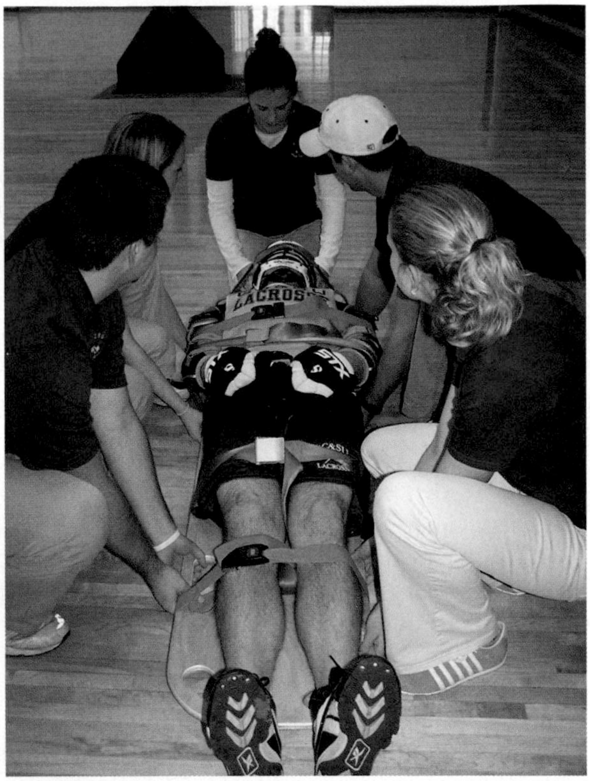

FIGURE 15-4 Whenever a severe spinal injury is suspected, the athlete's spine must be immobilized for transportation to a hospital for further medical evaluation.

Acute Injury Evaluation

After a nonlife-threatening acute injury that occurs in the playing area, the athletic trainer should continue to assess the athlete immediately after the primary survey. This aspect of the assessment underscores the importance of the athletic trainer's role during a practice or contest. Because the athletic trainer was most likely watching the activity when the injury occurred, the athletic trainer has the opportunity to examine the injured area before swelling ensues, which makes for a better assessment of the signs and symptoms. It is important to remember that swelling can provide false stability to a joint and affect range of motion. During an acute assessment, the HIPS formula must be followed again.

The following sections, which refer to the evaluation of the discus athlete from the opening scenario, highlight the assessment of an acute low back injury of this type.

dermatome area of skin's sensation controlled by a given nerve; loss of normal sensation in a particular area indicating injury to the nerve linked to that area

myotome specific muscle controlled by a given nerve; muscle weakness possibly indicating injury to the nerve controlling that particular muscle

History

During the history, the athletic trainer should not focus exclusively on the injury site. The athletic trainer should always observe the areas above and below the injury site well. The athletic trainer should ask the athlete to demonstrate the skill or mechanics (e.g., throwing a discus, driving a car, reaching for an item on the top shelf of a cabinet) that causes pain. The athlete should also be asked if she remembers the mechanism of injury and any previous injuries. The athletic trainer should ask questions to determine the type of pain, the duration of the pain, and previously taken measures to alleviate the pain. She should also be asked whether she has seen a physician; whether she has any numbness or burning sensations in her neck, shoulders, arms, hands, or legs; and whether she has equal muscle strength in her hands. She should be asked whether she has discovered any positions (e.g., standing, sitting, sleeping) that relieve or worsen the pain.

A history of the acute nonlife-threatening spine injury should include the following questions:

History
- What brought you to see the athletic trainer?
- How did your injury occur?
- When did your signs and symptoms start?
- Did you hear or feel anything when you hurt yourself?
- Have you ever hurt this part of your body before?
- How old are you?

Presentation of Signs and Symptoms
- Did your signs and symptoms start suddenly or gradually?
- Are your signs and symptoms constant or intermittent?
- What type of pain do you feel? Please describe it.
- Does the type of pain change at all?
- What can you do to increase or decrease the pain?
- Do you feel any unusual sensations (e.g., numbness, tingling)?

Location
- Where does it hurt?
- Is the pain confined to a particular area, or does it radiate?

Activity Information
- What is your sport, activity, position, or event?
- Do you warm up? If so, how?
- Have you changed your activity type, level, frequency, or duration recently?
- Do your signs and/or symptoms affect your participation?

Self-Treatment
- Have you done anything or taken any medications for your injury?
- Do you take any over-the-counter, prescription, or supplement medications?
- Are you currently on any medications?
- Do you have an idea as to what is wrong with you?

Inspection

When a potential injury occurs to the head and neck and the player is wearing a helmet, the question that always emerges is whether to remove the helmet before moving the athlete. In sports such as football, lacrosse, and ice hockey, numerous experts have concluded that the protective equipment should not be removed.[8] Removal of the helmet and pads may result in a significant increase in cervical spine extension; the back of the head rolls backward, further compressing the cervical vertebrae and causing increased trauma. In fact, spine board immobilization of helmeted players effectively limits cervical motion during transportation.[9,10]

Points to Ponder

When profuse bleeding is present, it must be addressed immediately to prevent shock. The bleeding is probably not directly related to the spine injury but rather to another injury that occurred at the same time (e.g., arm fracture, nosebleed). What measures would you take to control the bleeding while being careful not to move the cervical spine?

As the athletic trainer inspects the back, he or she should compare the side on which the athlete is injured with the other, noninjured side, checking for any swelling, bruising, redness, and posture abnormalities (e.g., whether hips and scapula are level, whether the arms are hanging evenly, whether the head is tilted to one side). Is the athlete leaning on the table or counter?

Inspection of acute nonlife-threatening spine injuries includes the following:
- The athletic trainer should examine the way in which the athlete is positioned on the field.
- If she approaches the athletic trainer after the injury occurs, the athletic trainer should observe how she is walking. Is she holding the injured area? Is she limping or carrying one arm differently? Has her normal gait pattern changed to favor the area, protecting it from further discomfort?
- The athletic trainer should look for swelling, discoloration, or unusual marks. The athletic trainer should ask to see the part of her back that she pointed out as painful. The athletic trainer should check for any bleeding.

Points to Ponder

In athletic accidents that involve the use of helmets—such as football or lacrosse—a controversy sometimes arises at the scene regarding whether the helmet should be removed or left in place during the evaluation on the scene. It is often necessary for emergency medical personnel to remove the helmet at a nonathletic accident scene (e.g., a motorcycle accident) to properly assess the head and neck. Removal of the helmet in this situation will be safer than in athletic situations, when removal of the helmet (or the shoulder pads) will result in significant movement of the cervical spine and increase the risk of permanent damage to the spinal cord. Modern athletic helmets are designed in such a way as to allow adequate assessment of the face, ears, and neck while eliminating the need to remove the helmet to conduct this assessment. How do the differences between athletic helmets and motorcycle helmets make it necessary and acceptable to remove the helmet at the scene of a motorcycle accident but not at the scene of a football accident?

Palpation

Palpation of the acute nonlife-threatening injury includes the following:

- To help rule out a fracture, the athletic trainer should palpate for **crepitus**. The fingertips should be used to palpate for the deformity, but it is inappropriate to "play piano" (i.e., tapping the fingertips on the injured area, which only tests sensation). When palpating the injured area, the athletic trainer should always assess the noninjured area first to let the athlete know what you are going to do on the injured area. The athletic trainer should ask her to take a deep breath and let it out slowly while the injured area is being palpated. The athletic trainer should be alert to any crunching sounds.
- Palpation also includes finding recognizable bony landmarks. In this case, the athletic trainer can certainly palpate the spinous process near the injured area. Areas for palpation might also include the posterior sacroiliac spine (PSIS) and iliac crest when the spine is assessed for injury.
- The athletic trainer should test skin temperature; an immediate increase in heat may indicate swelling. The athletic trainer should use the back of his or her hand to determine whether the noninjured side feels cooler than the injured area.

Palpation helps in the identification of the point of discomfort or whether pressure leads to increased pain; it also helps the athletic trainer to assess skin temperature, abnormal swelling, bony landmarks (e.g., spinous and transverse process of each vertebra), muscle tightness or rigidity (e.g., guarding or protecting of the area), and dermatomes. The athletic trainer should always start at the most proximal area of the injury site and move distally.

Range of Motion

Range of motion (ROM) testing should be performed with the client in different positions as tolerated, such as seated, standing, supine, and prone. The client's movements should be observed from various angles—anterior, posterior, and lateral—for better visualization of any limitations or deficits. As always, the athletic trainer should evaluate active ROM, passive ROM, and then resisted ROM. In this specific case scenario, the athletic trainer must determine active ROM. With the athlete still seated, the athletic trainer should see if she can reach forward toward the end of the treatment table without pain. Can she lean backward? Can she side-bend or reach to either side without pain? Can she rotate equally to both sides? When possible, these abilities should be assessed in the cervical and trunk regions, depending on the injury. As noted before, ROM assessment of the cervical spine is never assessed if the possibility of a cervical spine fracture exists.

Injury-Specific Special Tests

After identifying the painful areas through palpation, the athletic trainer should perform injury-specific special tests to assess trauma or damage to the ligaments, muscles, nerves, or bones. Functional or skill-related tests might also be completed on the client at this time. These special tests help confirm or rule out any potential pathological conditions that emerged during the history, observation/inspection, and palpation phases of the evaluation. Injury-specific special tests are discussed in greater detail later in the chapter.

Neurovascular Tests

The athletic trainer should perform neurological tests to determine whether any nerves have been injured and check myotomes and dermatomes for the area involved in the injury (Tables 15-1 and 15-2). A thorough evaluation includes assessment of circulation, or pulse, and reflexes. To properly diagnose the spine and neck injury, a bilateral comparison of both arms and legs is required.

DIAGNOSIS AND MANAGEMENT OF INJURIES TO THE SPINE

The mechanisms of injuries to the cervical, thoracic, and lumbar spine usually involve excessive motion such as hyperflexion, flexion, lateral flexion, rotation, or a combination thereof. These injuries typically result in sprains and strains to the involved soft tissue. The mechanism may also include violent

crepitus crackling sensation ("crunchies") noted with movement of an area indicating damage (e.g., dislocation, fracture) to the underlying tissue

TABLE 15-1 Assessment of Myotomes in the Evaluation of Low Back Injuries

MOTION TESTED	NERVE ROOT(S) TESTED
Hip flexion	L1 and L2
Knee extension	L3 and L4
Ankle dorsiflexion	L4
Great toe extension	L5
Knee flexion	S2

TABLE 15-2 Assessment of Dermatomes in the Evaluation of Low Back Injuries

AREA TESTED	NERVE ROOT TESTED
Anterior thigh	L2
Medial aspect of the knee	L3
Medial lower leg	L4
Lateral lower leg	L5

muscle contraction against resistance (stretching and tearing), a direct blow (contusion), compression of nerves (brachial plexus), **congenital** factors (repeated nerve syndromes), and body mechanics (gait, posture). Chronic spine and cervical injuries can be congenital or age related (arthritis, stenosis, and spurs). Following the HIPS formula allows the athletic trainer to identify the possible injury to the cervical, thoracic, and lumbar spine. Because most spine and neck injuries relevant to this discussion are acute injuries, they will all be addressed together. Chronic injuries will be identified when appropriate.

Cervical Spine Injuries

Cervical injuries are generally caused by **axial loading,** which causes cervical compression. Most athletic cervical spine injuries incurred in football are the result of an axial load applied with the cervical spine in flexion. In football, this position is generally assumed when the player incorrectly uses the crown of the head as the point of initial contact when tackling an opponent.[11] Thus this incorrect technique causes the player's normally curved cervical spine to straighten, which means that it cannot absorb the shock adequately at the time of impact.[12] In other words, the position of the head and neck upon impact determine whether an injury will occur. The alignment of the cervical vertebrae dictate how the force of the impact travels down the spine and whether the cervical spine is compressed between the rapidly decelerated (i.e., slowed down) head and the continued momentum of the body.[13] Examples in other sports might be a hockey player who is pushed into the boards head first, a wrestler who is lifted in the air and is pushed head first into the mat, or a diver who hits his or her head on the bottom of the pool.

With these types of injuries, the spinal cord may be crushed or torn and permanent paralysis may occur. However, in some cases, patients do regain some return of limited function. A direct blow to the cervical spine can cause muscular bruising; if the head is forced into an abnormal movement without the involvement of cervical vertebrae (i.e., muscle alone is involved), the patient will experience a contusion or sprain/strain.

Because the cervical muscular and ligamentous tissue is so complex, distinguishing between a sprain and a strain is challenging. The muscles and ligaments are often very small and located in the same general area, so differentiation of a single damaged structure is usually not possible without elaborate imaging tests such as a magnetic resonance imaging (MRI) or computed tomography (CT) scan. Moreover, the mechanisms of injury and the resulting symptoms are often very similar, regardless of which structure is injured. For this reason, clinicians often refer to a soft tissue (i.e., nonbone) injury as *sprain/strain* rather than simply *sprain* or *strain.*

Cervical Spine Dislocation and Fractures

Generally, cervical dislocations result from forceful flexion and rotation of the head and are more common than fractures. Fractures in this region are a consequence of compression forces. As previously mentioned, the normal curve, or lordosis, of the cervical spine straightens as impact occurs, and the force is transmitted directly through the spine. The result is a fracture of the vertebra or a vertebral dislocation (i.e., the articular facets slide away). Fractures or dislocations are classified as follows: transected, contused, and concussive. Sports such as wrestling, football, gymnastics, and diving expose the athlete to situations that potentially create axial loading, such as extreme cervical flexion or a blow to the top of the head. In such instances, the spinal cord can be transected, contused, or concussed, resulting in paralysis that can be temporary or permanent.

Transected Fractures. The spinal cord that is transected, or severed, exhibits **neuropraxia.** The fragments or edges of the fractured vertebrae cause the damage, which is usually irreversible.

congenital describes a characteristic present at birth and not caused by an injury or traumatic event

axial loading a vertical compressive load placed on top of the head that transmits through the vertebral column

neuropraxia cessation of nerve function through a complete tearing of the neurological tissue

Mechanism: The usual mechanism of injury for a transected spinal cord is axial loading of the cervical spine. The vertebrae compress together and usually fracture as they fail to dissipate the force placed on them. The sharp edges of the fracture slice through the spinal cord. A secondary trauma occurs as the swelling from the fracture builds and compresses the spine, destroying even more tissue.

Signs and symptoms: The client generally experiences any or all of the following:

- Burning cervical pain
- Numbness
- Tingling
- Loss of sensation
- Weakness
- Possible paralysis

Note that the location of increased or decreased sensation depends on the specific location in which the dislocation or fracture damages the spinal cord. The presence of any of these signs or symptoms is adequate reason to immediately refer the client to a physician for further evaluation.

The affected area is distal to the level of the fractured spine. This means that although the injury is in the cervical spine, the loss of function will be in the arms, trunk, and legs (i.e., beyond the spine). Areas of the body above or proximal to the level of transection will not show any dysfunction. The paralysis incurred from this type of injury usually is permanent.

Special tests: Special testing consists primarily of assessing sensation and very limited screening for movement (e.g., of fingers, toes, breathing in a way that will not move the cervical spine). Any paralysis or deficits in sensation in the arms or legs warrant transportation of the athlete by ambulance for further evaluation by a physician. Assessing sensation lets the athletic trainer know whether it is safe to assess motion. If sensation is abnormal (i.e., limited or absent), then motion/strength testing must be deferred and an ambulance summoned immediately. The athlete should be moved from the scene on a spine board for further diagnostic testing.

Immediate management: All episodes of neuropraxia require referral to a physician. The referral must be made quickly, avoiding excessive movement that would increase the extent of the symptoms or injury.

Intermediate management: Once the athlete is transported to a medical facility, X-ray scans and possibly other imaging techniques will be performed to determine the exact location of the fracture and the extent of the damaged spinal cord. Surgery is usually necessary to stabilize the area and prevent further damage to the cord caused by swelling.

Cervical Spine Sprains and Strains

As stated previously, cervical spine injuries involving trauma to the muscles and ligaments of the area are difficult to pinpoint or delineate. The signs and symptoms for each traumatized tissue are very similar, as is the treatment. It is nearly impossible to use palpation alone to differentiate the individual muscles. Discerning an individual muscle versus an individual ligament is challenging because the structures in this area are both deep (near the spine and not near the surface) and small (compared with larger muscles in other parts of the body). However, sprains are generally localized along the facets of the spine, whereas strains are generally farther away from the spine. Table 15-3 summarizes the complaints and recommendations associated with cervical spine sprains and strains.

TABLE 15-3 Classification of Cervical Spine Strains and Injuries

TYPE	COMPLAINTS	RECOMMENDATIONS
Grade I	Tenderness and pain during end points of range of motion (ROM)	Use modalities and mild stretching to diminish the symptoms and allow the athlete to play.
Grade II	Limited but not radiating pain in ROM without paresthesia	Refer to a physician who might order X-rays (usually negative) and perform a neurological evaluation to assess trauma to nerves.
Grade III	Experiences restrictive ROM accompanied by localized pain, muscle spasm, and the sensation that the cervical area is unstable	

Torticollis. **Torticollis**, commonly call *wryneck*, is an example of a nontraumatic muscle strain. It is usually caused by a peculiar position during sleep, a cold draft, or the head being held in an awkward position for a prolonged time.

Mechanism: This prolonged tightening and irritation of the muscle result in an involuntary contraction that tilts the head to one side. The muscle is contracted for a long period and becomes resistant to stretching or relaxation.

Signs and symptoms:

- The afflicted person typically cannot turn his or her head.
- Neck muscles are tender to the touch.
- The person tends to turn the head and shoulders at the same time, rather than just the head.

Irritation of the cervical spine musculature splints the head and prevents it from moving into those positions that increase pain. Usually not a traumatic or acute

torticollis nontraumatic muscle strain caused by incorrect positioning or cold draft; commonly called *wryneck* condition, torticollis typically occurs after a relatively long-term exposure (even less than an hour) to a situation requiring prolonged contraction.

Special tests: A person with torticollis exhibits difficulty moving the head, especially into rotation movements. The athletic trainer should ask the patient to actively attempt flexion, extension, and rotation of the spine to assess which specific muscles are affected. Use this opportunity to assess any neurological problems because movement of the cervical spine will amplify their effects.

Immediate management: With a sprain/strain, the client is treated **symptomatically** on the basis of ROM and level of pain. As long as the patient does not exhibit any neurological signs (e.g., numbness, burning, tingling) in the cervical spine or upper extremities, cold or hot modalities combined with stretching may return the individual to normal activities, including athletic participation. Ice massage and stretches help reduce the symptoms. These treatments decrease the client's pain and cause the muscle in spasm to relax and become less resistant to stretch.

Intermediate management: Finding the reason for the client's torticollis is key to preventing its recurrence. Once the condition is improved, the athletic trainer should identify the cause. If the offending situation cannot be avoided, the client should enter a supervised program of cervical spine strengthening and flexibility exercises to decrease his or her susceptibility to the condition in the future. If these steps have been taken already and the problem is still recurring frequently, further evaluation by a physician may be necessary to rule out a congenital condition that would predispose the client to this condition.

Brachial Plexus Injury (Burners or Stingers). Brachial plexus injury, or brachial nerve syndrome, is characterized by a burning sensation (hence the name *burner)* along the cervical region. Typically, the cervical spine is forced into lateral flexion, causing the nerve root of the brachial plexus to be stretched or impinged. Each spinal nerve connects to the spinal cord by way of a nerve root. Thus when the nerve root is stretched, it stretches the corresponding spinal nerve, creating the burning or stinging sensation.

Each of the 31 spinal nerves is named according to its starting point from the vertebral column. Because the nerves move out to the left and the right side of the spinal cord, they are considered to be in pairs. There are eight pairs of cervical nerves, twelve pairs of thoracic nerves, five pairs of lumbar nerves, and five pairs of sacral nerves.

Mechanism: Three general mechanisms can result in a brachial plexus injury. Excessive ROM that causes a brachial plexus stretch, excessive ROM that causes brachial plexus compression, and congenital defects all create the conditions in which this injury may occur. These mechanisms result from very different forces and situations, but they generally manifest in the same symptoms.

Excessive lateral movement takes the neck beyond its normal ROM and injures the nerves that exit the spine. This excessive lateral motion stretches the brachial plexus on the same side of the head as the impact or compresses it on the other side of the head (Figure 15-5).

Congenital defects in the formation of the spinal canal result in an opening that is too small to allow the normal freedom of movement of the spinal cord, a condition known as cervical stenosis. Normal movements that would not normally stretch the nerves as they exit the spine now produce injury. In effect, what would be normal lateral flexion for one person proves to be excessive lateral flexion for another because of the restricted space available for the spinal cord.

Signs and symptoms:

- Tingling or burning sensation
- Radiating pain along the neck, across the shoulder, and down the arm
- Sensations that generally subside in a few minutes as the nerve group recovers from the trauma

Special tests: The tests used to assess brachial plexus damage are those that gently reproduce the mechanism of injury. By reproducing the mechanism, the athletic trainer can make an educated guess as to what structures were injured and develop a treatment plan accordingly. Once the trauma is confirmed, myotome testing is performed to assess its resolution (Table 15-4). Finding weakness outside the brachial plexus—such as along the C4 dermatome—indicates an injury that is *not in the brachial plexus*, may not resolve as quickly, and may require further evaluation by a physician.

Brachial plexus stretch test: The patient is seated or standing while the athletic trainer passively flexes the cervical spine laterally. By placing a hand on the athlete's shoulder and moving the head away from that shoulder, the athletic trainer stretches the brachial plexus. Pain and tingling along the neck to the stabilized shoulder (possibly down the arm) confirm a brachial plexus stretch. Pain and tingling on the other side (toward the nonstabilized shoulder) indicate a brachial plexus compression. Testing of this type is not performed if either cervical spine fracture or dislocation is suspected. Also, this test may produce a false positive (i.e., indicating trauma when no trauma is present) if lateral flexion is performed too forcefully (Figure 15-6).

Immediate management: If the athlete has *pain-free* ROM and *full* muscle strength, he or she can return to play. If a specific dermatome area (i.e., an area of skin sensation supplied by a particular spinal nerve) remains

symptomatically term used to describe a method in which symptoms are treated rather than the cause of an injury; designed to restore function

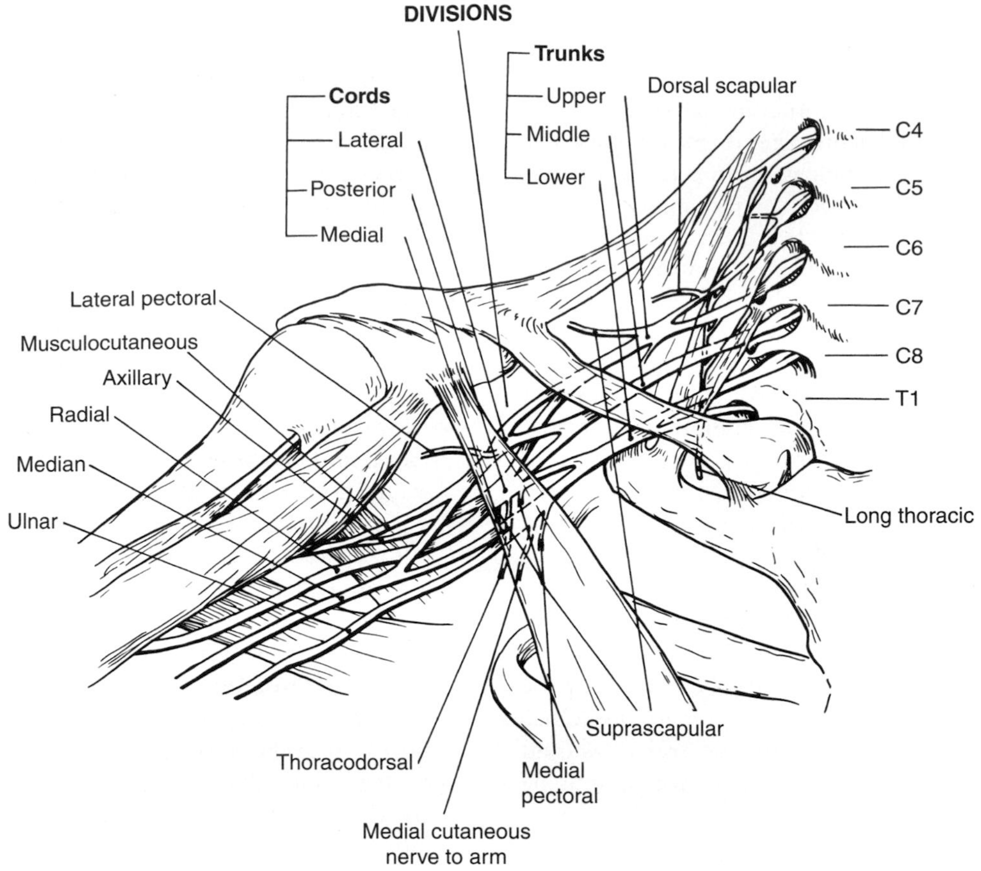

FIGURE 15-5 The brachial plexus is a bundle of nerves that extend from the neck across the shoulder. They can be compressed or stretched with abnormal cervical spine lateral flexion. (From Canale ST: *Campbell's operative orthopaedics,* ed 10, St Louis, 2003, Elsevier/Mosby.)

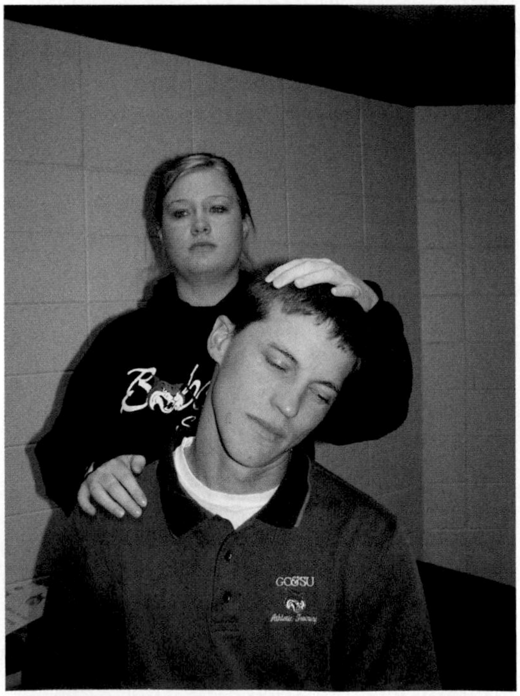

FIGURE 15-6 The brachial plexus stretch test reproduces pain along the brachial plexus when the cervical spine is flexed laterally.

TABLE 15-4 Myotomes Assessed in Brachial Plexus Testing

MOTION TESTED	NERVE ROOT ASSESSED
Shoulder shrug	C4*
Shoulder abduction	C5
Elbow flexion	C6
Elbow extension	C7
Finger flexion	C8
Finger abduction	T1

*C4 is not part of the brachial plexus, but testing it allows the athletic trainer to rule out more severe injuries that can occur with trauma in this area.

numb or seems otherwise abnormal, it is likely that a specific nerve root has been affected, and further evaluation by a physician is warranted. For example, if the athlete has decreased or no sensation when lightly touched along the medial aspect of the elbow, an injury to nerve root T_1 should be suspected.

Intermediate management: Repeated symptoms may indicate a congenital condition or a post-traumatic cervical spine abnormality. Identification of the cause is key to preventing further injuries. If no anatomical reason

BOX 15-1

Cervical Spine Injuries and Appropriate Special Tests

Dislocations and fractures
- Classifications: transected, contused, or concussive
- Transected fractures
  - Assess sensation.
  - Limit movement.

Sprains and strains
- Torticollis
  - Assess ROM.
- Assess neurological involvement.
- Brachial plexus injuries
  - Assess ROM.
  - Test myotomes.
  - Perform brachial plexus stretch test.

ROM, Range of motion.

is found for the incidence of burners, the athlete's sports technique should be assessed. Poor technique (e.g., blocking or tackling with the head as the primary point of contact in football) could increase the risk of injury by placing the cervical spine in an excessive laterally flexed position.

Box 15-1 summarizes the special tests used to help identify injuries to the cervical spine.

Thoracic Spine Injuries

Thoracic spine injuries are usually rare because the thorax is the most stable region of the vertebral column. Movements such as flexion, extension, rotation, and lateral bending allow only limited displacement of the vertebrae. Strong thoracic muscles lend support to the thoracic spine along with the anterior and posterior longitudinal ligaments. Thin intervertebral disks and overlapping of the spinous processes provide another layer of stability.

Thoracic Spine Contusions

A contusion, or a traumatic blow to the thoracic spine, usually affects the paraspinal muscles (i.e., the muscles that run lateral, or parallel, to the spinous processes), creating tenderness, muscle spasm, and increased pain. These injuries are usually not completely debilitating, but they can be quite painful and limit normal function and athletic participation. These muscle contusions act very similarly to muscle contusions in other parts of the body.

Mechanism: Contusions, or bruises, result from a traumatic blow to the thoracic region, causing the underlying structures to be forcefully compressed. This compression results in a black and blue discolored area that can be swollen and quite painful. Often, discomfort associated with contusions to the thoracic spine limits motion as well as function.

Signs and symptoms:
- The skin may become discolored, depending on the severity of the impact.
- The impact site is tender to palpation.
- The painful area is generally limited to the site of the traumatic blow.
- The amount of pain and stiffness is directly proportional to the size and extent of the blow.
- The symptoms usually last fewer than 3 days.

Special tests: No specific tests are indicated. Palpation will reveal the area of tenderness. No neurological deficits in strength or sensation will accompany the contusion. Special tests allow the athletic trainer to rule out more severe injuries and identify the relatively minor injury of contusion.

Immediate management: The use of a modality enhances recovery by reducing the pain and stiffness of this condition. Modalities such as ice massage or electric stimulation may enhance recovery by reducing pain and muscle spasm. When the client has pain-free ROM and full muscle strength, he or she can return to normal activities of daily living, including athletic participation.

Intermediate management: Thoracic spine contusions are usually not related to a problem in technique or abnormal motions. They simply happen as a consequence of a traumatic blow to an area that is not protected as well as other areas.

Thoracic Spine Sprains and Strains

A sprain or strain to the thoracic spinal area is caused by overstretching of the soft tissue surrounding the vertebrae and can be classified as grade I, II, or III (Table 15-5). Thoracic sprains and strains resemble cervical sprains and strains in that the treatment is dictated by the level of dysfunction. The greater the dysfunction, the more aggressive the treatment plan and greater the need for physician referral.

Thoracic Spine Fractures and Dislocations

Fractures and dislocations are also rare in the thoracic spine. However, when such a condition is present, the mechanism of injury is forced forward flexion that causes a compression of the anterior portion of the adjacent vertebral bodies; this might occur when a basketball player takes a charge that results in a hard fall on the buttocks. Usually, the athlete does not experience neurological symptoms (e.g., numbness, tingling, muscle weakness) even while walking but does experience constant localized pain, which is exacerbated by any movement of the spine. The athlete should be referred to a physician to rule out fracture or dislocation and provide medication for pain.

Box 15-2 summarizes the special tests that help identify injuries to the thoracic spine.

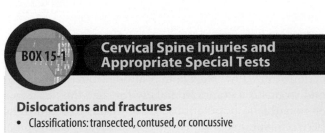

TABLE 15-5 Classifications of Thoracic and Lumbar Spine Strains and Sprains

TYPE	COMPLAINTS	RECOMMENDATIONS
Grade I	Tenderness and spasm with increased pain on active contraction or stretch	Use modalities and mild stretching to diminish the symptoms, and allow the athlete to play when full pain-free ROM returns.
Grade II	Limited but not radiating pain in ROM without paresthesia; complaints of stiffness and soreness	Modalities and stretching may allow the athlete to return to play if the athlete experiences no pain with ROM and has full muscle strength. However, if the pain persists, refer the athlete to a physician.
Grade III	Experiences restrictive ROM accompanied by intense localized pain, muscle spasm	A grade III sprain/strain is very rare and should be referred to a physician to assess other pathologies as well (e.g., fractures, internal injuries).

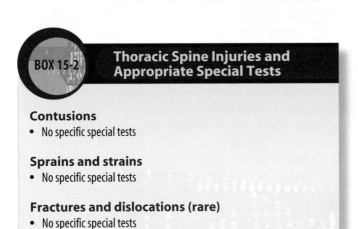

BOX 15-2 Thoracic Spine Injuries and Appropriate Special Tests

Contusions
- No specific special tests

Sprains and strains
- No specific special tests

Fractures and dislocations (rare)
- No specific special tests

Lumbar Spine Injuries

Back pain, especially in the lumbar region, can arise from many causes, including improper lifting techniques, decreased ROM, poor flexibility and tight hamstrings, and weak abdominal muscles or muscles surrounding the spine. Lumbar spine injuries are largely confined to the point where the fifth lumbar vertebra is joined with the sacrum (sacralization of the fifth lumbar vertebra). A very movable lumbar spine interacts with a very fixed and rigid sacrum below. The lower lumbar spine is susceptible to pain and injury because of poor conditioning, poor flexibility, congenital abnormalities, and poor posture habits.

Lumbar Spine Sprains and Strains

Acute trauma of the lumbar spine may be in the form of a sprain/strain. Low back pain resulting from these sprains and strains is a common malady for the athletic as well as nonathletic populations. Once again, distinguishing between sprains and strains is difficult with spinal injuries. A general guideline regarding the difference between a sprain and a strain is as follows: The closer the pain is to the vertebral column, the more likely it is to indicate a sprain because of possible ligament stretching. Pain farther away from the vertebral column is more likely to indicate a strain because more muscles are involved in this area (see Table 15-5).

Mechanism: Most of the time, low back pain is a result of repeated minor injuries occurring over months or even years that lead to cumulative damage to the musculature of the spine. Rarely is the back pain a result of a one-time incident, although a one-time error in lifting technique may be the so-called straw that broke the camel's back. This cumulative effect is why some people experience a sudden low back pain lifting something very light, such as a book or plate, whereas someone else can lift a very heavy object without injury. Proper lifting mechanics protect the spinal musculature, but poor lifting techniques abuse the musculature and contribute to poor posture as well (Figure 15-7). Generally, the cause of chronic low back strains is faulty posture or improper lifting, and the cause of acute low back strains is sudden extension in combination with rotation.

Signs and symptoms
- Localized pain
- No radiating pain down into the legs
- Muscle spasms
- Tenderness to palpation
- Involved tissue that is tight or hard to the touch

A simple muscle strain does not have a neurological component (e.g., tingling, burning, numbness in the legs), but the pain may be quite intense.

Special tests: As with most muscle injury assessments, testing for lumbar spine muscle strains involves placing the muscle under either tension (shortening contraction) or stretch (lengthening) to identify which major muscle group is affected. Also, as muscles are injured, they tend to tighten or spasm, and the stretches used to identify the injured muscles are also used to treat those muscles by reversing the localized muscle spasm. Some simple ROM and stretching tests include the following techniques:

Single knee to chest: While in a supine position, the client flexes one hip with the knee also flexed. The other leg should remain straight and extended on the table, floor, or ground. The hip flexion should be increased as much as possible without increasing the low back pain. The client should feel a stretch in the low back on the hip-flexed side and possibly a mild stretch on the front of the thigh of the hip-extended leg. The client may pull

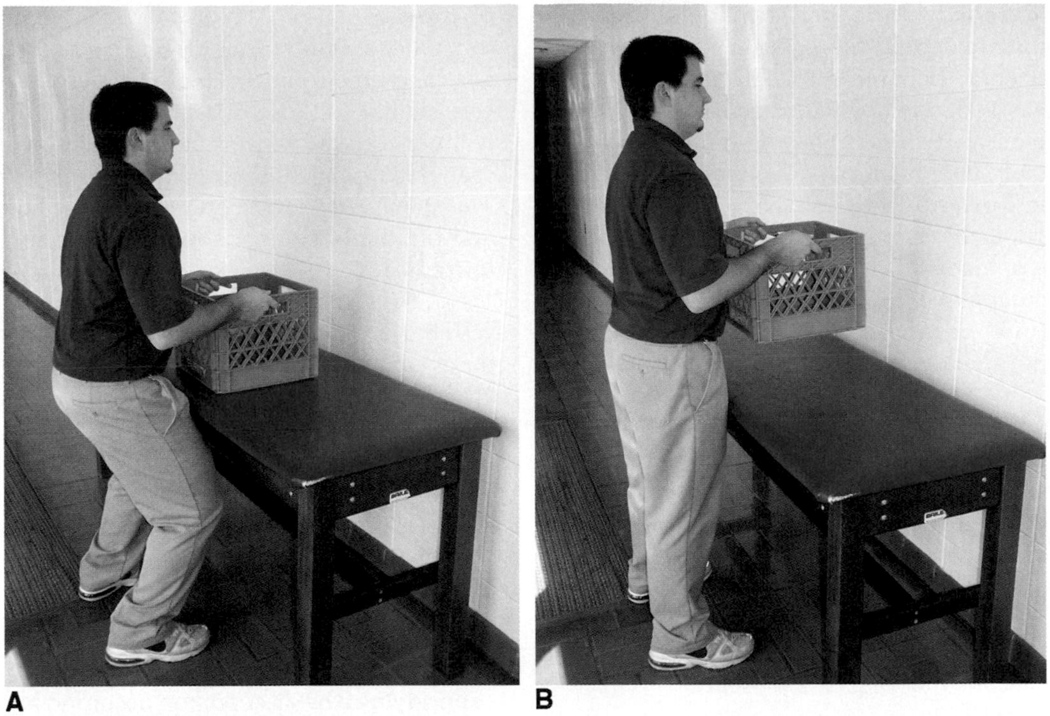

FIGURE 15-7 Proper lifting technique reduces the risk of low back strain and injury. **A,** The knees are flexed to lower the trunk to the level of the object being lifted. **B,** The knees are extended to lift the object while the elbows remain flexed.

the knee up to the chest independently or with the aid of a partner.

Double knee to chest: This stretching technique is performed with both hips flexed and both knees flexed at the same time to pull the knees to the chest. The client should feel a stretch in the lower back to a greater degree than when stretching either leg individually.

Immediate management: Modalities are useful to decrease the pain and spasm. Gentle stretching will also help to decrease these symptoms. The athlete should refrain from performing any movements that increase pain.

Intermediate management: Eliminating the cause of the pain, either in an acute or chronic situation, is the key to preventing recurrence. With acute injuries, the mechanism is easily identified, but with chronic low back pain, the cause may be harder to identify because there is no single clear-cut situation that leads to injury. As stated before, the problem is often brought on by years of poor lifting technique or poor posture.

A formal supervised program of strengthening and stretching exercises is often necessary to reverse the bad habits that led to the client's poor posture and improper lifting mechanics (Box 15-3).

Lumbar Spine Fractures and Dislocation

In rare cases, fractures and dislocations may occur because of a direct blow to the spinous or transverse process. In addition, hyperflexion or landing on the buttocks (e.g., taking a charge in basketball) can also produce compression on the spinous or transverse processes. The athlete will complain of low back pain or discomfort and point tenderness over the bony process. Assessing a fracture or dislocation is quite difficult because of the large musculature that protects the back and hides the deformities that often accompany other fractures. All suspected fractures and dislocations warrant referral to a physician for an X-ray examination.

BOX 15-3 Perspectives in Rehabilitation: Stretches for Low Back Strain

Two types of stretches have been recommended for low back strains: Williams's flexion exercises and McKenzie's extension exercises. When the athlete is in a supine "hook lying" (hips and knees flexed) position, Williams's flexion exercises provide a comfortable way for the athlete to begin a stretching program. While the athlete is prone, using the arms to extend the back (keeping the hips on the table), McKenzie's extension exercises bring the spine into a position of normal lordosis and produce a force that directs the vertebrae away from the spinal cord.[14] Either routine can relieve the symptoms; above all, the athlete should *not* resort to bed rest. Complete bed rest will only prolong the problem by postponing the strength and flexibility gains necessary to eliminate the problem in the first place. For more stubborn strains, referral to the physician is recommended to rule out conditions that are more serious.

Lumbar Spine Spondylolysis and Spondylolisthesis. **Spondylolysis** is a defect in the pars interarticularis of the lumbar vertebrae (Figure 15-8). This injury is commonly known as a "Scotty dog with a collar" because of its appearance on X-ray film (Figure 15-9). If the defect of the spondylolysis is bilateral, the vertebra with the defect will slip forward on the vertebra below. This is termed **spondylolisthesis**, and the resulting X-ray scan is described as a "Scotty Dog that has lost its head" or "Scotty Dog decapitated" (Figure 15-10). Spondylolysis may be congenital or the result of repeated stress. The latter may cause spondylolysis to turn into spondylolisthesis.

Mechanism: Either spondylolysis or spondylolisthesis may result from a congenital weakness or from continuous trunk extension maneuvers such as those required by gymnastics or football (the lineman being particularly vulnerable). Spondylolysis is a crack in the vertebra but only on one side. When the same injury occurs on both sides of the vertebra, the front half of the bone actually shifts away from the back half, like a boat floating away from a dock once the moorings are loosened.

Signs and symptoms:

- Low thoracic pain associated with activity that will be relieved during times of rest
- Pain commonly radiating into the buttocks and upper thigh region of the leg

If pain is tolerable and there is no radiating pain, the client may continue activities with no knowledge of their condition. Frequently, this injury is believed to be a common muscle strain that is taking an unusually long time to heal. The signs and symptoms may be very similar to those of a simple muscle strain, but they will not respond to normal treatment in a normal time span. Neurological damage to the lumbar region is rare. The spinal cord terminates at the first lumbar vertebra, and the **cauda equina** is relatively mobile and resistant to trauma.

Special tests: Tests to assess the presence of posterior vertebral fracture injuries (spondylolysis or spondylolisthesis) involve placing the spine in a position that will apply pressure to the injured area. The most common test to assess for this condition is the single-leg stance test, or stork test. For this test, the client stands on one

spondylolysis crack in the pars interarticularis of the lumbar vertebrae; commonly known as "Scotty dog with a collar"; can be congenital or result from trunk extensions performed in the course of athletics

spondylolisthesis condition occurring in bilateral spondylolysis in which the cracked vertebrae slip forward onto the vertebrae below; commonly known as "Scotty dog has lost his head"

cauda equina distal end of the spinal cord along the spinal cord canal in the vertebral column; so named because it resembles a horse's tail

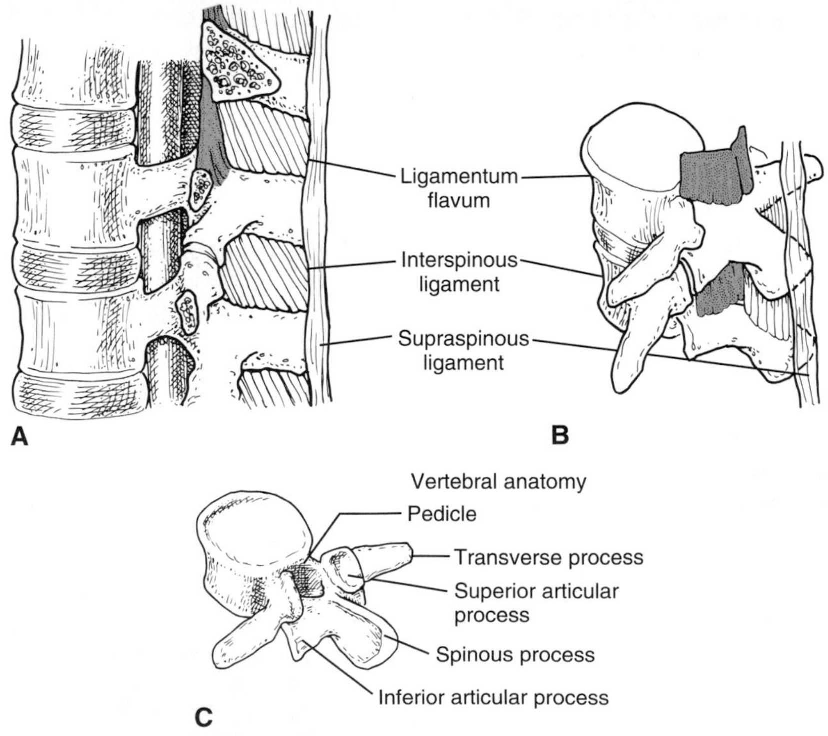

FIGURE 15-8 The normal lumbar vertebrae. **A**, Sagittal view. **B**, Oblique view **C**, Oblique view of single lumbar vertebra. (From Miller R: *Miller's anesthesia*, ed 6, Philadelphia, 2005, Elsevier/Churchill Livingstone.)

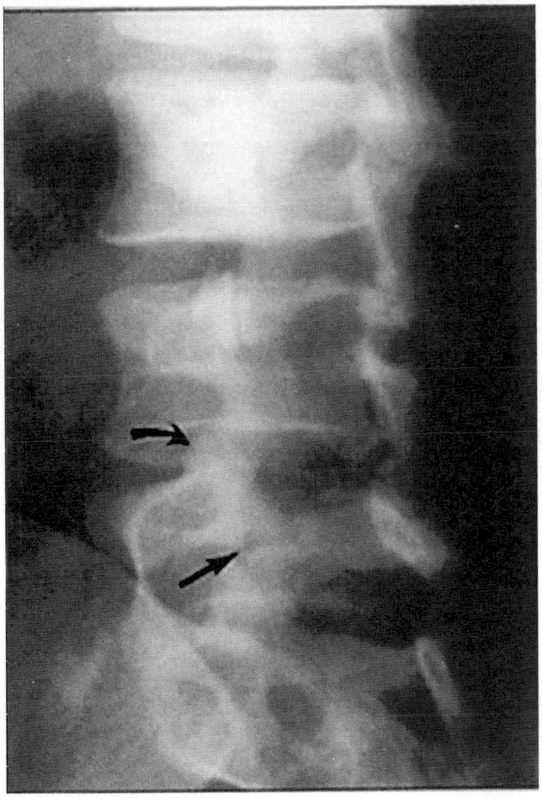

FIGURE 15-9 An oblique view of the vertebra with spondylolysis appears as a "Scotty dog with a collar," with the fracture line serving as a "collar." (From Katz DS, Math KR, Groskin SA: *Radiology secrets,* Chapter 48, Figure 2, Philadelphia, 1998, Hanley & Belfus.)

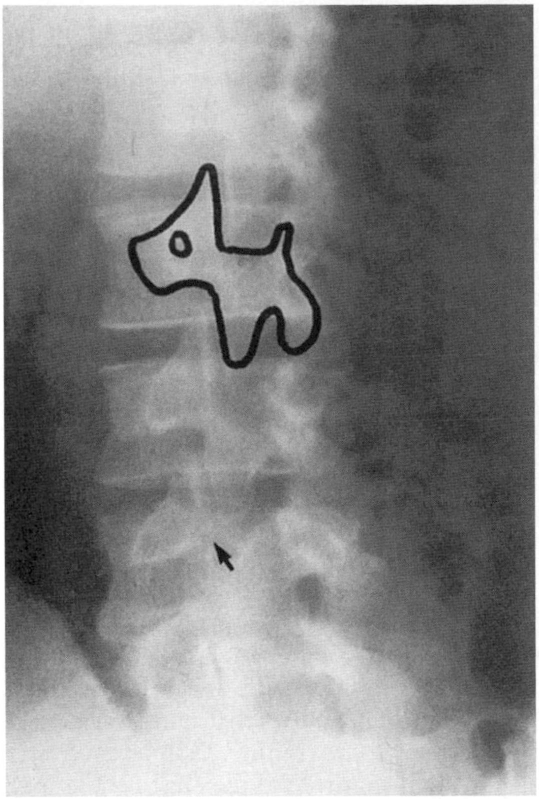

FIGURE 15-10 An oblique view of the vertebra with spondylolisthesis appears as "Scotty dog without a head," with the bilateral fracture line occurring at Scotty's "neck." (From Magee DJ: *Orthopedic physical assessment,* ed 4 [enhanced edition] Philadelphia, 2006, Saunders/Elsevier.)

leg with hands on waist. The athletic trainer stands behind the client and places a hand on the shoulder to assist with balance. The client extends, or leans back, causing compression of the posterior spine. Leaning back while standing on one leg causes the body to tilt to one side and compress only one side of the spine. The test should be repeated with the client standing on the other leg. A positive test results in significant pain at the point of the fracture site and possible tingling pain down the leg on that side (Figure 15-11).

Immediate management: At this point, the athlete should be referred to a physician. Referral should be made sooner in the event of low back pain that fails to improve or significantly worsens within 2 weeks of treatment. Modalities relieve pain and spasm. A rehabilitation program of gentle stretches and strengthening exercises is helpful but complicated by the fact that the motions that improve strength in the area—extension exercises—are also the motions that increase pressure on the fracture site(s).

Intermediate management: The client should be removed from the source of the spinal irritation, a change that will allow the area to heal and help prevent future injury. This measure may be temporary to treat the current injury or long-term to prevent future injury; in any case, failure to make a change will result in improper healing.

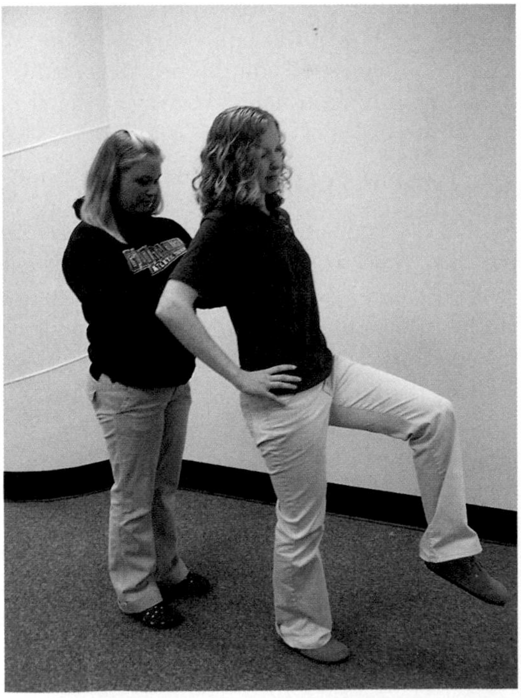

FIGURE 15-11 The stork test places pressure on the site of the vertebral fracture and causes significant pain at this site.

BOX 15-4 Lumbar Spine Injuries and Appropriate Special Tests

Sprains and strains
ROM tests
- Single knee to chest
- Double knee to chest

Fractures and dislocations
Spondylolysis and spondylolisthesis
- Stork test

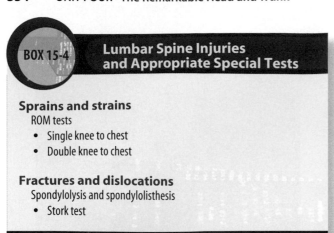

ROM, Range of motion.

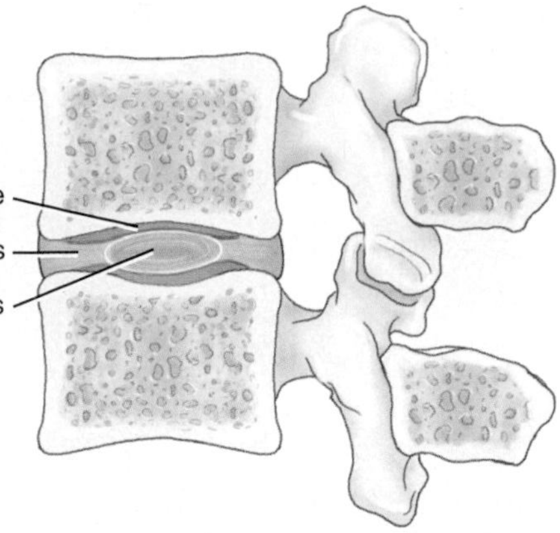

FIGURE 15-12 A vertebral disk consists of a dense outer covering and fluid-filled center. (From Muscolino JE: *Kinesiology: the skeletal system and muscle function,* p. 241, St Louis, 2006, Mosby/Elsevier.)

Box 15-4 summarizes the special tests used to help identify injuries to the lumbar spine.

THE AGE-GROUP ATHLETE

Age-group injuries to the spine include disk herniation, degeneration of the intervertebral disk, and spinal stenosis. Most conditions are the result of improper lifting mechanics and injuries that cause hyperextension, rotation, or compression of the vertebrae. Even smoking can play a significant role in the changes that occur to the disk over time. Just one cigarette cuts the amount of oxygen traveling to disks in half.[14] Usually, what is perceived to be a little back injury will be dismissed without proper care. Over time, body mechanics, agility, flexibility, and speed of movement change and lead to different—and sometimes less efficient and riskier—body mechanics. These new movements occur to compensate for discomfort or pain. Activity modification and postural adjustments minimize the pain. The aforementioned conditions can certainly occur acutely among young athletes. However, the condition is usually chronic.

Herniated Disk Problems

A herniated, or "slipped," disk is a problem that usually develops over time from repeated stresses but can also occur with a sudden twisting or extreme loading of the spine. Other names for the condition include prolapsed, bulging, or ruptured disk. The disk lies between each vertebra and is filled with gel-like fluid to maintain the separation between the vertebrae. The disk functions to assist with movement of the back and cushion the vertebrae during activity. The disk has a center nucleus composed of tissue and an outer ring of cartilage, the annulus (Figure 15-12). While compressive forces act on the disk, the annulus may bulge or even rupture and the nucleus tissue is forced outward against one or more of the spinal nerves. This displacement causes pain, numbness, or weakness in the lower back, leg, or foot. The disks in the lumbar spine are most susceptible to herniation, but disk injuries also occur in the cervical spine.

Mechanism: Disk trauma is rarely isolated and usually occurs when a section of the spine is traumatized through excessive ROM or axial loading. Generally, disk injuries occur with other injuries. The other injuries—muscle strains and even mild vertebral fractures—may heal and leave the disk trauma as a lingering injury. If the nucleus material bulges away from the spinal nerves, the individual will have no neurological symptoms. Unfortunately, the nucleus usually bulges or herniates toward the nerves, and this pressure ultimately leads to the dysfunction.

Signs and symptoms:
- Pain in the buttocks and the back
- Radiating pain down into the leg (sciatica)
- Numbness in the affected region
- Weakness in the affected muscles
- Sensation of "pins and needles"

Special tests: Several tests are used in the identification of disk-related problems. Some tests indicate disk injury by increasing the **intrathecal** pressure on the damaged disk and the associated nerves. Other tests indicate disk injury by stretching the nerve in that area and causing it to impinge on the bulging disk. *Please note that none of these tests should be used to evaluate an acute injury until a vertebral fracture has been completely ruled out by a physician.*

The Valsalva maneuver is performed with the subject seated with legs hanging off the table. The athletic trainer should ask the athlete to take a deep breath and exhale into a closed fist. If the athlete experiences pain in the low back and possibly even down the legs, the

intrathecal term used in reference to the interior of the trunk, usually indicating the cavity that contains the internal organs and the thoracic and lumbar spinal regions test is positive. This test increases the pressure on the involved disk and amplifies the pain (Figure 15-13).

The second test is the straight leg raise test, also known as Lasegue's test. The subject is supine with legs extended. The athletic trainer places the athlete's hip into internal rotation and adduction with the knee in full extension and then asks the athlete to slowly flex his or her hip to move the leg toward the head until tightness is felt in the hamstrings. The athletic trainer then stops and repositions the leg in slight hip flexion so that no tightness or pain exists. Next, the athletic trainer passively dorsiflexes the foot. If pain occurs while the straight leg is at 30 degrees, the test is positive for disk involvement. If the pain does not reappear with the ankle dorsiflexion, the pain in the leg is due to tight hamstrings (Figure 15-14).

The well-leg straight leg raise test also determines disk involvement. When the straight-leg raise test is performed on the uninvolved side, pain occurs on the involved side. Pain with this test indicates a more severe disk injury than that found with a straight leg raise test.

A final test to assess nerve root irritation is the bowstring test. For this test, the athlete is supine with the hip and knee both flexed to 90 degrees. The athletic trainer passively extends the knee while palpating the **popliteal** space of the knee. If the sciatic nerve is irritated, this passive knee extension will reproduce radiating pain down the leg. Once this radiating pain occurs, the knee should be passively flexed slightly to see if the pain disappears. (The same degree of hip flexion should be retained throughout the test.) With the client's knee in the new position, the athletic trainer then presses on the popliteal space to compress the sciatic nerve again. Resumed radiating pain indicates trauma to the sciatic nerve and lower lumbar spine (Figure 15-15).

The cervical compression test assesses damage to vertebral disks in the cervical spine. The client is seated, looking straight ahead, and the athletic trainer places gentle downward pressure on the head, increasing the axial load on the disk of the cervical spine. A positive test brings pain in the neck along with radiating pain down one or both arms and indicates that the disk is not maintaining the proper separation of the vertebrae, leading to increased pressure on the nerve roots exiting the cervical spine (Figure 15-16). The Spurling test also measures cervical disk trauma but only on one side at a time. The client is seated facing straight ahead. However, the cervical spine is placed in slight lateral flexion as the

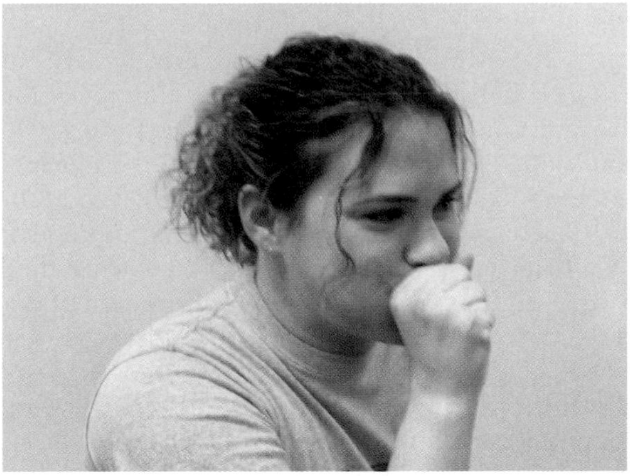

FIGURE 15-13 A Valsalva maneuver increases pressure on the involved disk and produces pain.

popliteal area behind the knee, generally between the hamstring tendon insertions where knee flexion occurs

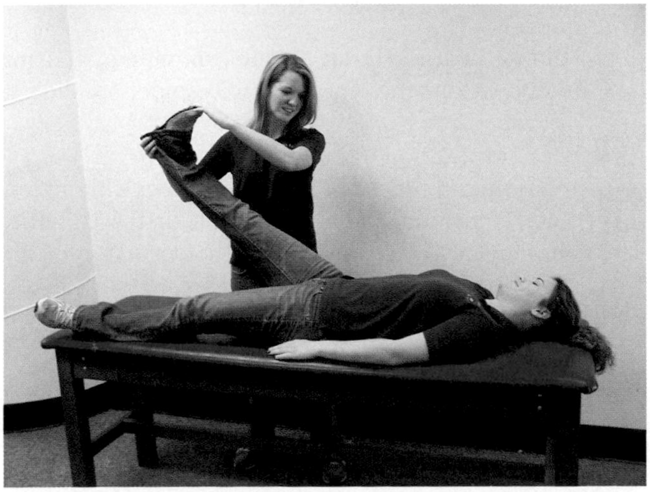

FIGURE 15-14 The straight leg raise test allows the athletic trainer to reproduce radiating pain in the legs and determine whether it is caused by disk injury or tight hamstrings.

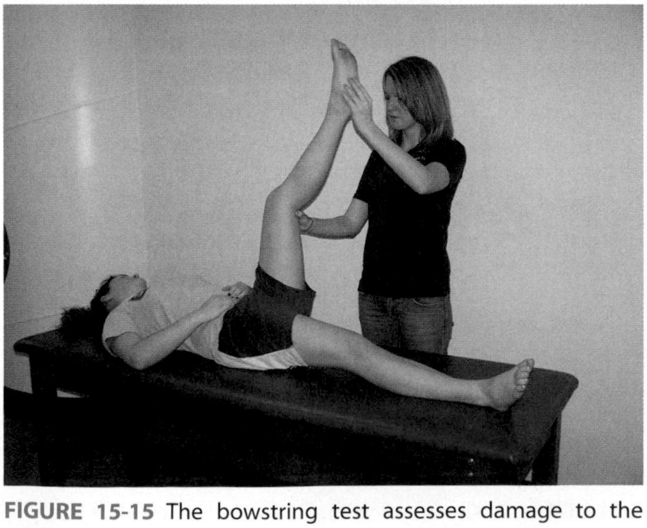

FIGURE 15-15 The bowstring test assesses damage to the sciatic nerve.

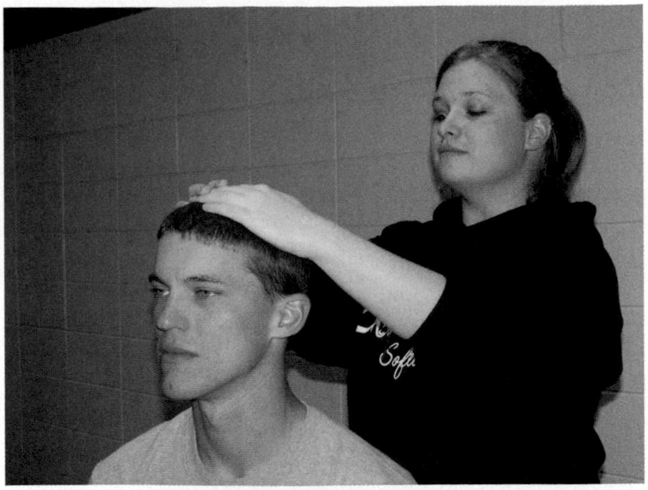

FIGURE 15-16 The cervical compression test reproduces pain to determine whether disk injury is present in the cervical spine.

athletic trainer again places gentle downward pressure on the top of the head. A positive test will produce a tingling pain down the arm on the side of the lateral flexion (Figure 15-17).

Immediate management: Modalities may help decrease pain and spasm in the area. The muscles of the area will tighten to prevent any motion that may worsen the injury; these treatments may decrease the pain of those spasms as well as the spasms themselves. Gentle stretching is sometimes beneficial as well, but care must be taken to avoid positions that exacerbate the disk irritation.

Intermediate management: Long-term management involves a plan of care that will help reduce the bulging or herniation of the disk. In some cases, surgery may be necessary. A formal rehabilitation plan may help delay the need for surgery and reduce the symptoms that accompany the disk problem.

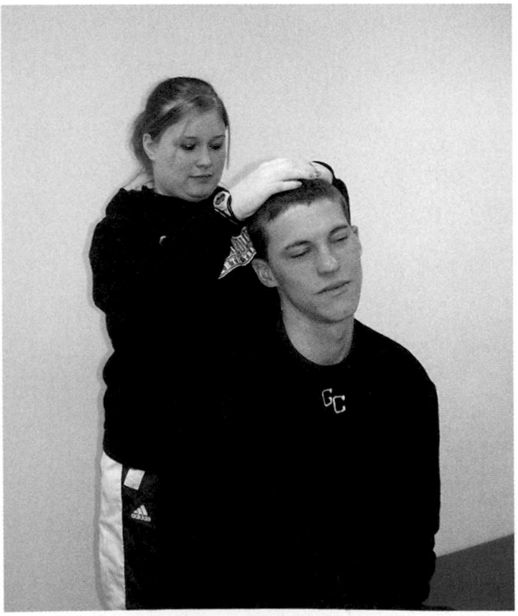

FIGURE 15-17 The Spurling test is used to assess disk injury in the cervical spine.

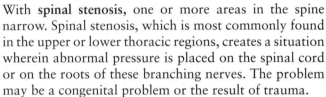

BOX 15-5 Special Tests to Assess Herniated Disk Problems

- Vertebral fracture ruled out first
- *Valsalva maneuver:* vertebral disk involvement
- *Lasegue's test:* vertebral disk involvement
- *Well-leg straight leg raise test:* vertebral disk involvement
- *Bowstring test:* nerve root irritation
- *Cervical compression test:* cervical vertebral disk involvement

Box 15-5 summarizes the special tests appropriate in the identification of problems related to a herniated disk.

Spinal Stenosis

With **spinal stenosis,** one or more areas in the spine narrow. Spinal stenosis, which is most commonly found in the upper or lower thoracic regions, creates a situation wherein abnormal pressure is placed on the spinal cord or on the roots of these branching nerves. The problem may be a congenital problem or the result of trauma.

Mechanism: Congenital stenosis occurs when the spinal canal is too small to allow normal freedom of movement as the trunk flexes, extends, and twists. The nerves are stretched or impinged as they pull tight against the walls of the spinal canal. Traumatic stenosis occurs as a complication of an earlier injury. Generally, the spine is injured and the healing structures produce excess amounts of bone, decreasing the diameter of the canal where the nerves exit the spine.

Signs and symptoms:

- Cramping in the legs, thoracic spine, shoulders, or arms
- Pain in the legs, thoracic spine, shoulders, or arms
- Numbness in the legs, thoracic spine, shoulders, or arms
- Loss of sensation in the extremities

In addition, problems with bladder or bowel function may occur, depending on the location of the stenosis. The neurological symptoms follow the dermatome patterns mentioned previously.

Special tests: Most neurological tests of the cervical spine will be positive even when no apparent mechanism

spinal stenosis condition in which one or more areas in the spine narrow, putting pressure on the spinal cord or the roots of the branching nerves; can be congenital or result from trauma is present. When the nerves are affected, the muscles controlled by those nerves are also affected. Therefore significant muscle weakness is apparent in the areas controlled by the affected nerves.

Immediate management: Because stenosis involves a structural problem, the only true way to reverse it is through surgery. The symptoms can be treated, but the problem cannot be corrected simply through a rehabilitation program. As the symptoms worsen and intensify, the chances of permanent neurological damage increase.

Intermediate Management: Because degenerative changes in the spine are caused by aging, spinal stenosis is not often seen in the athlete. The main cause of spinal degeneration is osteoarthritis, an arthritic condition that affects the cartilage that cushions the ends of bones in the joints. Over time, the cartilage begins to deteriorate and its smooth surface becomes rough. If the cartilage wears down completely, bone may rub painfully on bone. In an attempt to repair the damage, the body may produce bony growths called *bone spurs*. When these form on the facet joints in the spine, they narrow the spinal canal. Spinal stenosis is typically ignored by many sufferers, especially elderly people. If the client has leg pain that worsens during walking and improves during sitting or bending forward, referral to a physician for further evaluation is warranted.[15]

Box 15-6 summarizes the special tests associated with spinal stenosis.

SUMMARY

Excessive force and violent movement may result in serious injuries to the cervical, thoracic, and lumbar spine. Any potential head and cervical injury must be treated with the proper protocol for stabilization in preparation for transportation to a hospital.[16] Before the start of every season, the athletic training room staff, medical team, and local emergency medical services (EMS) personnel should review the athletic program's emergency plan. Repetitive sessions on stabilization and transport minimize any further trauma to the athlete. The most common injuries of the cervical, thoracic, and lumbar spine are sprains and strains. Because it is very difficult to differentiate between a sprain and a strain, the athletic trainer must rely on an accurate history of the mechanism of injury. Strict attention must be made to the signs and symptoms provided by the patient. Once the injury has been determined, rehabilitation (be it heat or cold therapy, ROM exercises and stretches, or electric stimulation) may commence immediately.

BOX 15-6 Special Tests to Assess Spinal Stenosis

- Neurological assessment
- Manual muscle testing to affected neurological areas

Revisiting the OPENING Scenario

The scenario at the beginning of the chapter involves a muscle strain of the lumbar spine. The injury may be quite debilitating and painful initially, but with proper care it can progressively improve. Active ROM is usually limited because of the pain that results from stretching of the strained muscles. Prolonged sitting or standing requires the muscles to tighten, and the muscles are simply too weak to stabilize the trunk efficiently. This type of injury is often ignored by athletes because it is not extremely painful at first. As the activity ends and the muscle begins to cool down, the muscle tightens and becomes increasingly painful. In the absence of any neurological signs (e.g., numbness, tingling), it is reasonable to suspect an isolated muscle injury and no disk or vertebral involvement.

Issues & Ethics

After being thrown to the mat by his opponent, Ben, a collegiate wrestler, lands on his head in a slightly flexed position. Ben is treated as if he had a potential head and cervical injury using in-line cervical stabilization and a spine board. After his return from the emergency room, the medical referral paperwork indicates a subluxation of the C6 vertebra, which means that the bone has moved out of alignment and the capsule surrounding the joint is stretched but not completely torn. The physician tells Ben that his collegiate career is over because he is at high risk of causing further injury to his cervical spine should he return to wrestling. Ben was lucky this time but may not be so lucky in escaping a paralyzing injury the next time he steps on the mat.

Ben seeks a second opinion, and the second physician agrees with the emergency physician. Ben is still not satisfied, and after three more trips to different physicians, he finally finds one who allows him to wrestle. His parents do not object to their son's decision to wrestle and give their consent. As the head athletic trainer, you decide not to allow Ben to wrestle. You feel strongly that this decision is in the best interest of the athlete. The athletic director also supports your decision. However, Ben and his parents are furious with you and are threatening to go to the president of the college and hire a lawyer if necessary.

1. Was the decision to prohibit Ben from wrestling incorrect or even unethical?
2. Should the decision change in light of the potential legal action?
3. What paperwork or guidelines should be in place to prevent litigation?

Web Links

National Athletic Trainers' Association: www.nata.org
The American Journal of Sports Medicine: www.ajsm.org or http://ajs.sagepub.com
The Mayo Clinic: www.mayoclinic.com
The Spine Journal: www.thespinejournalonline.com

References

1. Turner JA et al: Surgery for lumbar spinal stenosis: attempted meta-analysis of the literature, *Spine* 17: 1–8, 1992.
2. Boden BP et al: Catastrophic cervical spine injuries in high school and college football players, *The American Journal of Sports Medicine* 24: 1223–1232, 2006.
3. Horton J, Lindsay D, MacIntosh B: Abdominal muscle activation of elite male golfers with chronic low back pain, *Medicine and Science in Sports and Exercise* 33(10): 1647–1654, 2001.
4. Starkey C: Injuries and illnesses in the National Basketball Association: a 10-year perspective, *The Journal of Athletic Training* 35: 161–167, 2000.
5. Mueller F, Zemper E, Peters A: American football. In Caine D, Caine C, Lindner K, editors: *Epidemiology of sports injuries,* pp. 41–62, Champaign, Ill, 1997, Human Kinetics.
6. Banerjee R, Palumbo M, Fadale P: Catastrophic cervical spine injuries in the collision sport athlete. Part 2: Principles of emergency care, *Am J Sports Med* 32: 1760–1764, 2004.
7. Kleiner D et al: Prehospital care of the spine-injured athlete: A document from the Inter-Association Task Force for Appropriate Care of Spine-Injured Athlete, Dallas, 2001 (March), National Athletic Trainers' Association.
8. Palumbo M, Hulstyn M, Fadale P: The effect of protective football equipment on alignment of the injured cervical spine: radiographic analysis in a cadaveric model, *Am J Sports Med* 4: 446–453, 1996.
9. Waninger K: On-field management of potential cervical spine injury in helmeted football players: leave the helmet on, *Clin J Sport Med* 8: 124–129, 1998.
10. Donaldson W et al: Helmet and shoulder pad removal from a player with suspected cervical spine injury: a cadaveric model, Spine 23(16): 1729–1732, 1998.
11. Torg J et al: The epidemiologic, pathologic, biomechanical, and cinematographic analysis of football-induced cervical spine trauma, *Am J Sports Med* 18: 50–57, 1990.
12. Cross K, Serenelli C: Training and equipment to prevent athletic head and cervical injuries, *Clin Sports Med* 22: 639–667, 2003.
13. LaPrade R et al: Cervical spine alignment in the immobilized ice hockey player: a computed tomographic analysis of the effects of helmet removal, *Am J Sports Med* 28: 800–803, 2000.
14. Foster MR: *Backache: putting it behind you*, Danbury, Conn, 2001, Rutledge Books.
15. Mayo Clinic Staff: *Diseases and conditions: spinal stenosis,* Rochester, Minn, 2006 (March 10), Mayo Foundation for Medical Education and Research. Retrieved March 28, 2007, from www.mayoclinic.com/health/spinal-stenosis/DS00515.
16. Waninger K: Management of helmeted athlete with suspected cervical spine injury, *The American Journal of Sports Medicine* 32: 1331–1350, 2004.

16

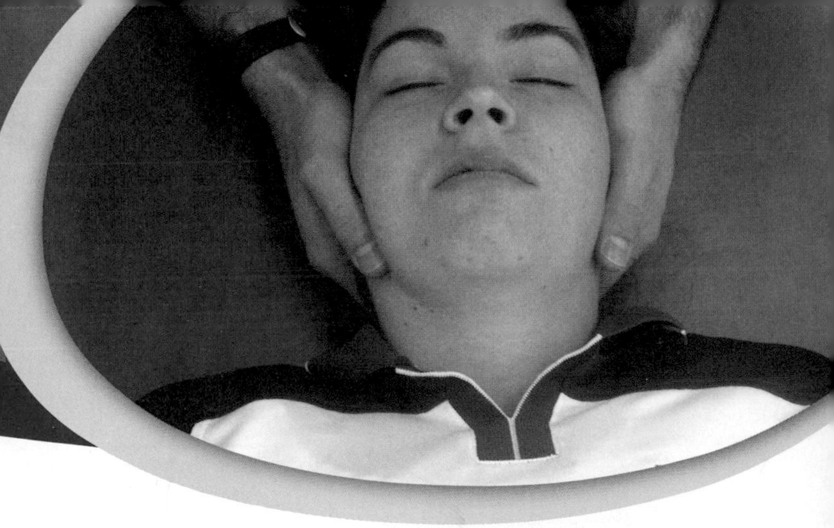

Anatomy of the Senses

PAUL HIGGS

Learning Goals

1. Understand the anatomy of the structures that contribute to the senses of sight, hearing, smell, taste, and touch.
2. Comprehend the physiology of the senses and the process of transmitting information to the brain.
3. Recognize the various pathological conditions that affect the senses.
4. Describe the way the senses interrelate.
5. Define the appropriate use of an ophthalmoscope and an otoscope.

This chapter covers the anatomy of the structures involved with the senses of the face: sight, hearing, taste, and smell. By understanding the relevant anatomy, the athletic trainer will be better prepared to evaluate injuries and illnesses that affect the senses of the face. Senses are invaluable in coordinating activities of daily living. In athletic activities, these structures are indispensable; even a mild injury to the senses is a great hindrance to normal activities. For example, a baseball player with a vision problem will suffer in his ability to hit or field a ball during a game. A diver with a hearing problem may not hear the starting gun and will be forced to rely on visual cues to start a race. Outside of athletics, a student with a vision or hearing problem will find it challenging to follow concepts taught in class. Someone with an altered sense of smell, dependent on visual and auditory cues, might not escape a burning building without injury. This chapter is the foundation for a solid understanding of the anatomical structures of the face and their sensory functions.

ANATOMY OF SIGHT

The sense of sight is a process that begins when an image, created by light from the local environment, enters the anterior chamber of the eye. The image then passes through the eye and is projected onto the highly innervated wall at the back of the eye. This neurological tissue interprets the colors, intensity, and shadows of the image. Once the data is interpreted, this information is passed along the optic nerve from the posterior eye to the visual centers at the back of the brain (Figure 16-1).

Bones

The bones that encase the eye are very important in that they serve to protect the structures that enable sight. Encasing the eye is the opening in the skull called the **orbit**. Three skull bones make up the orbit: the (1) frontal, (2) zygomatic, and (3) maxillary bones. The frontal bone is composed of the superior or upper rim and part of the lateral of the orbit. The zygomatic bone helps form the **lateral** border and, along with the maxillary bone, part of the inferior border of the orbit. The posterior or back of the orbit is formed by the sphenoid bone, along with parts of the lacrimal and ethmoid bones (Figure 16-2). An opening in the

lateral away from the midline or center of the body (outer aspect) relative to another landmark

Terms that appear in boldface green type are defined in the book's glossary.

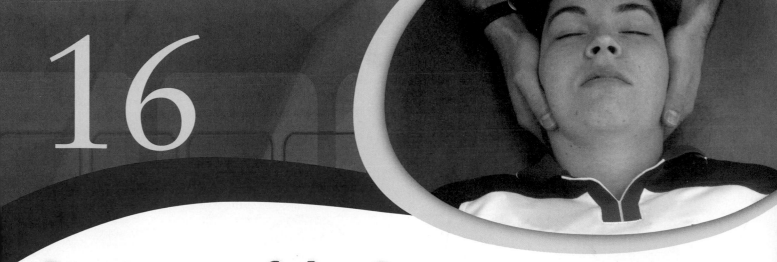

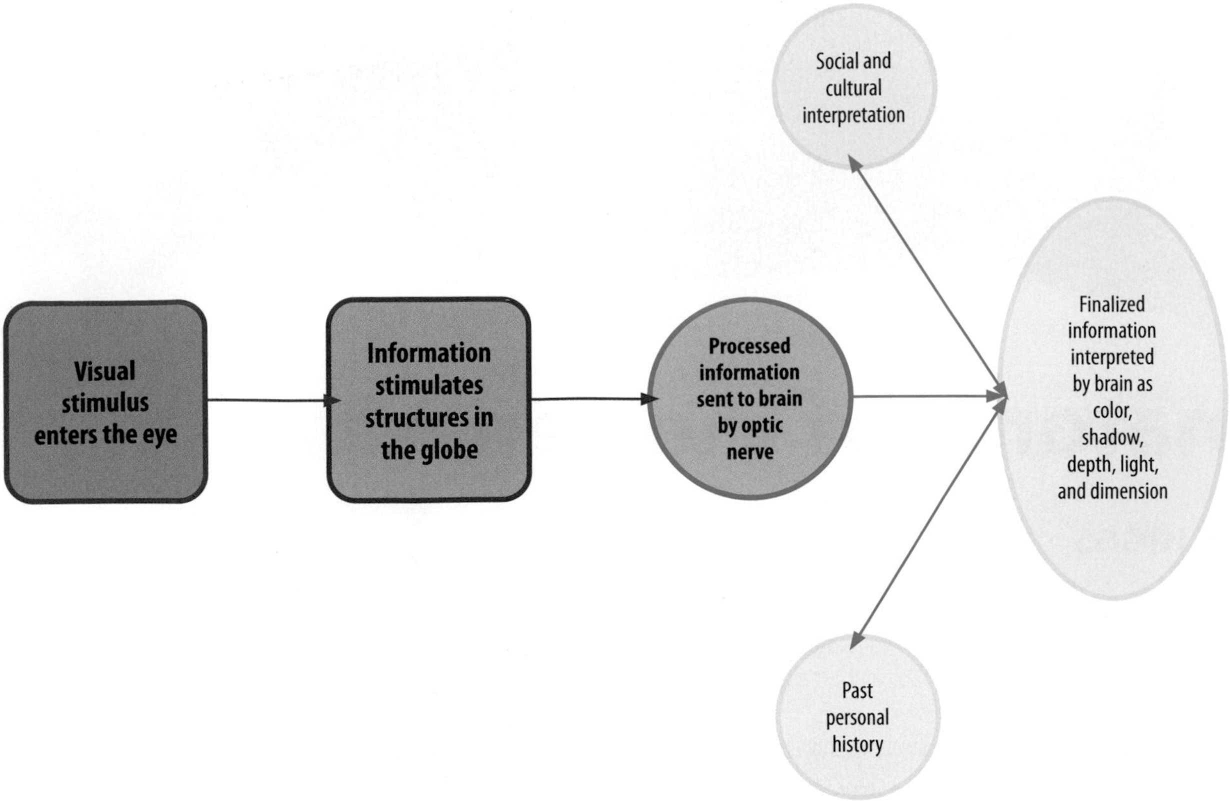

FIGURE 16-1 Conceptual drawing of the sense of sight.

sphenoid bone that allows for passage of the cranial nerves and blood supply to reach the eye is the superior orbital fissure. The optic nerve passes from the brain to the eye through an opening at the back of the orbit by way of the optic canal. The auditory center of the brain that interprets the information delivered by the optic nerve is located in the occipital lobe.

Surface Landmarks

The anterior borders of the orbit are easily palpated and give a great deal of information about the integrity of the skull in the event of facial trauma. Bones are very **superficial** and easily **palpated**, although differentiation into individual bones is generally not possible without an X-ray examination. The frontal bone is easily located just below the eyebrows. The **medial** border of the orbit also forms the lateral nasal region. The lateral border of the orbit, formed by the zygoma, or cheekbone, is easily palpated moving medially from the more prominent area of the bone.

superficial near the surface and easily noticed
palpated felt or noticed through touch
medial toward the midline or center of the body (inner aspect) relative to another landmark

Common Fractures

Fractures of the orbit can greatly affect the sense of sight. The bones of the face are generally very strong and protect the eye, but once a fracture occurs, the orbit's shape is easily distorted and the location of the globe changes, altering the ability of one eye to synchronize vision with the other eye. The primary danger of an orbital fracture is the threat of laceration of vital neurological and vascular structures by the edges of the fractured bone. All fractures of the face should be evaluated to determine how they affect not only the sense of sight but also the sense of smell because the bones of the face serve to protect both senses.

Globe

The fluid-filled ball-shaped structure of the eye is the globe. It is the globe that receives the sensory information from the local environment and passes it along to the brain by way of the optic nerve. The globe is divided into two chambers, anterior and posterior, by the lens. The clear lens is an elastic structure suspended across the globe that serves to focus the image entering the eye through the anterior chamber by placing it on the wall of the posterior chamber, much as a lens on a camera manipulates an image to bring it into focus for a photographer. The white covering of the globe, the sclera, extends over the majority of the globe and becomes part of the optic nerve sheath at the posterior eye (Figure 16-3).

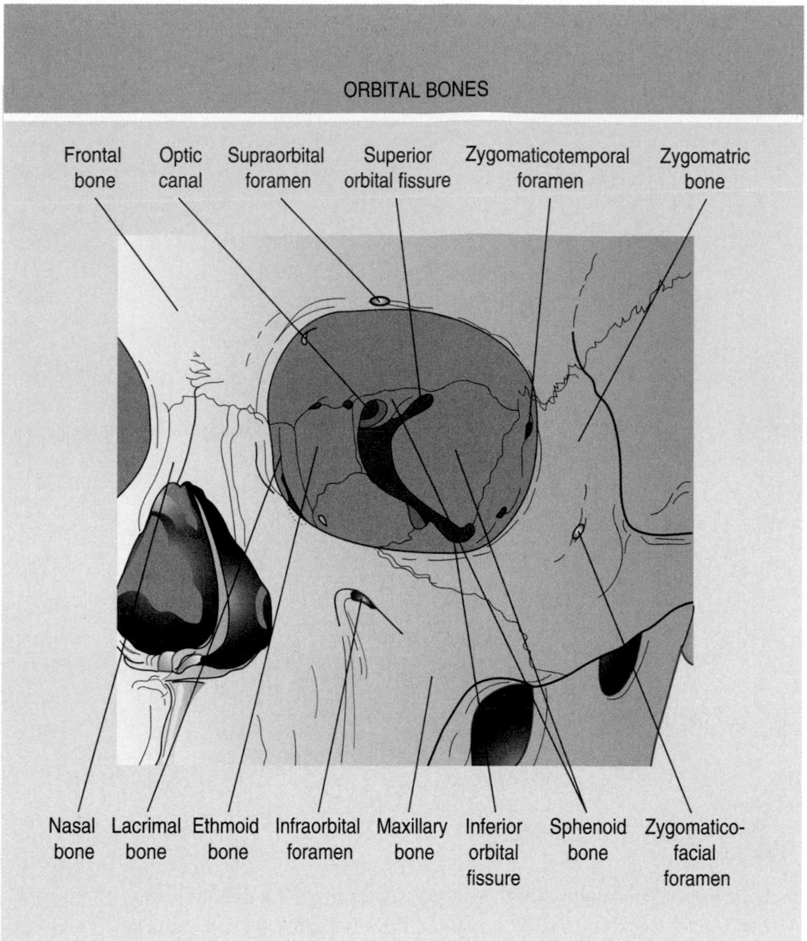

FIGURE 16-2 Bones of the eye orbit. (From Yanoff M, Duker J: *Ophthalmology,* ed 2, St Louis, 2004, Mosby. Redrawn from Dutton JJ: *Atlas of clinical and surgical orbital anatomy,* Philadelphia, 1994, Saunders.)

Anterior Chamber

The anterior chamber, the fluid-filled front part of the eye seen when the eyelids are open, initially receives stimulus from the local environment. The ring of color seen at the front of the globe, or iris, is a pigmented sphincter muscle that controls the amount of light entering the globe by way of the pupil, or dark central opening at the middle of the iris. In darker environments, the iris relaxes to allow more light to pass through the pupil. In brighter environments, the iris contracts to limit the passage of light. The pupils should be round and symmetrical in size when one eye is compared with the other. The speed or briskness of constriction and dilation should also be symmetrical in comparison.

symmetrical equal in size and shape
constriction process by which something becomes smaller in diameter
dilation process by which something becomes larger in diameter

Posterior Chamber

The posterior chamber of the globe processes the sensory information passed to it from the anterior chamber and prepares it for interpretation by the brain. The retina, or lining on the surface of the posterior chamber, contains a network of neurological tissue that eventually joins to form the optic nerve and exit the posterior eye. This neurological tissue is differentiated to respond to subtle differences in light and darkness to formulate an image to pass along to the visual centers of the brain. The image of the local environment that passes through the lens is focused on the retina and interpreted by this network to process colors, shades of light and darkness, and depth.

Muscles

It is important to assess the range of motion of the eye whenever it or the structures around it are injured. The rectus eye muscles—medial, inferior, lateral, and superior—provide movement of the globe in four directions, moving toward the contracting muscle. The oblique eye muscles—inferior and superior—contract to provide diagonal movement of the globe. When the rectus and oblique muscles work together, the globe

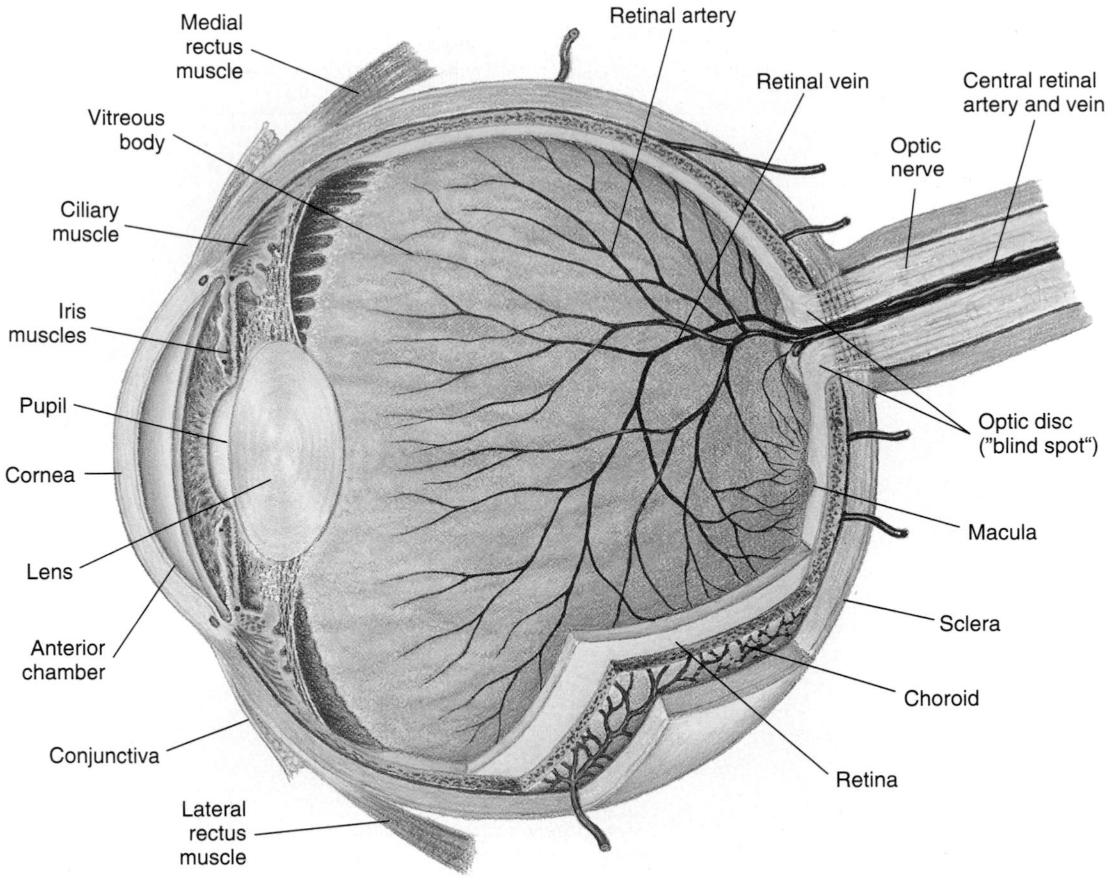

FIGURE 16-3 Pathway for the optic nerve. This diagram shows a cross-section of the eye, including the optic nerve as it exits the back of the eye going toward the brain. (From Seidel HM et al: *Mosby's guide to physical examination,* ed 6, p. 281, St Louis, 2006, Mosby/Elsevier.)

can be moved in circular motions. The two groups of extrinsic muscles give the globe a tremendous freedom of movement (Figure 16-4). Facial injuries near the eyes should be assessed for fractures that are often manifested by decreased range of motion of the eye. The small muscles of the eye can be trapped, and sometimes severed, by pieces of the fractured bone in the orbit surrounding the globe.

Eyelids

The eyelids serve to protect the globe from foreign bodies and keep the surface of the eye lubricated with the tears produced in the lacrimal gland. The highly vascular lining of the upper eyelid, the conjunctiva, reflects back to cover the front of the sclera and continues to reflect back to line the lower lid. Because the lids are highly vascular, the eyelids, like any other vascular area of the face, are subject to inflammation after trauma and can greatly distort the appearance of the eye region when they are injured.

Box 16-1 summarizes the major anatomy associated with sight.

ANATOMY OF HEARING

Like sight, the sense of hearing is the result of a complex process. As sound passes through the local environment, it is captured and funneled down the auditory canal. As the sound waves travel down the canal, they strike the eardrum, causing it to vibrate. These vibrations in turn cause the articulating chain of bones to vibrate and stimulate the neurological structures of the inner ear. Then, the mechanical energy of the sound waves converts to electrical energy and passes along the cochlear branch of the vestibulocochlear nerve to the brain (Figure 16-5).

Hearing may be affected at any point in this chain, and the problem may be either structural or neurological. Structural problems affecting the sense of hearing include the shape of the outer ear (e.g., the shape may prevent the sound waves from traveling to the eardrum) and damage to the eardrum itself (e.g., an injury may prevent vibrations from passing to the bones of the middle ear). Finally, neurological damage to the inner ear may prevent the passage of electrical signals from the ear to the brain.

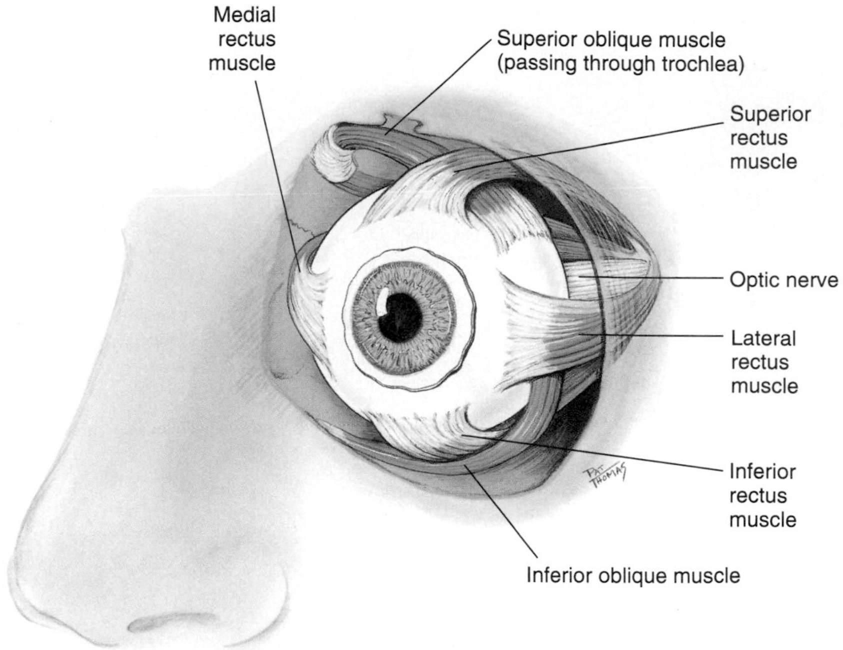

FIGURE 16-4 Muscles of the eye. (From Jarvis C: *Physical examination and health assessment,* ed 4, p. 299, Philadelphia, 2004, Elsevier/Saunders.)

Bones and Cartilage

The outer ear, or auricle, is composed of flexible cartilage. This cartilage funnels auditory stimulus to the inner ear by guiding it along the ridges and turns of the outer ear to the ear canal. The external cartilage is very flexible and easily deformed, but it returns to its normal shape quickly. This resilience allows the cartilage to maintain its shape and preserve its ability to aim sound waves correctly into the ear canal. When the shape of the outer ear is altered, the conduction of sound into the ear canal is also changed, which may result in hearing loss.

Three small bones—the malleus (hammer), incus (anvil), and stapes—form a chain extending from the tympanic membrane to the inner ear. These bones are extremely small and serve to pass along vibrations

BOX 16-1 Major Anatomy of Sight

Bones
- Orbit
  - Superior rim and part of lateral: frontal bone
  - Lateral border and some of inferior: zygomatic bone
  - Inferior border: maxillary bone
  - Posterior: sphenoid, lacrimal, and ethmoid bones

Globe
- Clear lens
- Sclera
- Anterior chamber
  - Iris
  - Pupil
  - Posterior chamber
  - Retina
  - Neurological tissue that forms optic nerve

Muscles
- Rectus muscles
  - Medial
  - Inferior
  - Lateral
  - Superior
- Oblique muscles
  - Inferior
  - Superior
- *Associated movements:* circular

Eyelids
- Conjunctiva

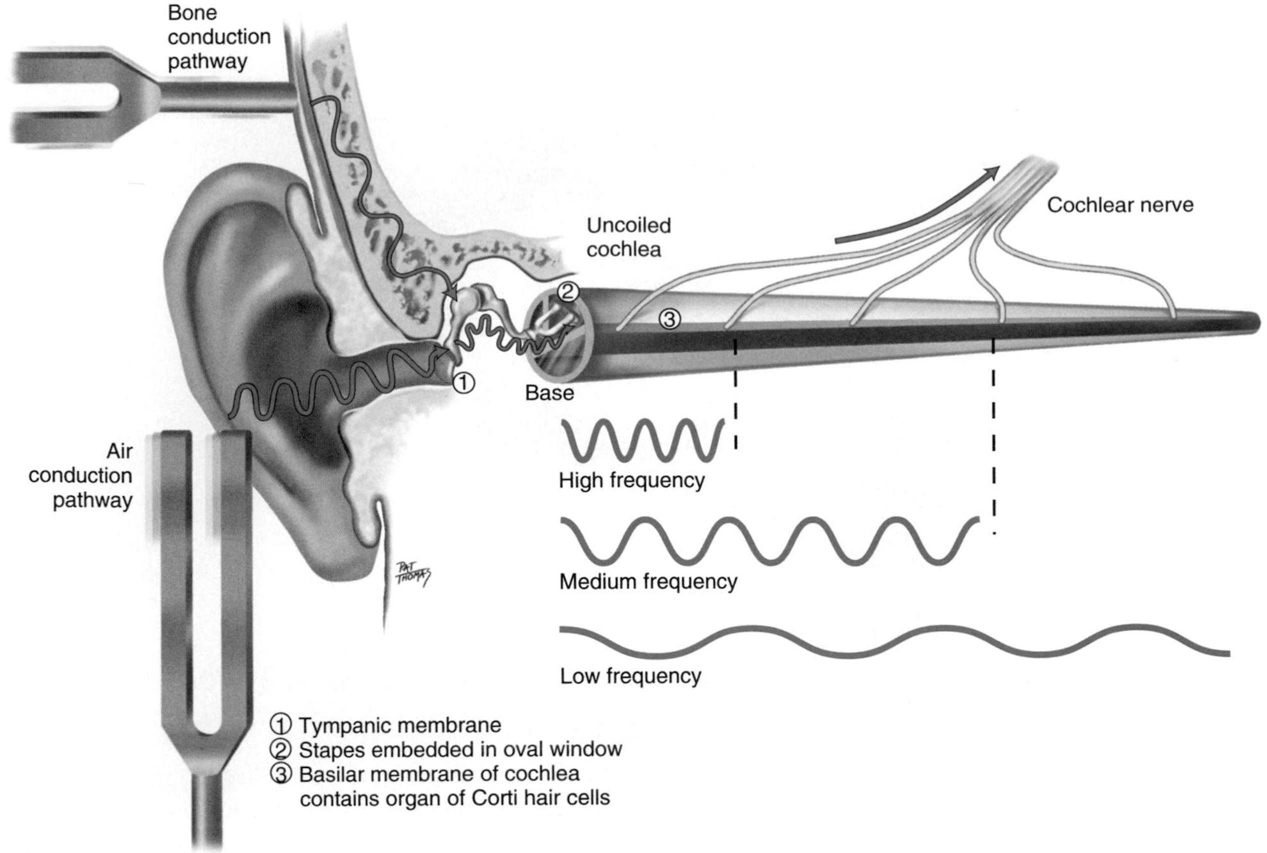

FIGURE 16-5 Diagram illustrating the pathways of hearing. (From Jarvis C: *Physical examination & health assessment,* ed 4, p. 344, Philadelphia, 2004, Elsevier/Saunders.)

from the membrane. As one bone vibrates, it triggers vibrations in the other bones in the chain until the vibrations are passed along to the vestibulocochlear system. (Figure 16-6).

Sections

The ear is divided into three sections, the outer, middle, and inner ear. The sections are discussed here in the order that sound impulses travel through them toward the brain.

Outer Ear

Known as the *auricle* or *pinna,* the outer ear is the part of the auditory system easily seen from outside the body. Sound is channeled down the auditory canal by way of the folds and ridges of the pinna and travels to the eardrum. The outer one third of the auditory canal contains hair follicles, sebaceous glands, and ceruminous glands. Ceruminous glands secrete a waxy reddish-brown substance called cerumen, commonly called *earwax.* This bacteriostatic substance protects the canal from excessive drying. The inner or more medial aspect of the canal does not contain the ceruminous glands, and this skin is more delicate than that which is more lateral in the canal (see Figure 16-6).

bacteriostatic not conducive to growth of bacteria

Points to Ponder

Given that the skin farther inside the ear is quite delicate and that the ceruminous glands are producing earwax to protect the auditory canal from infection and irritation, do you see why attempting to clean the ear canal with a cotton-tipped swab is potentially dangerous?

Middle Ear

The tympanic membrane, commonly called the *eardrum,* divides the outer ear from the middle ear. The eardrum is a thin membrane stretched across the auditory canal that vibrates as sound waves strike it. The vibration of the eardrum is passed along to the chain of bones in the ear. The eustachian tube extends inferiorly to connect the middle ear to the nasal passages and serves to regulate the pressure on the membrane from the middle ear (see Figure 16-6).

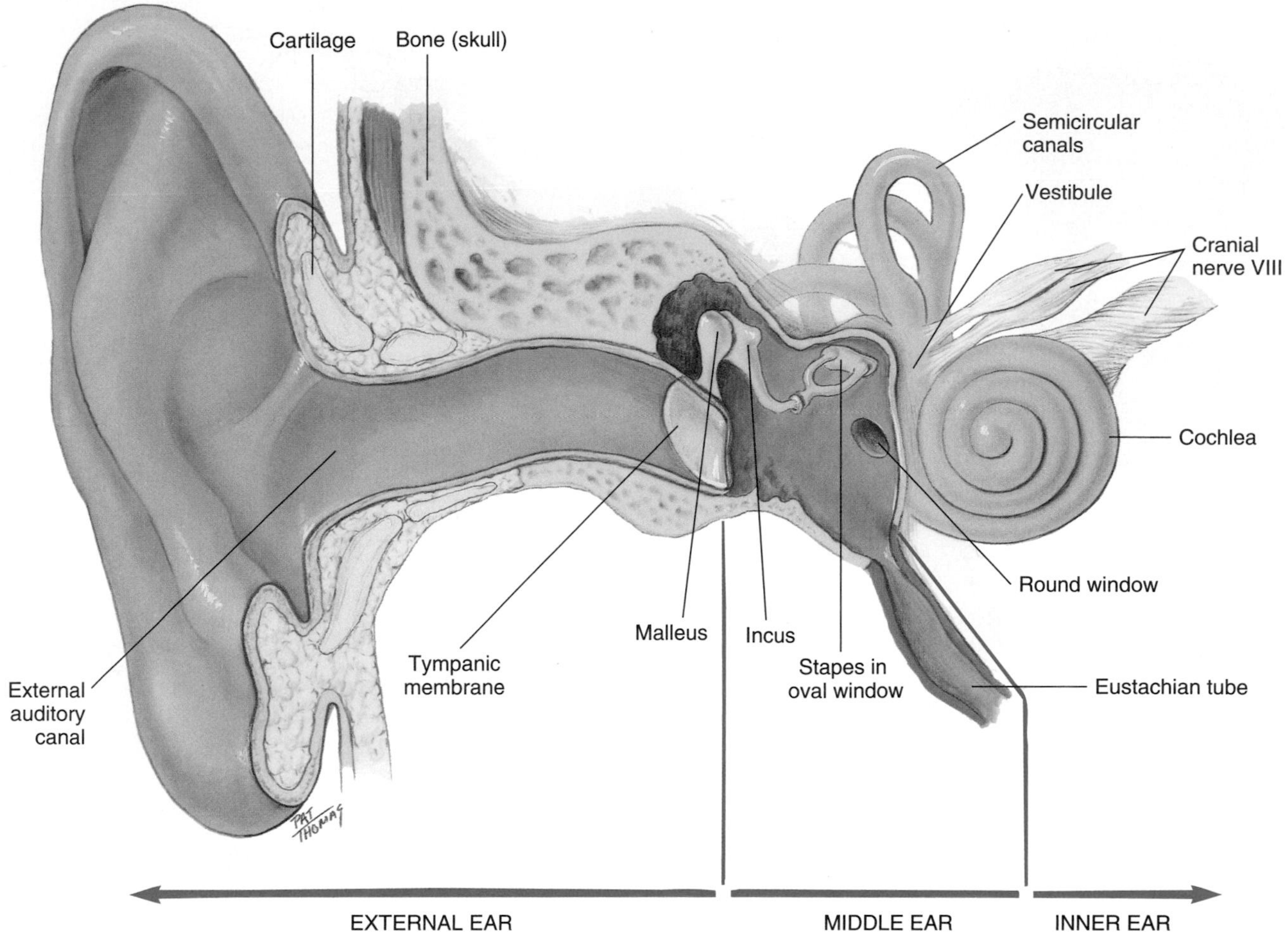

FIGURE 16-6 Internal anatomy of the ear. (From Jarvis C: *Physical examination and health assessment,* ed 4, p. 343, Philadelphia, 2004, Elsevier/Saunders.)

Inner Ear

In the inner ear, the mechanical energy generated in vibrations of the tympanic membrane and passed along the chain of bones is converted into electrical energy as their vibrations enter the neurological structures of the ear. The cochlea and semicircular canals are located within the temporal bone in a fluid-protected chamber. The stapes articulates with the cochlea, and its vibrations trigger impulses that travel to the brain for interpretation by way of the vestibulocochlear nerve. The semicircular canals are fluid-filled, and the fluid shifts with movement of the head. The location of the fluid in the canals is interpreted by the brain and assists in maintaining balance and proper posture of the head and body. As the fluid shifts, the pressure shifts inside the canals and informs the brain about the location of the head in relation to the ground (see Figure 16-6).

Box 16-2 summarizes the major anatomy associated with hearing.

ANATOMY OF TASTE

The surfaces in the mouth and throat known as taste buds control the sense of taste. The taste buds are

BOX 16-2 **Major Anatomy of Hearing**

Bones and Cartilage
- Flexible cartilage
  - Makes up outer ear
- Three small bones
  - Malleus (hammer bone)
  - Incus (anvil)
  - Stapes
  - Together, pass along vibrations from tympanic membrane to inner ear

Sections
- Outer ear
  - Folds and ridges
  - Hair follicles, sebaceous glands, ceruminous glands
- Middle ear
  - Tympanic membrane
  - Eustachian tube
- Inner ear
  - Cochlea
  - Semicircular canals

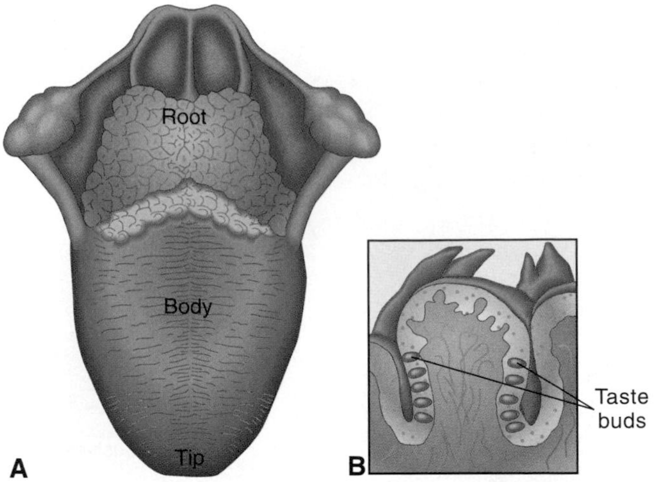

FIGURE 16-7 **A,** Parts of the tongue. **B,** A detailed site of a taste bud. (Modified from Thibodeau GA, Patton KT: *Anatomy & physiology*, ed 6, p. 562, St. Louis, 2007, Mosby/Elsevier.)

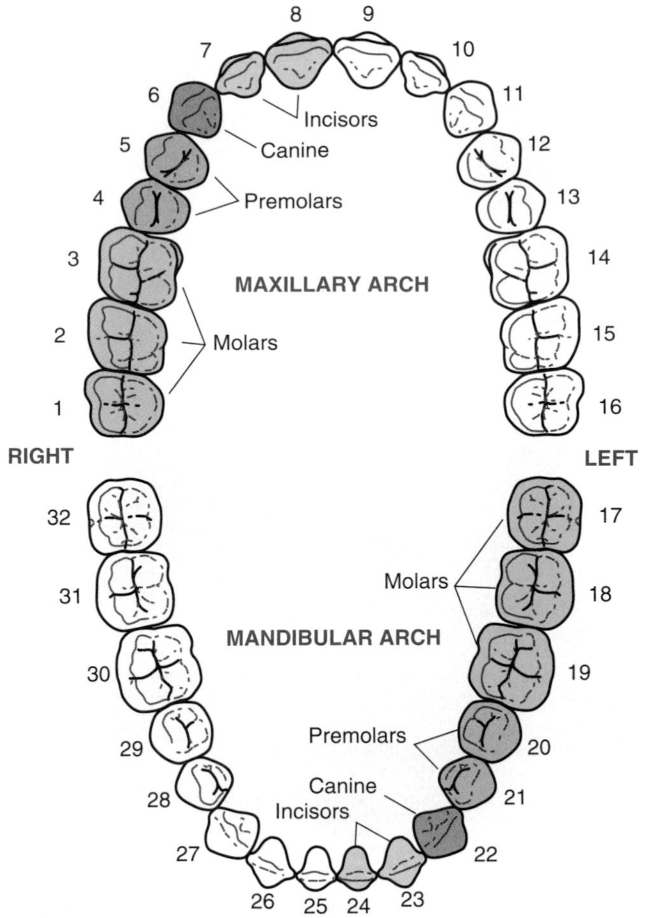

FIGURE 16-8 The adult typically has 32 teeth. (From Bath-Bahlogh, Fehrenbach MJ: *Illustrated dental embryology, histology, and anatomy*, ed 2, p. 234, Philadelphia, 2006, Saunders/Elsevier.)

located on the surface of the tongue, the soft palate, the uvula, and the first one third of the esophagus. These structures differentiate sweet, salty, and bitter flavors and relay this information to the brain. As substances pass over the taste buds, they trigger their respective interpretations, and this information is passed along to the brain and interpreted as a given taste. Taste buds are more abundant in childhood, and the number decreases in adulthood to around 10,000. The taste buds degenerate rapidly after age 45, and the sense of taste is dulled as the degeneration progresses (Figure 16-7). Much of the attributes of a food's taste are gained through smell, but the tongue provides a great deal of information to process with the information from the nose as all incoming stimuli are processed by the brain.

Bones

The primary bones of the mouth are the mandible, or lower jawbone, and the maxilla, or upper jawbone. Each bone holds a row of teeth that should approximate with its corresponding partner on the other bone. When the bones are damaged through fracture or dislocation, the alignment of the teeth will suffer. Mandibular fractures are the second most common facial fracture, second to nasal fractures. Because of the proximity to the nose, most maxillary fractures occur in tandem with nasal fractures.

Teeth

Adults generally have 32 permanent teeth, divided equally among the upper and lower jaws. Teeth are formed by dentin, a hard calcium-rich substance that is encased in an even harder enamel shell. The core of each tooth is known as the pulp and houses a neurovascular supply. The neurovascular vessels enter the tooth inferiorly through the root of the tooth that is embedded in the jaw. The teeth are divided into four groups: incisors, cuspids, bicuspids, and molars. The four incisors are used for cutting and are located at the front of the upper and lower rows. The two cuspids, also known as *canines*, are shaped for tearing and are located laterally from the incisors. The four bicuspids, or *premolars*, are farther back in the rows and are shaped for crushing and grinding as are the six molars, the teeth located farthest back in the jaw (Figure 16-8).

Muscles

Muscles in the mouth serve one of two functions: (1) chewing, or mastication, and (2) expression. The muscle with the primary action to close the mouth is the masseter, which stretches from the mandibular angle to the zygomatic arch. Several muscles act in concert to open the mouth, including the digastric, medial pterygoid, mylohyoid, and lateral pterygoid. Muscles of expression act on the lips and help form smiles, frowns, and other expressions as well as change the shape of the lips for enunciation of speech. These muscles generally act in symmetry, and any asymmetry should be evaluated as a possible injury or illness.

Box 16-3 summarizes the major anatomy associated with taste.

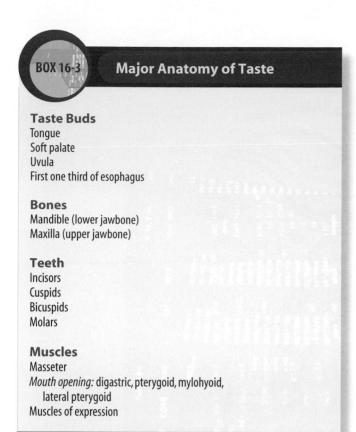

BOX 16-3 Major Anatomy of Taste

Taste Buds
Tongue
Soft palate
Uvula
First one third of esophagus

Bones
Mandible (lower jawbone)
Maxilla (upper jawbone)

Teeth
Incisors
Cuspids
Bicuspids
Molars

Muscles
Masseter
Mouth opening: digastric, pterygoid, mylohyoid, lateral pterygoid
Muscles of expression

ANATOMY OF SMELL

Receptors in the olfactory (smell-related) centers of the nose react to various stimulants in the inhaled air. Extremely small hairs, or cilia, line the interior of the nose, forming a mat in the mucous layer, but are still stimulated by the air that passes across them during inhalation. Various stimulants have different thresholds for recognition; therefore some smells seem stronger than others because they are recognized at a much lower threshold than others. As a person becomes accustomed to a smell, the threshold may be raised—in fact, the smell may not even be noticed when re-introduced at a later time. The cilia are stimulated in much the same way that taste buds are stimulated in the mouth and relay their message to the brain to be interpreted as a given smell (Figure 16-9).

Bones and Cartilage

The nasal bones are the most commonly fractured bones in the face. The **proximal** end of the nose is composed of bone, and the **distal** end of the nose is flexible cartilage. The nose is composed of two sections, right and left, that meet along their medial borders to form the nasion. The distal end of the nose is composed of cartilage covered in skin. Each section of the flaring cartilage is called an ala. The cartilage dividing the nose into two distinct longitudinal sections is the septum, which serves to divide the opening of the nose into two nostrils, or nares. The interior roof of the nose is separated from the rest of the skull by the cribriform plate. This plate is perforated with many small holes, which allow the olfactory nerve to pass information to the brain. This cribriform plate is the primary structure separating the cranial cavity from infection in the outside environment (Figure 16-10).

Blood Supply

The face in general is a very vascular part of the body, and the abundant vessels in the nose cause copious bleeding when a traumatic injury occurs. The area where these vessels converge in the anterior nose is known as Kiesselbach's area and is the source of profuse bleeding when a nosebleed or nasal fracture occurs (Figure 16-11). Controlling the bleeding from this area is the primary treatment goal after a traumatic injury. The athletic trainer may consider placing a rolled gauze under the top lip inside the mouth to decrease blood flow through this area and limit the scope of an injury.

Box 16-4 summarizes the major anatomy associated with the sense of smell.

INTERACTION OF THE SENSES

The senses all have their own identities and offer specific information to the brain, but they also work in concert to provide a "bigger picture" of our environment. Sight and hearing complement each other as do taste and smell. Interrelation of the senses ensures that a constant stream of information is available for the brain. This constant availability of information creates a more vivid and vibrant picture of the environment.

Sight and Hearing

The senses of sight and hearing both contribute to balance and coordination by processing information from the local environment and sending it to the brain for interpretation as to proper positioning and **proprioception** of the body. Each system contributes information, and the brain can function adequately without input from one system or the other, but when an injury or illness occurs, the information available from a single sense may be misleading. This inappropriate interpretation manifests itself as dizziness, or vertigo, or poor coordination. The eyes work together to process information regarding distance, depth perception, and shadows to give the brain a three-dimensional picture of the local environment. The ears, in the vestibulocochlear

proximal closer to the midline or center of the body relative to another landmark
distal farther away from the body's midline or center relative to another landmark
proprioception an individual's awareness of position, movement, and muscle tension

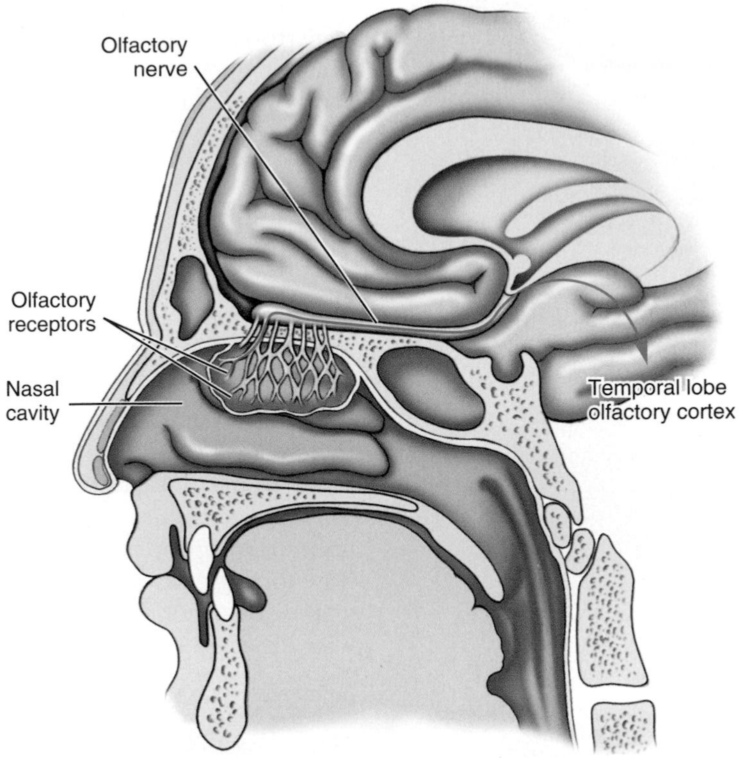

FIGURE 16-9 The sense of smell. (From Herlihy B: *The human body in health and illness,* ed 3, p. 221, Philadelphia, 2007, Saunders/Elsevier.)

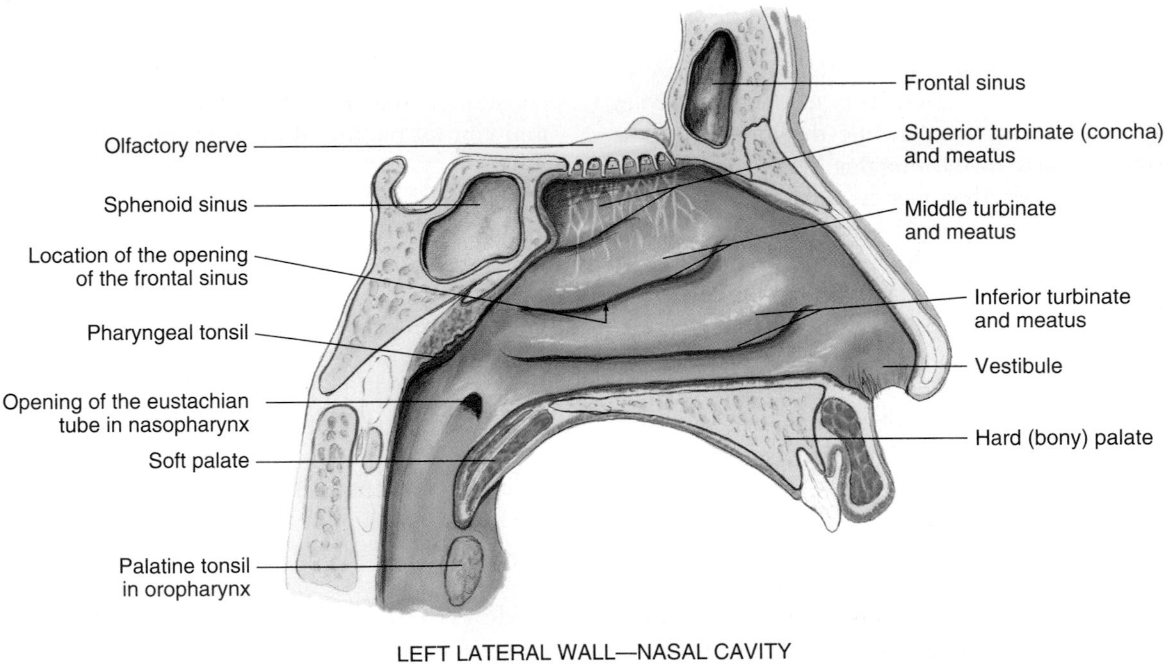

FIGURE 16-10 The interior anatomy of the nose. (From Jarvis C: *Physical examination and health assessment,* ed 4, p. 373, Philadelphia, 2004, Elsevier/Saunders.)

areas, give the brain information about the body's position, and the brain cross-references that information with the data received from the eyes.

Taste and Smell

The senses of taste and smell both process information about the food we eat and drink. Problems with adequate smell and taste affect our food choices and therefore can affect weight gain or loss. A person with a nose injury and diminished sense of smell will often report a decrease in taste as well. This decrease is not because of an injury to the sense of taste but because much of the stimuli present in the person's food choices were actually processed by the sense of smell. When

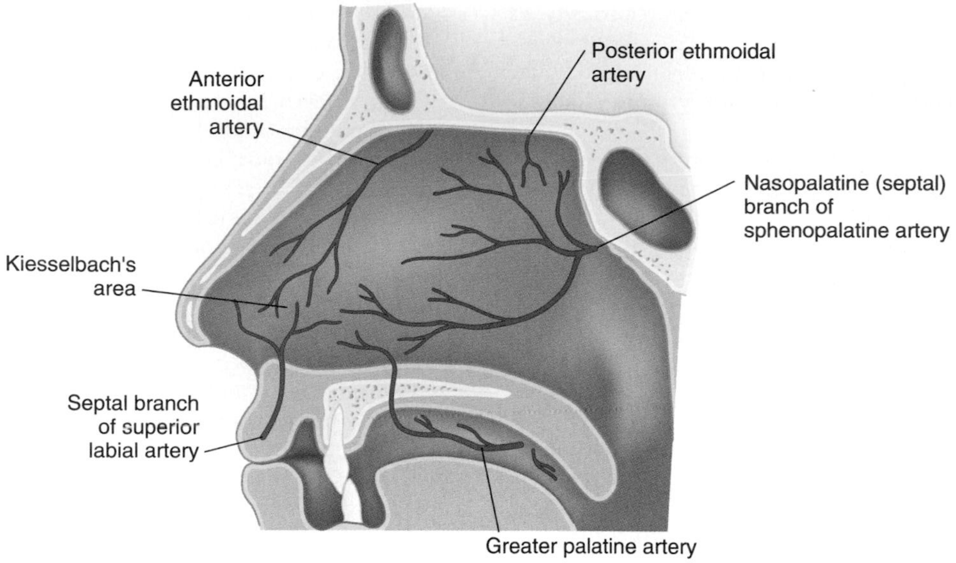

FIGURE 16-11 Kiesselbach's area of the nose as part of a drawing illustrating the arterial supply to the medial wall of the nose. (From Marx J, Hockburger R, Walls R: *Rosen's emergency medicine: concept and clinical practice,* ed 6, Figure 71-1, St Louis, 2006, Mosby.)

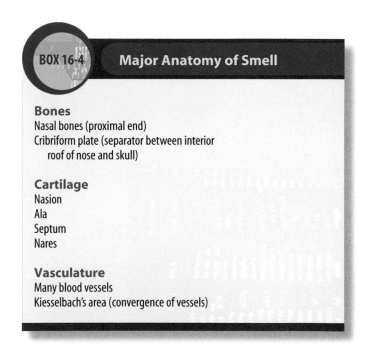

BOX 16-4 Major Anatomy of Smell

Bones
Nasal bones (proximal end)
Cribriform plate (separator between interior roof of nose and skull)

Cartilage
Nasion
Ala
Septum
Nares

Vasculature
Many blood vessels
Kiesselbach's area (convergence of vessels)

both systems are integrated in the information they process to the brain, the stimuli from the food are easily recognized and appreciated. If one system is affected, the overall deficit leads to a noticeable change in that recognition. For this same reason, a person with an upper respiratory infection will often complain that food is unappetizing.

SUMMARY

Injuries to the senses may seem mild, but they can be very debilitating when they disrupt activities of daily living. By understanding the anatomy of the senses, the athletic trainer will have a better appreciation of mechanisms of injury and be better prepared to map out a treatment plan. Physician referral is common, and the appropriate disciplines include otolaryngology (ear, nose, and throat physician), family practice, and sometimes even orthopedists or neurologists. Because of the dramatic presentation of injuries to these specialized structures (e.g., copious bleeding, obvious deformity, disruption of normal activities), underlying trauma is sometimes overlooked. By understanding the involved anatomy, the athletic trainer can assess the pathology of superficial and underlying structures and make more informed decisions about treatment, referral, and return to play.

Points to Ponder
How should the athletic trainer respond to an individual with an injury or illness that affects smell and/or taste who makes nutrition choices on the basis of an item's taste or lack thereof?

Web Links

American Academy of Otolaryngology—Head and Neck Surgery: www.entnet.org
The Anatomy Lesson: http://mywebpages.comcast.net/wnor/homepage.htm
American Dental Association: www.ada.org
American Ophthalmology Association: www.aao.org
Anatomy on the Internet: www.meddean.luc.edu/lumen/MedEd/GrossAnatomy/anatomy.htm
Body Worlds Project: www.koerperwelten.de/en/pages/home.asp

Medical Gross Anatomy Learning Resources (University of Michigan): http://anatomy.med.umich.edu/

Muscles of the Face (PowerPoint presentation): http://ferl.becta.org.uk/content_files/ferl/resources/colleges/filton/resources/facialmuscles.ppt

The Visible Human Project (National Library of Medicine, National Institutes of Health): www.nlm.nih.gov/research/visible/visible_human.html

WebAnatomy (University of Minnesota): www.msjensen.gen.umn.edu/webanatomy

Bibliography

Applegate E: *The Anatomy and physiology learning system*, ed 3, Philadelphia, 2006, Elsevier/Saunders.

Booher JM, Thibodeau GA: *Athletic injury assessment*, ed 4, Boston, 2000, McGraw-Hill.

Bromley SM: Smell and taste disorders: a primary care approach, *American Family Physician*, [serial online] 61(2), 2000. Retrieved March 6, 2007, from www.aafp.org/afp/20000115/427.html

Cuppett M, Walsh KM: *General medical conditions in the athlete*, St Louis, 2005, Elsevier/Mosby.

Drake RL, Vogl W, Mitchell ADM: *Gray's anatomy for students*, Edinburgh, 2005, Elsevier/Churchill Livingstone.

Guyton AC: *Human physiology and mechanisms of disease*, ed 4, Philadelphia, 1987, Saunders.

Herlihy B: *The human body in health and illness*, ed 3, Philadelphia, 2007, Saunders/Elsevier.

Moses KP, et al: *Atlas of clinical gross anatomy*, St Louis, 2005, Elsevier/Mosby.

Muscolino JE: *Kinesiology: the skeletal system and muscle function*, St Louis, 2006, Mosby/Elsevier.

Neumann D: *Kinesiology of the skeletal system: foundations for physical therapy*, St Louis, 2002, Elsevier/Mosby.

Pichichero ME: Acute otitis media. Part I: Improving diagnostic accuracy, *American Family Physician*, 61: 2051–2059, 2000.

Romeo SJ, et al: Facial injuries in sports: a team physician's guide to diagnosis and treatment, *The Physician and Sports Medicine* [serial online] 33(4) 2005. Retrieved March 6, 2006, from www.physsportsmed.com/issues/2005/0405/romeo.htm

Sander R: Otitis externa: a practical guide to treatment and prevention, *American Family Physician*, 63: 927–936, 2001.

Seidel HM, et al: *Mosby's guide to physical examination*, ed 6, St Louis, 2006, Elsevier/Mosby.

Starkey C, Ryan J: *Evaluation of orthopedic and athletic injuries*, ed 2, Philadelphia, 2002, FA Davis.

Thibodeau GA, Patton KT: *Anatomy and physiology*, ed 6, St Louis, 2007, Mosby/Elsevier.

17

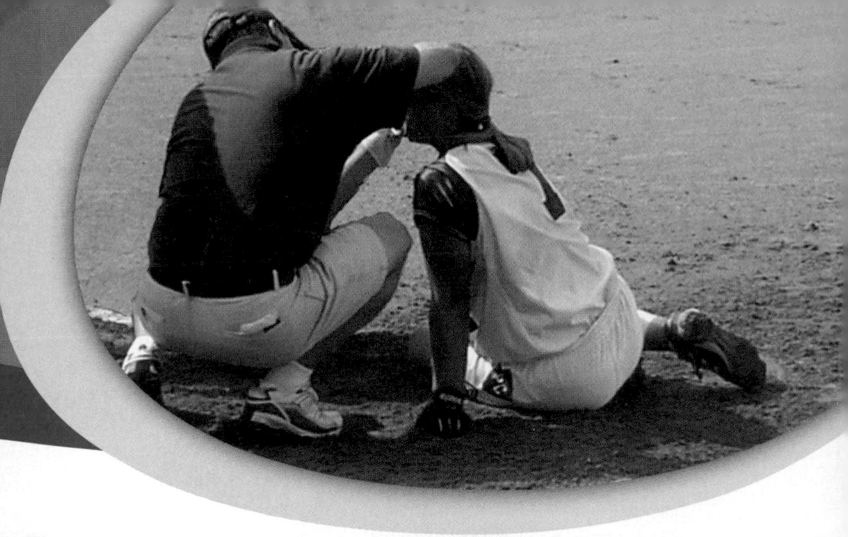

Diagnosis and Management of Injuries to the Senses

PAUL HIGGS

Learning Goals

1. Learn to assess injuries and illnesses of the face that involve the senses of sight, smell, taste, and hearing.
2. Learn proper techniques to triage these injuries during on-field evaluations and off-field management.
3. Learn proper techniques to care for these injuries, limit their scope, and promote healing.
4. Learn appropriate decision-making processes related to return to play criteria for injuries and illnesses involving the senses.
5. Learn when to refer these injuries to the appropriate physician.

This chapter covers the evaluation and treatment of injuries and illnesses that affect the senses, primarily the sense organs of the face. Athletic trainers should not underestimate the impact of these pathological conditions, which can greatly affect a person's daily activities in a completely different manner than most orthopedic injuries. It is imperative to understand that these problems must be evaluated accurately, treated properly, and referred appropriately when indicated. Injuries to the senses are often so striking that they distract the clinician from a less obvious, but possibly more serious, injury. The athletic trainer should be extremely careful to assess the entire face and all of the senses for any injury before allowing the athlete to return to full participation. Figure 17-1 summarizes the major types of injuries affecting sight, hearing, taste, and smell.

> **Points to Ponder**
> Injuries to the senses often have a shocking appearance, and the symptoms of some obvious injuries (e.g., copious bleeding, clear deformity) sometimes overshadow less obvious, but sometimes more serious, secondary injuries. How do you project a calm demeanor and professional outlook when you are really thinking, "Wow, that is really gross and must hurt a lot!"?

CLINICAL EVALUATION OF CONDITIONS THAT AFFECT THE SENSES

Conditions that affect the senses should be evaluated using a systematic evaluation very similarly to the scheme used in assessment of orthopedic injuries. Using the HIPS/HOPS model outlined in other chapters, the athletic trainer can ascertain valuable information about the condition and make the best decisions about caring for that condition.

The senses can be affected through traumatic injury or through a non-traumatic action such as an illness or infection. Both types of problems, traumatic and non-traumatic, should be thoroughly evaluated to prevent any long-term damage and disability to the senses.

History

As with any injury or illness, obtaining a thorough history in an efficient and systematic manner will result in an accurate diagnosis and the formulation of

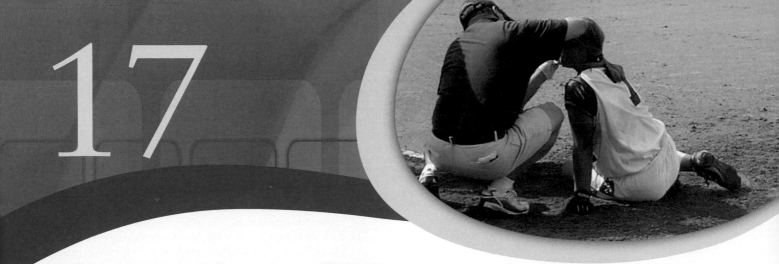

OPENING *Scenario*

In a close play at home, Karen is struck in the face as she successfully tags the opponent, forcing the last out in the final inning of a collegiate softball game. Because she has removed her catcher's mask at the beginning of the play, the collision at home has left her with a severely injured nose. It is her senior year, and this incredible play has secured her team its first-ever spot in the regional finals. On the basis of your evaluation, you suspect that Karen has suffered a fractured nose. A trip to the local emergency room confirms this suspicion. The physician tells Karen that she can continue to play the remainder of the season as long as her nose is protected. Although it is not a career-threatening injury by any means, performing the role of catcher will be difficult for her. The catcher's mask will protect her injured nose from further impact, but she must frequently remove her mask during the game to make certain plays that require a full field of vision. Because she must remove the mask quickly, it will be difficult to protect her nose. She wants to play very much, and her talent and leadership contribute greatly to the success of the team. The next game is less than 24 hours away.

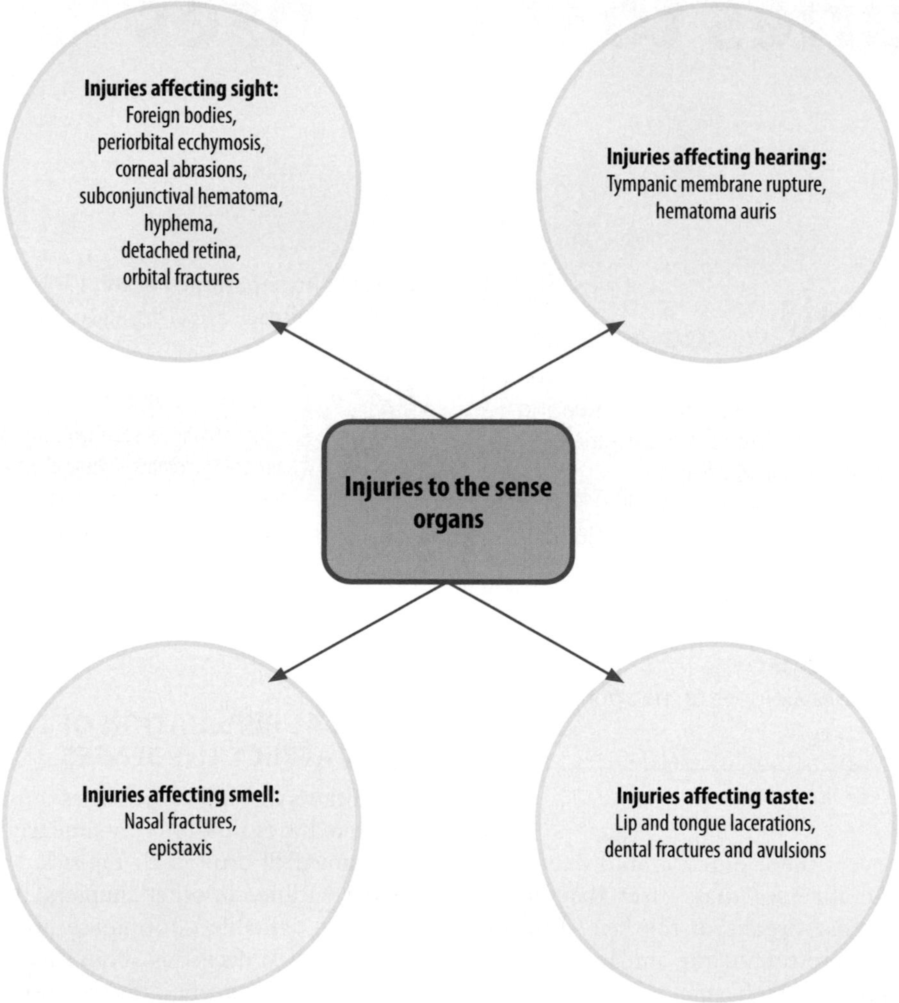

FIGURE 17-1 Concept map summarizing injuries to the senses of sight, hearing, smell, and taste.

an appropriate treatment or referral plan. The athletic trainer should use open-ended questions to determine any mechanism of injury or history of exposure to an irritant, illness, or other problem that would result in a condition that affects the senses. Most injuries that affect the senses have a readily identifiable mechanism and the cause and effect connection is very clear. However, in the case of an infection or other illness that affects the senses, the cause may not be so easy to identify. At times, no clear cause can be identified at all. However, the athletic trainer must make every attempt to determine the cause of the condition by questioning the patient about past medical history as well as current injury and illness risks and exposures.

Inspection and Observation

Inspection and observation of conditions that affect the senses can at times be overwhelming. Injuries and illnesses to the eyes, ears, nose, and tongue can have a tremendous "wow factor" and be quite startling at times with great swelling, discoloration, deformity, or bleeding. These symptoms are more common with acute injuries than with illnesses, yet the symptoms of even some illnesses can be quite surprising themselves. The athletic trainer should be aware of this possibility and not be distracted by the symptoms to the point that an underlying trauma or pathology is overlooked. Any trauma great enough to cause significant bleeding or deformity of the superficial sense organs and structures is often great enough to cause significant injury to other underlying structures of the face.

Most of the sense organs—eyes, ears, and nostrils of the nose– appear in pairs and the damaged side can easily be compared to the uninjured side to determine the extent of an injury or illness. Even the tongue has two sides that should appear symmetrical and damage to one side is easy to notice when compared to the uninjured side. As with most parts of the body, normal variations occur and the athletic trainer will need to appreciate the wide variety of "normal" presentations before referring a patient to a physician for evaluation of something that may be entirely normal.

Palpation

Palpation is a form of observation using the hands to assess the stability of the underlying structures in an area. Again, the presence of paired sense organs or structures makes it easy to determine normal from abnormal anatomy and appearance. The athletic trainer should palpate the injured side as well as the uninjured side to determine the presence of deformity, pain, crepitus, or altered sensation. Any of these symptoms should be further assessed to determine their cause and referred to a physician if they do not resolve quickly. Because the sense organs and structures are very close to each other, a condition involving one area may influence another area. Therefore, structures at the site of the condition should be assessed along with those structures nearby. An injury to the eye can impact the nose, and an injury to the nose can also have an impact on taste.

Range of Motion Testing

The eyes and tongue are the only sense organs that can be voluntarily moved in most people. When an injury or illness occurs to one of these structures, an assessment of normal motion can tell the athletic trainer about damage to muscles or nerves that supply the area. Measurement by instrumentation is not necessary. The athletic trainer can ask the patient to move the area all normal planes of motion and document any areas lacking full motion.

General Guidelines for Referral to Physicians

Many injuries to the senses can be treated without medical intervention, but some cases require referral for further evaluation and stabilization. In short, a physician should evaluate any illness or traumatic injury that diminishes the ability of the senses. If not appropriately and promptly treated, damage to the senses could be irreversible.

Any condition that lessens the field of vision or compromises sight should be referred to a physician. Pupils should be evaluated using the acronym *PEARL,* which stands for "pupils equal and reactive to light." In other words, the pupils constrict and dilate with the addition or removal of light, respectively, and the pupils always react as a pair (i.e., when one pupil is exposed to a bright light, the other should also constrict).

An ophthalmologist or neurologist should evaluate conditions of the eye that include **nystagmus**, anisocoria, or flashes/floaters; these symptoms may indicate a more serious condition and greater risk of permanent dysfunction. Complaints of double vision, blurred vision, or altered ability to focus warrant referral for further evaluation as well.

Any condition that forces the athlete to keep the eye closed for protection (e.g., foreign bodies) or closed because of pain (e.g., foreign bodies, corneal abrasion, conjunctivitis) warrants referral; such an injury prevents normal participation in activities of daily living and may actually increase the risk of further injury by creating a "blind side." This blind side interferes with the athlete's ability to react to normal situations in his or her sport and protect the rest of the body from further injury.

A physician should evaluate conditions that affect the sense of hearing. Any trauma that involves drainage of blood or cerebrospinal fluid from the ears should be evaluated as soon as possible because it could indicate serious internal injury to the brain. Any hearing impairment subsequent to trauma or illness should be further evaluated, as should any presence of vertigo, or dizziness. A physician should remove from the ear canal any foreign bodies that could not be easily removed by the athletic trainer. Battle's sign, or ecchymosis at the mastoid process following a head injury, indicates skull or brain trauma and warrants immediate referral to a physician.

nystagmus "dancing eyes"; a symptom of eye injury in which the globe moves erratically, appearing to bounce or shake when following an object moving across the field of vision

Injuries with bleeding that cannot be controlled, such as some lip or mouth lacerations, may require suturing. Conditions that limit the normal senses of smell or taste may not be catastrophic but nonetheless require medical evaluation because they may signal some type of neurological trauma or underlying pathology.

If the senses are unaffected, the degree of inconvenience and the risk of spreading any infection dictate the necessity of referral. A common cold is a nuisance, but with proper hygiene and good common sense, the risk of spreading the infection is minimized. Highly contagious infections warrant prompt referral to a physician so that they do not spread to others.

Diagnostic Tests and Imaging

Ophthalmoscope. An **ophthalmoscope** is an instrument used to view the interior of the eye. A light source shines through a variety of lenses to provide an optimal view of the eye structures. The magnification power of the lens is measured in positive or negative lenses, or diopters, and may be set by the clinician. The ophthalmoscope contains various types of lights and lenses that will allow assessment of the interior eye in a variety of ways. The athletic trainer looks through the lens into the eye of the athlete. The ophthalmoscope is held steady against the orbit of the clinician. The athletic trainer should use the right eye and hold the scope with the right hand when assessing the right eye of the athlete; similarly, the left hand and left eye are used when assessing the left eye of the athlete. The handle is normally held so that it is pointing laterally during assessment. (Figure 17-2).

The light of the ophthalmoscope should not be shined directly into the front of the eye but should be shined diagonally into the front chamber of the eye. The bright light may be slightly uncomfortable for the athlete, and the pupil will constrict to protect the eye and hinder visualization of the posterior chamber. The light should gradually be drawn closer to the eye from a distance of approximately 1 foot. If the light is shined into the posterior chamber from a lateral position, the pupil is less likely to constrict. By viewing the interior of the eye, the athletic trainer should be able to assess the integrity of the blood vessels on the retinal lining.

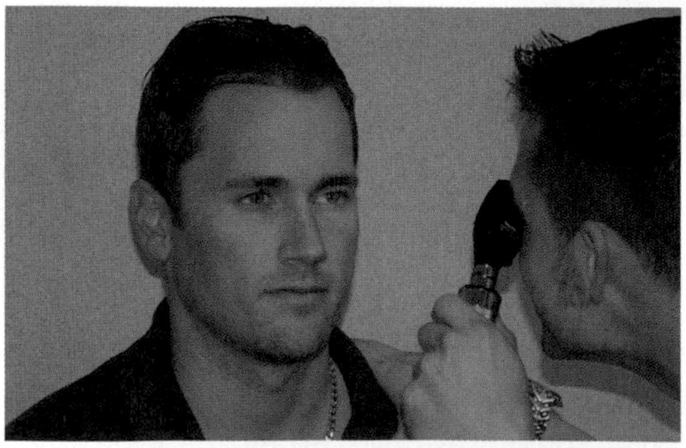

FIGURE 17-2 Proper assessment technique using an ophthalmoscope. (From Cuppett M, Walsh KM: *General medical conditions in the athlete,* p. 21, St Louis, 2005, Elsevier/Mosby.)

Otoscope. An **otoscope** is an instrument used to view the interior of the ear. It is used to confirm or rule out a clinician's opinion formulated during the history assessment. A light source is focused to view the auditory canal and tympanic membrane (Figure 17-3). Some otoscopes include an integrated pneumatic device that allows the clinician to test the integrity of the tympanic membrane. The tympanic membrane should be easily viewed with the otoscope and should appear a translucent pearly gray color, with no deformities such as tears, perforations, or bulging (Figure 17- 4). It is important to assess not only the color of the tympanic membrane but also its position and mobility. These factors, combined with color, give a better impression of the integrity and health of the tympanic membrane. Trauma to this delicate tissue is relatively easy to identify and should be assessed with any trauma or illness involving the ear.

In addition to searching for trauma to the tympanic membrane, the clinician should also use the otoscope to look for any abnormal nodes or lesions in the auditory canal. The presence of cerebrospinal fluid in the canal signifies an emergency and warrants immediate referral to a physician. Excessive buildup of cerumen

ophthalmoscope instrument used to view the interior of the eye
otoscope instrument used to view the interior of the ear

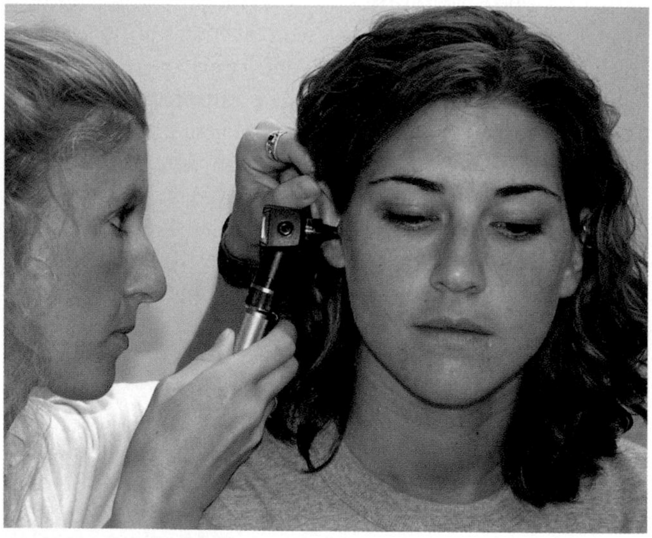

FIGURE 17-3 Proper use of an otoscope to examine the inner structures of the ear. (From Cuppett M, Walsh KM: *General medical conditions in the athlete,* p. 248, St Louis, 2005, Elsevier/Mosby.)

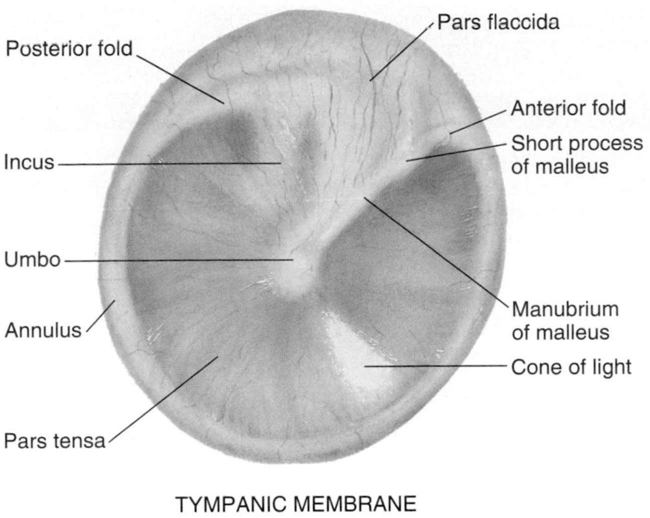

FIGURE 17-4 The anatomical landmarks of the normal tympanic membrane. (From Jarvis C: *Physical examination and health assessment,* ed 4, p. 343, Philadelphia, 2004, Saunders.)

can significantly impede the visualization of the canal and membrane. In the event of suspected infection, the uninvolved ear should be assessed first to prevent any cross-contamination from the involved ear.

Imaging. Most diagnostic imaging techniques, including plain film radiography, magnetic resonance imaging (MRI), and computed tomography (CT) scans can be beneficial in assessment of conditions affecting the senses. Plain film radiography, x-rays, is useful in determining damage to the bones of the area, but the other more sophisticated techniques of MRI and CT are useful in assessing the integrity and stability of the non-bone structures in the area such as neurological structures, blood vessels, and cartilage.

Functional Testing for the Senses

Injuries to the senses often cause loss of normal function. The only way to assess the degree of dysfunction is through functional testing. Just as evaluation of orthopedic injuries includes a series of drills or movements to determine the extent of trauma, evaluation of injuries to the senses must also be sufficiently thorough to assess loss of function.

Cranial Nerve Assessment

Assessment of the cranial nerves should be a part of every evaluation with injuries involving the senses. Because the cranial nerves control many functions of the face, they have a direct impact on the senses. Loss of a sense may be traumatic. Bleeding in the nose may block the sense of smell even when the neurological pathways to the brain from the nose are intact. Also, inflammation from facial trauma may cause the eyelid and other structures around the eye to swell to the point that vision is blocked. Other losses may be due to neurological damage. In these cases, nerves are damaged and the pathways to the brain are compromised. These nerves could be damaged by sharp fracture fragments or through the pressure of edema in the surrounding tissue.

The nerves primarily responsible for the senses in the face are the cranial nerves. By testing the reception of the sensory stimulus to the brain, the athletic trainer can assess the integrity of the cranial nerve system. Trauma that damages the cranial nerve system reveals itself in many ways, including **anisocoria**; dysfunctional pupil (e.g., **diplopia, photophobia**); and an altered sense of taste, smell, or hearing. Even slurred speech caused by uncoordinated tongue control could be a signal of an underlying neurological pathology. All of these symptoms indicate neurological damage involving the cranial nerves and should be assessed by a physician. Table 17-1 summarizes the cranial nerves and the functional testing associated with each.

Vision Assessment

Reflexes. Several reflexes exist in a healthy eye, and verification of these reflexes during an evaluation helps confirm the neurological integrity of the sense of sight. A **reflex** is a predictable, involuntary, neurological response to a stimulus. The reflexes of the eye are largely present to protect the eye from injury, but they also indicate the integrity of the neurological controls present in the eye. When a reflex is absent, diminished, or asymmetrical, the likelihood of significant injury increases. The most easily observed reflex is the blink reflex, which causes the eyelids to cover the globe whenever something either touches the anterior globe or threatens to touch it.

The pupil has its own set of reflexes. The most obvious reflex involving the pupil is the light reflex, also known as the *pupillary reflex*. As a penlight is shined into the eye from a close range, the pupil of that eye should constrict or become smaller. As the light is decreased or removed, the pupil should dilate or enlarge. The more quickly the light is introduced or reduced, the more quickly the pupils will respond by dilating or constricting. When testing this reflex, the athletic trainer should always shield the other eye from the light source because of the consensual reflex dictating that one pupil will mimic, or consent, to the actions of the other pupil. Shining

anisocoria unequal pupil size, usually indicating neurological damage to the eye or brain
diplopia medical term for double vision
photophobia literally "fear of light;" refers to intense eye discomfort during exposure to bright light
reflex a predictable, involuntary, neurological response to a stimulus

TABLE 17-1 Cranial Nerve Function and Testing

SOURCE	NAME	FUNCTION/SENSE	TESTING
CN I	Olfactory	Smell	Smell an alcohol prep pad, tape adherent spray, or analgesic ointment.
CN II	Optic	Sight	Snellen chart: Read the time or score on the game clock; read the print on a gauze or medication packet.
CN III	Oculomotor	Pupil reaction	Penlight is used to assess constriction and dilation of pupils.
CN IV	Trochlear	Eye movement	Eye movement is tracked.
CN V	Trigeminal	Chewing; facial and tongue sensation	Chewing and touch discrimination on forehead, lips, and lower jaw are assessed.
CN VI	Abducens	Eye movement	Lateral eye movement ability is noted.
CN VII	Facial	Taste; facial expression	Expressions (e.g., smiling, frowning) and taste (e.g., candy, sports drink, antacid) are assessed.
CN VIII	Vestibulocochlear	Balance; hearing	Balance (eyes open and closed) and hearing (e.g., paper crumpling; game sounds, cell phone ringers) are assessed.
CN IX	Glossopharyngeal	Taste	Taste (e.g., candy, sports drink, antacid) is assessed.
CN X	Vagus	Swallowing	Drinking ability is assessed.
CN XI	Accessory	Trapezius and sternocleidomastoid movement	Athlete shrugs shoulders.
CN XII	Hypoglossal	Tongue movement	Athlete sticks out the tongue.

From Cuppett M, Walsh KM: *General medical conditions in the athlete,* p. 27, St Louis, 2005, Elsevier/Mosby.

light into the right eye will also cause the left pupil to constrict. The left pupil reflex may appear intact simply because it is mimicking the actions of the right pupil to a light source.

Snellen Chart. Vision can be assessed through the use of a **Snellen chart** (Figure 17-5), a simple eye chart that features a series of characters (e.g., letters, symbols) The athlete is placed 20 feet away from the chart and instructed to read a designated row of characters. The degree of accuracy with which the characters are read indicates the level of visual acuity. Results are given in terms of two numbers that represent what most people with normal vision would see clearly at a given distance, usually at 20 feet. Therefore someone with great visual acuity, perhaps a major league baseball player, would score 20/15, which means that he or she would see normally at 20 feet what most people with normal vision would need to move to 15 feet to see clearly. Conversely, someone with 20/200 vision would need to stand 20 feet from an object to clearly see what most people with normal vision would see clearly at 200 feet.

Hearing Assessment

Hearing is assessed grossly on the sidelines through a discussion with the athlete. Often, hearing loss is self-evaluated and quickly reported. At other times, the loss may be subtle and unilateral and not easily recognized when it occurs in a loud environment such as a sports setting. The athlete should be moved to a quiet setting to evaluate the possible hearing loss. Hearing loss can be assessed using a tuning fork and the Weber and Rinne tests (Figure 17-6).

MANAGEMENT OF TRAUMATIC ACUTE INJURIES THAT AFFECT THE SENSES

Common Injuries Affecting Sight

Injuries that affect sight are probably the most difficult for the athlete to ignore because they are so disruptive to normal athletic activity. These injuries must be evaluated quickly and efficiently to prevent long-term, and even permanent, damage to the eye.

Most injuries to the eye that affect the sense of sight result from blunt force trauma mechanisms that damage the globe and prevent it from receiving sensory information from the local environment. These injuries include orbital fractures, detached retinas, hyphemas, foreign bodies, and corneal abrasions. Infections can occur in the conjunctiva that do not inhibit sight, but these can nevertheless inhibit the performance of normal activities of daily living. Some of these injuries, such as fractures, may be accompanied by other traumatic injuries to the head. Some injuries, such as infections, may occur with no associated trauma; these should be thoroughly screened for referral to a physician. As previously mentioned, the shocking appearance of many facial injuries, particularly traumatic ones, may overshadow

Snellen chart vision assessment tool containing a series of characters arranged in rows

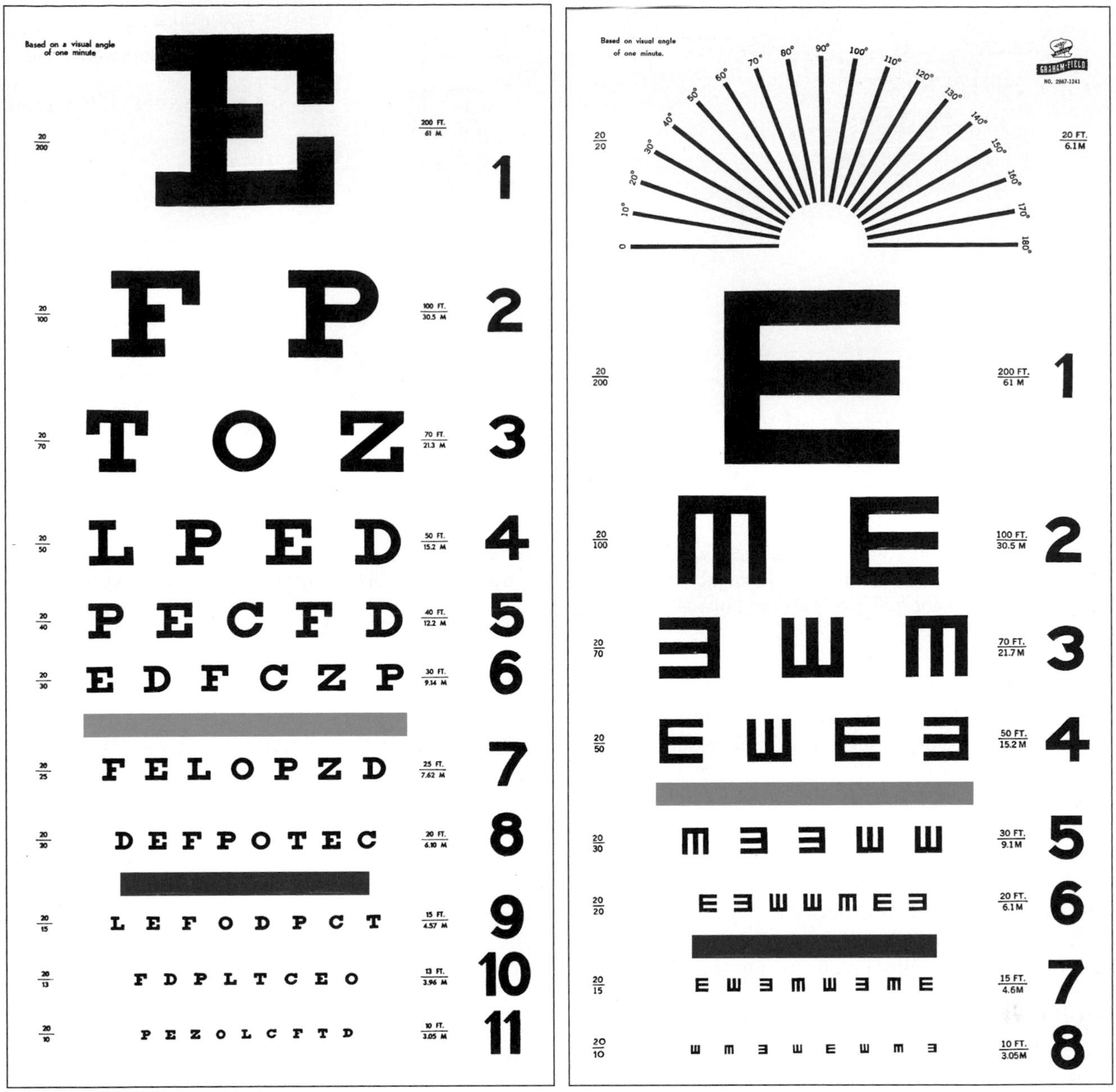

FIGURE 17-5 The Snellen eye chart is used to assess vision. (From Seidel HM et al: *Mosby's guide to physical examination,* ed 6, p. 73, St Louis, 2006, Mosby/Elsevier.)

a less conspicuous injury elsewhere on the face. Box 17-1 summarizes common injuries affecting the sense of sight.

Foreign Bodies

Foreign bodies range from minor nuisances to major pathological traumas (Figure 17-7). Most minor foreign bodies such as dust, dirt, and even small pieces of grass may be rinsed from the eye with water or saline. Foreign bodies in the eye may also include nonenvironmental factors. When an athlete is engaged in athletic pursuits, a foreign body may include an opponent's fingers, a teammate's foot, or even a bat or ball. These objects generally cause more than a simple irritation and will be discussed later in the chapter.

Mechanism: Foreign bodies may come into contact with the surface of the eye accidentally (e.g., dust, pollen) or intentionally (e.g., fingers, bats). The smallest speck of debris can cause great discomfort and halt any productive athletic activity.

Signs and symptoms: The affected eye is red and obviously irritated. Tear production increases in an attempt to flood the eye and thereby dislodge the irritant. These additional tears may further inhibit normal activity by affecting the ability of the eye to focus properly through the tears.

Immediate management: Copious amounts of saline or water mimic the eye's own mechanism of flooding the eye to clear itself of foreign bodies. If the foreign

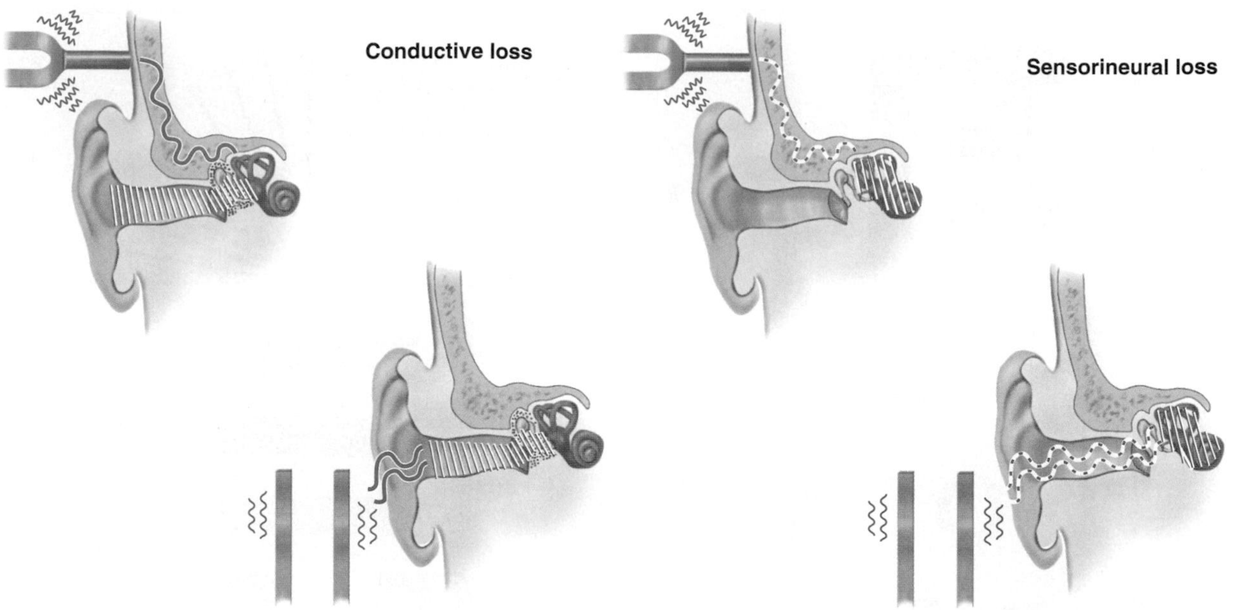

FIGURE 17-6 Weber and Rinne tests are used to distinguish between sensorineural and conductive hearing loss. (From Cuppett M, Walsh KM: *General medical conditions in the athlete,* St Louis, 2005, Elsevier/Mosby. Modified from Jarvis C: *Physical examination & health assessment,* ed 4, pp. 368–369, Philadelphia, 2004, Elsevier/Saunders.)

body can be identified and is not embedded in the eye, it generally can be flushed easily. Any irritant that is embedded or cannot be readily dislodged requires referral to a physician for removal.

Intermediate management: Before referring someone with an eye injury of this type, the athletic trainer should cover or patch the injured eye to keep it closed. This will protect the area and cause the injured eye to produce additional tears. Because the eyes move in tandem, it may be helpful to cover both eyes to prevent further irritation from movement of the uninjured eye.

Periorbital Ecchymosis

Periorbital **ecchymosis** often has a shocking presentation, but appearance does not necessarily correlate with the severity of the underlying pathology. However, every attempt should be made to evaluate the injury and not dismiss it as a simple black eye.

BOX 17-1 Common Sight-Related Injuries

Traumatic
- Orbital fracture
- Detached retina
- Hyphema
- Presence of a foreign body
- Corneal abrasion

Other
- Infections

Mechanism: Periorbital ecchymosis generally results from blunt force trauma to the face. Possible fractures can be evaluated through palpation of the periorbital area, including the nasal bones, orbital bones, and frontal bone.

Signs and symptoms: The discoloration is usually delayed by 12 hours or so, and depending on the source and area of the trauma, the eyelids may also be inflamed; the resulting weight may make fully opening the eye difficult (Figure 17-8). The structures outside the eye are primarily affected by this injury, and the bony border of the orbit is greatly discolored and painful to palpation.

Immediate management: The globe itself should be observed by gently easing the eyelid open with gloved hands. After observing the globe, the athletic trainer should assess pupillary response, which can indicate damage to the eye itself. The eye should be observed for any deformity of the pupil and iris and for any obvious blood pooling in the front chamber of the eye. If any of these problems are identified, the athlete should be referred to a physician for further evaluation.

Intermediate management: If fractures have been ruled out, the application of ice packs will decrease inflammation and discoloration. When cooling the surrounding

ecchymosis discoloration or bruising resulting from direct trauma

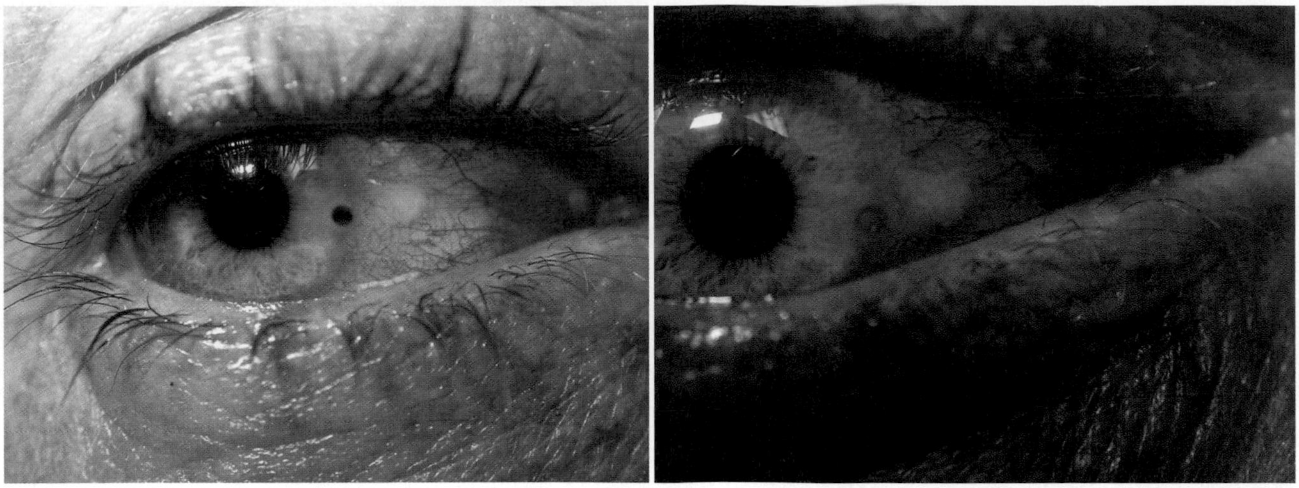

FIGURE 17-7 Corneal injuries resulting in a foreign body to the eye. (From Cuppett M, Walsh KM: *General medical conditions in the athlete,* St Louis, 2005, Elsevier/Mosby.)

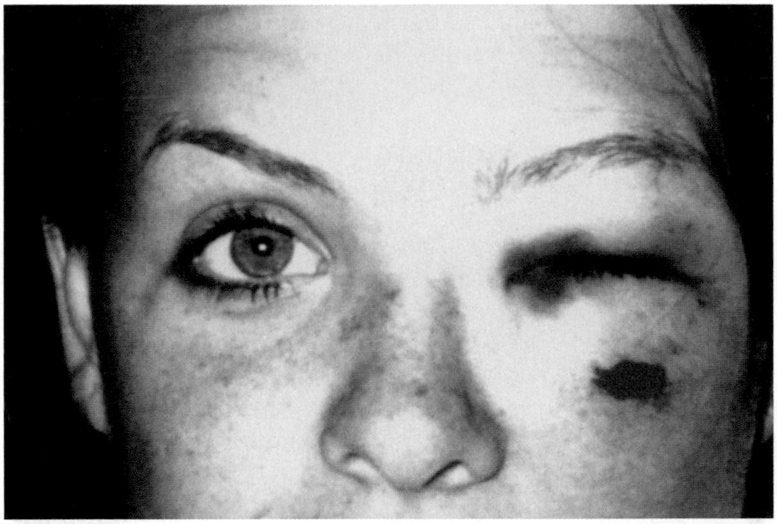

FIGURE 17-8 Periorbital ecchymosis.

tissues, the athletic trainer should apply a dry gauze pad over the closed eye to prevent cold damage. Vision is normally somewhat blurry after the application of ice packs because the cold temperature temporarily changes the shape of the eye and its ability to focus. As the eye warms, focusing should return to normal as well.

Corneal Abrasions

Corneal abrasions are among the most common eye injuries in sports.[1] This type of injury is often caused by damage incurred from a foreign body. Avascular and transparent, the cornea is the clear outer layer on the globe. Nutrition is obtained through atmospheric oxygen and from the **vascular limbus system** in the eye. Consequently, damage to this structure can be very painful and troubling to the athlete.

Mechanism: Corneal abrasions occur as a foreign object literally scrapes the outer protective coating of the eye. This abrasion exposes the underlying layers of the globe. The greater the size of the foreign object in the eye, the greater the pain and disability. Sometimes, even after the foreign body has been flushed from the eye, the damage remains.

Signs and symptoms: Athletes suffering from a corneal abrasion will complain of the physical sensation of a foreign body in the eye, although inspection will reveal no such problem. The sensation is very painful and disruptive to activities of daily living because of excessive tear production in the eye and associated spasm of the orbicularis muscle, which causes involuntary closing of the eye, limiting the visual field. The athlete will experience

vascular limbus system fine network of small blood vessels in the outer layers of the eye significant photophobia and sudden onset of pain. The pain is due to irritation of the nerve endings of cranial nerve V, which is located in the cornea.

Because of its location, an abrasion of the clear cornea is not as obvious as it would be on other parts of the body. Confirmation of a corneal abrasion is made through the use of fluorescein strips. These strips are coated with **fluorescein**, a material that glows under certain types of light. The fluorescein reveals the abrasion by illuminating the area when it is exposed to a black light (Figure 17-9). The fluorescein is green under normal light but turns yellow under blue light. It will not adhere to intact tissue, but it will stain the irritated area and reveal the injury. The staining is necessary because an area of transparent intact cornea appears the same as an area of missing, or abraded, cornea. The fluorescein stains the area of underlying tissue to reveal the missing corneal layer (Box 17-2).

Immediate management: Treatment for a corneal abrasion consists of topical antibiotic ophthalmic ointment to decrease pain and spasm. The affected eye may be patched for 24 to 48 hours as needed to decrease photophobia and further irritation of the eye caused by constant tears and blinking.

Intermediate management: Contacts should not be worn until the abrasion is fully healed. The athlete should be re-assessed daily and referred to an ophthalmologist if the abrasion is present after 48 hours. Most corneal abrasions will heal during this 48-hour window.

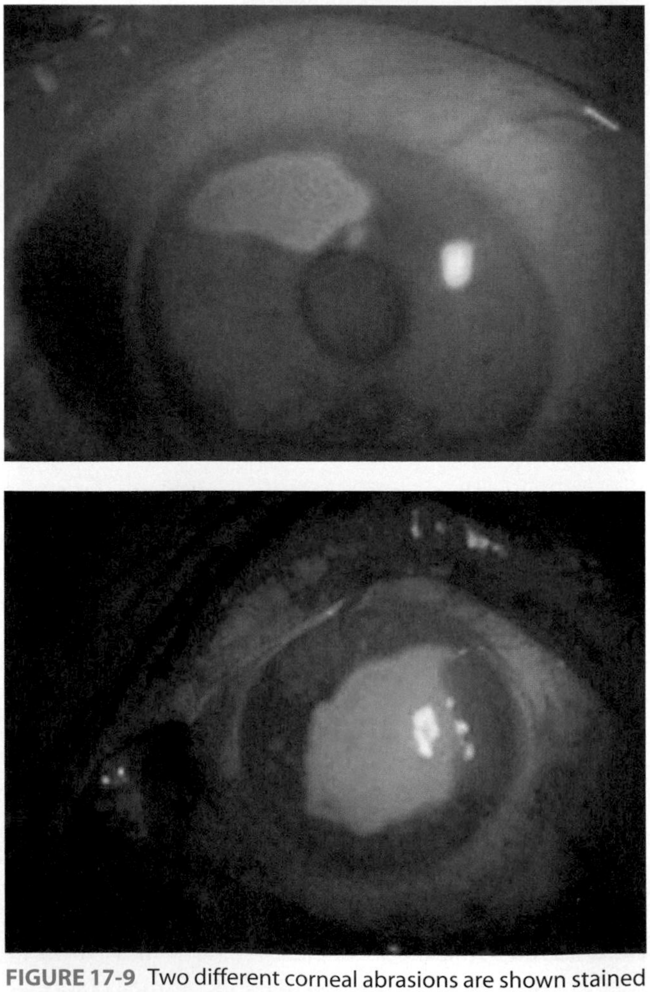

FIGURE 17-9 Two different corneal abrasions are shown stained with fluorescein dye. (From Cuppett M, Walsh KM: *General medical conditions in the athlete,* St Louis, 2005, Elsevier/Mosby.)

BOX 17-2 Technique for Fluorescein Strip Testing

1. Wet the strip with sterile saline to activate the fluorescein.
2. Pull the lower eyelid down, and touch the inner surface of the lid with the strip, passing the dye into the pouch made by the lower lid. To prevent further injury, do not touch the cornea itself with the strip..
3. Ask the athlete to blink to spread the dye across the cornea.
4. View the open eye with a penlight equipped with a blue filter or a black light to identify the corneal abrasion.

Modified from Street S, Runkle D: *Athletic protective equipment: care, selection, and fitting,* New York, 2000, McGraw-Hill.

Subconjunctival Hematoma

As the name implies, a subconjunctival hematoma is a collection, or pooling, of blood in the external layers of the eye (Figure 17-10). The sclera of the eye will be reddened secondary to blunt force trauma to the eye. The condition is generally benign, causing no real irritation or dysfunction.

Mechanism: This condition is usually a symptom of another injury (e.g., direct trauma to the eye and orbit)

fluorescein material that glows under certain types of lights

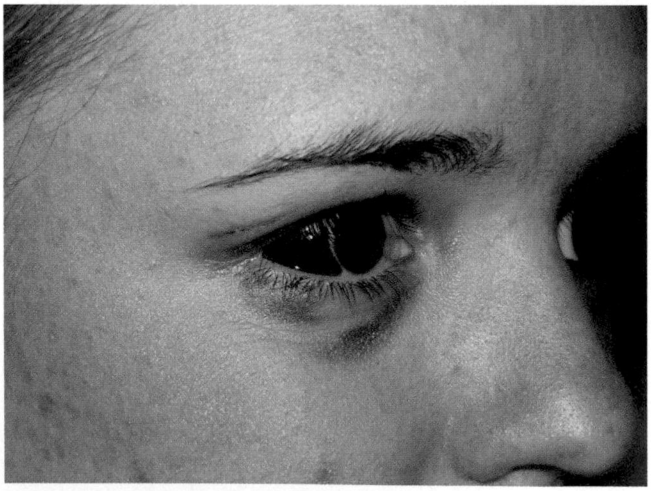

FIGURE 17-10 Subconjunctival hematoma.

rather than an isolated injury in itself. It may occur suddenly as an acute symptom or be delayed 12 to 24 hours after some type of facial trauma. The normally white sclera of the globe will become red as the blood from the trauma pools between the conjunctiva and sclera.

Signs and symptoms: The pooled blood is confined to the sclera and does not enter the iris. Subconjunctival hematomas are rarely painful and usually look far worse than they feel. The athlete should be warned of this fact to lessen any anxiety that he or she may experience when seeing the injury in a mirror for the first time. However, any trauma significant enough to cause this irritation may also be significant enough to cause damage to the other structures in the eye; therefore the athletic trainer should assess the athlete for other pathologies as well. Subconjunctival hematomas rarely affect vision.

Immediate management: The athlete should be monitored for pain and any signs of blood in the iris or across the pupil. Such symptoms indicate a more serious pathological condition. If an athlete with a subconjunctival hematoma complains of any pain or blurred vision, referral should be made to an ophthalmologist for further evaluation.

Intermediate management: Barring any additional injury, the hematoma should resolve completely in 1 to 3 weeks without treatment.[2] Monitor the eye over the next several days to make sure that the hematoma is still confined to the sclera and conjunctiva and not entering the iris.

Hyphema

A **hyphema** is a pooling of blood in the anterior chamber of the eye secondary to blunt force trauma. Often, it may accompany a subconjunctival hematoma. The major differences between a hyphema and a subconjunctival hematoma are the specific location and the presence of pain.

Mechanism: As with a subconjunctival hematoma, a hyphema may occur after blunt force trauma to the eye. Blows to the face are common in many sports, but blows to the eyes specifically are not especially common, given the increased use of face masks and goggles in high-risk sports.

Signs and symptoms: A hyphema occurs in the iris of the eye rather than the sclera. The amount of blood ranges from a few flecks of red in the iris to a growing pool that extends across the entire lower pupil (Figure 17-11). Symptoms usually appear 12 to 24 hours after the trauma. As the pressure increases in the anterior chamber of the eye, pain also increases. The hyphema may progress slowly over several hours and not affect vision until much later, or it may occur rapidly after a blow to the eye and quickly impair the athlete's vision by blocking the pupil. The greater the extent of the hyphema, the greater the internal pressure and resulting damage to the eye. The athlete will usually complain of a gradual decrease in the field of vision, which seems to close from the bottom up.

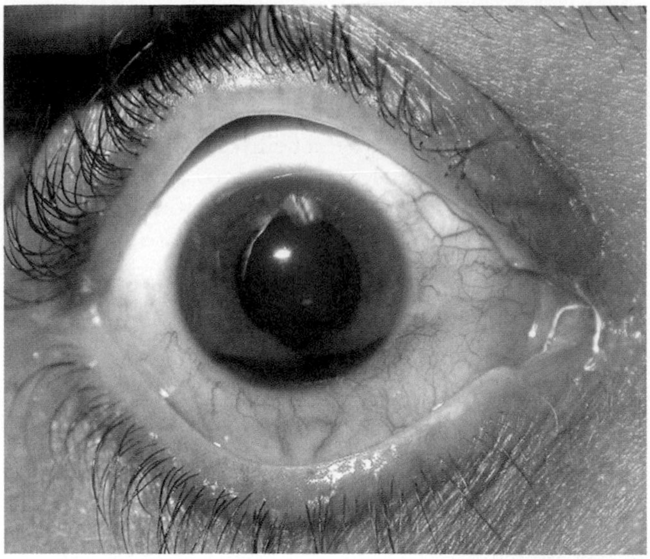

FIGURE 17-11 Hyphema. (From Cuppett M, Walsh KM: *General medical conditions in the athlete,* p. 225, St Louis, 2005, Elsevier/Mosby.)

Immediate management: Very minor hyphemas may heal without treatment and disappear completely in just a few days. A physician should assess the athlete with a hyphema to evaluate the damage to the eye. Any force great enough to cause a hyphema may also cause damage to other structures in the eye. Both eyes should be patched to prevent movement and possible exacerbation of the bleeding in the eye.

Intermediate management: The athlete should remain seated in an upright position while awaiting transportation to a physician. The athlete should not be allowed to add strain to the eye by lying down, bending forward, or moving excessively. Non-aspirin analgesics are permissible to alleviate the pain without raising the risk of increased bleeding into the eye.[2]

Detached Retina

A detached retina generally results from blunt force trauma to the face, but it may occur after any blunt force trauma to any part of the head. Any athlete with a head injury and associated complaints of vision loss should be screened for a detached retina.

Mechanism: Trauma causes fluid in the eye to seep behind the retina and loosen it from the wall of the eye itself. As it detaches, a "falling curtain" is seen

hyphema a pooling of blood in the anterior chamber of the eye secondary to blunt force trauma descending across the field of vision as it blocks light entering the pupil.

Signs and symptoms: The detachment may occur within minutes to weeks after the initial trauma.[2] The athlete suffering from a detached retina may also complain of flashing lights and "floaters" in the field of vision, signs that suggest early damage to the retina.

Immediate management: The only appropriate treatment option is to refer the athlete to an ophthalmologist for evaluation. Examination with an ophthalmoscope may reveal the falling retinal layer inside the eye, but nothing can be done on the sidelines to bring about an instant repair and return to play.

Intermediate management: Surgery is often required to repair the injury. During transportation to a physician for evaluation, it is very important to keep the athlete as calm and still as possible. Unnecessary changes to the pressure in the eye can accelerate the resulting damage to the retina.

Orbital Fracture

The orbit of the eye is the bony socket where the globe of the eye is located. Usually, this area is very stable and does an adequate job of protecting the eye.

Mechanism: As with most traumatic facial fractures, this injury is caused by blunt force trauma to the upper or lateral face. The injury may be quite disfiguring and affect tracking of the eye. The eye is literally trapped in position by the fracture fragments because the eye muscles that would normally move the eye are severed or impinged.

Signs and symptoms: The typical appearance is a sunken position of the eye in relation to the uninjured eye, an inability to move the eye, blurred vision, and possible facial numbness.

Immediate management: Treatment should begin with application of ice packs as soon as possible. The athletic trainer should be careful to not to increase pressure to the globe itself. The athlete should be referred to a physician as quickly as possible for evaluation of the extent and damage of the fracture. Both eyes should be patched during transportation to prevent eye motion that could further irritate or damage the injured eye.

> **Points to Ponder**
> In the event of imminent edema around the eye of an athlete wearing contact lenses, the contacts should be removed immediately to avoid painful maneuvers to the eyelid after the swelling builds.[2]

Common Injuries Affecting Hearing

Injuries that affect hearing are also difficult to ignore because of the impact they have on normal activities of daily living. They are sometimes quite painful and debilitating.

Common traumatic injuries that affect the sense of hearing are cauliflower ear (i.e., auricular hematoma), which decreases the ability to hear by restricting the passage of sound into the auditory canal, and eardrum (i.e., tympanic membrane) rupture, which affects hearing by altering the conversion of acoustic energy to mechanical energy as the soundwaves are passed across the membrane. Common illnesses include otitis externa (i.e., swimmer's ear) and otitis media. Swimmer's ear is an infection that often inhabits the auditory canal when the protective cerumen layer is compromised. Otitis media is an infection that occurs when the normal fluid present in the inner ear is not drained properly by way of the eustachian tube, creating pressure on the tympanic membrane. Although the condition can be quite painful, hearing is compromised minimally with the former illness, but hearing can be significantly altered with the latter illness because of the compromised ability of the eardrum to vibrate effectively. If the pressure becomes too great with otitis media, the tympanic membrane could rupture.

Box 17-3 summarizes the common injuries associated with the sense of hearing.

Tympanic Membrane Rupture

Mechanism: The tympanic membrane, or eardrum, can often be ruptured after a forceful pressure increase in the auditory canal (Figure 17-12). This pressure change could result from a sudden increase in environmental pressure, as in scuba diving or air travel, but it could also result from an increase in internal pressure behind the membrane caused by an upper respiratory infection or ear infection. A traumatic rupture may be caused by a blow to the head that forces a great amount of air pressure into the auditory canal. Some tympanic membrane ruptures are completely asymptomatic and may occur without obvious cause.[3]

Signs and symptoms: Whenever evaluation of the ear reveals fluid in the auditory canal, tympanic membrane rupture should be suspected. Tympanic membrane ruptures usually are very painful, so much so that the

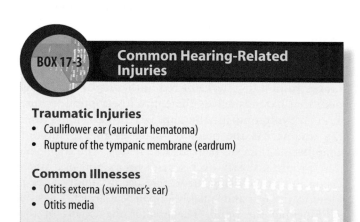

BOX 17-3 Common Hearing-Related Injuries

Traumatic Injuries
- Cauliflower ear (auricular hematoma)
- Rupture of the tympanic membrane (eardrum)

Common Illnesses
- Otitis externa (swimmer's ear)
- Otitis media

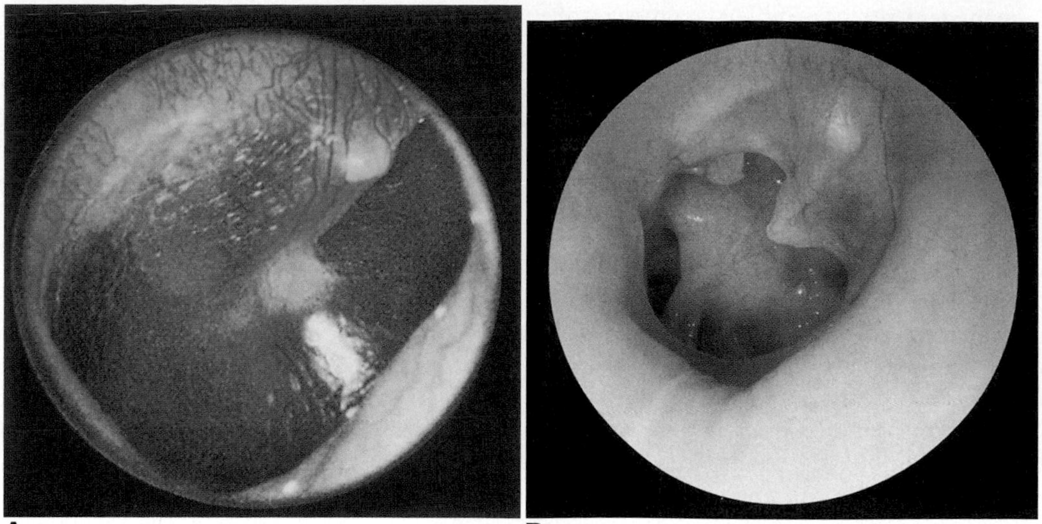

FIGURE 17-12 Normal **(A)** and ruptured **(B)** tympanic membrane. (**A** from Jarvis C: *Physical examination & health assessment*, ed 4, pp. 343, 351, Philadelphia, 2004, Elsevier/Saunders. **B** from Epstein O et al: *Clinical examination,* ed 3, p. 93, Philadelphia, 2003, Elsevier/Mosby.)

afflicted person may experience nausea. Because the ear houses structures that direct and guide our balance, this injury may lead to dizziness caused by a change in the structure of the ear. **Tinnitus**, or ringing in the ears, and hearing loss are directly related to the size of the tear. The more membrane left intact, the greater the remaining level of hearing. Large tears or ruptures often require surgical repair, but fortunately small tears often heal without surgical intervention.

Immediate management: The person with a suspected tympanic membrane rupture should be evaluated by a physician. Continued athletic participation immediately after the injury is difficult because of the pain and loss of balance.

Intermediate management: The physician will usually prescribe antibiotic drops to protect the inner ear while the membrane is healing. The membrane has a remarkable ability to heal itself and close the opening in just a few weeks. The athlete recovering from this injury should avoid submersion in water (swimming, diving, and even showering under some circumstances) until the membrane is fully healed.

Hematoma Auris

Mechanism: Hematoma auris is caused by repeated blunt force trauma to the ear that results in localized inflammation. The injury can result from one severe traumatic force to the ear, such as in basketball, or after a series of moderate blows to the ear, such as in wrestling.

Signs and symptoms: Commonly known as "cauliflower ear" because of its outward deformity of the pinna, the inflammation causes the skin covering the external ear to separate from the underlying cartilage (Figure 17-13). Left untreated, the hematoma filling the gap between the skin and cartilage turns into a fibrotic mass and is not absorbed. This mass can permanently deform the external ear and potentially interfere with hearing. If the inflammation is sufficiently great, the deformity of the external ear may actually impede the flow of sound into the auditory canal.

tinnitus ringing in the ears
hematoma auris "cauliflower ear;" localized inflammation of the external ear resulting from repeated blunt force trauma

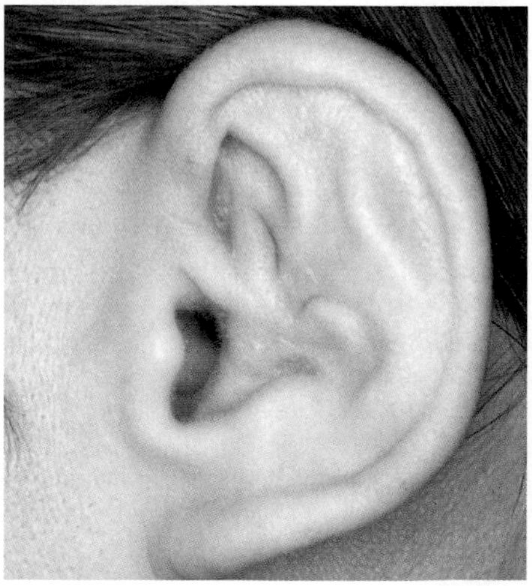

FIGURE 17-13 "Cauliflower ear," or hematoma auris. (From Bingham BJG, Hawke M, Kwok P: *Atlas of clinical otolaryngology,* St Louis, 1992, Mosby.)

Immediate management: Treatment consists of quickly reducing the hematoma to prevent deformity of the ear. The ear should be monitored for several days after treatment until the skin reduces back to the surface of the cartilage. This will ensure that the hematoma does not recur in the same area. Aspiration of the hematoma may be necessary and is most effective when performed promptly after the injury to remove the hematoma and prevent the risk of deformity as well as decrease the risk of tissue damage to the underlying cartilage.

Intermediate management: Oral or topical antibiotics are often used for 7 to 10 days after injury to prevent infection in the area. The use of nonsteroidal antiinflammatory drugs (NSAIDs) should be discouraged because they typically thin the blood and promote leakage of fluid into the injured area. Ice pack applications can be very effective in reducing the pain and swelling associated with this injury. If aspiration is required to promote healing, the athlete should not participate in the sport for 24 hours and should be required to wear protective headgear to prevent re-injury.

A popular adjunct treatment of auricular hematoma is the use of a flexible collodion cast. Liquid collodion, which hardens as it dries, is applied to the area of the hematoma.[4] This hardened shell splints the injured area as a cast would splint a fracture site (Box 17-4).

Athletes suffering from external ear injuries should be held from any high-risk activities that could possibly re-injure the ear for at least 24 to 48 hours. Athletes in low-risk or noncontact activities may return to participation immediately after the condition is treated and stabilized. Athletes treated for external trauma should also be evaluated for other pathological conditions, including tympanic membrane rupture and auditory canal inflammation, because these problems result from similar mechanisms.

BOX 17-4 Application of a Collodion Cast

1. Cut ½ inch strips of gauze 1 to 2 inches long.
2. Soak the strips in collodion.
3. Apply the gauze to the entire area of removed hematoma, including the back of the ear.
4. Paint the area with an additional layer of collodion.
5. Leave the splint in place for 5 days.
6. Add layers of collodion and/or gauze if the cast loosens.
7. Remove the cast by cutting the gauze along the helix of the ear, and remove each half.

Modified from Street S, Runkle D: *Athletic protective equipment: care, selection, and fitting*, New York, 2000, McGraw-Hill.

Common Injuries Affecting Taste

Injuries of the mouth and lips are especially painful because of the high sensitivity of the area. The tongue and lips are highly vascular, and even small lacerations often bleed copiously. However, this abundant vascular supply ultimately leads to quick healing, and most tongue lacerations rarely require sutures.[3] Dental injuries often have a shocking appearance, with great amounts of bleeding and immediate deformity.

The most common nose injury, other than a fracture, is an epistaxis, or nosebleed. Fractures generally display obvious deformity. An epistaxis may occur as an injury in its own right or as a symptom of some other trauma, such as a fracture. Both injuries involve copious amounts of bleeding and have a startling appearance, although neither is usually catastrophic. The entire face should be evaluated when a nasal injury occurs. The dramatic appearance of a severely bleeding face may distract the athletic trainer from less obvious, yet still very important, injuries of the face.

Box 17-5 summarizes common injuries associated with the sense of smell.

Lip and Tongue Lacerations

Mechanism: Lacerations are almost always caused by accidental self-inflicted biting accidents when the athlete's head undergoes some form of unexpected blunt force trauma. As the head is hit, the mouth snaps shut and sometimes the tongue or lip gets caught in the teeth.

Signs and symptoms: These injuries significantly affect the functions of the mouth, namely taste and speech. Complete loss of taste is rare because of the multiple neurological pathways innervating the tongue. Lacerations that extend completely through the tissue should be sutured, and the athlete should be placed on oral antibiotics as quickly as possible. Partial-thickness lacerations generally heal without suturing, although the long-term aesthetic results may be less than desirable.

Immediate management: Lacerations in these areas should be treated as they would be in any other place on the body. They must be cleaned, and the bleeding must be controlled. Initially, saline or a similar solution should be used to cleanse the area. The athletic trainer can control bleeding by applying direct pressure with a gloved hand through a gauze pad that is held against the laceration or by allowing the athlete to hold the gauze pad to his or her own tongue.

BOX 17-5 Common Smell-Related Injuries

Fracture
Epistaxis (nosebleed)

Dental Fractures and Avulsions

Mechanism: Dental fractures and avulsions result from blunt force trauma to the mouth. At times, the tooth is injured by direct impact, or it may fracture as the mouth slams shut and the teeth collide. The use of mouthpieces, both custom and off-the-shelf, has significantly decreased the frequency of dental injuries in sports. With proper care and immediate referral, the tooth can be saved. A dental fracture may occur independently or concurrently with an avulsion. If the tooth is fractured at the bottom one third, it usually cannot be salvaged. Fractures of the upper one third can usually be secured in place by a dentist and saved.[5]

Signs and symptoms: With a **dental avulsion**, the tooth is traumatically dislodged from its socket. The tooth may be twisted in the socket or completely knocked out, with the tooth being avulsed as it is fractured. An avulsed tooth is easily identified, especially if it is compared with its mate on the opposite side of the mouth. Athletes with an avulsed tooth usually recognize the avulsion themselves after feeling the asymmetry with his or her own tongue. In addition, the fractured tooth and the socket are very painful and sensitive to temperature changes. Bleeding may be minimal or copious, depending on how well the tooth blocks the flow of blood from torn vessels.

Dental fractures are very painful and sensitive to temperature extremes. The deeper the fracture, the more intense the symptoms. Bleeding is common with dental fractures, which open the blood supply to the tooth.

Dental fractures occur in various forms and are grouped into four different classes. Class I fractures are generally self-evaluated and affect only the enamel, or most superficial layer, of the tooth. Class II fractures affect a deeper level of the tooth, reaching to the dentin level. Class III fractures involve the crown and pulp of the tooth. Class IV fractures disrupt the root of the tooth and are clearly visible on X-ray examination. Pain is minimal with a class I fracture and increases significantly with each progressive level of fracture (Box 17-6).[6]

Immediate management: The success rate for dental re-implantation depends on the prompt replacement of the avulsed tooth in its socket. If the tooth can be replaced in its socket within 30 minutes, there is a 90% success rate for permanent implantation of the tooth, compared with a 95% failure rate if replacement takes over 120 minutes.[2] The tooth is connected to the surrounding jaw by the periodontal ligament, and protecting the remnants of this ligament is vital if the tooth is to be permanently implanted. When re-implanted, these remnants on the tooth will reattach to the remnants located in the socket.

The tooth should be *gently* rinsed with saline or another pH-balanced solution to remove any environmental debris. The tooth should not be scrubbed or scraped because this may remove remnants of the periodontal ligament from the tooth surface. Once the tooth is rinsed, it is reinserted into the socket and the injured person is immediately referred to a dentist.[5] If the tooth is completely knocked out of the socket and cannot be placed back into the socket, it should be located quickly and stored in **Hank's solution** or fresh whole milk.

Intermediate management: The dentist will check the tooth placement and will often prescribe oral antibiotics. Contact drills or other potentially traumatic athletic activities should be avoided for the next 7 to 10 days while fixation of the tooth progresses. If protected, the periodontal ligaments will reattach themselves to the surrounding socket tissue[2] (Figure 17-14).

With a dental fracture, a partial or full root canal may be required because of the damage to the internal structures of the tooth. All dental fractures should be referred to a dentist for repair. The greater the amount of tooth fractured, the greater the amount of repair required to save it. Very superficial fractures that affect only the dental enamel and not the interior structures may not be symptomatic but should also be referred to a dentist. The dentist can evaluate the structures below the gumline as well as smooth out any rough surfaces on the tooth to prevent potential damage to the tongue.

Common Injuries Affecting Smell

Athletic trainers should know which athletes under their care have a nontraumatic congenital deformity. Familiarity with the athlete's status before the onset of injury prevents confusion later. When in doubt as to the straightness of an injured nose, the athletic trainer should ask the athlete to assess his or her own nose with a hand-held mirror after the bleeding has been controlled and the face thoroughly cleaned.

BOX 17-6 Classes of Dental Fractures

Class I: Damage to the enamel only
Class II: Damage to the dentin
Class III: Damage to the pulp
Class IV: Damage to the root

dental avulsion traumatic dislodging of a tooth from its socket

Hank's solution a special commercially available pH-balanced liquid made for storage of avulsed teeth; prevents cell death of the periodontal ligament tissue during transport for dental treatment

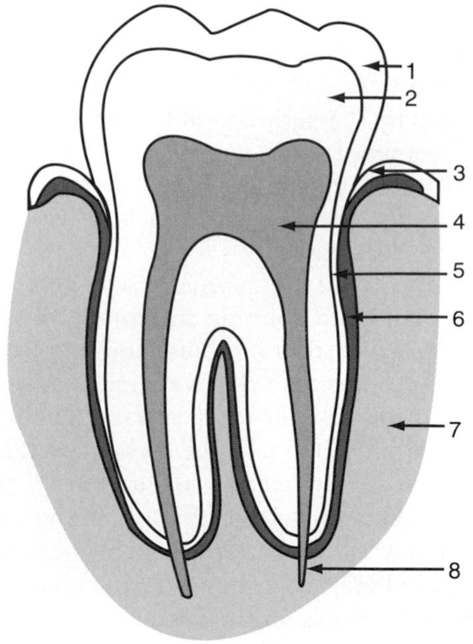

FIGURE 17-14 Basic dental anatomy. *1,* Enamel; *2,* dentin; *3,* gingival margin; *4,* pulp; *5,* cementum; *6,* periodontal ligament; *7,* alveolar bone; *8,* neurovascular bundle. (From Behrman R, Kliegman R, Jenson H: *Nelson textbook of pediatrics,* ed 17, Philadelphia, 2004, Elsevier/Saunders.)

Common injuries that affect taste include lacerations of the tongue and lips and fractures and avulsions of the teeth. Because of the presence of taste buds, any injury to the tongue will decrease the overall interpretation and processing of taste stimuli. If the injury is sufficiently traumatic, sensory nerves of the mouth may be severed, greatly affecting the conduction of information to the brain. Although the teeth do not directly process tastes, a dental injury can greatly diminish the ability to chew food, a dysfunction that results in decreased taste. Oral and upper respiratory illnesses can affect taste because they are often accompanied by increased mucus production, which masks the taste buds and dulls the conduction of taste stimulus to the brain.

Box 17-7 summarizes common injuries associated with the sense of taste.

Nasal Fracture

Mechanism: Nasal fractures may result from any type of blunt force trauma to the face. These fractures occur proximally, affecting the bone of the nose, not the cartilage. All traumatic injuries to the nose should be assessed for nasal fractures; possible deformities range from a greenstick depression to a total disruption of the cartilage-bone union. Lateral displacement is the most common deformity with nasal fractures (Figure 17-15).

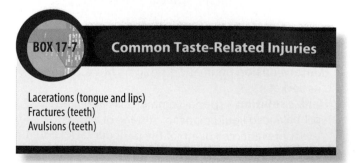

BOX 17-7 Common Taste-Related Injuries

Lacerations (tongue and lips)
Fractures (teeth)
Avulsions (teeth)

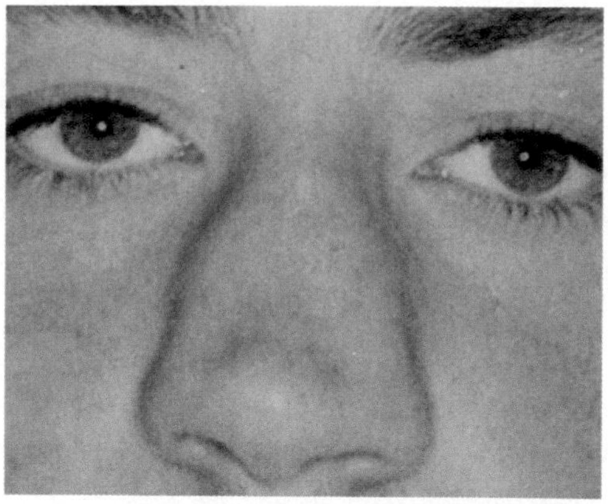

FIGURE 17-15 Nasal fracture. Note the bony deformity. (From Gallaspy JB, May JD: *Signs and symptoms of athletic injuries,* p. 64, St Louis, 1996, Mosby.)

Signs and symptoms: Common symptoms of nasal fractures include generalized pain, bleeding, immediate swelling, deformity, and compromised nasal breathing. The injury's tell-tale sign is nasal deformity. Deformity is self-evaluated by the athlete in a mirror, but the athletic trainer should also evaluate the nose by viewing it anteriorly and superiorly. The actual sense of smell is not directly affected, but it may be hindered if inflammation or deformity blocks the nasal passages and prevents the free flow of air from the outside environment. The severity of symptoms is directly related to the extent of the fracture and the degree of displacement. Displacement is determined through actual palpation of the nose. Palpation revealing crepitus, sharp edges, and pain may be accurately assessed as a fracture. The fracture may cause significant bleeding in the nose, but this bleeding may not always exit the nostrils because of blockage by septal inflammation and bone displacement. In that case, the bleeding will drain into the throat and possibly fill the sinus cavities of the face. In the days following the injury, ecchymosis often appears across the nose and under the eyes, a condition know as "raccoon eyes."

Immediate management: If the blood can easily from the nostrils, the flow will be copious and dramatic. To decrease anxiety, the athletic trainer should control the bleeding and clean the athlete's face before asking him or her to self-evaluate the nasal displacement. Any athlete with a suspected nasal fracture should also be assessed for concussion because the mechanisms are very similar and the dramatic nature of the bleeding may overshadow many neurological signs of the concussion (e.g., dizziness, disorientation, amnesia).

Treatment of a suspected nasal fracture or common epistaxis includes controlling the bleeding. The application of ice packs will reduce the hemorrhage and decrease the pain. Athletes with a suspected nose fracture should be referred to a physician for further evaluation, but they may return to noncontact activities when the bleeding ceases.

Intermediate management: The swelling in the nose may build quickly, which affects the treating physician's ability to reduce the displaced bone. Therefore reduction should be attempted within the first hour or delayed for 3 to 5 days until the swelling has subsided. In any case, a splint should be applied to protect the nose from further injury.[3] The maximum delay in reducing or setting the nose fracture is 4 days in children and 10 days in adults.[7] To prevent further injury, a noseguard should be worn for 4 weeks during contact sports.

Epistaxis

Mechanism: An epistaxis, or nosebleed, may be a symptom of another pathological condition, such as a nasal fracture, or it may be a distinct injury in itself. Trauma to the nose often results in epistaxis. Although a commonplace injury in some sports, an epistaxis should not be summarily dismissed as a minor injury. It should be evaluated appropriately, treated, and referred if signs of further pathology are present. If a nasal fracture is dismissed as "just another nosebleed," permanent deformity and disability may result.

Signs and symptoms: Symptoms of epistaxis are similar to those of nasal fracture, although deformity is rare with common epistaxis. Anterior epistaxis occurs with injury to the superficial blood vessels of the anterior septum and accounts for the majority of nosebleeds.[7] Posterior nosebleeds result from damage to the lateral walls of the nose. Anterior nosebleeds are common with trauma, but posterior nosebleeds are not. Some episodes of epistaxis are nontraumatic in origin and may be due to illness, dehydration, or other conditions that dry out the nasal mucosa. Viewing the septum and mucosal membranes of the nose will help in identifying the origin of the bleeding. Visualization of the septum will also help the athletic trainer determine whether a traumatic deviation or nasal fracture is present.

Immediate management: As with nasal fractures, the primary objective of treatment is hemorrhage control, which permits a better visual inspection of the injured tissue. Hemorrhage control is accomplished in a variety of ways and head positions, but the overriding principle is the comfort of the athlete.

Some health care professionals choose to tilt the head forward to prevent aspiration of the blood draining down the throat by redirecting it to drain from the nostrils. Other clinicians choose to tilt the head back to maintain an airway and protect the cervical spine. If a cervical spine injury is not suspected and a forward-tilting posture is equally comfortable, either may be safely implemented. Some athletes become dizzy as a result of the sudden blood loss and choose to tilt their heads back for comfort. Others become nauseated by the taste of blood draining down their throats and opt to tilt their heads forward. Either position is safe as long as it does not interfere with treatment or increase the scope of the injury.

Most nasal bleeding stops spontaneously or with the application of cold packs or direct pressure. If not, many techniques to control bleeding have been proved effective. The insertion of an absorbent plug will put pressure on the walls of the nose to slow the bleeding as well as absorb the blood. Commercial nose plugs are available, but gauze rolls and tampons may also be used. If the noseplug is saturated with a vasoconstricting medication such as an over-the-counter decongestant spray, the hemorrhage can be controlled even more efficiently. Using a thin layer of antibiotic ointment on the noseplug will control the hemorrhage and reduce the risk of infection.[3] Athletic trainers should be cautious when inserting the noseplug to make sure that it extends beyond the end of the nostrils about one-half inch to allow for easy removal. They should also be careful when removing a nose plug to keep from dislodging the newly formed clot and restarting the hemorrhaging.

A second method of treatment is to place a rolled gauze or noseplug in the mouth under the upper lip and against the gum. Placement under the upper lip controls hemorrhage by reducing blood flow to the nose through pressure on the blood vessels supplying the nose.[5] This method is especially effective in controlling hemorrhage in anterior epistaxis and allows better visualization of the nasal passages. Because many athletes are accustomed to seeing epistaxis treated by using a gauze roll *in* the nose, the athletic trainer must be very clear in instructing athletes to place this roll *under the lip*. If nasal bleeding cannot be stopped with one of these methods, cauterization by a physician may be necessary.

Intermediate management: Once the hemorrhage is stopped and the noseplug or gauze is removed, the athlete should be cautioned not to blow the nose for several hours to prevent a new hemorrhage. Other complications of epistaxis include sinusitis, otitis media, and pressure necrosis of the nasal mucosa.[7] Aspirin and other blood-thinning medications should be avoided until the risk of hemorrhage has passed. Saline sprays may be helpful to moisturize the nasal mucosa and prevent hemorrhage. Nasal decongestant sprays may help reduce inflammation in the nasal passages and improve airflow.

epistaxis medical term for a nosebleed

The athletic trainer should cautiously evaluate nasal injuries to rule out a septal hematoma, which results from hemorrhage between the cartilage and the overlying skin along the nasal septum. This complication of nasal trauma can form within hours of the initial injury or 2 or 3 days later if the hemorrhage is not controlled effectively. Failure to identify and treat the septal hematoma may result in infection, bone or cartilage necrosis, and permanent deformity.[3] Inspection of the nasal passage will reveal a bluish bulge inside the nose on the septum. Treatment consists of incision and drainage by a physician after any other hemorrhage in the nose has been controlled through the application of ice packs and direct pressure.

MANAGEMENT OF ILLNESSES AND NON-TRAUMATIC CONDITIONS THAT AFFECT THE SENSES

Illnesses and conditions are problems that result not from trauma but from other factors such as infection, stress, and even genetics. These problems can be just as debilitating as a traumatic injury. They can easily prevent normal activities of daily living.

Illnesses and Conditions Affecting Sight

Nontraumatic conditions that affect sight can be very debilitating as they greatly impact a person's ability to continue normal activities of daily living. Conditions affecting sight can increase the risk of other injuries as they prevent a person from seeing a potential risk and taking the measures necessary to avoid a problem. For example, a driver with a limited vision due to an eye problem or severe headache will be unable to see or effectively react to obstacles in the road, increasing the risk of injury to himself and others.

Headaches

Headaches can significantly disrupt activities of daily living for athletes and nonathletes alike. Although their origins vary widely, ranging from stress, allergies, sinus congestion, concussion, hypoglycemia, and other nontraumatic factors, this chapter will focus on two types of headaches: migraine headaches and tension headaches. A physician should evaluate all chronic headaches that do not respond to conservative treatment.

Migraine Headaches. **Mechanism:** According to the International Headache Society, a migraine is a "recurring headache disorder manifesting in attacks lasting 4 to 24 hours."[8] These debilitating headaches are more common in women than in men and usually occur for the first time in the early 20s. Some of the causes, or triggers, of migraines include lifestyle issues such as stress, fatigue, skipped meals, and sleep deprivation. Of female migraine headache sufferers, 60% report a relationship between the headache and their menstrual cycle, with the headache occurring either at menses, 2 days before menses, or 2 days after menses. Duration of headaches related to the menstrual cycle can be from 4 to 72 hours. Some foods, which are considered **vasoactive**, affect the bloodflow through the brain and trigger migraines in some people. These foods include chocolate, aged cheese, pickled foods, sour cream, yogurt, alcoholic beverages, and sometimes caffeinated items. Food additives such as monosodium glutamate (MSG) and aspartame sweetener are also believed to trigger migraines in certain people.[8] In some cases, exercise can trigger a migraine headache, a particularly problematic trigger for physically active individuals.

Signs and symptoms: The headaches are unilateral, which means that they affect only one hemisphere of the head. The pulsating pain is of moderate to severe intensity and can be significant enough to cause nausea and vomiting. Photophobia, **phonophobia**, and **osmophobia** are very common during the migraine headache. People who suffer from migraine headaches often have family members with the same condition.[9] Activity generally aggravates and prolongs migraine headaches. Because of the many exacerbating factors, migraine sufferers are often forced to retreat to a dark, quiet room, where they try to sleep as much as possible.[8]

Some types of migraine headaches have two characteristic phases that occur before the actual headache: prodromal phase and aura phase. The prodromal phase lasts for 10 to 20 minutes before the onset of the headache, and visual disturbances are common during this time (e.g., blurred vision, focusing problems). In the aural phase, experienced by about one third of migraine sufferers, visual disturbances are common, but vertigo and paresthesia are also common symptoms before the onset of the headache.[8] The aura phase serves as a warning phase of an imminent migraine headache. This warning phase may also include symptoms such as loss or increase of appetite, loss or increase in overall energy, increased or decreased urinary output, and mood changes such as irritability, depression, or even euphoria. Many migraine sufferers complain of difficulty concentrating during the aura phase.

Immediate management: The best course of treatment for migraine headaches is to identify their cause and prevent them. These triggers should be identified and avoided as much as possible to prevent the onset of migraines.

If exercise prompts a migraine, a change in frequency or intensity may be all that is necessary to avoid the

vasoactive causing constriction or dilation of blood vessels

phonophobia literally "fear of sound;" refers to intense ear discomfort during exposure to loud noise

osmophobia intense discomfort, even to the point of nausea, during exposure to intense smells headache. Proper warm-up and hydration are also beneficial in keeping exercise triggers to a minimum. Some migraine sufferers notice an increase in their headaches with increased exercise, whereas other sufferers notice a corresponding decrease. For individuals who routinely suffer migraines with increased activity, a referral to a physician may be warranted to rule out other arteriovenous malformation pathologies, such as an aneurysm.

Medications used for the treatment of migraines may be over-the-counter or prescription, and different medications are appropriate to different phases of the headache. Some medications are taken at the initial onset of symptoms during the prodromal or aura phase and are intended to reverse the onset of the headache. Other medications are taken after the headache is triggered and are intended to promote sedation and pain relief until the headache can run its course. Prophylactic, or preventive, medications may also be prescribed to be taken on a routine basis. These are often prescribed for those individuals who suffer migraines more than twice a month. The dosage is slowly increased over time until the migraines are brought under control.[8] Prophylactic medications may affect the person's ability to engage in routine heavy exercise, such as sports, and should also be closely monitored in those taking insulin, oral hypoglycemics, and certain antidepressants.

Intermediate management: Nonpharmacological treatments include the identification and elimination of specific triggers. Migraine sufferers should be vigilant to establish and maintain strict daily schedules for eating and sleeping. Too much or too little of either can trigger a migraine. Exercise sessions should be preceded by a long, slow warm-up period. Relaxation and other stress management techniques are usually helpful in decreasing the frequency of migraines.[8]

Tension Headaches. **Mechanism:** As the name implies, tension headaches are common in people with high-stress, tense lifestyles. Some studies show that these headaches are very common, affecting from 29% to 71% of patients.[10] These headaches are commonly caused by stress but can also result from high fevers, hypoglycemia, and the abuse of or withdrawal from alcohol or caffeine.[9]

Signs and symptoms: These headaches manifest as a diffuse, throbbing pain over the entire top of the head or possibly on only one side of the head. Nausea is not normally a symptom, although the pain can be very intense. Tension headaches usually last approximately 45 minutes and produce no systemic effects, but they have been known to last for several days.[10] If systemic symptoms, such as loss of function or sensation in the extremities, are present, immediate referral to a physician is necessary to rule out conditions such as a stroke.

Immediate management: As with migraines, triggers for tension headaches should be identified and avoided. Over-the-counter analgesics are generally helpful in treating these headaches. Stress management techniques, stretching routines for the neck and upper back, and relaxation techniques are helpful in preventing tension headaches.

Infections

Infections can occur nearly anywhere in the body. Infections that affect the senses result from a break in the skin or a weakening of the body's natural defense system of antibodies. These problems can affect vision because they often cause inflammation of the eye or related structures, which hinders the ability of the eye to open and sometimes to focus.

Styes. **Mechanism:** A **stye**, or hordeolum, is a *Staphylococcal* infection of the eyelid margin at the eyelash line occurring when the oil glands of that area become blocked.[6] The stye can be a minor nuisance, or it can progress to a painful lesion that appears as a raised pimplelike area with a yellow center on the margin of the eyelid at the base of the eyelashes (Figure 17-16).

Signs and symptoms: Inversion of the eyelid will reveal a small round lump at the eyelid margin.[9] The stye should be treated early to keep it from growing into a painful mass that obstructs the athlete's vision. A stye always occurs at the outer edge of the eyelid margin; a lesion anywhere else should be referred to a physician for evaluation.

Immediate management: Moist warm compresses applied for 10 minutes four times a day should help reduce the inflammation by opening the obstructed gland and neutralizing the infection.[2,9] If this conservative

stye also known as a *hordeolum; Staphylococcus* infection of the eyelid at the eyelash line that occurs from blockage of the area's oil glands

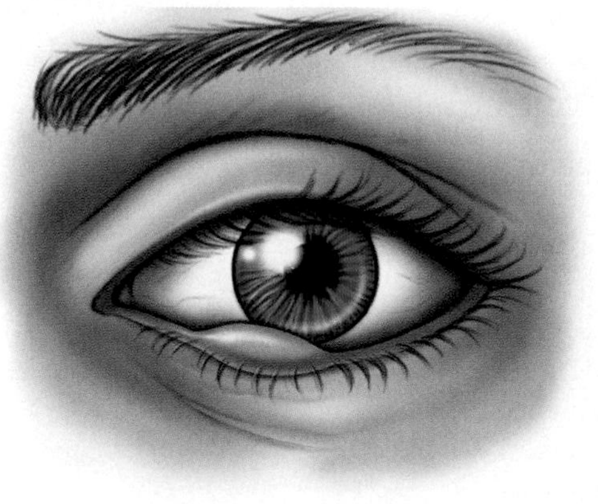

FIGURE 17-16 External stye. (From Herlihy B: *The human body in health and illness,* ed 3, p. 227, Philadelphia, 2007, Saunders/Elsevier.)

treatment is not effective after 48 hours, the athlete should be referred to a physician for topical or oral antibiotics. Antibiotics should be applied two or three times a day. Most styes resolve with application of the warm compresses and antibiotics within 10 days. In cases that either do not resolve or recur frequently, incision and drainage by a physician may be necessary.[11]

Chalazions. **Mechanism:** A **chalazion** is a lesion similar to a stye, but it occurs farther proximally on the eyelid than where a stye forms (Figure 17-17). It also forms when an oil gland is blocked, either through infection or localized inflammation from trauma. Because of its proximity to the globe of the eye, a secondary conjunctivitis infection may occur.[11]

Signs and symptoms: Chalazions initially manifest as a red and tender mass in the eyelid and gradually become a nontender lump.

Immediate management: Topical antibiotics and warm compresses applied several times a day can reduce the inflammation, although chalazions usually do not resolve as quickly as styes. Incision and drainage by a physician is not recommended until the lesion has been present for 4 weeks.[11] Incising the lesion increases the potential for generating scar tissue that could possibly obstruct the duct even longer.

Conjunctivitis. **Mechanism: Conjunctivitis** is an infection of the posterior eyelid lining, or conjunctiva, and is highly contagious.[9] Conjunctivitis may result from a systemic bacterial or viral illness and may be the initial symptom or the final symptom of the illness. In any case, the pathogen infects the conjunctiva and results in conjunctivitis.

Signs and symptoms: Conjunctivitis is usually accompanied by itchy, burning, red eyes and drainage (Figure 17-18). Symptoms may appear to be an allergic reaction at first, but they are more intense and do not have a supporting trigger or history. Conjunctivitis generally starts in one eye and spreads quickly to the other eye, whereas an allergic response affects both eyes simultaneously.

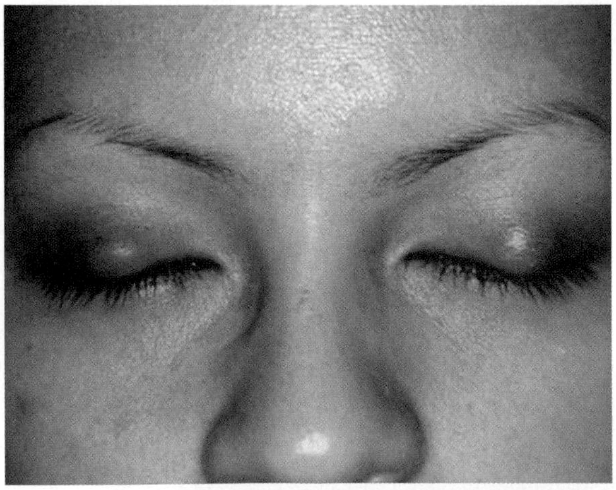

FIGURE 17-17 Bilateral chalazion. (From Goldman L, Ausiello D: *Cecil textbook of medicine,* ed 22, Philadelphia, 2004, Elsevier/Saunders.)

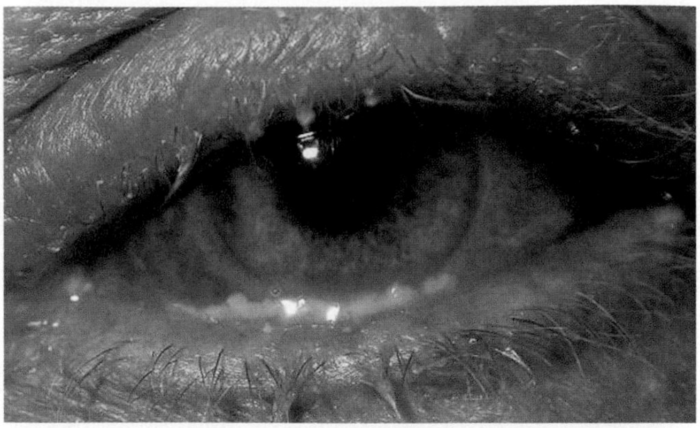

FIGURE 17-18 Bacterial conjunctivitis. (From Cuppett M, Walsh KM: *General medical conditions in the athlete,* p. 225, St Louis, 2005, Elsevier/Mosby.)

Immediate management: The only effective treatment is to refer the athlete to a physician for prescription antibiotic medication. To prevent further spreading of the infection, the athlete should be cautioned not to rub the eye and to wash the hands frequently.[2]

Intermediate management: It is extremely important that contact lenses not be worn during the time the eye is infected. Once the infection resolves, new contact lenses should be worn instead of the pair that was worn when the infection first occurred. Wearing contact lenses during an active infection will further irritate the conjunctiva and worsen the condition. Returning the infected contacts to the eye once the infection is resolved will infect the eye again.

Illnesses and Conditions Affecting Hearing

Illnesses that occur in the ear can be quite painful and may affect not only hearing but also balance. Infections of the ear are named for the location of occurrence, based on the names of the chambers of the ear.

Otitis Externa

Mechanism: Otitis externa is an infection of the lining of the auditory canal distal to the tympanic membrane, or eardrum. This bacterial or fungal infection in the

chalazion lesion similar to a stye but occurring proximally farther on the eyelid

conjunctivitis highly contagious bacterial infection of the posterior eyelid lining

otitis externa infection of the lining of the auditory canal distal to the tympanic membrane (eardrum); commonly known as "swimmer's ear"

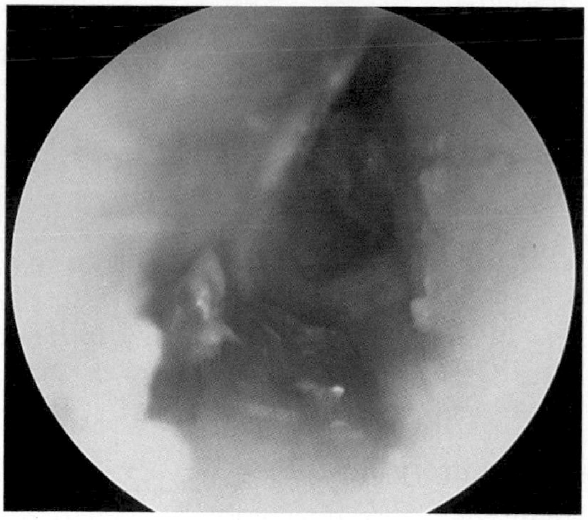

FIGURE 17-19 Otitis externa. (From Zitelli BJ, Davis HW: *Atlas of pediatric physical diagnosis,* ed 3, St Louis, 1997, Mosby.)

external part of the ear is commonly called "swimmer's ear" and occurs when the protective layer of earwax, or cerumen, is flushed out and can no longer protect the skin (Figure 17-19). As the name suggests, swimmers frequently experience this problem. The skin is easily irritated without the protective covering, and the infection readily establishes itself in the warm, dark, and moist environment of the ear.[9] Overcleaning may also compromise the protective cerumen layer and increase the risk of otitis externa.[5]

Signs and symptoms: Symptoms include itching and pain in the auditory canal. A discharge of pus may be present. Pain increases when the pinna is pulled. If left unchecked, the infection may easily spread.[2] Lymph nodes near the ear are usually swollen, and the mastoid area may be enlarged.[5] The cerumen layer usually replaces itself over the course of 3 days. Immersion of the ear may be resumed after symptoms resolve.

Immediate management: Swimmers who frequently suffer from otitis externa should focus on maintaining the protective layer of cerumen in the auditory canal. Over-the-counter solutions are available to properly clean the auditory canal without compromising the cerumen. One or two drops of a mixture of equal parts white vinegar (ascetic acid), 20% alcohol, and water can be used to rinse the canal after each session of swimming or other water activity.[2] This solution dries the auditory canal without removing the protective layer of cerumen. Earplugs are also beneficial in preventing accumulation of water in the ear.

Otitis Media

Mechanism: Otitis media, as the name implies, is an infection of the middle ear, that part of the ear between the eardrum and the inner ear. This infection is very common in children, yet some physicians believe that it is probably overdiagnosed.[12] Otitis media is usually a complication or symptom of a recent or current upper respiratory infection in which the mucous membrane is inflamed and the eustachian tube becomes blocked. Fluid naturally occurs in the ear but is usually drained off by way of the eustachian tubes (Figure 17-20). With those tubes obstructed by inflammation, pressure builds in the middle ear that often distends the eardrum. If the pressure becomes great enough, the eardrum can rupture.[5] The primary cause of tympanic membrane rupture is pressure from otitis media.[3]

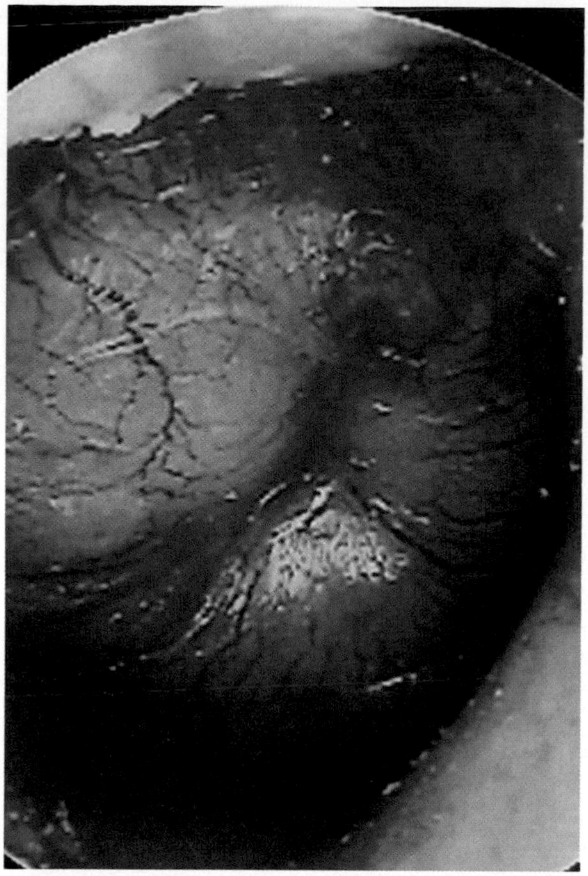

FIGURE 17-20 Otitis media. (From Behrman R, Kliegman R, Jenson H: *Nelson textbook of pediatrics,* ed 17, Philadelphia, 2004, Elsevier/Saunders.)

Signs and symptoms: The infection often follows a recent or current upper respiratory infection (URI); pain at the mastoid process; fever; earache; and a sensation of fullness in the ear. The athlete may complain of impaired hearing, which is caused by fluid that hinders the vibration mechanism of the tympanic membrane. When viewed with an otoscope, the tympanic membrane may appear red and distended (Figure 17-21).

otitis media infection in the middle ear, between the eardrum and inner ear; usually a complication of an upper respiratory infection in which the eustachian tube is blocked

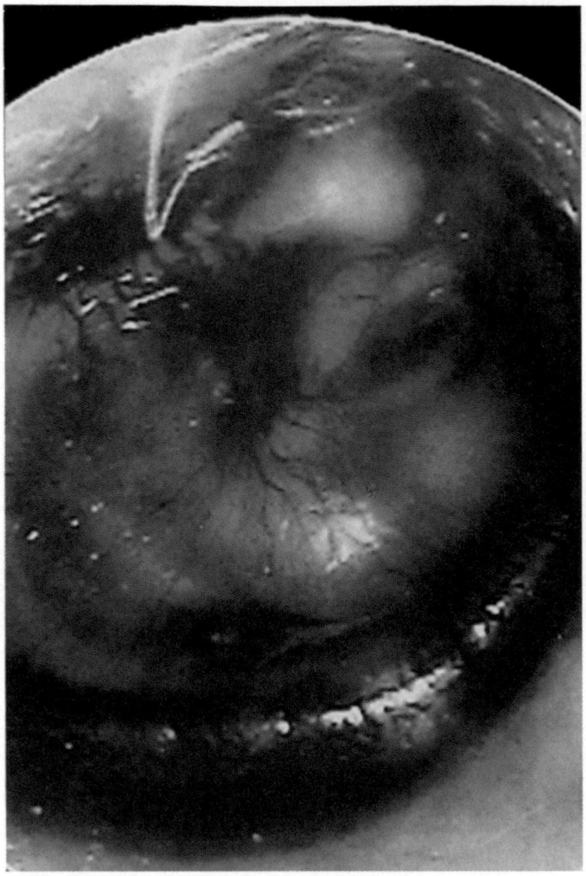

FIGURE 17-21 Distended tympanic membrane. (From Behrman R, Kliegman R, Jenson H: *Nelson textbook of pediatrics,* ed 17, Philadelphia, 2004, Elsevier/Saunders.)

Although the eardrum is normally opaque, a fluid level may still be visualized in a case of true otitis media. The color of the tympanic membrane does not correlate with the presence of pathogenic fluid in the ears.[12] Redness may be caused by fever, crying, or cerumen removal and not necessarily an infection. The bulging membrane and fluid border confirm the presence of an accumulated fluid. Oddly enough, about one third of those suffering from otitis media do not experience an earache.[12] In the other two thirds, the earache can become quite debilitating, depending on the amount of pressure building up behind the tympanic membrane. A positive Weber test, which calls for a use of a tuning fork, indicates the affected ear.[5] It should be noted that many children who display the classic symptoms of otitis media do not have a true otitis media infection but rather benign fluid in the ear.

Immediate management: Because the infection may be viral, prescribed oral antibiotics are not always effective. They are effective only in treating bacterial infections. Sinus decongestants, either prescription or over-the-counter, can reduce the inflammation of the mucous membranes and help in draining the excess fluid from the ear. Air travel and scuba diving can irritate otitis media by increasing the pressure in the ear and should be avoided to decrease the risk of tympanic membrane rupture during ascent or descent.[2]

Illnesses and Conditions Affecting Taste and Smell

The senses of taste and smell are so closely related that conditions affecting one sense tend to affect the other sense as well. Because the respiratory tract and digestive tract enter the body through the mouth, infection can enter either system and cross over to the other, affecting sense organs on both sides.

Upper Respiratory Infections

Mechanism: An upper respiratory infection (URI) is a diagnosis applied to conditions that affect the nasopharynx, trachea, and bronchi. Commonly known as a "common cold," these conditions are usually viral, self-limiting, and highly contagious. The droplets released through a cough or sneeze easily travel great distances and make an entire roomful of people capable of spreading the infection. An athlete suffering from an upper respiratory infection can easily infect an entire team in a very short time when that team is confined to the same dressing room, classroom, bus, or athletic training room.[13] Although URIs are more common in colder seasons, they are not caused by cold weather; instead, they are spread more easily among groups who are confined to close quarters for prolonged periods of time, which often correlates with colder temperatures. Regular exercise seems to increase resistance to the infection, although heavy training can have the opposite effect.[14]

Signs and symptoms: Sufferers of URIs usually exhibit cough, nasal congestion, sore throat, and runny nose. Headaches are common and accompany nasal congestion. Fever may be present, but it usually resolves in the first 24 to 48 hours. The other symptoms may last 7 to 10 days. The symptoms are annoying, but they rarely cause cessation of normal daily activities. Symptoms that last more than 10 days, or are accompanied by a high fever or dark, purulent nasal discharge should not be dismissed as inconsequential. Athletes with these symptoms should be evaluated by a physician.[13]

Immediate management: Treatment is primarily aimed at improving the person's level of comfort because the course of the common cold virus cannot be shortened by medication. Over-the-counter cough preparations, antihistamines, **analgesics**, and **antipyretics** are helpful in reducing the symptoms.

Intermediate management: The athlete suffering from an upper respiratory infection often becomes frustrated by the slow resolution and needs

analgesic medication taken to reduce pain
antipyretic medication taken to reduce fever

reassurance that the symptoms will not linger on indefinitely. Proper hydration is extremely important because it loosens secretions and helps the athlete feel better as the cold runs its course. Athletes involved in activities that lead to great fluid loss will need even more monitoring to ensure that they are properly hydrated.

Allergic Reactions

Mechanism: Hypersensitivity to inhaled environmental matter affects 10% to 20% of the population in the United States and is often seasonal, involving triggers such as pollen.[13] A runny nose, or rhinitis, may be triggered by perennial irritants such as dust, smoke, animal allergens, and some detergents.

Signs and symptoms: In addition to sneezing, the most common symptoms include a runny nose or nasal congestion, with the symptoms improving after the afflicted person leaves the troublesome environment. The symptoms can be very frustrating and exhausting.

Immediate management: Avoiding triggers is the best course of treatment whenever possible. Treating the symptoms with over-the-counter medication is the best course of action. Increased fluid intake will also help by thinning the nasal secretions and reducing the sinus congestion that often accompanies the allergic reaction.

Intermediate management: Allergy immunotherapy injections can raise the threshold at which environmental triggers cause a reaction and should be considered when the allergy symptoms are disruptive to activities of daily living or when the triggers are so common that simple avoidance is not practical.[15] Athletes should be cautious when considering any medications for allergic rhinitis because several preparations that are effective for this condition, such as certain antihistamines and nasal decongestants, are restricted or banned by many national or association sport governing bodies. Athletes with chronic rhinitis that lacks an apparent allergic trigger should be evaluated for other pathological conditions, such as a URI.

Asthma

Mechanism: Asthma is a disorder in which the bronchial passages are temporarily obstructed through inflammation and spasm. Anxiety, environmental allergic triggers, cold ambient temperatures, or dry ambient air can precipitate inflammation and spasm. An episode of asthma is usually short, lasting a few minutes or a few hours, but it can sometimes last for several days.

Signs and symptoms: Wheezing, shortness of breath, dry cough, and associated chest tightness are common symptoms. With prolonged episodes, breathing is difficult without enlisting the neck and upper thoracic muscles to expand the chest. The prolonged use of these muscles may cause generalized soreness in the trunk. Pulse and respirations are elevated during the asthmatic episode.[13]

Immediate management: Many asthma medications work to decrease the frequency of episodes or reverse an episode once it does occur. The medications come in many forms, including pills and aerosolized mists delivered through a metered-dose inhaler (Figure 17-22). For the most part, maintenance medications must be taken daily to prevent the onset of an episode and cannot reverse an episode once it is started. Rescue medications are used to reverse the inflammation and spasm of the airways and therefore reverse the asthma attack. It is important to educate the athlete who requires an inhaler in its proper use so that the medication actually reaches the lungs and is not sprayed onto the walls of the mouth or expelled out of the mouth without reaching the lungs. Box 17-8 summarizes the proper use of a metered-dose inhaler.

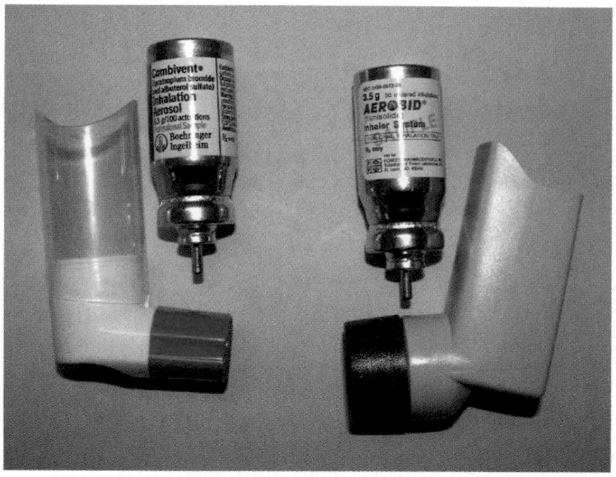

FIGURE 17-22 Metered-dose inhalers. (From Cuppett M, Walsh KM: *General medical conditions in the athlete,* p. 37, St. Louis, 2005, Elsevier/Mosby.)

BOX 17-8 Use of a Metered-Dose Inhaler

1. Shake the inhaler for several seconds to thoroughly mix the aerosol and the medication.
2. Exhale as much as possible through your mouth before placing the mouthpiece of the inhaler to the lips.
3. Close your lips tightly around the mouthpiece.
4. Inhale as the inhaler is activated, releasing the metered-dose of medication.
5. Hold your breath as long as possible.
6. Repeat as prescribed by your physician. You must wait at least 1 minute to allow the inhaler to reload the medication
7. Rinse your mouth after the prescribed number of inhalations.
8. Clean the inhaler casing and canister occasionally by rinsing it in warm water.
9. Replace the canister when the medication is exhausted or whenever it is no longer as effective as expected.

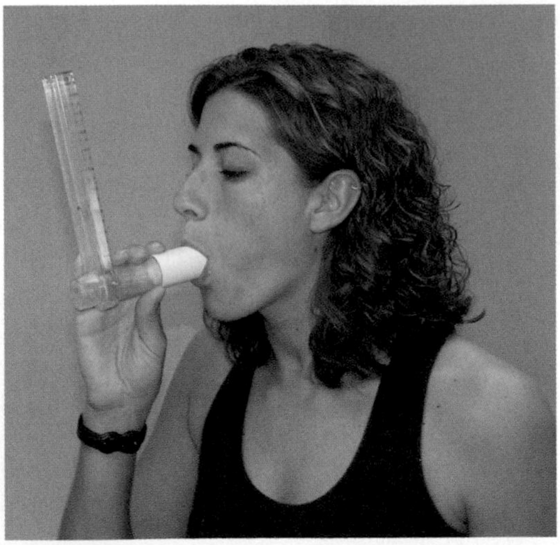

FIGURE 17-23 Peak flow meter. (From Cuppett M, Walsh KM: *General medical conditions in the athlete,* p. 83, St Louis, 2005, Elsevier/Mosby.)

Intermediate management: Athletes with asthma will need to take their maintenance medications daily to decrease the risk of attack. If maintenance medications are used consistently, the use of rescue medications may be decreased. A peak flow meter (Figure 17-23), a quick and simple way to measure pulmonary function, can allow the athlete and the clinician to assess the effectiveness of medication as well as the overall condition of the lungs. A change in seasons may bring an increase in environmental allergens or temperature changes, and the effect of these triggers on the lungs is apparent in peak flow readings long before a full-blown asthma episode occurs.

Aerobic exercise may cause some athletes to experience bronchospasm. These athletes suffer from the symptoms of asthma after only 10 to 15 minutes of vigorous activity. No other environmental triggers are present, but the athlete suffers prolonged shortness of breath, chest tightness and congestion, and a dry cough. The episode may be very subtle or very dramatic. Asthma triggered by exercise may be controlled effectively with metered-dose inhaler medications or through the use of a refractory period.

Using the refractory period to control the onset of asthma requires the athlete to modify the pre-event warm-up to include short bursts of activity at 80% to 90% of maximum workload after administration of a metered-dose inhaler. The warm-up period is lengthened, and the athlete works out to levels just short of inducing an asthma attack. When timed correctly, a refractory period of about 3 hours exists after the initial bronchospasm. During this refractory window, the athlete may compete without worrying that an impending bronchospasm episode will disrupt the event.[13]

Figure 17-24 is a concept map summarizing the various illnesses and conditions affecting the sense organs.

Return to Play Guidelines

Some physicians use the "above the neck" rule to determine an athlete's participation status.[16] For any symptoms located above the neck (e.g., a runny nose, nasal congestion, a sore throat), participation is initially limited to 50% of normal intensity, progressing as tolerated if the symptoms resolve within 15 minutes. If the symptoms remain or worsen, participation should be delayed until the next day. With symptoms that are not "above the neck" (e.g., fever above 100° F, shortness of breath, vomiting, extreme fatigue), participation should not be attempted until the next day.[16]

Because of the neurological basis of the senses, any damage to the senses generally includes a neurological pathology and should be taken seriously. With traumatic injury or with illness, sensory limitations preclude most athletic participation. Because a vast amount of athletic skill relies on information gained though the senses, athletic performance is usually hindered in direct proportion to the damage incurred to the senses. Once the damage is identified and thoroughly evaluated, decisions can be made about return to play; however, damage of any kind should prompt at least a short limitation in activity. With illnesses, the athlete may resume activity once the sensory limitations are minimized and the spread of infection is contained.

Points to Ponder

A multitude of physician specialists, including orthopedists, ophthalmologists, neurologists, family practice practitioners, and otolaryngologists (ENT), may be involved in the resolution of injuries and illnesses to the senses. Once you decide that a physician should see an injured or ill athlete under your care, how do you decide which physician to call?

SUMMARY

The athletic trainer often confronts injuries and illnesses that have an impact on the senses of sight, smell, hearing, and taste. For the most part, these conditions involve the face and should be assessed immediately for any long-term damage to the senses. This chapter gives an overview of the conditions that affect the senses and their management. The athletic trainer should be able to assess these conditions efficiently and promptly and, when indicated, make prudent decisions regarding the need for referral to an appropriate physician.

Revisiting the OPENING *Scenario*

In the opening scenario, the best option would be to limit Karen's participation until the pain and inflammation of her injury had fully resolved and her sense of smell had

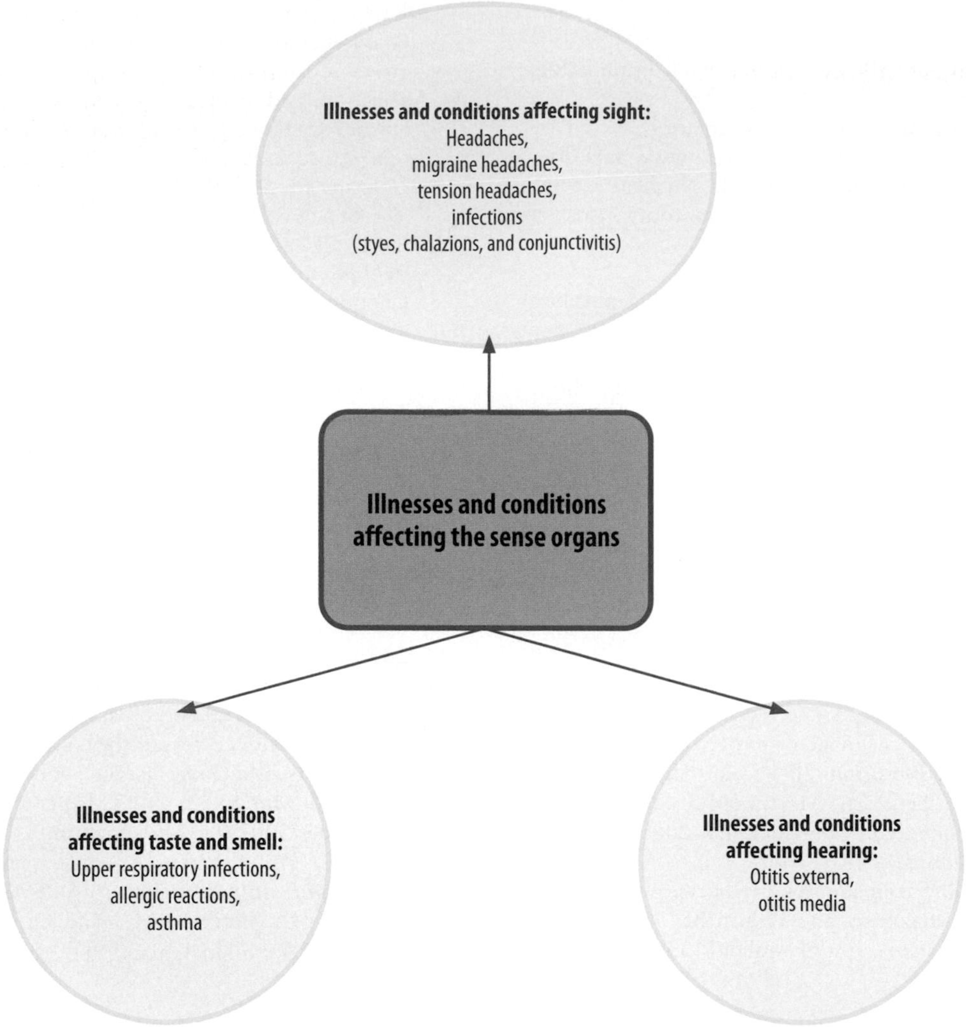

FIGURE 17-24 Concept map overview of illnesses and conditions affecting the senses.

fully returned. Although participation in a game of that magnitude is a goal for most athletes, the game cannot be the deciding factor for the medical staff in clearing or limiting an athlete's participation. The best option for Karen, the team, and the medical staff in this scenario would be to construct a low-profile splint for her nose to protect the current injury and to do as much as possible to prevent re-injury when removing the catcher's mask. Ideally, her participation in softball should be limited to playing only offense—that is, serving as a designated hitter and not playing her usual position of catcher. If a splint or protective face mask could be constructed that would protect Karen adequately, full participation could be allowed. In that case, the nose and the splint should be checked frequently during the game to make sure that the nose remains adequately protected. Karen should be warned to avoid any medications that could either affect reaction times or thin the blood. Both situations increase the risk of re-injury and exacerbation of the original injury.

Issues & Ethics

A few ethical dilemmas may emerge in the management of injuries and illnesses to the senses. Because the problems affecting the senses are rarely catastrophic, the athletic trainer may be tempted to ignore the severity of the situation in light of "the big game" and delay referral to a physician. The athletic trainer should always remember the duty to care for the athlete in a way that will be beneficial in the present as well as in the future. Winning the big game but losing the function of one of the senses is usually not a fair trade. Explaining the need for physician referral to a player for a nonorthopedic injury is sometimes difficult. The "big picture" of continued normal use of the senses is often overshadowed by the "immediate picture" of the big game or the perceived need to compete. How would you explain to a player, coach, or parent the necessity to forgo athletic participation after an injury to the senses?

Web Links

American Academy of Allergy Asthma and Immunology: www.aaaai.org
American Optometric Association: www.aoa.org
Asthma and Allergy Foundation of America: www.aafa.org
Eye and Ear Page (University of Kansas Medical Center): hwww.kumc.edu/instruction/medicine/anatomy/histoweb/eye_ear/eye_ear.htm
Eyeatlas Online: www.eyeatlas.com
Medline Plus: www.nlm.nih.gov/medlineplus/medlineplus.html
National Center for Drug Free Sport: www.drugfreesport.com
National Eye Institute: www.nei.nih.gov/index.asp
Otolaryngology Houston: www.ghorayeb.com/Pictures.html
Structure of the Human Body, Visible Human Cross-Sections (Loyola University Chicago): www.meddean.luc.edu/lumen/MedEd/GrossAnatomy/cross_section
The Physician and Sportsmedicine Online journal: www.physsportsmed.com/index.html
Video Otoscopy: http://rcsullivan.com/www/ears.htm
WebAnatomy (University of Minnesota): www.msjensen.gen.umn.edu/webanatomy

References

1. Wilson SA, Last A: Management of corneal abrasions, *American Family Physician.* 70(1): 123–128, 2004.
2. Anderson MK, Hall SJ, Martin M., editors: *Sports injury management*, ed 2, Philadelphia, 2000, Lippincott Williams & Wilkins.
3. Romeo SJ et al: Facial injuries in sports: a team physician's guide to diagnosis and treatment, *The Physician and Sports Medicine* [serial online] 33(4): 1, 2005. Retrieved March 13, 2007, from www.physsportsmed.com/issues/2005/0405/romeo.htm.
4. Street S, Runkle D: Athletic protective equipment: care, selection, and fitting, New York, 2000, McGraw-Hill.
5. Starkey C, Ryan J: *Evaluation of orthopedic and athletic injuries*, ed 2, Philadelphia, 2002, FA Davis.
6. Gallaspy JB, May JD: *Signs and symptoms of athletic injuries*, St Louis, 1995, Mosby.
7. Baker CL, editors: *The Hughston Clinic sports medicine field manual*, Baltimore, 1996, Williams and Wilkins.
8. Diamond S: Managing migraines in active people, *The Physician and Sports Medicine* [serial online] 24(12): 1, 1996. Retrieved March 13, 2007, from www.physsportsmed.com/issues/1996/12_96/diamond.htm.
9. O'Connor DP: Clinical pathology for athletic trainers: recognizing systemic disease, Houston, 2001, Slack.
10. Millea PJ, Brodie JJ: Tension-type headaches, *American Family Physician* 66: 797–804, 2002.
11. Carter SR: Eyelid disorders: diagnosis and management, *American Family Physician* 57: 2695–2704, 1998.
12. Pichichero ME: Acute otitis media. Part I: Improving diagnostic accuracy, *American Family Physician* 61: 2051–2059, 2000.
13. Cuppett M, Walsh KM, editors:. *General medical conditions in the athlete*, St Louis, 2005, Elsevier/Mosby.
14. Krane JW: Upper respiratory infection, *The Physician and Sports Medicine*, [serial online] 30(9): 1, 2002. Retrieved March 13, 2007, from www.physsportsmed.com/issues/2002/09_02/okane.htm.
15. Huggins JL, Looney RJ: Allergen immunotherapy, *American Family Physician* 70(4): 690–696, 2004.
16. Mellion MB, Putikian M, Madden C: *Sports medicine secrets*, ed 3, Philadelphia, 2003, Hanley & Belfus.

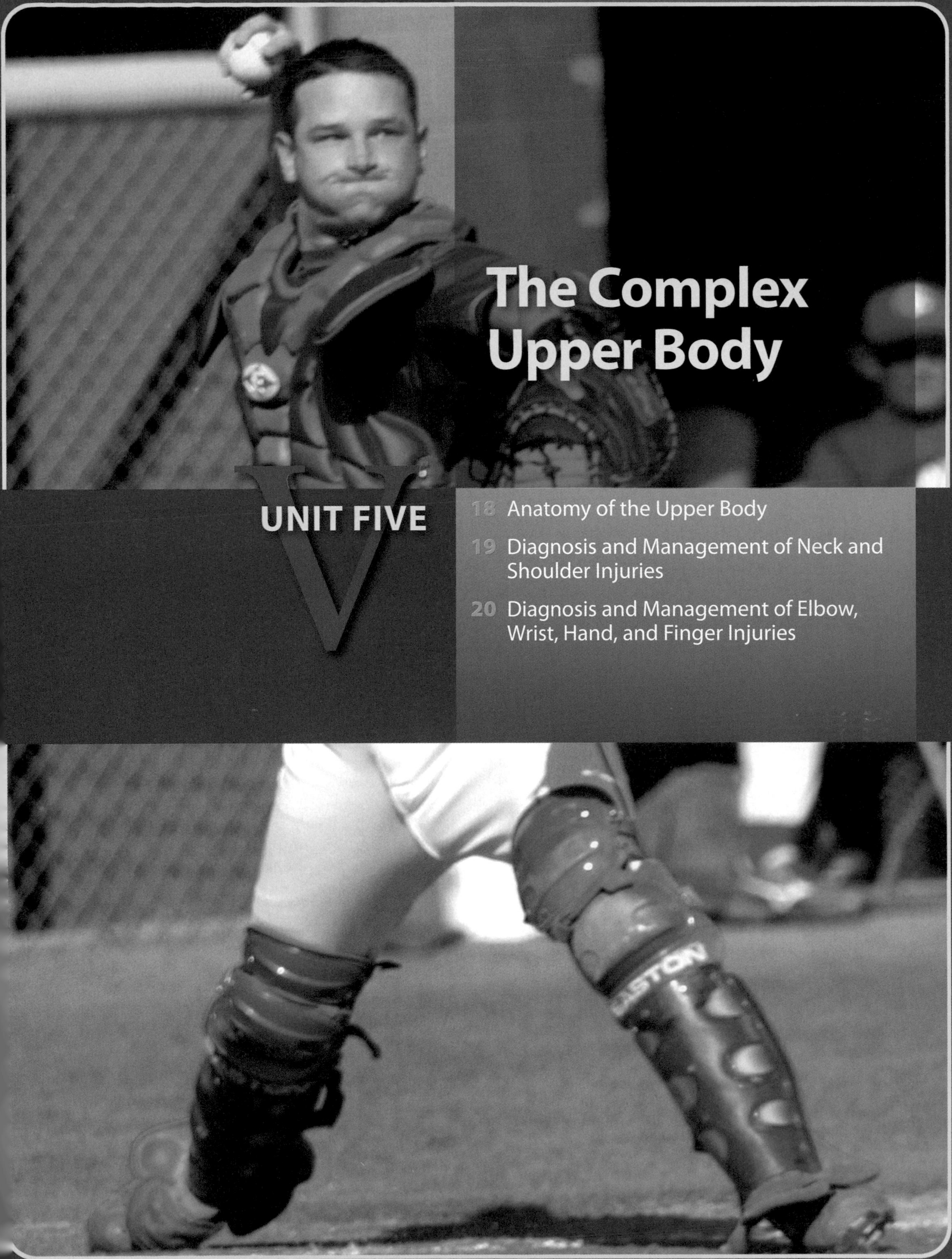

UNIT FIVE

The Complex Upper Body

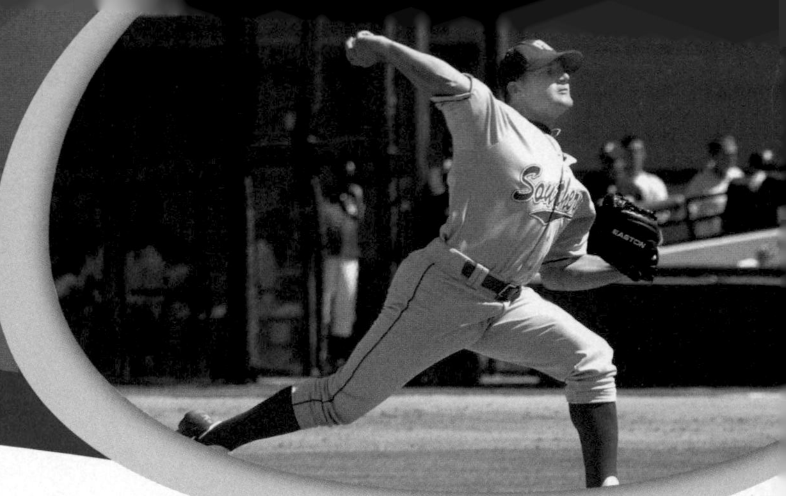

18 Anatomy of the Upper Body

ROBERT MOSS

Learning Goals

1. Name and describe the basic anatomical structures (i.e., bones, ligaments, muscles, tendons, nerves, arteries, veins), their unique aspects, and their locations relative to the upper body.
2. Use appropriate terminology when describing anatomical structures of the upper body.
3. Conceptualize the interdependence of the structures of the upper body.
4. Recognize the complexity of the structures of the upper body.
5. Identify how the role or function of each of the anatomical structures in the upper extremity may change as other parts of the upper extremity move.

The lower body is amazing not only for its own accomplishments but also for its often overlooked role in enabling the spine to be our workhorse. As the lower extremity goes, the spine must follow. Similarly, the workhorse aspect of the spine means that it must be stable while also being somewhat mobile to permit all the movements that happen below and above it. The transfer of forces created by the larger-muscled lower body must go up thorough the spine to the upper body so that the upper body may accomplish several highly complex movements. The spine never rests. Whether a person is standing, sitting, or lying down, the spine is absorbing forces and protecting the spinal cord so that appropriate movements may occur.

The complexity of the upper body is evident in the fine tuning of the articulating bones that form joints, the ligaments that provide stability but still allow mobility, the muscles that initiate and control movements, and the nervous system that supplies the sensory feedback and signals to fire the muscles. The upper body often moves as if it were the end of a whip because the major forces are generated by the legs, thighs, and gluteal and abdominal regions. Other times, movements are initiated within the upper body that result in powerful actions, moderating movements, or delicate dexterities. The complex and simple movements will be better understood as the anatomy is presented. In brief, a greater variety of movements is performed in the upper body than anywhere else in the body, and yet an appropriate amount of stability is necessary to allow the mobility to occur. This concept is made evident as the upper body serves as a platform to support movements in the hand.

FUNCTIONS OF THE UPPER BODY

The upper body is an extension of the upper thorax and spine in that many of the muscles that work on the upper body have attachments on the thorax, spine, and clavicle. These body parts were presented earlier in Chapter 13 (Figure 18-1). Here, these structures are discussed in the context of the upper body. The upper body is often broken down into three anatomical areas: (1) the shoulder and arm, (2) the elbow and forearm, and (3) the wrist, hand, and fingers. Each subsequent **distal** area works best as an

distal farther away from the body's midline or center relative to another landmark

Terms that appear in boldface green type are defined in the book's glossary.

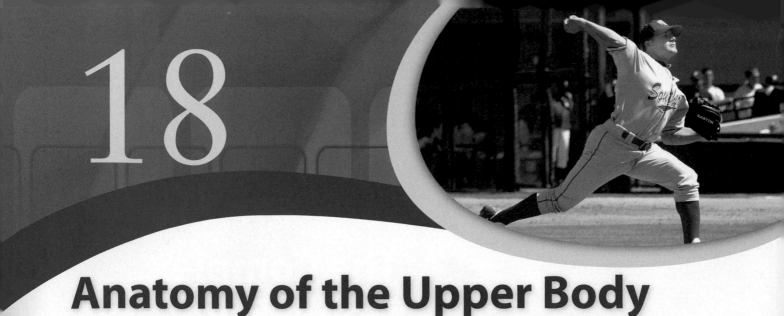

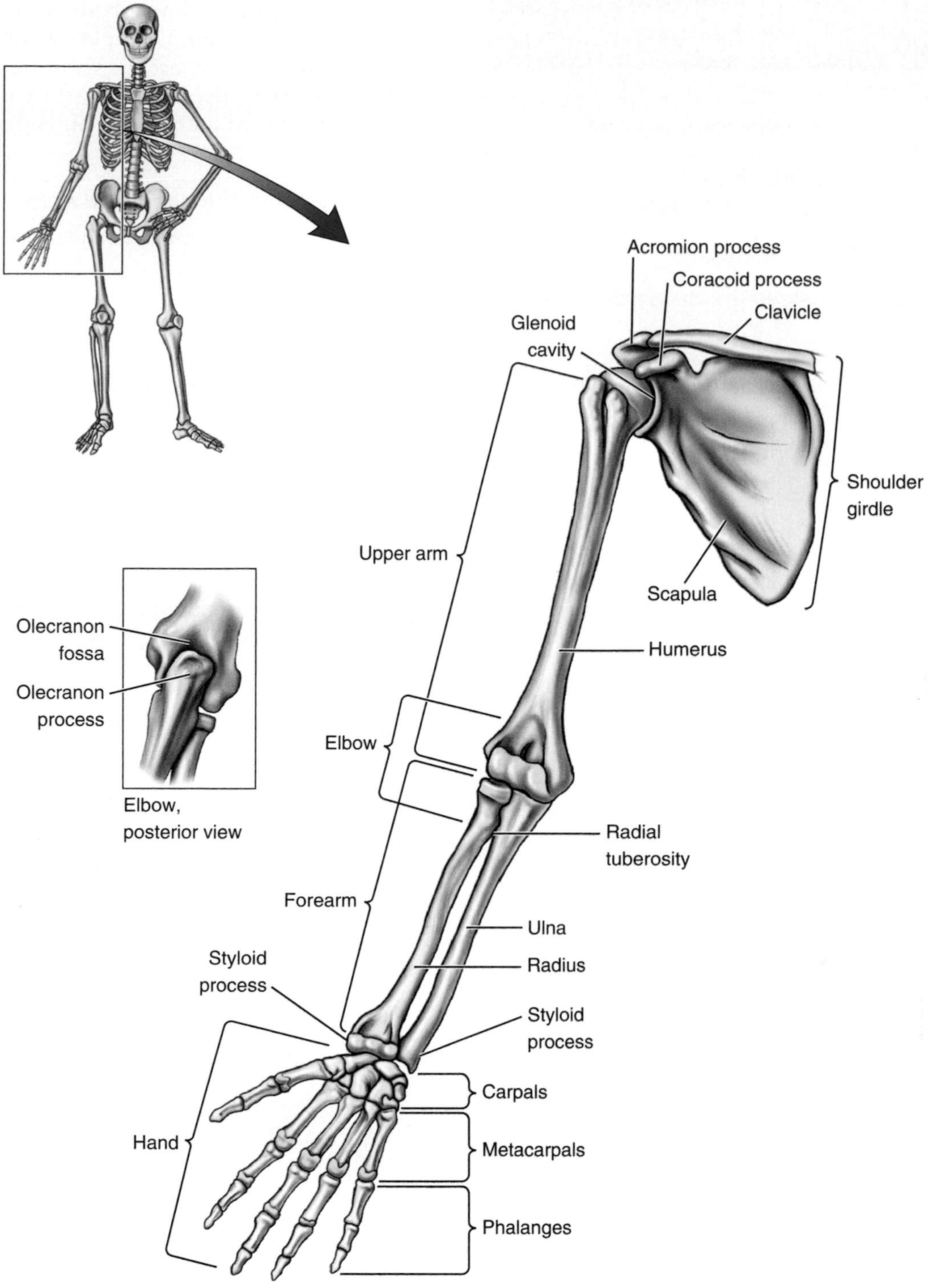

FIGURE 18-1 Bones of the upper body, anterior view. (From Herlihy B: *The human body in health and disease,* ed 3, p. 122, Philadelphia, 2007, Saunders/Elsevier.)

extension of a healthy working **proximal** area. This relative dependence demonstrates the complex interactions of the various components of the upper body.

Functions of the upper body, as summarized in Box 18-1, are often taken for granted. They include reaching in a multitude of directions to grab or pick up objects of many different sizes and shapes, pushing objects of many different sizes and shapes in a multitude of directions, and initiating a throwing motion in several directions with objects of various shapes and

proximal closer to the midline or center of the body relative to another landmark

BOX 18-1 Four Main Functions of the Upper Body

1. Reaching to pick things up, manipulate objects, and extend the length of the body
2. Pushing objects of different shapes and sizes
3. Perform a throwing motion, both overhand and underhand, to propel something though the air
4. "Catching" the body when it falls out of balance

sizes. The upper body also works to catch the weight of the body when falling or losing balance.

ANATOMY OF THE UPPER BODY

The anatomy of the upper body consists of bones, ligaments, joints, muscles, and nerves. This chapter covers only basic information about these structures, sufficient for an understanding of subsequent chapters that discuss the evaluation of upper body injuries.

Bones of the Upper Body

There are some similarities and some differences between the bones of the upper body and those of the lower body. For example, the bones of the upper body closely resemble the shape of their companion bones in the lower body, just on a smaller level and with the exception of the phalanges (i.e., the phalanges of the fingers are bigger than those of the toes). A difference between the two sets of bones is that the bones and joints of the upper body appear to face the opposite direction from the bones of the lower body, with the exception of the shoulder and hip. Examples of companion joints facing the opposite way are the knee and the elbow and the ankle and the wrist. Note how the palm of the hand faces up or forward but the sole of the foot faces down or backward.

Bones of the Shoulder and Arm Area

The three bones that form the foundation of the shoulder and arm are the clavicle, scapula, and humerus.

Clavicle. The clavicle is an S-shaped bone that protects the organs of the thorax; the upper part of the lungs and major vessels that arise off the heart are all located behind the medial aspect of the clavicle (Figure 18-2). The clavicle serves another important role of being a strut for the shoulder in that it actually keeps the shoulder complex, composed of the clavicle, scapula, and humerus, in its normal lateral position. Without the clavicle, the shoulder would collapse in on the chest. There are two key landmarks on the clavicle: the sternal end, which articulates with the sternum, and the acromial end, which articulates with the acromion process of the scapula. The S-shaped shaft of the clavicle lies between the two ends. The clavicle's S shape lends itself to another function, which is to absorb forces from the side. Excessive forces can be absorbed as the clavicle slightly bends along its S curve, similar to what the spine does as it absorbs forces that are transmitted up and down the spine. The shaft of the clavicle is a common site of fracture resulting from a direct force and from a force on the lateral aspect, such as that which would occur after a person falls on the shoulder or is shoved into the boards during ice hockey.

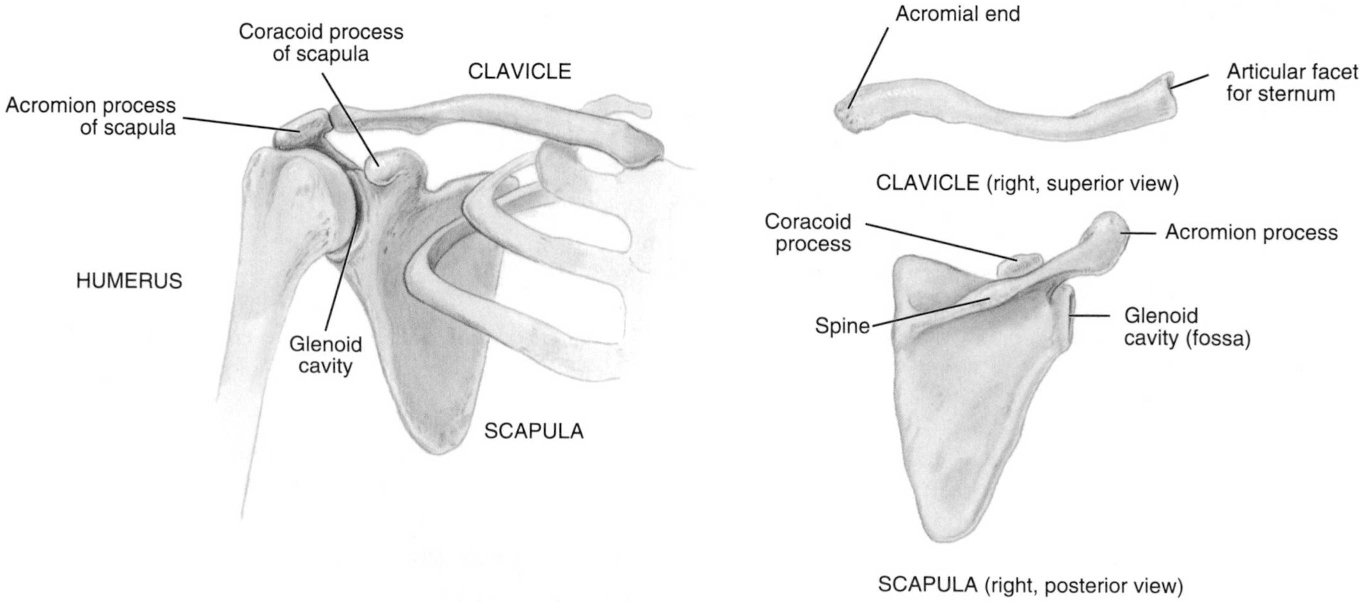

FIGURE 18-2 Scapula and clavicle. (From Applegate EJ: *The anatomy and physiology learning system,* ed 3, p. 102, Philadelphia, 2006, Saunders/Elsevier.)

Scapula. The scapula, a bone that is commonly called the *shoulder blade,* is found on the superior, posterior thorax (see Figure 18-2). It is triangular and has three borders, or sides (i.e., medial, lateral, and superior) and three irregularly shaped bony landmarks (i.e., the acromion process, the coracoid process, and a "spine" that resembles a ridge and runs across the posterior surface about one third of the way down from the top. The scapula is unique in that it appears to be suspended on the upper, posterior thorax by many muscles pulling in all different directions. By reaching behind your back with one hand, you can feel your scapula move in all directions as you move your arm up and down, forward, and backward.

Technically, the scapula's articulation with the posterior thorax does not form a joint, but the resultant movements that occur here are integral for the general movements that occur at the shoulder. All the muscles that attach to and cover the scapula also protect it if it is hit. Therefore the body of the scapula is rarely injured. The glenoid **fossa**, located at the lateral uppermost aspect of the scapula, is important because it forms the shallow cup in which the head of the humerus rests. This configuration forms what is often referred to as the *shoulder joint proper.* This fossa is actually rather shallow, but it is extended by a cartilaginous extension called the *glenoid labrum.* The role of the labrum will be explained in greater detail when the joints of the shoulder are presented.

Humerus. The longest bone in the body, the humerus spans the gap between the shoulder and the elbow (Figure 18-3). Proximally, it has a head that articulates with the glenoid fossa. The neck of the humerus connects the head of the humerus with the shaft of the humerus. On the lateral aspect of the point at which the neck connects to the shaft, there is a big bump called the greater tubercle. The lesser tubercle is located anterior and medial to the greater tubercle, with an intertubercular groove running vertically between the two tubercles. Following the shaft of the humerus down to the elbow, you can feel bumps on the medial and lateral aspects of the humerus just above the elbow. These bumps are called the medial and lateral **condyles.** The respective centers of these condyles are called **epicondyles.**

The distal aspect of the humerus is similar to the distal aspect of the femur in that they both have condyles and epicondyles. Behind the distal humerus, between the condyles, is a shallow depression called the olecranon fossa. The olecranon fossa accepts the olecranon of the ulna, which allows the elbow to be fully straightened. On the **medial** side of the olecranon fossa, still on the distal humerus, is the spool-shaped bony projection called the trochlea, and on the **lateral** side is the capitulum, a rounded bony projection. These two bony projections join with the proximal ulna and radius, respectively, to form the elbow. These projections, along with other sites on the humerus, also serve as muscle attachments.

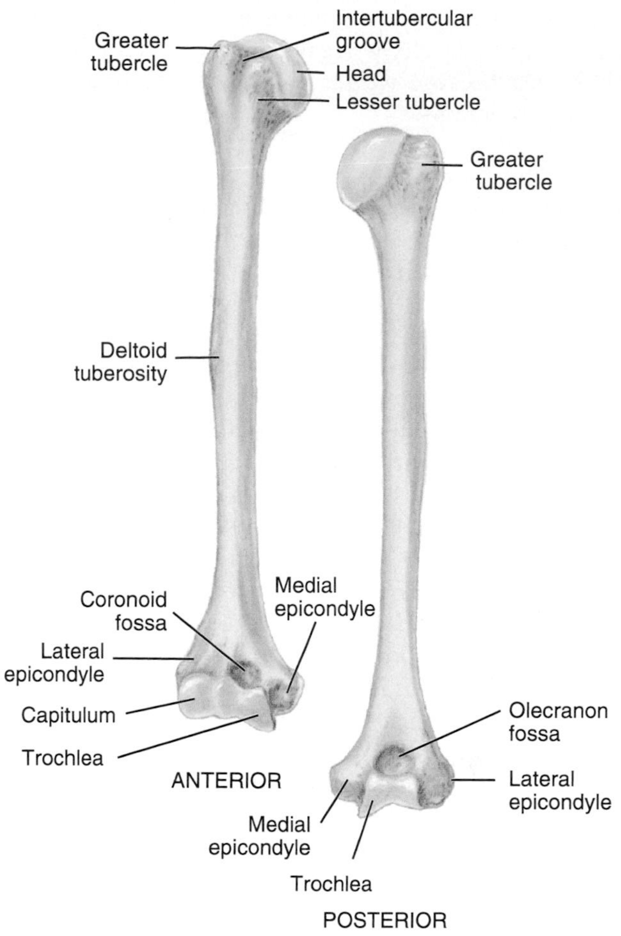

FIGURE 18-3 Humerus. (From Applegate EJ: *The anatomy and physiology learning system,* ed 3, p. 102, Philadelphia, 2006, Saunders/Elsevier.)

Bones of the Elbow

The elbow comprises three bones and is arranged similarly to the knee—one proximal bone that hinges

fossa a shallow, broad, round depression on a bone that serves as a base of articulation for the head or rounded surface of another bone in the same joint
condyle rounded prominence at the end of a bone to facilitate articulation with another bone
epicondyle rounded projection at the end of a bone and the center of a condyle that serves as an attachment point for tendons and ligaments
medial toward the midline or center of the body (inner aspect) relative to another landmark
lateral away from the midline or center of the body (outer aspect) relative to another landmark

with two distal bones running parallel to each other. The bones of the elbow are much smaller than the bones of the leg because weight bearing is not one of their primary functions.

Ulna. The ulna is one of two long thin bones in the forearm, the area between the elbow and the wrist (Figure 18-4). The proximal end of the ulna is larger than its distal end, and it has two distinguishing landmarks—the olecranon and the trochlear notch. They articulate with the olecranon fossa and the trochlea, respectively, of the distal humerus to form the elbow proper. When you place your elbow on your desk and cup your chin with your hand as you contemplate this material, it is your olecranon that makes contact with the desk. Distally, the ulna has a "head" with a concave surface that allows it to articulate with the wrist bones.

Radius. The radius is the other long thin bone in the forearm (see Figure 18-4). Its proximal end is smaller than its distal end. Proximally, it has a head that articulates with the capitulum of the humerus and an area called the *neck,* just below the head. Distally, it has a relatively large concave surface that articulates with the wrist bones. The ulna and radius are connected by an interosseous membrane. When palpated distally, the radius projects about a half inch farther than the ulna. The distal aspects of the radius and ulna are susceptible to fracture when a person falls on an outstretched arm and hand.

Bones of the Wrist, Hand, and Fingers

Continuing distally, you run into the wrist, hand, and fingers. There are eight carpals, or wrist, bones; five metacarpals, or hand bones; and 14 phalanges that make up the five fingers (Figure 18-5). The configuration is similar to that of the foot except that there are only seven tarsal bones. The carpals of the wrist are irregularly shaped bones that articulate with each other in such a way that subtle delicate movements of the wrist can take place and strong powerful movements can be supported. The proximal row of carpals from medial to lateral is composed of the pisiform, triquetrum, lunate, and scaphoid. The distal row, from medial to lateral, is composed of the hamate, capitate, trapezoid, and trapezium. The bone that receives the most attention is the scaphoid, which is commonly fractured and may have a poor healing outcome.

To consider all aspects of the wrist, the five metacarpals must also be included. They are small "long" bones

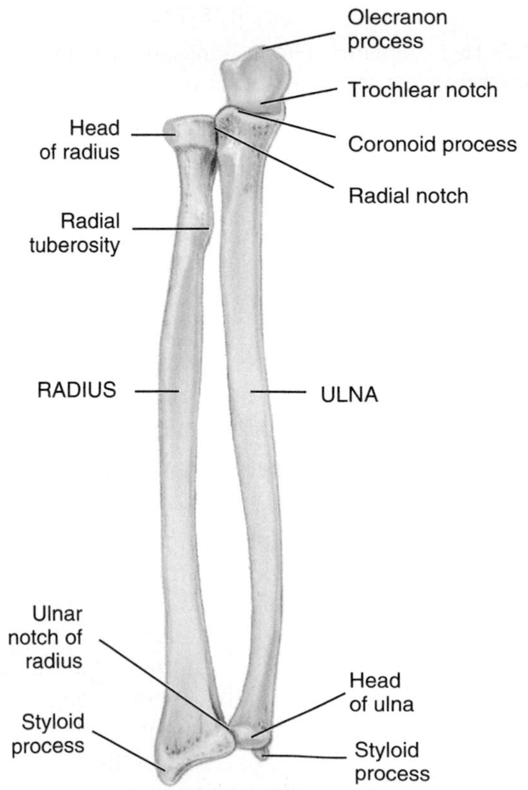

FIGURE 18-4 Radius and ulna. (From Applegate EJ: *The anatomy and physiology learning system,* ed 3, p. 103, Philadelphia, 2006, Saunders/Elsevier.)

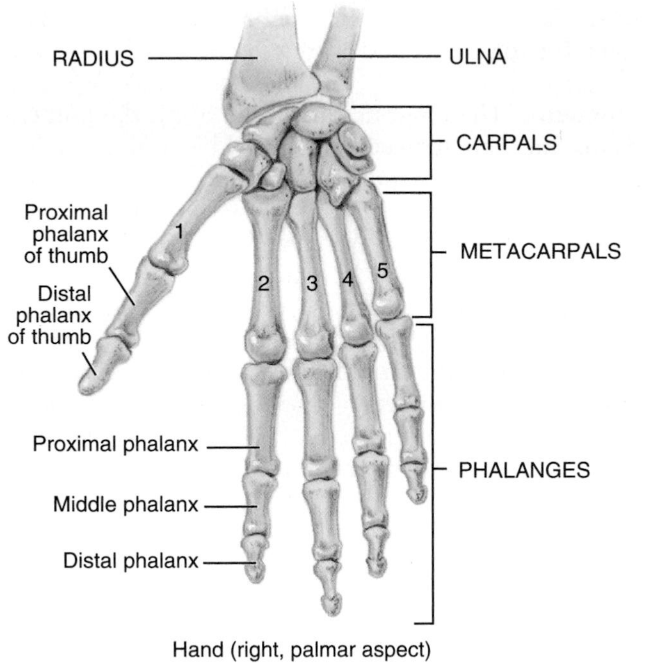

FIGURE 18-5 Bones of the hand and wrist. (From Applegate EJ: *The anatomy and physiology learning system,* ed 3, p. 104, Philadelphia, 2006, Saunders/Elsevier.)

interosseous membrane thin fibrous tissue separating bones at the joint

BOX 18-2 Bones of the Upper Body

Shoulder and Arm
Clavicle
Scapula
Humerus

Elbow
Ulna
Radius
Olecranon fossa

Wrist, Hand, and Fingers
Carpals (eight wrist bones)
Proximal row: pisiform, triquetrum, lunate, scaphoid
Distal row: hamate, capitate, trapezoid, trapezium
Metacarpals (five hand bones)
Phalanges (14 finger bones)

much like the metatarsals of the foot. Each metatarsal has a proximal base and a distal head. There are five metatarsals, which are numbered from one through five from lateral to medial when the hand is viewed in the anatomical position. The phalanges are even smaller "long" bones with proximal bases and distal heads.

Box 18-2 summarizes the bones of the upper body, which are discussed in detail in the following sections.

Joints and Ligaments of the Upper Body

The joints and ligaments of the upper body operate under different stressors than the joints and ligaments of the lower body. Although the lower body must absorb all the forces from landing on the ground when walking and running, the upper extremity absorbs forces from the ground less frequently. (An exception is when a person walks on his or her hands.) Therefore the joints and ligaments of the upper body are more concerned with allowing free-flowing movements than with absorbing significant forces.

Shoulder Joints

There are three synovial joints of the shoulder: the sternoclavicular, acromioclavicular, and glenohumeral. The ability of the scapula to move freely and yet be stabilized on the posterior thorax is also very important, but this scapulothoracic articulation, although it functions as a joint, is not generally considered a joint. It does play a vital role in stabilization and function of the shoulder complex and glenohumeral joint.

Glenohumeral Joint. The joint formed by the glenoid fossa and the head of the humerus is called the glenohumeral joint (GH joint; Figure 18-6). This joint is responsible for the majority of the movement that occurs at the shoulder. Most of its ligamentous support is in the front of the joint, but there are also muscles, primarily the rotator cuff, that provide dynamic support. When someone is told that he or she has a dislocated shoulder, the reference is to the glenohumeral joint. The most common mechanism of such an injury is when a person falls on an outstretched hand, forcing the arm back and levering the head of the humerus forward and out of the glenoid fossa. This type of injury will be covered in Chapter 19.

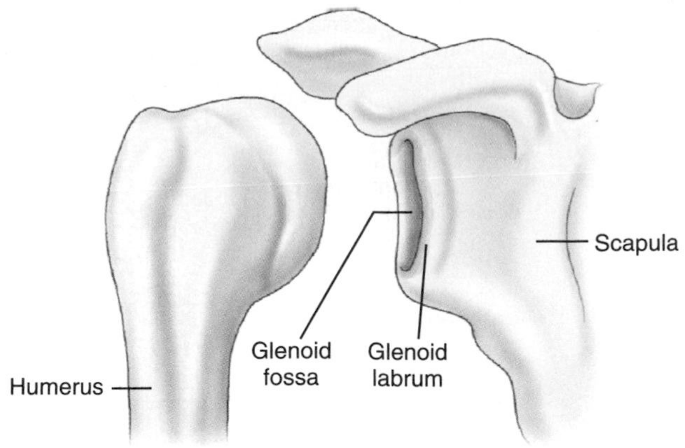

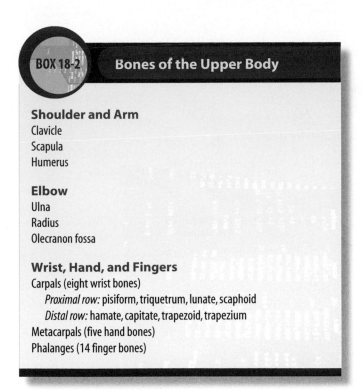

FIGURE 18-6 Glenohumeral joint. (From Muscolino JE: *Kinesiology: the skeletal system and muscle function,* p. 369, St Louis, 2006, Mosby/Elsevier.)

Sternoclavicular and Acromioclavicular Joints. Two joints, the sternoclavicular joint (SC joint) and the acromioclavicular joint (AC joint), are formed by the clavicle and articulate with the sternum and acromion of the scapula, respectively. The sternoclavicular is a relatively stable, somewhat immobile joint, but the clavicle does elevate, depress, and spin slightly when the arm is raised or rotated. Thick anterior and posterior sternoclavicular ligaments cover the front and back of the sternoclavicular joint, keeping it securely in place (Figure 18-7).

The acromioclavicular joint is more prone to injury than the sternoclavicular joint because it is exposed to a greater variety of forces and its three ligaments are not as strong. Also, the clavicle is positioned slightly superior of the center of the relatively flat acromion process, unlike many joints in which there often is a "reception" area on one bone (e.g., the olecranon fossa on the distal, posterior humerus for the olecranon of the ulna) in which the other bone fits. There are the two coracoacromial ligaments holding the

synovial joint a type of joint allowing some degree of free movement

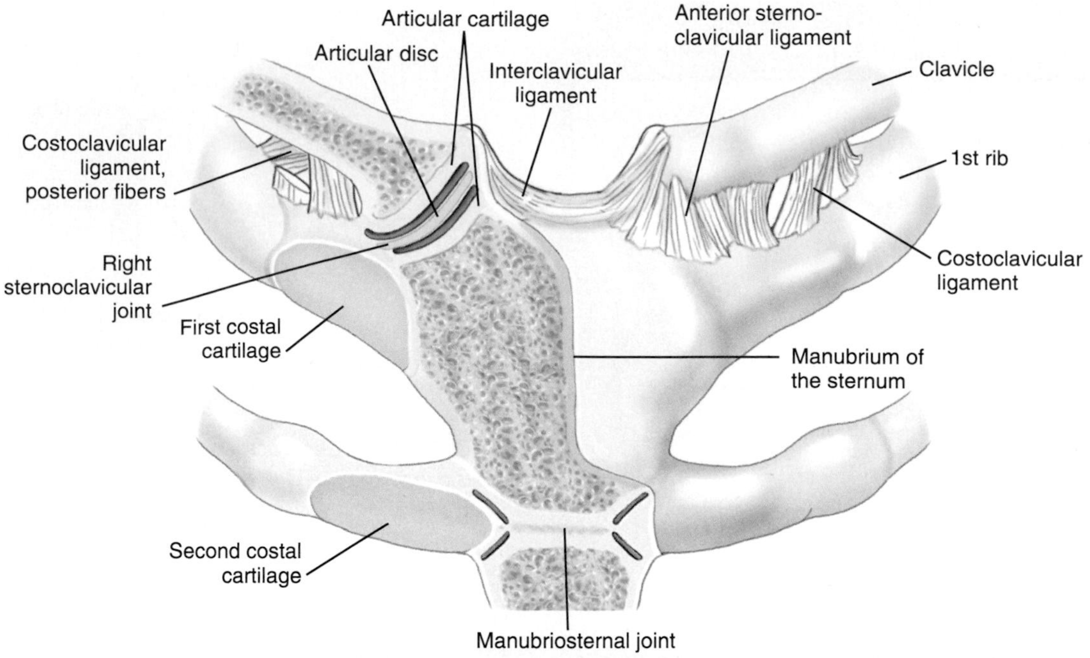

FIGURE 18-7 Sternoclavicular joint. (From Muscolino JE: *Kinesiology: the skeletal system and muscle function,* p. 376, St Louis, 2006, Mosby/Elsevier.)

clavicle down and an acromioclavicular ligament spanning the acromial end of the clavicle with the acromion process, but these ligaments are not particularly strong. The general injury mechanism for this structure is when a force is applied to the top of the joint. Injury to this joint is often classified as a shoulder separation (Figure 18-8).

Shoulder Kinematics

There are 13 movements that can occur at the shoulder area. Most of these movements rely on the interaction of the three shoulder joints and the scapula's articulation with the posterior thorax. *Complex* is a very apt term for these movements. Flexion and extension occur in the sagittal plane. Abduction and adduction occur in the frontal plane. Internal rotation, external rotation, horizontal flexion, and horizontal extension occur in the transverse plane. The movements of elevation, or shrugging the shoulders, and depression, or letting the shoulders sag, are often overlooked. Similarly, protraction, in which the scapula slides laterally and

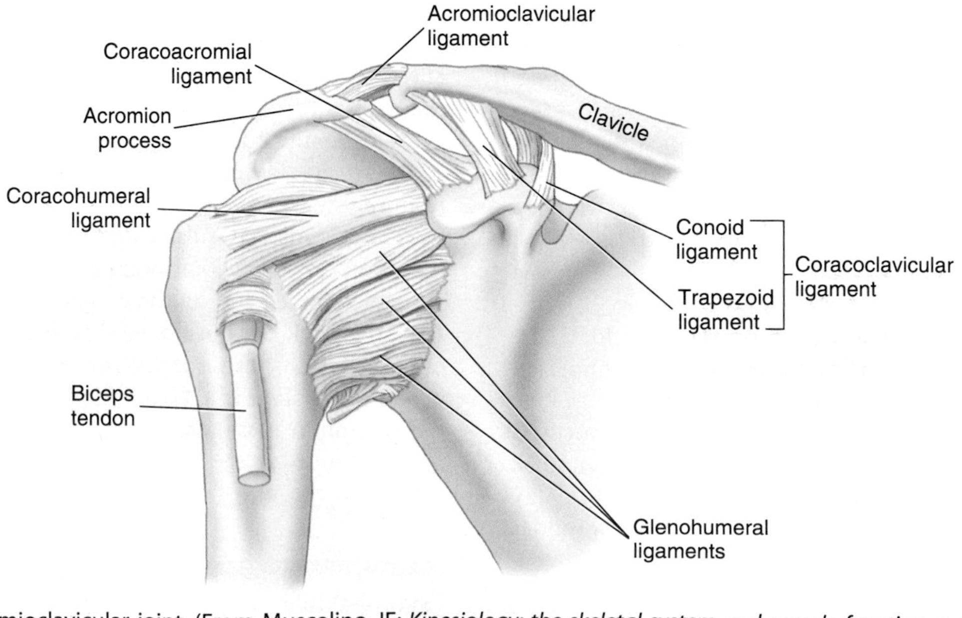

FIGURE 18-8 Acromioclavicular joint. (From Muscolino JE: *Kinesiology: the skeletal system and muscle function,* p. 378, St Louis, 2006, Mosby/Elsevier.)

forward as you reach straight out in front of your body as far as you can; and retraction, the action of pulling your scapula back and medially toward your spine, are also often overlooked. All four of these movements are rarely considered compared with more recognizable movements such as abduction and extension during the initiation of a throwing motion. The final movement, circumduction, is a combination of many movements; it happens when you swing your arm in a big circle, and it occurs in all three planes. The muscles that initiate and control these movements will be discussed later in this chapter.

Elbow Joints

Just as the shoulder can be thought of as group of three joints—the sternoclavicular, the acromioclavicular, and the glenohumeral—the elbow can be thought of as a group of two and possibly three joints (Figure 18-9).

Humero-Ulnar Joint. The actual hinge joint of the elbow is the humero-ulnar joint, which comprises the trochlea of the distal humerus and the trochlear notch of the proximal ulna. The elbow joint is stabilized on its medial aspect by the medial collateral ligament of the elbow. It can also be called the ulnar collateral ligament. This is a triangular ligament that works to prevent excessive **valgus** movement at the elbow, much like the lower extremity and the medial collateral ligament of the knee. The elbow actually has a valgus position in the frontal plane similar to that of the knee. This valgus position in the elbow is called the carrying angle and is generally a bit larger in women than in men (Figure 18-10).

Humero-Radial Joint and Annular Ligament. Lateral to the humerus-ulna articulation are the humerus and radius, or humero-radial joint. This joint is formed by the capitulum of the distal humerus and the head of the proximal radius. This lateral joint is stabilized on its lateral aspect by the lateral collateral ligament of the elbow. It can also be called radial collateral ligament. This ligament works to prevent excessive varus movement at the elbow—again, much like the lower extremity and the lateral collateral ligament of the knee. **Varus** means that the lower segment, in this case the forearm, is deviated medially or toward the inside. Because there are very few forces or stresses that place the arm in that position, the lateral collateral ligament is rarely injured. This scenario of function and form is also similar to the forces and stresses on the lateral collateral ligament of the knee.

There is one other ligament in this area, the annular ligament. It runs anteriorly from the medial anterior ulna to the medial posterior ulna. On the way, it encircles the head of the radius. The point at which the proximal radius and ulna meet is called the proximal radioulnar joint. This ligament allows the radius to rotate under the capitulum.

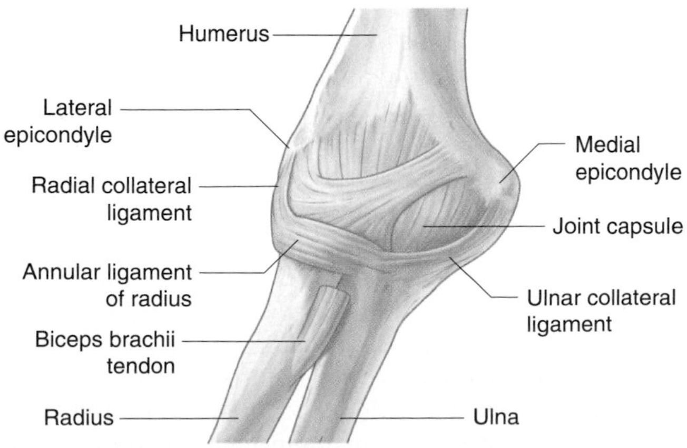

FIGURE 18-9 The elbow joint. (From Moses KP et al: *Atlas of clinical gross anatomy,* p. 224, St Louis, 2005, Elsevier/Mosby.)

Points to Ponder
Is it the shape of the bones that dictates the angle of the carrying angle, or is it the placement of the muscles that attach on and around the bones of the elbow?

Elbow Kinematics

There are four movements that occur at the elbow joint. The main two are flexion and extension. When viewed in an anatomical position, they occur in the sagittal plane. The other two movements are pronation and supination. **Pronation** is the movement of turning your hand to a palm down position while keeping your elbow flexed to 90 degrees, and **supination** is the movement of turning your hand to a palm-up position while keeping your elbow flexed to 90 degrees. A way to remember that supination is with the palm up is to imagine carrying a cup of soup. The muscles that initiate and control these movements will be discussed later in the chapter.

Wrist Joints

The wrist joint is really a host of many joints because wherever two bones articulate, there exists a ligament

valgus abnormal turning of a bone outward
varus abnormal turning of a bone inward
pronation movement of the forearm so that the palmar surface is downward
supination movement of the forearm so that the palmar surface is upward

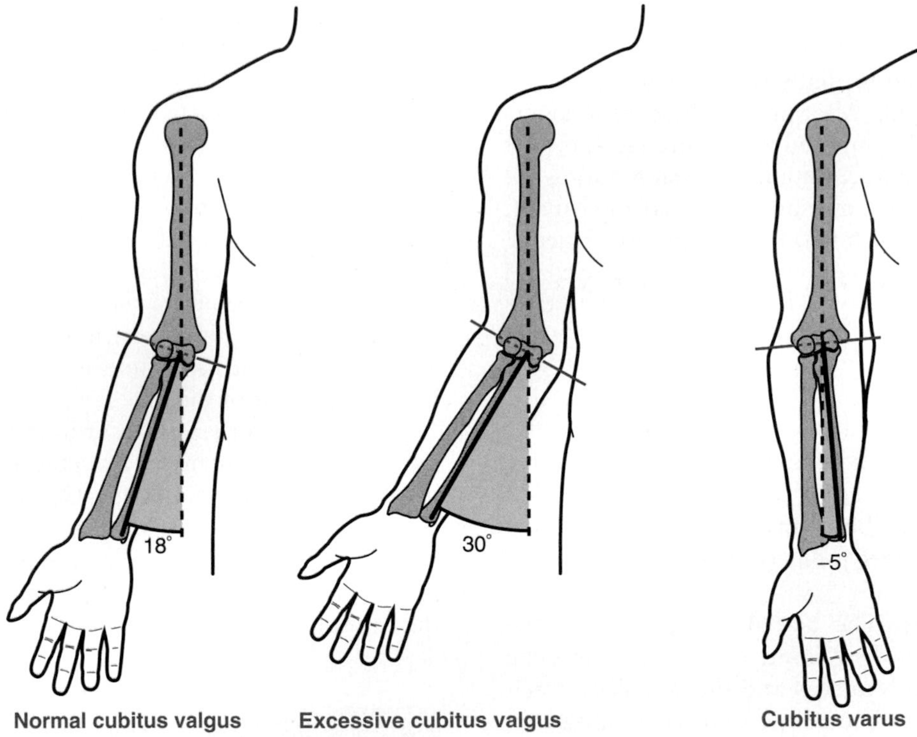

FIGURE 18-10 Carrying angle (cubitus valgus) of the elbow. (From Neumann D: *Kinesiology of the musculoskeletal system: foundations for physical rehabilitation,* p. 138, St Louis, 2002, Mosby.)

of sorts. With two forearm bones, eight carpal bones, and five metacarpals, many articulations are possible (Figures 18-11 and 18-12). The distal radioulnar joint, unlike the proximal radioulnar joint that was stabilized by an external annular ligament, is stabilized by an internal ligament and an articular disk. The articular disk

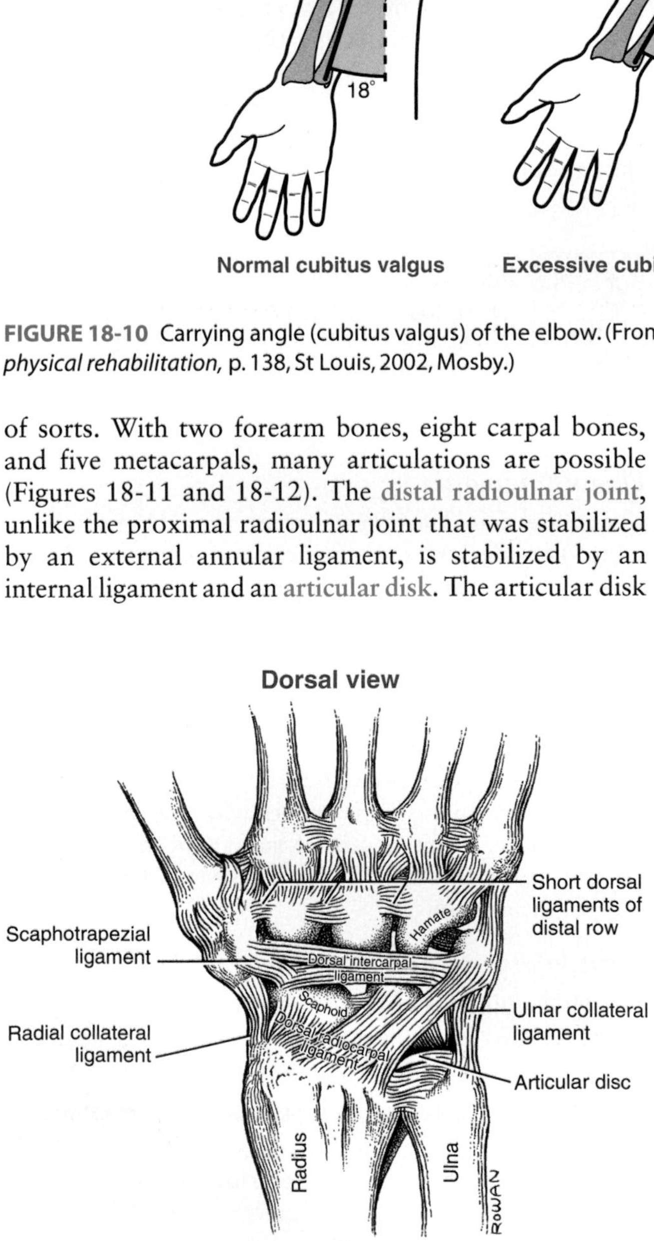

FIGURE 18-11 Dorsal wrist. (From Neumann D: *Kinesiology of the musculoskeletal system: foundations for physical rehabilitation,* p. 178, St Louis, 2002, Mosby.)

works similarly to the meniscus in the knee and plays an important role of buffering the forces when a person falls and lands on an outstretched hand. Medially at the wrist, just as at the elbow, there is an ulnar collateral ligament that helps prevent a valgus movement of the distal segment—in this case, the hand. It is called the *ulnar collateral ligament* because it connects the ulna to the carpal bones on the medial side of the wrist. The lateral wrist has a radial collateral ligament connecting the radius to the lateral carpal bones. This ligament works to prevent excessive varus movement, which is also called *ulnar deviation.*

Wrist Kinematics

It appears that the wrist has several movements because of the many bones and joints in the area. However, only five movements occur at the wrist. Two of the movements are flexion and extension, which occur in the sagittal plane. Two other movements, mentioned in the previous paragraph, are ulnar deviation and radial deviation. Both of those movements occur in the frontal plane. Varus motion at the wrist is called ulnar deviation because the hand moves up toward the ulnar side. Because a valgus movement at the wrist moves toward the radius bone, this motion is often called radial deviation. To understand these motions better, place your hand with your palm facing you about 12 to 18 inches away from your face. Bend your wrist as far as it goes toward your pinky side. Note how far

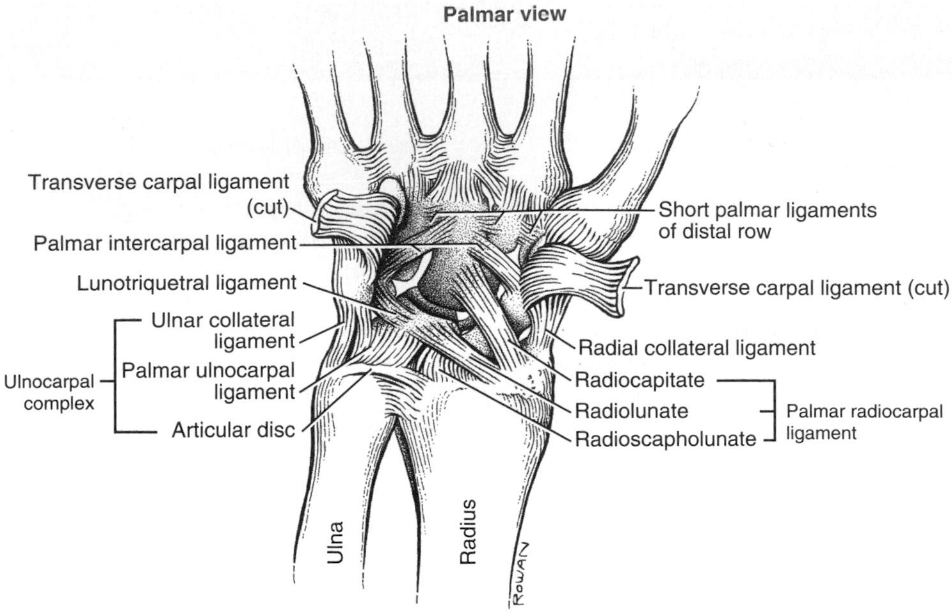

FIGURE 18-12 Palmar wrist. (From Neumann D: *Kinesiology of the musculoskeletal system: foundations for physical rehabilitation*, p. 179, St Louis, 2002, Mosby.)

it moves. This is called *ulnar deviation* because the hand is moving toward the ulna. Bend your wrist as far as it goes toward your thumb side. This is called *radial deviation* because the hand is moving toward the radius. In which direction does your hand move the most? (NOTE: It should be toward your ulna unless you have had a wrist injury in the past.) The fifth motion is circumduction, which occurs when you make circles with your hand. It occurs in all three planes.

Finger Joints and Kinematics

Metacarpophalangeal Joints. Distal to the carpometacarpal joints are the metacarpophalangeal joints. Flexion-extension and adduction-abduction occur at the metacarpophalangeal joints. Flexion and extension are easy to see, and adduction-abduction is evident when you spread your fingers and bring them back together. Adduction and abduction at the fingers are in relation to an imaginary line going down through the middle finger. When your fingers move toward your middle finger, they are adducting; when they move away from your middle finger, they are abducting. The metacarpophalangeal joints have medial and lateral collateral ligaments to stabilize them during valgus and varus movements, just as collateral ligaments do wherever they are located (Figure 18-13).

Interphalangeal Joints. Beyond the metacarpophalangeal joints are the interphalangeal joints. The thumb has only two phalanges, so it has only one interphalangeal joint. The four fingers have three phalanges, so they each have two interphalangeal joints. The proximal interphalangeal joint is made up of the proximal and middle phalanges, whereas the distal phalangeal joint is made up of the middle and distal phalanges. Medial and lateral collateral ligaments stabilize the interphalangeal ligaments on their sides. The interphalangeal joints have two motions, flexion and extension.

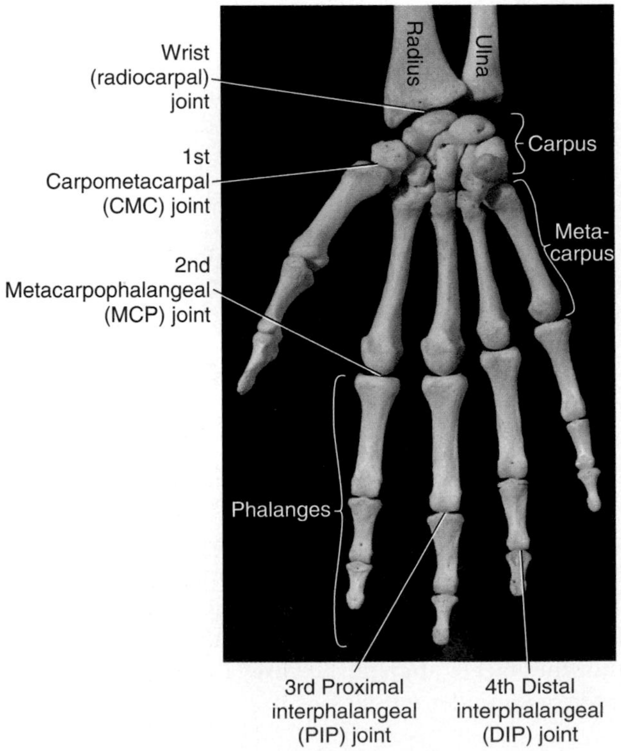

FIGURE 18-13 Joints of the fingers. (From Muscolino JE: *Kinesiology: the skeletal system and muscle function,* p. 389, St Louis, 2006, Mosby/Elsevier.)

BOX 18-3 Joints and Ligaments of the Upper Body

Shoulder
Glenohumeral joint
Sternoclavicular joint
Acromioclavicular joint
 Coracoacromial ligaments
 Acromioclavicular ligament
Associated movements: 13 total: flexion and extension (sagittal); abduction and adduction (frontal); internal rotation, external rotation, horizontal flexion, horizontal extension (transverse); elevation and depression; protraction and retraction; and circumduction

Elbow
Humero-ulnar joint
 Medial (ulnar) collateral ligament
Humero-radial joint
 Lateral (radial) collateral ligament
 Annular ligament: anterior from medial aspect of ulna to posterior ulna; encircles radial head
Associated movements: 4 total: flexion, extension, pronation, supination

Wrist
Host of many joints
Distal radioulnar joint
 External annular ligament
 Internal ligament
 Articular disc (buffers forces on wrist)
 Ulnar collateral ligament: connects ulna to carpal bones on medial side of wrist
 Radial collateral ligament: connects radius to lateral carpal bones
Associated movements: five total: flexion and extension (sagittal); ulnar deviation and radial deviation (frontal); circumduction (all three planes)

Finger
Metacarpophalangeal joints
 Medial and lateral collateral ligaments
 Associated movements: flexion, extension, abduction, adduction
Interphalangeal joints
 Thumb: one
 Fingers: two each (proximal and distal)
 Medial and lateral collateral ligaments
 Associated movements: flexion and extension

Box 18-3 summarizes the joints and ligaments of the upper body, which are discussed in detail in the following sections.

Muscles of the Upper Body

The muscles of the shoulder area may be grouped in a number of ways. They are presented in this text on the basis of their location.

Anterior Shoulder and Shoulder Girdle Muscles

The anterior shoulder girdle is the area that spans from the upper thorax over to the scapula and humerus. In this arrangement, muscles classified as the anterior shoulder girdle muscles will be the pectoralis major, pectoralis minor, subclavius, and serratus anterior. Although the serratus anterior is also located laterally, it is included in this group because it connects the thorax to the scapula. The anterior shoulder muscles are the coracobrachialis and the biceps brachii. Figure 18-14 illustrates the anterior shoulder muscles.

Pectoralis Major. *Pectoralis* is Latin for "chest," and the pectoralis major is the largest chest muscle. It has two proximal attachments and one distal attachment. The two proximal attachments are called the clavicular head, which comes off the proximal clavicle, and the sternocostal head, which comes off the anterior sternum and first six rib costal cartilages. The two heads come together in a common tendon that inserts on the lateral aspect of the intertubercular groove. Functions of the pectoralis major are to adduct and medially rotate the humerus. The "pecs" get a good workout when doing a push-up or a bench press as they pull the humerus forward (horizontal adduction).

Pectoralis Minor. The pectoralis minor is a smaller chest muscle that lies beneath the lateral aspect of the pectoralis major. It comes off ribs three, four, and five and runs up to the coracoid process of the scapula. The main function of the "pec" minor is to protract the scapula. It also stabilizes the scapula when acting in concert with the rhomboid muscles.

Subclavius. The name of the subclavius muscle indicates its location, which is below the clavicle. It actually runs from the first rib up to the middle third of the clavicle, anchoring the clavicle on its inferior aspect. Its function is depression of the clavicle.

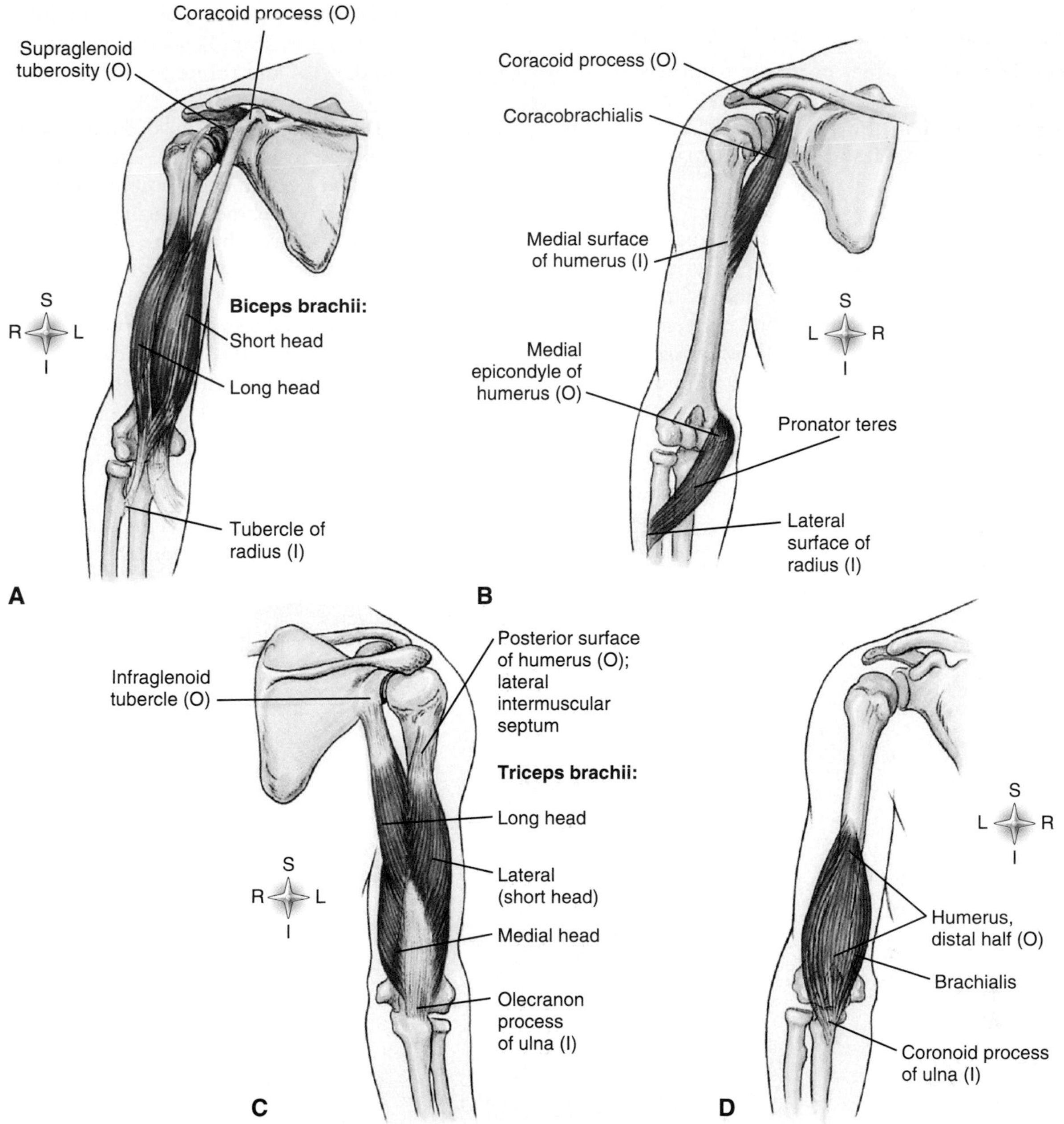

FIGURE 18-14 Anterior shoulder muscles. **A**, Biceps brachii. **B**, Triceps brachii. **C**, Coracobrachialis and pronator teres. **D**, Brachialis. *O*, Origin; *I*, insertion. (From Thibodeau GA, Patton KT: *Anatomy and physiology,* ed 6, p. 377, St Louis, 2007, Mosby/Elsevier.)

Serratus Anterior. The serratus anterior is the last muscle of this group. Like the other muscles, it has attachments on the ribs. In this case, it attaches on the lateral aspects of ribs one through eight and then proceeds to wrap around the rib cage to the posterior thorax, attaching to the anterior medial border of the scapula. Its main function is to protract the scapula. An example of protraction of the scapula is when someone performs a punching motion and reaches out with the fist. Protraction is when the scapula moves laterally and anterior around the ribs.

Coracobrachialis. The coracobrachialis runs from the coracoid process of the scapula to the medial aspect of the humerus about one third of the way down from the humeral head. It is one of three muscles that have attachments on the coracoid process. The function of the coracobrachialis is to help with shoulder flexion and adduction.

Biceps Brachii. The biceps brachii has two heads; *bi* means "two," and *ceps* means "heads." The short head comes off the coracoid process and merges with the long head, which comes off the superior aspect of the glenoid labrum, and then attaches to the medial, upper radius. The biceps acts on the shoulder to help with shoulder flexion, but it is better known for its action on the elbow, where it helps with flexion and supination.

Posterior Shoulder and Shoulder Girdle Muscles

Muscles classified as the posterior shoulder girdle muscles include the trapezius, latissimus dorsi, levator scapulae, rhomboid major, and rhomboid minor; the posterior shoulder muscles are the teres major and the triceps (Figure 18-15).

Trapezius. There are three parts to the trapezius: upper, middle, and lower. The upper "trap" actually comes off the middle, lower part of skull and a broad, thick ligament that runs over the spinous processes of the cervical vertebrae. The middle "trap" comes off the same ligament, where it runs over the first six thoracic vertebrae. Lastly, the lower trapezius comes off the spinous processes of thoracic vertebrae seven through twelve. All of these portions merge to form an attachment on the back of the lateral clavicle and the acromion and spine of the scapula. The angle of pull of each part of the trapezius determines its action. The upper trap elevates and upwardly rotates the scapula; the middle portion retracts, or pulls the scapula medially; and the lower trap tends to depress and rotate the scapula downward.

Latissimus Dorsi. The latissimus dorsi, as its name implies, covers almost the entire lateral dorsal (back) surface of the body. Specifically, it comes off the spinous process of thoracic vertebrae six through twelve, the thoracolumbar fascia, lower three ribs, and iliac crest. This large muscle then runs up under the arm, twists, and attaches on the floor of the intertubercular groove. The "lats" are often called the *swimmer's muscle* because they work to adduct, extend, and medially rotate the humerus, essentially pulling the swimmer through the water.

Levator Scapulae. The levator scapulae comes off the back of cervical vertebrae one through four and inserts on the superior, medial aspect of the scapula. As its name implies, this muscle elevates the scapula. However, because it elevates the scapula from the scapula's medial

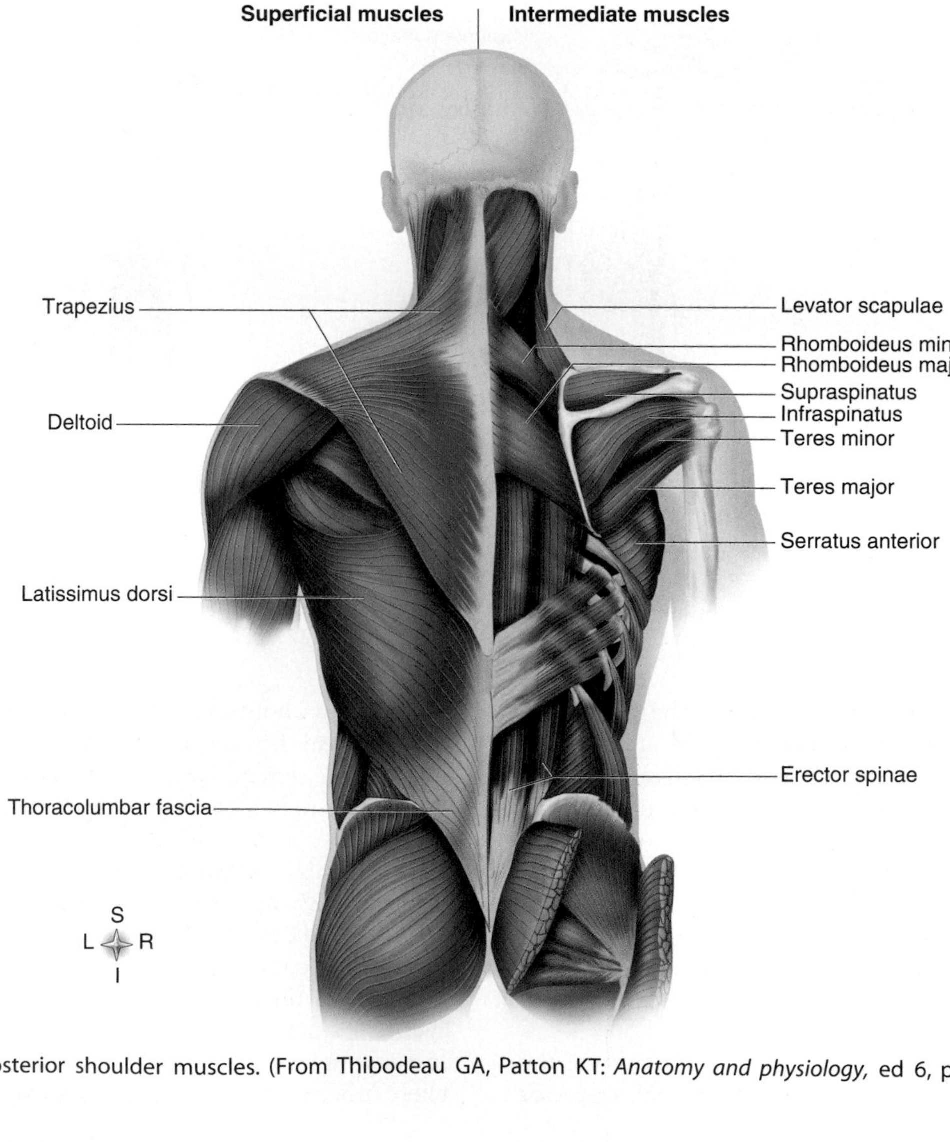

FIGURE 18-15 Posterior shoulder muscles. (From Thibodeau GA, Patton KT: *Anatomy and physiology,* ed 6, p. 367, St Louis, 2007, Mosby/Elsevier.)

aspect, this action ends up tipping the lateral part of the scapula down. You can picture this by looking at the scapula from the back and imagining a string pulling up on the medial aspect of the scapula. If the medial side goes up, then the lateral side has to go down.

Rhomboids Major and Minor. The last two muscles of this group are the rhomboid major and rhomboid minor. The rhomboid minor is smaller (hence "minor") and is located above the rhomboid major. It comes off the nuchal ligament and spinous processes of the seventh cervical and first thoracic vertebrae, and it runs down and laterally to the medial aspect of the scapular spine. The rhomboid major comes off the spinous processes of vertebrae two through five and then attaches on the medial border of the scapula below its spine. These two muscles work to retract the scapula, or pull it back toward the spine.

Teres Major. The teres major runs along the lower edge of the scapula, under the armpit, and attaches at the inner aspect of the intertubercular groove, near the insertion of the latissimus dorsi. It is an adductor and internal rotator of the humerus.

Triceps. The word triceps means "three heads" in Latin. Each head serves as a proximal attachment of this muscle. The long head comes off the back of the lower glenoid cavity. The lateral head comes off the back of the upper midhumerus. The short head comes off the inner half of the lower midhumerus. All three heads merge and form the resultant tendon that inserts on the olecranon process of the ulna. Extension of the humerus is one of the functions of the triceps because the long head inserts on the inferior glenoid fossa, but it plays a larger role in movement at the elbow.

Glenohumeral Muscles

In this presentation, there are five muscles classified as the glenohumeral muscles. They are classified as such because of their intimate relationship with the glenohumeral joint. These muscles include a superficial muscle (the deltoid), four deep muscles (the rotator cuff muscles). The deltoid is superficial and considered to be a prime mover of the glenohumeral joint. The rotator cuff muscles lie deep and are largely responsible for stability of the glenohumeral joint so that the deltoid and other large muscles can move it around. Two other muscles that were placed in other muscle groups, the pectoralis major in the anterior shoulder girdle muscles and the latissimus dorsi in the posterior shoulder girdle muscles, may also be considered glenohumeral muscles because they play an important role in the movements of the glenohumeral joint.

Deltoid. The most superficial muscle is the deltoid, which is composed of three parts: anterior, middle, and posterior. These three parts come off the lateral clavicle, acromion, and scapular spine and merge to attach approximately 2 centimeters below the greater tubercle of the humerus. When the three parts of the deltoid work together, the humerus is abducted, or brought above the head in the frontal plane. The anterior part of the deltoid flexes the humerus in the horizontal plane, and the posterior part of the deltoid extends the humerus in the horizontal plane. The other four muscles are deep to the deltoid, and together they make up the rotator cuff muscles. These four muscles form a "cuff" over the glenohumeral joint inserting on the greater tubercle of the humerus (Figure 18-16).

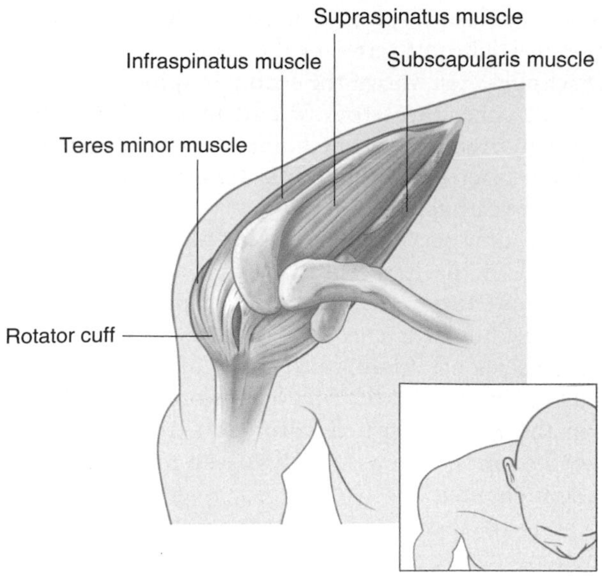

FIGURE 18-16 Rotator cuff muscles. (From Moses KP et al: *Atlas of clinical gross anatomy,* p. 197, St Louis, 2005, Elsevier/Mosby.)

Subscapularis. Covering the anterior aspect of the glenohumeral joint is the subscapularis. It comes off the anterior surface of the scapula and angles up to blend in with the three other rotator cuff muscles. This muscle internally rotates the humerus.

Infraspinatus and Teres Minor. The infraspinatus comes off the posterior scapula from under the scapular spine and merges with the teres minor. The teres minor runs parallel to and just below the infraspinatus and parallel to and just above the teres major. Both of these muscles merge with the supraspinatus and attach on the greater tubercle of the humerus. Both of these muscles work concentrically to externally rotate the humerus and work eccentrically to decelerate internal rotation of the humerus during the throwing motion. These two muscles cover the posterior aspect of the glenohumeral joint.

Supraspinatus. Covering the top of the glenohumeral joint and lying just below the deltoid in the supraspinous fossa is the supraspinatus muscle. The supraspinatus helps the deltoid to abduct the humerus. It comes off the scapula, just above the scapular spine, and merges with the other three rotator cuff muscles to insert on the greater tubercle of the humerus. The subscapularis actually inserts on the lesser tubercle. Individually, these are relatively small muscles, but when they work together, they serve the important function of keeping the head of the humerus stabilized and depressed in the glenoid fossa, letting the more powerful muscles move the humerus through its motions. The rotator cuff muscles are often called the "SITS" muscles, an acronym formed by the first letters of the muscles that form the rotator cuff. Rotator cuff injuries are relatively common and will be discussed more in the subsequent chapter.

Table 18-1 summarizes the names, locations, and functions of the anterior, posterior, and glenohumeral muscles.

Muscles of the Elbow Joint

Muscles that cross the elbow joint and initiate the volitional movements that occur at the elbow are the brachioradialis, biceps brachii, brachialis, triceps, anconeus, pronator teres, and supinator (Figure 18-17).

Brachioradialis. The brachioradialis comes off the middle third of the lateral humerus and travels laterally down to the distal lateral aspect of the radius. It helps flex the elbow, particularly in the "thumbs-up," or neutral, position of the elbow.

Biceps and Brachialis. Functionally, because the biceps crosses the anterior elbow joint, it works to flex the elbow. Further, because it attaches on the medial aspect of the proximal radius, it also spins the radius in such a way that the palm ends in the upward-facing position. This motion, as discussed previously, is called *supination*. The brachialis is another strong elbow flexor. It runs from the distal anterior humerus to the proximal anterior ulna and is deep to the biceps.

Triceps and Anconeus. The main extensors of the elbow are the triceps and the anconeus. The triceps was mentioned in the section dealing with the glenohumeral joint, but it is more active at the elbow and is the most powerful elbow extensor. The anconeus is a small muscle that runs from the lateral epicondyle of the humerus to the lateral olecranon. It is deep to the triceps and has more of a stabilizing role that actually extends the elbow. Like the biceps and triceps, many muscles cross two or more joints. This allows the muscle to multitask and work on each joint. Just as the biceps brachii works on the shoulder but is more active on the elbow, the same is true of the triceps. The anconeus works with the triceps to produce elbow extension.

Pronator Teres. The pronator teres is often included with the forearm muscles, but because it works on the proximal radioulnar joint, it is also relevant to the elbow (see Figure 18-20). It mainly comes off of the medial epicondyle and runs diagonally down and in front of the elbow joint to the mid lateral radius. It helps pronate the forearm by spinning the radius in such a way that the palm faces down.

Supinator. The supinator mainly comes off of the lateral epicondyle of the humerus and dives between the ulna and radius, attaching to the posterior aspect of the proximal radius. Following its path shows that when this muscle contracts, the radius is spun in such a way that the palm ends facing up, or in a supinated position.

Table 18-2 summarizes the names, locations, and functions of the elbow joint muscles.

Wrist Muscles (Flexors)

The muscles of the wrist are usually described as flexors or extensors. The muscles that lie on the anterior surface of the forearm are called the *flexor-pronator group* because they initiate wrist and finger flexion or pronation. Most of these muscles that act on the wrist come from a point fairly high up on the forearm, at the medial epicondyle of the humerus. They travel down the forearm to cross the front of the carpals and eventually attach to the metacarpals or phalanges. These muscles are often described according to their location relative to the skin surface.

The superficial group is composed of the pronator teres, which was discussed previously; the flexor carpi ulnaris; the palmaris longus; and the flexor carpi radialis. The entire superficial group arises from the medial epicondyle.

Flexor Carpi Ulnaris. The flexor carpi ulnaris attaches distally at the base of the second metatarsal. Individually, it flexes the wrist and flexes to the ulnar side, a movement that is sometimes called *ulnar deviation.*

Palmaris Longus. The palmaris longus inserts into the distal palmar **aponeurosis** and is absent in approximately 15% of the population. Although the lack of a palmaris longus may seem to be a disadvantage, no evidence supports such a theory. In fact, the palmaris longus tendon is often used to replace torn or injured ligaments and muscles, which suggests that its presence is inconsequential. If it is present, it is thought to help flex the wrist.

aponeurosis a tough, broad, fibrous sheet of connective tissue serving as a means to connect bone and muscle to bone

TABLE 18-1 **Muscles of the Shoulder**

MUSCLE(S)	LOCATION	FUNCTION*
	ANTERIOR SHOULDER MUSCLES (6)	
Pectoralis major	There are two pectoralis major muscles, and each has two parts: the clavicular and the sternal. The clavicular and sternal parts merge and form a triangular muscle that runs laterally across the chest to the upper lateral humerus.	Acting alone, each muscle adducts and internally rotates the humerus. Acting together, they are used in performing push-ups and the bench press. When they contract concentrically, they push the body or weight up; when contracting eccentrically, they control the body or weight as it is lowered.
Pectoralis minor	There are two pectoralis minor muscles. Each runs from ribs two through five up to the coracoid process of the scapula.	Acting alone, each muscle protracts, or pulls forward, the scapula.
Serratus anterior	There are two serratus anterior muscles. Each runs from ribs one through eight or nine around the ribs to the medial anterior border of the scapula.	Acting alone, each muscle protracts, or pulls forward, the scapula. This muscle allows a person to thrust the arm forward when making a punching motion.
Subclavius	There are two subclavius muscles. Each runs from the clavicle down to the first rib.	Acting alone, each muscle stabilizes the first rib and protects the vessels that run behind it.
Coracobrachialis	The coracobrachialis runs from the coracoid process to the medial aspect of the humerus about one third of the way down from the humeral head.	It serves to help with shoulder flexion and adduction.
Biceps brachialis	The biceps brachii has two heads. The short head comes off the coracoid process and merges with the long head, which comes off the superior aspect of the glenoid labrum. They attach to the medial radius.	The biceps acts on the shoulder to help with flexion, but it is better known for its role on the elbow. (See elbow muscles.)
	POSTERIOR SHOULDER MUSCLES (7)	
Trapezius	There are two trapezius muscles. Each has three parts that run from (1) the lower posterior skull, (2) the cervical spine , and (3) the thoracic spine out to the upper lateral back attaching onto the scapula.	Acting alone, each side-bends the head and neck to the same side as the muscle. Acting together, they extend the head and neck and control flexion of head and neck.
Latissimus dorsi	There are two latissimus dorsi muscles. Each runs from the lateral to the thoracic and lumbar spine below the trapezius out and under the axilla, attaching to the front of the upper humerus.	Acting alone, each adducts, or pulls the arm down, as when swimming. Acting together, they allow a person to perform pull-ups.
Levator scapulae	There are two levator scapula muscles. Each runs from the first four cervical vertebrae to the upper medial aspect of the scapula.	Acting alone, each can side-bend the head and neck to the same side as the muscle; however, as the name indicates, they primarily are used to elevate the scapula.
Rhomboid major	There are two rhomboid major muscles. Each runs from the first four thoracic vertebrae to the middle medial scapula. These muscles are deep to the trapezius.	Acting alone, each can retract, or pull back, the scapula closer to the spine.
Rhomboid minor	There are two rhomboid minor muscles. Each runs from the last two cervical vertebrae to the upper medial scapula. These muscles are deep to the trapezius.	Acting alone, each can retract, or pull back, the scapula closer to the spine.
Teres major	The teres major runs just below the teres minor, under the armpit, and attaches at the inner aspect of the intertubercular groove, near the insertion of the latissimus dorsi.	It is an adductor and internal rotator of the humerus.
Triceps	The triceps has three heads. The long head comes off the inferior glenoid fossa and merges with the lateral head, which comes off the lateral upper midhumerus and the short head, which comes off the medial, lower midhumerus. The resultant tendon inserts on the olecranon process of the ulna.	Extension of the humerus is one of the functions of the triceps because the long head inserts on the inferior glenoid fossa. It also plays an important role in movement at the elbow.
	GLENOHUMERAL MUSCLES (5)	
Deltoid	There are two deltoid muscles. Each has three parts that run form (1) the lateral clavicle, (2) the acromion, and (3) the scapular spine. They merge to attach just below the greater tubercle of the humerus.	The middle and three parts work together to abduct the humerus in the frontal plane. The anterior and posterior parts act alone to flex and extend, respectively, the humerus in the horizontal plane.

*Remember that all of these muscles cover an anatomical structure and thereby protect that underlying structure.

TABLE 18-1 Muscles of the Shoulder—Cont'd

MUSCLE(S)	LOCATION	FUNCTION*
	ROTATOR CUFF MUSCLES (4)	
Supraspinatus	Each supraspinatus muscle arises from the supraspinous fossa and merges with the infraspinatus and teres minor to attach to the greater tubercle of the humerus.	The supraspinatus helps the deltoid to abduct the humerus. It also works to eccentrically control the humeral head and keep it where it belongs in the glenoid fossa.
Infraspinatus and teres minor	The infraspinatus comes off the posterior scapula under the scapular spine and merges with the teres minor. It runs parallel and just below the infraspinatus. They merge with the two other rotator cuff muscles and attach on the greater tubercle of the humerus.	Both work concentrically to externally rotate the humerus, and they work eccentrically to decelerate the internal rotation of the humerus during the throwing motion. They also control the humeral head and keep it where it belongs in the glenoid fossa.
Subscapularis	There are two infraspinatus muscles. Each comes off the anterior surface of the scapula and angles up to attach to the lesser tubercle of the humerus.	This muscle internally rotates the humerus. Together with the other rotator cuff muscles, it works to keep the humeral head where it belongs.

Flexor Carpi Radialis. The flexor carpi radialis attaches to the pisiform, hamate, and fifth metacarpal base. Because of its lateral attachment, it can radially deviate the wrist when acting alone; when contracting with the other wrist flexors, it flexes the wrist distal to the carpals.

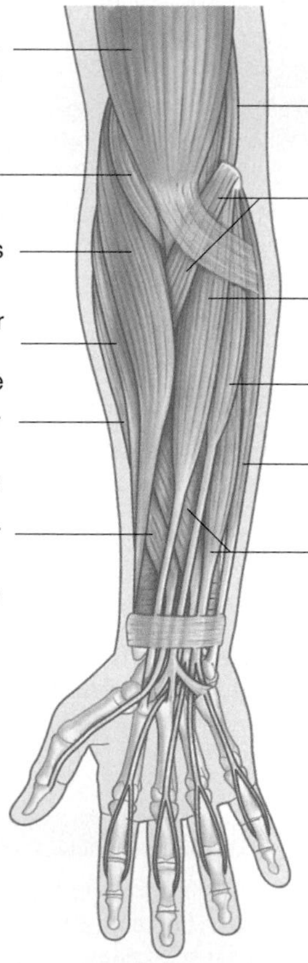

FIGURE 18-17 Muscles of the elbow, forearm, wrist, and thumb. (From Moses KP et al: *Atlas of clinical gross anatomy,* p. 240, St Louis, 2005, Elsevier/Mosby.)

Flexor Digitorum Superficialis. The intermediate group of muscles has one name, the flexor digitorum superficialis. Its name is derived from the fact there is another group of flexors that are deeper than this superficial group. The flexor digitorum superficialis arises from the medial epicondyle and runs distally to the middle phalanges of fingers two through five. This muscle helps flex the wrist and fingers, a function that is explained in more detail later in the chapter.

Flexor Digitorum Profundus, Flexor Pollicis Longus, and Pronator Quadratus. There are three muscles in the deep flexor group. The flexor digitorum profundus comes off the medial epicondyle and runs down to the bases of distal phalanges four and five. This muscle helps flex the wrist and also works on the fingers. The flexor pollicis (Latin for "thumb") longus comes off the anterior radius and runs to the base of the distal phalanx of the thumb. Although it crosses the wrist joint, it works primarily on the thumb. The last muscle included in the deep wrist flexor group is the pronator quadratus, a name that indicates both its function and its shape. Located more distally than the muscles of the anterior forearm, it runs from the distal quarter of the ulna to the distal quarter of the radius, and when it contracts, it pulls the radius toward the ulna, helping with pronation.

Points to Ponder
Consider all of the motions of the hand that involve the use of the thumb. When the thumb is injured, how disruptive to activities of daily living is this?

TABLE 18-2 Muscles of the Elbow

MUSCLE	LOCATION	FUNCTION*
Brachioradialis	It comes off the middle third of the lateral humerus and travels laterally down to the distal lateral aspect of the radius.	Although it is grouped with the extensor-supinator group, it actually helps to flex the elbow, particularly in the "thumbs-up," or neutral, position of the elbow.
Biceps brachialis	The biceps brachii has two heads. The short head comes off the coracoid process and merges with the long head, which comes off the superior aspect of the glenoid labrum. They attach to the medial radius.	The biceps acts on the elbow to help with flexion but is also an important supinator.
Brachialis	It runs from the distal anterior humerus to the proximal anterior ulna and is deep to the biceps.	It is a strong flexor of the elbow.
Triceps	The triceps has three heads. The long head comes off the inferior glenoid fossa and merges with the lateral head, which comes off the lateral, upper midhumerus and the short head, which comes off the medial, lower midhumerus. The resultant tendon inserts on the olecranon process of the ulna.	Extension of the humerus is one of the functions of the triceps because the long head inserts on the inferior glenoid fossa. It also plays an important role in movement at the elbow.
Anconeus	The anconeus is a small muscle that runs from the lateral epicondyle of the humerus to the lateral olecranon.	It is deep to the triceps and stabilizes more than actually extending the elbow.
Pronator teres	It mainly comes off of the medial epicondyle and runs diagonally down and in front of the elbow joint to the mid lateral radius.	It helps to pronate the forearm by spinning the radius in such a way that the palm faces down.
Supinator	It mainly comes off of the lateral epicondyle of the humerus and dives between the ulna and radius, attaching to the posterior aspect of the proximal radius.	Following its path shows that when this muscle contracts, the radius is spun in such a way that the palm ends facing up, or in a supinated position.

*Remember that all of these muscles cover an anatomical structure and thereby protect that underlying structure.

Table 18-3 summarizes the names, locations, and functions of the extensor muscles of the forearm and wrist.

Carpal Tunnel

An area of special interest in the area of the anterior wrist is the carpal tunnel. The carpal tunnel is defined as the area under a thickening in the palmar aponeurosis, called the *transverse carpal ligament,* and over the carpal bones (Figure 18-18). Traveling through this area are many of the flexor tendons and the median nerve. Because this is a relatively small area, it is possible for the median nerve to be traumatized, which leads to pain, numbness, and tingling in the wrist, hand, and fingers. The pain often becomes debilitating. This condition will be discussed in more detail in Chapter 20.

Wrist Muscles (Extensors)

The muscles that lie on the posterior surface of the forearm are called the *extensor-supinator group* because they initiate wrist and finger extension or supination. Most of the muscles that act on the wrist come from a relatively high point in the body, at the lateral epicondyle of the humerus, and travel down the forearm to cross behind the carpals and eventually attach to the metacarpals or phalanges. These muscles are often described according to their location relative to the skin surface. The superficial group is composed of the extensor carpi radialis longus, extensor carpi radialis brevis, extensor digitorum, extensor digiti minimi, and extensor carpi ulnaris.

Extensor Carpi Radialis Longus. The extensor carpi radialis longus arises just proximal to the lateral epicondyle and travels along the back of the forearm (dorsal aspect) down to the second metacarpal. It works to extend the wrist and radially deviate it.

Extensor Carpi Radialis Brevis. The extensor carpi radialis brevis arises from the lateral epicondyle and travels along the back of the forearm to the base of the third metacarpal. It also works to extend the wrist and radially deviate it.

Extensor Digitorum and Extensor Digitorum Minimi. The extensor digitorum arises off the lateral epicondyle and runs dorsally to the backs of fingers two through five. It is the primary extensor of the fingers at the metacarpal phalangeal joints and also helps with wrist extension. The extensor digiti minimi arises from the lateral epicondyle and continues down to the back of finger five, working to extend it at the metacarpal phalangeal joint.

Extensor Carpi Ulnaris. The last muscle of this group is the extensor carpi ulnaris. It arises off of the lateral epicondyle and runs down to the dorsal base of

TABLE 18-3 Flexor Muscles of the Forearm and Wrist

MUSCLE	LOCATION	FUNCTION*
Pronator teres	It mainly comes off the medial epicondyle and runs diagonally down and in front of the elbow joint to the mid lateral radius.	It helps to pronate the forearm by spinning the radius in such a way that the palm faces down.
Flexor carpi ulnaris	It comes off the medial epicondyle and attaches distally at the base of the second metatarsal.	It flexes the wrist to the ulnar side, a movement that is sometimes called *ulnar deviation.*
Palmaris longus	It comes off the medial epicondyle and inserts into the distal palmar aponeurosis.	It helps flex the wrist.
Flexor carpi radialis	It comes off the medial epicondyle and attaches to the pisiform, hamate, and fifth metacarpal base.	It can radially deviate the wrist when acting alone, and when contracting with the other wrist flexors, it flexes the wrist.
Flexor digitorum superficialis	It arises from the medial epicondyle and runs distally to the middle phalanges of fingers two through five.	This muscle helps flex the wrist and fingers.
Flexor digitorum profundus	It comes off the medial epicondyle and runs down to the bases of distal phalanges four and five.	This muscle helps flex the wrist and fingers.
Flexor pollicis longus	It runs from the mid-anterior radius and to the base of the distal phalanx of the thumb.	It flexes the thumb.
Pronator quadratus	It runs transversely from the distal quarter of the ulna to the distal quarter of the radius.	When it contracts, it pulls the radius toward the ulna, helping with pronation.

*Remember that all of these muscles cover an anatomical structure and thereby protect that underlying structure.

the fifth metacarpal. It extends and deviates the wrist toward the ulna.

Supinator and Extensor Indicis. There are two muscles in the deep extensor group: the supinator and the extensor indicis. The supinator, found in the proximal forearm, helps supinate the forearm. The extensor indicis comes off of the back of the distal third of the ulna and inserts on the back of the proximal phalanx of the second finger. It works to extend the index finger at the metacarpal phalangeal joint and helps extend the wrist.

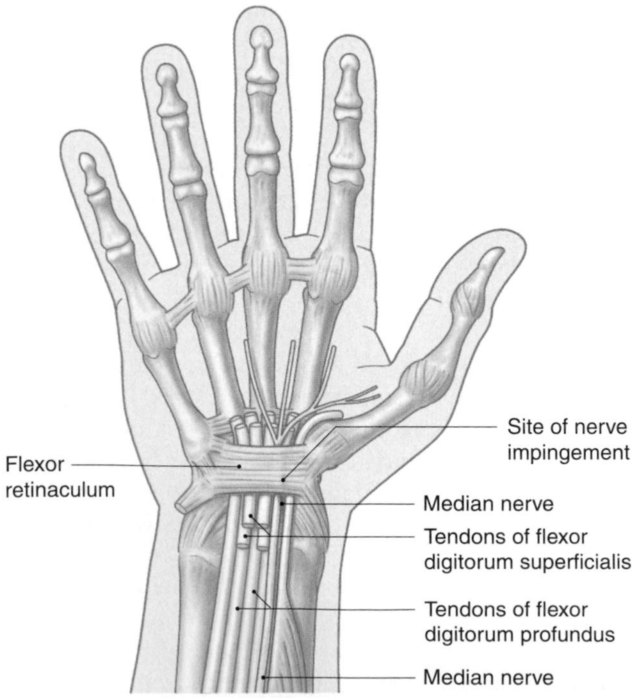

FIGURE 18-18 Carpal tunnel syndrome. (From Moses KP et al: *Atlas of clinical gross anatomy,* p. 261, St Louis, 2005, Elsevier/Mosby.)

Abductor Pollicis Longus, Extensor Pollicis Longus, and Extensor Pollicis Brevis. There are three muscles in the deep extensor group that work on the thumb: the abductor pollicis longus, the extensor pollicis longus, and the extensor pollicis brevis. The abductor pollicis longus arises off the posterior middle radius and ulna and continues down to insert on the base of the first metacarpal. It abducts the thumb. The extensor pollicis longus comes off of the posterior middle ulna and runs down to the back of the distal phalanx of the thumb. It extends the thumb at all the joints it crosses—carpometacarpal joint (where the carpals contact the metacarpals), metacarpophalangeal joint (where the metacarpals contact the phalanges), and interphalangeal joint (where the two phalanges of the thumb make contact). The thumb is unique in that it has only two phalanges, whereas the four fingers have three phalanges. The extensor pollicis brevis comes off of the posterior distal radius and runs down to the back of the proximal phalanx of the thumb. It extends the thumb at the carpometacarpal and metacarpophalangeal joints. Be aware that flexion and extension at the thumb do not occur in the sagittal plane as is the case with the fingers, wrist, elbow, shoulder, and other joints. Flexion and extension of the thumb occur in the frontal plane because, when viewed in the anatomical position, the thumb is rotated

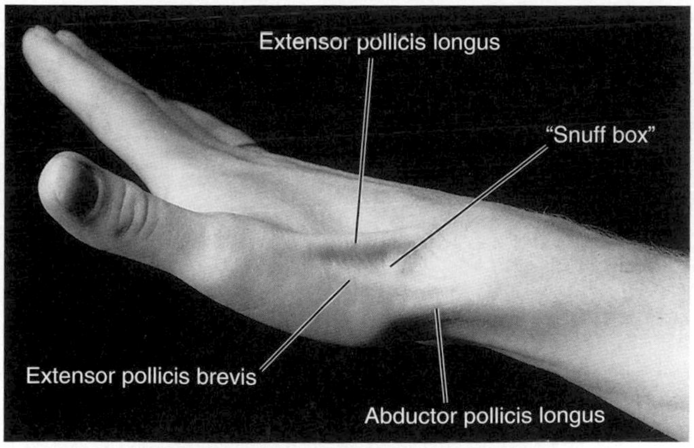

FIGURE 18-19 Anatomical snuffbox. (From Neumann D: *Kinesiology of the musculoskeletal system: foundations for physical rehabilitation*, p. 223, St Louis, 2002, Mosby.)

90 degrees medially from the fingers, wrist, elbow, and shoulder. Similarly, abduction and adduction at the thumb do not occur in the frontal plane as with the fingers, wrist, and shoulder, but instead occur in the sagittal plane.

As the tendons of the abductor pollicis longus, extensor pollicis longus, and extensor pollicis brevis cross the carpals, they form the "anatomical snuffbox" when fully extended or abducted (Figure 18-19). Try putting your thumb in a hitchhiker position, and look at the tendons that cross the carpals and run down to the thumb. The little depression that forms between the tendons is the snuffbox. Deep to the snuffbox is the scaphoid carpal bone.

Flexion and extension at the wrist occur between rows of bones. The rows are the distal aspects of the radius and ulna, the proximal carpals (i.e., pisiform, triquetrum, lunate, and scaphoid), the distal carpals (i.e., hamate, capitate, trapezoid, and trapezium), and the bases of the five metacarpals. Therefore there are three lines of flexion and extension. The carpal bones glide on each other as the wrist flexes and extends. Small ligaments limit the carpal movements.

Several other small muscles in the hand allow the hands and fingers to perform many delicate and precise movements (Figure 18-20). There is a small group of muscles for the thumb called the **thenar muscles**. They form the pad just medial to the first metacarpal. In addition, there is a small group of muscles for the fifth finger called the **hypothenar muscles**. They are found in the pad just lateral to the fifth metacarpal. Deep in the hand are two groups of small muscles found between the metacarpals, the **interossei**. The dorsal interossei abduct the fingers, and the palmar interossei adduct the fingers. The last muscles to be mentioned are the **lumbricals**. The term *lumbrical* is Latin for "wormlike." These muscles come off the tendons of the flexor digitorum profundus. Their unique

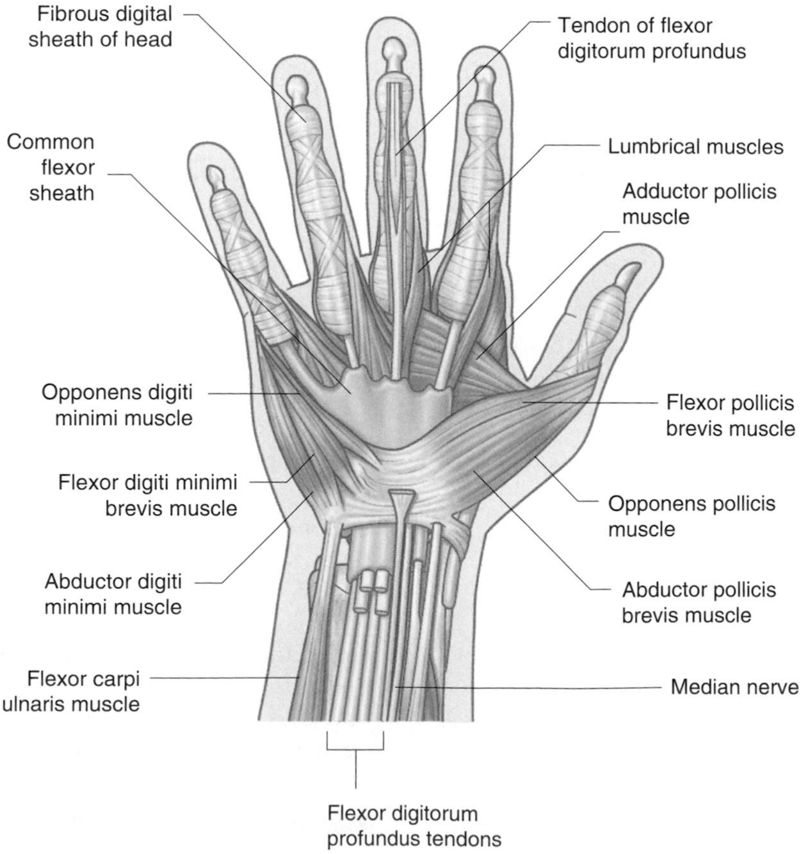

FIGURE 18-20 Small muscles of the hand. (From Moses KP et al: *Atlas of clinical gross anatomy*, p. 275, St Louis, 2005, Elsevier/Mosby.)

TABLE 18-4 Extensor Muscles of the Forearm and Wrist

MUSCLE	LOCATION	FUNCTION*
Extensor carpi radialis longus	It arises just proximal to the lateral epicondyle and travels along the back of the forearm (dorsal aspect) down to the second metacarpal.	It works to extend the wrist and radially deviate it.
Extensor carpi radialis brevis	It arises from the lateral epicondyle and travels along the back of the forearm to the base of the third metacarpal.	It works to extend the wrist and radially deviate it.
Extensor digitorum	It arises off the lateral epicondyle and runs dorsally to the backs of fingers two through five.	It is the primary extensor of the fingers at the metacarpal phalangeal joints and also helps with wrist extension.
Extensor digiti minimi	It arises from the lateral epicondyle and continues down to the back of the fifth finger.	It extends the fifth metacarpal phalangeal joint.
Extensor carpi ulnaris	It arises off of the lateral epicondyle and runs down to the dorsal base of the fifth metacarpal.	It extends and deviates the wrist toward the ulna.
Supinator	It mainly comes off the lateral epicondyle of the humerus and dives between the ulna and radius, attaching to the posterior aspect of the proximal radius.	Following its path shows that when this muscle contracts, the radius is spun in such a way that the palm ends facing up, or in a supinated position.
Extensor indicis	It comes off the back of the distal third of the ulna and inserts on the back of the proximal phalanx of the second finger.	It works to extend the index finger at the metacarpo-phalangeal joint and helps extend the wrist.
Abductor pollicis longus	It arises off the posterior middle radius and ulna and continues down to insert on the base of the first metacarpal.	It abducts the thumb.
Extensor pollicis longus	It comes off the posterior middle ulna and runs down to the back of the distal phalanx of the thumb.	It extends the thumb at all the joints it crosses.
Extensor pollicis brevis	It comes off the posterior distal radius and runs down to the back of the proximal phalanx of the thumb.	It extends the thumb at the carpometacarpal and metacarpophalangeal joints

*Remember that all of these muscles cover an anatomical structure and thereby protect that underlying structure.

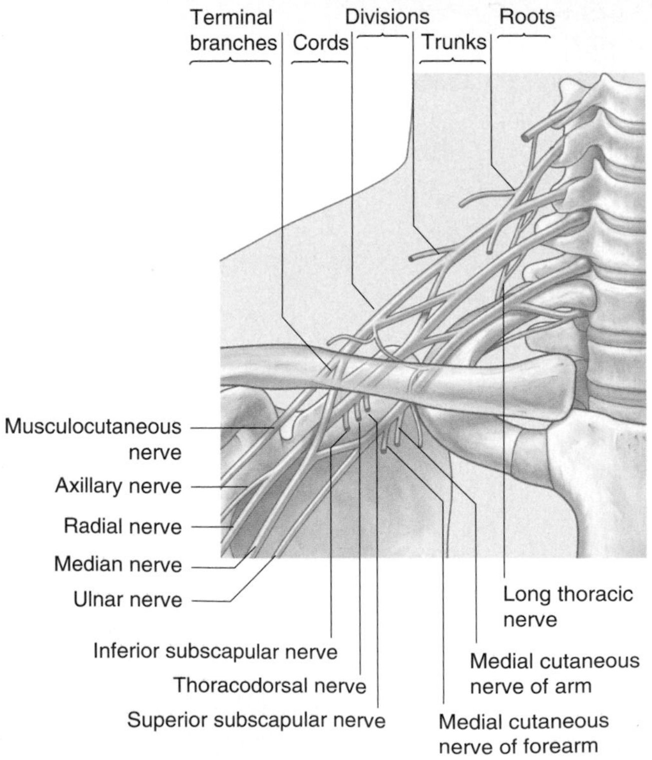

FIGURE 18-21 Brachial plexus. (From Moses KP et al: *Atlas of clinical gross anatomy,* p. 172, St Louis, 2005, Elsevier/Mosby.)

path allows them to flex the metacarpophalangeal joints and extend the interphalangeal joints.

Table 18-4 summarizes the names, locations, and functions of the extensor muscles of the forearm and wrist.

NEUROLOGICAL CONSIDERATIONS

The brachial plexus is a group of nerves coming off the spinal cord that travels laterally under the clavicle through the **axilla** and then down the arm (Figure 18-21). *Brachial* means "arm," and *plexus* means "a group"—in this case, a group of nerves. Three of these nerves eventually end up down in the hand. The ulnar nerve runs down the arm just behind the medial epicondyle of the humerus. When you hit your elbow on something and feel a shooting, tingling pain down your arm to your small finger, it is usually because you hit your ulnar nerve. Another nerve that goes down into your hand is the median nerve. It is the nerve involved in the carpal tunnel of your anterior wrist. The last nerve that goes down to your hand is the radial nerve. It ends up crossing over to the back of the hand.

axilla anatomical term for armpit

SUMMARY

A thorough understanding of anatomy is critical to understanding injuries as they occur. By understanding normal anatomy, the athletic trainer can easily identify any deviation during an injury evaluation.

The complexity of the upper body is difficult to comprehend. The upper extremity is capable of performing some amazing feats: virtuosic guitar playing, championship dart throwing, and typing 200 words a minute, to name a few. From gymnasts who can walk 100 yards on their hands to pitchers who can throw baseballs over 100 mph, to track-and-field stars who can pole vault 18 feet, the upper extremity allows the human body to function in amazing ways.

Web Links

Body Worlds Project: www.koerperwelten.de/en/pages/home.asp

Medical Gross Anatomy Learning Resources (University of Michigan): http://anatomy.med.umich.edu/

The Anatomy Lesson: http://mywebpages.comcast.net/wnor/homepage.htm

Web Anatomy (University of Minnesota): www.msjensen.gen.umn.edu/webanatomy/

The Visible Human Project (National Library of Medicine, National Institutes of Health): www.nlm.nih.gov/research/visible/visible_human.html

Bibliography

Applegate E: *The Anatomy and physiology learning system*, ed 3, Philadelphia, 2006, Saunders/Elsevier.

Caine CG, Caine DJ, Lindner KJ: *Epidemiology of sports injuries*, Champaign, Ill, 1996, Human Kinetics.

Cuppett M, Walsh KM: *General medical conditions in the athlete*, St Louis, 2005, Elsevier/Mosby.

Drake RL, Vogl W, Mitchell ADM: *Gray's anatomy for students*, Edinburgh, 2005, Elsevier/Churchill Livingstone.

Herlihy B: *The human body in health and illness*, ed 3, Philadelphia, 2007, Saunders/Elsevier.

Moses KP, et al: *Atlas of clinical gross anatomy*, St Louis, 2005, Elsevier/Mosby.

Muscolino JE: *Kinesiology: the skeletal system and muscle function*, St Louis, 2006, Mosby/Elsevier.

Neumann D: *Kinesiology of the skeletal system: foundations for physical therapy*, St Louis, 2002, Elsevier/Mosby.

Seidel HM, et al: *Mosby's guide to physical examination*, ed 6, St Louis, 2006, Mosby/Elsevier.

Standring S., editor: *Gray's anatomy: the anatomical basis of clinical practice*, Edinburgh, 2005, Elsevier/Churchill Livingstone.

Thibodeau GA, Patton KT: *Anatomy and physiology*, ed 6, St Louis, 2007, Mosby/Elsevier.

19

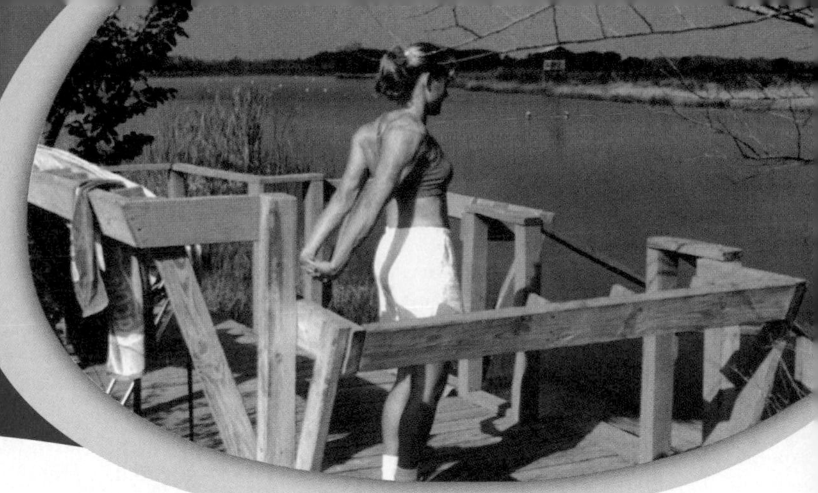

Diagnosis and Management of Neck and Shoulder Injuries

ROBERT C. MANSKE AND MICHAEL P. REIMAN

Learning Goals

1. Describe assessment and diagnostic procedures for evaluation of common acute injuries to the neck and shoulder.
2. Explain common signs and symptoms of acute athletic injuries occurring to the neck and shoulder.
3. Describe assessment and diagnostic procedures for evaluation of common chronic injuries to the neck and shoulder.
4. Explain common signs and symptoms of chronic athletic injuries occurring to the neck and shoulder.
5. Understand the purpose of a systematic assessment in the management of neck and shoulder athletic injuries.
6. Develop a differential diagnosis system to properly identify the injury and provide proper first aid and immediate care for management of acute or chronic injuries to the neck and shoulder.
7. Identify risk factors for neck and shoulder injuries associated with athletic participation.
8. Develop methods to identify and employ injury prevention procedures for athletic injuries to the neck and shoulder.

Terms that appear in boldface green type are defined in the book's glossary.

Neck and shoulder injuries sustained by individuals in various settings range from minor and mundane to severe and life threatening. The athletic trainer must always remain on high alert for potential life-threatening situations. This chapter covers numerous cervical spine and shoulder injuries that are frequently encountered in athletic, recreational, and industrial settings.

CLINICAL EVALUATION AND DIAGNOSIS OF NECK AND SHOULDER INJURIES

The evaluation of neck and shoulder injuries must be comprehensive, with a primary emphasis on determining whether a serious condition exists. A systematic evaluation process will assist in providing the requisite information for diagnosis of both acute and chronic injuries. Starting with an in-depth history, information obtained during the evaluation will ultimately guide the management of neck and shoulder injuries. The management of the injury influences how and when the athlete can return to activity. The goal is to return the athlete to activity as safely and as quickly as possible.

History

A detailed history is paramount to eliciting a mechanism of onset, as well as to providing information regarding the extent of trauma, the possible structures involved, and the areas on which to focus during the objective portion of the evaluation. The goal of the subjective portion of the history is to make an assessment of the area or structure(s) involved, the nature of the injury, the irritability of the condition, factors that aggravate

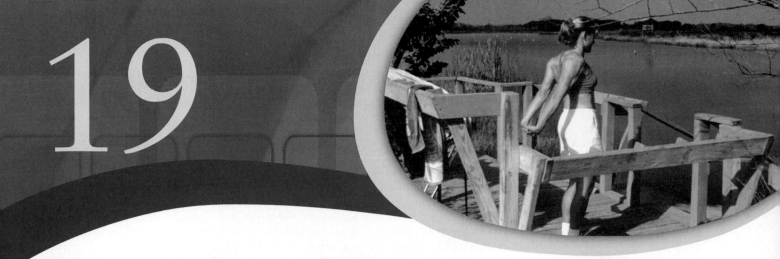

Opening *Scenario*

Matthew, a 31-year-old motocross rider, comes to the Saturday morning free injury clinic. Last night was a major race for him. He reports that while he was jumping over a series of small mounds along the course, his front tire landed while it was slightly turned, which caused him to wreck the cycle and land directly on his side, with barely enough time to remove his hands from the handlebars. He felt immediate pain in his left shoulder. He was able to drive the cycle back to the starting point but was unable to continue racing. Now Matthew exhibits an almost total inability to move his shoulder; even the simplest activities of daily living are difficult to perform. He is fully dressed but unable to undress on his own because of pain with active shoulder movements. On removal of his shirt, moderate swelling can be seen throughout the posterior lateral shoulder. He has noticeable ecchymosis along the lateral scapular border and axilla. Elevating his shoulder to 10 degrees results in pain. He can actively internally and externally rotate his shoulder in an antigravity position, but he offers no additional resistance to either motion during manual muscle testing. Palpation of all areas surrounding the left scapular region produces exquisite tenderness.

or alleviate the injury, characteristics of the symptoms, and a general idea of the prognosis. Specific questions should address the description, intensity, duration, and pattern of the pain or dysfunction. The athletic trainer should always be alert to subjective cues that suggest the possible presence of a more serious pathological condition, such as systemic-type complaints, complaints of nausea or vomiting, and respiratory difficulties.

Although an accurate history of any injury will generally suffice, more information can be gleaned by an athletic trainer who actually observes the injury as it occurs on the field of play. Determining whether the injury occurred as a result of direct contact is as important as determining the position of the neck and shoulder and the remainder of the upper extremity.

Observation/Inspection

The observation/inspection portion of the examination should be systematic and detailed. At this time, the athletic trainer should focus on any obvious deformities, especially those that necessitate referral to a physician. Opposing players, safety equipment, and protective padding may all interfere with adequate observation and inspection. For full appreciation of any abnormalities of bony or soft tissue structures, the client must be properly exposed. The neck and shoulder should be visualized from all angles if possible. If visual inspection is not possible, the athletic trainer should use his or her hands to palpate structures that cannot be seen. Palpation of unseen structures requires bilateral comparison. The trainer should look for any unusual or irregular prominences or discoloration.

Athletes in acute discomfort often display a physical appearance that can assist the athletic trainer in formulating a diagnosis and treatment plan. Pain posturing and slow, guarded movements are signs that the athletic trainer should proceed cautiously with the rest of the examination and that a serious pathological condition should be ruled out first.

A structural examination of the neck and shoulder region should include static and active positioning of the head, neck, and shoulder. The athletic trainer should monitor for any postural deviations from normal, including head and neck tilting/rotation, forward head posturing, bilaterally rounded shoulders, increased muscle tone/guarding, and abnormal spinal curvature.

Palpation

The athletic trainer should begin palpation proximally and cranially, progressing distally as necessary. The focal area of signs and symptoms should be palpated last to avoid irritating the involved area, which could potentially affect the rest of the evaluation. Palpation of the cervical and upper thoracic spine should include palpation for temperature changes to assess possible sympathetic nervous system involvement, as well as tissue texture abnormalities. During an activity, palpation of the acutely injured shoulder should be performed as quickly and efficiently as possible; a more thorough palpatory examination may be performed later, when the athlete has left the field. Box 19-1 provides a complete list of relevant soft tissue and bony structures that should be palpated during the shoulder examination.

Range of Motion Testing

Once a serious pathological condition has been ruled out, a physical examination should be performed. Active range of motion (AROM) of the neck and shoulders, bilaterally, should include assessment of degrees of motion, the client's willingness to move throughout the available range of motion (ROM), the point at which pain appears in the ROM (if applicable), and any pattern of ROM restrictions.

Passive range of motion (PROM) of the same regions should be performed next. The athletic trainer should perform all PROM testing cautiously to keep from exacerbating the injury. With clients who cannot move their arms because of severe pain or deformity, PROM may not be warranted before fractures and dislocations are ruled out. If PROM is allowed, gentle overpressure can be given to end ROM, if this is not painful, in an attempt

BOX 19-1 Soft Tissue and Bony Palpation of the Shoulder

Bony Structures	Muscular Structures	Other
Clavicle	Deltoid	Joint capsule
Acromion	Anterior	Transverse humeral ligament
First rib	Medial	Subdeltoid bursa
Acromioclavicular joint	Posterior	Subacromial bursa
Coracoid process	Trapezius	Sternoclavicular ligaments
Greater tubercle	Upper third	Acromioclavicular ligaments
Lesser tubercle	Middle third	
Bicipital groove	Lower third	
Humerus	Pectoralis major	
Sternoclavicular joint	Pectoralis minor	
Manubrium	Serratus anterior	
Ribs	Rhomboid major	
Sternum	Rhomboid minor	
Scapula	Latissimus dorsi	
Scapular spine	Supraspinatus	
Medial border of scapula	Infraspinatus	
Lateral border of scapula	Teres major and minor	
	Subscapularis	
	Biceps brachii	
	Triceps	
	Levator scapulae	

From Manske RC, editor: *Postsurgical orthopedic sports rehabilitation: knee and shoulder,* p. 69, St Louis, 2006, Mosby.

to assess the joint end-feel. A significant improvement in PROM compared with AROM signals that the surrounding contractile tissues may be involved to some degree.

Special Tests

Special tests for the neck and shoulder are performed to reproduce the client's symptoms so that the condition may be better understood and the diagnosis further defined. In many cases, these tests are provocative in nature, meaning that pain or renewed symptoms will result. If any of the following special tests are positive, which indicates a severe pathological condition, an immediate referral may be necessary. Special tests are dependent on and specific to the injuries that have occurred. An overall head, neck, and shoulder assessment should be performed for any client who complains of or demonstrates upper cervical instability or another serious condition. Upper cervical instability should be ruled out by testing the transverse ligament, alar ligaments, and C1-C2 instability and testing for a Jefferson fracture. Of particular importance is the client's ability to recognize the progressive worsening of his or her symptoms. In this case, referral for additional evaluation and diagnostic testing is mandatory.

Points to Ponder

How can the position of the individual—sitting or standing versus lying supine or prone—affect the results of special tests?

Transverse Ligament Stress Test

The transverse ligament stress test is performed with the client in the supine position and the athletic trainer at the client's head. The athletic trainer palpates the bilateral lamina of C1 with the index fingers and the occiput with the other fingers. The index fingers also palpate the spinous process of C2 to monitor for movement. The athletic trainer lifts the head and C1 in a ventral direction while preventing flexion or extension of the neck. A normal finding would reveal the C2 vertebra moving along with the C1 vertebra, with a hard end-feel being detected (Figure 19-1). Abnormal findings, or a positive sign, would include soft end-feel; muscle spasm; dizziness; nausea; paresthesia of the lip, face, or limb; **nystagmus**; or a lump sensation in the throat.

Alar Ligament Stress Test

The alar ligament stress test is performed with the client in an upright sitting position with the athletic trainer standing to the client's side. The athletic trainer palpates the spinous process of C2 and passively side-bends the head minimally. Normal findings with side-bending to the left present the spinous process immediately kicking to the right with a

nystagmus abnormal eye movements; possibly jerking or jumping

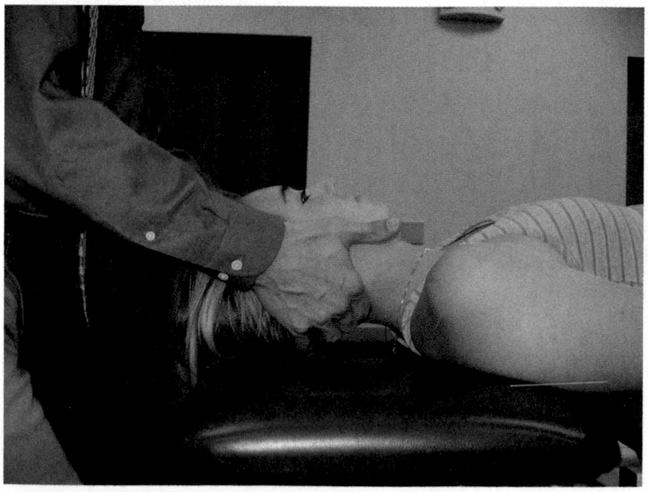

FIGURE 19-1 Transverse ligament stress test.

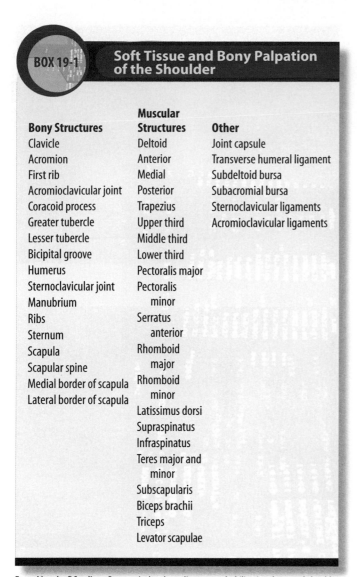

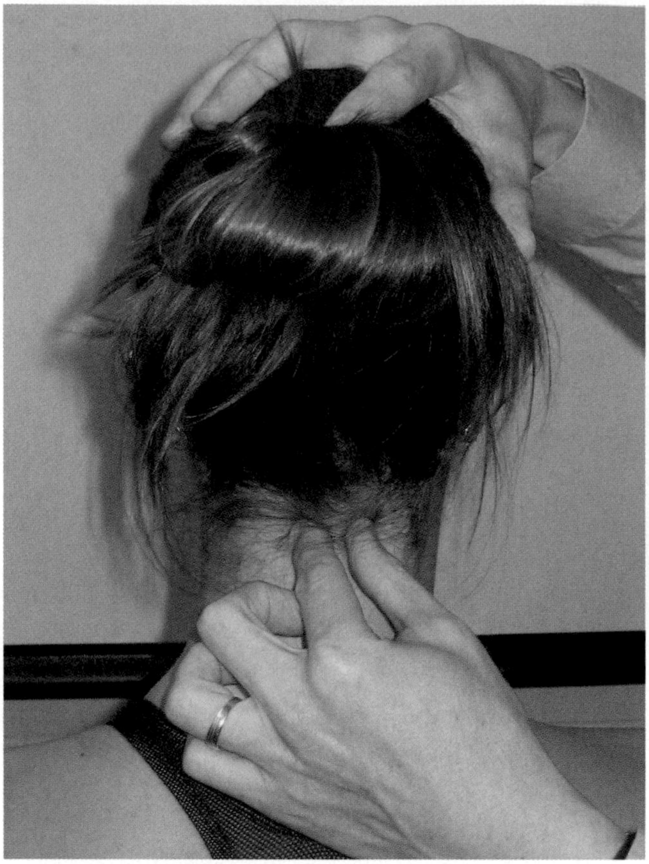

FIGURE 19-2 Alar ligament stress test.

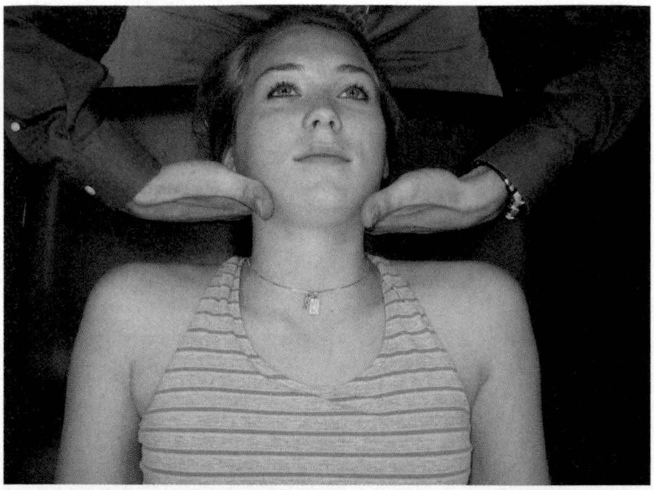

FIGURE 19-3 C1-C2 stress test.

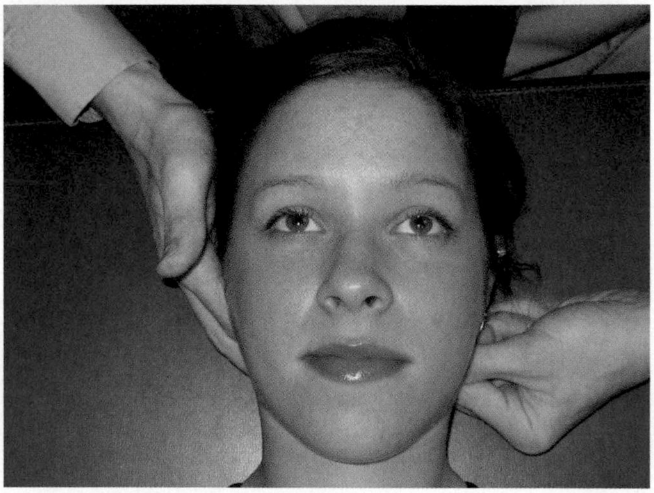

FIGURE 19-4 Test for Jefferson fracture.

strong end-feel—testing the right alar ligament. Normal side-bending of the head to the right assesses the left alar ligament, with the findings corresponding to those of side-bending to the left (Figure 19-2). This test can be performed with the client in a supine position to allow for maximum relaxation and minimization of muscle guarding.[1–3]

C1-C2 Stress Testing

C1-C2 stress testing involves the client being placed in a supine position with the arms relaxed at the sides and the athletic trainer standing at the client's head. The athletic trainer's right metacarpophalangeal joint (the soft part) is placed on the client's transverse process and arch of C1 (as well as supporting occiput) while the athletic trainer's left metacarpophalangeal joint region is placed on the transverse process and arch of C2, providing stabilization to this region. The athletic trainer then attempts a lateral shear of the atlas (C1) and occiput on the axis (C2) to the right while stabilizing the inferior segment. A parallel directed force to the other hand is used. The test is then reversed so that the superior segment is stabilized and the inferior segment is translated under it (Figure 19-3). If excessive movement or reproduction of the client's symptoms occurs, the test is positive, suggesting lateral instability of the atlantoaxial joint. A firm end-feel and no reproduction of symptoms is a negative result.

Jefferson Fracture Test

The Jefferson fracture test is best performed with the client lying supine with arms relaxed at the sides and the rest of the body still. The athletic trainer stands at the client's head, palpating both transverse processes of C1. The athletic trainer stabilizes one side and provides a medial directed force on the opposite side. The test is then reversed so that a medial directed force is applied in the other direction to assess both sides of C1 (Figure 19-4). A normal test results in a hard, nonyielding end-feel. A positive test indicates a disruption in the ring of the atlas.

Reflexive Tests

Ruling out upper motor neuron involvement is critical. Assessments should minimally include testing for **Hoffmann's sign**,[4] deep tendon reflex response, and **clonus**.

Hoffmann's sign reflex test finding that indicates the presence or absence of corticospinal problems
clonus sudden, reflexive twitches

Hoffmann's sign is the upper extremity equivalent to the Babinski test. The athletic trainer holds the client's hand that is to be tested and briskly flicks the distal phalanx of the third digit. If the test is positive, the thumb and index finger of the same hand will produce an "OK sign" (i.e., interphalangeal joints flex and both fingers touch at their distal components). Deep tendon testing is performed on the jaw, brachioradialis, biceps, and triceps. Normal reflexive responses, an immediate withdrawal, or kickback signifies a normal and intact neurological status. Clonus is an involuntary contraction of muscle after stimulus.

Functional Positional Testing

Functional positional testing is an attempt to compromise arterial blood flow by passively maintaining the cervical spine in a particular position. Possible positions include extension; combined extension and rotation; a premanipulation position; and rotation alone, the most common choice.[5] The Australian Physiotherapy Association's clinical guidelines for premanipulative procedures for the cervical spine recommend a 10-second hold of rotation or the position or movement that provokes symptoms.[6]

Neurovascular Tests

Evaluation of neurovascular (NV) function in an individual with a suspected injury to the neck, shoulder, or arm is paramount. Because many crucial nerves and vessels to the upper extremity are in close proximity to the neck and shoulder, these structures are easily compromised by injuries such as fractures and dislocations. The athletic trainer should perform an initial NV evaluation and monitor status at a minimum of every 30 minutes.[7] To perform this evaluation, the athletic trainer will palpate for pulses, check superficial sensation, and assess muscular strength. To establish specific neurological involvement, the athletic trainer should also perform palpation of specific cutaneous innervation, reflex testing, and myotome testing (Table 19-1).

Pulse

The client's pulse should be assessed distally from the site of injury. With most shoulder or upper extremity injuries, the location of choice for pulse assessment is the radial artery. The athletic trainer should always remember that a pulseless limb is dying until circulation is returned; therefore it is a medical emergency that should receive high priority.[7]

Capillary Filling Time

Capillary filling time may be assessed with firm pressure on either a nail bed or the skin near a nail bed. Pressure to the nail or skin in this area causes the nail to blanch, or turn white. Once pressure is released, a quick return to normal pink should occur within approximately 2 to 3 seconds. Capillary refill that takes longer than 2 to 3 seconds indicates impaired circulation, a potential medical emergency.[7]

Sensation

An individual's ability to perceive light touch sensation to the limb distal to the site of injury is a good indication that the nerve supply is intact. All dermatomes in the upper extremity distal to the site of injury should be assessed for light touch sensation.

Motor Function

The client's ability to actively move the injured limb using muscles or groups of muscles may indicate motor

TABLE 19-1 Innervation for Neurological Evaluation of the Cervical Spine

NERVE ROOT	PERIPHERAL NERVE	MYOTOMES	CUTANEOUS INNERVATION	REFLEX
C1		Head flexion	Vertex of head	
C2		Head extension	Posterior auricular	
C3		Head lateral flexion	Supraclavicular area	
C4-C5	Axillary (shoulder abduction)	Shoulder girdle elevation (C4) Shoulder abduction (C5)	Anterolateral shoulder and arm	Biceps (C5)
C5-C6	Musculocutaneous (elbow flexion) Radial (wrist extension)	Shoulder abduction (C5) Elbow flexion and wrist extension (C6)	Lateral forearm and hand (C5) Posterior thumb (C6)	Biceps (C5) Brachioradialis (C6) Pronator teres
C6-C7	Radial (elbow extension)	Elbow flexion and wrist extension (C6) Elbow extension (C7)	Posterior thumb (C6) Posterior aspect of middle finger (C7)	Triceps (C7)
C7-C8	Radial (elbow extension) Median (wrist flexion) Median (finger flexion) Ulnar (finger abduction)	Elbow extension and wrist flexion (C7) Thumb extension (C8)	Posterior aspect of middle finger (C7) Medial forearm and hand and little finger (C8)	Triceps (C7)
T1-2	Median (finger flexion) Ulnar (finger abduction)	Hand intrinsics	Medial forearm (T1) and axilla (T2)	

TABLE 19-2 **Manual Muscle Testing**

FUNCTION OF MUSCLE	GRADE	SYMBOLS				
No Movement						
No contraction felt in muscle	Zero	0	0	0	(0)	(0.0)
Tendon becomes prominent or feeble contraction felt in muscle, no visible movement	Trace	T	T	1	(1)	(1.0)
Movement in Horizontal Plane						
Movement through partial range of motion	Poor -	P-	1	2-	(1½)	(1.5)
Moves through complete range of motion	Poor	P	2	2	(2)	(2.0)
Moves to completion of range against resistance or moves to completion of range and holds against pressure	Poor +	P+	3	2+	(2 1/3)	(2.33)
Antigravity Position						
Moves through partial range of motion	Poor +	P+	3	2+	(2 1/3)	(2.33)
Gradual release from test position	Fair -	F-	4	3-	(2 2/3)	(2.66)
Holds test position (no added pressure)	Fair	F	5	3	(3)	(3.0)
Holds test position against slight pressure	Fair +	F+	6	3+	(3 1/3)	(3.33)
Holds test position against slight to moderate pressure	Good -	G-	7	4-	(3 2/3)	(3.66)
Holds test position against moderate pressure	Good	G	8	4	(4)	(4.0)
Holds test position against moderate to strong pressure	Good +	G+	9	4+	(4½)	(4.5)
Holds test position against strong resistance	Normal	N	10	5	(5)	(5.0)

From Kendall FP, McCreary EK, Provance PG: *Muscle testing and function with posture and pain*, ed 4, Baltimore, 1993, Williams and Wilkins.

function. Another method of assessment is manual muscle testing. Grades of manual muscle testing are listed in Table 19-2. If strength testing reveals full strength with no discomfort, the pathology is probably minimal. If the strength testing is significantly weak or painful, further testing is necessary. Repeated movements should be performed, especially if the client complains of gradual worsening or improvement of pain or disability. Repeating specific movements may gradually reproduce symptoms that were not evident during single movement testing.

Referrals and Diagnostic Testing

If not managed properly, many neck and shoulder injuries lead to long-term disability. Referring or transporting clients with these injuries in a timely manner may prevent exacerbation of the injury and sometimes permanent loss of function. Radiographs, or X-ray scans, are typically used first to rule out any bony abnormalities or dislocations. X-ray scans may also be used to rule out potential fractures. When radiographs are negative but symptoms persist, magnetic resonance imaging (MRI) and other advanced forms of imaging may be used to diagnose soft tissue injuries. Athletic trainers should pay particular heed to any injury accompanied by severe pain or loss of pulse, sensation, or function; clients with these symptoms should always be immediately referred to a physician.

MANAGEMENT OF ON-FIELD/ACUTE NECK AND SHOULDER INJURIES

The cervical spine is responsible for a large amount of mobility for various reasons. Anatomically, mobility is provided by a large intervertebral disk in relation to the vertebral body height, orientation of the facet joints, and the large diameter of the spinal canal. This increased mobility of the neck, combined with the small amount of surrounding musculature, makes the cervical spine especially vulnerable to injury. In addition, neck injuries frequently cascade and incite shoulder injuries (Figure 19-5). The athletic trainer's primary concern when confronted by a neck and shoulder injury is to rule out major trauma as soon as possible.

Acute Neck Injuries

Cervical spine and spinal cord injury is a small but inherent risk associated with any contact or collision sport. Sporting events are the fourth most common cause of spinal cord injury (after motor vehicle accidents, violence, and falls).[8] During the first three decades of life, sports injuries are the second most common cause of spinal cord injury,[9] with a mean age of 24 years.[10] American football and ice hockey are two sports involving helmeted athletes that have been extensively researched. Other sports in which athletes routinely wear equipment, such as lacrosse, rugby, equestrian sports, baseball and softball, kayaking, skiing, bicycling, skateboarding, cricket, and bull riding, have been less extensively studied.

A 204% increase in cervical spine fractures, subluxations, and dislocations, as well as a 116% increase in the rate of cervical spine injuries associated with permanent quadriplegia, was noted between 1959 and 1963 and again between 1971 and 1975 in a study by the National

Football Head and Neck Injury Registry.[11] Because axial loading (typically a vertical compression force from the top of the head through the cervical spine) was identified as the predominant mechanism of injury, rule changes were adopted in 1976 to prohibit the use of the head in tackling or spearing an opponent (Figure 19-6). As a result of the implementation of these rule changes, fractures, subluxations, and dislocations of the cervical spine progressively decreased between 1976 and 1984.[11] Along with the National Football Head and Neck Injury Registry, another campaign in the prevention of neck injuries is the STOP patch. This patch serves as a reminder to be mindful of safety toward other players (STOP).

Dislocations

Cervical dislocations occur more frequently than cervical fractures. However, both are equally serious. Dislocations in the cervical spine, as with other regions of the body, involve separation of one bony segment from the other. In the case of the cervical spine, there can be various dislocations, but most likely the facet joints separate and lose contact with each other. An obvious risk and potential complicating factor is the potential for pressure to be placed on the spinal cord or the nerve roots as they exit the spinal cord.

axial loading a vertical compressive load placed on the top of the head that transmits through the cervical spine

facet joints articulations between the two levels of the respective vertebrae

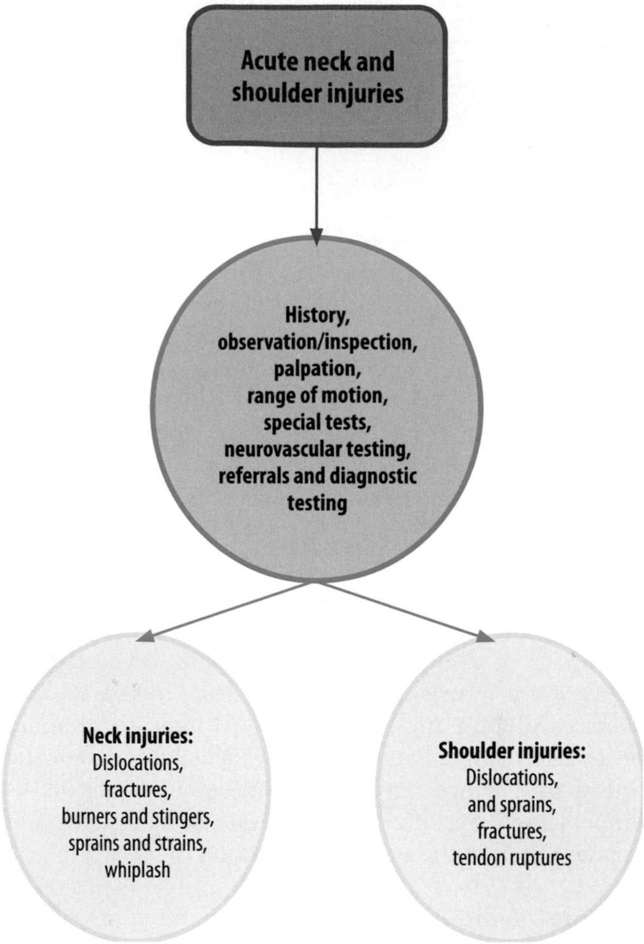

FIGURE 19-5 Concept map overview of acute neck and shoulder injuries.

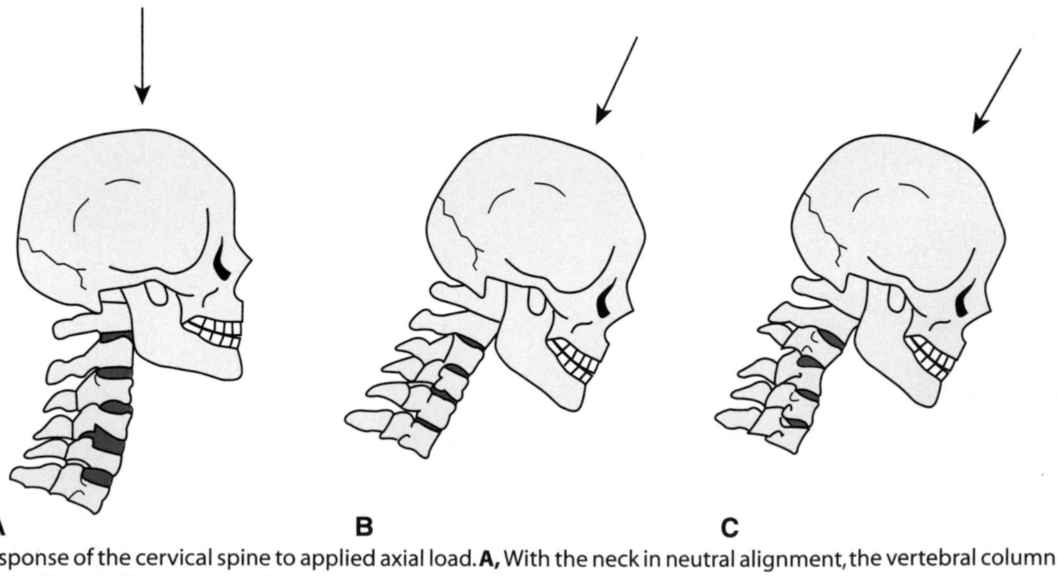

FIGURE 19-6 Response of the cervical spine to applied axial load. **A,** With the neck in neutral alignment, the vertebral column is extended, and the compressive force is dissipated by the spinal musculature and ligaments. **B,** With the neck in a flexed position, the spine straightens out and becomes collinear with the axial force. **C,** At the time of an impact, the straightened cervical spine undergoes a rapid deformation and buckles under the compressive load. (Redrawn from Banerjee R, Palumbo MA, Fadale PD: Catastrophic cervical spine injuries in the collision sport athlete. Part 1: Epidemiology, functional anatomy, and diagnosis, *Am J Sport Med* 32: 1077–1087, 2004.

Neural damage resulting from dislocations and fractures ranges from none to complete severance of the spinal cord.

Mechanism: Cervical dislocations involve flexion and rotation of the head.

Signs and symptoms:
- Pain
- Numbness
- Muscle weakness
- Muscle tightness and spasm
- Visible tilting of the neck toward the dislocated side with a unilateral dislocation

Special tests: No special tests are applicable.

Immediate and intermediate management: Clients with suspected cervical dislocations should be immobilized and prepared for immediate transport. Diagnostic testing and medical intervention will most likely be warranted. This is a medical emergency.

Fractures

Recognition of a cervical fracture is sometimes quite difficult, and great care must be taken if the client complains of deep and sharp neck pain. Some clinical indicators of a cervical fracture are listed in Box 19-2. A client exhibiting any of these clinical indicators should be referred immediately to a physician for diagnostic follow-up before any conservative intervention is implemented. Specific cervical fractures are discussed in greater detail in the subsequent sections.

Fracture of the Axis. Three types of fractures of the axis (C2 vertebra) can be observed in active individuals. **Hangman's fracture** involves bilateral traumatic spondylolisthesis of the pars interarticularis (Figure 19-7).

BOX 19-2 Clinical Indicators of a Craniovertebral Fracture

- Painful neck splinting
- Neck and occipital numbness
- Pain and stiffness in the neck, with reluctance to move the head
- Presence or absence of neurological signs and symptoms

Data from Greene KA, Dickman CA, Marcianno FF: Acute axis fractures: analysis of management and outcomes, *Spine* 22: 1843–1852, 1997; Lui TN et al: C1-C2 Fracture-dislocations in children and adolescents, *J Trauma-Injury Infect Crit Care* 40: 408–411, 1996; and Wong DA, Mack RP, Craigmile TK: Traumatic atlanto-axial dislocation without fracture of the odontoid, *Spine* 16: 587–589, 1991.

Odontoid fractures involve trauma to the dens, or odontoid process. Various other types of fractures are also possible (Figure 19-8).

Mechanism: The most commonly described mechanisms of a hangman's fracture include hyperextension combined with distraction, (for example, a supine hold in wrestling), hyperextension combined with vertical compression, (for example, a fall during a gymnastics dismount), and forceful hyperextension of an already extended neck (for example, contact made during a football tackle).

Signs and symptoms:
- Pain
- Neck splinting

hangman's fracture bilateral traumatic spondylolisthesis of the pars interarticularis; fracture at the axis (C2 vertebra)

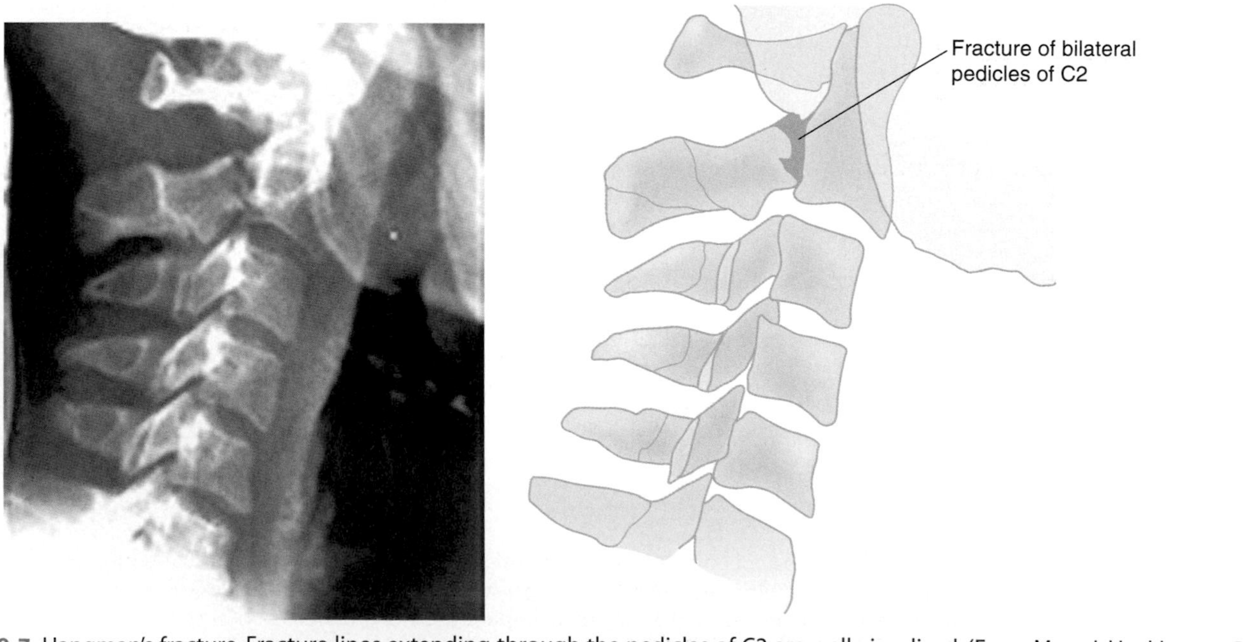

FIGURE 19-7 Hangman's fracture. Fracture lines extending through the pedicles of C2 are well visualized. (From Marx J, Hockberger R, Walls R: *Rosen's emergency medicine: concepts and clinical practice,* ed 6, Figure 40-14, St Louis, 2006, Mosby.)

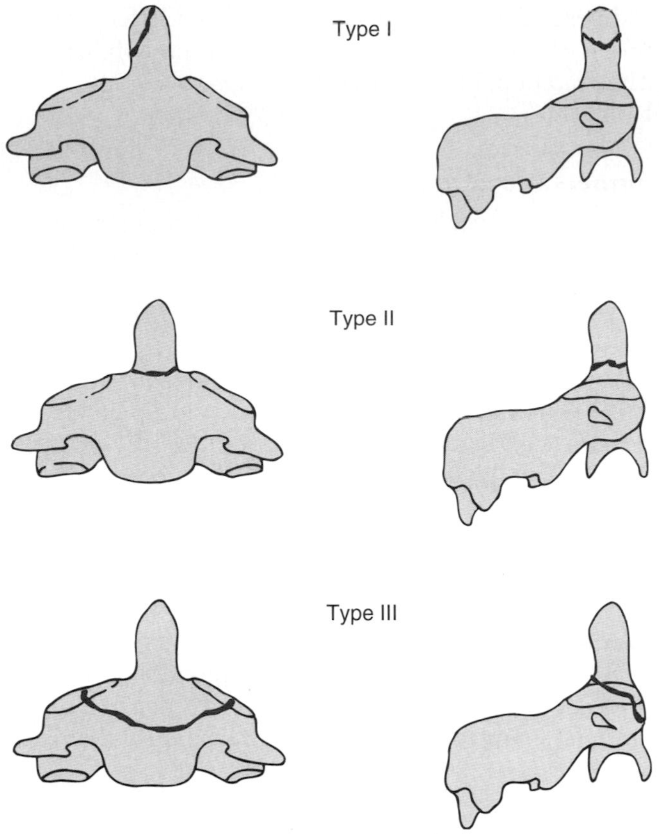

FIGURE 19-8 Classification of fractures of the atlas. Three types of odontoid fractures as seen in the anteroposterior (*left*) and lateral (*right*) planes. Type I is an oblique fracture through the upper part of the odontoid process itself. Type II is a fracture at the junction of the odontoid process and the vertebral body of the second cervical vertebra. Type III is actually a fracture through the body of the atlas. (Redrawn from Anderson LD, D'Alonzo RT: Fractures of the odontoid process of the axis, *J Bone Joint Surg* 56: 1663–1674, 1974.)

- Numbness in the neck and occipital regions
- Reluctance to move the head
- Unusual neurological symptoms

Special tests: Alar ligament test, transverse ligament stress test, and the lateral stability stress test can be used to assess for axis fractures.

Compression and distraction test: For the compression and distraction test, the client is preferably in the supine position with the athletic trainer standing at the client's head. The athletic trainer cups the client's occiput and rests the anterior aspect of the ipsilateral shoulder on the client's forehead. The other hand provides stabilization at a level close to the base of the neck [12] A traction-compression-traction force is applied (Figure 19-9). The athletic trainer notes the quality and quantity of motion. Pain reproduced with compression suggests a positive finding for injury, including the following: vertebral body fracture, disk herniation, vertebral end plate fracture, acute arthritis or joint inflammation of the facet joint, and nerve root irritation (if radicular pain is produced).[13] Reproduction of pain with cervical distraction suggests a positive finding, with the possibility for spinal ligament tear, tear or inflammation of the annulus fibrosus, muscle spasm, large disk herniation, and dural irritability (if nonradicular arm or leg pain is produced).[13]

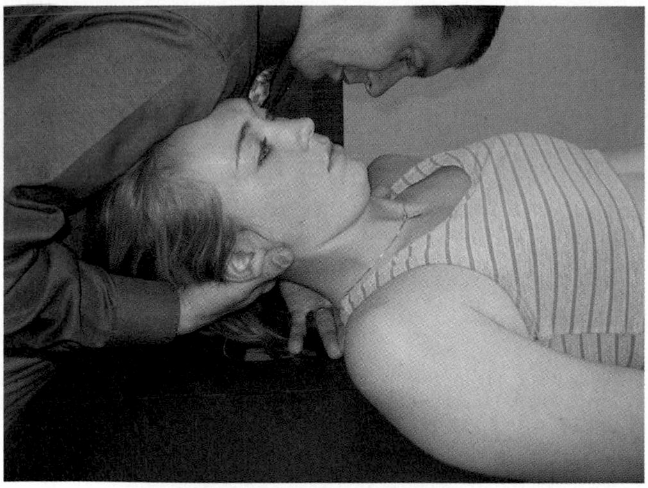

FIGURE 19-9 Compression and distraction test.

Immediate and intermediate management: Immediate transport to an emergency room after standard spine board stabilization procedures is indicated for fractures of the axis.

Odontoid Fractures. Fractures to the odontoid process, a toothlike projection from the upper surface of the body of the second cervical vertebra, are a relatively common upper cervical spine injury. They make up almost 60% of all fractures of the axis and between 10% and 18% of all cervical spine fractures.[14,15]

Mechanism: High-energy trauma, especially that resulting from motor vehicle accidents, is responsible for the majority of odontoid injuries in younger individuals.[14,16]

Signs and symptoms:

- Pain
- Neck splinting
- Numbness in the neck and occipital regions
- Reluctance to move the head
- Unusual neurological symptoms

Special tests: Cervical instability testing can be used to assess for odontoid fractures.

Immediate management: Immediate management for odontoid fractures is referral to a physician or emergency room after standard spine board stabilization procedures.

Intermediate management: Management of odontoid fractures is currently based on three principles: timely diagnosis, reduction of the fracture, and sufficient immobilization to permit healing.[17] Several treatment strategies have been implemented to achieve optimal alignment and stability, including cervical orthoses, halo-thoracic vests, posterior cervical fusion, and direct anterior dens screw fixation.[18]

Jefferson Fracture. **Jefferson fractures** occur to the ring of C1. These fractures are typically associated with minimal neurological deficit and good prognosis for neurological recovery.[19]

Mechanism: Jefferson fractures are typically the result of compression caused by a blow on top of the head, such as with a spearing motion in football or landing on top of the head after a fall or stumble in any sport.

Signs and symptoms:

- Pain
- Neck splinting
- Numbness in the neck and occipital regions
- Reluctance to move the head
- Unusual neurological symptoms

Special tests: The Jefferson fracture test is performed to assess for this specific fracture.

Immediate management: After a suspected Jefferson fracture, immediate transport to an emergency room, preceded by standard spine board stabilization procedures, is customary.

Intermediate management: An isolated Jefferson fracture is effectively treated with external immobilization. The traditional form of cervical immobilization is the halo vest.[20]

Burners and Stingers

A **burner** is typically a cervical nerve pinch injury, while a **stinger** is an upper trunk brachial plexus injury (Figure 19-10). Both are unilateral upper extremity neurological injuries that frequently occur in contact sports. Whether a burner is primarily a brachial plexus or a cervical nerve root injury is still unknown. The sagittal diameter of the canal where the spinal cord lies (i.e., the spinal canal) reaches adult dimensions by about the age of 13 years.[21] Approximately 50% of collegiate-level football players sustain a burner during their careers, and 30% of these

Jefferson fracture fracture to the ring of the C1 vertebra; typically involves minimal neurological deficit
burner injury in which a cervical nerve is pinched
stinger injury to the upper trunk of the brachial plexus

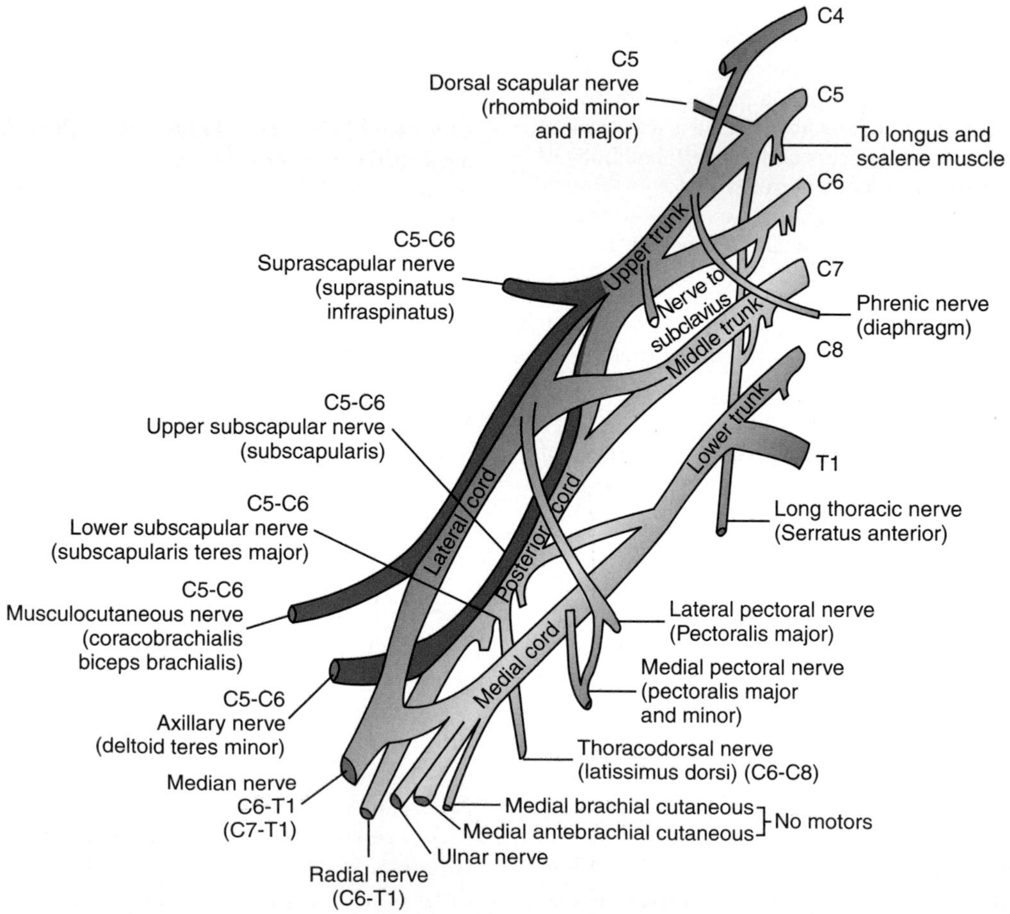

FIGURE 19-10 The brachial plexus. (Redrawn from Clancy WG Jr, Brand RL, Bergfield JA: Upper trunk brachial plexus injuries in contact sports, *Am J Sports Med* 5:209–216, 1977.)

players sustain their first injury in high school.[22] The overall reported annual incidence of a stinger is between 49% and 65% in collegiate-level football players.[23]

Mechanism: Three different mechanisms have been proposed: (1) stretch or traction injury to the brachial plexus, (2) extension of the cervical spine resulting in nerve root compression within the neural foramina, and (3) a direct blow resulting in injury to the brachial plexus. The precipitating event for a traction injury is typically as follows: The shoulder is pushed down, and the neck and head are forced laterally toward the contralateral shoulder. The upper cervical nerve roots (C5-C6) or upper trunk of the brachial plexus becomes stretched and injured.[24-26] The same traction-type mechanism has been reported to result in injury to the C5 or C6 nerve roots.[27] Forceful oblique cervical extension has also been suggested as a mechanism contributing to ipsilateral cervical nerve root injury.[28,29] This type of movement may result from a block or tackle when the head and neck are driven backward at impact.

Signs and symptoms:

- Pain in the upper arm that resolves in 1 or 2 minutes
- Paresthesia in the upper arm that resolves in 1 or 2 minutes
- Circumferential tingling, burning, or numbness around the extremity
- Localized symptoms or pain radiating down the affected extremity
- Possible weakness
- Localized trapezius tenderness, possibly for several days

Special tests:

Brachial plexus tension test: For the brachial plexus tension test, the client abducts and then laterally rotates the arms until symptoms are felt (Figure 19-11). Then, the client lowers the arms until symptoms disappear while the athletic trainer holds the client's arms in that position (see Figure 19-11, *A*). While the shoulders are held in position, the client flexes both elbows and places the hands behind the head (see Figure 19-11, *B*). Replication of symptoms indicates a positive test.

Shoulder depression test: For the shoulder depression test, the client is in the sitting position and the athletic trainer laterally flexes the client's head to one side while applying a downward pressure on the opposite shoulder (Figure 19-12). If the pain is increased, irritation or compression of the nerve roots is indicated.[30]

Spurling's test: A variation of the shoulder depression test is Spurling's test. The client is positioned as for the shoulder compression test. The athletic trainer applies overpressure into lateral flexion while stabilizing the contralateral shoulder. Replication of, or an increase in, pain indicates a positive response for brachial plexus injury.

Immediate management: The use of a soft collar can be implemented to protect the area and prevent exacerbation of the symptoms. Athletic trainers should consider the use of a shoulder sling if the client has increased sensitivity to passive traction of the upper extremity in normal resting positions.

Intermediate management: Burners and stingers are usually self-limiting but are commonly recurrent. Treatment involves removing the athlete from activity as long as symptoms or weakness to manual muscle testing persists. The gradual progression of a neck and shoulder strengthening program is implemented depending on the client's response to treatment. A special emphasis should be placed on correction of any postural imbalances and implementation of a cervical and upper quadrant stabilization program focusing on strength-endurance training of postural type I muscles (e.g., deep cervical neck flexors, scapular retractors and depressors) and stretching

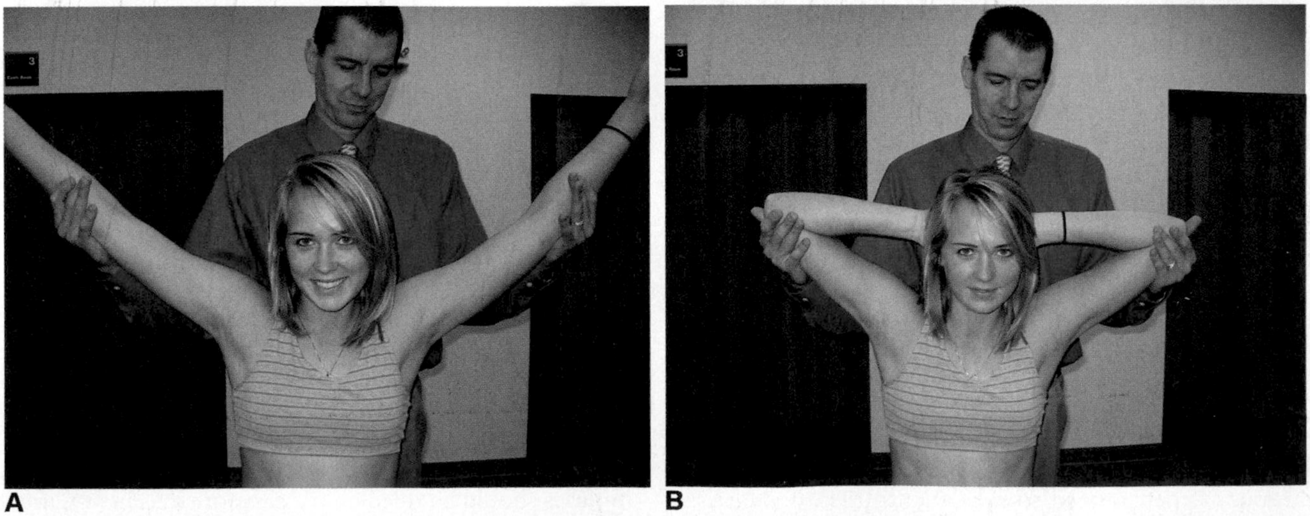

A B

FIGURE 19-11 Brachial plexus tension test. **A,** The client first lowers the arms until symptoms disappear while the athletic trainer holds the arms in that position. **B,** With the athletic trainer still holding the arms in position, the client flexes the elbows and places his or her hands behind the head.

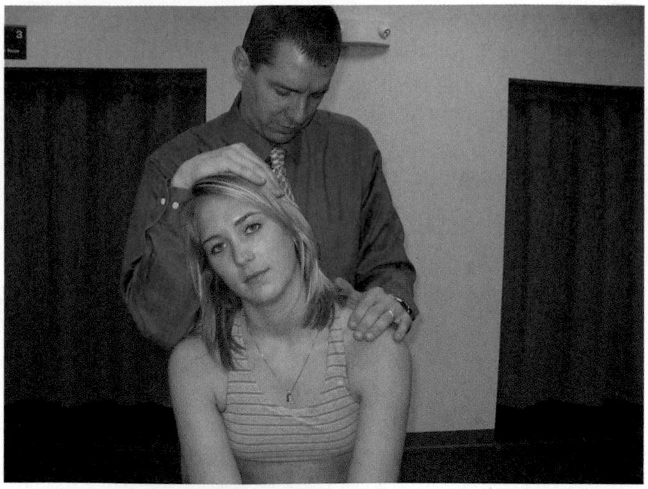

FIGURE 19-12 Shoulder depression test.

of any muscles determined to be shortened and contributing to the postural imbalances.

Sprains and Strains

Acute cervical strains typically occur at the extremes of ROM. Having the head and neck forcefully positioned at the end ROM by a playing surface or another player can injure the musculature and **inert** (noncontractile soft tissue, including ligaments, tendons, capsules, etc.) tissue of the head and neck region. Cervical sprains and strains are often caused by the same mechanism of injury and therefore often appear together.

Mechanism: Often hyperflexion, hyperextension, or excessive rotation of the cervical spine in association with either external trauma or violent muscle contractions causes sprains and strains.

> **Points to Ponder**
>
> Football players often wear external equipment known as "collars," hoping to prevent neck injuries. If these horseshoe-shaped pads are attached to the top of the shoulder pads, fitting around the neck to prevent cervical spine extension, can they potentially be increasing the risk of injury in other directions?

Signs and symptoms:
- Generalized aches
- Generalized stiffness
- Loss of motion
- Possible muscle spasms on palpation
- Pain with active movement or passive stretching

Special tests: Manual muscle and PROM/AROM tests are used to determine whether musculature or inert tissue are involved.

Immediate management: In severe cases, if pain or numbness is determined to radiate into the extremities, referral to a physician is warranted. This is necessary to rule out a possible spinal fracture, dislocation, or disk injury. If a serious pathological condition is ruled out, initial treatment typically includes PRICES.

Intermediate management: Physician-prescribed nonsteroidal antiinflammatory drugs and the possible use of a cervical collar for support and unloading of the involved spinal musculature and ligamentous tissue may be implemented once a serious pathological condition has been ruled out. A postural correction training program, as discussed in the section on burners and stingers, may also be implemented. After the athlete returns to activity, use of a neck roll or collar for additional protection and prevention may be appropriate.

Whiplash Injury

Damage resulting from a whiplash injury in the cervical spine frequently includes tears to the ligaments, muscles, and disks. More serious involvement must be ruled out, including any complaints of radiating pain; fracture or dislocation; upper cervical instability; and damage to the neurological, vestibular, and vascular systems.

Mechanism: A whiplash injury can be either a cervical flexion injury or an extension-type injury. The latter includes injuries resulting from motor vehicle and sports accidents; direct trauma to the head; and falls on the head, trunk, or shoulder. Extension-type injuries can be the most disabling type of whiplash injury.[31]

Signs and symptoms:
- Muscle spasm
- Varying degrees of pain
- Possible loss of cervical motion
- Headaches
- Possible anxiety or depression

Special tests: Upper cervical instability and central nervous system (CNS) involvement must be ruled out through the use of the transverse ligament test, alar ligament test, C1-C2 stress testing, Jefferson fracture test, and reflexive tests. Vertebral artery testing should not be performed for the first 4 to 6 weeks, nor should any treatment that might threaten this artery.

Immediate management: A soft collar may be used to provide stability and reduce the risk of aggravating any existing symptoms.[32]

Intermediate management: After ruling out instability and CNS involvement, the athletic trainer should emphasize pain management and pain-free rehabilitation of motor deficits.[32]

Acute Shoulder Injuries

Unlike cervical spine injuries, acute injuries to the shoulder are rarely life threatening. As with all injuries, an accurate and thorough history is necessary to determine the diagnosis. The athletic trainer should examine the client's shoulder as soon as possible, preferably during the acute phase. Serious conditions such as cervical spine and head injuries should be ruled out first, before the client is moved to another location for a more thorough evaluation.

inert noncontractile tissues

Dislocations and Sprains

The glenohumeral joint has several major ligaments that help provide stability. These ligaments include the fibrous joint capsule proper, the superior glenohumeral ligament, the middle glenohumeral ligament, and the inferior glenohumeral ligament. In some people, these are not so much strong ligaments in their own right as they are mere thickenings of the fibrous joint capsule. Because of its extreme mobility and relative thinness of the stabilizing structures, the shoulder may already be predisposed to ligamentous injuries. With active individuals, dislocations and instability can result from trauma as well as a congenital laxity.

Glenohumeral Joint. Glenohumeral instability can occur in any one of four directions (anterior, posterior, inferior, superior) or a combination of several directions. Usually, dislocations occur in the anterior or anterior inferior direction.[33–35] Dislocations are usually traumatic injuries that cause disruption of multiple layers of soft tissue and occasionally a bony avulsion of the glenoid fossa. If the dislocation is complete, multiple structures such as the joint capsule, ligaments, labrum, and tendons may be torn. Several concomitant injuries commonly occur with a glenohumeral dislocation. The **Bankart lesion** is a detachment of the capsule from the labrum or labrum from the glenoid fossa. When an actual avulsion of the glenoid fossa's bony surface occurs, it is called a **bony Bankart.** The other common injury involved with a dislocated glenohumeral joint is a **Hill-Sachs lesion,** which manifests as an osteochondral compression fracture on the posterior surface of the humeral head as it comes into contact with the anterior glenoid fossa while the muscles surrounding the shoulder contract in an attempt to guard or relocate the dislocated humeral head.

Mechanism: An anterior dislocation can occur when an individual is directly hit in the posterior aspect, causing the shoulder to move anterior. A more common mechanism is that of a powerful motion of the shoulder from the abduction and externally rotated position, such as when throwing or getting the arm blocked during acceleration, as in a volleyball spike. A final mechanism is when the arm is pulled posteriorly while in full elevation, as might occur when someone is going for a rebound or falls on an outstretched hand.

Less than 5% of all shoulder injuries are posterior glenohumeral dislocations.[36] Nonetheless, they can still cause significant shoulder morbidity. Posterior dislocations can be caused by nonsports-related injuries such as the violent muscular contractions seen during seizures and electrocutions. They can also result from sports activities such as falling onto a flexed and internally rotated arm.

Signs and symptoms:

- Guarded carrying position of affected arm in adduction and internal rotation
- If still dislocated, guarded position in slight external rotation
- Extreme pain
- Pronounced muscle spasm
- Numbness or tingling in arm
- Possible loss of motion
- *Anterior dislocations*: flat appearance of the top of the shoulder because of the humeral head being underneath either the glenoid fossa or the coracoid process
- *Posterior dislocations*: arm carried in internal rotation and adduction

Special Tests:

Apprehension test: The apprehension test can be performed while the client is either seated or supine. When the client is in the supine position, the scapula is stabilized against the floor, ground, or examination table, allowing the individual to better relax. The athletic trainer stands beside the client and uses his or her outside arm to grasp the client's elbow, abducting the arm to 90 degrees and flexing the elbow to 90 degrees. The shoulder is then slowly externally rotated while the athletic trainer's inside hand is placed at the level of the anterior shoulder to guard against any sudden loss of stability (Figure 19-13). Pain is not always an indicator of a positive test because the client may become sufficiently apprehensive to develop the sensation that the shoulder is about to come out of place again. When testing an overhead athlete, pain with the arm placed in the apprehension position is consistent with underlying glenohumeral instability even if the apprehension portion is absent.[37]

Bankart lesion detachment of the capsule from the labrum or the labrum from the glenoid fossa
bony Bankart actual avulsion of the glenoid fossa bony surface
Hill-Sachs lesion osteochondral compression fracture on the posterior surface of the humeral head; associated with a dislocation of the glenohumeral joint

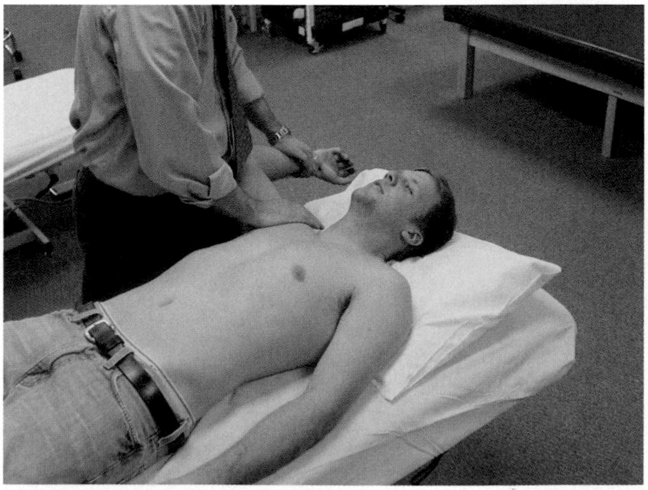

FIGURE 19-13 Apprehension test.

Immediate management: Because of the close proximity of the glenohumeral joint to various NV structures, a thorough NV examination should be performed. In most instances, reduction of shoulder dislocations is performed by the attending physician. If the client is not seen acutely or is unable to self-reduce the dislocation, he or she should be sent immediately to the hospital for radiographs and reduction. If the shoulder can be reduced immediately, the client should be immobilized in a sling and treated with cryotherapy. Even after reduction, the client will require follow-up radiographs to rule out fracture or osteochondral insult and to ensure anatomical reduction.

Intermediate management: A brief period of immobilization is generally recommended after a first-time shoulder dislocation.

Acromioclavicular Joint. Injury to the acromioclavicular (AC) joint is very common in sports. Although most AC joint injuries result from contact sports such as football, hockey, and rugby, they also occur in noncontact sports such as cycling, skiing, and skateboarding.[38–46] Probably the most recognizable classification of AC joint injuries is documented in Box 19-3.

Mechanism: The most common mechanisms of injury for an AC joint sprain are a fall directly onto the lateral shoulder, which forces the scapula away from the clavicle; however, the AC joint can also be injured by a fall onto an outstretched hand, or FOOSH'ing.

Signs and symptoms:

- Localized pain
- Tenderness to palpation over the AC joint
- Lateral displacement of the clavicle

Special tests:

Active compression test: Also known as the O'Brien test, the active compression test assesses for both superior labral tears and AC joint integrity. To perform this test, the athletic trainer stands near the client's injured extremity. The athletic trainer asks the client to flex his or her shoulder to 90 degrees and then horizontally adduct the shoulder about 15 degrees across the body, medial to the sagittal plane. The athletic trainer then maximally internally rotates the client's shoulder while maintaining

BOX 19-3 Rockwood Acromioclavicular Joint Injury Classification

Type I
Sprain of the acromioclavicular (AC) joint
AC joint intact
Coracoclavicular (CC) ligaments intact
Deltoid and trapezius muscles intact

Type II
AC joint disrupted
AC joint wider; may be a slight vertical separation when compared with the normal shoulder
Sprain of the CC ligaments
CC interspace perhaps slightly increased
Deltoid and trapezius muscles intact

Type III
AC ligaments disrupted
AC joint dislocated and the shoulder complex displaced inferiorly
CC ligaments disrupted
CC interspace greater than in the normal shoulder (25% to 100% more than in normal shoulder)
Deltoid and trapezius muscles usually detached from the distal end of the clavicle

Type IV
AC ligament disrupted
AC joint dislocated and clavicle anatomically displaced posteriorly into or through the trapezius muscle
CC ligaments completely disrupted
CC space perhaps displaced but may appear to be the same as the normal shoulder
Deltoid and trapezius muscles detached from the distal end of the clavicle

Type V
AC ligaments disrupted
CC ligaments disrupted
AC joint dislocated and gross disparity between the clavicle and the scapula (100% to 300% more than in the normal shoulder)
Deltoid and trapezius muscles detached from the distal half of the clavicle

Type VI
AC ligaments disrupted
CC ligaments disrupted in subcoracoid type and intact in subacromial type
AC joint dislocated and the clavicle displaced inferior to the acromion or the coracoid process
CC interspace reversed in the subcoracoid type (clavicle inferior to the coracoid) or decreased in the subacromial type (clavicle inferior to the acromion)
Deltoid and trapezius muscles detached from the distal end of the clavicle

From Rockwood CA Jr., Williams GR, Young DC: Disorders of the acromioclavicular joint. In Rockwood CA et al, editors: *The shoulder*, vol 1, ed 3, pp. 533–534, Philadelphia, 2004, Saunders/Elsevier.

the previously described position. An inferior directed force is applied to the client's distal forearm and the client is questioned about pain during this maneuver. If no pain occurs, the test is negative. Pain deep in the shoulder is assumed to be a superior labral anterior to posterior lesion (SLAP), and pain that occurs superiorly is thought to originate in the AC joint. If pain has been noted in one of the previously mentioned sites, the client's shoulder is then externally rotated and the forearm supinated while the same horizontally adducted initial position is maintained. Resistance is again given to the distal forearm, and the client is again questioned about pain. If the pain in either location is reduced or eliminated, the test is positive. A worsening of pain in either location indicates that some pathology other than the AC joint is at fault.

AC posterior shear test: The AC posterior shear test is performed with the athletic trainer seated alongside the client's injured side. The athletic trainer's anterior hand is placed slightly medial to the distal portion of the clavicle, and the posterior hand is located at the posterior lateral edge of the acromion. A compressive force is given along the anterior clavicle in a posterior direction in an effort to shear the clavicle (Figure 19-14). Although the positive test is reproduction of pain, inadequate or excessive mobility at the involved AC joint also may indicate a pathological condition.

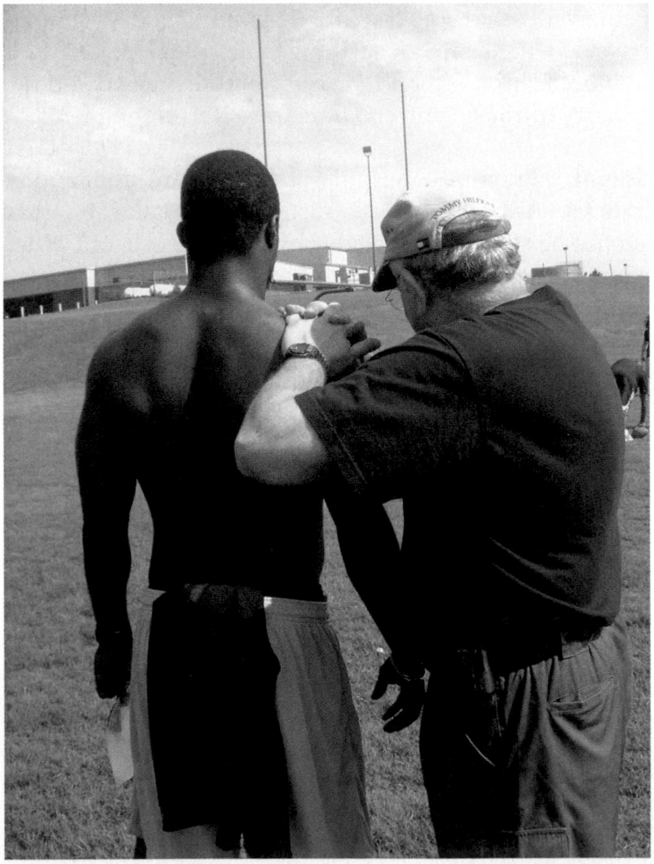

FIGURE 19-14 Acromioclavicular (AC) posterior shear test.

Piano key test: The piano key test may also be used to test for AC joint integrity.[47] For this test, the client sits with the arms at the sides and faces the athletic trainer. The athletic trainer then applies a downward-directed force to the distal end of the clavicle while watching for a depression of the distal end followed by an elevation once the pressure is removed. Excessive translation of the distal end of the clavicle compared with the uninvolved side or pain with testing is considered a positive finding.

Immediate and intermediate management: Because AC joint injuries are common, especially in contact sports, an understanding of the client's pre-injury anatomy is critical. If the AC joint has been previously injured, it may be indistinguishable from an acute injury on observation. Its severity determines whether the client may continue to participate in activity. If the injury is a minor first-degree injury, the client may be able to continue participation. Strength and ROM should be assessed. If ROM is full and only a mild, if painful, injury has occurred, the client may be able to continue participating in his or her chosen sport. With injuries that are more severe, discontinuing competition may be the best treatment. The arm should be placed in a protective sling, and radiographs probably should be obtained to rule out fracture if pain is severe and ROM and strength appear to be hindered.

Sternoclavicular Joint.

Although considered rare, occurring at a rate four to ten times less frequent than that of AC joint injuries, injuries to the sternoclavicular (SC) joint are possible.[48,49]

Mechanism: Although the most common cause of SC dislocation by far is motor vehicle accidents, the second most common cause is sporting activities.[50–52] An anterior dislocation of the SC joint can result from forces that retract and depress the shoulder displacing the clavicle on the first rib, and a posterior dislocation can result from a direct blow or a force acting on the posterolateral aspect of the shoulder. In sports such as football and soccer, an athlete may suffer SC dislocation when an opponent falls or steps directly on the athlete's clavicle after the athlete has fallen on his or her back.

Signs and symptoms:

- Hoarseness of voice with posterior dislocations
- Difficulty swallowing and breathing with posterior dislocations
- Pain
- Swelling
- Tenderness to palpation
- Possible joint laxity
- Possible loss of motion

Special tests: The only special test for the SC joint is general joint mobility testing to determine the degree of joint laxity.

Immediate and intermediate management: Because of the close proximity of the large vessels, esophagus, and trachea to the SC joint, it is reasonable to assume that posterior dislocation represents a medical emergency. Multiple problems such as cardiopulmonary collapse, occlusion of large vessels, and tracheal compression have been reported.[53] Posterior dislocations are obviously a medical emergency if cardiopulmonary compromise occurs. Reduction is performed as a surgical procedure under sufficient anesthesia. A closed reduction is performed using a towel clip to pull the clavicle anterior. A pillow is placed under the upper back of the supine client. Gentle traction is applied, with the shoulder held in 90 degrees of abduction and maximum extension.[7] If this does not work, an open reduction may be required. If the reduction can be accomplished conservatively, the athlete is placed in a figure-8 bandage to help maintain the reduction.

After reduction, cold therapy should be used judiciously. The shoulder should be held in a figure-eight dressing technique, or a similar type of brace should be used to stabilize the shoulders and allow ligament healing. This form of bandaging should be maintained for up to 6 weeks. The time frame may be decreased to only 3 or 4 days with a grade I injury.

Fractures

Although not extremely common, fractures to the upper extremity can occur. Fractures during sporting activities usually result from either falls or person-to-person contact (e.g., a direct blow). Most acute fractures are extremely painful and may be accompanied by swelling. They are generally tender to palpation.

Clavicle Fractures. Athletes who fracture their clavicles generally report feeling a painful popping sensation. Clavicle fractures are generally grouped and described by their location: middle third, medial third, or distal third. Most clavicular fractures occur in the middle third.

Mechanism: Clavicle fractures commonly occur when the athlete falls on an outstretched hand.

Signs and symptoms:

- Pain
- Tenderness to palpation
- Swelling
- Crepitus and extraneous movement
- Uninvolved arm supporting the arm that has sustained the clavicle fracture

Special tests: The tap or percussion test may be used to assess clavicular fractures.

Immediate and intermediate management: Anyone who has sustained a clavicle fracture should be immobilized and transported to the emergency room for diagnostic testing and possible medical intervention. Once further injury is ruled out, the arm on the involved side should be placed in a sling. If necessary, surgery is performed to pin the clavicle to prevent unnecessary movement. After immediate care has been provided, PRICES may be used to promote healing. A conservative comprehensive rehabilitation program addressing postural strengthening and stabilization and ROM should be implemented before the client is allowed to return to activity.

Humeral Fractures. Although somewhat rare in sports, proximal humeral fractures are possible. They often involve the joint surface, the anatomical or surgical neck, the greater and lesser tuberosities, and the shaft. With fracture, significant soft tissue damage also exists, in addition to possible NV compromise. Careful attention to NV status is always warranted with any high-energy humeral fracture. If a severe deformity is found and NV status is compromised, immediate referral to a physician is appropriate.

Mechanism: Humeral fractures are generally the result of high-energy trauma.[54] A fall on an outstretched hand, a fall on an elbow, and a fracture or dislocation of the shoulder are common mechanisms of injury for a humeral fracture.

Signs and symptoms:

- Loss of motion
- Pain
- Possible swelling
- Possible deformity

Special tests: The tap or percussion test, as well as compression and capillary refill tests, may be used to assess humeral fractures.

Immediate and intermediate management: Immediate management for any fracture is splinting and a visit to a physician to ensure an accurate diagnosis. The length of immobilization after a humeral fracture depends on the severity of the fracture and the physician's judgment.

Scapular Fractures. Scapular fractures are uncommon injuries. A client with a suspected scapular fracture should be sent to the emergency room to rule out other complications and injuries to thorax.

Mechanism: Scapular fractures are generally caused by high-energy trauma, such as a motorcycle accident, or any other type of trauma in which the posterior or posterior lateral thorax is forcefully driven into the ground (Figure 19-15).

Signs and symptoms:

- Inability to elevate the affected arm for several weeks
- Moderate to severe swelling
- Ecchymosis along posterolateral thorax
- Tenderness to palpation

Special tests:

In the scapular compression test the client is either sitting down or standing and the scapular spine is tapped. If tapping elicits a painful response, the test is positive.

Immediate management: Immediate management for a scapular fracture is splinting and physician intervention to ensure an accurate diagnosis. Early management of the scapular fracture includes a brief immobilization period and cold compression for up to 48 hours.

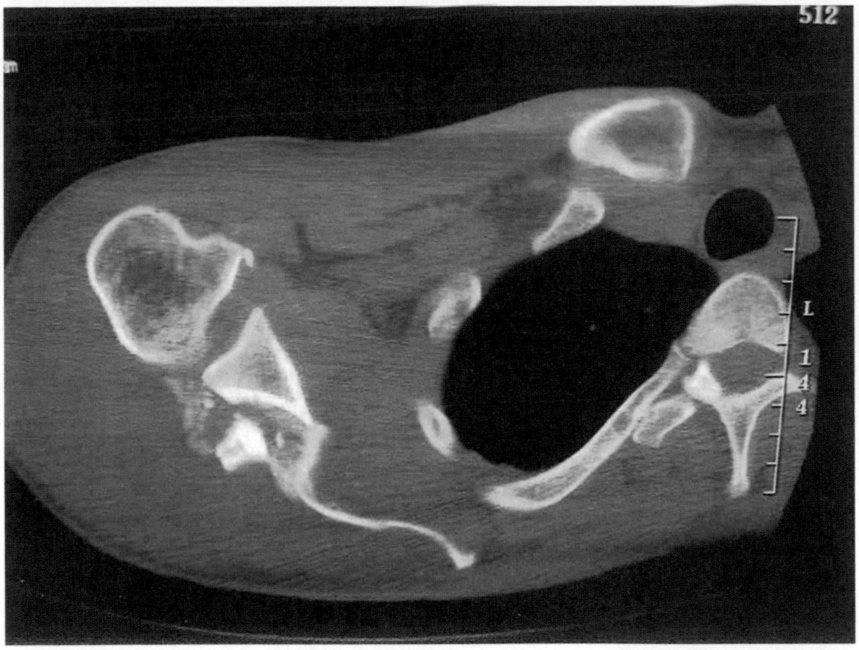

FIGURE 19-15 Computed tomography scan of displaced scapular fracture.

Intermediate management: After 48 to 72 hours, treatment may be changed to moist heat followed by active and passive mobilization. Although pain may be quite severe at the time of injury, significant displacement does not necessarily correlate with loss of function. Conservative return to activity is recommended.

Tendon Ruptures

Complete tendon ruptures of the shoulder are not especially common. However, sometimes a pectoralis major tendon rupture is reported, usually a consequence of overzealous weight training. Occasionally, the long head of the biceps ruptures during grasping and lifting activities. The rotator cuff is the most common site of tendon rupture. The rotator cuff is usually injured because of attritional factors and overuse rather than acute trauma.

Box 19-4 summarizes acute injuries to the neck and shoulder and the appropriate special tests used in diagnosis.

Prevention of Acute Neck and Shoulder Injuries

Prevention of acute neck and shoulder injuries rests with the athlete, who must strive to be in top physical condition and consistently wear appropriate equipment that fits properly. Conditioning and warm-up activities should include components of muscular strength, muscular endurance, and muscle tendon unit flexibility as well as other fitness components, such as power, speed, agilities, and reaction time. Barring accidents, most acute injuries to this area are preventable.

BOX 19-4 **Acute Neck and Shoulder Injuries and Appropriate Special Tests**

Neck Injuries

Dislocations
- No appropriate special tests

Fractures
- Fracture of the axis
  - Alar ligament test
  - Transverse ligament stress test
  - C1-C2 stress test
  - Compression and distraction test
- Odontoid fractures
  - Cervical instability testing
- Jefferson fractures
  - Jefferson fracture test

Burners and stingers
- Brachial plexus tension test
- Shoulder depression test
- Spurling's test

Sprains and strains
- Manual muscle testing
- Passive/active range of motion exercises

Whiplash injury
- Transverse ligament test
- Alar ligament test
- C1-C2 stress test
- Jefferson fracture test
- Reflexive tests

Shoulder Injuries

Dislocations
- Glenohumeral joint
  - Apprehension test
- Acromioclavicular joint
  - Active compression test (O'Brien test)
  - Acromioclavicular posterior shear test
  - Piano key test
- Sternoclavicular joint
  - General joint mobility testing

Fractures
- Clavicle
  - Tap or percussion test
- Humeral
  - Tap or percussion test
  - Compression test
  - Capillary refill test
- Scapular
  - Scapular compression test

Tendon ruptures
- No appropriate special tests

Depending on the activity, knowledge of rules and equipment can go a long way in reducing the risk of a neck or shoulder injury.

MANAGEMENT OF CHRONIC/OVERUSE NECK AND SHOULDER INJURIES

Clinical evaluation and diagnosis are different for chronic overuse neck and shoulder injuries than for acute neck and shoulder injuries (Figure 19-16). When evaluating chronic injuries, the athletic trainer is not under immediate time constraints and can usually perform a more thorough and detailed assessment.

Chronic/Overuse Neck Injuries

Many chronic injuries or dysfunctions are the result of repetitive microtrauma or poor posture. Mobility of the cervical spine makes this area susceptible to chronic soft tissue and joint injuries. Repetitive microtrauma and increased mobility expose the athlete to degenerative joint changes. Microtrauma can also lead to neurological involvement.

Cervical Myelopathy

Cervical **myelopathy** is the most serious condition of cervical spondylosis and is the most commonly acquired cause of spinal cord dysfunction among people over 55 years of age.[55] Although the exact pathophysiology underlying myelopathy remains uncertain, it is generally thought to be a disorder that involves compressive forces on the spine, likely caused by multiple factors.

Mechanism: Cervical cord compression, or myelopathy, may occur as a result of a disk herniation alone; degenerative changes that occur in the spine, such as degeneration of the joints, intervertebral disks, ligaments, and connective tissue of the cervical vertebrae; and bone spur growth in the spinal canal (spondylosis).[56] Infolding of the ligamentum flavum and facet joint capsule can create decreased space within the spinal canal, contributing to the myelopathy.[57]

Signs and symptoms:
- Spastic weakness
- Paresthesia
- Possible uncoordination in one or both lower limbs
- Possible proprioceptive dysfunction
- Possible sphincter dysfunction
- Possible muscle wasting bilaterally
- Possible decreased sense of vibration in the upper extremities
- Possible limitations in cervical ROM

Special tests: Clonus, Babinski, and Hoffmann's tests may be used to assess for cervical myelopathy.

Immediate management: The use of a cervical collar, rest, and nonsteroidal antiinflammatory medications has been shown to provide limited relief.[58–60]

Intermediate management: The continued use of cervical collar, rest, and nonsteroidal antiinflammatory drugs, with the addition of controlled ROM exercise in the pain-free range, is recommended. The use of a cervical collar for intermediate immobilization has also been advocated.[58–60]

Sprains and Strains

Cervical sprains and strains may also have a slow, progressive onset for chronic pain. The most common injuries are muscle strains and postural dysfunctions.[30]

Mechanism: The client may sustain cervical sprains or strains as a result of minor repetitive microtrauma, such as by maintaining the head in an awkward posture or sleeping position for a prolonged time.

Signs and symptoms:
- Pain
- Localized tenderness
- Possible loss of motion
- Swelling

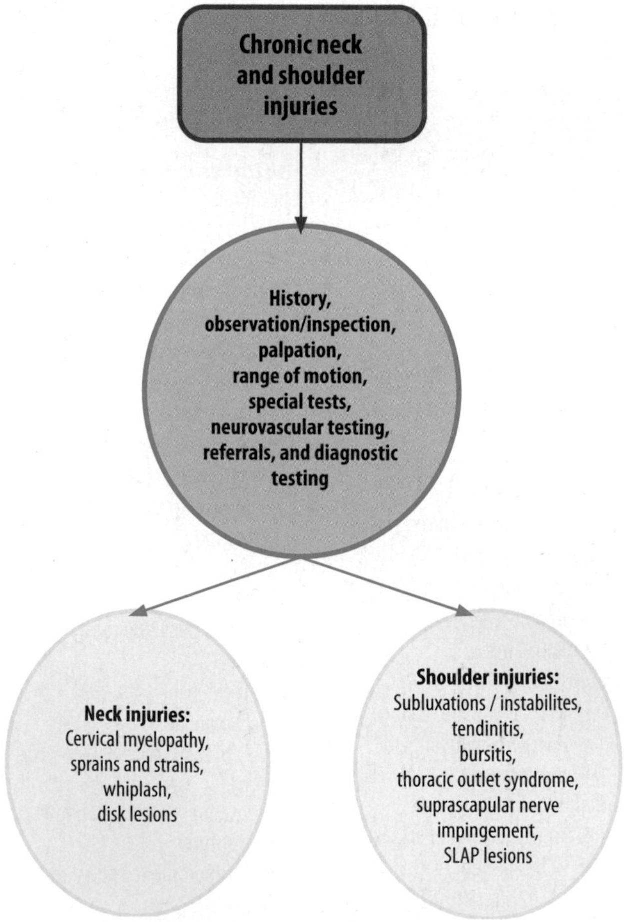

FIGURE 19-16 Chronic neck and shoulder injuries.

cervical myelopathy disorder that involves compressive forces on the spine, likely caused by multiple factors; the most serious condition of cervical spondylosis

Special tests: Performing manual muscle testing and putting the involved structure on a passive stretch are ways to identify sprain or strain to a specific structure or structures.

Immediate management: The structure at fault should determine the intervention. If ligamentous tissue damage or intra-articular lesion is suspected, the safest initial approach would be to help unload the joint and control the extremes of motion with a soft collar for a 7- to 10-day period [61] PRICES may be used to manage initial pain and swelling.

Intermediate management: The athletic trainer should gradually emphasize helping the athlete regain normal functional status of the involved structure or structures and the cervical spine as a whole.

Whiplash Injury

If the neck is held in a hyperextended position and exposed to cumulative microtrauma, whiplash may result. Multiple sudden jarring motions are absorbed by the cervical tissues, producing progressive pain and an inability to hold the neck in an extended position.[61]

Mechanism: A sudden or unexpected impact that forces the head back is a frequent cause of whiplash injuries in sports. Another mechanism is repetitive trauma over a period of time while the neck is in a sustained extension position.

Signs and symptoms:

- Aching pain in the posterior occipital muscles
- Possible radiating pain down into the shoulder girdle
- Generalized headaches in the frontal region or behind the eye

Special tests: Same as acute injury.

Immediate management: As with the cervical sprain, immediate management includes unloading the joint and controlling the extremes of motion with a soft collar for a 7- to 10-day period.

Intermediate management: Gradual progression of deep neck flexor strengthening precipitated by the increased co-activation of the superficial neck flexors is recommended. Also, because it is likely that a compensatory movement pattern has developed over time, reduced deep neck flexor function may result.[62] Therefore middle and lower trapezius strengthening, postural imbalance corrections, and cervical extensor muscle stretching should be implemented as tolerated.

Cervical Disk Lesions

The structure of the intervertebral disk in the cervical region is distinctly different from that in the lumbar region. Even with the anatomical variations assisting with movement and function, cervical disk lesions are fairly common in active populations. A disk herniation is extremely rare before the age of 30.[63]

Mechanism: Various mechanisms—including acute traumatic onset involving cervical extension, side-bending, or rotation and axial loading, as well as progressive onset as a result of repetitive microtrauma caused by cervical loading—can predispose someone to disk herniation.

Signs and symptoms:

- Variances in pain ranging from dull aches to severe burning
- Possible referred pain to the medial scapula, then down into the arm

Special tests: The cervical compression and distraction test and sensory and motor nerve testing (dermatomal and myotomal testing) may be performed to assess for cervical disk lesions.

Cervical distraction test: For the cervical distraction test, the client is supine on the table. The athletic trainer grasps the client under the chin and occiput and flexes the client's neck to a position of comfort. Then, the athletic trainer gradually applies a distraction force of 10 to 15 kilograms (Figure 19-17). If relief or reduction of cervical radicular symptoms occur, the test is positive.[64]

Spurling's test: With the client sitting down, the athletic trainer can perform this test in three stages. The first stage involves compression with the head in a neutral position as performed when assessing burners and stingers (Figure 19-18, *A*). The second stage involves compression with the head in extension (see Figure 19-18, *B*). The final stage is with the head in extension and rotation (see Figure 19-18, *C*), first to the unaffected side, then to the affected side. The athletic trainer applies slight compression through the top of the head in an effort to further narrow the intervertebral foramen. If pain radiates into the upper extremity on the same side that the head is rotated, the test is positive.[65] The test is stopped if a positive test result occurs in an earlier stage.

Bakody's test: For Bakody's test, the client's involved upper extremity is positioned on top of his or her head. If significant relief of the symptoms occurs, the test is positive.

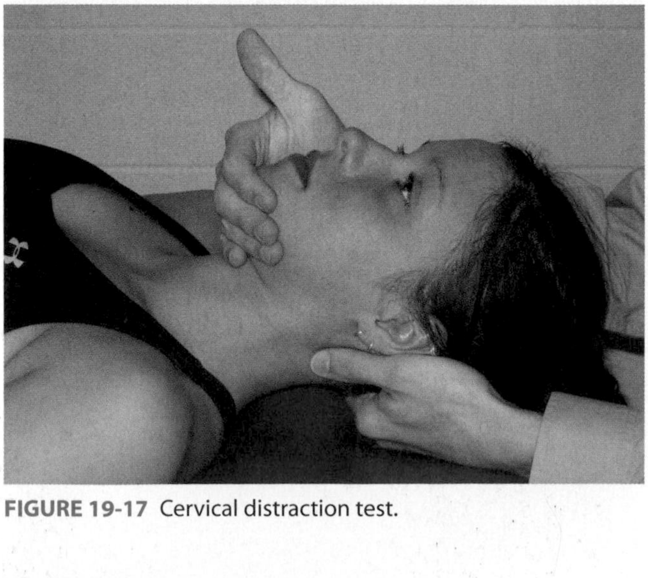

FIGURE 19-17 Cervical distraction test.

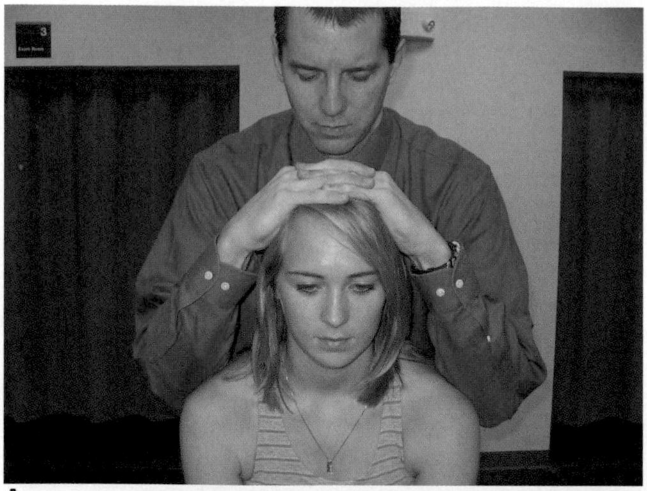

A

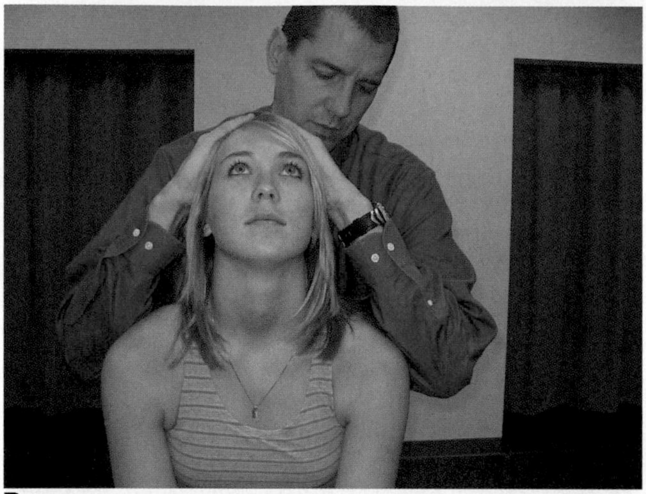

B

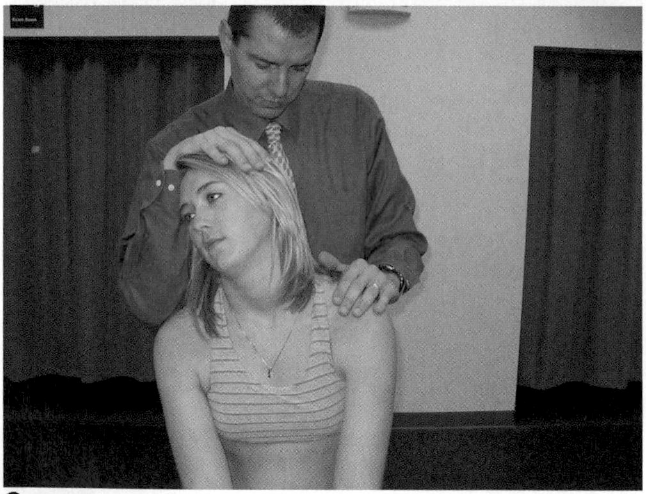

C

FIGURE 19-18 Spurling's test. **A,** The athletic trainer compresses the client's head while it is in the neutral position. **B,** Compression is again performed, but with the head in extension. **C,** Slight compression is applied to both the affected and unaffected sides with the head in extension and rotation.

Immediate management: Treatment includes modified rest, limiting painful ranges of motion, and possibly ice for pain control.

Intermediate management: The client should continue with modified rest, physician-prescribed nonsteroidal antiinflammatory medications or oral corticosteroids, and possible use of cervical collar. Manual therapy and soft tissue and joint mobilization techniques (dependent on individual tolerance) should also be implemented at this time. If appropriate, a progressive rehabilitation program focusing on correction of postural imbalances and cervical/upper quadrant stabilization should be initiated at this stage of rehabilitation.

Chronic/Overuse Shoulder Injuries

Chronic overuse injuries to the shoulder are extremely common in athletic activities. Sports such as baseball, softball, tennis, and swimming are particularly demanding in that they require high levels of forces to the shoulder and high numbers of repetitions of shoulder movements. A simple 20- to 30-minute swimming practice, for instance, may require thousands of arm strokes.

Chronic shoulder injuries include various forms of shoulder instability, tendonitis, and bursitis. With continued activity, the pathological condition is likely to worsen. For example, a chronic impingement may ultimately lead to a partial rotator cuff tear, which can progress to a full thickness labral tear. Therefore proper diagnosis, assessment, and intervention of these conditions are imperative.

Subluxations/Instability

A combination of static and dynamic structures in and around the shoulder are required to allow maximal movement and ROM at the glenohumeral joint. Glenohumeral instability may exist in any or all directions of movement, including anterior, posterior, inferior, and any combination thereof.

Laxity simply describes asymptomatic translation, or movement, of the humeral head on the glenoid fossa. This normal translation is required for adequate and **osteokinematic** motion at the glenohumeral joint. **Instability,** on the other hand, is a clinical diagnosis that results from excessive translation of the humeral head on the glenoid fossa during active or passive motion and is frequently associated with the sensation that the

laxity asymptomatic movement within a joint
osteokinematics classic movements of bones, such as flexion and extension
instability excessive movement

TABLE 19-3 Signs and Symptoms of Chronic Glenohumeral Instability

	ANTERIOR INSTABILITY	POSTERIOR INSTABILITY	MULTIDIRECTIONAL INSTABILITY
Onset	Chronic	Chronic	Insidious or chronic
Pain	Diffuse ache during ADLs accompanied by the sensation that the shoulder is loose when brought into abduction with external rotation	Diffuse ache during ADLs; complaint that the shoulder feels unstable when it is brought across the body	Pain in the shoulder that increases with ADLs; complaint that the shoulder feels loose with positions in the extremes of rotation motions
Mechanism	A specific mechanism of injury sometimes described, but chronic anterior instability often caused by repetitive microtrauma involving external rotation when the GH joint is abducted to 90 degrees	Possible report by patient of specific mechanism, but chronic posterior instability generally caused by repetitive microtrauma involving longitudinal force on the length of the humerus while glenohumeral joint is internally rotated and the flexion of GH joint to 90 degrees while also horizontally adducted	Instability multidirectional, but chief complaint typically pain during external rotation with the shoulder abducted to 90 degrees; possible sensation of instability during the midrange of motion
Predisposition	Joint hypermobility	Joint hypermobility	Joint hypermobility
Inspection	As flattened as possible because chronic cases can cause atrophy of the deltoid muscle group and the scapular muscles; possible atrophy of the rotator cuff muscles	Chronic cases sometimes lead to atrophy of the deltoid muscle group, rotator cuff muscles, and scapular muscles	Chronic cases sometimes lead to atrophy of the deltoid muscle group and the scapular muscles
Palpation	Tenderness of the anterior GH joint	Tenderness of the posterior GH joint	Tenderness in the anterior GH joint
Range of motion			
AROM	Decreased external rotation secondary to sensation of instability and/or pain	Decreased internal rotation	Possible limitation at the end ranges of motion secondary to a sensation of instability
PROM	Decreased external rotation secondary to sensation of instability and/or pain	Decreased internal rotation	Limited end range because of pain and instability
RROM	Decreased external rotation secondary to sensation of instability and/or pain	Pain and weakness during internal rotation in advanced cases	Pain and weakness during internal and external rotation
Ligamentous tests	Increased anterior glide, although may not appear increased to the contralateral side because of the bilateral nature of instability in chronic cases	Increased posterior glide, although may not appear increased to the contralateral side because of the bilateral nature of instability in chronic cases	Increased glide in all directions
Special tests	Apprehension test, relocation test	Posterior apprehension test; test for posterior instability in the plane of the scapula	Apprehension test; relocation test; posterior apprehension test; test for posterior instability in the plane of the scapula
Comments	With chronic cases, possible predisposition to bilateral involvement; chronic atraumatic instability usually occurring in patients younger than 30 years	With chronic cases, possible predisposition to bilateral involvement; chronic atraumatic instability usually occurring in patients younger than 30 years	With chronic cases, possible predisposition to bilateral involvement; multidirectional instability usually occurring in patients younger than 30 years

ADLs, Activities of daily living; *GH*, glenohumeral; *AROM*, active range of motion; *PROM*, passive range of motion; *RROM*; resistive range of motion.
From Starkey C, Ryan J, editors: *Evaluation of orthopedic and athletic injuries*, ed 2, p. 464, Table 13-9, Philadelphia, 2002, FA Davis.

shoulder is coming out of place or slipping. The key finding differentiating the two conditions is that instability includes the client's subjective report that the shoulder is unstable. *Multidirectional laxity (MDL)* means that the instability occurs in two or more planes.

Mechanism: Subluxations or shoulder instabilities may be caused by several means. Acute trauma, such as a direct blow, may prompt the instability. Microtrauma resulting from repetitive overuse caused by improper technique and mechanics may also cause the instability.

Signs and Symptoms:

- Dependent on the primary direction of the instability
- See Table 19-3

Special tests: Several tests are used to determine the extent and direction of shoulder instability. Special testing procedures are critical in determining shoulder joint instability through various humeral translation testing procedures. Special tests for the different directions of the more common instabilities are listed in the following sections.

Inferior Instability

The sulcus sign test: The sulcus sign test should be one of the first special tests performed to assess for increased laxity of the shoulder. The sulcus sign is the hallmark test for MDL.[66] It is commonly believed that

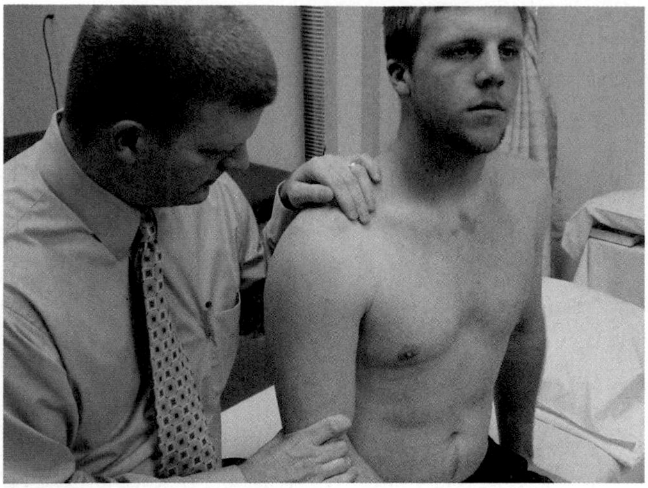

FIGURE 19-19 Sulcus sign test.

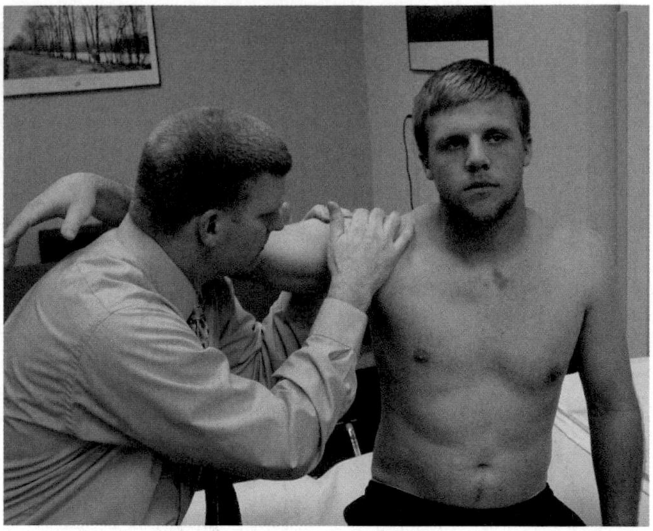

FIGURE 19-20 Feagin test.

inferior glenohumeral instability is a prerequisite for the diagnosis of MDL.[67] The sulcus sign test is performed with the client sitting in a relaxed position with his or her arms resting on the thighs. The athletic trainer stabilizes the shoulder with one hand while the other hand gives a gentle inferior traction force by grasping at the bicondylar axis of the humerus (Figure 19-19). When present, MDL manifests as a shallow depression above the humeral head and just beneath the acromion. Grading of this depression or sulcus is determined by recording the amount of translation between the lateral acromion and the humeral head[68,69] (Tables 19-4 and 19-5). When positive, extensive shoulder rehabilitation may be indicated to help improve the dynamic stabilizers and compensate for the increased capsular mobility noted during a positive test.

TABLE 19-4 Sulcus Sign Grading System

GRADE	TRANSLATION AMOUNT
I	<1.0 cm
II	1.0 to 1.5 cm
III	>1.5 cm

From Mallon W, Speer KP: Multidirectional instability: current concepts, *J Shoulder Elbow Surg* 4:55–64, 1995.

TABLE 19-5 Sulcus Sign Grading System

GRADE	TRANSLATION AMOUNT
1+	0.5 to 1.0 cm
2+	1.0 to 2.0 cm
3+	2.0 to 3.0 cm or greater

From Wilk KE, Andrews JR, Arrigo CA: The physical examination of the glenohumeral joint: emphasis on the stabilizing structures, *J Orthop Sports Phys Ther* 25(6): 380–389, 1997.

The Feagin test: The Feagin test is simply the sulcus sign tested in varying degrees of shoulder abduction; it may be performed at either 45 or 90 degrees of shoulder abduction.[70] The Feagin test is performed with the client seated and the shoulder passively taken to 90 degrees of glenohumeral abduction (Figure 19-20). The athletic trainer's hands are wrapped around the client's superior shoulder with fingers interlocked so that the ulnar sides of the digits are just distal to the lateral acromion. The athletic trainer then translates the humerus in an inferior direction while the glenohumeral joint is at 90 degrees of abduction. The athletic trainer watches and feels for inferior translation and compares this amount with that of the contralateral extremity. Because the grading schemes described for inferior translation are designed for testing in 0 degrees of abduction, testing at either 45 or 90 degrees of abduction requires greater experience and skill on the athletic trainer's part to appreciate and palpate slight translations in these positions. It is not uncommon to see up to a full centimeter of inferior glenohumeral translation in an individual with a stable shoulder. It must be emphasized that assessment of the sulcus sign is simply one piece of a diagnostic puzzle comprising various signs and symptoms of shoulder instability.

Anterior and Posterior Instability. Anterior and Posterior Drawer Tests: The preferred methods for assessing anterior and posterior instability are the anterior and posterior drawer tests. These are also known as the anterior and posterior load and shift, or the push-pull test. To perform this test in the seated position, the athletic trainer sits alongside or slightly behind the client. The client's hands rest comfortably in his or her lap,

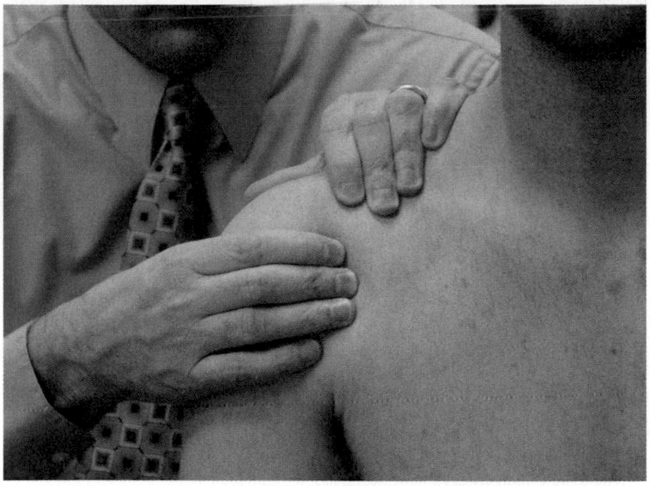

FIGURE 19-21 Proper hand and finger placement for anterior and posterior load and shift.

which helps promote relaxation. The athletic trainer's inside hand stabilizes the scapula and shoulder girdle, with the hand and fingers over the top of the shoulder positioning the thumb on the posterior acromion and the index finger on the anterior humeral head, while the third and fourth fingers are located on the clavicle. The athletic trainer's outer hand gently grabs the proximal humeral head, with the thumb on the posterior humeral portion and the fingers flat along the anterior portion of the humerus. The fingers on the anterior humeral head should be flat to enhance surface area contact along the anterior portion of the humerus (Figure 19-21). While gently stabilizing the scapula with one hand, the athletic trainer directs a load medially using the hand on the proximal humerus, which is thought to center the humerus in the glenoid and provides a neutral starting position. From this neutral position, the humerus is gently loaded or "shifted" in an oblique anterior and medial direction (Figure 19-22) for assessment of anterior glenohumeral displacement. The rationale for the oblique plane of movement has to do with glenohumeral joint geometry. The scapula sits on the chest wall and faces up to 30 degrees anterior and about 20 degrees forward relative to the sagittal plane.[71] A clinical pearl for performing the posterior load and shift is that it is done in a manner quite similar to that used for the anterior portion, but the load is applied in a posterolateral direction, following the plane of the scapula.

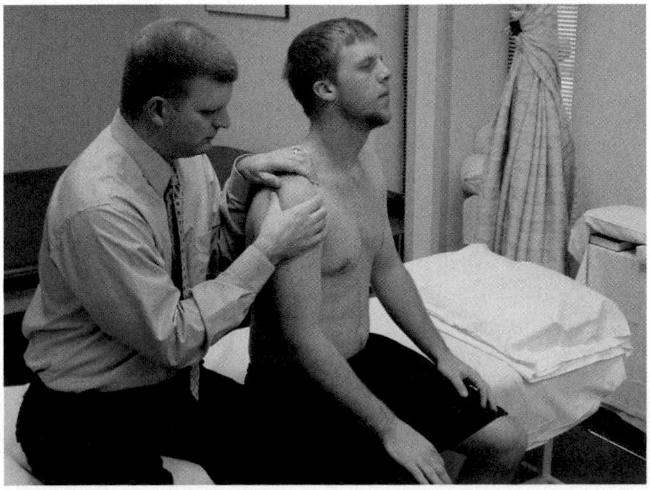

FIGURE 19-22 Anterior and posterior load and shift.

Points to Ponder

What anatomical structure causes posterior instability to be less common than anterior instability?

Grading anterior and posterior translation of the humeral head is done by documenting the amount of translation relative to the glenoid fossa[69] (Tables 19-6 and 19-7).

Immediate and intermediate management: Conservative nonsurgical management for glenohumeral instability emphasizes functional stabilization of the shoulder joint. Specific intervention involves using the rotator cuff musculature to apply force couples around the shoulder. A force couple is defined as two groups of synchronously contracting muscles that enable specific motions to occur.[72] With a concomitant contraction of all the rotator cuff muscles, the force created

TABLE 19-6 Load and Shift Grading System

GRADE	TRANSLATION AMOUNT
1+	Humeral head translates farther than contralateral shoulder but not over rim.
2+	Humeral head translates over rim but spontaneously reduces when force is removed.
3+	Humeral head is locked over glenoid rim.

From Warren RF: Physical examination of the shoulder for instability. Presented at the 14th Annual Team Concept Meeting, Williamsburg, Va., October 15, 1995.

TABLE 19-7 Load and Shift Grading System

GRADE	GLENOHUMERAL TRANSLATION
Trace	Small amount of humeral head translation
I	< 50% of humeral head translating over glenoid rim
II	> 50% of humeral head translating over rim but does not completely sublux
III	Entire humeral head translating over glenoid rim

From Wilk KE, Andrews JR, Arrigo CA.: The physical examination of the glenohumeral joint: emphasis on the stabilizing structures, *J Orthop Sports Phys Ther* 25(6): 380–389, 1997.

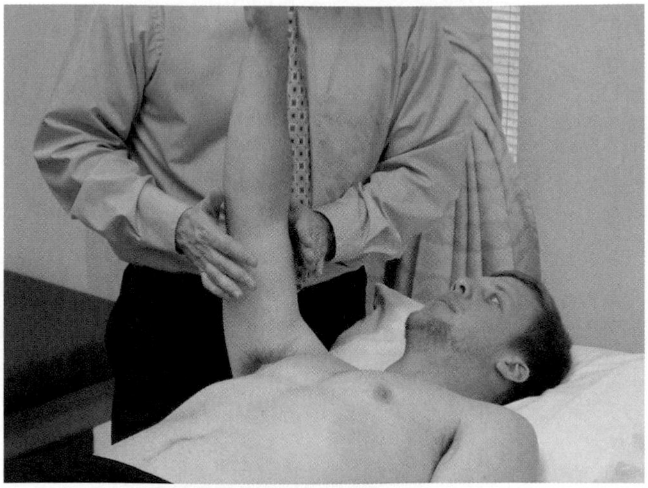

FIGURE 19-23 Proactive neuromuscular training of the glenohumeral joint (eyes open, known patterns).

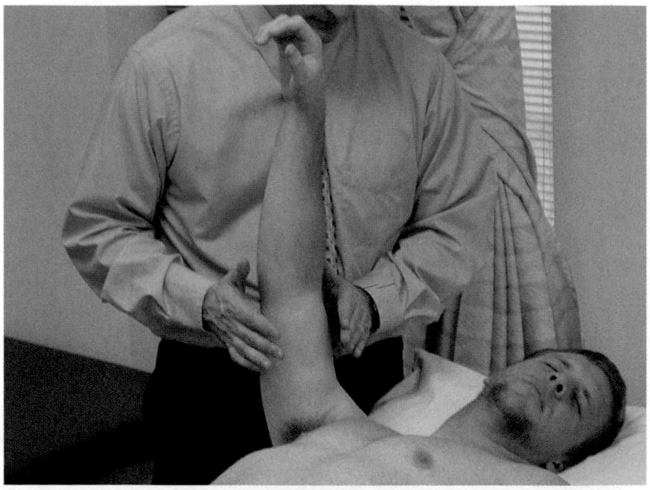

FIGURE 19-24 Reactive neuromuscular training of the glenohumeral joint (eyes closed, random patterns).

causes compression, which assists in the resistance to the superiorly directed force created by the deltoid muscle. The direct effect of these agonistic/antagonistic muscle groups is glenohumeral joint compression. Thus one of the most important roles of a fully functioning rotator cuff muscle group is to assist with glenohumeral compression. If rotator cuff weakness exists, a program of endurance training should be instituted immediately. Because these muscles are not made for pure strength development, use of a higher repetition and a lower load is recommended to enhance function of the rotator cuff through specificity of training effects.

The entire shoulder, including the rotator cuff groups and the scapular muscles, will benefit from reactive neuromuscular control, or neuromuscular dynamic stability. The focus of neuromuscular dynamic stability is on mechanoreceptors in various structures, such as muscle spindles and Golgi-tendon organs, and the sensors in the capsule and ligaments, which control joint proprioception and kinesthesia. When these dynamic exercises are performed, each is broken into two categories. The first category, proactive neuromuscular stabilization, should be practiced and mastered before the client moves on to the next category. Reactive neuromuscular stabilization is the second category. Proactive neuromuscular stabilization is used to create neuromuscular stability that is much more controlled. The athletic trainer can manage these exercises by providing submaximal manual resistance in known or visually recognized patterns (Figure 19-23). This form of exercise incorporates rhythmic stabilization exercises with a practiced and familiar pattern of resistance. The proactive response is one in which the client has control over the exercises being performed. Because these exercises are performed in a predictable pattern, the client knows what motion or resistance is coming next.

The reactive neuromuscular stabilization exercises take away some of the control that the client previously had. This type of exercise is thought to improve muscular power and endurance by improving reactive neuromuscular abilities.[73] In this series of exercises, the client is given random patterns of resistance. These exercises are still progressed from submaximal to maximal effort, but they are performed with eyes closed to stress the neuromuscular system to a greater degree by reducing visual input to the proprioceptive system[73] (Figure 19-24).

Tendonitis

The most prevalent form of tendonitis of the shoulder is rotator cuff tendonitis, also termed *rotator cuff impingement syndrome* or *subacromial impingement syndrome (SAIS)*.

Mechanism: There does not appear to be any single known cause for SAIS.[74] Athletes who participate in overhead activities (e.g., baseball, softball, tennis, swimming) appear to be at greater risk for rotator cuff tendonitis–type problems.

Signs and symptoms:

- Pain with overhead activity
- Possible loss of motion
- Possible weakness
- Possible discomfort with external rotation

Special tests: Diagnosis of tendinopathy of the glenohumeral joint may involve multiple special tests, including those used to assess subluxations and instabilities as well as those listed in the following sections.

Neer impingement test: The Neer impingement test is used as a provocative maneuver to compress the supraspinatus or the long head of the biceps tendon into the acromial undersurface.[75] To perform this test, the athletic trainer grasps the client's arm at the level of the elbow and passively elevates the shoulder to end range of flexion. With the arm in neutral rotation, a gentle passive overpressure is given at the end of elevation ROM (Figure 19-25). This test is done in a position that closely mimics the client's end range of reaching or lifting overhead. A positive test replicates the pain or symptoms.

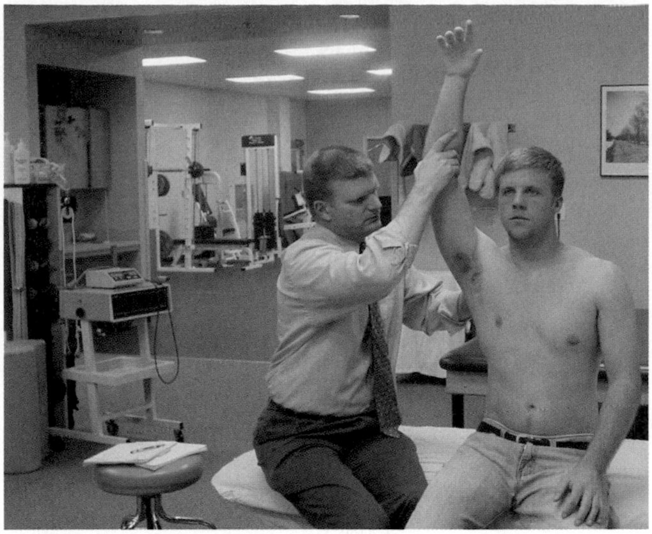

FIGURE 19-25 Neer impingement test.

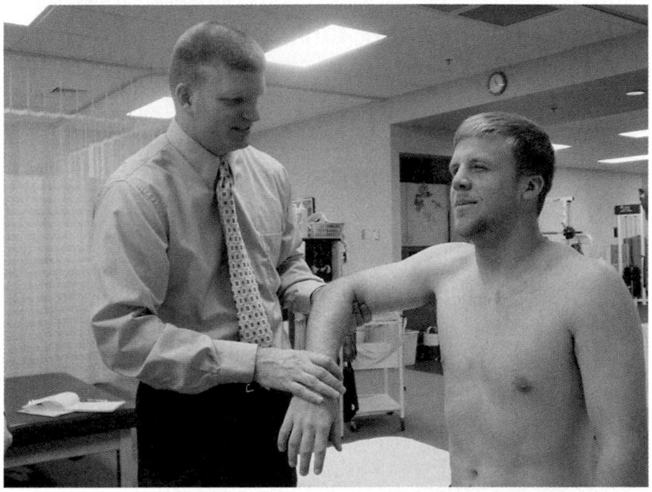

FIGURE 19-26 Hawkins-Kennedy impingement test.

Hawkins-Kennedy impingement test: To perform the Hawkins-Kennedy impingement test, the athletic trainer elevates the client's shoulder to 90 degrees of flexion in the plane of the scapula with the elbow also flexed to 90 degrees (Figure 19-26). From this position, the shoulder is gently internally rotated in an attempt to compress the supraspinatus under the coracoacromial arch. A positive test replicates the pain.

Coracoid impingement test: To perform the coracoid impingement test, the athletic trainer stands directly in front of the client, who assumes the same position as in the Hawkins-Kennedy test. However, this test is performed in the frontal plane rather than the scapular plane. The shoulder is again gently internally rotated in an attempt to compress soft tissue structures. Medially located pain indicates compression of the long head of the biceps or subscapularis, and lateral pain indicates supraspinatus impingement.

Immediate management: Immediate management requires proper evaluation, as described in the instability section, to determine whether the condition is related to glenohumeral joint hypomobility or hypermobility of the rotator cuff. If the problem is due to a lack of mobility, treatment should begin by increasing capsular motion so that normal joint **arthrokinematics** return to the glenohumeral joint. If the tendonitis is due to hypermobility, dynamic control of the rotator cuff and the scapular muscles should be instituted.

Intermediate management: If the problem is related to overuse, relative rest from the offending activity will generally resolve the issue. If the condition is not properly managed, the weakness created by the initial offending activity will disrupt the normal force couples of the rotator cuff, leading to a superior migration of the humeral head during activities requiring shoulder elevation. These offending activities lead to microtrauma, which results in pain and inflammation that lead to further rotator cuff damage and ultimately perpetuate the dysfunction. Unfortunately, what often begins as a simple case of overuse tendonitis becomes a complex issue involving multiple structures. Such a situation requires careful thought and consideration in formulating the proper treatment approach to return athletes to their full unrestricted activities.

Bursitis

Bursitis of the shoulder is an inflammatory condition of the bursa in or around the shoulder.

Mechanism: Bursitis can be caused when the shoulder is brought into forceful contact with the ground or when the humerus is forcefully driven into the acromion. Although isolated bursitis can occur in traumatic contexts, bursitis is usually a secondary condition of SAIS. In most instances, the signs and symptoms of bursitis almost entirely parallel those of SAIS.

Signs and symptoms:

- Possible thickened "boggy" sensation during palpation around the area of the lateral acromion
- Pain with overhead activity
- Possible loss of motion
- Possible weakness
- Possible discomfort with external rotation

Special tests: There are no known tests that differentiate true bursitis from SAIS. Testing for SAIS will also elicit a positive response for bursitis.

Immediate and intermediate management: As with treatment of SAIS, immediate management of bursitis includes decreasing the offending activity. Once normal glenohumeral arthrokinematics have returned, the offending activity and irritation that is occurring will be resolved and the bursa will return to its normal state. If the bursitis is caused by overuse, the same treatment

arthrokinematics movement of the joint surfaces, such as rolls, slides, and glides
bursitis inflammatory condition of the bursa (in and around the shoulder)

approaches mentioned in the tendonitis section should be implemented.

Thoracic Outlet Syndrome

Thoracic outlet syndrome (TOS) refers to a collection of signs and symptoms that are attributed to compression of the NV bundle, including the lower trunk of the brachial plexus and the subclavian and axillary arteries at the location of the thoracic inlet. Central to the discussion of TOS is the first thoracic rib, which is frequently recognized as a contributing factor.[76–79]

Mechanism: TOS typically results from compression of one of the numerous structures inserting onto the first rib in one or more of three locals. Most proximal TOS results from compression entrapment between the middle and anterior scalene muscles.[80] The second location of entrapment occurs at the location between the first rib and the lower border of the clavicle. The final location occurs at the area of the coracoid process directly behind the attachment of the pectoralis minor. These problems are fairly common among people who participate in sports that require repetitive overhead activities. Activities such as pitching create additional rotational torques about the shoulder that repetitively stretch the axillary artery, thus creating a tethering effect that damages the affected structures.[81] Additionally, poor posture about the neck and shoulders with drooping, sagging, or sinking of the shoulder girdle is a potential cause, one that appears to be more common in women than in men.[82]

Signs and symptoms:

- Symptoms depend on the type of TOS that occurs.
- Two forms are classified as either neurological TOS or arterial and vascular TOS.
- Neurological TOS is much more common.
- Neurological TOS symptoms are as follows:
  - Paresthesia on the inside of the forearm and hand in the C8-T1 dermatome distribution
  - Difficulty with fine motor skills
  - Cramping in the forearm and hand
  - Intermittent numbness and tingling in the forearm and hand
- Vascular TOS symptoms are as follows:
  - Swelling
  - Discoloration
  - Vascular distention of the superficial venous distribution of the hand
  - Possible deep, boring toothachelike pain in the neck, shoulder, and arm
- If the client has venous distention that does not decrease rapidly, ruling out a venous effort thrombosis (analogous to the deep venous thrombosis in the lower extremity) is of immediate concern.
- Delayed or untreated cases of effort thrombosis have resulted in grave outcomes, including gangrene of the fingers, aneurysm rupture, and stroke.[82–84]

Special tests: It is simply not enough to determine whether an athlete has TOS. To increase the likelihood of identifying a conservative treatment that will alleviate symptoms, the athletic trainer should be able to determine the exact location of the TOS.

Roo test: The **Roo test** is also known as the positive abduction and external rotation position test and the elevated arm stress test. For this test, the client abducts the shoulder to 90 degrees and then brings it into lateral rotation.[85–88] From this position, the client is asked to slowly and repeatedly open and close the hands for up to 3 minutes (Figure 19-27). A return of symptoms indicates a positive test. Minor numbness and tingling or fatigue that occurs bilaterally may not be pathological. An increase and replication of the athlete's symptoms unilaterally may be more important.

thoracic outlet syndrome (TOS) collection of signs and symptoms that are attributed to compression of the neurovascular bundle at the thoracic inlet

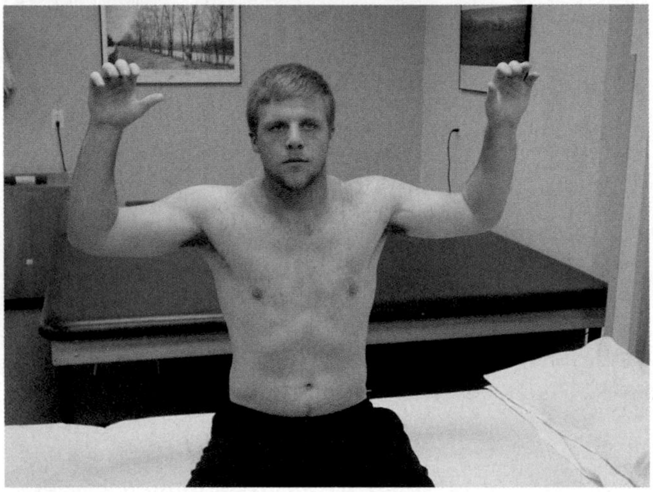

FIGURE 19-27 Roo test.

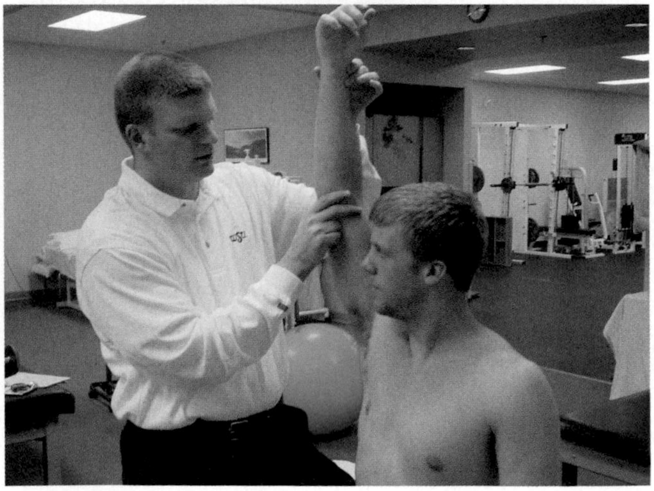

FIGURE 19-28 Wright test.

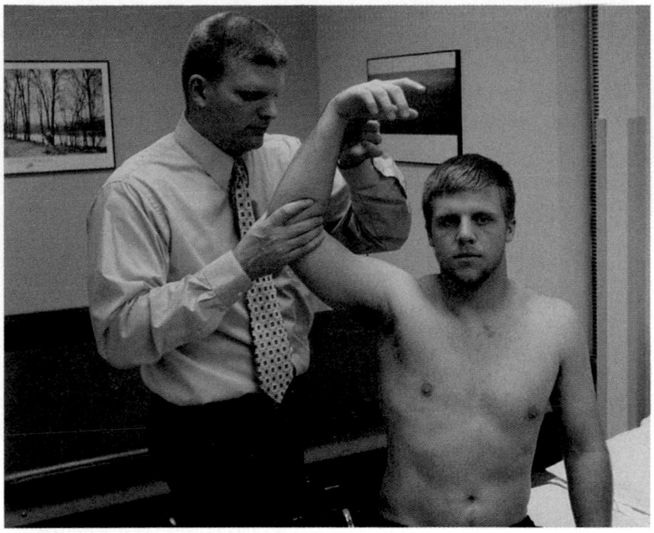

FIGURE 19-29 Allen test.

Wright test: During performance of the Wright test, the client's arm is taken into full passive elevation and lateral rotation by the athletic trainer (Figure 19-28). The athletic trainer is also palpating for a pulse at the radial artery. After finding the pulse, the athletic trainer asks the client to take a deep breath and then rotate or extend the cervical spine to produce additional effects. If the test is positive, a change in pulse and reproduction of symptoms will be evident.

Allen test: The Allen test is essentially the same as the Wright test except that the shoulder is abducted to approximately 100 degrees and the elbow is flexed to 90 degrees (Figure 19-29). While palpating for the radial pulse, the athletic trainer asks the client to rotate the head away from the side being tested. If the test is positive, a diminished pulse and return of symptoms will be evident.

Costoclavicular test or sign: The costoclavicular test is used to produce compression between the clavicle and the first rib. The client is placed in an exaggerated military-type position in which the scapulae are retracted and depressed. The athletic trainer assesses the radial pulse for 1 minute. Like all other tests to this point, an alteration in pulse and return of symptoms indicate a positive test.[4]

Adson maneuver: The Adson maneuver is probably the most conventional of TOS special tests and is used to implicate the scalenes as a sight of entrapment. For this test, the client actively rotates his or her head toward the examined side while taking a deep breath. The athletic trainer extends and laterally rotates the shoulder while assessing for the radial pulse. If the test is positive, a diminished pulse and return of symptoms will be evident.

Immediate management: Luckily for most, nonoperative treatment of TOS has been shown to be successful in 67% to 90% of cases.[86,89] As with most chronic conditions, relative rest is the first line of defense against TOS. Because slouching may decrease the space available for NV structures in the shoulder, postural training is critical for successful treatment.[89] Reports indicate that physical therapy directed at strengthening the shoulder muscles, including the scapular and rotator cuff muscles, is helpful.[90–92]

Intermediate management: Because of pain, compensatory patterns commonly occur in the shoulder, causing overuse and tightness of the upper trapezius, the levator scapulae, and the pectoralis minor muscles. These muscles typically need to be lengthened to maintain proper muscle length symmetry in the shoulder girdle. Manual techniques that are preceded by heating agents to the soft tissue are sometimes helpful. Strength imbalances must be thoroughly assessed and addressed to strengthen weakened muscles around the shoulder before return to activity.

Suprascapular Nerve Impingement

Because it is fairly uncommon, suprascapular nerve impingement or suprascapular neuropathy is often overlooked as a potential cause of shoulder pain and dysfunction.

Mechanism: Suprascapular neuropathy occurs when either compression or traction is applied at one of two locations: the suprascapular notch or the spinoglenoid notch of the scapula. Repetitive microtrauma or a single traumatic event is more likely to cause pathology at the suprascapular notch.[93] Compression by a ganglion cyst is more often the culprit at the level of the spinoglenoid notch.[94]

Signs and symptoms:

- Minimal pain
- Possible dull ache in the posterior shoulder region
- Weakness with manual muscle testing of shoulder external rotators and abductors
- Possible supraspinatus or infraspinatus atrophy

Special tests: There are no special tests specific to suprascapular neuropathy, although electromyography and nerve conduction studies are essential in the diagnosis and treatment of this condition.[93]

Immediate management: The success of rehabilitation greatly depends on the severity and cause of the suprascapular nerve impingement. Surgery may be required to repair a labral tear that is causing the cyst formation. Without surgical repair, intra-articular swelling may continue and the cyst will remain. Regardless, strengthening exercises are appropriate for muscles that have atrophied. The athletic trainer must remember that if the client is treated conservatively, great gains in strength may not be seen because the cyst will continue to put pressure on the neurological structures that are innervating the weakened muscles. With continued pressure on the nerves, the muscles cannot gain the appropriate strength. Ensuring full shoulder ROM is beneficial.

Intermediate management: Once the cause of the impingement is resolved, a gradual progression of strengthening may be implemented. Beginning rotator cuff strengthening with the arm in a position below shoulder height is usually recommended. This positioning decreases the risk that weakened supraspinatus and infraspinatus muscles will produce SAIS, because weakness of these muscles drastically alters normal force couples in the shoulder.

Superior Labral Anterior to Posterior Lesions

A superior labral anterior to posterior (SLAP) lesion involves the superior aspect of the glenoid labrum. It can begin posterior to the biceps tendon and extend anteriorly to the biceps tendon, stopping at or above the midglenoid notch. This area of the superior labrum is important because it serves as the anchor for the insertion of the long head of the biceps tendon on the glenoid rim.

Mechanism: SLAP lesions may result from occult trauma[95] or an eccentric deceleration mechanism in the overhead throwing athlete.[96]

Signs and symptoms:

- Pain with overhead activities, especially throwing or serving
- Instability
- Locking, clicking, or popping with activity

Special tests: Several special tests exist to assess for SLAP lesions in the shoulder.

The active compression test: This test is used to assess for either a SLAP lesion or acromioclavicular joint pathology.[97] To perform the active compression test, the athletic trainer stands alongside the client's affected shoulder. The client's shoulder is taken into 90 degrees of flexion, followed by 15 degrees of horizontal adduction medial to the sagittal plane. The athletic trainer then maximally internally rotates the client's shoulder and provides resistance with an inferior directed force at the distal forearm. The client is asked whether this recreates pain and symptoms. If pain occurs during the first part of this test, the shoulder is then externally rotated while still maintaining 15 degrees of horizontal adduction. Resistance is again applied. If pain is diminished or no longer present, the test is considered positive. The pain may occur at one of two locales: superiorly for the AC joint and deep in the shoulder for a SLAP lesion.

Crank test: The crank test is performed with the athletic trainer at the client's head on the side of the injured shoulder. The athletic trainer takes the client's arm into 150 to 160 degrees of elevation in the scapular plane. Next, the athletic trainer gives a compressive force along the long axis of the humerus, while internally and externally rotating the upper extremity in an attempt to catch a piece of torn labrum. A positive finding is reproducible pain, clicking, clunking, pseudolocking, or any combination of these symptoms.

BOX 19-5 Chronic Neck and Shoulder Injuries and Appropriate Special Tests

Neck Injuries

Cervical myelopathy
- Clonus, Babinski, and Hoffmann's tests

Sprains and strains
- Manual muscle testing

Whiplash injury
- Same as acute whiplash injury

Cervical disc lesions
- Cervical distraction test
- Spurling's test
- Bakody's test

Shoulder Injuries

Subluxations/Instability
- *Inferior instability:* Sulcus sign, Feagin test
- *Anterior and posterior instability:* Anterior and posterior drawer test

Tendonitis
- Neer's impingement test
- Hawkins-Kennedy impingement test
- Coracoid impingement test

Bursitis
- No tests to differentiate from SAIS

Thoracic outlet syndrome
- Roo's test
- Wright test
- Allen test
- Costoclavicular test or sign
- Adson maneuver

Suprascapular nerve impingement
- No appropriate special tests

Superior labral anterior to posterior (SLAP) lesions
- Active compression test
- Crank test

Immediate and intermediate management: Conservative rehabilitation is often appropriate. Its success depends on the severity of the labral injury, however. Some of the pain and symptoms associated with a labral tear may actually be caused by other concomitant injuries. Affected individuals commonly exhibit SAIS, posterior capsule tightness, and scapular asymmetry. Immediate treatment is dictated by presenting symptoms. Not much can be done in terms of conservative treatment to repair a labral tear. Instead, treatment must focus on other problems, such as lack of mobility and decreased strength and endurance of the cuff and scapular stabilizers.[98]

Box 19-5 summarizes chronic injuries to the neck and shoulder and the appropriate special tests used to help diagnose each.

Prevention of Chronic/Overuse Neck and Shoulder Injuries

Prevention of chronic neck and shoulder injuries rests again with the athlete, who must strive to be in top physical condition, consistently wear appropriate equipment that fits properly, and follow proper technique. Proper posture in sitting, standing, and ambulation enhances the ability of this area to avoid muscle strength imbalances and thereby avoid chronic pain conditions. Chronic injuries often occur gradually over a long time of minor incidents

BOX 19-6 **Return to Play Guidelines and Recommendations**

No Contraindications to Participation in Contact/Collision Sports

- Congenital conditions, such as type 2 Klippel-Feil anomaly
- Spina bifida occulta
- Patients with healed stable nondisplaced fractures without sagittal malalignment
- Patients with asymptomatic disk herniations treated conservatively in the past
- Asymptomatic patients after a one-level anterior or posterior cervical fusion for miscellaneous reasons who are neurologically intact and pain free and who have a solid fusion

Relative Contraindications to Returning to Contact/Collision Sports

Patient with full cervical motion, no pain, and a normal neurological examination with:

- A previous upper cervical spine fracture, such as:
  - A healed nondisplaced Jefferson fracture
  - A healed type 1 or 2 odontoid fracture
  - A healed lateral mass fracture of C2
  - A healed stable, minimally displaced, vertebral body compression fracture without sagittal malalignment
- A healed stable fracture of the posterior elements, excluding spinous process fractures
- The presence of minimal residual facet instability after surgical or conservative treatment of cervical disk disease
- After a healed two- or three-level cervical fusion

Absolute Contraindications to Returning to Contact/Collision Sports

- Odontoid anomalies
- An atlantooccipital fusion
- Atlantoaxial instability
- Atlantoaxial rotary fixation
- Certain Klippel-Feil anomalies
- Radiographic presence of a spear tackler's spine
- Subaxial spinal instability
- Acute fracture of either the body or posterior elements with or without ligamentous instability
- Healed subaxial vertebral body fractures with sagittal malalignment
- Acute fracture of the vertebral body with associated posterior arch features and/or ligamentous laxity
- Residual bony canal compromise from retropulsed bony fragments
- Continued pain, abnormal neurological findings, or limited motion from a healed cervical fracture
- The presence of a symptomatic acute soft or chronic disk herniation with associated neurological findings, pain, or limited motion
- After a successful one-level fusion in the presence of diffuse congenital narrowing of the cervical canal

From Torg JS, Ramsey-Emrhein JA: Suggested management guidelines for participation in collision activities with congenital, devolopmental, or postinjury lesions involving the cervical spine, *Med Sci Sports Exerc* 29:S256–272, 1997.

and compromises that eventually lead to a condition that limits normal activities of daily living. By intentionally working to avoid unnecessary strain on these areas, an athlete can help prevent chronic or overuse injuries.

TAPING, BRACING, AND RETURN TO PLAY

In general, taping and bracing are done to rest or stabilize the shoulder after an acute injury. Acute injuries are prevented with progressive ROM exercises and a maintenance regimen emphasizing adequate flexibility, muscular strength, and muscular endurance.

Returning the client with a neck or shoulder injury to his or her previous functional level of activity is often a difficult decision, one that can cause the athletic trainer an undue amount of stress and uneasiness. Box 19-6 outlines previously established guidelines and recommendations that should be consulted when making such a decision.

THE AGE GROUP ATHLETE

Because the neck and shoulder are so highly involved in most activities, it is no surprise that neck and shoulder injuries affect both young and mature populations. Humeral stress fractures, or "Little Leaguer's shoulder," are quite common among children and adolescents. Because of the nature of these injuries, early diagnosis and management is critical to ensure that involvement in future activities and sports will not be compromised or prevented. Active mature individuals tend to be more prone to sustaining a frozen shoulder following injury than other age populations.

Humeral Stress Fracture

In the adolescent athlete, Little Leaguer's shoulder is an injury to the proximal humeral epiphyseal plate that results in a stress fracture. This condition usually affects athletes who have not yet reached skeletal maturity.

Mechanism: This injury is caused by repetitive overuse conditions. Sometimes, poor mechanics and technique are direct causative factors as well.

Signs and symptoms:

- Pain with active motion, especially throwing
- Diffuse pain
- Pain that worsens with increased activity
- Pain that frequently decreases with rest

Special tests: No special tests are applicable.

Immediate and intermediate management: Initial treatment for proximal humeral stress fractures is relative rest. Therefore the youngster should refrain from performing any offending activity. In most cases, stopping the offending activity while remaining physically active is more beneficial for both conditioning and psychological reasons. Certain shoulder exercises are still permissible, depending on symptoms. ROM exercises for the shoulder are continued to maintain flexibility of the numerous muscle tendon units that coordinate shoulder function. Strengthening of the scapula is maintained because it does not place excessive stress on the proximal portion of the shoulder. Most glenohumeral exercises may be performed if they do not cause pain. Wrist, forearm, and hand exercises are maintained as tolerated to sustain or enhance total arm strength. Only if the client reports severe pain with any active movement should the shoulder be placed in an immobilizer. The immobilization period should be brief, if at all possible.

Frozen Shoulder

Not as common in the younger athlete but seen regularly in the older athlete is a condition known as frozen shoulder, or adhesive capsulitis. Frozen shoulder is a very challenging injury to treat.

Mechanism: Idiopathic frozen shoulder occurs when there is a global deterioration of ROM that is accompanied by slow onset of pain with movements, especially shoulder abduction and external rotation. Secondary frozen shoulder is more common in the active individual because it is generally marked by an acute onset of trauma followed by immobilization of the shoulder. Affected individuals commonly exhibit a specific direction of shoulder limitation rather than the global loss seen among those with the primary version.[99]

Signs and symptoms:

- Pain with movement in all directions
- Loss of motion both actively and passively

Special tests: No special tests are applicable.

Immediate and intermediate management: No definitive treatment approach for frozen shoulder has yet been described. Eclectic approaches seem to work best. Because people afflicted with frozen shoulder go through multiple stages, treatment must be stage specific. The first line of defense is usually some form of antiinflammatory medication, in the form of either oral agents or intra-articular injections. Because a primary symptom of this condition is loss of motion, regaining motion is a huge component of the treatment plan. Joint mobilizations to the glenohumeral and scapulothoracic joints followed by gentle PROM exercises are beneficial. In some cases, it is helpful to administer heat through the use of moist hot packs or ultrasound treatments before attempting joint mobilizations. These mobilizations should not cause dramatic increases in subacromial pain and thereby exacerbate an already painful condition. Strengthening exercises are also beneficial, although significant strength loss is generally not among the sequelae of frozen shoulder.

SUMMARY

Proper management of acute and chronic neck and shoulder injury requires careful evaluation to ensure proper diagnostic categorization. Once a proper diagnosis is reached, every attempt should be made to use intervention approaches that have been proved effective. This chapter has reviewed numerous neck and shoulder injuries and the evaluation and management schemes that are appropriate for those conditions. When solid evidence does not clearly dictate the best treatment approach, clinical intuition and experience

OPENING *Scenario Differential Diagnosis*

		DIFFERENTIAL DIAGNOSIS	
EVALUATION TECHNIQUE	ROTATOR CUFF TEAR	SCAPULAR FRACTURE	AXILLARY NERVE INJURY
History	Generally overuse	Trauma	Trauma
Inspection	Mild swelling	Moderate to severe	Depends on severity
Palpation	Diffuse	Point tenderness	Minimal
AROM	Depends on severity	Decreased	Decreased
PROM	Full	Decreased	Full
RROM	Weakness	Severe weakness	Severe weakness
Neurological	Normal	Normal	Normal
Special Tests	Positive	Positive compression test	No special tests
Diagnostic Test	Radiographs (−) MRI (+)	Radiographs (+) MRI (−)	Radiographs (−) MRI (+)

AROM, Active range of motion; *PROM*, passive range of motion; *RROM*, resistive range of motion; *MRI*, magnetic resonance imaging.

usually prevail. The ultimate goal of rehabilitation is to return the athlete to the highest level of function in the shortest amount of time possible.

Revisiting the OPENING *Scenario*

Matthew was immediately placed in a shoulder sling and sent to a local orthopedic surgeon. Radiographic and computed tomography scans revealed a significantly displaced scapular fracture with soft tissue involvement. Because of multiple fractures, the rotator cuff muscles surrounding the scapula were unable to function properly, which made it impossible for Matthew to use his upper extremity for active movements. He was told to wear his shoulder sling and immobilizer for 4 weeks, at the conclusion of which he was gradually removed from immobilization. Matthew's athletic trainer instituted progressive range of motion and strengthening exercises. The differential diagnosis is traumatic rotator cuff tear, fracture, or deltoid rupture.

Issues & Ethics

John is a senior forward on the university's lacrosse team. He dislocated his shoulder in the first half of this game. To your knowledge, he has dislocated the same shoulder three other times in his career. He informs you that he is fine and can continue to play. Because of some team violations off the field, several players are ineligible for this game and the next five games. Coming out of the halftime, your team is down by two goals. As the leading scorer for both the team and conference, John expects to stay in the game so he can attempt to break another school scoring record. Reminding you that he has popped his shoulder back in before, he begs you to help him reduce the dislocation on the field so he can continue to play. What do you do?

Web Links

American Journal of Sports Medicine: www.ajsm.sagepub.com
American Society of Shoulder and Elbow Therapists: http://webteach.mccs.uky.edu/khp781/asset.htm
Cramer Products: www.cramersportsmed.com
Journal of Orthopaedic & Sports Physical Therapy: www.jospt.org
Journal of Shoulder and Elbow Surgery: www.jshoulderelbow.org
North American Spine Society (NASS): www.spine.org/
SpineUniverse: www.spineuniverse.com
The Visible Human Project: nlm.nih.gov/research/visible/getting_data.html

References

1. Olson KA et al: Radiographic assessment and reliability study of the craniovertebral sidebending test, *J Man Manipul Ther* 6: 87–96, 1998.
2. Meadows JJ, Magee DJ: An overview of dizziness and vertigo for the orthopedic manual therapist. In Boyling JD, Palastanga N, editors: *Grieve's modern manual therapy: the vertebral column*, ed 2, Edinburgh, 1994, Churchill Livingstone.
3. Pettman E: Stress tests of the craniovertebral joints, In Boyling JD, Palastanga N, editors, *Grieve's modern manual therapy: the vertebral column*, ed. 2, Edinburgh, 1994, Churchill Livingstone.
4. Magee DJ: *Orthopedic physical assessment*, ed 4, St Louis, Saunders, 2006.
5. Kerry R, Taylor AJ: Cervical arterial dysfunction assessment and manual therapy, *Man Ther* 11: 243–253, 2006.
6. Australian Physiotherapy Association: Clinical guidelines for assessing vertebrobasilar insufficiency in the mangement of cervical spine disorders. APA, August 22, 2006; [http://apa.advsol.com.au/]
7. *Athletic Training and Sports Medicine*, ed 2, Rosemont Ill, 1991, American Academy of Orthopedic Surgeons.
8. National Spinal Cord Injury Statistical Center: *Spinal Cord Information Network: facts and figures at a glance*, Birmingham, Ala, 2003, University of Alabama at Birmingham.
9. Nobunga AI, Go BK, Karunas RB: Recent demographic and injury trends in people served by the model spine cord injury care systems, *Arch Phys Med Rehabil* 80: 1372–1382, 1999.
10. DeVivo MJ: Causes and costs of spinal cord injury in the United States, *Spinal Cord* 35: 809–813, 1997.
11. Torg JS et al: The national football head and neck injury registry. Fourteen-year report on cervical quadriplegia, 1971–1984, *JAMA* 254(24): 3439–3443, 1984.
12. Lee DG: *A workbook of manual therapy techniques for the upper extremity*, Delta, Canada, 1989, Delta Orthopaedic Physiotherapy Clinics.
13. Dutton M: The cervical spine. In *Orthopaedic examination, evaluation, and intervention*, New York, 2004, McGraw-Hill Medical Companies.
14. Appuzo ML et al: Acute fractures of the odontoid process: an analysis of 45 cases, *J Neurosurg*, 48: 85–91, 1978.
15. Marchesi DG: Management of odontoid fractures, *Orthopaedics* 20: 911–916, 1997.
16. Clark CR, White AA: Fractures of the dens: a multicenter study, *J Bone Joint Surg* 67A: 1340–1348, 1985.
17. Heller J, Levy M, Barrow D: Odontoid fracture malunion with fixed atlantoaxial subluxation, *Spine*, 18: 311–314, 1993.
18. Seybold EA, Bayley JC: Functional outcome of surgically and conservatively managed dens fractures, *Spine*, 23: 1837–1846, 1998.
19. Hadley MN et al: Acute traumatic atlas fractures: management and long-term outcome, *Neurosurgery* 23: 31–35, 1998.
20. Lee TT, Green BA, Petrin DA: Treatment of stable burst fracture of the atlas (Jefferson fracture) with rigid cervical collar, *Spine* 23: 1963–1967, 1998.

21. Clancy WB, Brand R, Bergfeld J: Upper trunk brachial plexus injuries in contact sports, *Am J Sports Med* 5: 209–216, 1977.
22. Wang JC et al: Growth and development of the pediatric cervical spine documented radiographically, *J Bone Joint Surg* 83-A: 1212–1218, 2001.
23. Vacarro AR et al: Return to play criteria for the athlete with cervical spine injuries resulting in stinger and transient quadriplegia/paresis, *Spine J* 2: 351–356, 2002.
24. Bateman JE: Nerve injuries about the shoulder in sports, *J Bone Joint Surg* 49A: 785–792, 1967.
25. Hoyt W: Etiology of shoulder injuries in athletes, *J Bone Joint Surg* 49A: 755–766, 1967.
26. Robertson WC Jr, Eichman PL, Clancy WG: Upper trunk plexopathy in football players, *JAMA* 241: 1480–1482, 1979.
27. Chrisman OD et al: Lateral-flexion neck injuries in athletic competition, *JAMA* 192: 117–119, 1965.
28. Levitz CI, Reilly PJ, Torg JS: The pathomechanics of chronic, recurrent cervical nerve root neurapraxia, *Am J Sports Med* 25: 73–76, 1997.
29. Watkins RG: Neck injuries in football players, *Clin Sports Med* 5: 215–246, 1986.
30. Dutton M: *Orthopaedic examination, evaluation, and intervention*, New York, 2004, McGraw Hill.
31. Kroon P, Kruchowsky T: *Manual therapy course handbook* [unpublished manuscript], San Marcos, Tex, 2006, The Manual Therapy Institute.
32. Meadows J: *A rational and complete approach to the acute and sub acute post-MVA cervical patient* [course Manual], Alberta, Canada, 1995, Swodeam Consulting Inc.
33. Burkhead WZ, Rockwood CA: Treatment of instability of the shoulder with an exercise program, *J Bone Joint Surg* 74: 890–896, 1992.
34. Liu SH, Henry MH: Anterior shoulder instability. Current review, *Clin Orthop* 323: 327–337, 1996.
35. Rowe CR: Prognosis in dislocations of the shoulder, *J Bone Joint Surg* 38A: 957–977, 1956.
36. Samilson RL, Prieto V: Posterior dislocation of the shoulder in athletes, *Clin Sports Med* 2: 369–378, 1983.
37. Jobe FW, Bradley JP: The diagnosis and nonoperative treatment of shoulder injuries in athletes, *Clin Sports Med* 8: 419–438, 1989.
38. Stuart MJ et al: Injuries in youth football: a prospective observational cohort analysis among players aged 9 to 13 years, *Mayo Clin Proc* 77(4): 317–322, 2002.
39. Stuart MJ, Smith A: Injuries in junior A ice hockey. A three-year prospective study, *Am J Sports Med* 23(4): 458–461, 1995.
40. Webb J, Bannister G: Acromioclavicular disruption in first class rugby players, *Br J Sports Med* 26(4): 247–248, 1992.
41. Kocher MS, Dupre MM, Feagin JA Jr: Shoulder injuries from alpine skiing and snowboarding. Aetiology, treatment and prevention, *Sports Med* 25(3): 201–211, 1998.
42. Kocher MS, Feagin JA Jr: Shoulder injuries during alpine skiing, *Am J Sports Med* 24(5): 665–669, 1996.
43. Molsa J et al: Injuries to the upper extremity in ice hockey: analysis of a series of 760 injuries, *Am J Sports Med* 31(5): 751–757, 2003.
44. Kelly BT et al: Shoulder injuries to quarterbacks in the National Football League, *Am J Sports Med* 32(2): 328–331, 2004.
45. Axe MJ: Acromioclavicular joint injuries in the athlete, *Sports Med Arthroscopy Rev* 8: 182–191, 2000.
46. Clark HD, McCann PD: Acromioclavicular joint injuries, *Orthop Clin N Am* 31: 177–187, 2000.
47. Konin JG et al, editors: *Special tests for orthopedic examination*, ed 3, Thorofare, NJ, 2006, SLACK.
48. Cave AJE: Surgical anatomy in sternoclavicular dislocation of the shoulder. In Rockwood C, Green D, editors: *Fractures*, Philadelphia, 1975, J.B. Lippincott.
49. Sadr B, Swann M: Spontaneous dislocation of the sternoclavicular joint, *Acta Orthop Scand* 50: 269–274, 1979.
50. Nettles JL, Linscheid R: Sternoclavicular dislocations, *J Trauma*, 8: 158–164, 1968.
51. Omer GE: Osteotomy of the clavicle in surgical reduction of anterior sternoclavicular dislocation, *J Trauma* 7: 584–590, 1967.
52. Waskowitz WJ: Disruption of the sternoclavicular joint: an analysis and review, *Am J Orthop* 3: 176–179, 1961.
53. Wickiewicz TL: Acromioclavicular and sternoclavicular joint injuries, *Clin Sports Med* 2: 429–438, 1983.
54. Blaine TB, Biglinani LU, Levine WN: Fractures of the proximal humerus, In Matsen FA, Lippitt SB, editors: *The shoulder*, Philadelphia, 2004, Saunders.
55. Fehlings MG, Skaf G: A review of the pathophysiology of cervical spondylotic myelopathy with insights for potential novel mechanisms drawn from traumatic spinal cord injury, *Spine* 23: 2730–2737, 1998.
56. Baptiste DC, Fehlings MG: Pathophysiology of cervical myelopathy *Spine J*, 6: 190S–197S, 2006.
57. Rao R: Neck pain, cervical radiculopathy, and cervical myelopathy: pathophysiology, natural history, clinical evaluation, *J Bone Joint Surg* 84A, 1872–1881, 2002.
58. Sampath P et al: Outcome of patients treated for cervical myelopathy: a prospective, multicenter study with independent clinical review, *Spine* 25: 670–676, 2000.
59. Resnick D et al: Guidelines for the performance of fusion procedures for degenerative disease of the lumbar spine. Part 2: Assessment of functional outcome, *J Neurosurg Spine* 2: 639–646, 2005.
60. Kadanka Z et al: Approaches to spondylotic cervical myelopathy: conservative versus surgical results in a 3-year follow-up study, *Spine* 27: 2205–2211, 2002.
61. Mellion MB: Neck and back pain in bicycling, *Clin Sports Med* 13: 137–164, 1994.
62. Jull G: Deep cervical flexor muscle dysfunction in whiplash, *J Muscul Pain* 8: 143–154, 2000.
63. Kondo K et al: Protruded intervertebral cervical disc: incidence and affected cervical level in Rochester, Minnesota, 1950 through 1974, *Minn Med* 64: 751–753, 1981.
64. Viikari-Junutura E, Porras M, Laasonen EM: Validity of clinical tests in the diagnosis of root compression in cervical disease, *Spine* 14: 253–257, 1989.
65. Jahnke RW, Hart BL: Cervical stenosis, spondylosis, and herniated disc disease, *Radiol Clin North Am* 29: 777–791, 1991.
66. Warren RF: Subluxation of the shoulder in athletes, *Clin Sports Med* 2(2): 339–354, 1983.

67. Neer CS, Foster CR: Inferior capsular shift for involuntary and multidirectional instability of the shoulder, *J Bone Joint Surg* 62A: 897–908, 1980.
68. Mallon W, Speer K: Multidirectional instability: current concepts, *J Shoulder Elbow Surg* 4: 55–64, 1995.
69. Wilk KE, Andrews JR, Arrigo CA: The physical examination of the glenohumeral joint: emphasis on the stabilizing structures, *J Orthop Sports Phys Ther* 25(6): 380–389, 1997.
70. Rockwood CA: Subluxations and dislocations about the shoulder, In Rockwood CA, Green DP, editors: *Fractures in adults*, Philadelphia, 1984, JB Lippincott.
71. O'Brien SJ et al: Developmental anatomy of the shoulder and anatomy of the glenohumeral joint, In Rockwood CA, Matsen FA, editors: *The shoulder*, Philadelphia, 1990, Saunders.
72. Speer KP, Garrett WE: Muscular control of motion and stability about the pectoral girdle, In Matsen FA, Fu FH, Hawkins RJ, editors, *The shoulder: a balance of mobility and stability*, Rosemont, Ill, 1993, American Academy of Orthopaedic Surgeons.
73. Ellenbecker T, Davies GJ, editors: *Closed kinetic chain exercise: a comprehensive guide to multiple joint exercise*, Champaign, Ill, 2001, Human Kinetics.
74. Neer CS: Anterior acromioplasty for the chronic impingement syndrome of the shoulder, *J Bone Joint Surg*, 54A: 41–50, 1972.
75. Neer CS III: Impingement lesions, *Clin Orthop* 173, 70–77, 1983.
76. Leffert R: Thoracic outlet syndrome, In Gelberman RH, editor: *Operative nerve repair and reconstruction*, Philadelphia, 1991, JB Lippincott.
77. Nehler MR et al: Upper extremity ischemia from subclavian artery aneurysm caused by bony abnormalities of the thoracic outlet, *Arch Surg* 132: 527–532, 1997.
78. Durham JR et al: Arterial injuries in the thoracic outlet syndrome, *J Vasc Surg* 21: 57–69, 1995.
79. Yao JS: Upper extremity ischemia in athletes, *Semin Vasc Surg* 11: 96–105, 1998.
80. Rayan GM: Thoracic outlet syndrome, *J Shoulder Elbow Surg* 7: 440–451, 1998.
81. Todd GJ et al: Aneurysms of the mid axillary artery in major league baseball pitchers: a report of two cases, *J Vasc Surg* 28: 702–707, 1998.
82. McCready RA et al: Recurrence and rupture of an axillary aneurysm, *Am Surg* 48: 241–242, 1982.
83. Brooks A, Fowler SB: Axillary artery thrombosis after prolonged use of crutches, *J Bone Joint Surg* 46A: 863–864, 1964.
84. Fields WS, Lemak NA, Ben-Menachem Y: Thoracic outlet syndrome: review and reference to stroke in a major league pitcher, *AJR* 146: 809–814, 1986.
85. Roos DB: Transaxillary first rib resection to relieve thoracic outlet syndrome, *Ann Surg* 163: 354–358, 1966.
86. Roos DB: Congenital anomalies associated with thoracic outlet syndrome, *Am J Surg* 132: 771–778, 1976.
87. Liebenson CS: Thoracic outlet syndrome: diagnosis and conservative management, *J Manip Physiol Ther* 11: 493–499, 1988.
88. Ribbe EB, Lindgren SH, Norgren NE: Clinical diagnosis of thoracic outlet syndrome: evaluation of patients with cervicobrachial symptoms, *Manual Med* 2: 82–85, 1984.
89. Leffert RD: Thoracic outlet syndrome, *J Am Acad Orthop Surg* 2: 317–325, 1994.
90. Aligne C, Barral X: Rehabilitation of patients with thoracic outlet syndrome, *Ann Vasc Surg* 6: 381–389, 1992.
91. Britt L: Nonoperative treatment of thoracic outlet syndrome symptoms, *Clin Orthop* 51: 45–48, 1967.
92. Kenny R et al: Thoracic outlet syndrome: a useful exercise treatment option, *Am J Surg* 165: 282–284, 1993.
93. Romeo AA, Rotenberg DD, Bach BR: Suprascapular neuropathy, *J Am Acad Orthop Surg* 7:, 358–367, 1999.
94. Inokuchi W, Ogawa K, Horiuchi Y: Magnetic resonance imaging of suprascapular nerve palsy, *J Shoulder Elbow Surg* 7: 223–227, 1998.
95. Snyder SJ, Karzel RP, Del Pizzo W: SLAP lesions of the shoulder, *Arthroscopy* 6, 274–279, 1990.
96. Andrews JR, Carson WG, Mcleaod WD: Glenoid labrum tears related to the long head of the biceps, *Am J Sports Med* 13: 337–341, 1985.
97. O'Brien SJ et al: The active compression test: a new and effective test for diagnosis labral tears and acromioclavicular (AC) abnormality, *Am J Sports Med* 26: 610–613, 1998.
98. Manske RC: Electromyographically assessed exercises for the scapular muscles, *Athlet Ther Today*, 11: 19–23, 2006.
99. Malone T, Hazle C: Rehabilitation of adhesive capsulitis, In Ellenbecker TS, editor: *Shoulder rehabilitation: non-operative treatment*, New York, 2006, Thieme.

20

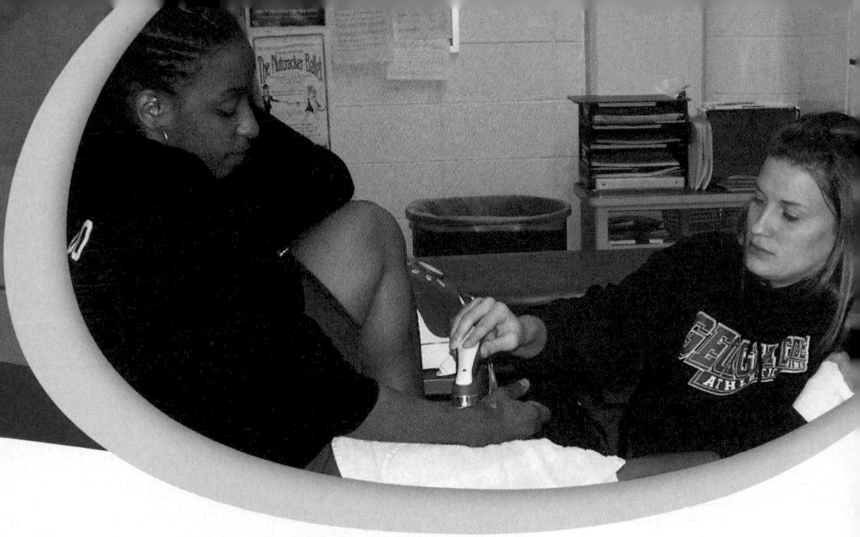

Diagnosis and Management of Elbow, Wrist, Hand, and Finger Injuries

KATHY TAYLOR REMSBURG

Learning Goals

1. Describe appropriate procedures for the evaluation and diagnosis of common acute and chronic injuries to the elbow, wrist, hand, and fingers.
2. Discuss the importance of a systematic assessment in the management of acute and chronic athletic injuries.
3. List common acute athletic injuries occurring to the elbow, wrist, hand, and fingers.
4. Explain the proper interventions for managing acute injuries to the elbow, wrist, hand, and fingers.
5. List common chronic athletic injuries occurring to the elbow, wrist, hand, and fingers.
6. Describe the proper management of common chronic injuries to the elbow, wrist, hand, and fingers.
7. Identify principles and concepts that can be used to prevent athletic injuries to the elbow, wrist, hand, and fingers.
8. Identify precautions and risks associated with athletic participation by the age group athlete to the elbow, wrist, hand, and fingers.

The elbow, wrist, and hand are routinely used to perform many activities of daily living. Some of the daily functions these body parts perform include throwing, lifting, carrying, gripping, bending, flexing, holding, and twisting. In many activities of daily living and work, these functions are necessary to perform tasks efficiently and without restriction. Unfortunately, the repetitive nature of many of these movements increases the risk of injury to the elbow, wrist, or hand.

Some of the most frequently reported injuries are incurred to this area of the body. Research indicates that between 3% and 9% of all athletic injuries and 14% of all high school football injuries involve the wrist and hand.[1] Athletes who engage in sports in which the arm is used for throwing, catching, or swinging (e.g., baseball, softball, tennis) are particularly susceptible. Some of the injuries sustained to the elbow, wrist, and hand are acute injuries, but these injuries also can be chronic. The goal of the athletic trainer is to recognize, diagnose, and properly treat both acute and chronic injuries. Completing this goal requires a thorough understanding of human anatomy and the ability to systematically evaluate an injury. After completing the evaluation, the athletic trainer must interpret the findings, decide on an appropriate course of action, completely and thoroughly treat the athlete, and prevent secondary injuries. This chapter presents the information that an athletic trainer needs to competently perform these tasks for elbow, wrist, hand, and finger injuries.

Terms that appear in boldface green type are defined in the book's glossary.

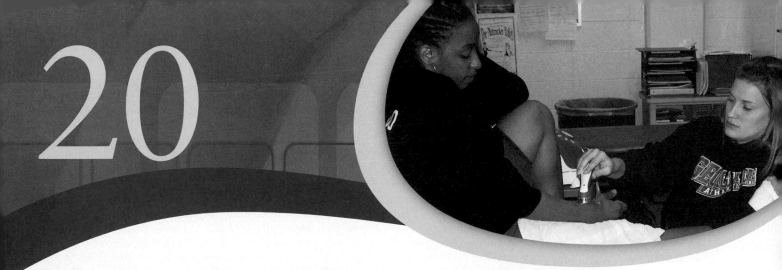

OPENING *Scenario*

Paul, an 18-year-old college freshman, goes to see the athletic trainer after football practice. He complains of right wrist pain caused by performing blocking drills in practice. Paul initially hurt his wrist last year during football season when he was in high school. He states that this injury does not hurt as much as the last one. Evaluation of Paul's wrist reveals pain with active range of motion (AROM) and passive range of motion (PROM) into wrist and thumb extension, swelling on the dorsum (back) of his hand, point tenderness in the anatomical snuffbox, decreased grip strength, and atrophy of the thenar eminence (the fleshy mass on the palmar side of the hand at the base of the thumb). He is sent to the hospital for an X-ray examination to rule out a fracture. The X-ray scans come back negative, and the wrist injury is treated as a sprain. After 2 weeks, Paul stops coming in for treatments. He is subsequently released from treatments in the athletic training room. A few months later, Paul re-injures his wrist while wrestling in his dorm room. During the history portion of the new evaluation, the athletic trainer discovers that Paul's wrist pain never went away after the initial injury in high school. His presenting symptoms now include pain and decreased AROM into wrist extension and radial deviation, point tenderness in the anatomical snuffbox, decreased PROM with wrist extension and ulnar deviation, and decreased grip strength. Differential diagnosis: triangular fibrocartilage complex injury versus wrist sprain versus scaphoid navicular fracture.

CLINICAL EVALUATION AND DIAGNOSIS OF ELBOW, WRIST, HAND, AND FINGER INJURIES

The elbow's role in the upper extremity is to position the hand and wrist so that they may effectively perform the actions required of them. If elbow motion is altered in any way, whether through incorrect throwing mechanisms, falling on an outstretched hand (**FOOSH**), or overuse, injury to the elbow, wrist, hand or fingers may result.[2] Most acute elbow, forearm, wrist, hand, and finger injuries are the result of FOOSH caused by contact or collision-related mechanisms.[2] Frequently, these injuries do not require the athletic trainer to rush to conduct an evaluation, because most individuals with these injuries will be able to get to them on their own accord. Exceptions are elbow dislocations and forearm fractures. Because deformity and swelling are usually superficial and therefore easily detected in the elbow and forearm, acute injuries are easily identified. Evaluations of chronic injuries are more challenging because the outward signs and symptoms are not as easily detected. The disabling effect of both acute and chronic injuries usually accounts for lost participation time and varies according to the athlete's activity and hand dominance.

The goals of an acute or on-field evaluation are to quickly rule out life- or limb-threatening injuries, profuse bleeding, fractures, joint dislocations, neurovascular injuries, and other emergency situations; to perform the evaluation as quickly as possible to prevent undue delays; and to determine the safest way to move the client away from the activity. Once removed, the client may be evaluated more thoroughly to help determine a diagnosis. On the basis of the evaluation findings and the injury diagnosis, proper management of the injury, the type of first-aid required, and the need for further diagnostic tests should be determined next. In the case of acute injuries, the evaluation process must be second nature because time is of the essence. The athletic trainer must have emergency protocols in place for communicating and responding before an actual emergency occurs. Most acute evaluations are limited to taking a brief history while also observing the athlete and injured body part, palpating bony and soft-tissue structures, conducting functional range of motion (ROM) and neurovascular testing, and performing specific special tests.

A chronic injury is an injury that has occurred over a period of time. Unfortunately, chronic injuries are becoming more common not only in athletics but also in professional settings.[3] Overuse injuries are caused by repetitive stress and insufficient time for the stressed area to return to normal between practices or competitions. In short, the individual or body part is required to do too much too quickly. The evaluation of a chronic injury is essentially the same as that of an acute injury. A thorough and expanded evaluation is necessary for a full understanding of the injury, especially given that signs and symptoms of chronic injuries are not as obvious as those of acute injuries. Also, there is more time for evaluation of chronic injuries, which are usually assessed in the athletic training room or another clinical setting.

History

The first and most important step in conducting an injury evaluation is taking a history. When taking a history, athletic trainers must listen carefully, ask questions that are easily understood by the client, ask questions that do not lead to a particular answer (i.e., open-ended questions), take the answers at face value, refrain from interrupting, show empathy by looking at the client when he or she answers, and not show emotions of surprise,

FOOSH falling on an outstretched hand

fear, or amazement through telltale facial expressions.[4] If the history is taken correctly, the athletic trainer will have a good idea of the diagnosis without the need for additional information.

During an acute evaluation, the athletic trainer should strive to keep the history taking brief so as to minimize any delays in the game or competition. History questions should center on determining the mechanism, symptoms, and any pertinent medical history.[5] As previously mentioned, the most common mechanisms of acute elbow, forearm, wrist, hand, and finger injuries are FOOSH and direct trauma.[2] If the athletic trainer actually witnesses the mechanism of injury, performing the acute injury evaluation will take even less time.

It is impossible to ask too many questions during the history section of a chronic injury evaluation. Some questions are always asked during the history, whether the injury is acute or chronic. Evaluation of a chronic injury usually calls for more questions, however.

Inspection/Observation

Observation begins the minute that the injured athlete and the athletic trainer meet and continues throughout the entire evaluation process. Ideally, observation of signs and symptoms should occur while the athletic trainer is taking the history so that the client does not become self-conscious. The goal of observation is to rule out obvious signs of severe injury or any limb-threatening conditions such as joint dislocations and fractures (Figure 20-1). Signs are easy to observe; the symptoms affecting the client must be determined now. The athletic trainer should watch the client remove his or her clothing and shoes to see whether the client exhibits any reluctance to use the injured body part. It is important to see how the client holds the elbow, arm, and hand. The arm as a whole should be examined, and bony and muscular structures should be compared bilaterally. Signs or symptoms may be visible on the dorsal aspect but not on the palmar side. All observations must be conducted bilaterally to establish the client's unique baseline. Because everyone varies slightly in structure and mechanics, the athletic trainer must know what "normal" is for each client.

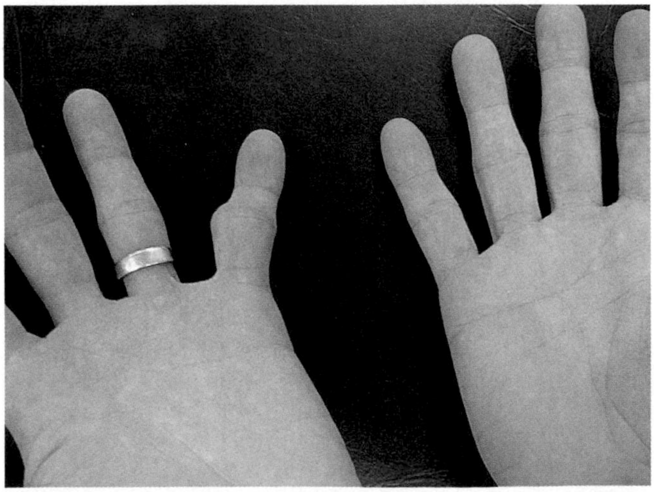

FIGURE 20-1 An obvious finger deformity, or sign, that can be seen during bilateral comparison. This hand has sustained an injury to the fifth finger that has permanently deformed the finger at the proximal interphalangeal joint.

Because of their superficial nature, most acute injuries of the elbow, wrist, and hand are easily determined. All sides of the injured body part must be observed as well as the position of the body part, deformity or loss of bony continuity, open wounds or bleeding, **ecchymosis**, swelling, and the client's willingness to use the body part. Obvious deformity indicates the possibility of a fracture or dislocation and warrants immediate referral.

Palpation

After completing the history and observation, the athletic trainer palpates specific body structures to rule out severe injury and help determine the correct diagnosis. The goal of palpating is to detect bony abnormalities, soft tissue injuries, and neurovascular (i.e., arteries, veins, nerves) compromise. As with the entire evaluation process, it is critical that palpations be conducted systematically to rule out any signs and symptoms. Start with light circular patterns away from the injured area and work toward the specific injury location. Gradually work deeper into the tissues. Palpate the injured area last so that pain is not referred or worsened before a determination can be made. Palpate both bony and soft tissue structures bilaterally and at the same time, if possible. When palpating bony tissue, feel for any **ipsilateral** signs such as **crepitus**, abnormal bending of a body part, point tenderness (diffuse or pinpoint), deformity, and swelling. Any positive signs of the aforementioned necessitate a referral to a physician. When palpating soft tissue, determine any changes in skin texture or temperature, swelling, lumps, muscle tightness, muscle or tendon deficits, differences in shape, and loss of sensation. As previously noted, it is important to palpate the entire arm to rule out possible secondary injuries and compare structures bilaterally to determine a baseline.

Range of Motion Testing

If the aforementioned evaluation steps were not sufficient to determine the presence of a fracture or joint dislocation, bilateral ROM tests are conducted. Each joint has a specific ROM that is available for movement (Table 20-1).

ecchymosis bruising or discoloration
ipsilateral same side
crepitus crunchy or crackling sound heard with movement of a body part or felt with palpation

TABLE 20-1 Elbow, Wrist, and Hand Active Range of Motion

JOINT	ACTIVE RANGE-OF-MOTION AVAILABLE	PRIMARY MUSCLES INVOLVED
Elbow: humeroulnar	Extension: 0 to −10 degrees Flexion: 140–150 degrees	Extension: triceps brachii Flexion : biceps brachii
Elbow : humeroradial	Extension: 0 to −10 degrees Flexion:140–150 degrees Supination: 90 degrees Pronation: 80–90 degrees	Extension: triceps brachii Flexion : biceps brachii Supination: supinator Pronation: pronator quadratus
Elbow: proximal radioulnar	Supination: 90 degrees Pronation: 80–90 degrees	Supination: supinator Pronation: pronator quadratus
Wrist: distal radioulnar	Supination: 85–90 degrees Pronation: 85–90 degrees	Supination: supinator Pronation: pronator quadratus
Wrist: radiocarpal	Extension: 70–90 degrees Flexion: 80–90 degrees Abduction (radial deviation): 15 degrees Adduction (ulnar deviation): 30–45 degrees	Extension: extensor carpi radialis longus and extensor carpi ulnaris Flexion : flexor carpi radialis and flexor carpi ulnaris Radial deviation: extensor carpi radialis longus and brevis Ulnar deviation: extensor carpi ulnaris
Thumb: carpometacarpal	Extension: 0 degrees Flexion: 45–50 degrees Abduction: 60–70 degrees Adduction: 30 degrees Opposition: opposing the thumb and fifth fingers	Extension: extensor pollicis longus and brevis Flexion: flexor pollicis longus and brevis Abduction: abductor pollicis longus and brevis Adduction: adductor pollicis Opposition: opponens pollicis and opponens digiti minimi
Thumb - metacarpophalangeal	Extension: 0 degrees Flexion: 50–55 degrees	Extension: extensor pollicis longus and brevis Flexion : flexor pollicis longus and brevis
Hand – metacarpophalangeal	Extension: 30–45 degrees Flexion: 85–90 degrees Abduction: 20–30 degrees Adduction: 0 degrees	Extension: extensor digitorum communis Flexion: flexor digitorum profundus and superficialis Abduction: dorsal interossei and abductor digiti minimi (fifth finger) Adduction: palmar interossei
Thumb: interphalangeal	Extension: 0 to −5 degrees Flexion: 80–90 degrees	Extension: extensor pollicis longus and brevis Flexion: flexor pollicis longus
Hand: proximal interphalangeal	Extension: 0 degrees Flexion: 100–115 degrees	Extension: extensor digitorum communis Flexion : flexor digitorum profundus and superficialis
Hand: distal interphalangeal	Extension: 20 degrees Flexion: 80–90 degrees	Extension : extensor digitorum communis Flexion: flexor digitorum profundus

ROM testing is designed to determine what motions are restricted, how much motion is restricted, and what type of tissue is affected. ROM testing consists of active, passive, and resistive methods and should always be conducted in that order. Any motions that aggravate the injury should have been discovered during the history section. The motions that aggravate should be performed last during the evaluation of ROM and only performed if necessary to make an accurate decision about the condition.

AROM is used to determine the integrity of contractile tissues that have contraction capabilities, such as muscles and tendons. During AROM testing, the client is instructed to move the affected body part through the available joint ROM. AROM determines the client's willingness to move the body part, his or her ability to move the body part, and the presence of any injuries or lesions to the contractile tissues.

PROM should be performed after AROM. PROM should exhibit more motion than with AROM. PROM requires the examiner, not the client, to move the respective body part through all of its available motions. PROM is used to determine the integrity of noncontractile tissues that do not have contraction capabilities. These tissues are ligaments, fascia, bones, joint capsules, and nerves. The goal of PROM is to determine an end-feel or limitation of a particular joint motion. Normal end-feels found during PROM consist of the following: soft or tissue approximation, tissue stretch or firm, or bone-to-bone or hard depending on the particular joint motion being conducted. Abnormal end-feels that can be found during PROM are empty, spasmodic, loose, or springy. It is important for all athletic trainers to know what normal ROM is for every joint in the body. If normal is not known, determining whether the end-feel being felt is abnormal is much more difficult. Pain is not an end-feel. It is important to physically elicit one of the normal or abnormal end-feels previously mentioned. If an injured person reports pain before a normal passive end-feel has been reached, inflammation is usually the culprit. If a passive end-feel occurs before the normal available joint

ROM is completed, blockage, injury, or tissue inflammation is possible.

Finally, the strength of the **contractile** tissues should be assessed to identify any strength deficits in the affected joint or body part. There are two methods for determining contractile tissue strength: RROM or manual muscle tests (MMTs). When testing RROM, the individual is asked to move the body part through the available joint ROM while the examiner applies resistance. During MMT, the body part is moved into the midway point of the joint's available ROM, whereupon a **break test** may be performed. This is a test that attempts to break the strength of a particular tissue or muscle. It involves an isometric contraction that is performed at the joint's midway point and resisted for a minimum of 5 seconds. MMTs are graded according to how well the client resists a force on the muscle (Table 20-2). The client is asked to move the body part through the full available joint motion while the athletic trainer resists that motion. An acute injury typically exhibits a weak and painful contraction, whereas a chronic injury typically exhibits a strong but painful contraction. A weak and painless contraction indicates a complete rupture of a muscle or tendon, or an MMT of 0/5 or 1/5.

Special Tests

Injury-specific special tests are used to confirm a diagnosis and rule out other possible injuries. Special tests reproduce the injury mechanism to stress specific structures in an attempt to evaluate the integrity of contractile and noncontractile tissues. Special tests help identify laxity, tightness, instability, or fractures within the structures. Each body part or joint has specific special tests that are unique to it. Only the applicable special tests should be performed with each diagnosis, and these should be performed bilaterally. Caution must be used when performing any special test that could exacerbate the injury.

A few special tests are available to help confirm a diagnosis of an injury to the elbow, wrist, hand, and fingers.[4,5,6] In the presence of an obvious or suspected joint dislocation or fracture (open, in which bone breaks through the skin, or closed, in which bone does not penetrate the skin) caused by visual deformity, loss of bony continuity, palpable defects, or loss of sensation, only the special tests that are necessary to determine how to immobilize and move the injured person to safety should be performed. If any of the aforementioned signs are present, immediately immobilize the body part and refer the client to a physician. Defer any other special tests at this time.

TABLE 20-2 Manual Muscle Test Grading

MMT GRADE	RESPONSE FELT DURING TESTING
5/5	The athlete is able to perform the break test, against gravity, with full resistance.
4/5	The athlete is able to perform the break test, against gravity, with some resistance.
3/5	The athlete is able to perform the break test, against gravity, with no resistance. The athlete can get the body part into position but is not able to provide any resistance.
2/5	The athlete is able to get into position, without gravity resistance, but cannot provide any resistive strength.
1/5	The athlete is not able to move the body part into position, even after gravity resistance is removed. The muscle is contracting but with insufficient strength to move the body part.
0/5	No muscle contraction is occurring visibly or through palpations.

Neurovascular Testing

A thorough evaluation of the neurovascular status of acute and chronic injuries includes testing **myotomes** (a nerve's innervation of a muscle), **dermatomes** (a nerve's innervation of the skin), circulation or pulse, and reflexes. A bilateral evaluation of the client's neurovascular status is imperative to properly determine the extent of the injury. A quick and easy way to test the neurovascular status of any upper extremity injury is to have the client simultaneously squeeze each of the examiner's index fingers. This will help determine any loss of strength or sensation in the upper extremity. If the neurological evaluation shows any bilateral or unilateral loss of strength, the situation should be treated as an emergency, one that warrants immediate referral to the emergency room. If necessary, a more thorough neurovascular exam may be conducted once the client is removed from the activity.

Myotomes are tested by manually resisting a muscle or group of muscles that a particular nerve innervates. The method used is similar to that of a manual muscle test. Dermatomes are tested by running a finger or soft object over the client's arm while the client's eyes are closed. Any difference in sensation between one arm and the other should be noted. If no loss or difference in sensation is found, the test is considered normal. If a difference in strength or sensation is detected, the client should be seen by a physician as quickly as possible.

contractile tissues that have contraction capabilities
break test a test designed to break the athlete of a particular position
myotomes a nerve's innervation of a muscle
dermatomes a nerve's innervation of the skin

The next component of a neurovascular examination involves monitoring vascular status by checking the distal pulse. In the upper extremity, vascular status may be evaluated by performing a capillary refill test. A normal capillary refill test allows the nail bed to refill within 2 or 3 seconds (Box 20-1 and Figure 20-2). A pulse in the upper extremity may be taken at either the brachial (upper arm) or radial (wrist) artery, with the latter being the most common site. A normal radial pulse rate is between 60-80 beats per minute. Finally, reflexes are evaluated by striking the distal tendon of a specific muscle with a neurological hammer or other solid object (Table 20-3). Normal reflexes will result in the involuntary contraction of the affected muscle after the tendon is struck. If the neurovascular exam shows any bilateral loss of strength, sensation, circulation, or reflexes, immediate referral to the emergency room is warranted.

Referrals and Diagnostic Tests

Many of the injuries discussed can cause long-term disability if they are not properly managed. For example, carpal tunnel syndrome is not a common athletic injury but always warrants referral to a physician. Ganglion cysts should be examined by a physician only if the signs and symptoms persist or cannot be tolerated. Physicians generally first use radiographs as a diagnostic tool to detect abnormalities in bones and rule out acute or chronic bony injuries. In adolescents, X-rays are used to rule out potential avulsion or epiphyseal fractures. If the radiographic examination is inconclusive but signs and symptoms persist, the physician may opt to use magnetic resonance imaging (MRI), which produces a detailed picture of the body part or joint to reveal abnormalities in the body's soft tissues as opposed to the bony tissues that are evaluated on X-ray film.

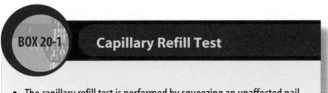

BOX 20-1 Capillary Refill Test

- The capillary refill test is performed by squeezing an unaffected nail bed for several seconds.
- Upon release, the nail bed should refill or "pink up" within 2 seconds.
- Capillary refill that takes longer than 3 seconds may indicate compromised blood flow and the possible presence of a severe injury.

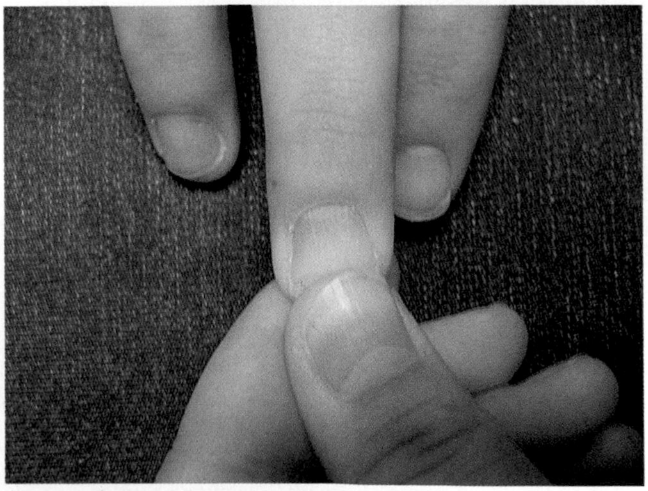

FIGURE 20-2 Capillary refill test.

TABLE 20-3 Common Upper Extremity Reflexes

NERVE ROOT LEVEL	REFLEX	REFLEX LOCATION
C5–C6	Biceps	Tap distal biceps brachii tendon in cubital fossa.
C5–C6	Brachioradialis	Tap distal brachioradialis tendon just proximal to radial styloid process.
C7–C8	Triceps	Tap distal triceps brachii tendon just proximal to olecranon process.

MANAGEMENT OF ON-FIELD/ACUTE ELBOW, WRIST, HAND, AND FINGER INJURIES

Acute evaluation decisions must be made immediately. The athletic trainer must decide what first-aid is warranted, whether immediate immobilization is required, how the injured person will be transported, and whether referral to a physician is necessary. Most acute on-field injuries are best diagnosed by taking a history, performing a thorough visual inspection, and conducting injury-specific special tests. All evaluation findings must be thoroughly documented. If a referral is necessary for further evaluation or testing, a copy of the evaluation notes should be sent with the client for the physician to read. Figure 20-3 is a concept map overview of the issues involved in diagnosis and management of acute injuries to the elbow, wrist, hand, and finger.

Elbow Injuries

Most acute injuries to the elbow will pose problems during activity. Typical acute elbow injuries include dislocations and sprains. In most cases, dislocations occur as a result of traumatic injury, whereas elbow sprains are often caused by falls. For proper care, appropriate special tests and injury management are crucial. The following injures are commonly associated with the elbow.

Elbow Dislocation

A tremendous amount of force is required to separate the humerus from the radius or ulna at the elbow joint.

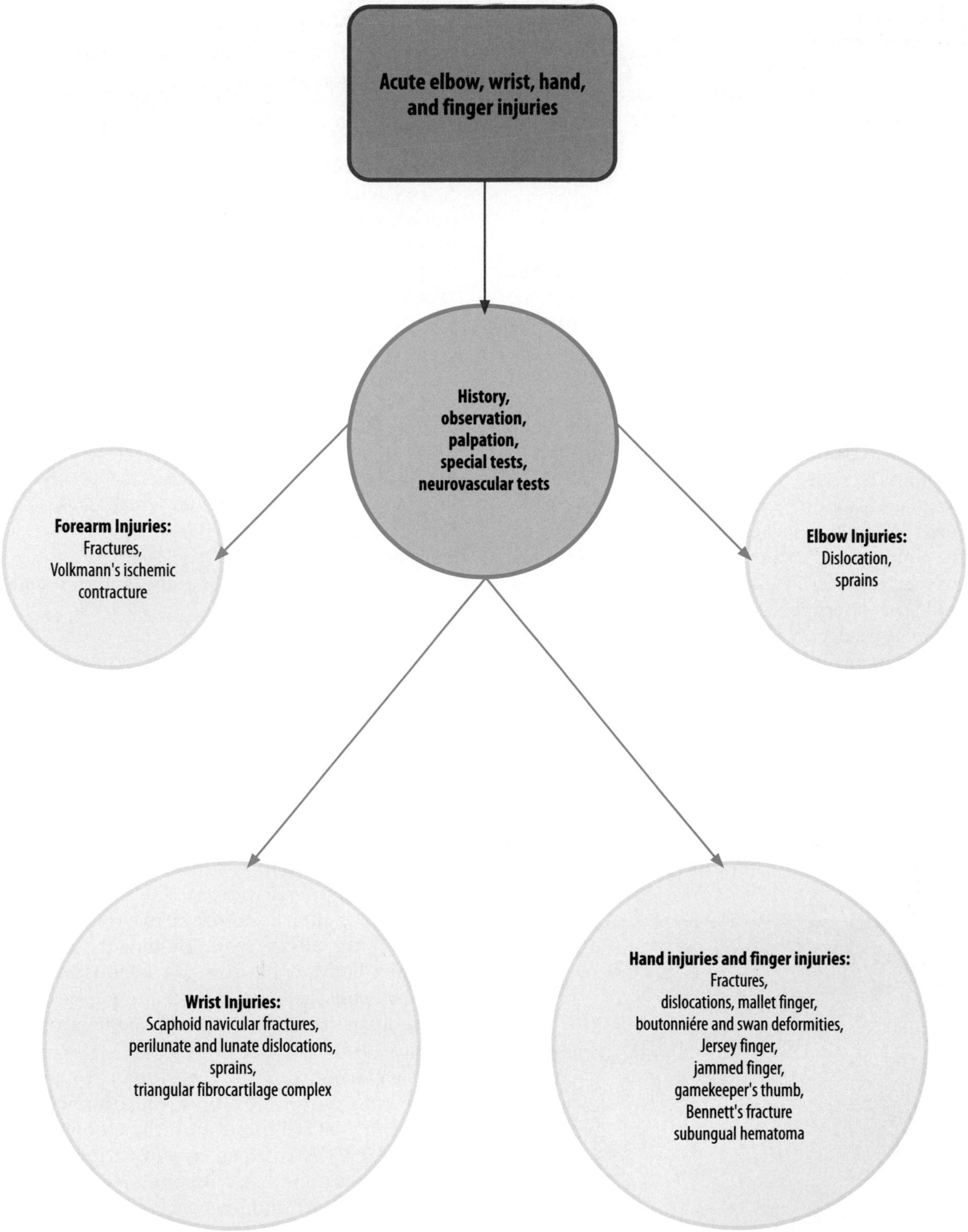

FIGURE 20-3 Concept map overview of acute injuries to the elbow, wrist, hand, and finger.

An elbow dislocation is one of the most traumatic injuries that an athletic trainer will assess. Posterior dislocations account for more than 90% of all elbow dislocations.[7] Careful management of this injury is critical to ensure that the client does not sustain any long-term disability.

Mechanism: Most elbow dislocations occur from FOOSH, with the elbow extended, or direct trauma.[6] This injury is commonly seen in gymnasts who perform certain floor moves and in football players whose elbows get caught between players during tackling.[8]

Signs and symptoms:

- Obvious deformity
- Extreme pain
- Distinctly palpable olecranon process with accompanying deformity either posteriorly or posterolaterally
- Inability to actively move the elbow and arm
- Immediate swelling
- Numbness or tingling
- Possible snapping or cracking sensation

Some elbow dislocations have an associated fracture of the olecranon as a result of the trauma[2,7,8] (Figure 20-4).

Special tests: No special tests are applicable to this injury.

Immediate management: This injury represents an emergency situation because of the potential for neurovascular compromise of the arm. As a result, emergency medical service personnel should be called immediately. It is not within the realm of an athletic trainer to reduce an elbow dislocation. The dislocated elbow should be immobilized as found, including the joint above and below the elbow, using vacuum splints, a soft aluminum splint, pillows, or other available materials. Immobilization should never interfere with the ability of medical staff to check the client's neurovascular status. Immediate referral to a physician or the emergency room is required.

Intermediate management: An X-ray examination is necessary to determine the direction of the dislocation, whether surgery is required to reduce the elbow, and what type of stabilization is warranted. Once the elbow has been reduced, a posterior splint must be applied to protect and immobilize the elbow. A compression wrap is also applied to minimize the tremendous amount of swelling that occurs as a result of this injury.

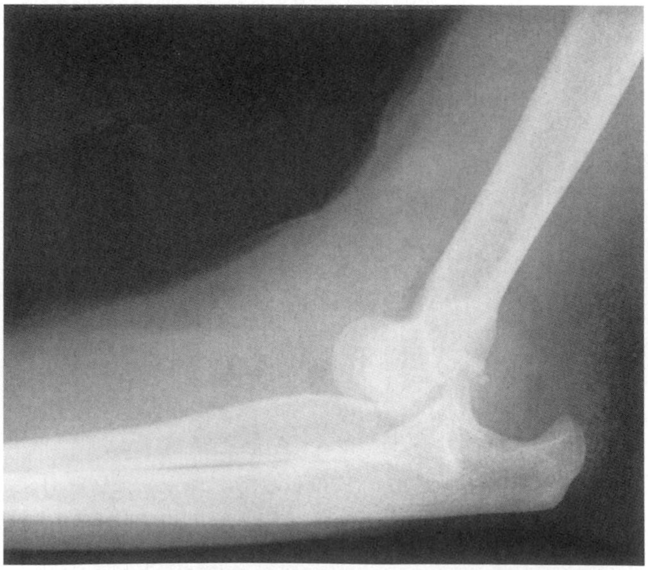

FIGURE 20-4 A lateral radiograph (X-ray) of a posteriorly dislocated elbow. (From O'Donoghue DH: *Treatment of injuries to athletes*, ed 4, p. 227, Philadelphia, 1984, WB Saunders.)

Points to Ponder

Why is it not in an athletic trainer's scope of practice to reduce an elbow dislocation?

Elbow Sprains

A collateral ligament sprain of the elbow may be considered both an acute and a chronic injury. Such sprains are much more common as acute injuries in people who participate in activities in which FOOSH is common, such as football or wrestling. Chronically, this injury is common in athletes who participate in throwing sports.[2,8–12]

Mechanism: Acutely, the collateral ligament (typically the ulnar collateral ligament) is most commonly injured by FOOSH. Chronically, it is much more common to injure the ulnar collateral ligament through overuse; repetitive tensile forces; or repetitive overhead throwing, pitching, or hitting, which causes the elbow to hyperextend.

Signs and symptoms:

- Point tenderness along the anterior and medial aspects of the elbow
- Swelling
- Pain with active and resisted **pronation** and elbow extension

Special tests:

Valgus stress test of the elbow: To perform the **valgus stress test of the elbow**, the athletic trainer asks the client to stand or sit with the affected elbow flexed to 20 degrees and the forearm supinated. The athletic trainer places one hand on the lateral aspect of the elbow joint (fulcrum) and the other hand on the medial aspect of their wrist (force). The athletic trainer then gradually applies a valgus stress toward the medial aspect of the elbow while pulling the forearm away from the body. A positive test produces pain or laxity when stress is applied, indicating a possible sprain to the ulnar (medial) collateral ligament of the elbow (Figure 20-5).

Varus stress test of the elbow: To perform the **varus stress test of the elbow**, the athletic trainer asks the client to stand or sit with the elbow flexed to 20 degrees and the forearm in **supination.** The athletic trainer places one hand on the medial aspect of the elbow (fulcrum) and the other hand on the lateral side of the client's wrist (force). Then, the athletic trainer gradually applies a varus stress toward the lateral aspect of the elbow while pulling the forearm toward the body. A positive test results in pain or

pronation turning the palm of the hand down
supination turning the palm of the hand up

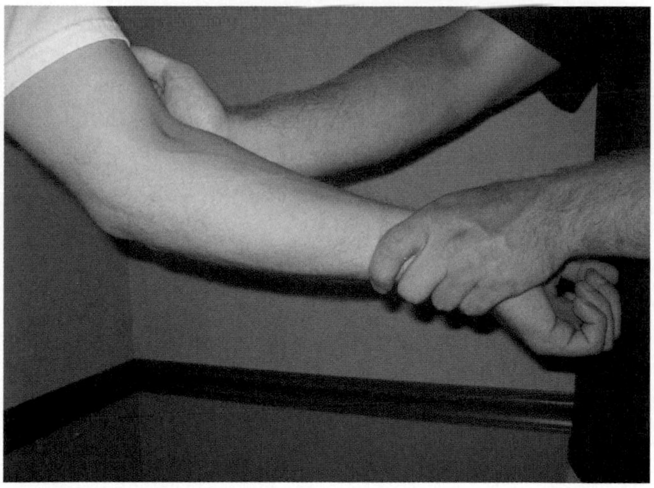

FIGURE 20-5 A valgus stress test of the elbow to assess laxity of the ulnar (medial) collateral ligament of the elbow.

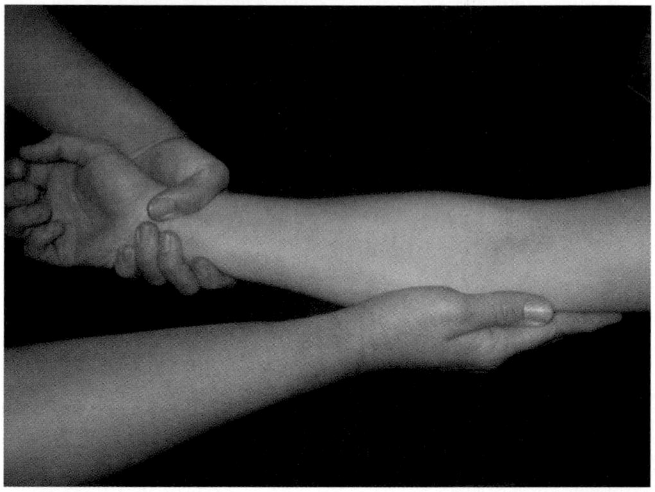

FIGURE 20-6 A varus stress test of the elbow to assess laxity of the radial (lateral) collateral ligament of the elbow.

laxity when stress is applied, indicating a possible sprain of the radial (lateral) collateral ligament of the elbow (Figure 20-6).

Tinel test: To perform the Tinel test, the athletic trainer asks the client to sit with the elbow flexed to 75 degrees and the forearm supinated. The athletic trainer uses his or her index finger to tap along the ulnar groove between the olecranon process and the medial epicondyle of the humerus. If the client experiences tingling or radiating pain into the forearm and hand along the fourth and fifth fingers, the test is considered positive for an injury involving the ulnar nerve.

Immediate management: Treatment includes implementing rest by decreasing activity until the pain diminishes, application of ice packs, compression through use of an Ace wrap or compressive sleeve, and above-the-heart elevation in a sling to minimize swelling and inflammation.

Intermediate management: Treatment includes nonsteroidal antiinflammatory medications, a sling to rest the elbow, and continued application of ice and compression.

Forearm Injuries

One of the most common acute forearm injuries is a fracture. Fractures are either **displaced** or nondisplaced. A displaced fracture, in which the bone separates into two pieces, is easily detected on account of its obvious deformity. A nondisplaced fracture, in which the bone does not separate into distinct pieces, usually does not exhibit deformity. Special tests are necessary for the accurate assessment of a possible nondisplaced fracture. A displaced fracture warrants immobilization and immediate referral to a physician or an emergency room.

Forearm Fractures

Distal radial and ulnar fractures occur either individually or together. These fractures are not associated with as many complications as other fractures but still warrant a thorough evaluation. A true **Colles' fracture** is a fracture to the distal aspect of the radius that displaces toward the dorsal aspect of the hand (Figure 20-7). A **Smith's fracture** (reverse Colles') is a fracture to the distal aspect of the radius that displaces to the palmar aspect of the hand (Figure 20-8). Both normally occur within 1½ to 2 inches from the wrist joint. Fractures to the ulna commonly occur when the forearm is used defensively, such as when blocking the face from harm. Ulnar fractures are sometimes called "blocker's fractures" because they typically occur in football or hockey.

Mechanism: Forearm fractures are caused by FOOSH, a direct blow to the medial or lateral aspect of the forearm, or a sudden force that hyperextends the hand.[13]

Signs and symptoms[14]:

- Visible deformity in the forearm in the shape of a "silver spoon" (Colles')
- Pinpoint point tenderness
- Crepitus
- Pain
- Swelling
- Tenderness around the wrist
- Limited wrist or thumb movement
- Possible neurovascular impairment

displaced a fracture that separates into two pieces
Colles' fracture a fracture to the distal aspect of the radius
Smith's fracture (reverse Colles') a fracture to the distal aspect of the radius that displaces to the palmar aspect

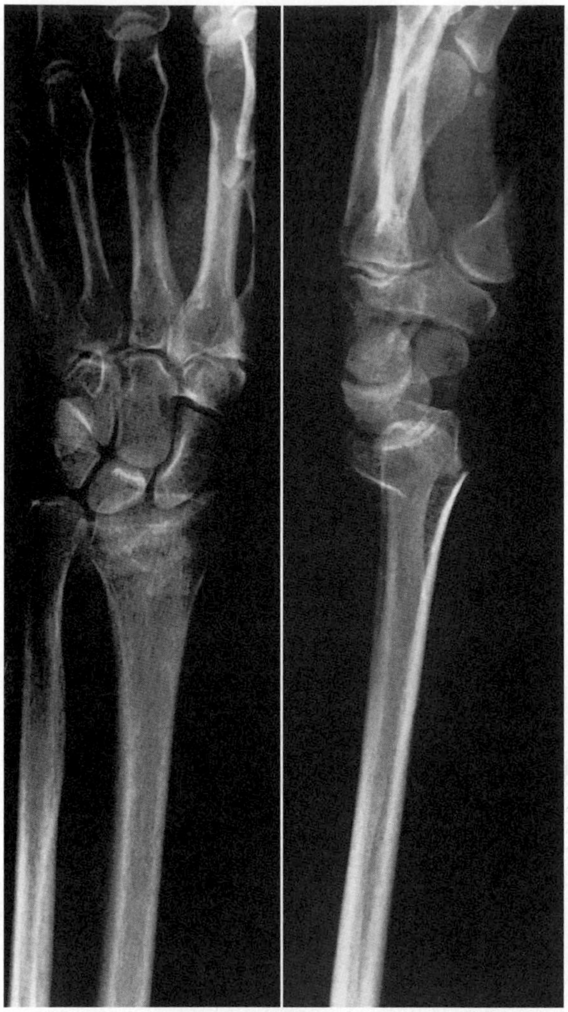

FIGURE 20-7 A Colles' fracture of the distal radius. Note that the displacement goes toward the dorsal aspect of the wrist. **A**, Posteroanterior view shows fracture and shortening of radius. **B**, Lateral view. (From Propp DA, Chin H: Forearm and wrist radiology: Part I, *J Emerg Med* 7:393, 1989.)

Special tests:

Long bone compression test: To perform the long bone compression test, the athletic trainer asks the client to stand or sit with the hand and wrist relaxed and the forearm pronated. One hand is placed behind the elbow of the affected limb, and the other hand is placed on the dorsal aspect of the client's flexed wrist. A compressive force is applied through the length of the forearm, gently at first and then with progressively greater pressure. Crepitus or pinpoint pain in the forearm or elbow may indicate a fracture to the lower arm. If the test is positive, the client should be referred to a physician for further evaluation (Figure 20-9).

Immediate management: The fracture should be immobilized as it was found, one joint above and one joint below the injured area, using vacuum splints, air splints, a SAM splint, pillows, towels, or other materials that would limit the injured body part's ability to move. Once the fracture has been immobilized, the client should be transported to a physician's office or the emergency room for further evaluation. Continued monitoring of the client's neurovascular status is imperative.

Intermediate management: An X-ray examination is necessary to determine the displacement of the fracture, whether open or closed reduction is warranted, and whether surgical stabilization or casting is required.

Volkmann's Ischemic Contracture

Volkmann's ischemic contracture is a complication that can result from a displaced fracture. (Figure 20-10). A displaced fracture puts pressure on the brachial artery, inhibiting circulation to the rest of the arm. Affected individuals typically complain of forearm pain that worsens with passive finger extension. Volkmann's ischemic contracture represents an emergency situation that warrants immediate referral.

Points to Ponder
Which sports carry the greatest risk for forearm fractures?

Wrist Injuries

Wrist, hand, and finger injuries are very common in athletics, especially in ball-handling sports.[15] Between 3% and 9% of all athletic injuries and 14% of high school injuries involve the wrist or hand.[1,16] Fortunately, most do not require acute evaluations. Individuals who injure their wrists or hands usually visit the athletic trainer on their own volition. Unfortunately, however, wrist and hand injuries are often overlooked. Long-term or permanent damage may result if these injuries are not properly evaluated. Therefore athletic trainers must take all wrist and hand injuries seriously. A thorough and careful evaluation must be conducted for each injury; none is too small to receive attention.[15]

Scaphoid Navicular Fracture

A **scaphoid navicular fracture** is a break in the carpal bone located on the thumb side of the wrist[9] (Figure 20-11). It is the most common type of wrist fracture, accounting for 60% of all wrist fractures, especially in adolescent and college-age athletes.[16]

Volkmann's ischemic contracture a complication resulting from a displaced fracture that puts pressure on the brachial artery and inhibits circulation; an emergency situation

scaphoid navicular fracture break in the carpal bone on the thumb side of the wrist

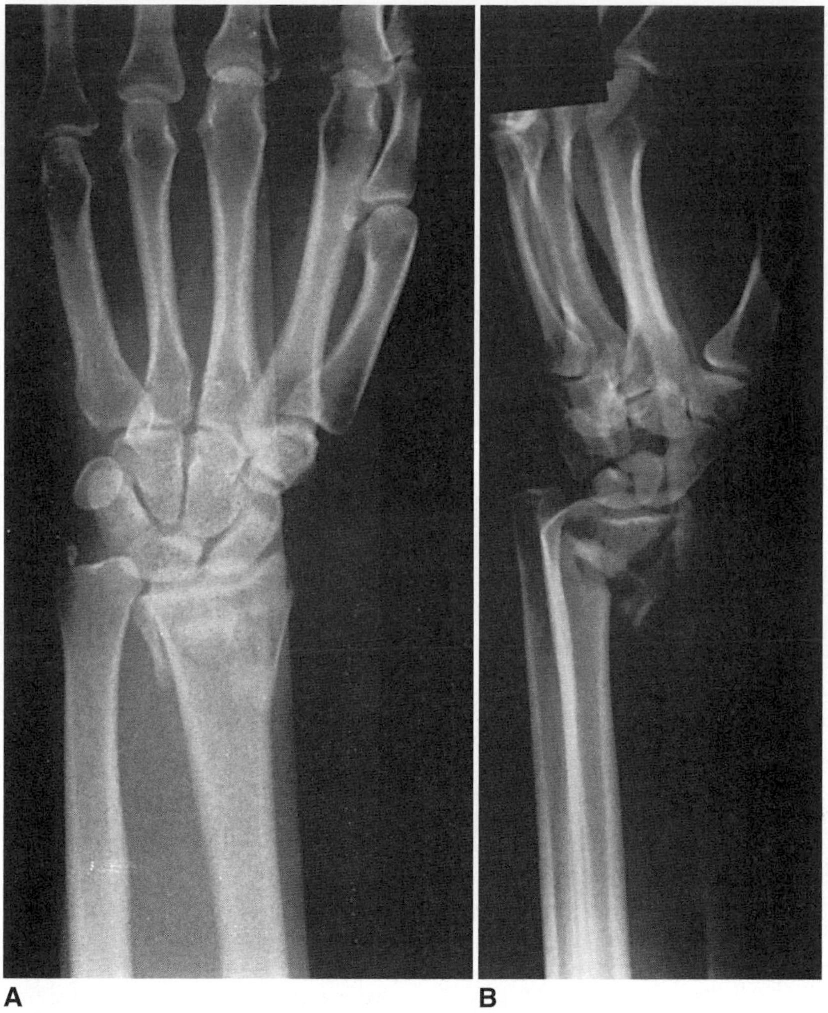

FIGURE 20-8 A Smith's fracture of the distal radius. Note that the displacement goes toward the palmar aspect of the wrist. **A**, Posteroanterior view. **B**, Lateral view. (From Propp DA, Chin H: Forearm and wrist radiology: Part I, *J Emerg Med* 7:393, 1989.)

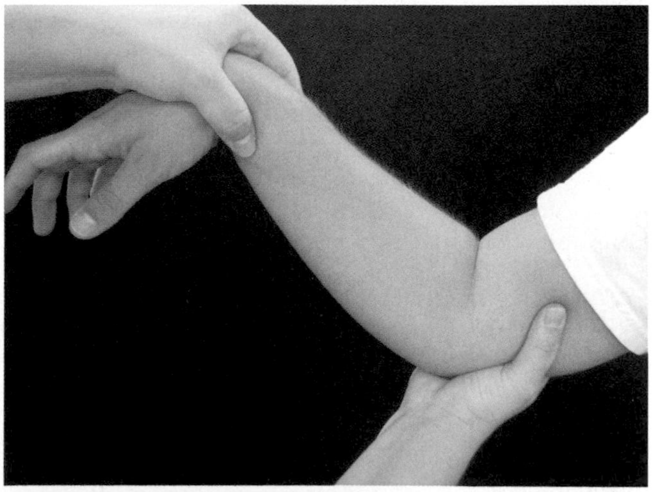

FIGURE 20-9 A long bone compression test of the forearm to rule out possible fractures.

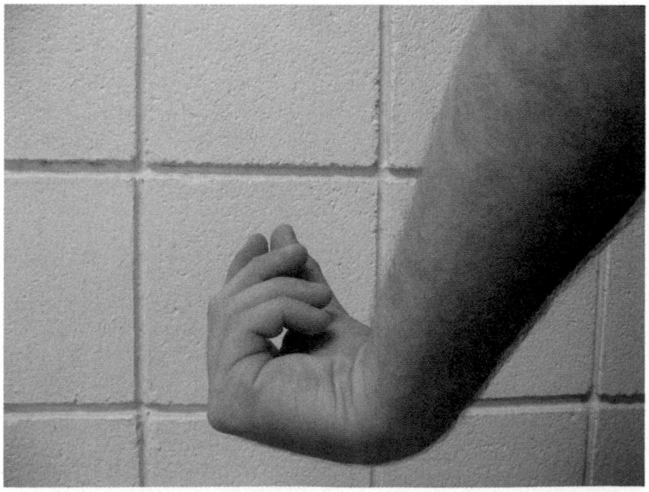

FIGURE 20-10 Volkmann's ischemic contracture is an obvious deformity that can occur as the result of decreased blood flow to the area after fracture.

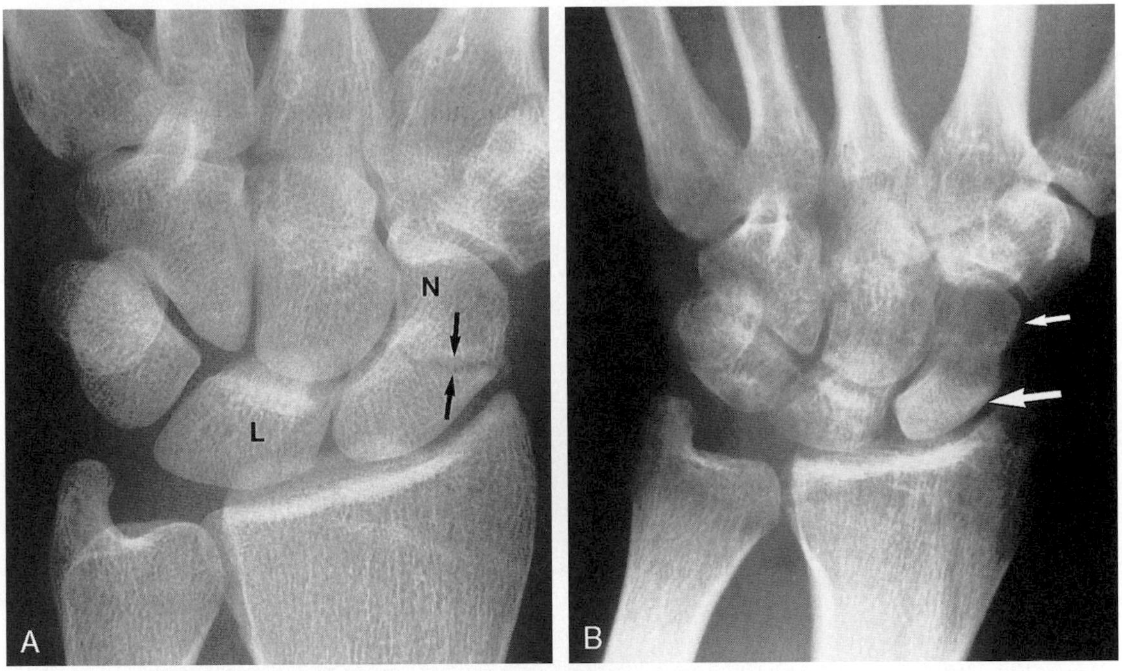

FIGURE 20-11 A radiograph (X-ray) of a scaphoid navicular fracture. **A**, Posteroanterior view of the wrist of a patient who fell on his outstretched hand. **B**, A later complication in this patient is aseptic necrosis of the proximal fragment (*large arrow*). (From Mettler FA: *Essentials of radiology,* ed 2, Figure 8-70, Philadelphia, 2005, Saunders/Elsevier.)

Mechanism: A scaphoid navicular fracture can be caused by FOOSH, a direct blow to the wrist, or a force that causes the wrist to hyperextend with the thumb extended.

Signs and symptoms[14,17]:

- Pain
- Point tenderness in the anatomical snuffbox
- Swelling
- Possible crepitus
- Delayed ecchymosis
- Possible loss of function.

Special tests: Palpation in the anatomical snuffbox (Figure 20-12) and a thumb long bone compression test may be used.

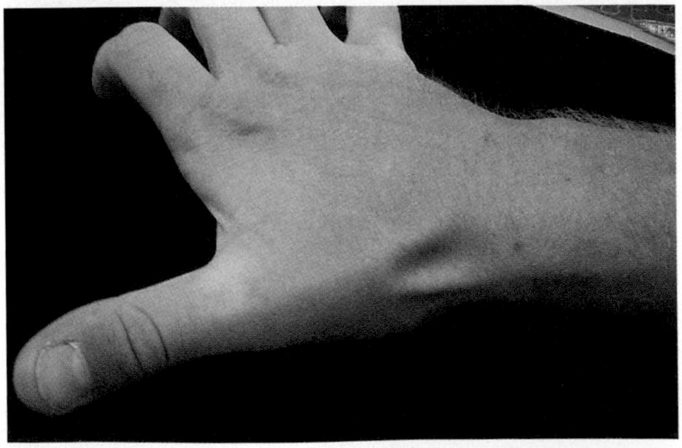

FIGURE 20-12 The dorsal surface of the hand showing the tendons that make up the anatomical snuffbox.

Immediate management: A physician should perform an evaluation and X-ray examination. The X-ray images should include a dedicated scaphoid view because these fractures often appear normal at first in other views. If signs and symptoms persist, the radiographs should be repeated in 10 to 14 days and the wrist should be re-evaluated.[14,15,17] If repeat X-rays are negative but the athlete still exhibits wrist pain and muscle atrophy, an MRI or bone scan may be necessary to reveal the fracture.[15]

Intermediate management: The fracture is immobilized with a full arm cast that goes superior to the elbow and distally to include the thumb.[17] The cast is worn for a minimum of 3 months to ensure that the bone heals completely. Unfortunately, the scaphoid navicular does not have a good blood supply so the fracture commonly becomes **nonunion**, which means that the two pieces of bone do not heal together. If nonunion occurs, surgical stabilization is required. If the two parts of the bone fail to heal, **avascular necrosis** or bone death may occur. This situation also requires surgery to remove the dead bone and repair it using a bone grafting technique.[17]

Perilunate and Lunate Dislocations

Another injury that can occur with FOOSH is a perilunate or lunate dislocation. Injuries to the lunate, the most

nonunion two pieces of bone that do not heal together
avascular necrosis bone death

commonly dislocated carpal bone, are associated with many long-term complications. During FOOSH, all the force is placed on the radial side of the wrist, which forces the scaphoid-navicular to strike the radius and rupture the ligaments on the volar side of the wrist that connect the scaphoid-navicular to the lunate. With the volar ligaments compromised, the lunate bone rotates and moves dorsally; this is a perilunate dislocation. If the force is strong enough, the dorsal ligaments are also ruptured and cause the lunate to shift further and rest in a more volar direction than the other carpal bones; this is a lunate dislocation. Perilunate dislocations are two to three times more likely than lunate dislocations and are usually associated with a fractured scaphoid-navicular. If the perilunate or lunate dislocation is not caught early or is treated improperly, it can cause a slow degeneration of the lunate bone or Kienböck's disease. A common sign of Kienböck's disease is pain with PROM into extension at the metacarpophalangeal (MCP) joint of the third finger.[4,5]

Mechanism: A perilunate or lunate dislocation can be caused by FOOSH or forced wrist extension or hyperextension.

Signs and symptoms[4,5]:

- Pain on the radial side of the wrist, both palmarly and dorsally
- Numbness or tingling in the second through fourth fingers along the median nerve distribution
- Deformity on the dorsal (perilunate) or volar (lunate) side of the wrist
- Point tenderness over the lunate, crepitus, and a third knuckle that now is even with the other knuckles when the hand is flexed

Special tests:

Watson's test: For **Watson's test**, the client is seated with the affected elbow resting on the table and the forearm pronated. The examiner passively forces the wrist into extension and ulnar deviation. The distal aspect of the scaphoid is then pushed dorsally to keep it from moving in a palmar direction while the examiner flexes and radially deviates the wrist. If the scaphoid and lunate shift, creating pain, the test is positive for an unstable wrist and indicates injury to the scapholunate ligament complex.[6]

Immediate management: Treatment includes application of ice packs, immediate referral to a physician, and radiographic examination. A definitive diagnosis can be made only through an X-ray examination.

Intermediate management: A perilunate or lunate dislocation that is caught early can usually be treated nonoperatively by casting it in slight flexion for 6 to 8 weeks. If at any time during this period the reduction is lost, surgery is necessary to pin the lunate back in place.

Wrist Sprains

There are many ligaments in the wrist, any of which can be injured. The most commonly injured ligaments in the wrist are the scapholunate, distal ulnar, radial collateral, and triangular fibrocartilage complex.

Mechanism: Wrist sprains are caused by FOOSH or forced wrist extension or hyperextension.

Signs and symptoms:

- Pain with wrist AROM, PROM, and RROM
- Localized swelling
- Localized point tenderness
- Possible instability

Special tests:

Valgus stress test of the wrist: For the **valgus stress test of the wrist**, the client is seated with the affected elbow flexed to 90 degrees, the forearm pronated, and the wrist and fingers in a neutral, relaxed position. The athletic trainer grasps the client's distal forearm with one hand and the client's hand with the other hand as if shaking hands. The athletic trainer then gradually applies a valgus force to the medial aspect of the wrist by pulling the hand toward the thumb side. Remember, with the forearm pronated it will look as if the lateral aspect of the wrist is being tested. If the test is positive, pain or laxity occurs when stress is applied, indicating a possible injury to the ulnar (medial) collateral ligament of the wrist.

Varus stress test of the wrist: For the **varus stress test of the wrist**, the client is seated with the affected elbow flexed to 90 degrees, the forearm pronated, and the wrist and fingers in a neutral, relaxed position. The athletic trainer grasps the client's distal forearm with one hand and the client's hand with the other hand. The athletic trainer then gradually applies a varus force to the lateral aspect of the wrist by pulling the hand toward the pinky side. Remember, with the forearm pronated, it will look as if the medial aspect of the wrist is being tested. If the test is positive, pain or laxity occurs when stress is applied, indicating a possible injury to the radial (lateral) collateral ligament of the wrist.

Immediate management: Immediate management includes rest from activity, application of ice packs, compression of the injured part with use of a compressive wrap, and elevation of the injured part above the heart with use of a sling.

Intermediate management: Scapholunate instability resulting from ligamentous damage is difficult to recognize and diagnose. Two of the three scapholunate ligaments must be injured for instability to occur.[1,15] If an individual's pain and other signs and symptoms do not resolve in 2 to 3 weeks, further testing and evaluation may be necessary to rule out scapholunate injury.

Triangular Fibrocartilage Complex Injuries

The triangular fibrocartilage complex (TFCC) is located on the ulnar side of the wrist between the ulna and the triquetrum and pisiform. The TFCC is the stabilizer of the distal radioulnar joint and supports 18% of the

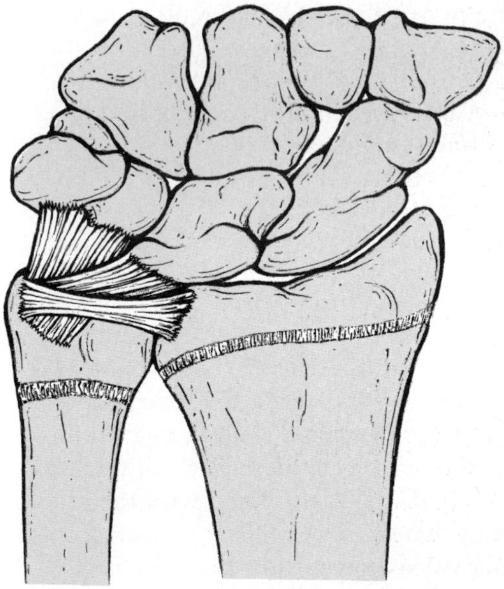

FIGURE 20-13 The triangular fibrocartilage ligament complex of the wrist. (From Bowers WH: Fractures of the forearm, wrist, and hand. In Green DP, editor: *Operative hand surgery,* ed 2, New York, 1988, Churchill Livingstone.)

wrist compressive load.[1] Injuries to this complex are a common source of ulnar-sided pain but are typically diagnosed as wrist sprains (Figure 20-13).

Mechanism: Injuries to the TFCC are caused by forced ulnar deviation of the wrist (hitting a tennis ball with a top-spin), forced hyperextension of the wrist, or FOOSH.

Signs and symptoms:

- Pain and swelling on the ulnar side of the wrist
- Point tenderness distal to the ulna
- Decreased ROM, especially with wrist extension and ulnar deviation
- Decreased wrist extension and ulnar deviation strength

Special tests: The valgus stress test of the wrist and push-off test (the pain is recreated when the client pushes up from an armchair with the wrist extended, forcing the wrist to ulnarly deviate[1]) can be used.

Immediate management: Ice, compression, and physician referral are the immediate management techniques.

Intermediate management: This injury may require further evaluation using diagnostic imaging procedures, most commonly MRI. An MRI machine uses radiofrequency waves to take pictures of the inside of the body. Another common diagnostic tool is an arthrogram. An arthrogram is an X-ray that is taken after injecting dye or air into the joint, which allows the technicians to see the soft tissue structures. Conventional X-rays allow the technicians to see only bony structures.

Other management techniques used for this injury are splinting the wrist to protect and prevent rotation and taking antiinflammatory drugs (e.g., ibuprofen, naproxen sodium) to help reduce inflammation. Because this injury may lead to long-term permanent disability, surgical intervention may be necessary.[15]

Hand and Finger Injuries

Fractures and dislocations of the metacarpals and phalanges and extensor mechanism injuries of the fingers are common in athletics, especially in ball-handling sports.[1,15] A common fracture of the hand is a **boxer's fracture**, which is a fracture to the fifth metacarpal bone (Figure 20-14). This fracture occurs as the result of striking an immovable object, such as a wall, dashboard, door, or face, with a closed fist.

Finger Fractures

Finger fractures usually result from trauma. Typically, the finger is injured by direct contact with an object. Immediate and appropriate evaluation and management will determine the outcome and function of the finger (Figure 20-15). Because this type of fracture is not considered to be a medical emergency, many finger fractures go untreated.

Mechanism: Fingers are fractured as a result of direct trauma to the end of the finger, a direct blow to the metacarpals, or punching an immovable object with a closed fist.

Signs and symptoms:

- Pain
- Loss of ROM
- Possible deformity
- Crepitus
- Rapid localized swelling
- Point tenderness

Special tests:

Tap/percussion test: For the tap, or percussion, test, the client is seated with the elbow flexed to 90 degrees, the forearm pronated, and the wrist and fingers relaxed. Using the index finger, the athletic trainer taps the bony and soft tissue surrounding the injured area (Figure 20-16). The tapping should start away from the area that is most tender and then slowly moved toward the site of suspected injury. A positive test produces pinpoint or radiating pain or crepitus caused by associated vibrations and could indicate a possible fracture to either the metacarpals or phalanges. The client should be referred to a physician for further evaluation and radiographic assessment if a fracture is suspected.

Long bone compression test of the metacarpals or phalanges: For the long bone compression test of the metacarpals or phalanges, the client is seated with the elbow flexed to 90 degrees, the forearm pronated, the wrist

boxer's fracture a fracture to the fifth metacarpal bone

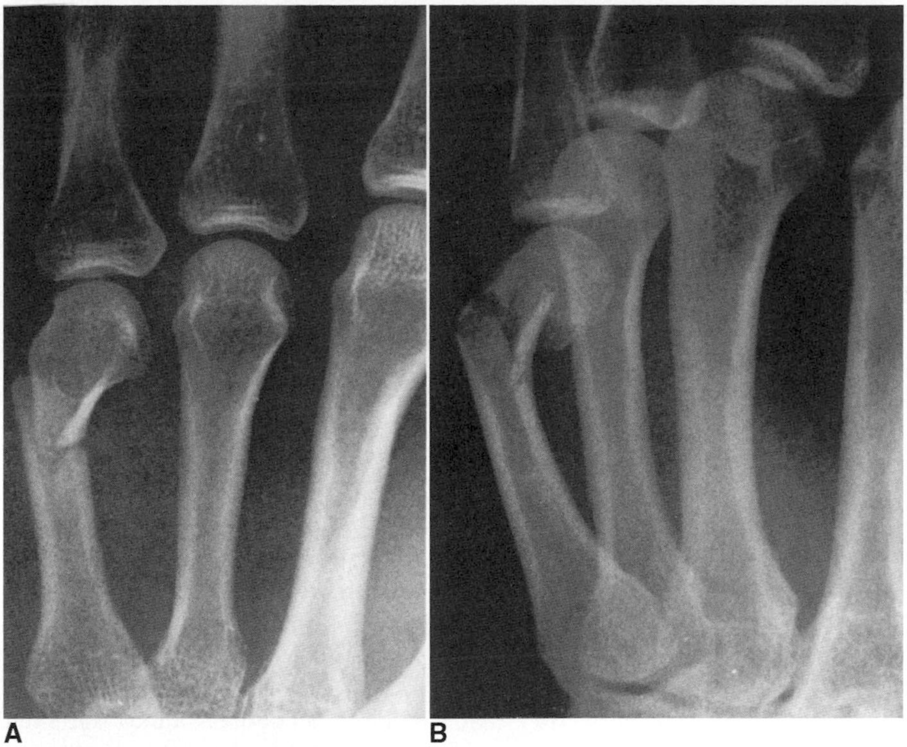

FIGURE 20-14 A "boxer's fracture" of the fifth metacarpal. **A**, Anteroposterior view of a fracture through the neck of the fifth metacarpal. **B**, The same fracture seen in a lateral view in 10 degrees of supination. (From DeLee JC, Drez D, Miller MD: *DeLee & Drez's orthopaedic sports medicine,* ed 2, Figure 24B1-37, Philadelphia, 2003, Saunders/Elsevier.)

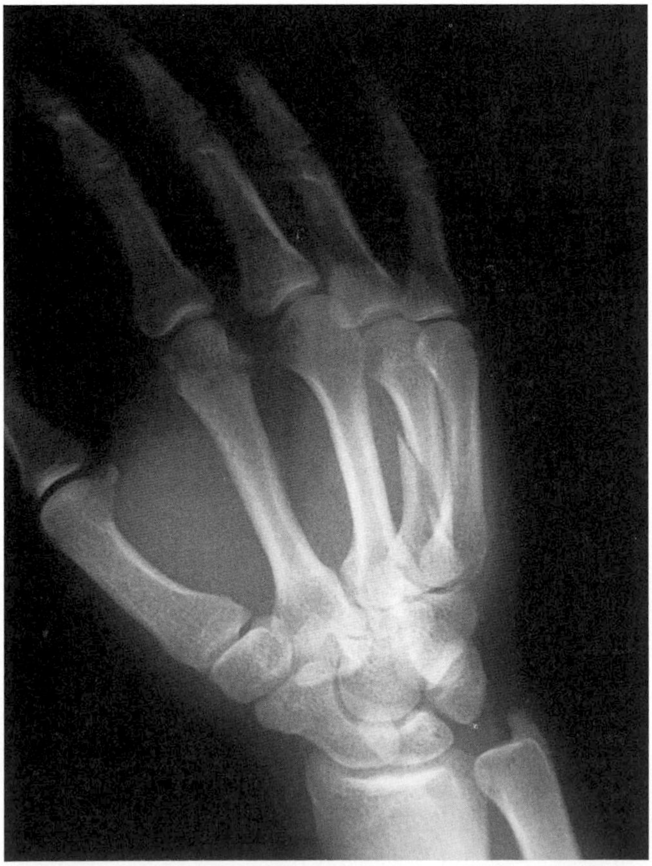

FIGURE 20-15 A spiral fracture of the fourth metacarpal caused by a blow to the end of the fingers.

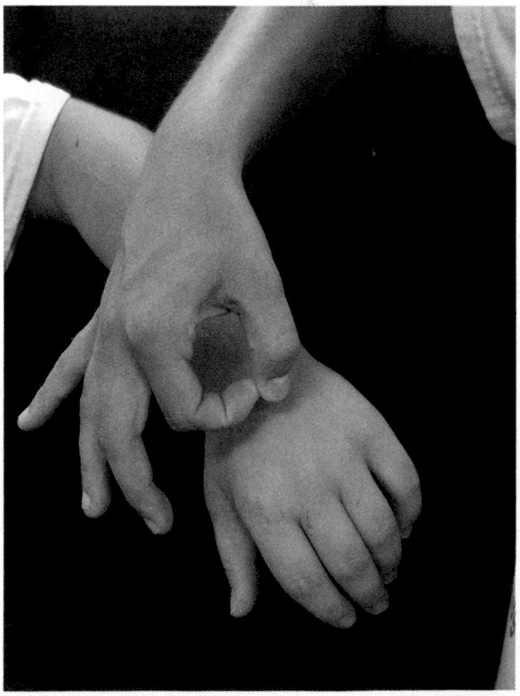

FIGURE 20-16 Tap or percussion test for a possible fracture of the metacarpals or fingers.

slightly extended, and the fingers relaxed. The athletic trainer places one hand at the wrist of the affected hand and the other hand at the MCP joint or distal aspect of the fingers. The athletic trainer then applies compression through the length of the hand, gently at first and then gradually increasing the amount. A positive test produces pinpoint or radiating pain and possibly crepitus and could indicate a possible fracture. If the test is positive, the client should be referred to a physician for further evaluation and radiographic assessment.

NOTE: To rule out the possibility of a fracture to a specific finger, this test should be performed on each affected finger individually to properly isolate the finger or specific phalanx.

Immediate management: The hand or finger should be splinted as found, ice should be applied, and the client should be referred to a physician for an X-ray examination.

Intermediate management: Depending on its severity and type, the fracture should be immobilized for approximately 4 weeks by casting the hand or using an aluminum finger splint. After 4 weeks, the hand should be protected with foam or another form of protection during all activities. After the initial 4 weeks of protection in a soft aluminum splint, a healing finger should then be splinted 2 to 3 more weeks in 20 to 30 degrees of flexion to ensure complete bone healing.

NOTE: Rotation of a fractured finger is not uncommon. It can be detected by observing the line of the finger to see if the fingernail of a particular finger is not lined up as the other fingers are. In cases of rotation, surgical intervention may be warranted.

Finger Dislocations

Because of the nature of most sports and some occupations, finger dislocations occur fairly often. Falls and the grasping of heavy or moving objects are associated with many finger dislocations.

Mechanism: Finger dislocations are caused by direct trauma to an extended finger, a violent twist to the end of the finger, forced hyperextension, or FOOSH.[18,19]

Signs and symptoms:

- Pain
- Loss of function
- Visible deformity
- Swelling
- Point tenderness

Special tests: No special tests are applicable for this injury.

Immediate management: The dislocation should be reduced, either by the athletic trainer (with the physician's permission) or by a physician. If the athletic trainer is allowed to perform the reduction, it should be done immediately, before muscle spasm occurs. Once the dislocation has been reduced, the client should be referred to a physician for further evaluation and testing to rule out associated fractures. If the dislocation cannot be reduced, it should be splinted as found and the athlete referred to a physician for X-ray examination.

Intermediate management: The finger should be splinted for 3 to 4 weeks in 30 degrees of finger flexion. Additional splinting during competition will also be required for another 3 to 4 weeks to properly protect the injured joint.

Mallet Finger

A **mallet finger** injury occurs when the extensor tendon of the finger is **avulsed,** which is a fracture at the tendinous attachment instead of a tear of the tendon, at the distal interphalangeal joint (DIP) of the finger (Figure 20-17).

Mechanism: A mallet finger injury is caused by a compressive force through the long axis of the finger, forced flexion of the distal phalanx, or a blow to the tip of the finger.

Signs and symptoms:

- Deformity
- Inability to extend the finger at the DIP joint
- Pain
- Point tenderness along the extensor tendon and the distal phalanx flexed

Special tests: The inability of the client to complete AROM into extension at the DIP joint is a positive finding for a mallet finger injury.

mallet finger injury in which the extensor tendon of the finger is avulsed at the tendinous attachment
avulsed a fracture at the tendinous attachment instead of the tendon tearing between structures

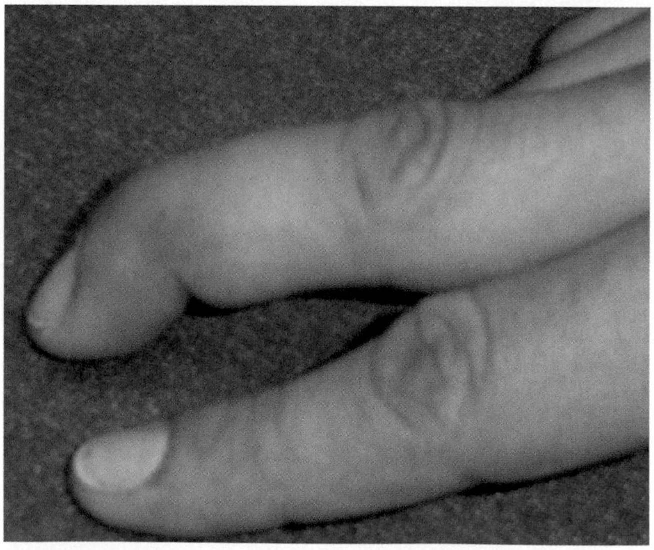

FIGURE 20-17 A mallet finger deformity caused by an avulsion of the extensor digitorum longus tendon at the distal interphalangeal joint.

Immediate management: The client should be referred to a physician for an X-ray examination to determine the location of the avulsion, the DIP joint should be splinted in hyperextension to **approximate the injury** or bring the edges of an injured structure close together and ice packs and compression should be applied.

Intermediate management: The DIP joint should be splinted in hyperextension for 6 to 8 weeks, with an additional 6 to 8 weeks of taping or splinting required for return to activity.

Boutonnière and Swan Neck Deformities

A **boutonnière deformity** is a rupture of the extensor tendon on the dorsal aspect of the finger. Observation of this injury reveals that the proximal interphalangeal (PIP) joint is in a flexed position and the MCP and DIP joints are in extended positions (Figure 20-18).

Mechanism: The extensor tendon on the dorsal side of the PIP joint is ruptured or torn.

Signs and symptoms:

- Deformity
- Finger in extension at the MCP and DIP joints and flexion at the PIP joint
- Pain
- Swelling
- Point tenderness
- Inability to extend the finger at the PIP joint.

Special tests: If the client is unable to perform AROM at the PIP joint but can perform PROM, a boutonnière deformity injury is possible.

Immediate management: The PIP joint of the finger should be splinted in extension, ice and compression should be applied, and the client should be referred to a physician for further evaluation.

Intermediate management: Continued splinting of the finger for 6 to 8 weeks is recommended, with an additional 6 to 8 weeks of follow-up splinting during activity.

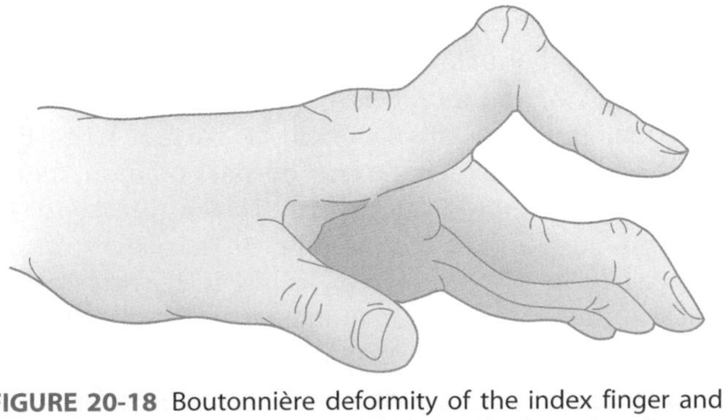

FIGURE 20-18 Boutonnière deformity of the index finger and also swan neck deformities exhibited with the other fingers. (From Marx JA, Hockberger R, Walls R: *Rosen's emergency medicine: concepts and clinical practice,* ed 6, Figure 47-52, St Louis, 2006, Mosby/Elsevier.)

> **Points to Ponder**
> What is a pseudo-boutonnière or swan neck deformity?

Flexor Digitorum Profundus Tendon Rupture (Jersey Finger)

In an injury to the flexor digitorum profundus tendon, the flexor tendon of the finger, most commonly the fourth finger, is avulsed from its origin at the DIP joint. This injury is commonly called **jersey finger** because it often occurs as a result of grabbing a jersey with a flexed finger and having that finger forcibly extended when the person wearing the jersey moves away (Figure 20-19).

Mechanism: This injury is caused by forced extension at the flexed DIP joint of the finger.

Signs and symptoms:

- Swelling along the palmar aspect of the finger at the DIP joint
- Inability to flex the finger at the DIP joint (sweater finger sign)

approximate the injury bring the edges of an injured structure close together

boutonnière deformity rupture of the extensor tendon on the dorsal side of the finger

jersey finger injury to the flexor digitorum profundus tendon that sometimes occurs when an athlete uses a flexed finger to grab the jersey of another athlete

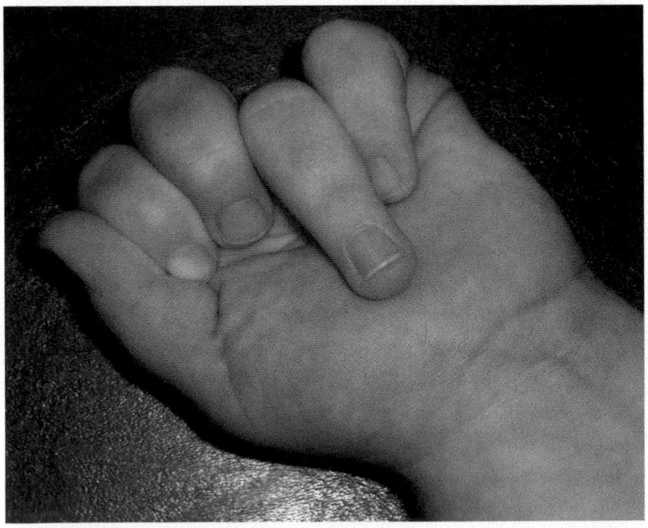

FIGURE 20-19 A positive sweater finger sign showing a rupture of the flexor digitorum profundus tendon at the distal interphalangeal joint. This injury is commonly called a *jersey finger* and usually occurs in the ring finger.

- Pain
- Point tenderness along the flexor tendons

Special tests: The sweater finger test can be used.

Immediate management: Techniques include ice, compression, splinting the DIP and PIP joints in 30 degrees of flexion using an aluminum splint, and referral to a physician for further care.

Intermediate management: If the tendon retracts into the palm, surgical reattachment within 7 to 10 days is required. If not, surgery is required within 3 months.

Collateral Ligament Sprain (Jammed Finger)

A collateral ligament sprain, also known as a "jammed finger," is a very common injury in basketball, football, and wrestling.[20] The name "jammed finger" refers to the mechanism of the injury.

Mechanism: A jammed finger is caused by hyperextension of the PIP joint, excessive valgus or varus force, or an axial force to the distal aspect of the finger.

Signs and symptoms:

- Point tenderness over the PIP joint
- Swelling
- Ecchymosis
- Laxity (in severe injuries only)
- Pain with AROM and PROM of the PIP joint

Special tests:

Valgus/varus stress test of the fingers: For the valgus or varus stress test of the finger, the client is seated with the affected elbow flexed to 90 degrees, the forearm pronated, and the wrist and fingers in a neutral and extended position. The finger is grasped distal and proximal to the injured joint with the athletic trainer's thumb and index finger, respectively. The athletic trainer gradually applies a valgus force to the medial aspect of the injured joint or a varus force to the lateral aspect of the injured joint by pulling the distal aspect of the finger away from the midline. A positive valgus stress test produces pain or laxity when stress is applied to the ulnar (medial) collateral ligament of the respective MCP, PIP, or DIP joint (Figure 20-20).

A positive varus stress test would also produce pain or laxity when stress is applied but to the radial (lateral) collateral ligament of the respective MCP, PIP or DIP joint (Figure 20-21).

A valgus stress test may also be performed on the MCP and IP joints of the thumb. The medial collateral ligament of the thumb is commonly injured in sports.

Immediate management: Immediate management should include ice, compression, immobilization with an aluminum splint in 30 degrees of flexion at the PIP joint, referral to a physician, and X-rays to rule out an avulsion fracture.

Intermediate management: Intermediate management should include splinting in 30 degrees of flexion for 2 to 3 weeks. After that, buddy or check rein taping is suggested for another 3 to 4 weeks.

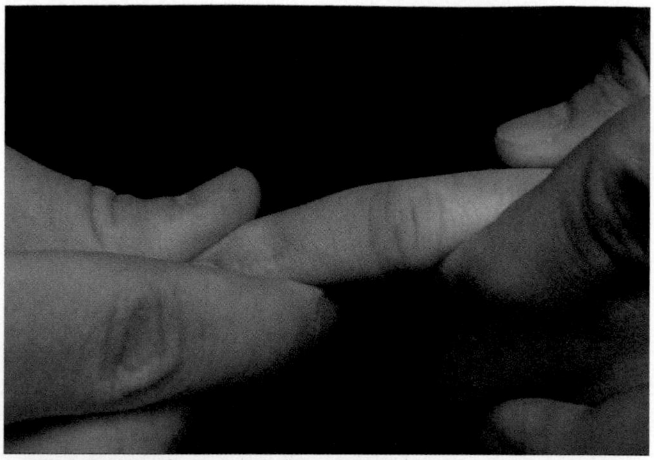

FIGURE 20-20 A valgus stress test of the second proximal interphalangeal joint of the finger to determine laxity of the medial collateral ligament.

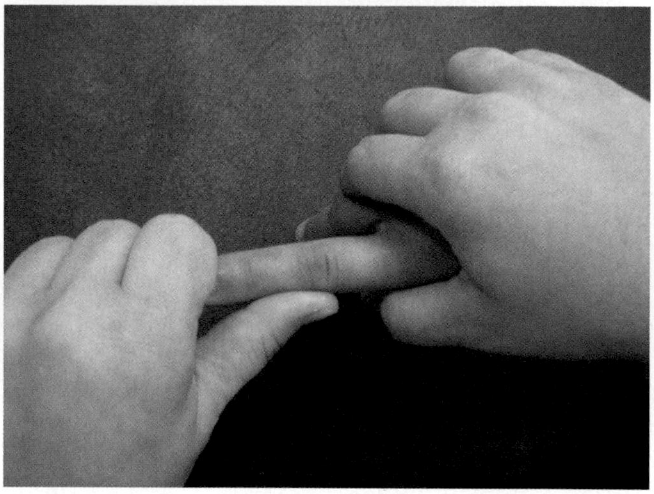

FIGURE 20-21 A varus stress test at the proximal interphalangeal joint testing to determine laxity of the lateral collateral ligament of the finger.

Ulnar Collateral Ligament Sprain (Gamekeeper's/Skier's/Bowler's Thumb)

Integrity of the ulnar collateral ligament (UCL) of the MCP joint of the thumb is required for normal hand function. Injury to this ligament will cause some loss of hand function. The roots of its common name, **gamekeeper's thumb**, can be traced back to early days, when hunters used their thumbs to snap the neck of the game they caught, thereby killing it. It is also called *skiers thumb* because of the manner in which ski poles

gamekeeper's thumb injury to the ulnar collateral ligament of the MCP joint of the thumb; also called *skier's thumb* are jammed in the web space between the thumb and index finger, causing injury to this ligament.

Mechanism: This sprain of the thumb is caused by hyperextension of the thumb, forceful abduction of the thumb, or a combination of the two.

Signs and symptoms:
- Swelling and point tenderness into the thenar eminence of the thumb
- Laxity with a valgus stress test
- Loss of thumb function
- Possible ecchymosis

Special tests: The valgus stress test of the thumb may be used.

Immediate management: Immediate management should include ice, compression, elevation, immobilization, and referral to a physician.

Intermediate management: If significant laxity is present, surgical intervention may be required. If laxity is not significant, a thumb splint should be worn for 6 to 8 weeks, with taping required for athletic competitions for 4 weeks thereafter.[15]

Bennett's Fracture

A **Bennett's fracture** is a fracture and dislocation that occurs at the carpometacarpal joint near the base of the thumb. This is the most common type of thumb fracture, especially in fist fights and ball-handling sports such as football.[15,21,22]

Mechanism: Striking an object with a closed fist, a direct blow to the thumb, and axial loading caused by a blow with a closed fist can cause this fracture.

Signs and symptoms:
- Immediate swelling and pain centered over the CMC joint
- Loss of function
- Point tenderness
- Crepitus
- Increased pain with longitudinal compression

Special tests: The long bone compression test may be used.

Immediate management: Immediate management should include ice, compression, elevation, immobilization of the thumb and wrist, and referral to a physician for X-ray examination.

Intermediate management: Surgery is usually warranted because of the unstable nature of this injury.[21,23]

Subungual Hematoma

A subungual hematoma is a collection of blood underneath a fingernail (Figure 20-22).

Mechanism: A subungual hematoma can be caused by direct trauma to the fingernail or a blow to the end of the finger.

Signs and symptoms:
- Ecchymosis under the fingernail
- Pain and throbbing

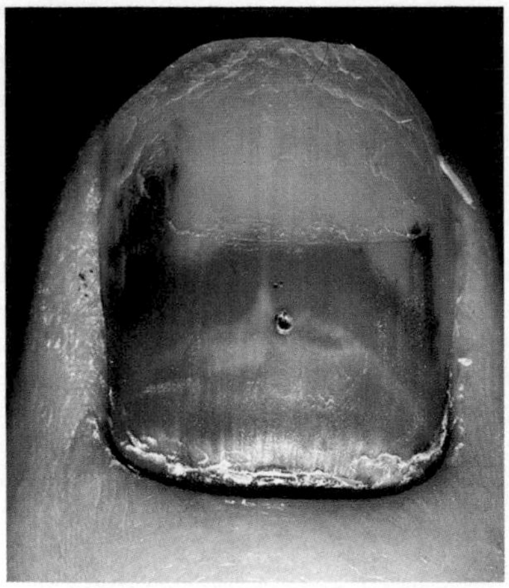

FIGURE 20-22 Blood underneath the fingernail of the hand, commonly called a *subungual hematoma.* (From Habif TP: *Clinical dermatology: a color guide to diagnosis and therapy,* ed 4, Figure 25-36, St Louis, 2004, Mosby/Elsevier.)

- Possible tingling
- Increased pressure within the distal phalanx

Special tests: No special tests are applicable.

Immediate management: An associated fracture should be ruled out. Ice and compression should be applied.

Intermediate management: If absolutely warranted, the hematoma can be drained. Box 20-2 details the procedure for draining blood from underneath a fingernail. After blood is drained, it is imperative to monitor for signs and symptoms of infection afterward.

Box 20-3 summarizes acute injuries of the elbow, forearm, wrist, hand, and finger and the appropriate special tests used in the diagnosis of each.

Bennett's fracture dislocation occurring at the CMC joint near the base of the thumb

BOX 20-2 Procedure for Draining Blood from Underneath a Fingernail

- Numb the area with ice.
- Before starting the procedure, wash your hands and the affected fingernail thoroughly.
- Apply mild pressure to the fingernail by using a sterile surgical blade or a heated paper clip to drill a hole through the distal aspect of the fingernail.
- Once the blood has been removed, soak the fingertip in warm soapy water for 10 minutes, cover it with a sterile dressing, and apply a protective splint.
- Make sure to follow up with the athlete to monitor for signs of infection.

Data from Anderson MK, Hall SJ, Martin M, editors: *Sports injury management,* ed 3, Philadelphia, 2004, Lippincott Williams & Wilkins.

BOX 20-3

Acute Injuries to the Elbow, Forearm, Wrist, Hand, and Finger and Appropriate Special Tests

Elbow Injuries
Dislocations
- No appropriate special tests

Sprains
- Valgus stress test of the elbow
- Varus stress test of the elbow
- Tinel test

Forearm Injuries
Fractures
- Long bone compression test

Volkmann's ischemic contractures
- No appropriate special tests

Wrist Injuries
Scaphoid navicular fracture
- Palpation in the anatomical snuffbox
- Long bone compression test

Perilunate and lunate dislocations
- Watson's test

Sprains
- Valgus stress test of the wrist
- Varus stress test of the wrist

Triangular fibrocartilage complex injuries
- Valgus stress test of the wrist
- Push-off test

Hand and Finger Injuries
Finger fractures
- Tap or percussion test
- Long bone compression test of the metacarpals or phalanges

Finger dislocations
- No appropriate special tests

Mallet finger
- AROM into extension at the DIP joint

Boutonnière and swan neck deformities
- AROM and PROM at the PIP joint

Flexor digitorum profundus rupture (jersey finger)
- Sweater finger test

Collateral ligament sprain (jammed finger)
- Valgus stress test of the fingers
- Varus stress test of the fingers

Ulnar collateral ligament sprain (gamekeeper's thumb)
- Valgus stress test of the thumb

Bennett's fracture
- Long bone compression test

Subungual hematoma
- No appropriate special tests

AROM, active range of motion; *DIP*, distal interphalangeal; *PROM*, passive range of motion; *PIP*, proximal interphalangeal.

Prevention of Acute Injuries

As noted with most of the previously described elbow, wrist, and hand injuries, FOOSH usually results in an injury to one of these areas. The best way to prevent such an injury is to learn how to fall properly. It is a natural reaction to try to catch oneself with an outstretched hand when falling. However, the proper way to fall is to tuck the arm into the body and fall onto the posterior aspect of the shoulder while rolling onto the ground. This technique is known as "tuck and roll."

Another way to prevent injuries is to maintain strength in the muscles being used. In the event that an athlete does fall incorrectly, muscles that are sufficiently strong to compensate or bear the brunt of the load may minimize the severity of the injury. Some common exercises used to strengthen the elbow, wrist, and hand are as follows: gripping exercises, biceps curls, triceps extensions, wrist curls into flexion and extension, and finger extensions with rubber bands. The biceps curls and triceps extensions are used to strengthen the muscles surrounding the elbow. The wrist curls and the gripping exercises strengthen the muscles in the forearm that control the wrist. The finger extensions work the small muscles of the fingers.

Other methods used to prevent injuries to the elbow, wrist, and hand include the following: wearing proper padding and safety equipment; maintaining proper physical conditioning and flexibility; working on balance and proprioception; maintaining a positive attitude on and off the field; having coaches who are well-versed in the rules and regulations of the game; and allowing athletic trainers and other allied health care personnel to educate coaches, parents, and athletes in injury prevention.[15,23,24] Providing guidelines for safe participation prevents many injuries. If athletes learn correct playing techniques as adolescents, they will use them later in their careers.[24] It is imperative that all involved personnel work together to learn mechanisms that cause injury, incorporate injury prevention methods, and watch for warning signs of an impending injury. Prevention is everyone's responsibility.

MANAGEMENT OF CHRONIC ELBOW, WRIST, HAND, AND FINGER INJURIES

Chronic injuries of the elbow, wrist, hand, and fingers are very common, especially as more and more people participate in overhand sports. As with acute injuries, correct management of chronic injuries requires a comprehensive knowledge of anatomy; an accurate assessment; possibly preventive padding, wrapping, or taping; and, especially for adolescent athletes, follow-up with a physician.

Elbow Injuries

Unfortunately, individuals with chronic injuries usually do not seek an evaluation until they have had the injury for some time. In most cases, they do not obtain medical treatment soon enough, waiting until the pain starts impairing their performance.[10,24] A typical history reveals that the client with a chronic injury has had pain for days, weeks, or months that initially went away with rest but will not go away now. The pain is typically severe enough to affect the client's ability to participate fully in his or her activity. The client does not recall a particular mechanism or incident that started the injury, when the injury started, or any other details about it. The client does know, however, what aggravates the injury and what can no longer be done without pain. Parents and coaches can help by being alert to the complaints of their sons, daughters, or players during or after participation. Athletic trainers can help by educating their clients about the importance of immediately communicating any problems or signs and symptoms. Figure 20-23 provides an overview of the diagnosis and management of chronic injuries to the elbow, wrist, hand, and fingers.

Elbow Sprains

Collateral ligament sprains of the elbow may occur as either acute or chronic injuries. Because sprains of these ligaments typically occur in throwing athletes, the injuries are usually encountered as repetitive chronic rather than acute ones.[2,3,8,10,24,25]

Mechanism: The most common mechanism for chronic injury to an elbow collateral ligament (typically the ulnar collateral ligament) is overuse or repetitive

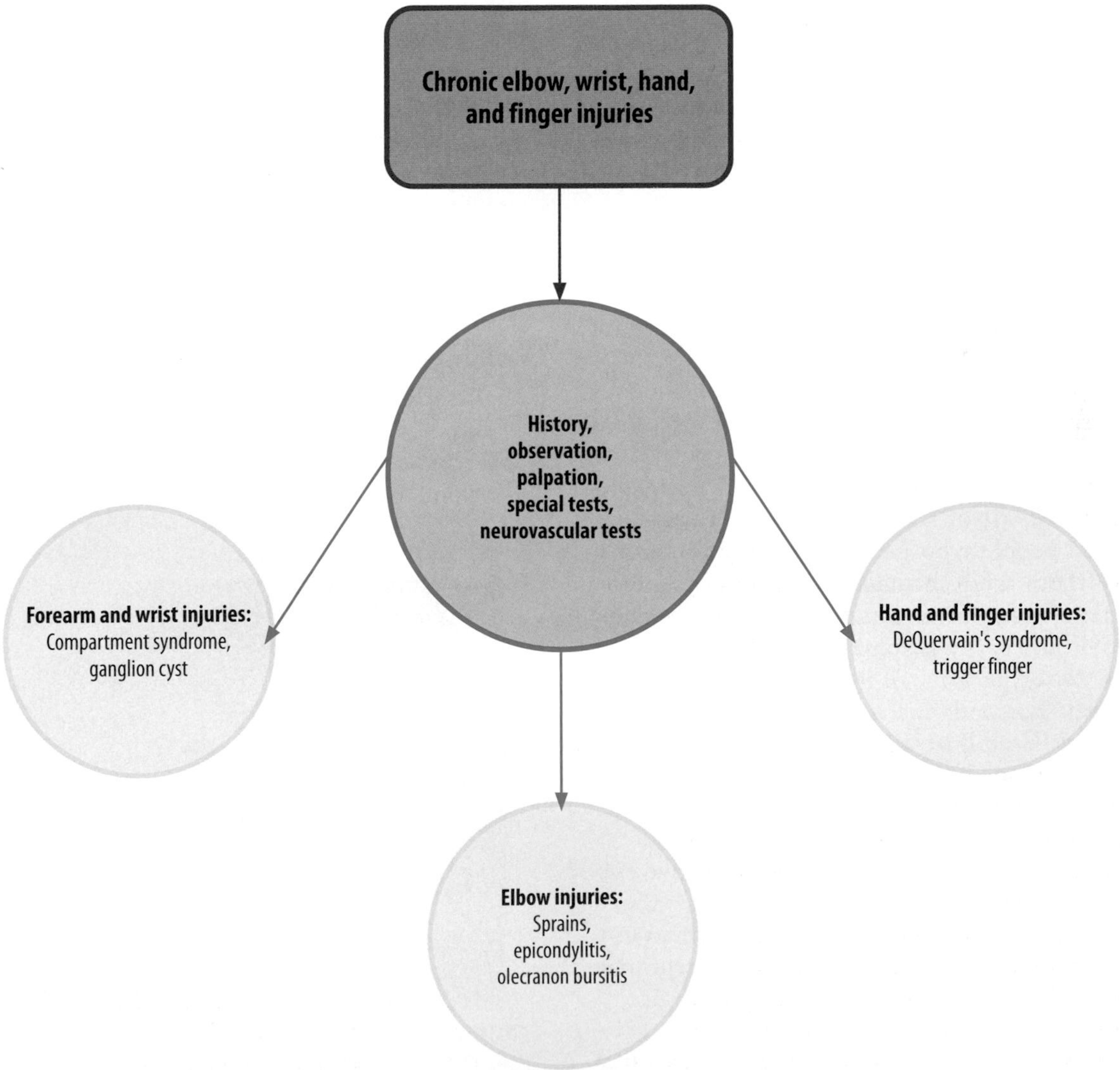

FIGURE 20-23 Concept map overview of chronic elbow, wrist, hand, and finger injuries.

tensile forces through throwing biomechanics or repetitive hyperextension of the elbow (e.g., throwing overhand, pitching, hitting).

Signs and symptoms:

- Point tenderness along the anterior and medial aspects of the elbow
- Swelling
- Pain with AROM and PROM into pronation and elbow extension

Special tests: The valgus stress test of the elbow may be used.

Immediate management: Rest, ice, compression, and elevation may be used to minimize swelling and inflammation.

Intermediate management: Nonsteroidal antiinflammatory medications, a sling to rest the elbow, and continued ice and compression are helpful intermediate techniques.

Epicondylitis

The epicondyles of the humerus are origin points for many forearm and wrist muscles. With overuse, these origins are easily inflamed, causing pain with motions of the wrist. If the inflammation persists for an extended period or the tension is too much for the origin, an avulsion fracture or stress fracture may occur. **Epicondylitis** most commonly occurs in the dominant arm or hand of people older than 40 years of age.[2,5]

Lateral epicondylitis, commonly called *tennis elbow,* is one of the most common overuse injuries in the upper extremity.[2] Lateral epicondylitis is caused by motions particular to a sport, a patient's occupation, or overuse around the house (e.g., gardening). The wrist extensors and supinators originate on the lateral epicondyle and become inflamed when repetitive motions or forces are brought to bear.

Medial epicondylitis is often called *Little Leaguer's elbow, golfer's elbow,* or *swimmer's elbow.* It is a common injury in people who perform overhead motions, particularly those who participate in throwing sports. The wrist flexors and pronators originate on the medical epicondyle and easily become inflamed as a result of the repetitive stress or force of those motions.

Mechanism: Epicondylitis is caused by excessive or repetitive varus (lateral) or valgus (medial) stress, forced extension or flexion of the wrist, and repetitive wrist motions into extension or flexion.

Signs and symptoms:

- Pain and point tenderness over the respective epicondyle
- Pain with the respective valgus or varus stress test
- Pain with AROM and RROM into the respective wrist motions
- Pain with PROM into the opposite motion

Special tests: Tests to be used are the valgus or varus stress tests of the elbow, RROM into wrist flexion (medial epicondylitis), or wrist extension (lateral epicondylitis).

Immediate management: Immediate management should include application of ice, nonsteroidal antiinflammatory drugs, and rest.

Intermediate management: The client should avoid activities that reproduce the pain, alter activity to avoid those particular motions, and participate in a rehabilitation program to increase the strength of the related wrist muscles and a stretching program to increase the flexibility of the wrist muscles. The athletic trainer should evaluate all equipment being used to make sure that the grip size and the weight of the implement are appropriate for the athlete, especially in cases of lateral epicondylitis.

Olecranon Bursitis

Olecranon bursitis is an inflammation of the bursa that sits behind the elbow—the olecranon bursa (Figure 20-24).

Mechanism: Olecranon bursitis is typically caused by receiving a traumatic blow to the posterior elbow or consistently resting an elbow on a hard surface.

Signs and symptoms:

- Localized swelling
- Redness
- Point tenderness over the olecranon process
- Pain with ROM into elbow extension and flexion

Special tests: No special tests are applicable.

Immediate management: Application of ice packs, compression using an Ace wrap, and antiinflammatory drugs such as ibuprofen and naproxen sodium can help reduce the inflammation.

epicondylitis inflammation of the epicondyles of the humerus

olecranon bursitis inflammation of the bursa that sits behind the elbow (olecranon bursa)

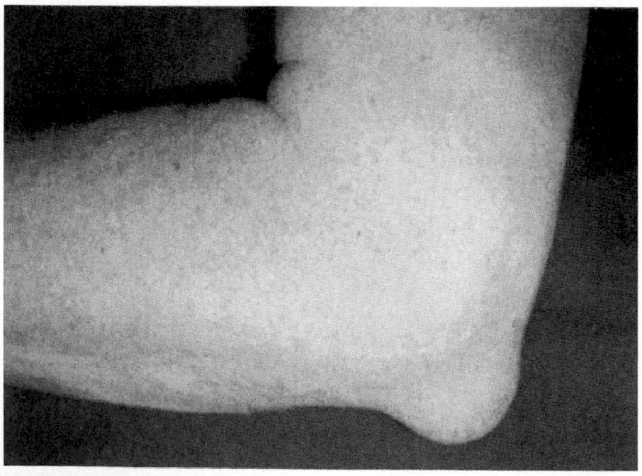

FIGURE 20-24 Olecranon bursitis of the elbow. (From DeLee JC, Drez D, Miller MD: *DeLee & Drez's orthopaedic sports medicine*, ed 2, Figure 23D-3, Philadelphia, 2003, Saunders/Elsevier.)

Intermediate management: The athlete should be monitored for possible signs of infection (e.g., redness, swelling, warmth, pain, loss of normal ROM) and referred to a physician for draining, if needed. Ice and compression should be continued, and the athlete should be adequately protected on return to participation.

Forearm and Wrist Injuries

Overuse forearm and wrist injuries are most common in football and other contact sports, gymnastics, racquet sports, and activities that involve repetitive motions or FOOSH.[1,4,5] Fortunately, most of these injuries are relatively minor, with no long-term effects.[15] Because of pressure from coaches, athletic trainers often minimize or overlook a wrist injury and return an athlete to play too quickly. Chronic injuries of the elbow, wrist, and hand may go unevaluated for extended periods, which may lead to permanent, long-term consequences. When evaluating a chronic injury, the athletic trainer should strive to be thorough and not minimize its importance in an effort to return the athlete to play more quickly.

Compartment Syndrome

The forearm contains three compartments that each contain numerous muscles, blood vessels, and nerves.[5] **Compartment syndrome** is an increase in pressure within any of the three compartments caused by bleeding, fractures, or muscle **hypertrophy.**[5] Any increase in pressure within one of these compartments increases the risk of injury to the blood vessels and nerves within it and could allow Volkmann's ischemic contracture to develop. Surgery is usually required to reduce the pressure within the respective compartment (Figure 20-25).

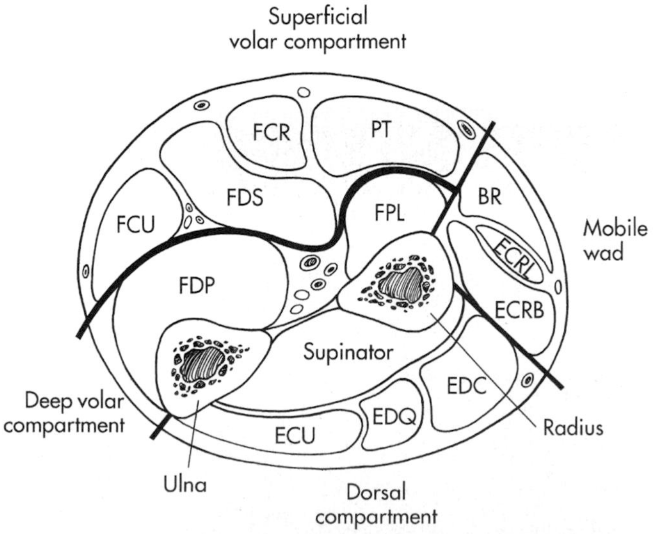

FIGURE 20-25 Compartments of the forearm. (Redrawn from Rowland SA: Fasciotomy: the treatment of compartment syndrome. In Green DP, ed: *Operative hand surgery,* ed 3, New York, 1993, Churchill Livingstone.)

Mechanism: Compartment syndrome is caused by hypertrophy, swelling within a compartment, or a fracture.

Signs and symptoms:

- Dull ache within the forearm
- Loss of sensation
- Loss of function of the wrist, hand, and fingers
- Complaints of pressure in the arm
- Pain with forearm stretching

Special tests: No special tests are applicable.

Immediate management: Immediate management should include ice, monitoring of pulses, and referral to a physician.

Intermediate management: Surgery is usually warranted.

Carpal Tunnel Syndrome

Carpal tunnel syndrome affects an estimated 3% of adult Americans and is three times more common in women then men[11] (Figure 20-26). The carpal tunnel is an osseous structure formed by the proximal row of carpal bones on the floor and the transverse carpal ligament on the roof. It has 10 structures passing through it, nine of which are tendons: four tendons of the flexor digitorum profundus, four tendons of the flexor digitorum superficialis, the flexor pollicis longus tendon, and the median nerve. If any of these structures hypertrophies or becomes inflamed, space in the tunnel decreases. As the space decreases, the median nerve is compressed, causing numbness and tingling to radiate into the hand and fingers, specifically fingers two through four.

compartment syndrome syndrome involving increased pressure in any of the three forearm compartments

hypertrophy increase in size

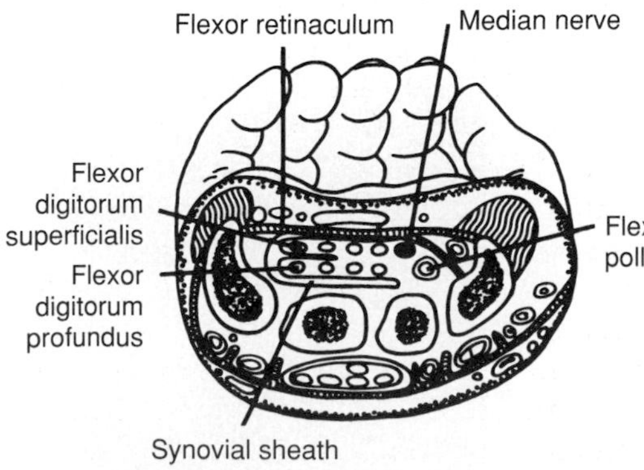

FIGURE 20-26 Carpal tunnel of the wrist. (From Noble J: *Textbook of primary care medicine,* ed 3, Figure 126-20, St Louis, 2001, Mosby/Elsevier.)

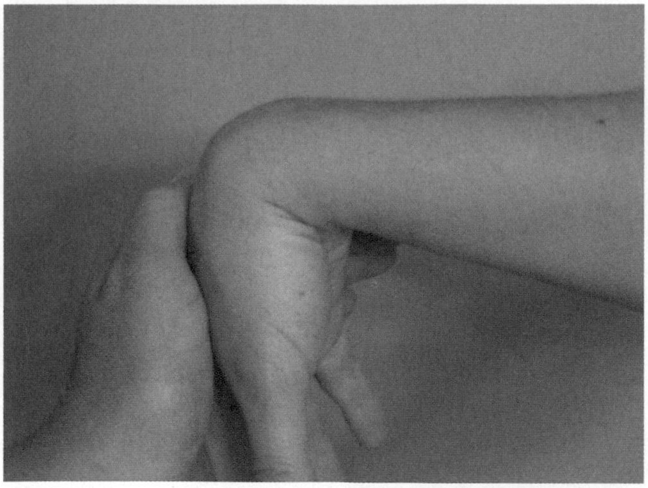

FIGURE 20-27 Phalen's test to detect signs of carpal tunnel syndrome.

Mechanism: Immediate management should include repetitive wrist motion into flexion and extension.

Signs and symptoms:

- Pain
- Numbness
- Tingling into the hand and fingers that worsens at night
- Radiating pain into the elbow and shoulder
- Atrophy of the thenar muscles
- Decreased ability to perform activities of daily living (e.g., driving a car, opening a door, brushing hair, drinking from a glass)
- Decreased grip strength

Special tests:

Phalen's test: Phalen's test is designed to determine the presence of carpal tunnel syndrome by reproducing the signs and symptoms associated with it (Figure 20-27). The client should either stand or sit with his or her wrist passively flexed while the athletic trainer applies overpressure to the flexed wrist for a minimum of 1 minute. A positive test elicits tingling or numbness that radiates into the hand and into the second through the fourth fingers.

Tinel's test: Tinel's test is another test used to determine the presence of carpal tunnel syndrome (Figure 20-28). The client is in a seated position with his or her forearm supinated and resting on the table. The athletic trainer taps or flicks the palmar aspect of the wrist over the carpal tunnel area. If positive, the client will complain of tingling or numbness radiating into the second, third, and fourth fingers and possibly the thumb.

Immediate management: Ice and nonsteroidal antiinflammatory drugs may be used to reduce inflammation, and a wrist extension splint may be applied.

Intermediate management: Intermediate management should include avoidance of repetitive wrist motions, anti-inflammatory medication, evaluation of sport or workplace ergonomics, an extension wrist splint, and possibly a corticosteroid injection.

Ganglion Cyst

A **ganglion cyst** is a soft tissue tumor most commonly found on the dorsal aspect of the wrist (Figure 20-29). The signs and symptoms of ganglions are not consistent from person to person. Most people do not seek out treatment until symptoms become troublesome.

Mechanism: Repeated wrist extension causes a herniation of the wrist joint capsule.

ganglion cyst soft tissue tumor commonly located on the dorsal side of the wrist

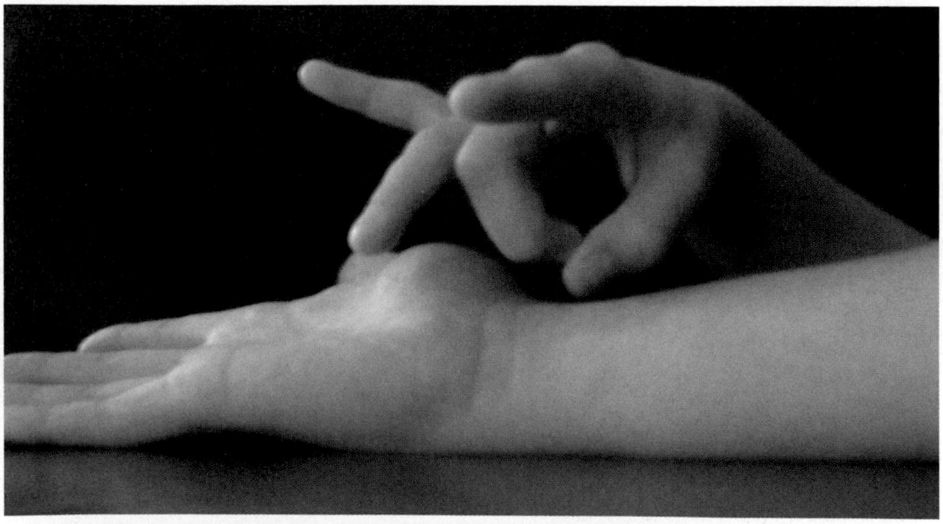

FIGURE 20-28 Tinel's test also may be used to detect signs of carpal tunnel syndrome.

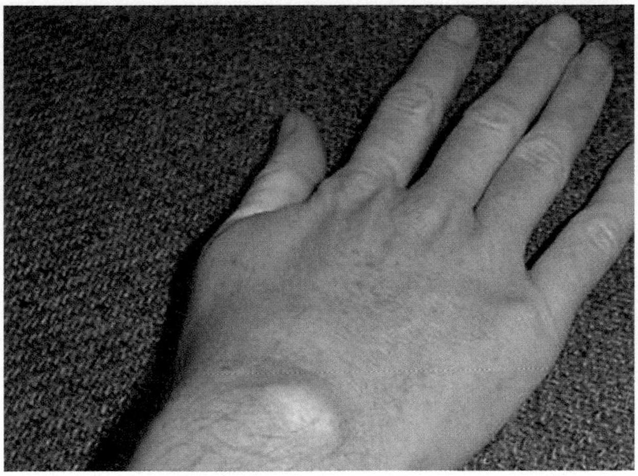

FIGURE 20-29 A ganglion cyst on the dorsal aspect of the wrist.

Signs and symptoms:

- Some loss of wrist motion, especially with flexion
- Pain with wrist extension
- Noticeable deformity on the dorsum of the hand that appears intermittently
- Point tenderness on deformity
- Discomfort or pressure

Special tests: No special tests are applicable.

Immediate management: Immediate management should include applying ice and limiting motions of extreme flexion.

Intermediate management: Minor surgery to aspirate or excise the mass if warranted.

Hand and Finger Injuries

Most overuse hand and finger injuries occur as the result of racquet sports, excessive training, repetitive motions, or specific sport demands.[1,12,20,25,26] Using proper prevention, warming up, stretching before and after exercising, gradually increasing stresses and intensity, learning proper techniques, using proper equipment, and identifying the injury early will go a long way in minimizing lost time.[12,25,26]

De Quervain's Syndrome

De Quervain's syndrome occurs when the sheath or tunnel that surrounds the thumb tendons becomes irritated or inflamed (Figure 20-30).

Mechanism: The syndrome is caused by repetitive stress involving ulnar deviation and thumb extension.

Signs and symptoms:

- Swelling over the radial styloid process and thumb tendons
- Point tenderness over the radial styloid process and dorsal thumb tendons
- Pain with AROM of the wrist into radial deviation and with PROM of the wrist into ulnar deviation
- Pain with AROM and RROM into flexion, extension, and abduction of the thumb

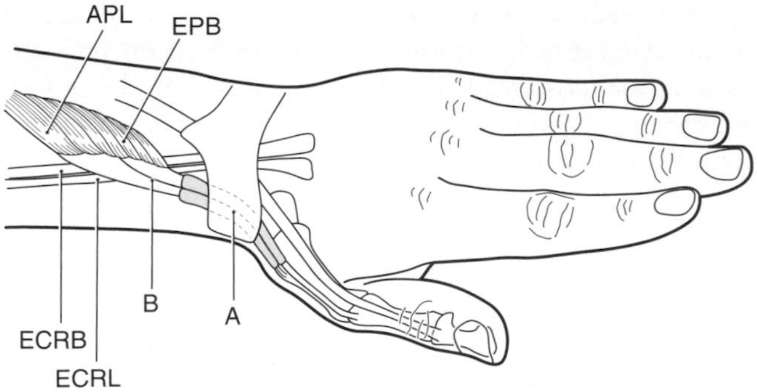

FIGURE 20-30 *A*, Site of de Quervain disease at the extensor pollicis brevis (*EPB*) and abductor pollicis longus (*APL*) tendons. *B*, Site of intersection syndrome at the extensor carpi radialis longus (*ECRL*) and extensor carpi radialis brevis (*ECRB*) tendons. (From Roberts JR, Hedges JR: *Clinical procedures in emergency medicine,* ed 4, Figure 53-17, Philadelphia, 2004, Saunders/Elsevier.)

Special tests:

Finkelstein's test: Most sports and upper extremity activities require repetitive thumb motions that could lead to overuse and tendonitis. Finkelstein's test is used to determine the presence of tenosynovitis of the thumb (de Quervain's syndrome; Figure 20-31). The client is seated with his or her thumb flexed into the palm of the hand. The client then closes the fingers over the thumb to make a fist. The athletic trainer asks the client to forcibly move the wrist into ulnar deviation, which moves the wrist toward the pinky side while keeping the thumb in the fist position. Increased pain in the wrist along the thumb side is considered positive and indicates the presence of tenosynovitis of the thumb muscles.

Immediate management: Ice and nonsteroidal anti-inflammatory drugs may reduce inflammation, and a splint may limit ulnar deviation.

de Quervain's syndrome stress injury occurring when the sheath or tunnel surrounding the thumb tendons becomes irritated or inflamed

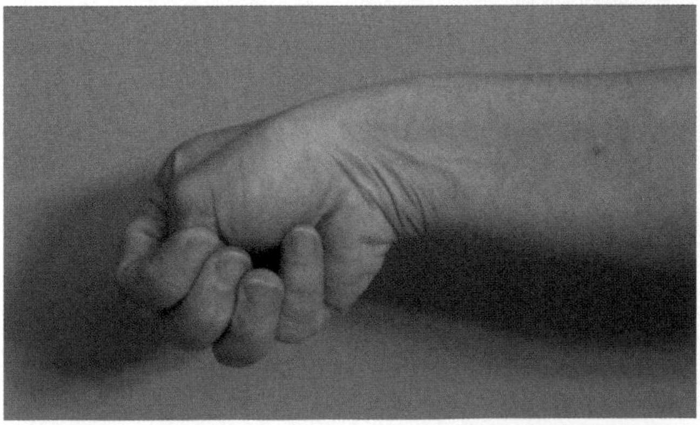

FIGURE 20-31 Finkelstein's test to detect tenosynovitis of the thumb or De Quervain's syndrome.

Intermediate management: **Iontophoresis**, the use of a direct electrical current to push medication into the body; corticosteroid injection; activity modification; continued splinting; and possible surgical intervention are all used in intermediate management.

Trigger Finger

Trigger finger is caused by repetitive gripping action with the flexed fingers. The most common symptom is a mechanical "locking" of the finger when going from a flexed to an extended position. To alleviate this problem, the client usually has to "unlock" the finger by passively extending the respective finger, which produces a popping sensation, analogous to pulling a trigger (Figure 20-32).

Mechanism: Overuse or repetitive motions cause swelling and inflammation of the tendinous sheath.

Signs and symptoms:

- Catching or locking during flexion and extension of the affected finger
- Pain
- Minor swelling

Special tests: No special tests are applicable.

Immediate management: Ice and nonsteroidal antiinflammatory drugs may reduce inflammation.

Intermediate management: Intermediate management includes avoidance of the aggravating cause and possible splinting.

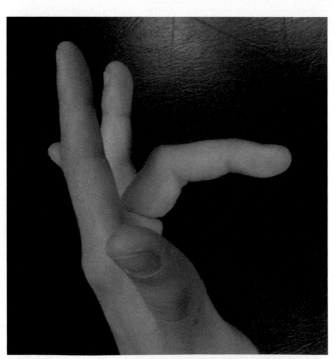

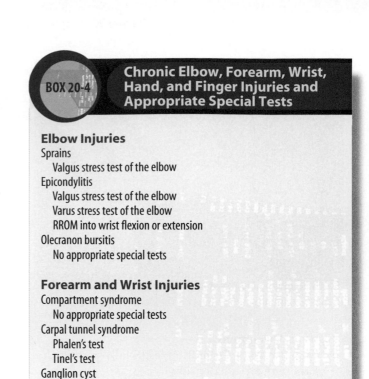

FIGURE 20-32 A picture of an index finger "stuck" in flexion. This is commonly called trigger finger and is result of inflammation of the sheath surrounding the extensor tendon. The only way to "unstick" this finger is to passively put it into extension.

BOX 20-4 Chronic Elbow, Forearm, Wrist, Hand, and Finger Injuries and Appropriate Special Tests

Elbow Injuries

Sprains
- Valgus stress test of the elbow

Epicondylitis
- Valgus stress test of the elbow
- Varus stress test of the elbow
- RROM into wrist flexion or extension

Olecranon bursitis
- No appropriate special tests

Forearm and Wrist Injuries

Compartment syndrome
- No appropriate special tests

Carpal tunnel syndrome
- Phalen's test
- Tinel's test

Ganglion cyst
- No appropriate special tests

Hand and Finger Injuries

DeQuervain's syndrome
- Finkelstein's test

Trigger finger
- No appropriate special tests

RROM, Resistive range of motion.

Box 20-4 summarizes chronic injuries to the elbow, forearm, wrist, hand, and finger and the appropriate special tests used to help diagnose each.

Prevention of Chronic Injuries

There are many reasons for the greater number of chronic injuries that are reported today: an increase in organized sports, decreased free play, early sport specialization, year-round training, and simply doing too much too soon. The most significant factor in developing chronic injuries is the individual's training or activity.[25] Properly warming up and stretching the body, completing an easy throwing progression or series of exercises to warm up the arm, and practicing good mechanics are important for all athletes and workers who rely on the upper

iontophoresis the use of a direct electrical current to push medication into the body

trigger finger stress injury caused by repetitive gripping action with flexed fingers extremity. Also, for throwing athletes in particular, limiting pitching to 4 to 10 innings per week, 80 to 100 pitches per game, and 30 to 40 pitches per practice will go a long way in preventing chronic elbow, wrist, and hand injuries.[26]

Another way to prevent overuse injuries is to develop good strength in the muscles involved, retain flexibility as one ages, and maintain cardiovascular fitness. Flexibility exercises should be included in any exercise or fitness program to prevent injury, improve strength, and minimize the occurrence or recurrence of injuries. Stretches for the elbow, forearm, wrist, and hand should focus on elbow and wrist motions (i.e., flexion and extension). It is important to keep the elbow straight when stretching the forearm muscles because this will increase the amount of stretch felt. Each stretch should be held for a minimum of 20 seconds and repeated two or three times each day.

TAPING, BRACING, AND RETURN TO PLAY

Most athletes want to return to activity as soon as possible. Even though they might disagree with you, their activities should always take a back seat to the proper treatment and care of any elbow, wrist, or hand injury.[1] Long-term disability can result from many wrist and hand injuries. No return to play decision should be made at the expense of the athlete's future functional abilities. Recognition of common injury patterns, early activity modification, and initiation of comprehensive treatment programs can go a long way in preventing long-term disability. The age of the athlete and his or her level of play are also important factors in making return to play decisions.[1]

Most athletes can continue participating in their chosen sport while undergoing treatment for the injury, unless it is affecting their level of participation. Generally, when the client has full ROM, minimal pain or soreness with AROM and RROM, minimal pain with palpation of the injured area, and at least 80% strength of the injured side compared with the contralateral side in terms of gripping and pinching abilities,[15] the athlete can return to play. Most elbow, wrist, and hand injuries are not life-threatening, although they can cause considerable problems with activities of daily living. Therefore it is important to specify physical restrictions so that clients fully understand the activities that must be avoided.

Athletic trainers may choose from a few protective equipment options to assist in the client's return to play. Most of these methods are used to prevent re-injury or re-aggravation of an injury. Participation with a protective splint or brace is regulated by the rules of the sport or the governing bodies (e.g., NCAA, state high school federations) and depends on the level of participation. When deciding whether to have an athlete participate in a splint or brace, the athletic trainer should first determine what body part requires protection and what the rationale is for using the device.[9] Because most, if not all, activities require the unrestricted use of the elbow, wrist, hand, and fingers, protective equipment is rarely used. Box 20-5 lists general guidelines for using protective splints or braces for the upper extremity.

Most elbow, wrist, and hand braces or splints are designed to provide immobilization, limit ROM, or provide compression. The counterforce brace is very common. Designed to help alleviate signs and symptoms of either medial or lateral epicondylitis, it is more often worn by athletes or patients who suffer from lateral epicondylitis or participate in racquet sports. The brace is designed to put pressure on the proximal forearm near the origins of the wrist muscles. This pressure decreases the pull on the respective wrist tendons and reduces the inflammatory pain.[9] An athlete with olecranon bursitis may use a protective pad on return to play to prevent re-injury. Patients with carpal tunnel syndrome or de Quervain's syndrome may use wrist splints as part of their rehabilitation programs to restrict wrist motion. The availability of custom-made and specialty braces for particular injuries has decreased the amount of time that individuals must refrain from activity. Proper education regarding the use and application of these braces is the responsibility of physicians, coaches, athletic trainers, and the athlete.[9]

THE AGE GROUP ATHLETE

Upper extremity injuries among adolescent athletes are becoming more prevalent as participation and competition levels increase.[20] Approximately 35 million children and young adults between the ages of 6 and 21 participate in sports, including 6 to 8 million who participate in school programs.[10] Of these injuries, most (80%) are minor contusions, abrasions, and lacerations.[27] Despite these numbers, school age sports are still relatively safe. Sports camps are a common source of overuse problems because they place high

BOX 20-5 General Guidelines for Using Protective Splints or Braces for the Upper Extremity

- Obtain a note from the supervising physician authorizing use of the device.
- Understand how the device will affect the athlete in the specific position or sport in which he or she participates.
- Know the proper use of the device.
- Ensure that the athlete is aware that the device may cause other injuries.
- Ensure that the athlete understands that no brace or splint will protect a body or joint 100% of the time.
- Ensure that the athlete is aware of the risks associated with using the splint or brace.

demands on athletes who typically are not prepared to meet those demands.[27] Overuse injuries are the most common adolescent sports injuries.[10]

Injuries to the upper extremities are unique to the growing musculoskeletal system of an adolescent athlete and specific to the demands of the sport.[20] Injuries are typically proportional to the athlete's size, age, maturity level, and chosen sport. Adolescent athletes have a greater chance of injuring themselves because they are primarily skeletally immature, with open epiphyseal growth plates. These athletes have unossified cartilage, and their muscles, tendons, and ligaments are still growing. The most common acute adolescent injuries to the upper extremity are epiphyseal or avulsion fractures. Fractures typically occur in the growing part of a bone because it is only one third as strong as the ligaments that attach to that area. As a result, most children sustain epiphyseal fractures, such as clavicular fractures or distal radial fractures, and not ligament sprains.[21,27] About 75% of all adolescent fractures occur in the upper extremity as a result of FOOSH.[28] The hand and wrist are also exposed to possible injury every day through sports and daily activities, increasing the vulnerability of these areas. Injuries to the hand are especially common in basketball, football, snowboarding, softball, and skateboarding.[20] Because of the possibility of long-term disability if these injuries are not handled properly, proper recognition and treatment are mandatory. Careful and accurate diagnosis is imperative to assist in developing rehabilitation goals, treatment protocols, and proper referral.

Elbow, wrist, and hand injuries are not limited to adolescent athletes. Older people are also susceptible to injuries to these areas.[29] Statistically, older athletes are likely to injure themselves as the result of unavoidable facts of aging: loss of bone, loss of strength and muscle mass, a decrease in flexibility, and an overall decline in cardiovascular output.[29,30] Injuries particular to the aging athlete are very similar to those affecting the adolescent athlete: fractured arms related to falls, tendonitis as the result of overuse, and musculoskeletal injuries such as sprains and strains. Prevention measures are also quite similar. Most injuries can be prevented, regardless of the age of the athlete, by incorporating warm-up and cool-down periods, stretching exercises, proper conditioning, weight training, balance training, and a good dose of common sense. There is no reason for the aging athlete to avoid physical activity. Almost all studies suggest that the more active older athletes are, the more enjoyment they will get from life, as well as the possibility of a better and longer life.[29,30]

Most injuries in the adolescent population are due to overtraining and become chronic injuries because the athlete tried to do too much too soon. With overhead throwing athletes, it is the number of pitches thrown in a specific amount of time that matters, not necessarily the type of pitches thrown. Young athletes have a higher susceptibility to injury because their bones, muscles, tendons, and ligaments are still growing. Approximately 60% of children and adolescents between the ages of 11 and 18 experience elbow injuries during or after pitching or throwing in organized games.[10] This process usually begins with a repetitive activity that fatigues a tendon or bone and causes inflammation. It is combined with inadequate recovery time and a lack of preventive measures. All these factors lead to chronic soreness, pain, loss of flexibility, and weakness. Recurrent elbow pain in young throwing athletes should not be ignored because it can cause long-term damage to the elbow, affecting future throwing ability.

Common mistakes that occur in the treatment of injuries to the elbow, wrist, and hand among children are as follows: failing to identify related injuries; failing to correctly splint the injured extremity; attempting to reduce a dislocation before obtaining radiographs; confusing a growth plate injury with an avulsion fracture; and failing to include the joints above and below the injured area in a physical exam.[28] Recognition of common injury patterns, a thorough evaluation, and proper treatment of all injuries are essential in preventing short- and long-term disability.

Supracondylar Elbow Fracture

A supracondylar elbow fracture is an acute injury that is particular to the age group athlete. This type of fracture occurs superior to the distal condyles of the humerus or between the condyles. Of all elbow fractures in children, 65% are supracondylar fractures.[28] Children are more susceptible to this type of fracture because their ligaments and joint capsules are hypermobile, which means that they move more than the corresponding structures in adults. Supracondylar elbow fractures are also more common in boys between the ages of 5 and 8 years.[28] Surgical intervention is usually necessary for this fracture. Improper assessment and treatment may result in a **gunstock deformity,** in which the elbow exhibits a varus angle instead of a valgus angle (Figure 20-33). This deformity results in a loss of the normal carrying angle, producing a gunstock appearance.

Mechanism: FOOSH (Figure 20-34) is the most common mechanism, but this fracture can also be caused by falling onto a flexed elbow.

Signs and symptoms:

- Possible visible deformity
- Swelling
- Muscle spasm

gunstock deformity an elbow with a varus angle instead of a valgus angle

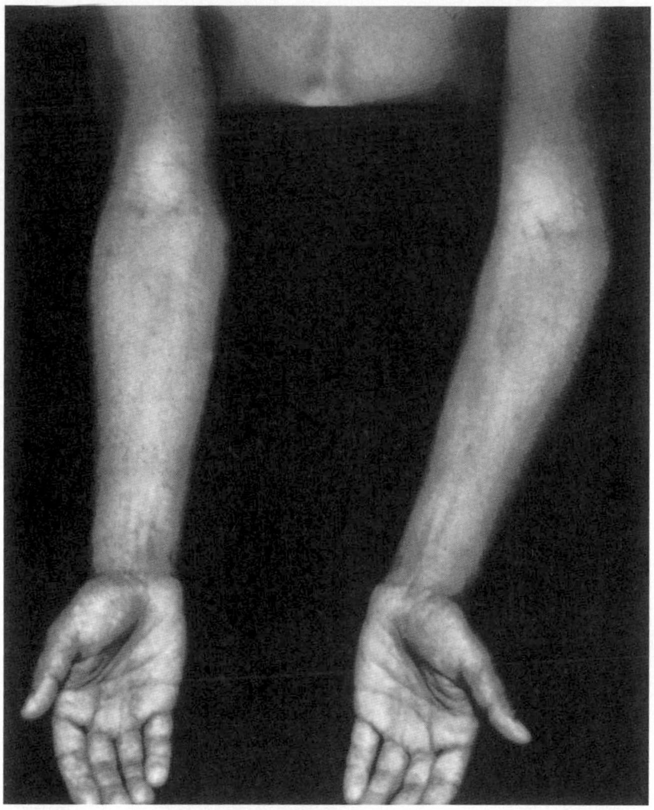

FIGURE 20-33 Cubital varus deformity, or "gunstock deformity," at the elbow caused by elbow and humeral fractures. (From Regan WD, Morrey BF: The physical examination of the elbow. In Morrey BF: *The elbow and its disorders*, ed 2, p. 74, Philadelphia, WB Saunders.)

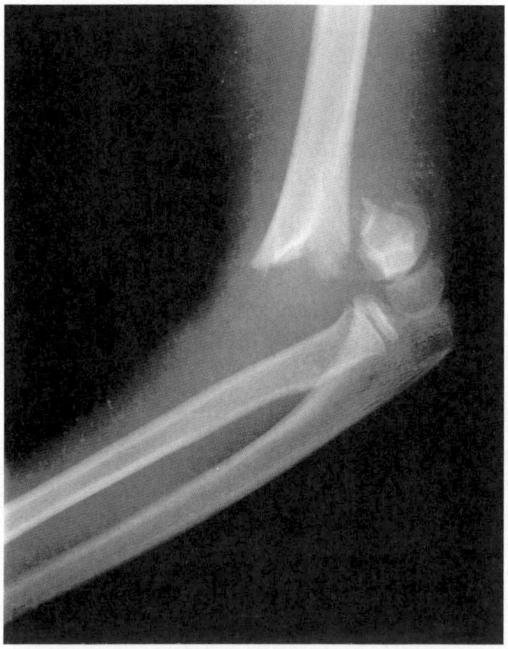

FIGURE 20-34 A supracondylar elbow fracture caused by falling on an outstretched hand (FOOSH).

- Loss of arm function
- Possible neurovascular compromise

Special tests: The long bone compression test and tap test may be used.

Immediate management: The elbow should be immobilized in a splint in 20 to 30 degrees of flexion, and the client should be transported to the emergency room. This elbow position often releases the brachial artery from the distal humerus and could help restore blood flow to the remainder of the arm, possibly preventing Volkmann's contracture. Continued monitoring of the neurovascular status is imperative. If neurovascular status is compromised, ice and compression should NOT be applied because these could cause further complications. If the fracture is open, the wound should be cleaned and covered immediately.

Intermediate management: Intermediate management includes further evaluation by a physician, X-ray assessment to determine the direction of displacement, and open or closed reduction followed by surgical stabilization or casting. Once stabilization has occurred, the elbow must be splinted.

Epiphyseal Fracture (Little Leaguer's Elbow)

Little Leaguer's elbow is an all-inclusive term for medial elbow pain in adolescent baseball players. An epiphyseal fracture occurs when the stress becomes too much for the wrist flexor and pronator origin points. Although the condition was first documented in baseball pitchers, the throwing motion is common to the nonpitcher's throw, the tennis serve, and the football pass.[20] Consequently, this type of fracture is also common in golfers, javelin throwers, racquetball players, tennis players, gymnasts, bowlers, and wrestlers.

Throwing too many pitches or throwing the wrong types of pitches puts great stress on a young pitcher's elbow ligaments and growth plates.[26] The growth plates are the weakest aspect of an adolescent's bone, and too much stress makes them susceptible to injury. **Osteochondritis**, in which a piece of articular cartilage and underlying bone is dislodged from its origin, can occur when the tension placed on the growth plate becomes too taxing. If a young athlete exhibits medial elbow pain that increases with throwing, decreased elbow movement, and decreased throwing velocity and the athlete is an overhead thrower (as opposed to a fast-pitch softball pitcher), an epiphyseal fracture or osteochondritis should be suspected until proved otherwise (Figure 20-35).

Mechanism: Overuse injury, valgus stress with throwing, too many pitches, and coming back too soon after an off-season are all causes of epiphyseal fractures.

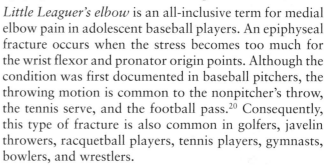

osteochondritis a piece of articular cartilage and underlying bone that has been dislodged from its origin

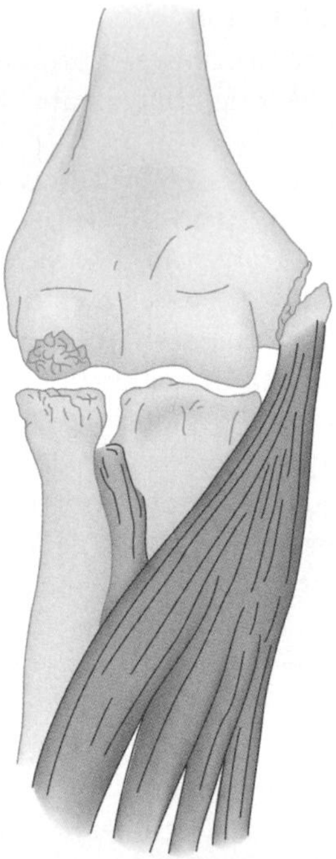

FIGURE 20-35 A schematic drawing of a stress fracture of the medial epicondyle of the humerus, commonly called *Little Leaguer's elbow*. (From Connolly JF: *DePalma's management of fractures and dislocations,* Philadelphia, 1981, WB Saunders.)

Signs and symptoms:

- Point tenderness and swelling over the medial elbow and epicondyle
- Pain with throwing, gripping, or carrying heavy objects
- Pain with AROM and RROM into wrist flexion or pronation
- Ulnar nerve symptoms
- Possible flexion contracture
- Possible clicking in the elbow

Special tests: The valgus stress test is used.

Immediate management: Immediate management includes ordering the client to stop all throwing, applying ice and compression, administering nonsteroidal antiinflammatory drugs to reduce inflammation, and referring the client to a physician.

Intermediate management: Intermediate management includes keeping the athlete from throwing until symptoms have ceased. The athlete should also participate in a rehabilitation program that increases elbow and wrist strengthening and flexibility and improves or corrects throwing mechanics. On return to play, the number of throws should be limited, and a functional throwing progression should be implemented[31] (Box 20-6).

Chronic Injuries

Chronic injuries to the elbow, wrist, hand, and fingers are also quite common in the aging population. Although increasing numbers of older people are staying in shape and forestalling the aging process, the decline in physical fitness is inevitable, even among dedicated athletes.[29] It is estimated that ¼ of the U.S. population will be 55 years of age or older by the year 2010.[32] Given the propensity of baby boomers to be more physically active than previous generations, the possibility of suffering an injury, especially a musculoskeletal injury, will be at an all-time high.[32] Aging brings decreases in maximum heart rate, overall lung capacity, muscle strength and mass, and reaction time and balance. As a result, muscles, tendons, and ligaments are more prone to wear and tear, leading to chronic or overuse injuries. People 60 years of age and older account for approximately 70% of chronic injuries in veteran athletes, compared with 41% of athletes ages 21 to 25.[32] The most common chronic injuries affecting the older population are muscle strains (hamstrings), tendonitis (elbow epicondylitis), stress fractures (lower extremities), osteoarthritis (wear-and-tear arthritis), back problems (disk), and torn rotator cuffs.[29,32] Despite the increased risk of injury, older people still need to stay active. Research has shown that with appropriate exercise, many of the normal aging processes can be slowed or even reduced.

SUMMARY

Upper extremity injuries are specific to the demands and stresses of the activities in which people participate. Competitive, recreational, and adolescent athletes as well as certain workers sustain a wide array of injuries to their upper extremities. Most are related to direct trauma or repetitive stress. Recognition of the common injury mechanisms, patterns, and types will assist an athletic trainer in preventing injuries, making a correct diagnosis, and guiding the athlete through the proper treatment and care of the injury, particularly those athletes who participate in throwing, catching, or swinging sports. It is important for athletic trainers to evaluate these injuries early and prescribe the correct rehabilitation for a complete recovery without limitations.

Revisiting the OPENING *Scenario*

Paul, who has a history of injury to his wrist, experienced re-injury while playing football. He has pain with AROM and PROM into extension, which suggests that the injury is affecting noncontractile tissue (e.g., ligaments, fascia, bone). The atrophy of the muscle on the thenar eminence demonstrates that the injury is not an acute one because atrophy occurs over time. Most of Paul's pain is located on the radial side (which eliminates injury to the TFCC) in the anatomical snuffbox. Point tenderness found in the area indicates a possible injury to the

BOX 20-6 Sample: 13/14-Year-Old Baseball Pitcher's Interval Throwing Program

After medical clearance, begin throwing at step 1. For steps 1 through 3, advance no more than 1 step every three days with two days of active rest (warm up and long tosses) after each workout. For steps 4 through 8, advance no more than 1 step every three days with two days active rest after each workout. Advance to steps 9 through 16 daily as soreness allows.

Phase I: Return to throwing – all throws are at 50% effort

STEP 1
Warm-up toss to 60 ft
15 throws at 30 ft
15 throws at 30 ft*
15 throws at 30 ft
20 long tosses to 60 ft

STEP 2
Warm-up toss to 75 ft
15 throws at 45 ft
15 throws at 45 ft*
15 throws at 45 ft
20 long tosses to 75 ft

STEP 3
Warm-up tosses to 90 ft
15 throws at 60 ft*
15 throws at 60 ft*
15 throws at 60 ft*
20 long tosses to 90 ft

Phase II: Return to pitching: Fastballs are from level ground

STEP 4
Warm-up toss to 105 ft
20 fastballs at 50%*
16 fastballs at 50%*
16 fastballs at 50%*
25 long tosses to 105 ft

STEP 5
Warm-up toss to 120 ft
20 fastballs at 50%*
20 fastballs at 50%*
20 fastballs at 50%*
25 long tosses to 120 ft

STEP 6
Warm-up toss to 120 ft
16 fastballs at 50%*
20 fastballs at 50%*
20 fastballs at 50%*
16 fastballs at 50%*
25 long tosses to 160 ft

Phase III: Intensified Pitching: Pitches are from mound with normal stride

STEP 7
Warm-up toss to 120 ft
20 fastballs (50%)*
20 fastballs (75%)*
20 fastballs (75%)*
20 fastballs (50%)*
25 long tosses at 160 ft

STEP 8
Warm-up toss to 120 ft
20 fastballs (75%)*
21 fastballs (50%)*
20 fastballs (75%)*
21 fastballs (50%)*
25 long tosses at 160 ft

STEP 9
Warm-up toss to 120 ft
25 fastballs (50%)*
24 fastballs (75%)*
24 fastballs (75%)*
25 fastballs (50%)*
25 long tosses at 160 ft

STEP 10
Warm-up toss to 120 ft
25 fastballs (75%)*
25 fastballs (75%)*
25 fastballs (75%)*
20 fastballs (75%)*
25 long tosses at 160 ft

STEP 11
Active Rest
Warm-up toss to 120 ft
20 throws at 60 ft (5%)
15 throws at 80 ft (75%)*
20 throws at 60 ft (7%)
15 throws at 80 ft (75%)*
20 long tosses at 160 ft

STEP 12
Warm-up toss to 120 ft
20 fastballs (100%)*
20 fastballs (75%)
6 off speed pitches (75%)*
20 fastballs (100%)*
20 fastballs (75%)
6 off-speed pitches (75%)*
25 long tosses at 160 ft

STEP 13
Warm-up toss to 120 ft
20 fastballs (75%)
4 throws to first (75%)*
15 fastballs (100%)
10 off-speed pitches (100%)*
20 fastballs (100%)
5 off-speed pitches (100%)*
20 fastballs (75%)
4 throws to first (75%)*
25 long tosses at 160 ft

STEP 14
Warm-up toss to 120 ft
20 fastballs (100%)
5 throws to first (100%)*
15 fastballs (100%)
10 off-speed pitches (100%)*
20 fastballs (100%)
5 off-speed pitches (100%)*
20 fastballs (75%)
5 throws to first (75%)*
25 long tosses at 160 ft

STEP 15
Batting practice
90–100 pitches
10 throws to first
Field bunts and comebacks

Simulated Game

1. 10-minute warm-up of 50–80 pitches with gradually increasing velocity
2. 4 innings
3. 22–27 pitches per inning, including 15–20 fastballs
4. 6 minutes of rest between innings

From Axe MJ, Wickham K, Snyder-Mackler L: Databased interval throwing programs for Little League, high school, college, and professional baseball pitchers, *Sports Med Arthro* 9(1):24, 2001 Available at www.lww.com

* Rest 6 minutes after these sets.

scaphoid-navicular carpal bone. Even though initial X-rays scans were negative, a second set is warranted. Scaphoid-navicular fractures are easily overlooked in initial X-ray examination because swelling conceals a potential carpal fracture. With any wrist injury accompanied by signs and symptoms that do not disappear, it is imperative to obtain a second (or even third) set of X-rays to completely rule out the possibility of a scaphoid-navicular injury. It is also imperative that this injury be recognized early and treated properly because of its tendency to become nonunion or progress into avascular necrosis (bone death). An unresolved scaphoid-navicular fracture may result in Preiser's disease (osteoporosis of the scaphoid-navicular bone) if left untreated for any length of time.

Differential diagnosis: a scaphoid-navicular fracture.

Issues & Ethics

The starting point guard on the men's basketball team, Stephen, comes to see you with his right hand cradled against his body. You quickly notice that he has sustained a boxer's fracture to his shooting hand. He pleads with you to tell his coach that he did this during the game last night and didn't realize it was broken until later in the evening. Unfortunately, Stephen broke it during a fight last night after the game. The athletic training staff has worked really hard to gain the trust and respect of all the athletes and coaches. When you were hired this year, the head athletic trainer made it very clear that this is the philosophy of the entire staff. You also understand that you have an ethical responsibility to tell the truth. Not doing so would negatively affect your relationship with the head athletic trainer and defraud the school's insurance carrier. However, not telling the truth in this case would keep the athlete on the team and foster his trust. What do you tell to whom?

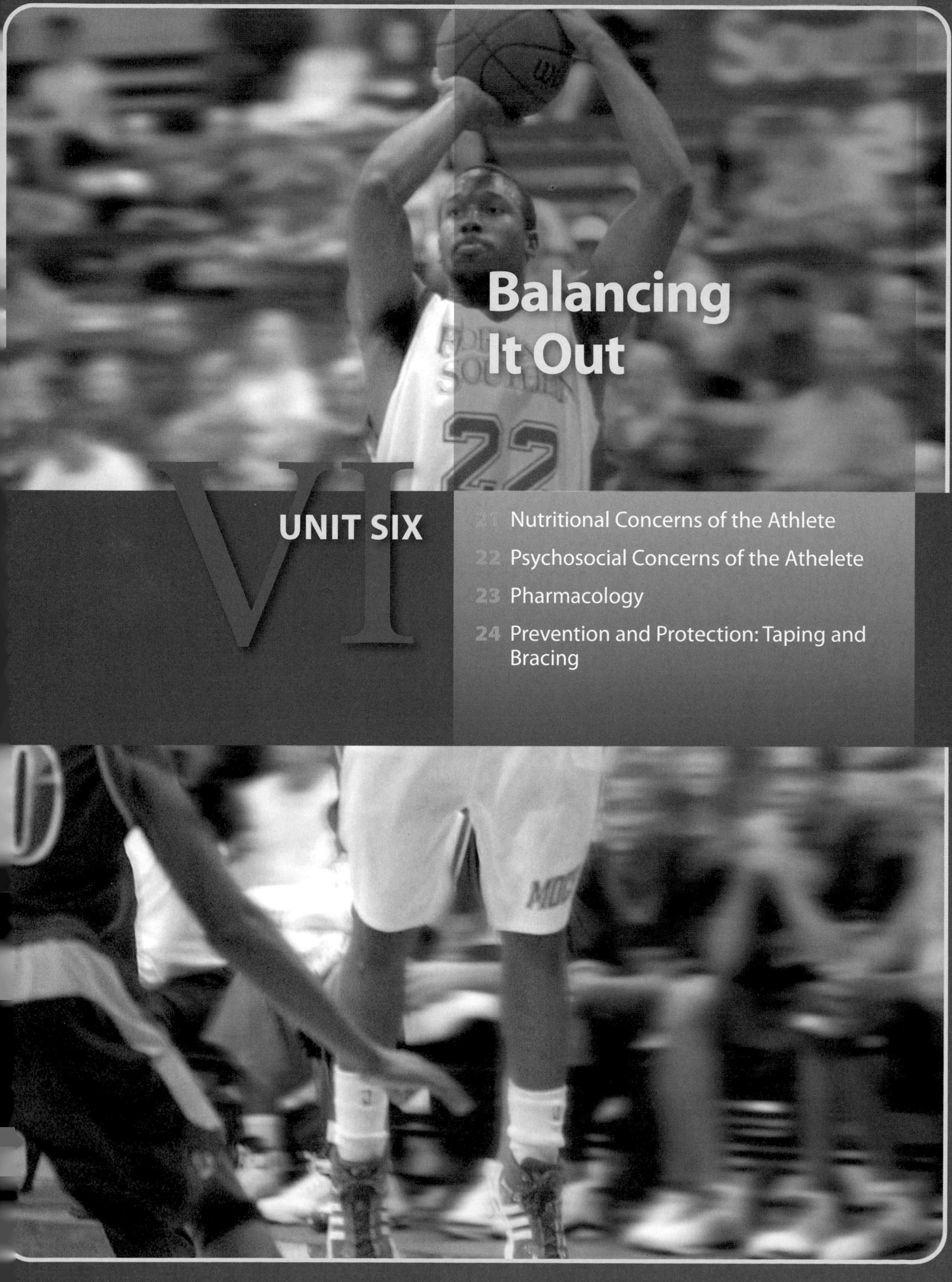

Balancing It Out

UNIT SIX

VI

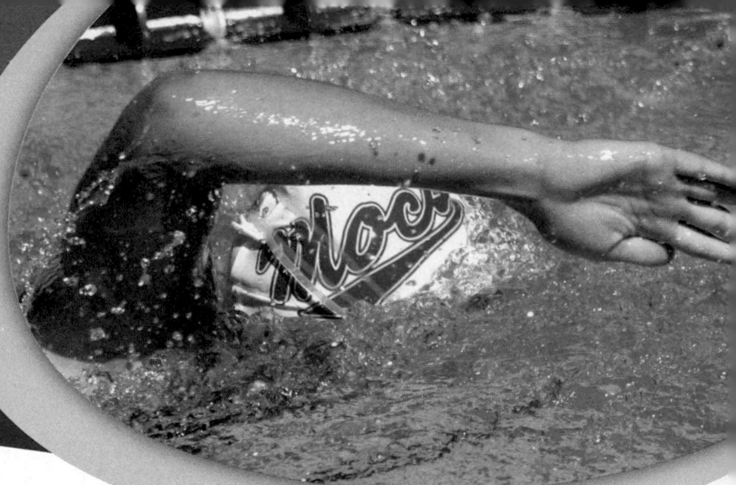

21

Nutritional Concerns of the Athlete

KATHLEEN M. LAQUALE

Learning Goals

1. Describe the key points regarding the six nutrients.
2. List the general nutritional demands for sports-related activity.
3. Identify methods to assess an athlete's dietary intake.
4. Illustrate the issues surrounding the use of performance enhancement substances by athletes.
5. Identify methods to evaluate performance enhancement substances.
6. List the characteristics of eating disorders.
7. Describe the team management approach to eating disorders in athletes.

A New England farmer was asked how his produce was performing this year. He replied, "The top soil is rich, but the deep soil, which nourishes the roots of the plants, is poor. Therefore my overall produce production is poor." This statement is an excellent analogy to describe the way athletes typically view sports nutrition. Athletes are quick to try a supplement or fad diet that looks good on the surface and promises great results. However, they may not realize the long-term effect of these products on their overall health performance. Other athletes simply disregard the basic guidelines for healthy nutrition, choosing a fast food meal or an energy bar for lunch instead of a turkey sandwich on whole wheat bread with a juice drink and an apple.

According to Barbara Day, RD, "nutrition is the bridge between ability and performance."[1] Likewise, energy intake from the six basic nutrients is the cornerstone of the athlete's performance. A proper balance of protein, carbohydrates, and fats is necessary to ensure sufficient energy. In addition, vitamins and minerals from fruits and vegetables are essential for recovery and injury prevention. Lastly, ingestion of fluids and adequate hydration can prevent fatigue and poor performance. To obtain proper nutrition, athletes should meet with a registered dietitian (RD) or a licensed dietary nutritionist (LDN) who is familiar with the unique nutritional demands of athletes. The RD or LDN should determine the athlete's specific energy intake (including energy expenditure) and the number of servings he or she requires daily from MyPyramid (formerly the Food Guide Pyramid; Figure 21-1). These professionals should also advise the athlete regarding good choices for pre-event and post-event meals as well as hydration.

According to Dr. Linda Houtkooper, a nutritionist should also educate the athlete about the three components of a healthy diet: variety, individualized meal planning, and moderation, or VIM (Box 21-1). Choosing a variety of foods during the week helps athletes make good food choices, prevents excessive intake of certain nutrients, and prevents boredom during mealtime[2] (Figure 21-2). Individualized meal planning allows athletes to customize their own dietary plans. An athlete is more likely to adhere to a self-created meal plan than one that has been imposed on him or her. Moderation in any dietary plan is critical to maintaining desired weight. Even ice cream may fit into someone's diet as long as the

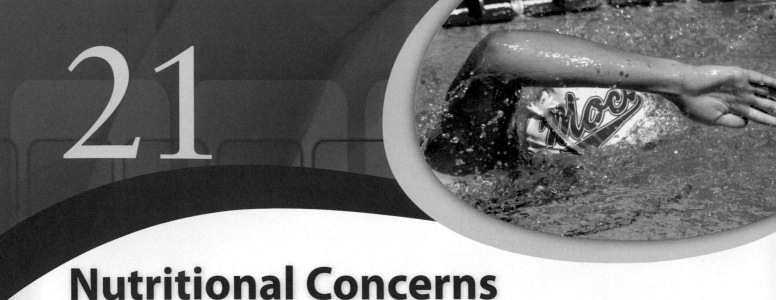

OPENING *Scenario*

Jim, a 19-year-old collegiate wrestler, is 20 pounds over his desired 126-pound weight classification. He has only 3 weeks to make his weight. He begins his weight loss program with a drastic reduction of energy intake (**calories**) and a large increase in energy expenditure (exercise). His daily diet consists of an 8-ounce glass of water and a banana for breakfast, a low-fat yogurt for lunch, and a salad with a piece of bread for dinner. His daily exercise program includes a 2-mile run in the morning before breakfast and a 2-mile run before dinner. He trains with weights 3 days a week for approximately 45 minutes per session.

After 5 days, Jim has lost 4 pounds. He is discouraged that he has not lost more weight. His fatigue level has increased, and his muscle endurance has decreased. After discussing the situation with his teammates, he purchases and tries creatine to help his endurance. Although the creatine seems to help his fatigue level a little, he is not losing weight quickly enough. He purchases another product that promises to burn fat. After a week on the fat-burning product, he has lost more weight but he begins to have headaches and develops insomnia. He attributes this to his weight loss, which is now at 12 pounds. He is still 6 pounds overweight 3 days before the weigh-in. He cuts out all water and finally makes the weight classification. The first practice of the season is the next day. The 2-mile run with the team before practice leaves him exhausted. The headaches are a daily occurrence now; he cannot focus in class, and he experiences heart palpitations whenever he exerts himself during exercise. He exhibits the same symptoms during the next few days of practice. After awhile, he develops the habit of bingeing whenever he eats, and the pounds start to accumulate again. During the season, he develops a stress fracture in his right lower leg. As a result of all the maladies he has suffered, Jim is forced to quit the wrestling team. Two weeks later, he has gained back every pound he lost.

basic nutrimental requirements have been met. Making healthier food choices during the competitive years will instill a pattern of healthier food choices later.

Points to Ponder

A competitive triathlete comes to you stating that he eats a can of tuna fish every day, along with other protein sources, to fulfill his protein requirements. Aside from the fact that his protein intake is excessive, how do you think this regimen affects his overall compliance and satisfaction with his diet plan?

THE SIX BASIC NUTRIENTS

The six basic nutrients are composed of the following elements: carbohydrates, proteins, fats, water, vitamins, and minerals (Table 21-1). Carbohydrates, protein, and fats (**macronutrients**) are the only nutrients that provide the body with energy. Water, vitamins, and minerals (**micronutrients**) do not provide energy but are involved in numerous chemical and physiological reactions that assist with the release of energy. For example, vitamin B_1, or thiamin, plays a critical role in the metabolism of glucose and is essential for the normal function of the nervous system. The body is kept in a delicate natural balance when all six basic nutrients are part of a consistent healthy diet.

Carbohydrates

Carbohydrates are organic compounds that contain carbon (C), hydrogen (H), and oxygen (O) molecules to form ($C_6H_{12}O_6$). There are two types of carbohydrates: simple carbohydrates (sugars) and complex carbohydrates (starches and fiber). **Simple carbohydrates** can be composed of simple sugars (monosaccharides), which are glucose (dextrose is the most abundant simple sugar), fructose (fruit sugar, the sweetest of all sugars), and galactose (sugar found in milk when linked to a glucose). In the body, energy supplied to the cells comes from glucose. Brain function also depends primarily on glucose for fuel. When two monosaccharides combine chemically, they form disaccharides. Common table sugar (sucrose) is a combination of two monosaccharides: glucose and fructose. Lactose, known as milk sugar, is a combination of glucose and galactose. Malt, or maltose, is a combination of two units of glucose. **Complex carbohydrates** are chains of two or more sugar

calorie energy intake in the form of food substances

macronutrients the nutrients that collectively provide most of the body's energy—carbohydrates, proteins, and fats

micronutrients substances necessary to the body in small amounts—vitamins and minerals

carbohydrates organic compounds that contain carbon (C), hydrogen (H), and oxygen (O) molecules to form ($C_6H_{12}O_6$)

simple carbohydrates substances composed of simple sugars, which are glucose, fructose and galactose; commonly considered empty calories

complex carbohydrates chains of two or more sugar molecules

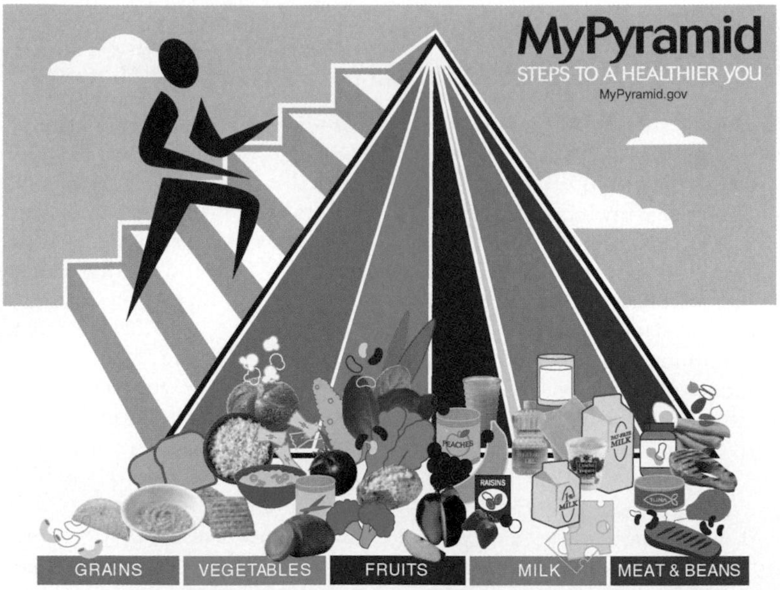

GRAINS Make half your grains whole	VEGETABLES Vary your veggies	FRUITS Focus on fruits	MILK Get your calcium-rich foods	MEAT & BEANS Go lean with protein
Eat at least 3 oz. of whole-grain cereals, breads, crackers, rice, or pasta every day 1 oz. is about 1 slice of bread, about 1 cup of breakfast cereal, or ½ cup of cooked rice, cereal, or pasta	Eat more dark-green veggies like broccoli, spinach, and other dark leafy greens Eat more orange vegetables like carrots and sweetpotatoes Eat more dry beans and peas like pinto beans, kidney beans, and lentils	Eat a variety of fruit Choose fresh, frozen, canned, or dried fruit Go easy on fruit juices	Go low-fat or fat-free when you choose milk, yogurt, and other milk products If you don't or can't consume milk, choose lactose-free products or other calcium sources such as fortified foods and beverages	Choose low-fat or lean meats and poultry Bake it, broil it, or grill it Vary your protein routine – choose more fish, beans, peas, nuts, and seeds
For a 2,000-calorie diet, you need the amounts below from each food group. To find the amounts that are right for you, go to MyPyramid.gov.				
Eat 6 oz. every day	Eat 2½ cups every day	Eat 2 cups every day	Get 3 cups every day; for kids aged 2 to 8, it's 2	Eat 5½ oz. every day

Find your balance between food and physical activity

- Be sure to stay within your daily calorie needs.
- Be physically active for at least 30 minutes most days of the week.
- About 60 minutes a day of physical activity may be needed to prevent weight gain.
- For sustaining weight loss, at least 60 to 90 minutes a day of physical activity may be required.
- Children and teenagers should be physically active for 60 minutes every day, or most days.

Know the limits on fats, sugars, and salt (sodium)

- Make most of your fat sources from fish, nuts, and vegetable oils.
- Limit solid fats like butter, stick margarine, shortening, and lard, as well as foods that contain these.
- Check the Nutrition Facts label to keep saturated fats, *trans* fats, and sodium low.
- Choose food and beverages low in added sugars. Added sugars contribute calories with few, if any, nutrients.

MyPyramid.gov
STEPS TO A HEALTHIER YOU

U.S. Department of Agriculture
Center for Nutrition Policy and Promotion
April 2005
CNPP-15
USDA

USDA is an equal opportunity provider and employer.

FIGURE 21-1 MyPyramid: Steps to a Healthier You. This miniposter provides an overview of MyPyramid, a customized version of the former Food Guide Pyramid, released in 2005. (From Center for Nutrition Policy and Promotion: *MyPyramid food guidance system mini-poster,* Washington, DC, 2005, U.S. Department of Agriculture. Accessed March 30, 2007, from www.mypyramid.gov/downloads/MiniPoster.pdf.)

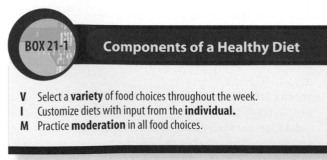

BOX 21-1 Components of a Healthy Diet

V Select a **variety** of food choices throughout the week.
I Customize diets with input from the **individual.**
M Practice **moderation** in all food choices.

Data from Dr. Linda Houtkooper, RD, University of Arizona, Tucson, Ariz.

molecules. There can be as few as three monosaccharides (short carbohydrate chains) or as many as one hundred to a thousand (long carbohydrate chains). Commonly known as polysaccharides, they include compounds such as glycogen (the storage form of carbohydrates in the liver and muscles) and starch.

Simple carbohydrates are commonly known as empty calories because they do not provide nutrients, just sugar. Examples of simple carbohydrates are soft drinks, white breads, and candy (Figure 21-3).

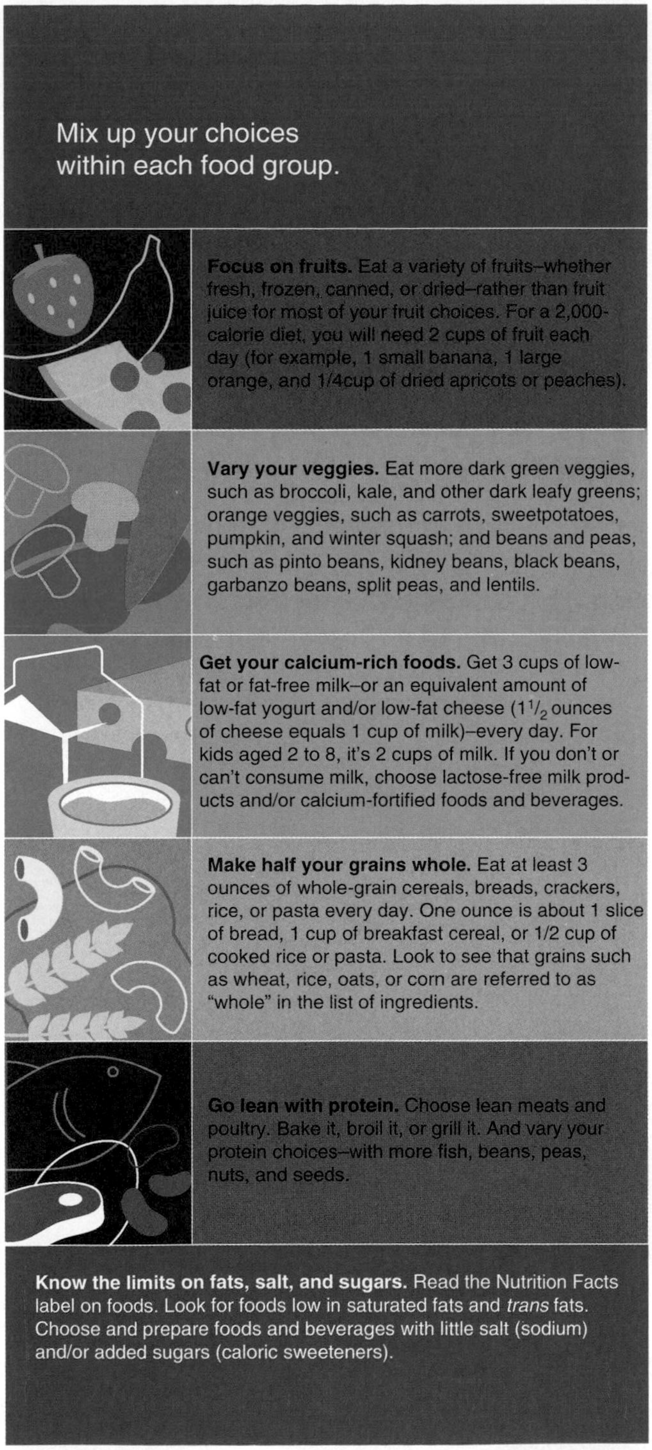
Mix up your choices
within each food group.
Focus on fruits. Eat a variety of fruits–whether fresh, frozen, canned, or dried–rather than fruit juice for most of your fruit choices. For a 2,000-calorie diet, you will need 2 cups of fruit each day (for example, 1 small banana, 1 large orange, and 1/4cup of dried apricots or peaches).
Vary your veggies. Eat more dark green veggies, such as broccoli, kale, and other dark leafy greens; orange veggies, such as carrots, sweetpotatoes, pumpkin, and winter squash; and beans and peas, such as pinto beans, kidney beans, black beans, garbanzo beans, split peas, and lentils.
Get your calcium-rich foods. Get 3 cups of low-fat or fat-free milk–or an equivalent amount of low-fat yogurt and/or low-fat cheese (1 1/2 ounces of cheese equals 1 cup of milk)–every day. For kids aged 2 to 8, it's 2 cups of milk. If you don't or can't consume milk, choose lactose-free milk products and/or calcium-fortified foods and beverages.
Make half your grains whole. Eat at least 3 ounces of whole-grain cereals, breads, crackers, rice, or pasta every day. One ounce is about 1 slice of bread, 1 cup of breakfast cereal, or 1/2 cup of cooked rice or pasta. Look to see that grains such as wheat, rice, oats, or corn are referred to as "whole" in the list of ingredients.
Go lean with protein. Choose lean meats and poultry. Bake it, broil it, or grill it. And vary your protein choices–with more fish, beans, peas, nuts, and seeds.
Know the limits on fats, salt, and sugars. Read the Nutrition Facts label on foods. Look for foods low in saturated fats and *trans* fats. Choose and prepare foods and beverages with little salt (sodium) and/or added sugars (caloric sweeteners).

FIGURE 21-2 Variety in food choices keeps the diet interesting and helps a person consume all the required nutrients. (From U.S. Department of Health and Human Services, U.S. Department of Agriculture: *Dietary guidelines for Americans 2005*, Washington, DC, 2005, Authors. Accessed March 30, 2007, from www.health.gov/dietaryguidelines/dga2005/document/media/FoodGroups.pdf).

TABLE 21-1 The Six Basic Nutrients

NUTRIENT	ENERGY RELATIONSHIP
Carbohydrates	Provides body with energy
Proteins	Provides body with energy
Fats	Provides body with energy
Water	Helps body produce energy
Vitamins	Helps body produce energy
Minerals	Helps body produce energy

Because simple carbohydrates enter the bloodstream very quickly with minimal digestion required, blood sugar levels tend to rise as well. With the release of insulin, a hormone produced in the pancreas, blood sugar levels can return to normal. When blood sugar levels drop, this is known as hypoglycemia. Alternatively, when blood sugar levels rise, this is known as *hyperglycemia*.

Ingestion of complex carbohydrates rather than simple sugars helps maintain blood sugar levels, which is particularly important for the athlete. Complex carbohydrates prevent the spiking of blood sugars that is often followed by an extreme drop in blood sugars. Because fructose does not require insulin for transportation into the cell, it is an exception. Thus fruits are a great travel food for athletes because they will not cause the peaks and valleys of blood sugar associated with glucose.

Complex carbohydrates, known as starches, provide many of the B vitamins necessary for energy metabolism. They are found in grains, breads, legumes, and fruit and are also known as **fiber** (Figure 21-4). Fiber is an indigestible complex carbohydrate. Complex carbohydrates have many health benefits. For example, a diet high in fiber promotes weight control by imparting a feeling of satiety without a correspondingly high number of calories. Soluble dietary fiber can slow glucose absorption in the small intestine and inhibit the absorption of cholesterol in the small intestine. Also, if enough fiber is consumed, the stool will be larger, thus stimulating the muscles of the large intestine and causing less strain during defecation.

The recommended intake of carbohydrates for the average person makes up 50% to 55% of the total daily energy intake. Some athletes, especially endurance athletes, may ingest as much as 65% to 70% of their total energy intake per day in carbohydrates, depending on their activity. Each carbohydrate provides 4 calories per gram.

fiber an indigestible complex carbohydrate

Protein

Proteins function in the body in numerous ways, including as enzymes and antibodies. They also transport key substances such as oxygen, vitamins, and minerals to the cells. **Amino acids** are the building blocks of protein. The body has 20 amino acids available to assist with bodily functions. Of the 20, nine are essential amino acids because the body must obtain them exclusively from food. Dietary sources of essential amino acids (i.e., histidine, isoleucine, leucine, lysine, methionine, phenylalanine, threonine, tryptophan, and valine) include eggs, dairy products, and meats (Figure 21-5). The body produces the remaining 11 when sufficient levels of nitrogen, carbon, hydrogen, and oxygen are available (Table 21-2).

Incomplete proteins are generally found in the form of plant proteins. These proteins lack one or more of the essential amino acids or contain insufficient amounts of one or more of the essential amino acids. The exception to this is soy protein, which is a complete protein. It was once falsely assumed that vegetarians needed to consume complementary proteins (two incomplete proteins) to create a whole protein. Although we do not store protein, the body has an amino acid pool that provides amino acids daily for the body to use. The protein in this amino acid pool can be used for protein synthesis, energy production, or the formation of new glucose through gluconeogenesis.

The **Dietary Reference Intake** (DRI) for protein intake is 0.8 gram per kilogram of body weight. For example, a 125-pound female would require 46 grams of protein per day. This equates to roughly 12% to 15% of her total energy intake per day. Protein is synthesized in the body at the rate of 300 grams per day. The amount of protein athletes require is somewhat controversial. Although some experts believe levels of 1.2 to 1.4 are adequate for the body builder and endurance athlete, others maintain that levels of 1.7 to 2.0 are appropriate. However, amounts greater than 1.4 grams/kg/body weight do not contribute to muscle building but rather to energy production, which is not favorable for these athletes. Each gram of protein contains four calories.

Despite the debate, one fact seems certain: Most people, weekend athletes and competitive body builders alike, consume far too much protein. A typical diet

proteins amino acids that assist with enzymes, antibodies, and the transportation of key substances such as oxygen, vitamins, and minerals to the cells

amino acids the building blocks of protein; there are nine essential ones

Dietary Reference Intake framework of nutrient standards that has replaced the old RDAs (recommended daily allowances)

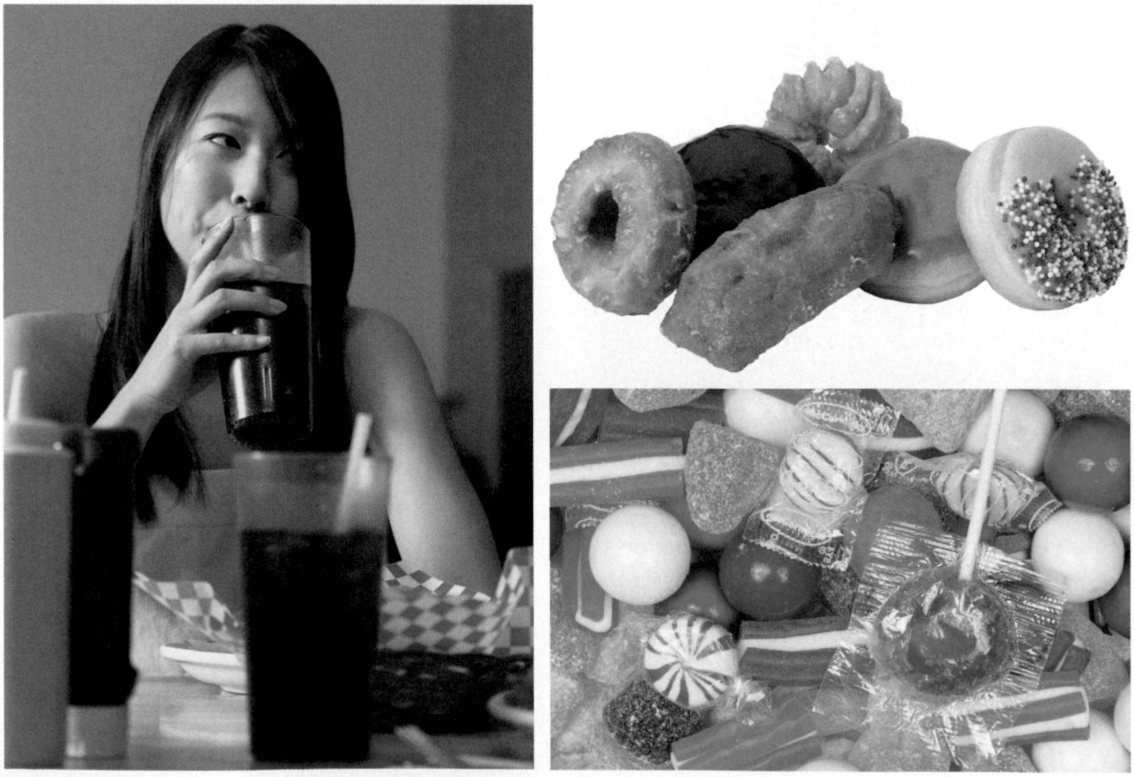

FIGURE 21-3 Simple carbohydrates are frequently referred to as *empty calories* and mainly consist of sugars and white breads. (Copyright 2007 JupiterImages Corporation.)

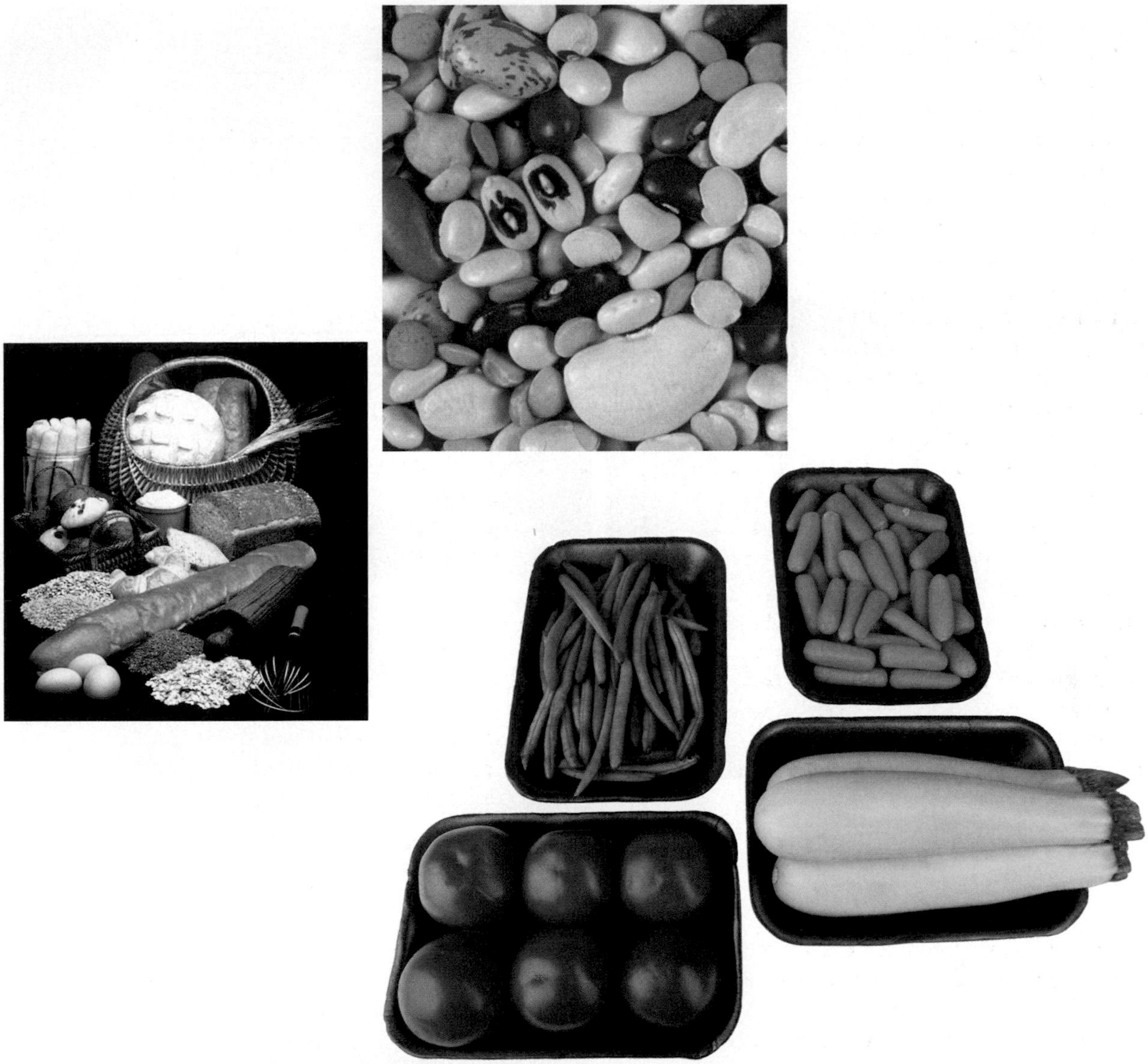

FIGURE 21-4 Complex carbohydrates are known as *starches* and mainly consist of grains, legumes, and fruits. (Copyright 2007 JupiterImages Corporation.)

usually provides more than enough protein for most people; the concern should be with the quality of protein intake. High-quality protein provides all of the essential amino acids in the amounts that the body needs, offers sufficient additional amino acids to serve as nitrogen sources for synthesis of nonessential amino acids, and is easy to digest. Because protein supplements are not regulated, their protein quality is questionable.

Fats

Known as **lipids**, fats perform several functions within the body, from insulation to neurotransmission and provision of energy for muscle contractions. Fatty acids, which make up a typical lipid, are attached to a glycerol base. The fatty acids differ in chain length and saturation. Structurally, if all the double bonds on the chain are full, the fatty acid is called a *saturated fatty acid*. A fatty acid with one double bond available is a **monounsaturated fatty acid** (MUFA). A fatty acid with two or more double bonds is a **polyunsaturated fatty acid** (PUFA).

Food fats are classified by the mixture of fatty acid types (saturated or unsaturated) and overall fatty acid content. Thus a food fat would not contain only MUFAs or only PUFAs. A food fat that contains higher amounts of MUFAs, such as olive oil, is classified as a MUFA. Corn

lipids fats

monounsaturated fatty acid a fatty acid with one double bond available; MUFA

polyunsaturated fatty acid a fatty acid with two or more double bonds; PUFA

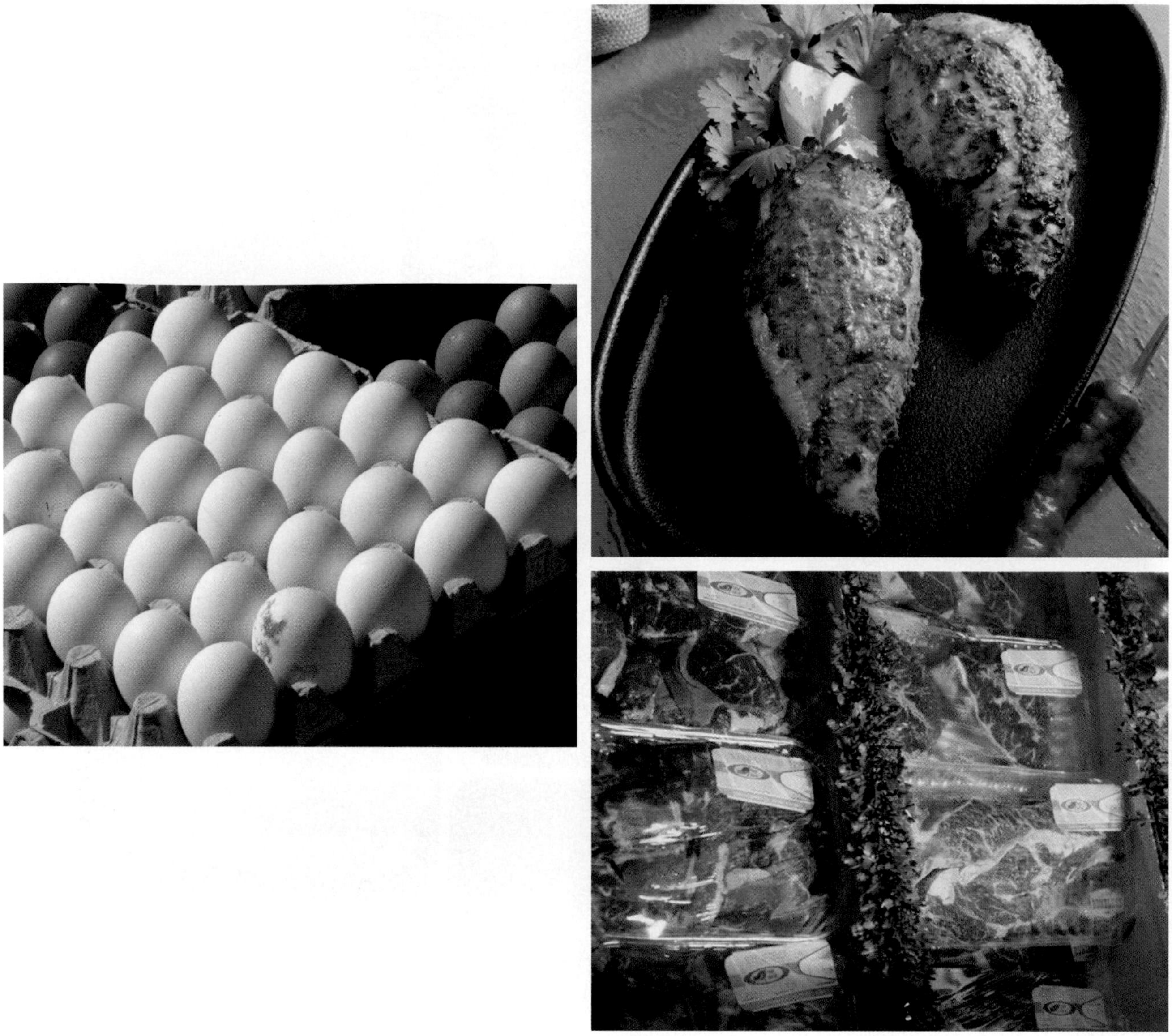

FIGURE 21-5 Protein selections containing the nine essential amino acids include foods such as eggs, meats, and soy. (Copyright 2007 JupiterImages Corporation.)

TABLE 21-2 Amino Acids

AMINO ACIDS	SOURCES
Essential (9)	From the diet: eggs, dairy, meat
Others (11)	Produced in the body: require the presence of nitrogen, carbon, hydrogen, and oxygen

oil has higher amounts of PUFAs and is therefore classified as a PUFA. Chocolate and butter have higher amounts of saturated fats and are classified as saturated fats. Saturated fats should be used in moderation to reduce the risk of cardiovascular disease. Unfortunately, many athletes are so fat-phobic that they do not consume any types of fat, even the ones that perform necessary functions. Two of the most important essential fatty acids are linoleic (omega-6) and linolenic (omega-3) fatty acids. Omega 3 is important because it has the potential to reduce the risk of vascular disease (Figure 21-6).

The amount of fat from the diet should be roughly 30% of the daily dietary intake. This can be broken down to 10% saturated fatty acids, 10% MUFAs, and 10% PUFAs. Each gram of fat contains 9 calories, nearly twice the amount of energy of carbohydrates.

Table 21-3 summarizes the three basic food groups. The recommended daily intake is for the average person; variances will occur depending on the specific demands of the sport or activities of daily living. The number of calories derived from each food group illustrates the energy balance between carbohydrates, proteins, and

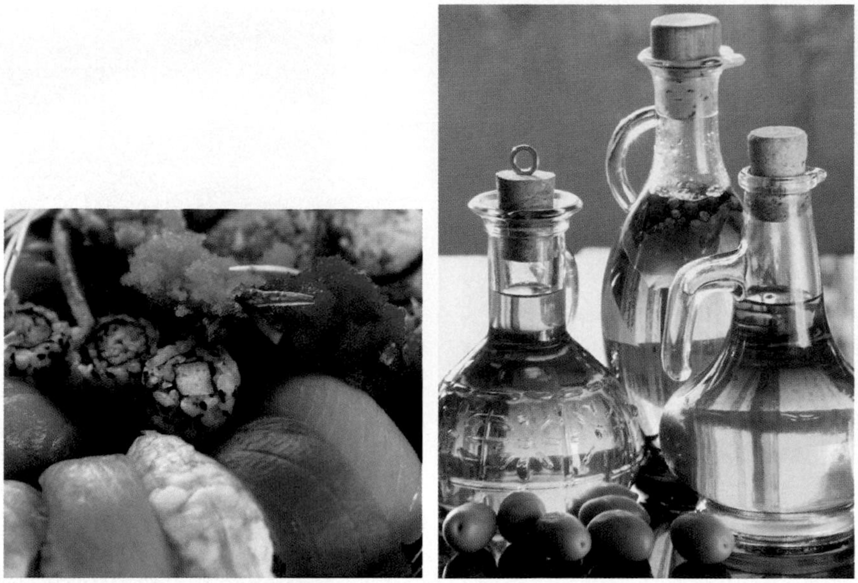

FIGURE 21-6 Fats that should be included in the daily diet include fish and olive oil. (Copyright 2007 JupiterImages Corporation.)

TABLE 21-3 Three Basic Food Groups

FOOD GROUP	FUNCTION	SOURCES	% DAILY DIET	CALORIES/GRAM
Carbohydrates	Provide energy or fuel; energy metabolism; fiber to aid in digestion	*Simple:* sugars in soft drinks, white breads, candy *Complex:* grains, bread, legumes, fruits	50–55	4
Proteins	Enzymes; antibodies; transportation of key substances such as oxygen, vitamins, and minerals to the cells	Eggs, dairy, meats, soy	12–15	4
Fats	Insulation; neurotransmission processes; energy for muscle contractions	Oils, nuts, avocado	30	9

fats. Athletic trainers should remember to incorporate the VIM approach in daily and weekly meal planning.

Water

The one nutrient without which the body cannot live is water; it is used in every physiological process of the body. Water performs many other functions, from cooling the body in warm weather or illness to facilitating metabolism. Approximately one third of our body is water. Muscles contain roughly 75% water. Because men tend to have more lean tissue and less fat than women, men also tend to have more body water. Electrolytes (i.e., sodium, potassium, and magnesium) bathe in water. To survive, each cell must contain a balance of electrolytes and water. Although many people have survived without food for weeks, no one can live without water for more than a few days.

Hydration refers to the amount of water that the body contains at any given moment. It can affect physical and mental performance either positively or negatively. If the body is **dehydrated**, or low on water, by as little as 3%, performance can be affected. Blood sugar and blood pressure levels rise during dehydration. Thirst may indicate dehydration, but it is not always reliable because fluid levels can be depleted long before a person actually feels thirsty. Athletic trainers should advise their clients to anticipate their water needs throughout their activities, particularly when they are exercising in new surroundings or in areas with unfamiliar altitudes, temperatures, or humidity levels. The use of a rehydration drink or sports drink also may help prevent dehydration in these environments (Figure 21-7).

Normal body functions such as sweating, elimination of wastes, and breathing cause water to be lost on

hydration the amount of water that the body contains at any given moment

dehydration a state in which the body is low on water

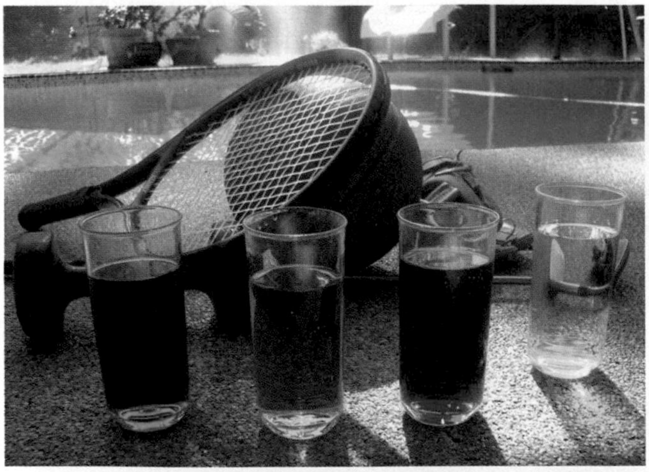

FIGURE 21-7 Rehydration drinks can help prevent dehydration.

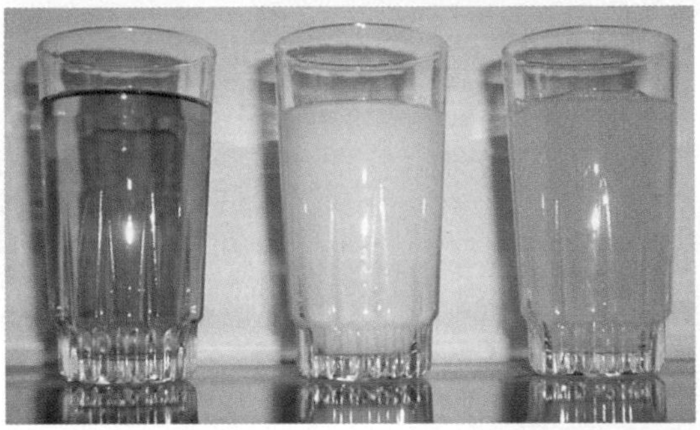

FIGURE 21-8 Color grades in urine help identify dehydration and range in color from apple juice (darkest) to lighter than lemon juice (lightest). Dark urine may indicate dehydration.

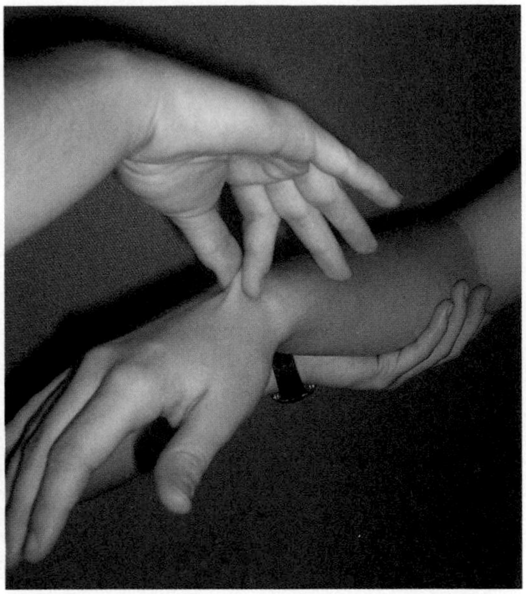

FIGURE 21-9 Pinching the skin on the back of the hand may help assess dehydration. Skin that quickly responds and returns to normal indicates proper hydration.

an ongoing basis. For example, exercising generates metabolic heat, which travels from the core through the blood to the skin for evaporation. Approximately 2 or more liters of water may be lost from the body during these functions. This water loss must constantly be replaced. Generally, drinking six to eight glasses of water (2.5 liters of water) is required for the average person, but athletes clearly need more. The NATA Position Paper, "Fluids and hydration for specific guidelines for athletes" (www.nata.org/publicinformation/position.htm), provides more information on this subject[3]

One way to tell whether you are properly hydrated is to check the color of your urine to see whether it is the color of apple juice or lemon juice or if it is lighter than lemon juice (Figure 21-8). The darker the color of the urine (apple juice), the more dehydrated you are; the lighter the color (lighter than lemon juice), the more hydrated you are. Be aware that some medications and vitamins can darken the urine. If you are not taking drugs or vitamins and your urine is dark in color, you may be dehydrated. Another method to check for dehydration is to pinch the skin on the back of your hand with your index finger and thumb and then release it. If it is still standing or raised after you release it, you may be dehydrated. The faster your skin snaps back to normal, the more hydrated you are (Figure 21-9).

Vitamins

Vitamins are classified as water-soluble or fat-soluble. The main difference between the two types lies in the way the body absorbs, transports, and then stores the vitamins. Water-soluble vitamins are identified as the B-complex vitamins as well as vitamin C. As water-soluble vitamins, they are absorbed in the intestinal cells and delivered directly to the bloodstream. Fat-soluble vitamins, which are vitamins A, D, E, and K, are absorbed or soluble in fat. Vitamins play a major role in the function, growth, and maintenance of numerous body tissues. As with anything else, however, they must be used in moderation; Table 21-4 lists the safe limits of intake for the various vitamins.

Vitamins do not provide energy to the body during activity because they do not contain any calories. Many athletes believe that vitamins are a safety net—if they skip a meal, all they need to do is take a daily vitamin and they will meet their nutritional requirements. However, vitamins require food to be absorbed, especially the fat-soluble vitamins. Athletes and nonathletes alike also believe that if one vitamin is good, then ten are better. Taking vitamins in amounts greater than the DRI as noted in Table 21-4 may elevate existing levels, which could lead to toxicity. If an athlete is eating three meals a day, a daily multivitamin should be taken every other day to prevent toxic buildup.

Minerals

Minerals are classified as major (100 mg/day or more required) or trace (less than 100 mg/day required) on the

TABLE 21-4 Safe Limits for Vitamins

VITAMIN	FUNCTION	DAILY VALUE	TOLERABLE UPPER INTAKE LEVEL
Vitamin A (retinol)	Vision Bone growth	5000 IU	10,000 IU
Vitamin B1 (thiamine)	Energy production Bone growth Heart functions Nervous system Digestive system	1.5 mg	None set
Vitamin B2 (riboflavin)	Energy production Red blood cell formation Antibody production Skin Hair Nails Thyroid regulation	1.7 mg	None set
Vitamin B3 (niacin)	Energy metabolism DNA repair	20 mg	35 mg
Vitamin B6 (pyridoxine)	Red blood cell production Na/K balance	2 mg	100 mg
Vitamin B9 (folic acid)	Cell production Cell maintenance DNA replication	400 mcg	1000 mcg (1 mg)
Vitamin B12 (cyanocobalamin)	Energy production	6 mcg	None set
Vitamin C (ascorbic acid)	Antioxidant Metabolic reactions Prevents scurvy	90 mg	2000 mg
Vitamin D (ergocalciferol and cholecalciferol)	Bone functions Regulates blood Immune system	400 IU	2000 IU
Vitamin E (tocopherol)	Antioxidant Protects cells from free radicals	30 IU (synthetic)	1100 IU (synthetic)
Vitamin K (naphthoquinone)	Blood clotting Bone functions	80 mcg	None set

Data from Food and Nutrition Board, Institute of Medicine: Dietary reference intakes for calcium, phosphorus, magnesium, vitamin D, and fluoride (1997); Dietary reference intakes for thiamin, riboflavin, niacin, vitamin B_6, folate, vitamin B_{12}, pantothenic acid, biotin, and choline (1998); Dietary reference intakes for vitamin C, vitamin E, selenium, and carotenoids (2000); and Dietary reference intakes for vitamin A, vitamin K, arsenic, boron, chromium, copper, iodine, manganese, molybdenum, nickel, silicon, vanadium, and zinc (2001), Washington, DC, National Academies Press [www.nap.edu].

basis of the amount needed in the diet and the amount of the mineral in the body. Whether the mineral is a major or trace mineral, the amount does not diminish its importance in the body. Calcium, sodium, iron, and potassium are some of the minerals that athletes in particular require. Unlike vitamins, minerals are not changed during digestion or when the body uses them. Like vitamins, taking in levels above the DRI will not improve performance. In fact, taking higher amounts of one mineral may affect the absorption of another mineral. For example, excessive amounts of iron inhibit the absorption of copper, which plays an important role in energy metabolism. Table 21-5 summarizes the recommended allowances for minerals.

Points to Ponder

An athlete believes that the supplements he is taking are the only reason his performance has improved. What do you tell him and why?

PHYSICAL DEMANDS OF SPORT

As discussed in Chapter 8, each sport exerts a physiological (aerobic or anaerobic) demand on the body. These demands vary according to the sport, the athlete's sex, and the number of minutes that the athlete performs during a given work-out or competition. For example, the energy expended, or calories burned, by a woman during a marathon is different from the energy expended by a male during a 100-meter sprint. Many textbooks on exercise physiology provide tables to determine the number of calories burned per minute during a certain activity. Quite often, the athlete's energy intake is well below the energy intake needed for their normal daily activities, never mind the energy expended during the activity itself. Matching the appropriate energy intake in calories with the physical or physiological demands of the activity is challenging, but it is the only way to maintain body weight.

Maintaining Ideal Body Weight

Ideal body weight is influenced by two factors: physiological concerns and the specific demands of the activity. Physiological concerns include the individual's muscle size, bone density, and subcutaneous fat. The demands of the activity take into account factors such as the size, strength, power, and energy required for successful participation in the activity. In all sports, success depends on the athlete's ability to sustain anaerobic and aerobic power as well as the athlete's ability to overcome resistance or drag. Athletes strive to achieve the ideal body weight with the hope of achieving optimal performance. However, ideal body weight does not always guarantee optimal performance.[4] Weight alone is not the precursor to athletic success. The truly accomplished athlete excels in speed, agility, balance, core strength, flexibility, neuromuscular control, and many other components of athleticism.

Several formulas may be used to determine ideal body weight (IBW), two of which are discussed here. The first

TABLE 21-5 Safe Limits for Minerals

MINERAL	FUNCTION	DAILY VALUE	TOLERABLE UPPER INTAKE LEVEL
Calcium	Muscle contractions Blood clotting Bone functions Nerve impulses Fluid balance Heartbeat regulation	1000 mg	2500 mg
Chromium	Cellular catalyst Weight control	120 mcg	None set
Copper	Blood enzymes Electron transport	2 mg	10 mg
Iron	Enzymes Cellular respiration Oxygen transport	18 mg	45 mg
Magnesium	Enzymes DNA synthesis RNA synthesis	320 mg (RDA/woman)	350 mg
Phosphorus	ATP transport Bone functions DNA functions RNA functions	1000 mg	4000 mg
Selenium	Thyroid function	70 mcg	400 mcg
Zinc	Enzymes	15 mg	40 mg
Potassium	Cell mortality Fluid balance Electrolyte balance Muscle contractions Nerve impulses	3000 mg	None
Sodium	Blood regulation Fluid regulation Nerve impulses Heart activity Metabolism	2400 mg	None
Boron		None set	20 mg
Iodine		150 mcg	1100 mcg
Manganese		2 mg	11 mg
Molybdenum		75 mcg	2000 mcg
Nickel		5 mcg	1 mg
Vanadium		10 mcg	1.8 mg

Data from Food and Nutrition Board, Institute of Medicine: Dietary reference intakes for calcium, phosphorus, magnesium, vitamin D, and fluoride (1997); Dietary reference intakes for thiamin, riboflavin, niacin, vitamin B_6, folate, vitamin B_{12}, pantothenic acid, biotin, and choline (1998); Dietary reference intakes for vitamin C, vitamin E, selenium, and carotenoids (2000); and Dietary reference intakes for vitamin A, vitamin K, arsenic, boron, chromium, copper, iodine, manganese, molybdenum, nickel, silicon, vanadium, and zinc (2001), Washington, DC, National Academies Press [www.nap.edu].

BOX 21-2 **Calculating Gender-Specific Ideal Body Weight with Height**

Female athletes: 100 lbs + 5 lbs for each inch over 5 feet in height
Male athletes: 105 lbs + 6 lbs for each inch over 5 feet in height

method calculates IBW according to gender-specific formulas using height (Box 21-2). First, the athletic trainer measures the height of the client. The formula for IBW for women is calculated starting from 5 feet in height. For every inch in height over five feet, add 5 pounds to 100 pounds. For example, the IBW for a woman who is 5′3″ is 115 pounds (Figure 21-10). The formula to calculate the IBW for men is much the same. With men, however, it is necessary to add six pounds to 105 pounds for every inch in height over 5 feet.

The second method to determine IBW is known as **body mass index** (BMI). This method is calculated using height and weight (Box 21-3). BMI is determined by dividing a person's weight by his or her height squared. For example, a person who weighs 180 lbs and is 5′11″ would have a BMI of 25.3.

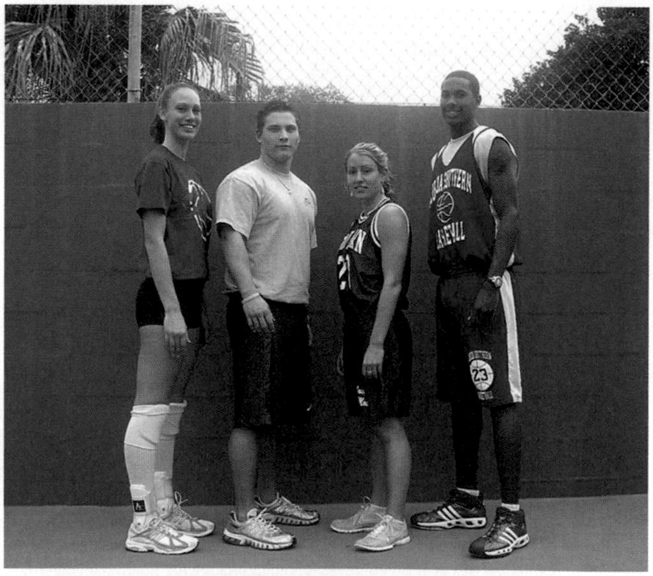

FIGURE 21-10 These athletes clearly show the range of dramatic physical differences between male and female athletes, as well as differences among same-gender athletes.

body mass index measure in which body weight is divided by height; BMI

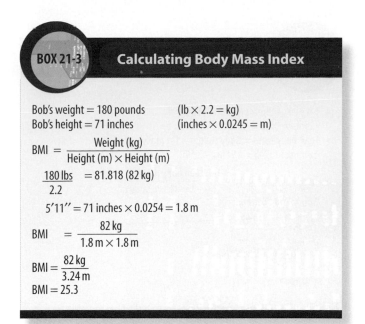

BOX 21-3 Calculating Body Mass Index

Bob's weight = 180 pounds (lb × 2.2 = kg)
Bob's height = 71 inches (inches × 0.0245 = m)

$$\text{BMI} = \frac{\text{Weight (kg)}}{\text{Height (m)} \times \text{Height (m)}}$$

$$\frac{180\ \text{lbs}}{2.2} = 81.818\ (82\ \text{kg})$$

$$5'11'' = 71\ \text{inches} \times 0.0254 = 1.8\ \text{m}$$

$$\text{BMI} = \frac{82\ \text{kg}}{1.8\ \text{m} \times 1.8\ \text{m}}$$

$$\text{BMI} = \frac{82\ \text{kg}}{3.24\ \text{m}}$$

$$\text{BMI} = 25.3$$

Once the BMI is obtained, that number is used to determine the person's weight status. Table 21-6 shows the weight status for BMI ranges. This individual would be classified as overweight, with an increased risk for heart disease and other conditions as defined by the guidelines published by the Centers for Disease Control and Prevention (CDC; see Appendix E).

Note that these two methods are not accurate for individuals who work out daily and have a greater muscle density. For example, Shaquille O'Neal, of the Miami Heat, stands at 7′1″, weighs 335 pounds, has a BMI of 32.7. Simply stated, muscle weighs more than fat. Technically, because fat tissue is approximately 20% less dense than muscle, it takes up more space. Muscle burns 19 times more calories than fat. Therefore a pound of muscle takes up less space and burns more calories than a pound of fat. An athlete who is 5′3″ and weighs 135 pounds may be overweight but not excessively fat. Advising that athlete to lose weight could put her at risk for disordered eating patterns, a loss of muscle mass and strength, increased potential for injury, and a decrease in performance. Generally speaking, however, athletes should stay within 2.3 kilograms (5 pounds) of their IBW.

TABLE 21-6 Body Mass Index Weight Status

BMI	WEIGHT STATUS
Below 18.5	Underweight
18.5–24.9	Normal
25.0–29.9	Overweight
30.0 and above	Obese

From Centers for Disease Control and Prevention: *BMI—Body mass index: About BMI for adults*, Bethesda, Md, [no date], U.S. Department of Health and Human Services. Accessed March 30, 2007, from www.cdc.gov/nccdphp/dnpa/bmi/adult_BMI/about_adult_BMI.htm.

Regular Exercise

Regular exercise helps a person achieve and maintain IBW. In addition, regular exercise provides the following benefits:

- It enhances the body's ability to use fat for fuel and helps maintain muscle, both factors in achieving optimal body composition.
- It improves blood circulation and lowers the risk for high blood pressure and osteoporosis.
- It improves the body's blood-sugar tolerance, which reduces the risk for heart disease and diabetes.
- It reduces stress, improves quality of sleep, creates higher levels of energy, and suppresses appetite.
- It increases self-confidence, self-esteem, and emotional well-being.

An athlete who participates in a varsity sport or another competitive activity usually exercises daily (Figure 21-11). This daily activity maintains the athlete's body weight because their energy expenditure is greater than or equal to their energy intake. Regular participation can also set the stage for a lifelong commitment to regular exercise. For the nonathlete, exercise recommendations take into account the frequency, intensity, and duration of activity (Table 21-7).

THE HEALTHY DIET

A healthy diet or meal plan provides adequate energy intake (calories), supplies nutrients in the needed amounts, and maintains hydration. No single food or supplement can do any of the aforementioned.[4] Energy intake from the six basic nutrients is the cornerstone of the athlete's performance. A proper balance of protein, carbohydrates, and fats is needed to ensure sufficient energy. In addition, vitamins and minerals from fruits and vegetables are essential for recovery and injury prevention. Lastly, ingestion of fluids and adequate hydration can prevent fatigue and poor performance. Athletes should refer to MyPyramid, mentioned earlier in this chapter, for the recommended number of daily servings per food group for the average person.[5]

TABLE 21-7 Activity Recommendations for the Non-Athlete

EXERCISE CHARACTERISTIC	AMOUNT
Frequency	Three to five times per week
Intensity	60% to 80% of maximum heart rate
Duration	30 to 60 minutes per session

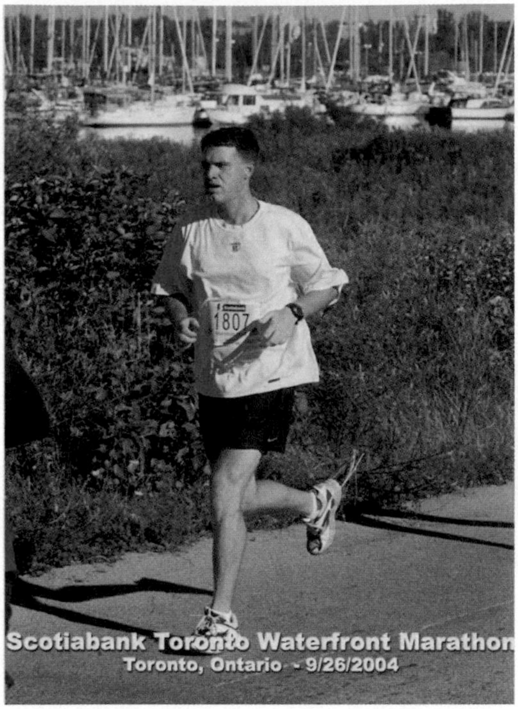

FIGURE 21-11 The average person interested in maintaining a healthy lifestyle needs to balance exercise frequency, intensity, and duration when planning an exercise regimen.

Determining Healthy Weight

A healthy body weight, or target weight, can be determined using the body-fat percentage as the guide to weight loss. Once the athlete's percentage of body fat and lean body mass (LBM) has been calculated, a target body weight formula can be determined. Target body weight is calculated according to body weight, percentage of body fat, and LBM in pounds. For example, an athlete who weighs 154 pounds and has 24% body fat should compete with a target body fat between 20% and 21%, with target body weights being 146 and 148 pounds, respectively. Box 21-4 provides a sample calculation of fat mass, lean body mass, and target body weight. This example shows that the athlete's target body weight, in accordance with the predetermined LBM goals, would range from 146 pounds to 148 pounds.

Determining Energy Intake

When determining an athlete's required energy intake or calories, the athletic trainer should take into consideration the age, gender, and weight of the athlete along with his or her level of daily activity. A calorie is a unit of energy equivalent to the amount used to raise the temperature of a gram of water 1 degree centigrade. Food is measured in kilocalories. There are a thousand calories in one kilocalorie. Kilojoules (kJ) are used to measure the energy contained in food items. One calorie equals 4.18 kilojoules, even though the standard term is *calorie*.

BOX 21-4 Calculating Target Body Weight with Lean Body Mass

- Fat mass = Body weight × % Body fat
  Example: 37 lb = 154 lb × 0.24
- Lean body mass = Body weight − Fat mass
  Example: 117 lb = 154 lbs − 37 lb
- $\text{Target body weight} = \dfrac{\text{Lean body mass}}{1.0 - \text{Desired \% body fat}}$

  Example at 20% body fat

  $146 \text{ lbs} = \dfrac{117 \text{ lbs}}{1.0 - 0.20}$

  Example at 21% body fat

  $148 \text{ lbs} = \dfrac{117 \text{ lbs}}{1.0 - 0.21}$

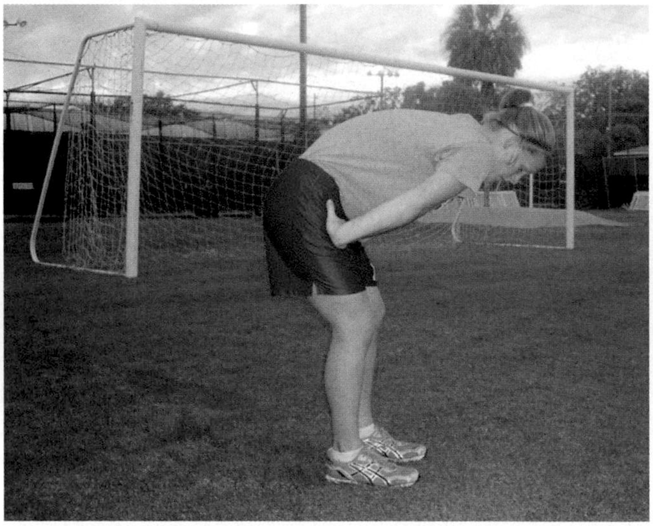

FIGURE 21-12 Maintaining an energy balance is one factor that allows athletes to perform at peak levels.

Energy balance, or caloric balance, is when energy intake from food and fluids equals energy expenditure (Figure 21-12). **Energy expenditure** is the sum of all energy expended as basal metabolism, the thermic effect of food, and any voluntary physical activity.[6] Just meeting the caloric intake required for daily activity is a common misconception. In fact, many athletes eat far below their necessary energy intake. Surveys completed by athletes indicate their food choices include low intakes of carbo-

energy balance caloric balance; when energy intake from food and fluids equals energy expenditure

energy expenditure the sum of all energy expended as basal metabolism, the thermic effect of food, and any voluntary physical activity hydrates and fiber and a lowered intake of salads and vegetables. Protein intake was found to be higher than the recommended amount for athletes.[7]

Studies have indicated that a lowered energy intake can affect an athlete's health and performance.[8] As energy intake decreases, fat and LBM are used for fuel. When muscle levels decline, decreases in power and endurance also occur. The effects of acute reduced energy availability and chronic energy deficiency on reproductive function can affect the female athlete. Intense training programs that are insufficiently fueled by energy intake may lead to fatigue, impaired performance, and a broad spectrum of menstrual disturbances in women.[9] For the competitive athlete, the consumption of energy nutrients can help fuel physical efforts and promote efficient recovery and adaptation.[10] However, basic nutrient requirements (i.e., water, carbohydrates, protein, fat, vitamins, and minerals) must first be met, whereupon adjustments may be made in the meal plan for additional energy expenditure during a practice or competition.

In the calculation of energy intake for an athlete, it is the intensity, frequency, and duration of the exercise that determines the overall energy expended during an activity. Greater body mass increases the work required to perform weight-bearing activities, whereas skills developed in training reduce the energy cost of exercise by increasing efficiency and conserving energy expended during activity. Adjustment of the athlete's energy intake will change when energy expenditure decreases (e.g., during injury rehabilitation or before and after the playing season).[11] An athlete's energy intake must be at least 1500 kilocalories daily to prevent a vitamin or mineral deficiency.[12].

The Harris Benedict formula is one method to determine daily energy intake (Box 21-5).[13] It uses the athlete's gender, height, weight, and age to determine the **basal metabolic rate** (BMR). BMR is the amount of energy in calories needed on a daily basis when the body is at rest. The BMR is then multiplied by an activity multiplier to determine the total daily energy intake. This formula is more accurate than using total body weight (TBW) alone. TBW determined on a scale can tell the athlete only how much resistance his or her body is providing against gravity. TBW does not take into account the athlete's bone and muscle density, frame size, gender, or activity level. Because muscle mass is denser and weighs more than fat, TBW often represents an overestimation of the athlete's weight. An increase in TBW can be due to an increase in dense muscle tissue but is often blamed on an increase in fat tissue.

One drawback to the Harris Benedict formula is the absence of LBM in the calculation. Because leaner bodies require more calories, the formula will underestimate the daily caloric needs for athletes who are very muscular. This calculation is merely an estimate of the energy needs required by an athlete. Depending on the sport and intensity, the energy intake may vary with regard to specific nutrients. For example, female marathon runners require at least 5 grams of carbohydrates per kilogram of body weight to maintain glycogen stores.[14] During intense activity (≥90 min/day), endurance athletes may require 8 to 10 grams per kilogram of body weight daily for men and 6 to 8 grams per kilogram of body weight daily for women. Protein intake will vary as well. The DRI for protein is set at 8 grams per kilogram of body weight daily. A power lifter or endurance athlete may require 1.2 to 1.4 grams of protein per kilogram of body weight daily. The increased amount of carbohydrates or protein required may change the number of servings from the food groups.

It is important to note that the aforementioned amount does not include the energy intake required for the athlete's wrestling practice itself. Thus an activity factor or activity multiplier must be used in the calculation as well. This multiplier depends on the athlete's particular activity (see Box 21-5). The activity multiplier of 1.2 to 1.9 must then be factored into the formula. The wrestler has daily practices for 2 hours each day; in addition, he runs 2 to 3 miles every morning. His activity multiplier would be 1.5. The result from the energy intake determined in the previous equation (1682.5 kcal/d) is then multiplied by 1.5 (activity multiplier). His total energy intake, including his energy expenditure for daily practice, would be

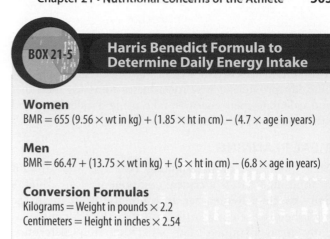

BOX 21-5 Harris Benedict Formula to Determine Daily Energy Intake

Women

BMR = 655 (9.56 × wt in kg) + (1.85 × ht in cm) − (4.7 × age in years)

Men

BMR = 66.47 + (13.75 × wt in kg) + (5 × ht in cm) − (6.8 × age in years)

Conversion Formulas

Kilograms = Weight in pounds × 2.2
Centimeters = Height in inches × 2.54

Example

A wrestler is 5′7″ (67″× 2.54 = 170 cm), 16 years old, and weighs 140 pounds. According to this formula, he requires 1682.5 kcalories per day.

Activity Multipliers

Sedentary activity	1.2
Moderate activity	1.3
Very active	1.5
Very heavy daily activity	1.9

basal metabolic rate the amount of energy in calories needed on a daily basis when the body is at rest; BMR

2523.8 kilocalories daily, or 2500 kilocalories daily. The final total of daily kilocalories is what the body requires to maintain its current weight. The Web site www.nat.uiuc.edu provides a way for athletes to assess their diet and calculate their energy intake using a calculator and other automated methods.[15]

MEAL PLANNING

Meal planning, or determining the type and amount of food ingested, is a critical component of an athlete's daily routine. Remember, it is not the meal eaten the night before the competition but the athlete's consistent daily meal planning that will ultimately determine performance. Good meal planning consists of strategies that provide a variety of foods from the food guide pyramid; healthy food choices; and well-planned meals and snacks before, during, and after the competition or practice. If done properly, meal planning will set the stage for a lifetime of healthy eating.

MyPyramid

Most athletes do not like to count calories and prefer to be told that they need to eat a set number of servings from each of the food groups in the food guide pyramid.[4] The United States Department of Agriculture (USDA) released the 2005 MyPyramid food guidance system to replace the 1992 Food Guide Pyramid. It represents a personalized approach to healthy eating; accessing the Web site—www.mypryamid.gov—allows the athlete to obtain customized guidelines and advice on energy intake and expenditure. For example, if an athlete requires 2200 kilocalories daily, the servings from each of the food groups would be as follows: 9 servings from the bread group, 4 servings from the vegetable group, 3 servings from the fruit group, 2 to 3 servings from the milk group, and 6 servings from the meat group. Athletes are encouraged to limit their calories from fats, oils, and sweets (73 grams of fat and 12 teaspoons of sugar per day).

What Is a Serving?

A serving is a certain portion or amount of food. When calculated into a daily meal plan, a serving equals a certain number of calories. The recommended number of servings depends on a person's daily caloric needs. For example, if a person's calorie needs are 2200 calories daily, serving requirements comprise nine servings from the bread, cereal, rice and pasta group from MyPyramid. A serving size from this group would be 1 slice of bread or ½ cup of cooked cereal, rice, or pasta (Table 21-8 and Figure 21-13). After energy intake is calculated, an athlete can create a meal plan from the pyramid for daily practices or contests. As long as the athlete knows how many servings are needed from each of the food groups per day, he or she can feel free to choose a variety of foods from each category that meet these needs.

TABLE 21-8 MyPyramid Descriptions of Serving Sizes

FOOD GROUP	SINGLE SERVINGS
Bread, cereal, rice, and pasta	1 slice of bread 1 oz ready-to-eat cereal ½ cup cooked cereal, rice, or pasta
Vegetable	1 cup raw leafy vegetables ½ cup cooked vegetables ¾ cup vegetable juice
Fruit	1 medium apple, banana, or orange ½ cup chopped, cooked, or canned fruit ¾ cup fruit juice
Milk, yogurt, and cheese	1 cup milk or yogurt 1½ oz natural cheese 2 oz processed cheese
Meat, poultry, fish, dry beans, and nuts	2-3 oz cooked lean meat ½ cup cooked dry beans 1 egg or 2 Tbsp peanut butter (counts as 1 oz lean meat)

Data from U.S. Department of Agriculture: *MyPyramid: Inside the pyramid,* Washington, DC, 2005, Author. Accessed March 30, 2007, from www.mypyramid.gov/pyramid/index.html.

Several Web sites provide tools to help athletes calculate a healthy eating index and determine whether they are meeting the recommendations from the food guide pyramid. For example, MyPyramid Tracker (www.mypyramidtracker.gov/), an online interactive self-assessment tool, provides a quick measure of the quality of a person's overall diet. The athlete can enter his or her daily food intake, including portion size, amount of food, and brand names. Once the data are entered, the program analyzes the athlete's diet in terms of nutrients, calories, and servings and then compares this dietary intake with a healthy diet. The athlete can easily assess his or her daily nutritional intake.[16]

Through the Web site for the National Heart Lung and Blood Institute, part of the National Institutes of Health (http://hp2010.nhlbihin.net/menuplanner/menu.cgi), athletes can obtain a personal food guide pyramid graphic. The Web site allows users to select a calorie level and plan meals with correct portion sizes.[17]

Following MyPyramid is an important way that athletes can assess whether their nutritional intake is sufficient. Athletes have modified the pyramid by placing fluids at the bottom of the pyramid below the grain group as a new food category to emphasize the importance of daily fluid replacement. Similar food guide pyramids may also be found for vegetarians and people with other dietary needs on the Web site of the U.S. Department of Agriculture's Food and Nutrition Information Center (http://fnic.nal.usda.gov). Vegetarian food guides work by adjusting specific diets to focus on protein, iron, calcium, zinc, and vitamin B from nonanimal sources.

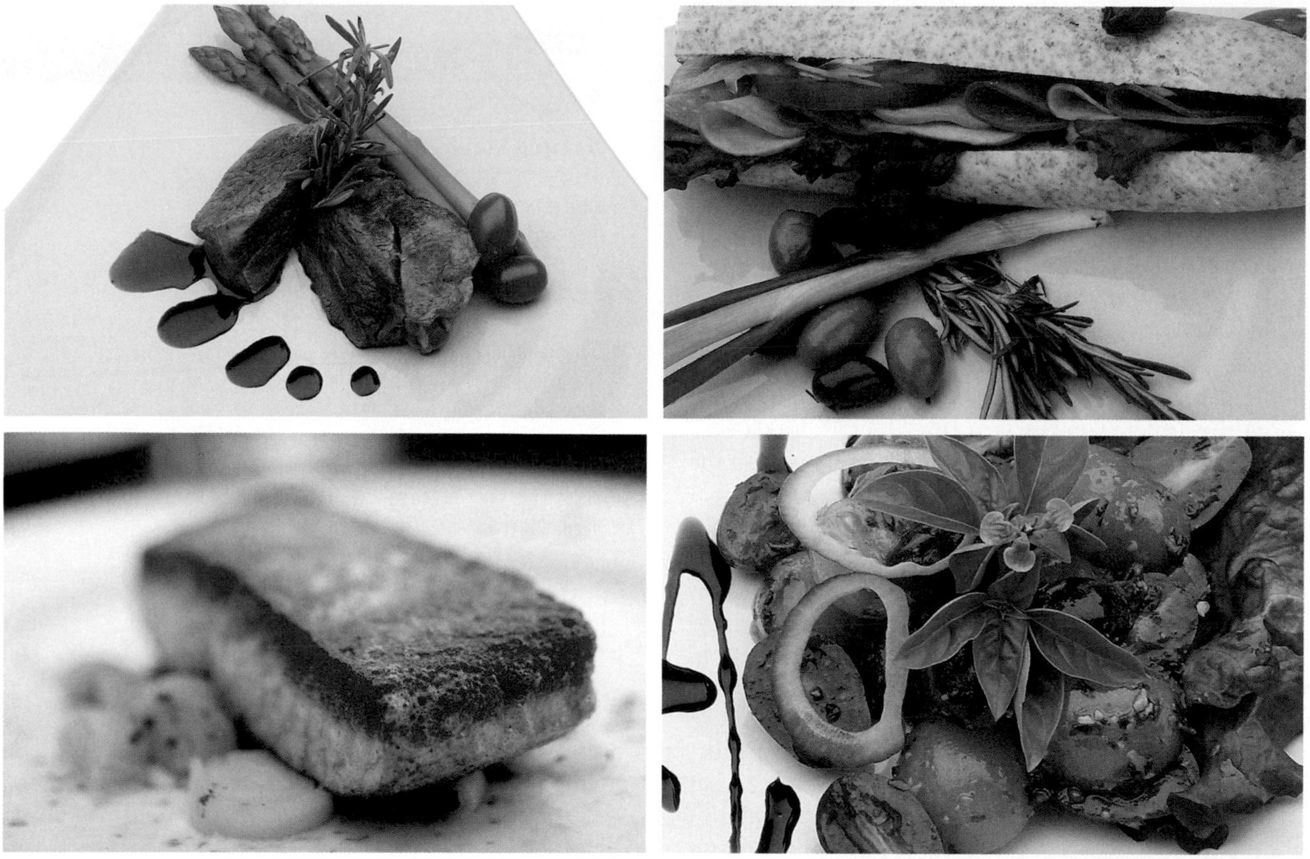

FIGURE 21-13 Understanding portion sizes helps maintain energy balance and ideal body weight. (Copyright 2007 JupiterImages Corporation.)

Precompetition and Postcompetition Meals and Practice Days

Meal planning for precompetition, postcompetition, and practice days is an ongoing process. The athlete's performance is not solely dependent on the pre-event meal strategy. Rather, it depends on three factors: the overall nutritional, physiological, and psychological status of the athlete; the unique circumstances of the individual and the event; and the amount of food consumed and the time of its consumption.

General recommendations for precompetition meals correspond to specific guidelines. Energy intake should be adequate to ward off any feelings of hunger or weakness during the entire period of the competition. Although precompetition food makes only a minor contribution to the immediate energy expenditure, it is essential to maintain an adequate level of blood sugar and prevent hunger and weakness. Many athletes prefer to abstain from food immediately before competition because they are nervous. The pregame meal should offer foods that will minimize upset in the gastrointestinal tract. Eating before practice provides the energy needed for a workout. Athletes prone to gastric distress should experiment with liquid meals to prevent fatigue. The NATA Position Paper recommends drinking 400 to 600 ml of fluid 2 to 3 hours before exercise (Figure 21-14). Taking in food and fluid before and during prolonged competition should ensure an optimal state of hydration. Optimal delivery of fluid from the stomach can be achieved by beginning exercise with a comfortable volume of fluid in the stomach and adopting a pattern of periodic

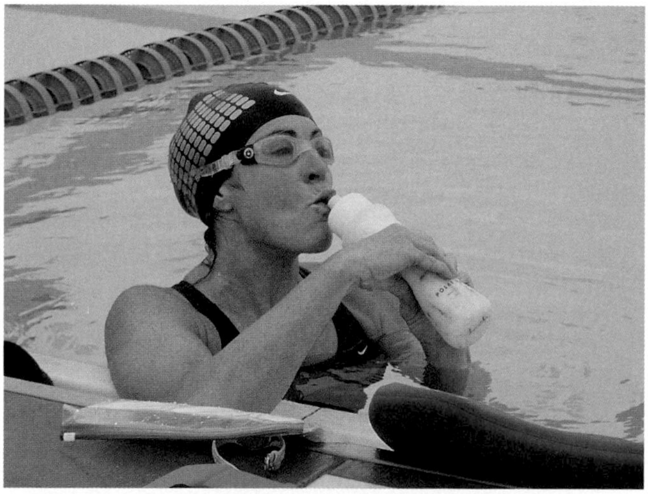

FIGURE 21-14 Hydration is important before, during, and after activity to prevent dehydration and maintain energy levels.

fluid intake during the actual exercise. The athlete will need to determine his or her ideal volume of fluid by experimenting with different types of drinks, amounts consumed, and even the time at which the drinks are consumed.[18]

The pre-event meal should include foods that the athlete has successfully ingested before the day of the competition. It is important that the intensity of the practice mimic the intensity of the contest when the athlete experiments with his or her pre-event meal. An athlete's food preference can be influenced by superstition. However, as long as the athlete has suffered no adverse effects after experimenting with the food during a practice session, the athlete is free to eat this "lucky" food.

Consuming foods as a pre-event meal depends on the timing of the meal relative to the practice or competition time. The optimal pre-event meal provides some protein, minimal amounts of fat, and liberal amounts of complex carbohydrates. Foods high in protein and fat are not digested quickly; they can delay gastric emptying and cause gastrointestinal upset during competition. Athletes should avoid pre-event meals that include foods such as fatty meats, sausage, processed lunch meats, and peanut butter, as well as fried foods such as doughnuts, chips, french fries, and fried meats.

Foods composed of mostly complex carbohydrates are more rapidly digested than high-protein and high-fat foods. Carbohydrates provide the most efficient source of energy. The recommendation that carbohydrates be consumed within 1 hour of activity has become controversial. It was previously believed that this practice would lead to hypoglycemia and premature fatigue.[19] More recent studies indicate that the decline of insulin during the first 20 minutes of exercise is self-corrected, with no apparent effects on the athlete.[20] Timing guidelines for carbohydrates are as follows: Amounts of 1 to 4.5 g/carbohydrate/kg/body weight can be ingested 1 to 4 hours before the event. Every hour an intake of 1 g/carbohydrate/kg/body weight is suggested. For meals that take place at least 4 hours before the event, 4.5 grams per kilogram of body weight is recommended.

Simple sugars such as candy, soda, honey, and sugar should be avoided because they provide only rapid, temporary increases in blood sugar. About an hour after a simple sugar is consumed, blood glucose and insulin levels spike. After 3 or 4 hours, blood glucose levels drop below fasting levels, leading to hunger. Slowly digested carbohydrates reduce the fluctuation in blood glucose levels. Ingestion of sugar before competition may produce negative side effects, including gastrointestinal upset, diarrhea, and hypoglycemia (low blood sugar), all of which can decrease athletic performance.

If the precompetition travel time is 1 hour or less, the athlete should take along bottled water or a bottle of juice. The juice will provide carbohydrates and calories. If the ride is 1 to 2 hours, the athlete should drink the water or juice and also have a banana or bagel, or some cereal. Having these types of food items may settle the stomach and prevent a feeling of hunger and weakness during competition. Fast-food restaurants can provide a nourishing meal. However, athletes should refrain from ordering double servings, mayonnaise, and dill spread. They should also opt for grilled rather than fried food. For breakfast at a fast food restaurant, the athlete might select two beverages to enhance hydration and one breakfast entrée among higher carbohydrate choices, such as pancakes with syrup (no bacon or sausage), an English muffin with jelly, or a raisin bran muffin.[21]

Box 21-6 illustrates a sample menu for a low-fat, high-carbohydrate precompetition meal that provides no more than 500 calories. A meal of this nature should be consumed approximately 2 hours before competition. The athlete should remember to drink plenty of water with the precompetition meal.

Meal consumption during a practice or training session depends on the event, duration of the event, and the environment. The athlete should consider the amount of time between events, bring healthy food choices, and plan accordingly. During endurance exercise, carbohydrate availability is limited; consuming 0.1 to 0.2 gram of a solution containing 6% to 8% carbohydrate per kilogram of body weight at 15 to 20 minute intervals has been shown to extend endurance performance. To determine the carbohydrate concentration of a drink, determine the number of grams of carbohydrates in the container. Generally, an 8-ounce container has 240 milliliters; divide the number of grams by 240 milliliters, and multiply by 100. Many athletes like energy bars and gels. These products are pure complex carbohydrates in a very small volume. One energy bar is generally equivalent to half of a bagel or half of a slice of bread. Energy bars and gels contain fructose, sucrose, maltodextrin,

BOX 21-6 Low-Fat, High-Carbohydrate Precompetition Options

Sample Meal

1 cup skim milk
2 slices bread
1–2 cups beverage (100% juice)
2 oz lean meat
1 serving fruit

Suggested Light Meals

Cereal with skim milk and banana
Poached egg on dry toast
Peaches with low-fat cottage cheese
Low-fat or nonfat yogurt with applesauce and cinnamon
Sliced turkey or chicken sandwich with fat-free mayonnaise
Vegetable soup with crackers

potassium, chloride, and sodium chloride. Because of their high fiber content, 2 cups of water should be ingested with each bar.

What an athlete eats after a strenuous workout or competition can dramatically affect his or her recovery. If the athlete chooses the post-exercise meal wisely, less recovery time will be needed for the next workout. In addition, the level of exercise intensity and time sequence of the workout will dictate the type of fluid replacement required. Fluids are the priority after exercise. The goal should be to immediately replace all fluids lost during exercise. As previously discussed, dehydration impairs performance more than any other factor. Water is also important for carrying oxygen and nutrients to cells and removing waste from the body. For every pound of weight lost during activity, 2 to 3 cups of fluids should be consumed. The following options are appropriate: plain water, fruit juice (100%), watery foods (e.g., watermelon, grapes), and high-carbohydrate drinks.

Carbohydrates are the next most important nutrient that should be consumed within 1 to 4 hours after the workout, ideally within 2 hours after activity to provide 1 gram carbohydrate per kilogram of body weight (CHO/kg/bw). This is the optimal time because it is when the enzymes that make glycogen are most active. Ingesting carbohydrates at this time enhances glycogen resynthesis and prevents fatigue from setting in the following day. Box 21-7 lists some food choices that are high in carbohydrates (50 grams or 200 calories) and low in fat, all good choices for postexercise consumption.

For athletes who do not engage in endurance sports and power lifting, 1gm CHO/kg/body weight is adequate. For example, if a nonendurance athlete weighs 70 kilograms, his or her postworkout carbohydrate intake would be 70 grams, or a food item that contains 280 calories. Two breakfast bars and one cup of cranberry juice would be 300 calories. For an endurance athlete or power lifter, the amount of carbohydrate consumed after the workout will vary. These athletes would require 1.2 to 2 grams of carbohydrates per kilogram of body weight. For example, if an endurance athlete weighs 70 kilograms, his or her postworkout carbohydrate requirement would be 140 grams (5 g/kg/body weight = 2 × 70 g = 140 g). One gram of carbohydrate contains 4 calories; thus 140 grams equals 560 carbohydrate calories that must be ingested as tolerated over the first 1 to 4 hours after the workout. Suggested food choices are as follows: 1 cup of orange juice (105 calories), one banana (105 calories), and a bagel (300 calories) with one tablespoon of strawberry jam (50 calories) for a total of 560 calories.

Proteins are the third nutrient that should be consumed after exercise or activity. Adding protein to the meal after the competition does not enhance glycogen resynthesis. However, including protein with the meal may supply the amino acids required for muscle protein repair.[22] If energy intake is inadequate, protein will be used as an energy source. Examples of foods that contain 50 grams of CHO and 10 grams of protein are as follows: one bowl of cereal, 1½ cup of fruit salad with ½ carton of fruit-flavored yogurt, or one large piece of thick-crust pizza.

The mineral potassium should also be ingested after a competition. Approximately 300 to 800 milligrams of potassium can be lost during 2 or 3 hours of hard exercise. Most commercially prepared fluid replacement beverages are poor potassium sources. Box 21-8 lists potassium-rich foods ranked in descending order.

During nonendurance conditions, sodium chloride replacement is not necessary. However, drinking a sports beverage that contains sodium chloride may promote fluid retention in the extracellular compartment, help maintain the osmotic drive to drink, and improve the palatability of the drink. The use of salt tablets is obviously not necessary, although replacing lost sodium may be recommended for athletes who do not acclimatize properly during their workouts.

WEIGHT-LOSS OR WEIGHT-GAIN GUIDELINES

Weight-loss and weight-gain strategies do not always go as planned. Some athletes believe that by limiting their energy intake (i.e., calories in) and increasing their energy output (i.e., calories out), they will enhance their weight loss. Healthy weight loss should be only 1 to 2 pounds per week. An athlete should not try to lose weight during the athletic season. Trying to cut calories and increase exercise during

BOX 21-7 Low-Fat, High-Carbohydrate Postexercise Options

Two breakfast bars or cereal bars
2 cups cranberry juice
1 cup of fruit yogurt with a bagel

BOX 21-8 Potassium-Rich Foods

Potato, 3-inch	750 mg
Yogurt, 1 cup	500 mg
Banana, medium	500 mg
Orange juice, 1 cup	420 mg
Pineapple juice, 1 cup	360 mg
Raisins, ½ cup	300 mg

the season may lead to negative consequences such as decreases in metabolism, muscle loss, fatigue, and illness. The athletic trainer should advise the athlete to get in shape for the sport, not use the sport to get in shape.

Dietary Guidelines

Every 5 years, the U.S. Department of Agriculture (USDA) and the Department of Health and Human Services (HHS) jointly issue new dietary guidelines. The most recent version, *Dietary Guidelines for Americans 2005,* provides nine recommendations:[23]

1. Consume a variety of foods within and among the basic food groups while staying within energy needs.
2. To maintain body weight in a healthy range, balance calories from foods and beverages with calories expended.
3. Engage in regular physical activity and reduce sedentary activities to promote health, psychological well-being, and a healthy body weight.
4. Increase daily intake of fruits and vegetables, whole grains, and nonfat or low-fat milk products.
5. Consume less than 10% of calories from saturated fatty acids and less than 300 milligrams of cholesterol daily, and keep total fat intake between 20% and 35% of total calories.
6. Choose and prepare foods and beverages with little added sugars or caloric sweeteners.
7. Consume less than 2300 milligrams of sodium (approximately 1 teaspoon of salt) per day.
8. If you drink alcoholic beverages, do so in moderation.
9. To avoid microbial food-borne illness, keep food safe to eat by storing it at the appropriate temperature until eaten.

The aforementioned guidelines certainly apply to all athletes attempting to maintain a healthy meal plan (Figure 21-15). Additional guidelines on weight loss for athletes include establishing energy intake and energy expenditure (total calories/day) and then deducting 500 calories daily from the total to lose 1 pound per week. Remember, 1 pound of fat equals 3500 calories. If, for example, an athlete is currently consuming 2500 calories per day, they would need to consume 2000 calories per day to lose 1 pound per week. A pound of fat is equivalent to 3500 calories consumed over the course of 7 days, which equals 500 calories per day.

There are limits as to the minimum number of calories per day that an athlete should consume. Dietary intake should not be restricted to less than 80% of their total calculated energy intake. For example, if an athlete's energy intake is 2000 calories per day, the athlete should not ingest fewer than 1600 calories per day. Overall, the athlete's diet should never include a caloric intake that is less than 1500 calories per day. As previously stated, a lowered energy intake of less than 1500 calories per day can lead to vitamin or mineral deficiency. The main aim of dietary change is to promote a moderate total energy restriction without compromising carbohydrate intake or other nutritional and performance goals, such as protein status and micronutrient needs. According to Dr. Louise Burke, energy restriction is best achieved by the implementation of a low-fat diet (15% to 25% of energy) and a moderate-to-high carbohydrate intake (6 to 8 g/kg/body weight/day). Protein intake should be approximately 1.5 to 2 grams per kilogram of body weight daily to assist in the maintenance of lean body mass and help promote satiety.[24,25]

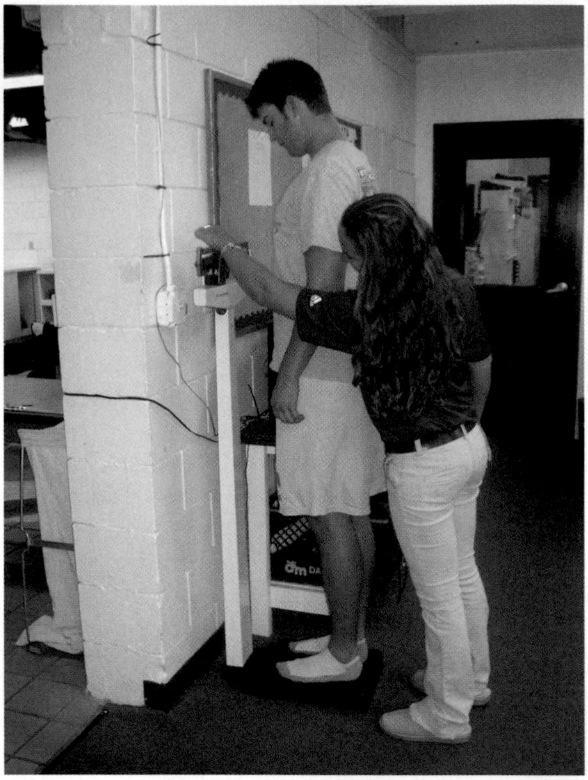

FIGURE 21-15 Monitoring weight helps athletes maintain or lose weight as needed for optimal performance.

Negative Consequences of Rapid Weight Loss in Athletes

Rapid weight loss is associated with many negative consequences, including the following: decreased aerobic and anaerobic performance, glycogen depletion, dehydration, impaired thermoregulation, impaired oxygen and nutrient exchange, impaired buffering capacity, and increased loss of fat-free mass. Recommendations for weight-conscious athletes may include the following: initiate a weight-control program well in advance of the competitive season; determine body fat levels so that realistic weight goals can be set; establish a range of acceptable body fat and weight values, and then monitor health and performance within this range; and determine a specific target level for body weight associated with optimal performance.[26]

Weight-Gain Guidelines

Weight gain for athletes can be very complicated. The athlete's strategy for gaining weight may include ingesting foods that are high in fat (e.g., doughnuts and french fries) and high in protein. Athletes who are already consuming excess calories may not feel hungry enough to consume additional calories. The athlete's schedule and budget constraints may interfere with the consumption of adequate healthful foods. Some athletes believe that ordinary food is not sufficient to help them gain weight, so they turn to sports supplements. Suggested guidelines for a successful weight gain program are as follows: Set realistic weight-gain goals, allow adequate time to reach these goals, and assess daily energy expenditure. Increase energy intake, emphasizing a high-carbohydrate diet of roughly 60% and a low fat intake of 20% to 25%.[27] Consumption of a high-carbohydrate diet should prevent excessive gains in body fat. Protein intake of 12% to 15% (or 1 to 2 g/kg/body weight) should be adequate to assist with lean tissue accretion. Therefore consuming an additional 1000 to 3500 calories should result in a weight gain of 1 pound (or 454 g) of muscle mass when incorporating strength training into the exercise regimen.

Points to Ponder

Why is it so challenging to convince athletes to eat more food when they believe "cutting out" food is better?

Ergogenic Aids to Manage Weight

Ergogenic aids are simply work-enhancing devices. In the athletic realm, they include any nutritional manipulation that improves performance. An ergogenic aid is a supplement containing a substance that is a component of a normal physiological or biochemical process. Most athletes believe taking the supplement will improve their performance, develop muscle, prevent or treat illnesses, and prevent fatigue. However, some supplements or ergogenic aids can also produce an ergolytic response, which means that they may impair performance.

The National Collegiate Athletic Association (NCAA) regulates the use of supplements among athletes. According to by-law 16.52.2, "an institution may provide only non-muscle building nutritional supplements to a student athlete at any time for the purpose of providing additional calories and electrolytes, provided the supplements do not contain any NCAA-banned substances."[28] Permissible nonbuilding nutritional supplements are identified according to the following classes: vitamins and minerals, energy bars, calorie-replacement drinks, and electrolyte-replacement drinks.

Athletes can take supplements on their own as long as they do not contain banned substances. Physicians can prescribe supplements for medical reasons as long as they are documented and reported to the appropriate agencies. Care should be taken to educate athletes regarding permissible substances. For example, a supplement that contains protein may be classified as a nonmuscle-building supplement, provided that it is included in one of the four permissible categories set forth in by-law 16.52.2, does not contain more than 30% of calories from protein based solely on the package label, and does not contain additional ingredients that are designed to assist in the muscle-building process.

Teaching athletes about supplements requires a delicate touch. The athletic trainer first must be familiar with the general guidelines of supplement use. Does the performance claim of the product make sense? What is the supporting evidence for its effectiveness (testimonials versus scientific evidence)? What are the consequences of taking the supplement in terms of safety, legal issues, and ethics? If the athletic trainer is asked about a supplement by an athlete, the first rule of thumb is not to tell the athlete that it doesn't work. The athlete must be presented with concrete evidence of the supplement's potential benefits or consequences.

The following steps may be helpful when advising the athlete about supplements. Investigate all of the ingredients in the supplement. What are the active ingredients? What is the existing information about the product and the recommended amount? Are any side effects associated with the product? What does it do? Determine the claims and benefits identified by the company. What is the delivery system (powder, pill, or liquid)? Look at the label. How many milligrams or grams per serving? How many servings are required per day, and how many servings are in the container? What is the cost per container? What is the suggested use? Should the product be taken in the morning or evening? Should it be taken on an empty or full stomach, with meals or during the workout?

Consult with the regulatory agencies governing the sport (NCAA, IOC, USADA) to determine the use of the product. Look up basic physiological claims of the product to determine if the improvement in performance does occur as a result of the supplement. Consult with the FDA to make sure the product has not been taken off the market. If time allows, investigate scientific studies regarding the product. Finally, because the use and recommendation of certain ergogenic aids remain controversial, it is in the best interest of the athlete that the athletic trainer not recommend the use of an ergogenic aid for weight gain or weight loss. Following the aforementioned guidelines will help the athlete make the best decision regarding ergogenic supplementation.

ergogenic aid a product that is work-enhancing; potentially improves performance

DISORDERED EATING AND EATING DISORDERS

Among athletes, eating-related problems are a universal concern, difficult to challenge and correct. Stress and pressures common to the athletic experience often engender eating-related problems, which can be classified as disordered eating and eating disorders. Disordered eating is not as severe as an eating disorder. However, disordered eating can still affect the athlete's performance and potentially lead to an eating disorder. Eating disorders are medically recognized conditions that must be medically diagnosed. As defined by the *Diagnostic and Statistical Manual of Mental Disorders* (DSM-IV) criteria of the American Psychiatric Association, eating disorders are difficult to detect and diagnose because of their complex and secretive nature. The key functional requirements for behavior to be clinically defined as an **eating disorder** are that the behavior must no longer be under personal control and must cause significant adverse changes in psychological, social, or physical functioning.[29,30]

Many athletes and nonathletes skip a meal during the day or binge on food during the holidays. This type of behavior is quite common and can be identified as **disordered eating**. Athletes who must meet a specific weight class or present a certain body type or shape may appear to have a disordered eating pattern (e.g., cutting out meals), but they represent neither a psychological nor a health risk at this time. They simply do not have healthy eating habits. Athletes who binge or purge twice a week are not suffering from clinical bulimia. However, an increase in this type of behavior, a decrease in self-esteem, and other psychological changes may increase their chance of developing an eating disorder. This serious behavior signals a problem that requires intervention.

Disordered eating and eating disorders are significant problems for many athletes. Female athletes who participate in sports that emphasize a thin body or appearance, such as gymnastics, ballet, figure skating, swimming, and distance running, are at particular risk. Male athletes who participate in body building and wrestling are also at risk. A greater risk is associated with sports in which anaerobic activities take precedence over aerobic activities.[30]

Many athletes may exhibit signs and symptoms of an eating disorder such as anorexia nervosa and bulimia nervosa but do not fully meet the criteria for these conditions. The American Psychiatric Association has established a separate category for such cases: eating disorder not otherwise specified (EDNOS). Consider the athlete who has a negative body image and is fasting regularly but appears to still be menstruating, or the athlete who tells everyone that she purges after large meals and believes that she is fat but turns out not to be purging at all. In both cases, the athlete has the symptoms of an eating disorder and can possibly be stopped before the disorder fully manifests. The term **anorexia athletica** has been used to describe a subclinical eating disorder syndrome characterized by disordered eating and compulsive exercising. Athletes who suffer from this condition exhibit an intense fear of gaining weight or becoming fat, even though they weigh at least 5% less than the expected normal weight for their age and height. Weight loss is achieved by restriction of food intake, extensive compulsive exercise, or both.[30,31]

Fatigue, weakness, lightheadedness, fractures, cramping, and irregular heart rates are some of the symptoms of eating disorders that may impair athletic performance. Physiological complications such as low levels of thyroid hormones, poor cardiac and circulatory function, osteoporotic changes, and electrolyte imbalances can also develop. The risk of morbidity and death will increase as the athlete's eating disorder progresses.

The female athlete who attempts to reach an unrealistically low body weight through disordered eating and exercise practices risks developing two associated disorders: amenorrhea and osteoporosis. This condition is known as the Female Athlete Triad.[32] Each of the disorders can be a medical concern in itself. Collectively, they present a greater risk for health problems and even death if left untreated. **Amenorrhea** (delayed menarche) is the absence of menstruation by age 16 in a girl with secondary sex characteristics. Secondary amenorrhea is the absence of three or more consecutive menstrual cycles after menarche, the time of the first menstrual period. If an athlete has her menstrual period and then skips three or more consecutive menstrual cycles, she is said to have secondary amenorrhea.

Amenorrhea associated with exercise and anorexia nervosa is hypothalamic in origin and is associated with decreased bone mineral density.[33] **Osteoporosis** is a bone condition characterized by a low bone mass and microarchitectural deterioration of bone tissue, which leads to enhanced skeletal fragility and increased risk of fracture.[34] The World Health Organization has identified four diagnostic criteria for the stages of osteoporosis, all of which pertain to bone mineral density. The framers of the criteria concluded that the principal cause of

eating disorder pattern of eating behavior that is no longer under personal control and causes significant adverse changes in psychological, social, or physical functioning

disordered eating pattern of eating behavior that can negatively affect an athlete's performance and potentially lead to an eating disorder

anorexia athletica a subclinical eating disorder syndrome characterized by disordered eating and compulsive exercising

amenorrhea delayed menarche

osteoporosis disease in which the bones become abnormally thin, porous, and subject to fracture premenopausal osteoporosis in active women is decreased ovarian hormone production and hypoestrogenemia as a result of hypothalamic amenorrhea.[35]

The NCAA provides educational material for coaches, athletes, and athletic officials (www.ncaa.com). One such document identifies the warning signs for eating disorders. After the disorder has been identified, a team made up of people experienced in the management of eating disorders should develop the best approach and treatment plan. Members of the team should include a physician; a registered dietitian or a licensed dietary nutritionist; a psychologist, psychiatrist, or counselor; and the athletic trainer and coach. Of utmost concern is the client's physical and psychological outcome. Reversing an eating disorder can help the client regain a healthy, normal lifestyle.

SUMMARY

In general, athletes tend to seek advice on nutrition from their teammates or friends. Unfortunately, nutrition practices that may work for one athlete may have adverse effects on another. The athletic trainer's role is to teach athletes about preferred dietary practices. It is important that the athletic trainer first find out what the athletes are saying about nutrition among themselves. What they think they know about nutrition may be inaccurate or even harmful. Food and fluid restriction, use of laxatives and diuretics, and excessive exercise are inappropriate methods for weight management. The initial team meeting is an opportune time to convey important nutritional facts, and athletes should be encouraged to discuss nutritional concepts openly. It is the athletic trainer's responsibility to be honest with

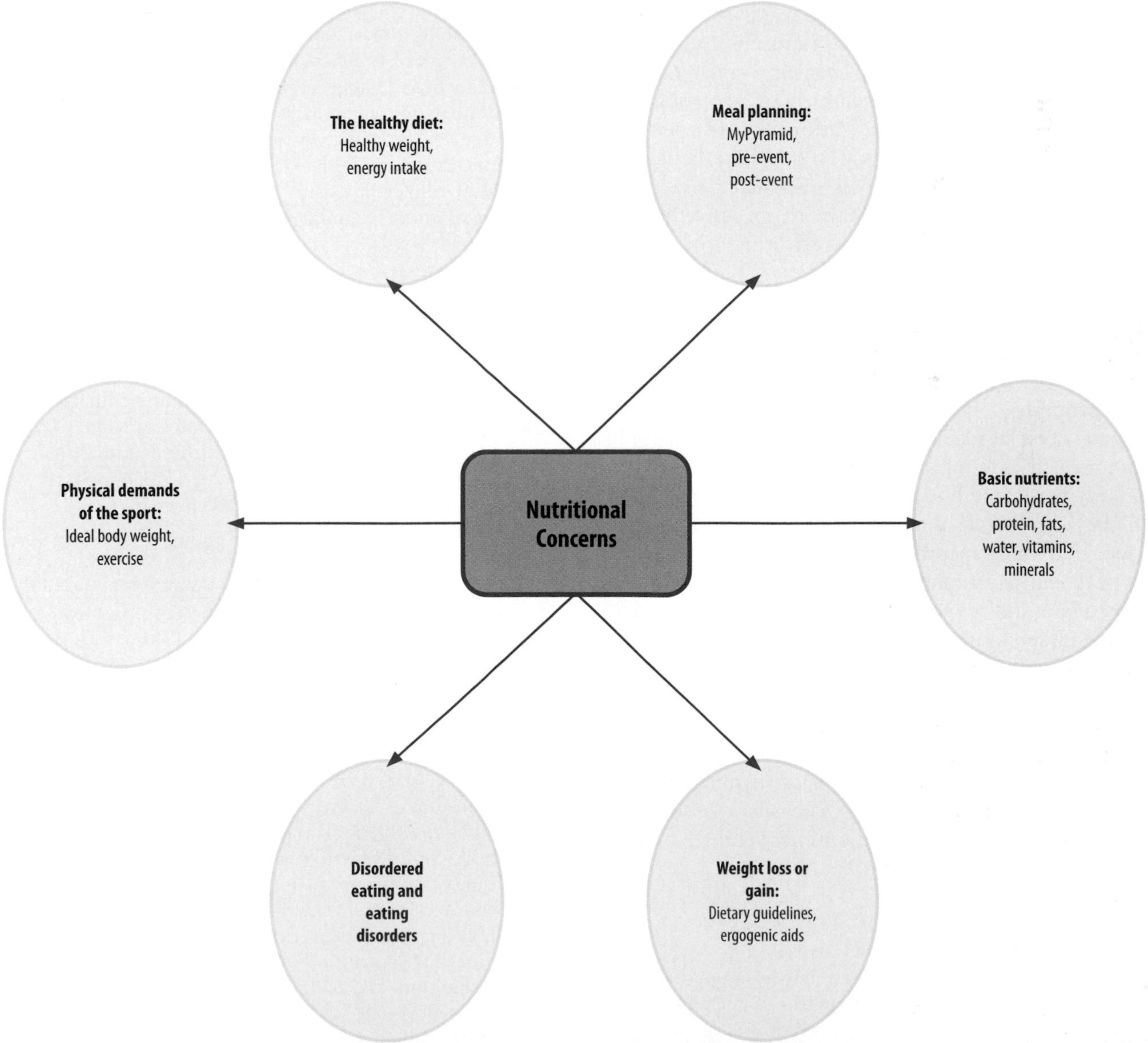

FIGURE 21-16 Concept map showing the multifaceted approach to the nutritional concerns of the athlete.

the athletes, give up-to-date advice, and thoroughly understand the nutritional and physiological demands of their sports (in addition to the rules governing weigh-in procedures, if applicable).

The athletic trainer should know when to refer the athlete to another experienced professional. An RD or LDN whose specialty is sports nutrition may be enlisted to provide a lecture to a specific team or all participants in varsity sports. When the athlete meets with the RD, LDN, or athletic trainer, the athlete's energy intake—including energy expenditure, the required number of servings per day from the food guide pyramid, and choices for pre-event and post-event meals—should be discussed. Guidelines for weight loss, weight maintenance, and weight gain should be established early in the offseason or preseason. Using sound techniques, the athletic trainer should calculate the athlete's weight and body composition and then determine whether the athlete needs to maintain, gain, or lose weight. The athlete's muscle mass (gain) and fat mass (loss) should be measured over time to ensure healthy adherence to weight-management goals. The athletic trainer's watchful, informed presence will help athletes achieve success on and off the field. The concept map in Figure 21-16 is designed to help the athletic trainer become familiar with the multifaceted approach to nutritional concerns affecting athletes.

Revisiting the OPENING Scenario

To properly counsel Jim, the young male wrestler, you must do several things. First, you should obtain an accurate measurement of his height, weight, lean body mass, and body fat. You can then provide him with the appropriate diet to fuel his body. In light of the fact that Jim expends a large amount of calories in both practicing and maintaining his weight, explaining energy intake and expenditure will help tremendously. Once he understands the delicate balance between his diet and exercise, he will be better equipped to make good choices in his food and supplement selection as well as in his weight management program. Keep in mind that nutrition provides the foundation for solid physical performances. Good choices in nutrition can propel an athlete to the top just as easily as poor ones can precipitate an athlete to an untimely end.

Issues & Ethics

A cross-country runner has been trying to make the third team spot for the last 2 years. She decides that it is her weight that is holding her back. You find out from one of her teammates that she is binge eating, purging after meals, and running 4 to 6 additional miles every morning before practice. Even after you implement a mandatory daily weigh-in before and after practice, her behaviors continue. Now she is complaining of chronic shin splints and serious mood swings. What do you do? What is your role in her care at this point?

Web Links

American Dietetic Association: www.eatright.org
American Diabetes Association: www.diabetes.org
American Heart Association: www.amhrt.org
American Society for Nutrition: www.nutrition.org
Beefnutrition.org: www.beefnutrition.org
Body by Milk: www.whymilk.com
Center for Food Safety and Applied Nutrition: www.cfsan.fda.gov
Center for Nutrition Policy and Promotion: www.cnpp.usda.gov
ConsumerLab.com: www.consumerlab.org
Dairy Council of California: www.dairycouncilofca.org
David Mendosa (diabetes specialist): www.mendosa.com
Fifty50 (diabetes research): www.Fifty50.com
Gatorade Sports Science Institute: www.gssiweb.com
Glycemic Index and GI Datatbase (The University of Sydney): www.glycemicindex.com
Institute of Food Technologists: www.ift.org
MyPyramid: www.MyPyramid.gov
National Cattlemen's Beef Association: www.beef.org
National Collegiate Athletic Association (NCAA): www.1.ncaa.org
National Heart Lung and Blood Institute, Obesity Education Initiative, Interactive Menu Planner: http://hp2010.nhlbihin.net/menuplanner/menu.cgi
National Institute of Diabetes & Digestive & Kidney Diseases, Nutrition: www.niddk.nih.gov/health/nutrition.htm
NetWellness (University of Cincinnati, The Ohio State University, Case Western Reserve University): www.netwellness.org
Teachfree: www.teachfree.com
United States Olympic Committee: www.olympic-usa.org

References

1. Day B: *Fast facts on fast food for fast people*, 1992. Apple a Day. Copyright Barbara Day.
2. Houtkooper L: *Winning sport nutrition training manual*, Tucson, Ariz, 1994, University of Arizona Cooperative Extension.
3. National Athletic Trainers' Association: *Position paper: Fluids and hydration*, Dallas, 2004, National Athletic Trainers Association.
4. Benardot D: *Nutrition for serious athletes*, Champaign, Ill, 2000, Human Kinetics.
5. Center for Nutrition Policy and Promotion: *MyPyramid*, Washington, DC, 2005, U.S. Department of Agriculture. Accessed March 30, 2007, from www.cnpp.usda.gov.
6. Jeukendrup A, Gleeson M: *Sport nutrition*, Champaign, Ill, 2004, Human Kinetics.

7. Burke L et al: Eating patterns and meal frequency of elite Australian athletes, *Int J Sport Nutr Ex Spo Sci Rev* 13(4): 521–538, 2003.
8. Manore M, Thompson J: *Sport nutrition for health and performance*, Champaign, Ill, 2000, Human Kinetics.
9. Haber V: Menstrual dysfunction in athletes: an energetic challenge, *Exerc Sport Sci Rev* 28: 19–23, 2000.
10. Burke L, Keins B, Ivy J: Carbohydrates and fat for training and recovery, *J Sport Sci.* 22(1): 15–30, 2004.
11. Peterson M, Peterson K: *Eat to compete*, Chicago, 1988, Yearbook.
12. Grandjean A: Diets of elite athletes: has the discipline of sport nutrition made an impact?, *Nutr* 127(suppl): 874S–877S, 1997.
13. Weight Loss Information: *Calorie needs: Harris-Benedict calculation*, 2003–2005, Author. Accessed March 30, 2007, from www.weight-loss-i.com/calorie-needs-harris-benedict.htm.
14. Hargreaves M, Hawley J, Jeukendrup A: Pre-exercise CHO and fat ingestion: effects on metabolism and performance, *Journal of Sport Sciences* 22: 31–38, 2004.
15. Nutrition Analysis Tools & System: Dietary assessment and energy intake calculation, Mundelein, Ill, 2007, FiberGel Technologies, Inc. Accessed March 30, 2007, www.nat.uiuc.edu.
16. Center for Nutrition Policy and Promotion: *MyPyramid*, Washington, DC, 2005, U.S. Department of Agriculture. Accessed March 30, 2007, from http://www.cnpp.usda.gov/MyPyramid-breakout.htm.
17. National Heart Lung and Blood Institute: *Obesity Education Initiative: Interactive menu planner*, Bethesda, Md, National Institutes of Health. Accessed March 30, 2007, from http://hp2010.nhlbihin.net/menuplanner/menu.cgi.
18. Noakes T, Rehrer N, Maughn B: The importance of volume in regulating gastric emptying, *Med Sci Sport Ex* 23: 307–313, 1991.
19. Foster C, Costil D, Fink W: Effects of pre-exercise feedings on endurance performance, *Med Sci Sport Ex* 11: 1–5, 1979.
20. Hawley J et al: Carbohydrate-loading and exercise performance: an update, *Sport Med* 24: 73–81, 1997.
21. Clark N: *Nutrition guidebook*, ed 3, Champaign, Ill, 2003, Human Kinetics.
22. Volek J: Influence of nutrition on responses to resistance training, *Med Sci Sports Ex* 36: 689–696, 2004.
23. U.S. Department of Health and Human Services, U.S. Department of Agriculture: *Dietary guidelines for Americans 2005*, Washington, DC, 2005, Authors. Accessed March 30, 2007, from http://www.healthierus.gov/dietaryguidelines/.
24. William MH: *Nutrition for health, fitness, and sport*, ed 7, New York, 2005, McGraw-Hill.
25. Burke L, Deakin V: *Clinical sports nutrition*, ed 2, New York, 2000, McGraw-Hill.
26. Fogelholm M: Effects of body weight reduction on sports performance, *Sports Med*, 18: 249–267, 1994.
27. Manore M, Thompson J, Russo M: Diet and exercise strategies of a drug-free world class bodybuilder, *Int J Sport Nutr* 3: 76–86, 1993.
28. National Collegiate Athletic Association (NCAA): NCAA Division II Manual. Indianapolis, Author.
29. Ravaldi C et al: Eating disorders, *Psychopathology*, 36(5): 247–254, 2003.
30. American Psychiatric Association: Diagnostic and statistical manual of mental disorder IV (DSM-IV), ed 5, text revision, Washington, DC, 2000, American Psychiatric Association.
31. Sundgot-Borgen J, Torstein M: Prevalence of eating disorders in elite athletes is higher than in the general population, *Clin J Sport Med* 14(1): 25–32, 2004.
32. Lo BP, Herbert C, McClean A: The female athlete triad: no pain, no gain, *Clin Pediatr* 42(7): 573–580, 2003.
33. Khan K et al: New criteria for female athlete triad syndrome? *Br J Sport Med* 36(1): 10–13, 2002.
34. Warren MP, Shantha S: The female athlete, *Baillieres Best Pract Res Clin Endocrinol Metab* 14: 37–53, 2000.
35. Nakamura T: World Health Organization criteria for osteoporosis and trends in Europe and USA, *Nippon Rinsho* 62(suppl 2): 235–239, 2004.

22

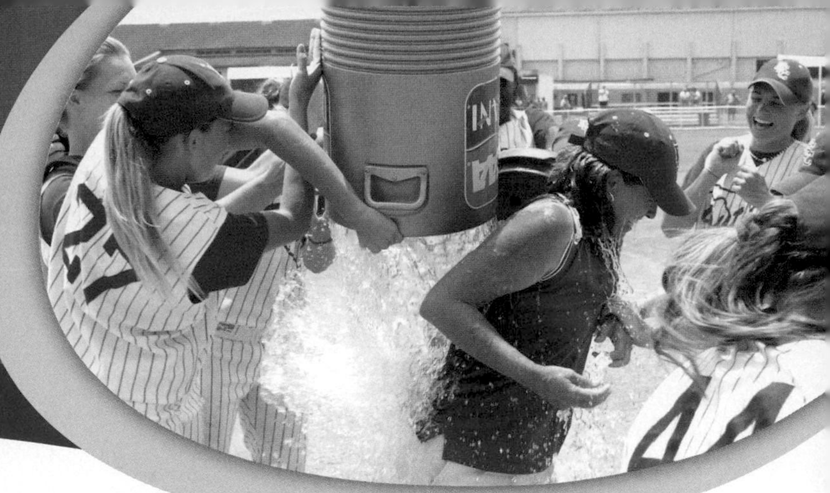

Psychosocial Concerns of the Athlete

WILLIAM N. MILLER

Learning Goals

1. List the major factors that predispose a person to sports-related injury.
2. Define the primary psychosocial concerns of the athlete that affect the athletic trainer.
3. Describe the factors that can improve sports rehabilitation adherence.
4. Describe the psychosocial perspective of eating disorders, substance abuse, and other self-injurious behaviors.
5. Identify the counseling role of athletic trainers and the importance of establishing a network of mental health professionals for referral purposes.
6. Describe the various psychological intervention skills that can be used to prevent injury and during the rehabilitation process.

As discussed in previous chapters, injury is common in sports, with an estimated 3 to 17 million sports-, exercise-, and recreation-related injuries occurring annually in the United States alone.[1] Because care of the injured athlete focuses on physical attributes, the athletic trainer may not hear much about the psychosocial consequences of sports injuries. Many people incorrectly assume that when an athlete is physically rehabilitated, he or she is fully prepared to safely return to physical activity. Athletes are at risk for suffering psychosocial consequences as a result of injury, and in fact, rehabilitation can and often is hampered by the athlete's emotional state. For example, one study reported that 47% of 482 athletic trainers surveyed indicated that *every* injured athlete suffers from psychological as well as physiological trauma[1]. For this reason, researchers have suggested that physical and psychological aspects of rehabilitation must be addressed in the future and that athletic trainers will play a central role in this relationship.[2]

Athletic trainers are in an ideal position to assist patients with the psychosocial consequences of athletic injury and rehabilitation. As health care providers, athletic trainers are central to the athlete's care from the onset of injury until the return to sport.[3] There is no question that athletic trainers should be as competent in the recognition of psychosocial concerns as they are in the recognition of physical concerns. However, most athletic trainers have a limited background in sport psychology and few resources whereby they might acquire such skills. This chapter covers several techniques and skills that athletic trainers can use to address the very important psychosocial aspects of athletics.

PREDISPOSING FACTORS TO SPORTS INJURY

Understanding the psychosocial factors that might make some athletes more susceptible to injury can help athletic trainers prevent injuries through the use of psychological intervention strategies (Figure 22-1). The following model is one of the more commonly used frameworks that explains why some athletes are at higher risk for injury than others.

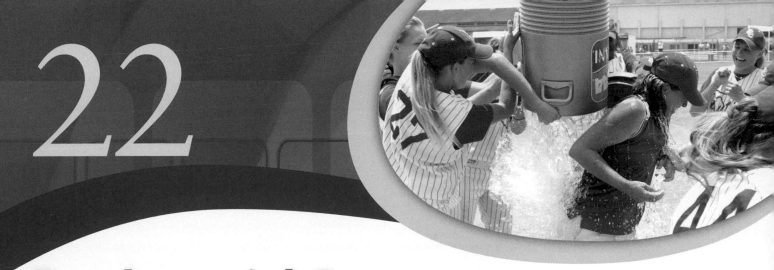

OPENING *Scenario*

Celeste and Jacob are student-athletes at a small New England college. Celeste recently sprained her left ankle for the first time during field hockey practice. Likewise, Jacob recently sprained his left ankle for the first time during soccer practice. For both, this was the first time that they had ever been injured. The diagnosis by Wade, the athletic trainer at their college, was a first-degree sprain of the anterior talofibular ligament for both student-athletes. Celeste and Jacob had similar treatment and rehabilitation regimens. Celeste, a happy go-lucky, well-rounded student, was able to return to field hockey in 5 days. Jacob, a fiercely competitive person without a lot of friends, did not return to the soccer team for close to 6 weeks. From a psychosocial perspective, how do you explain this difference?

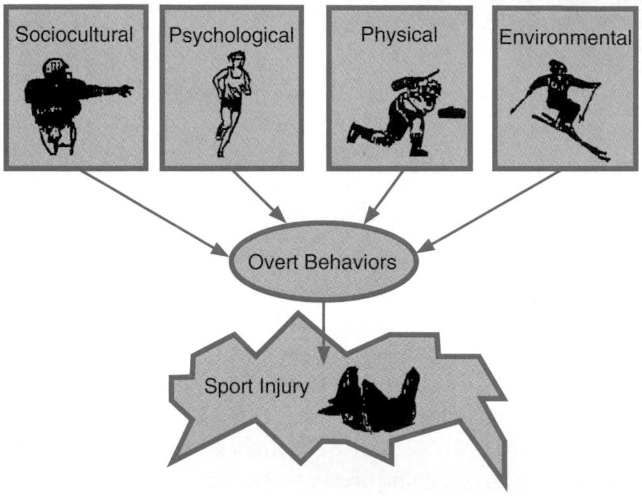

FIGURE 22-1 Precursors to sport injury. (From Williams JM: How to identify and prevent injuries resulting from psychosocial factors, *Athl Ther Today* 5(6): 36, 2000. Modified from Wiese-Bjornstal D, Shaffer S: Psychosocial dimensions of sport injury. In Ray R, Weise-Bjornstal D, eds: *Counseling in sports medicine,* p. 30, Champaign, Ill, 1999, Human Kinetics.)

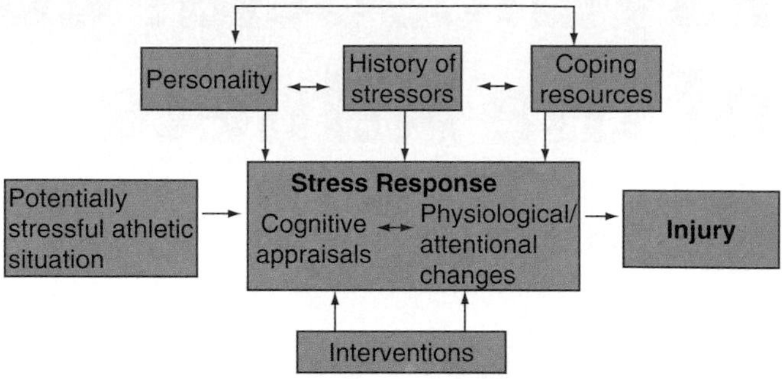

FIGURE 22-2 Stress and injury model. (From Williams JM, Andersen MB: Psychosocial antecedents of sport injury: review and critique of the stress and injury model, *J Appl Sport Psychol* 10:7, 1998.)

Model of Stress and Athletic Injury

One of the major models used to explain why certain individuals are more prone to injury is the stress-injury model. This model classifies individuals into different risk categories and shows why individuals with a high risk profile are more injury prone. Perhaps more important, this model also shows how specific interventions can help reduce injury risk[4] (Figure 22-2).

Stress Response

An athlete's response to stress is really the core of the stress-injury model.[5] The way an athlete responds to stress can affect his or her perception (cognitive appraisal) of a potentially stressful situation, which in turn affects his or her physical reaction. For example, an athlete with increased anxiety caused by stress may be increasingly distracted, with a subsequent narrowing of visual field and decreased coordination and flexibility. Imagine how this could possibly affect a linebacker in football. An effective linebacker takes in a tremendous amount of cues before and after the ball is snapped. When stress is lower, the linebacker will have a wider (normal) field of peripheral vision. If the linebacker's peripheral vision narrowed as a result of stress, he would be vulnerable to getting hit and sustaining injury without ever seeing the opponent coming.

Personality

The top left section of the model in Figure 22-2 refers to personality. *Personality* may be defined as the characteristics, or blend of characteristics, that make a person unique.[6] Personality differences influence whether individuals are likely to perceive situations as stressful, as well as their vulnerability to the effects of stressors. Box 22-1 provides some examples of positive personality traits that help some athletes deal better with stressful situations, resulting in a lower stress response and a decrease in injury risk.

Athletic trainers need to pay attention to athletes who appear to lack some of these personality traits. Under stress, these athletes would be more predisposed to injury. An athletic trainer can identify these individuals and use

BOX 22-1 Personality Traits Influencing the Stress Response

Hardiness	A configuration of beliefs involving a sense of control, commitment, and challenge that could protect physical health even under stressful circumstances. Hardiness has been proposed to affect the stress response by altering the appraisal of a stressor and by effective coping. Essentially, hardy individuals are more resilient.
Locus of control	The extent to which individuals feel they have control over their own lives.[9] A person with a high internal locus of control would feel in control over the events in his or her life, whereas a person with high external locus of control would attribute these events to be outside of their control (e.g., the fault of others, fate, bad luck).[10]
Sense of coherence	A construct that predicts effective coping measures against stressful conditions. Sense of coherence is a way of seeing the world that facilitates successful coping with stressors.
Trait anxiety	*Trait anxiety* refers to a general disposition or tendency to perceive situations as threatening and to react with an anxiety response.
Achievement motivation	Having a strong motive to succeed
Sensation seeking	The need for varied, novel, and complex sensations and experiences and the willingness to take physical and social risks for the sake of such experience
Tough-minded	A more assertive, independent, and self-assured personality type
Optimism	The tendency to expect positive outcomes and to "look for the silver lining in every cloud."[64]
Self-esteem	Having confidence and satisfaction in oneself
Self-concept	The way in which one perceives oneself
Introversion or extroversion	The tendency to direct one's thoughts and feelings toward oneself. Extroversion is interest in or behavior directed toward others or one's environment rather than oneself.
Positive mood states	Characterized by high levels of vigor and low levels of tension, depression, anger, fatigue, and confusion.

relaxation techniques to help them manage stress more efficiently and thereby prevent injury. Information on relaxation techniques and other psychological intervention strategies are discussed later in this chapter.

History of Stressors

The top middle section of the model in Figure 22-2 refers to the history of stressors. The history of stressors includes the following three factors[7–10]:

1. *Life events stress:* Life events stress consists of major changes in a person's life, such as the death of a family member, divorce of parents, break-up with a boyfriend or girlfriend, or extended illness. Major positive life events such as marriage, birth of a child, or starting a new job can also contribute to life events stress.
2. *Daily hassles:* Daily hassles can include disagreements with friends, roommates, and coaches; minor annoyances with school or work; sleep difficulties; transportation concerns; and financial problems. Daily uplifts are the more positive aspect of daily hassles; these represent positive minor daily events that make people feel good and can counteract the negative effects of daily hassles.
3. *Previous injuries:* If athletes return to sport when physically, but not psychologically, prepared, they could be worried about their ability to perform, still have concerns about their level of recovery and the possibility of re-injury, and feel anxious about their lack of sport-specific training over the rehabilitation period. The fear of re-injury may in itself lead to a significant stress response and increase the risk of injury.

Coping Resources

The top right section of the model in Figure 22-2 refers to coping resources. Coping resources include general coping skills and strategies, stress management, social support, proper nutrition and sleep habits, and mental skills such as the ability to stay positive and focused under pressure. Those who are low in coping resources are prone to more sports-related injuries.[11,12] Therefore the presence of good coping resources may directly protect the individual against injury.

Role of Interventions

Intervention strategies such as stress management techniques can help decrease the risk of injury as well as during the recovery period after the injury. These interventions should focus on altering or lowering the perceived threat of potentially stressful events and on modifying the physiological and awareness aspects of the stress response.[12] Athletic trainers working with potentially stressed athletes should watch the athlete's behavior closely. In some instances, the athletic trainer may want to talk with the coach and suggest that the athlete cut back on the activity. Athletes with significant life stress who do not appear to have personality characteristics that provide good coping skills should be observed closely.

Sociocultural Factors Influencing Injury

Social and cultural aspects of sports injury must be addressed with the psychological consequences. While the psychology of injury has received significant attention over the past 30 years, research regarding social and cultural aspects of sports injury is in its early stages of development.

The Sport Ethic

The *sport ethic* refers to what many participants in sport have come to use as the criteria for defining what it means to be a real athlete. Accepting the risks of participating in sport and playing with pain are inherent to the sport ethic. The acceptance of pain in sport has been termed *positive deviance*. **Positive deviance** in sport does not involve a disregard or rejection of social values; it refers to overconformity to the goals and norms of sport.[13]

Culture of Risk: Playing With Pain and Injury. Playing with pain and injury is a common and normal consequence of competitive sports participation. **Culture of risk** refers to the unquestioned tolerance of pain and injury for those who accept the potential negative (risky) consequences of sports participation. Those who conform to this ethic receive praise, whereas those who question the tolerance of pain and injury in sport are often degraded.[14] Within the sport culture, the rewards of participation far outweigh the negative consequences.

Athletes are often rewarded by compliments for sacrificing their body and playing with pain. Similarly, they are encouraged to be tough and take risks.[14] In following the "no pain, no gain" creed, male and female athletes alike view injury in sport, within the rules, as being a legitimate part of the game.[15] This encourages athletes to play hurt or take undue risks. How effectively the athlete manages pain influences performance and can ultimately determine athletic success. This is not limited to contact sports; many athletes in general are socialized to "train through pain" and that "more is always better." They subsequently overtrain, which results in a variety of overuse injuries.[16]

As a result of playing with pain and injuries over time, many former athletes are subjected to a life of discomfort and disability well beyond the playing years. No one dramatizes this scenario better than Jim Otto, who played for the Oakland Raiders and was inducted into the Pro Football Hall of Fame in 1980. Jim Otto is arguably the best center who has ever played. To many, Jim Otto is better known for being the iron man of iron men because he never missed a game while playing for the Raiders, a remarkable span of 210 consecutive games. He has paid dearly for playing with pain and injury, however, having undergone 40 major surgeries, 28 of which were on his knees. He has had eight artificial knees, and both shoulders have been replaced. His back has been broken, fused, rebroken, re-fused, and so on. His nose was broken more than 20 times. His condition is so fragile that he nearly died on three occasions in the 1990s from football-related injuries.[17]

Influence of the Media. The media frequently celebrate the willingness of an athlete to endure extreme amounts of pain and injury even at the youth sport level, which suggests that the "culture of risk" is evident in all levels of sport. The culture of risk normalizes pain and injury experiences. Athletes at all levels appear to be ingrained with the expectation that they must play as long as possible with pain and injuries and must try to come back as soon as possible after injury.[18] There is a high degree of cultural tolerance with regard to injury in sport, and particularly professional sports, that is not seen to the same degree in other professions. Television, radio, and the print media sensationalize injuries. Descriptions of injuries by television announcers are extremely graphic at times. Members of the media favorably compare athletes who have the ability to play while injured with those who do not. For example, Tedy Bruschi returned to practice with the New England Patriots on October 19, 2005, just 8 months after suffering a mild stroke. Jim Rome, host of a nationally syndicated sports radio show, called Bruschi's decision courageous but reckless. He went on to describe Bruschi as a warrior, suggesting that this was the rationale for his return.[19] Although current research examining pain and injury has been more focused on male athletes, a similarity that has emerged between male and female athletes is the willingness to play with pain and injury and return to sport before complete recovery.[15] For example, in women's ice hockey, the general opinion is that injury is part of the game and should be accepted as such.[20]

> **Points to Ponder**
> Have you noticed a gender difference among athletes regarding their willingness to play with pain?

Influence and Role of Sports Medicine Practitioners. Sports medicine is a unique aspect of medicine in which the concept of rest is the last resort when someone is injured. This concept is difficult for people outside of sports to understand, and the ethics of sports medicine practitioners is often questioned on the basis of the notion

positive deviance overconformity to the goals and norms of sport
culture of risk unquestioned tolerance of pain and injury for those who accept the potentially negative (risky) consequences of sports participation

that injured athletes are allowed to play when they do not seem physically or medically able. In sports medicine, the goal is to treat signs and symptoms of injury early so that the athlete does not have to "lose time." Even when the athlete is not cleared to participate, as part of the treatment and rehabilitation protocol the athlete is kept active. Whereas the nonathlete with a hamstring strain is advised to rest, ice, compress, and elevate the injured limb, the athlete or physically active patient will be advised to engage in "active rest." Active rest may include light exercises such as riding a stationary bike, walking on the treadmill, or working out in the pool.

Sports medicine practitioners can be influenced by the culture of risk. When deciding whether to allow a recently injured athlete to participate in a sport, the athletic trainer must weigh the perceived risks and benefits. These negotiations are affected by a variety of factors, such as the nature of the particular sport, the status of the athlete, the time of the season, the level of competition, whether it is a practice or a game, and the importance of a particular competition.[14]

Another element of this culture is that athletes may be unwilling even to seek medical care because they fear being labeled as weak.[6] The decision to seek medical care for a significant injury is fairly straightforward. However, with less serious injuries, a multitude of circumstances determines the manner in which athletes make decisions about their need to seek medical advice. Some athletes engage in self-diagnosis and self-prognosis as part of intrapersonal negotiation. If they believe that they will get treatment that will help them and that they will not be asked to decrease participation, then they will seek care. Other athletes will not seek care until they suffer an injury repeatedly.[14]

Athletes may also "self-doctor," or seek the advice of a teammate who has had a similar injury. If a teammate is not able to help, then they may seek the care of a sports medicine practitioner.[14] Obviously, not all athletes adhere to this philosophy. Many athletes have learned that if they take care of an injury right away, the medical staff can keep it from getting to a point at which they will miss time. In fact, many athletes wait too long before disclosing their injuries, leaving athletic trainers no choice but to discontinue all activity for a period of time.

Athletic trainers play a significant role with the social support networks of injured athletes. Athletic trainers who express a sympathetic or caring attitude about pain and injuries have a direct effect on whether injured athletes may seek their care.[18] Athletic trainers must develop a caring and trustful relationship with athletes, providing social support to them. Athletic trainers may exchange stories or jokes with athletes and convey to them the importance of courage, toughness, and dedication, an attitude that corresponds to the culture of the athletic training room. At the same time, however, they must make it clear to athletes that they should be forthright about their pain so that they can be properly examined, advised, and treated[18] (Figure 22-3).

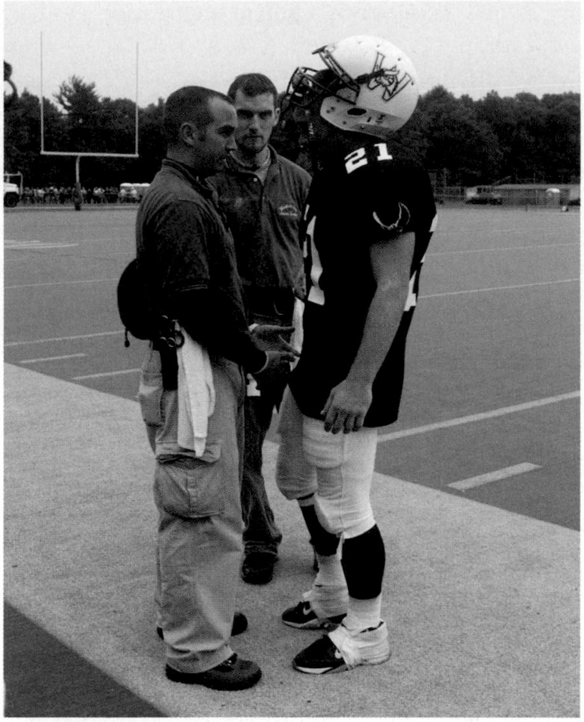

FIGURE 22-3 Rapport and trust must be established between the athletic trainer and the athlete so that athletes feel comfortable seeking out medical care when they need it.

Athletes tend to avoid athletic trainers who do not strike them as sympathetic or caring; they may also do this if they feel pressured by teammates to play hurt. Athletic trainers must not be coerced by coaches, athletic administrators, or anyone else to encourage injured athletes to play when it is not warranted. For athletic trainers, this directive should be taken only from a physician. Athletic trainers must focus on the health of the athlete and strive to resist the win-at-all-cost mentality. Ideally, the coach will support the athletic trainer's decision in front of the athlete. An environment of mutual respect between athletic trainers and coaches can have a significantly positive impact on the social support network and psyche of injured athletes. Team physicians and athletic trainers must remain independent in deciding what treatment an injured athlete should receive and when the athlete should be allowed to return to competition. Physicians and athletic trainers should not allow themselves to be unduly influenced by others regarding the disposition of an injured athlete.

PSYCHOLOGICAL RESPONSES TO SPORTS INJURY

Sports injuries are the unwanted side effects of sports participation. Restricted mobility and a perceived loss of independence can unleash an emotional roller coaster as athletes attempt to deal with and adapt to being injured.[21] Although most injured athletes cope well after injury, some experience clinical depression and even suicidal thoughts. Between 5% and 13% of injured athletes exhibit clinical levels of distress.[22]

Significant emotional responses after injury are normal. After all, a highly active individual has been rendered inactive and must face the uncertainty of his or her immediate future. For athletes who might derive significant amounts of self-esteem and personal competence from their ability to perform, the injury process can be emotionally devastating.[23] The greater the extent to which the athlete identifies with sport, the more difficult the transition from athlete to nonathlete will be. A host of negative psychological responses may occur after a sports-related injury, the most common being frustration, depression, anger, and anxiety (Box 22-2).[23]

Many factors influence the athlete's psychological reaction to sport injury. These factors may also influence the athlete's ability to adhere to a rehabilitation program. The major considerations are as follows:[24]

- *Injury influences:* Cause, onset, and severity of injury; body part injured (upper/lower); potential impact on athletic career and life
- *Sport influences:* Nature of the particular sport, status of the athlete (starter or backup), individual versus team sports, timing of the injury, coach
- *Personal influences:* Age, sex, and maturity of the athlete; previous injury experience; availability of sports medicine practitioners; pain tolerance and expression
- *Social influences:* Social support of friends, predisposing conditions and life experiences, ethnic background, family support

Athletic trainers can expect to see a wide range of psychological reactions to injury. Normal responses to injury may include the following: (1) anger, frustration, sadness, and a strong desire to compete again; (2) some denial and minimization of the injury; (3) concern about pain; (4) feeling discouraged about the injury; and (5) concerns about the loss of conditioning.[25] The critical issue for the athletic trainer is being able to distinguish between athletes who are just blowing off steam and those who are exhibiting signs and symptoms of poor adjustment to injury. Athletes who fall into the latter category should be referred to a mental health professional. Athletic trainers should be concerned when psychological reactions appear to be escalating or do not resolve with time and physical recovery.[26] Athletic trainers are in an excellent position to determine when athletes are having difficulty adjusting to an injury. Establishing a rapport with injured athletes will help them feel understood and more willing to share their fears and insecurities. Warning signs of poor adjustment to injury include the following:[27]

- Evidence of anger, depression, confusion, or apathy with little or no progress in rehabilitation
- Obsession with the question "When will I be able to play again?"
- Denial, reflected in remarks such as "Things are going great," "The injury is no big deal," and anything else that suggests the athlete is making an extraordinary effort to convince the athletic trainer that the injury does not really matter
- A history of coming back too soon after injuries
- Exaggerated storytelling or bragging about accomplishments in or out of sport
- Dwelling on minor aches and sensations, a possible indication that the athlete is overly anxious about returning to activity
- Remarks about letting the team down or feeling guilty about not being able to contribute
- Dependence on the athletic trainer or the therapy process or a tendency to spend too much time in the athletic training room
- Withdrawal from teammates, coaches, friends, family, or the athletic trainer
- Rapid mood swings or striking changes in affect or behavior
- Statements that indicate a feeling of helplessness to affect recovery

These warning signs do not automatically indicate major adjustment problems, but they do suggest that something is going on with the athlete that warrants a closer look.

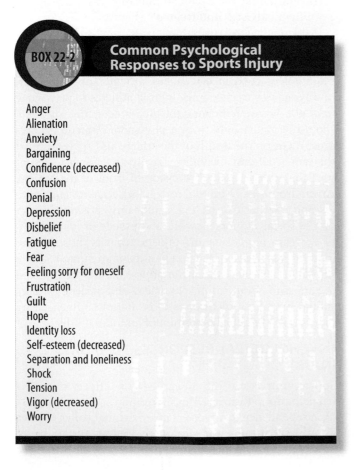

BOX 22-2 Common Psychological Responses to Sports Injury

Anger
Alienation
Anxiety
Bargaining
Confidence (decreased)
Confusion
Denial
Depression
Disbelief
Fatigue
Fear
Feeling sorry for oneself
Frustration
Guilt
Hope
Identity loss
Self-esteem (decreased)
Separation and loneliness
Shock
Tension
Vigor (decreased)
Worry

Models of Psychological Response to Sports Injury

The emotional consequences of sports-related injury can be explained by way of two models. The first is the integrated model of psychological response to the sports injury and rehabilitation process.[6,8] This model provides an understanding of the various factors that influence athletes' cognitive, emotional, and behavioral responses to injury.[8,28] The second model is the biopsychosocial model of sport injury rehabilitation. This model is aimed at combining medical and psychological approaches to sports injury rehabilitation and places a greater emphasis on rehabilitation processes and outcomes.[29]

Integrated Model of Psychological Response to the Sports Injury and Rehabilitation Process

The integrated model of psychological response to the sports injury and rehabilitation process (Figure 22-4) is the most comprehensive example of a cognitive appraisal model. The main premise of the model is that emotional and behavioral responses to sports-related injuries are directly influenced by the way the injured athlete interprets or perceives the injury. During the cognitive appraisal, athletes assess the demands of the injury to see if they have the resources to cope with it in an effective manner. If the appraisal of the injury is relatively positive and the athlete feels confident about the possibility of successful rehabilitation and full recovery, the model predicts that a positive emotional reaction will be more likely. The athlete's attitude has a direct impact on his or her ability to adhere to a rehabilitation plan.[30]

Rehabilitation adherence simply refers to compliance with a rehabilitation program. Because favorable sports injury rehabilitation outcomes presumably depend on the successful completion of therapy regimens, rehabilitation adherence has emerged as an area of interest in the psychology of sports injury. Compliance with a program can be the difference between a quick recovery and a long period of frustration.[31]

Despite the widespread belief that athletes who adhere to their prescribed rehabilitation program will have a more successful outcome, rehabilitation adherence is frequently a challenge for the health care professional. Not all patients show up regularly for scheduled appointments or participate fully in the rehabilitation session. Depending on the injury and type of rehabilitation program, the specific behaviors of rehabilitation adherence will vary. Adherence behaviors relevant to athletic training include the following: (1) attending and actively participating in rehabilitation appointments, (2) avoiding potentially harmful activities, (3) wearing therapeutic devices (e.g., orthotics), (4) consuming medications as prescribed, and (5) completing home rehabilitation activities (e.g., exercises, therapeutic modalities).[63] Box 22-3 provides some recommended *dos* and *don'ts* regarding rehabilitation for athletic trainers and physical therapists.

With regard to the opening scenario of the chapter, is it possible that Celeste and Jacob are appraising their injuries much differently? Perhaps Celeste's appraisal of the injury is that "it's no big deal; I'll get treatment and be back in no time." On the other hand, maybe Jacob thinks his injury is catastrophic, that he will never be able to return to his previous level of play.

The integrated model proposes that responses to injury are influenced by both pre-injury and postinjury factors. Pre-injury factors of the integrative model (see Figure 22-4) consist of personality, history of stressors, coping resources, and interventions that are extended from the stress-injury model discussed in the previous section of the chapter. Postinjury factors include personal issues (e.g., the type and severity of the injury, the athlete's general health status, demographic variables) and situational factors (e.g., the sport played, the athlete's social support system and access to rehabilitation).[30,31]

Biopsychosocial Model of Sports Injury Rehabilitation

The biopsychosocial model of sports injury rehabilitation is an interactive approach aimed at combining medical and psychological approaches (Figure 22-5). The biopsychosocial model incorporates existing models of sports injury rehabilitation into an integrative framework to widen the focus of research.[29] The seven components of the model are as follows:

1. Characteristics of the injury
2. Sociodemographic factors
3. Biological factors
4. Psychological factors
5. Social/contextual factors
6. Intermediate biopsychological outcomes
7. Sport injury rehabilitation outcomes

A primary benefit of the biopsychosocial approach in sports injury rehabilitation is the ability to enhance quality of care by implementing interventions directed at any one of the components of the model, because they all have a direct or indirect effect on rehabilitation outcomes.

Points to Ponder

Can you think of a way that you could enhance care for your athletes by implementing an intervention that would focus on biological factors? What would that be?

COMMON PSYCHOLOGICAL CONDITIONS

Athletic trainers regularly confront a plethora of common psychosocial issues such as academic concerns,

rehabilitation adherence committing to and following through with a rehabilitation program

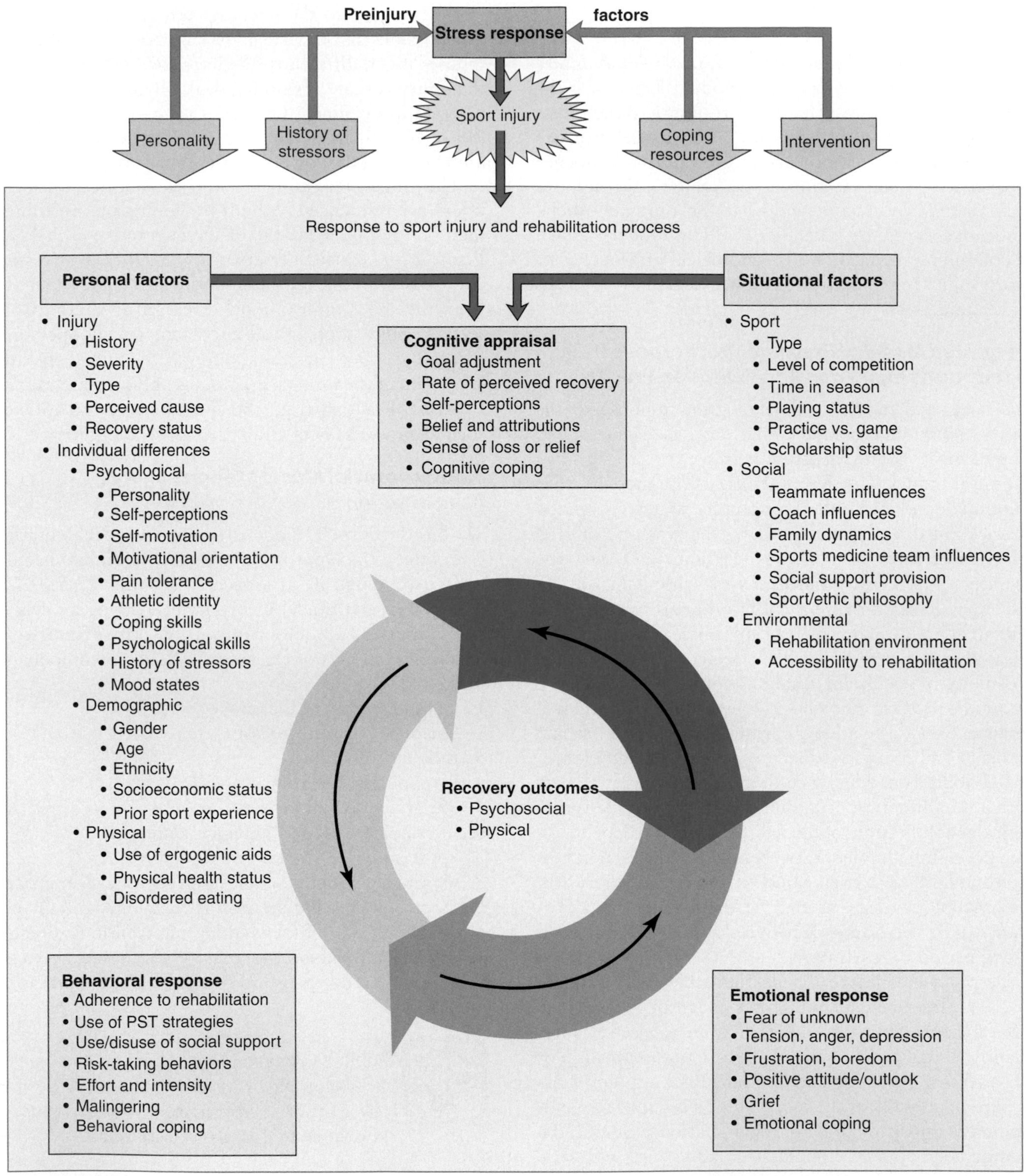

FIGURE 22-4 The integrated model of psychological response to the sports injury and rehabilitation process. (From Wiese-Bjornstal DM et al: An integrated model of response to sport injury: psychological and sociological dynamics, *J Appl Sport Psychol* 10(1): 49, 1998.)

career dilemmas, conflicts with coaches and teammates, drug and alcohol abuse, eating disorders, family-related problems, physical abuse, self-destructive behavior, social pressures, sport demands, and transition difficulties. Because individuals often confide in them, athletic trainers are usually in a position to learn a great deal about the people under their care. Athletic trainers must understand their limitations and know when and where to refer a patient. An updated referral list is of the utmost importance.

BOX 22-3 **Do's & Don'ts for Athletic Trainers/Sports Physical Therapists**

Do's

1. Let athletes know what to expect from their rehabilitation (e.g., soreness, tightness).
2. Educate athletes about their injuries, the prescribed rehabilitation, and the prognosis.
3. Focus more on the plan for rehabilitation and on future outlook than on the injury.
4. Explain the reality of human motivation; total commitment and effort all the time is difficult.
5. Establish a rapport with injured athletes to create a rehabilitation partnership.
6. Be realistic about the injury but put a positive spin on rehabilitation outcomes.
7. Make athletes take responsibility for their progress and hold them accountable for the outcome.
8. Reinforce important points.
9. Use handouts to supplement verbal instructions.
10. Listen when injured athletes talk about their injuries and rehabilitation regimens.
11. Assess every injured athlete's likelihood of adhering to rehabilitation.
12. Monitor the progress of rehabilitation.
13. Be firm and set ground rules so that the injured athletes know what to expect.
14. Involve the athlete's significant others to create a social support system.
15. Tailor the rehabilitation program to the injured athlete's particular circumstances.
16. Be ready to recognize individual differences in the athletes you treat.
17. Set short-term goals (e.g., complete the full range of motion) as well as long-term goals (e.g., return to play in 2 weeks).
18. Make all goals as specific and measurable as possible.
19. Create opportunities for athletes to rehabilitate in their sport environment where possible.
20. Share rehabilitation success stories of previous injured athletes with current ones.
21. Allow injured athletes to express their emotional responses to injury openly.
22. Base the return to play on specific criteria in order to clarify the expected outcome.
23. Set challenging but realistic goals.
24. Use functional progressions to monitor rehabilitation progress.
25. Reinforce injured athletes for their daily efforts regardless of the outcome.
26. Share some significant decision-making with injured athletes (e.g., choice of exercise).
27. Build in opportunities for success early in the rehabilitation.
28. Design exercises to keep discomfort at a minimum.
29. Help foster the injured athlete's commitment to rehabilitation, because commitment is the key to rehabilitation adherence.
30. Understand how significant in injury can be to an athlete, empathize with him or her.
31. Explain the relevance of particular exercises to the rehabilitation goals.
32. Be confident in your presentation of the rehabilitation process so as to establish credibility early.
33. Use humor in your interactions with injured athletes, but use it appropriately.

Don'ts

1. Don't give injured athletes too much information at once.
2. Don't allow injured athletes to give up on themselves.
3. Don't give up too soon on an athlete who shows lack of interest in the rehabilitation.
4. Don't be forced into categorical answers about exact date of return to play.
5. Don't use overly technical language when describing an injury or the rehabilitation regimen.
6. Don't use threats or scare tactics as your motivational approach.
7. Don't spend a lot of time on specifics of the injury unless the athlete asks.
8. Don't coddle or pity injured athletes.
9. Don't overassess the rehabilitation outcome.

From Fisher AC, Bitting LA: Rehabilitation adherence: dos and don'ts for both parties, *Athl Ther Today* 1(5):43, 1996.

Eating Disorders

Disordered eating behaviors have been classified as anorexia nervosa, bulimia nervosa, and eating disorders not otherwise specified.[32] Eating disorders are one of the most common reasons that athletes are referred to mental health practitioners. Athletic trainers must be able to identify these eating disorders, identify athletes at risk, help prevent the development of eating disorders, and intervene as necessary.[33] Eating disorders are thought to be more extensive and problematic in athletes than in the general population.[34] In part, this may be attributed to the culture of sport, in which appearance is very important.

Generally, athletes who are engaged in activities that emphasize being thin or small (e.g., gymnastics, diving, figure skating, ballet), have weight classifications (e.g., wrestling, rowing, weight lifting, martial arts), or focus on endurance (e.g., distance running, swimming, cross-country skiing) are most likely to develop eating disorders.[35,36] Both male and female athletes are influenced by social pressures to have a certain body appearance that is considered the norm for the sport in which they participate.[35,36] Box 22-4 contains additional information regarding the focus on weight in sports.[37]

Each specific sport and each position within that sport have an ideal body type. On the one hand, this

disordered eating behaviors anorexia nervosa, bulimia nervosa, and eating disorders not otherwise specified

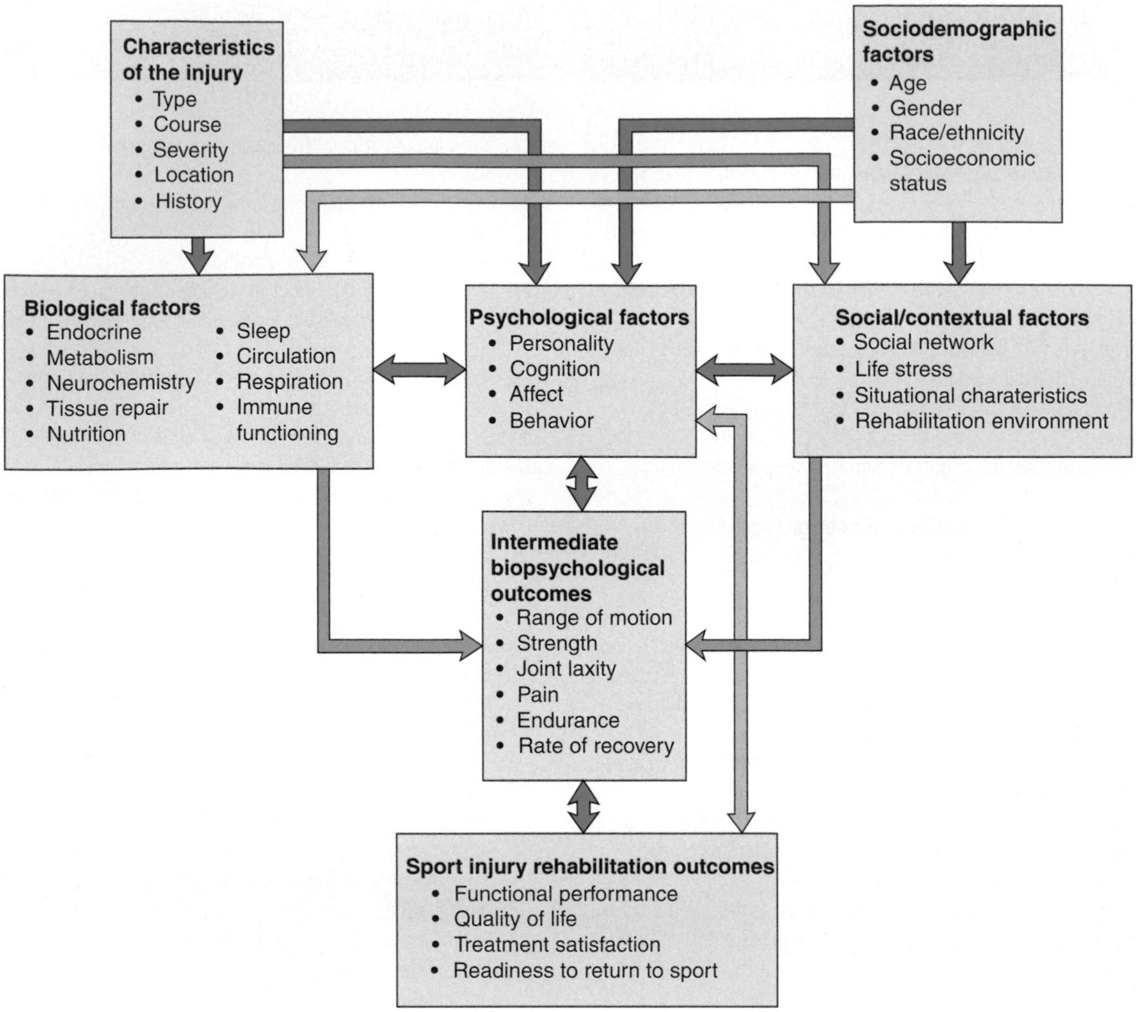

FIGURE 22-5 Biopsychosocial model of sport injury rehabilitation. (From Brewer BW, Andersen MB, Van Raalte JL: Psychological aspects of sports injury rehabilitation: toward a biopsychosocial approach. In Mostofsky DI, Zaichkowsky LD, editors: *Medical and psychological aspects of sport and exercise,* p. 48, Morgantown, W. Va, 2002, Fitness Information Technology.)

ideal is a purely practical matter, which is why we do not see 95-pound football players or 260-pound gymnasts.[37] On the other hand, the media tend to emphasize the relationship between physical appearance and performance. Such influences create a context wherein people place undue value on the size and shape of their bodies.[34] Many athletes, particularly female athletes, believe that they must conform to a specific body type to attain excellence in their chosen sport.[38] Additionally, eating disorders are influenced by certain styles of uniforms and are common in sports where more of the body is exposed.

Athletes with eating disorders commonly report a disturbance in body image (body dissatisfaction), depression, low self-esteem, anxiety, lack of assertiveness, obsessive-compulsive behavior, perfectionism, dietary restraint, sexual dysfunction, and lack of perceived control.[36,39] In addition, behavioral risks such as excessive exercise and steroid use are common.[39]

Psychological-behavioral signs of an eating disorder include the following:[16]

- Excessive dieting
- Excessive eating without weight gain
- Guilt about eating
- Claims of feeling fat at normal weight despite reassurance from others
- Preoccupation with food
- Avoidance of eating in public and denial of hunger
- Hoarding food
- Disappearing after meals
- Frequent weighing
- Binge eating
- Evidence of self-induced vomiting
- Use of drugs such as diet pills, laxatives, and diuretics to control weight

Early recognition and referral are key to a positive outcome for athletes with eating disorders. Athletic trainers can help ensure success by recognizing the signs

BOX 22-4 Focus on Weight in Sports

- Weight restrictions (classifications) exist in boxing, wrestling, weightlifting, rowing, judo, and tae kwon do. They can cause athletes to resort to unhealthy practices to lose weight, such as use of laxatives, diuretics, and diet pills; fasting; crash dieting; purging (self-induced vomiting) and fluid restriction.
- Judging criteria that emphasize thin and stereotypically attractive body build exist in sports such as diving, figure skating, gymnastics, and synchronized swimming. Perceived judging biases based on weight contribute to this factor.
- Performance demands encourage a very low percentage of body fat in sports such as swimming, speed skating, long-distance running, and cross-country skiing.
- Coaches sometimes urge their players to lose weight. They have a tremendous amount of influence in shaping the attitude and behavior of athletes, whether they are aware of it or not.
- Peer pressure sometimes inspires athletes to try pathogenic weight-loss techniques. Athletes may follow unhealthy eating behaviors on the basis of unsound advice from peers.

and symptoms of eating disorders and making a sensitive referral. Treatment of this multidimensional disorder must be multidisciplinary and include the following professionals: a psychologist (preferably someone with expertise in both eating disorders and sport psychology), a physician, a psychiatrist, a nutritionist, and the athletic trainer.[40]

Athletes suspected of having an eating disorder should be encouraged to see a mental health professional. If possible, the athletic trainer should make the appointment and accompany the athlete to the first session. People with eating disorders often deny that they have a problem. For this reason, focus on their feelings rather than eating behaviors as you counsel them.[34] If the athlete maintains his or her denial, solicit the advice of the team physician or a mental health professional.

Substance Abuse

Athletes from all sports and levels of competition have been known to use and abuse drugs. Athletes take drugs to enhance performance, alleviate pain, and self-medicate for injuries and other medical conditions, as well as for recreational purposes. College athletes may take drugs to combat the demands and pressure of performing well both as a student and as an athlete. These academic and athletic pressures may produce problems such as depression, anxiety, and burnout that may result in substance abuse if the athlete has no other mechanism with which to cope with the pressures.

Several theories have been employed to account for a person's predisposition to substance abuse. These theories include genetic predisposition, obsessive-compulsive personality type, addictive personality, and simply that substance abuse is a learned behavior.[41] Another perspective is that the undue emphasis on winning at all costs at all levels of sports participation influences athletes to take performance-enhancing drugs.

Points to Ponder
Why do you think substance abuse is so prevalent among college athletes?

One substance commonly abused by athletes is **anabolic steroids**. Anabolic steroids are chemical derivatives of testosterone and are used to increase muscle mass, which helps improve strength and power. Anabolic steroids have a host of side effects, one of the most serious and well-publicized of which is **roid rage**. Roid rage involves sudden outbursts of aggressive and violent behavior that is often uncontrollable. This behavior may be witnessed by family members, friends, classmates, teammates, coaches, athletic trainers, and other people who spend time with the affected athlete. Athletic trainers are likely to observe these behaviors because they are often around athletes during practice and conditioning and in the athletic training room. Athletic trainers should recognize abnormally aggressive behavior as a warning sign of substance abuse and then wait until the athlete is in a normal state of mind to discuss the problem. An appointment should be made for the athlete to meet with a mental health professional.[42]

As with eating disorders, athletic trainers must be able to prevent and recognize substance abuse and then intervene appropriately. Many warning signs exist to alert athletic trainers to a possible substance abuser. Early warning signs may include the inability to maintain normal commitments with school or employment. The student may start getting lower grades and missing classes, practice, and work shifts. Other signs include excessive fluctuations in mood, changes in groups of friends, and withdrawal and secretiveness[42] (Box 22-5).

After raising the issue of substance abuse, the athletic trainer should make the appropriate referral. The athletic trainer should schedule a time to meet with the athlete privately and discuss his or her recent physical, emotional, and behavioral changes. Recovery is a complex process that affects all aspects of a person's life.

anabolic steroids chemical derivatives of testosterone used to increase muscle mass, which helps improve strength and power

roid rage sudden outbursts of aggressive and violent behavior that is often uncontrollable and is caused by steroid misuse

BOX 22-5 Common Signs and Symptoms of Substance Use and Abuse

Physical Signs and Symptoms

- Acting intoxicated
- Bloodshot or red eyes, droopy eyelids
- Inaccurate eye movement
- Wearing sunglasses at inappropriate times
- Abnormally pale complexion
- Impaired motor skills
- Repressed physical development
- Loss of or increased appetite

Emotional-Cognitive Signs and Symptoms

- Moodiness
- Depression
- Anxiety
- Mood swings
- Emotional outbursts
- Irritability
- Confusion
- Denial that problem exists
- Belief that individual is in control

Behavioral Problems

- Inappropriate overreaction to mild criticism
- Decreased interaction and communication with others
- Change in speech or vocabulary patterns
- Preoccupation with self
- Neglect of personal appearance
- Loss of interest in sport
- Loss of motivation and enthusiasm
- Lethargy
- Blackouts
- Loss of ability to assume responsibility
- Need for instant gratification
- Changes in morals, values, and beliefs
- Change in friends (peer groups)

Data from Bacon VL et al: Substance abuse. In Taylor J, Wilson GS, editors: *Applying sport psychology: four perspectives*, pp. 240–241, Champaign, Ill, 2005, Human Kinetics.

Therefore a variety of mental health professionals, such as addiction counselors, licensed professional counselors, licensed psychologists, psychiatrists, and sport psychologists, may be involved. In educational settings, referral to the school guidance counselor or counseling center may be the first logical step in the process.[42]

As with eating disorders, it is not uncommon for athletes to deny that they have a drug problem. However, in this case, if their drug of choice is an illegal or banned drug, there could be legal ramifications associated with their abuse, which complicates the situation. The first step in treatment is for the athlete to admit that he or she has a problem. Family and friends may also recognize the problem; in this case, the athletic trainer and the athlete's loved ones should work together to help the athlete understand the importance of seeking treatment from a mental health professional.[41]

Self-Injurious Behavior

You have so much pain inside yourself, you try and hurt yourself on the outside because you need help.—Princess Diana, 1996[43]

Self-injury is an alarming trend among adolescents and young adults. Increasing numbers of adolescents and young adults are hurting themselves on purpose. Although self-injury has existed for quite some time, public interest in self-injurious behaviors (SIB) has increased significantly over the past decade. Self-injury is also called self-harm, self-mutilation, self-wounding, or self-abuse. **Self-injurious behavior** is defined as a voluntary, deliberate, repetitive, impulsive, nonlethal harming of one's own body. A common myth is that self-injury is failed suicide, when in fact self-injury is the deliberate damage to one's body with no conscious intent to commit suicide. The most common form of adolescent and young adult self-injury is cutting oneself with a razor blade or knife or using matches. Areas of the body that are easiest to conceal with clothing are generally preferred. Other common methods of self-injury are listed in Box 22-6.[44]

It is estimated that self-injurers represent nearly 1% of the population, with a higher proportion of female subjects. The behavior typically first emerges during puberty, and it can persist into adulthood. However,

self-injurious behavior a voluntary, deliberate, repetitive, impulsive, nonlethal harming of one's body

BOX 22-6 Common Methods of Self-Injury

- Cutting, scratching, self-biting, gouging
- Carving words or symbols into skin
- Sticking needles or pins into skin
- Picking scabs or interfering with wound healing
- Burning
- Punching self or objects
- Infecting oneself
- Inserting objects in body openings
- Bruising or breaking bones
- Some forms of hair pulling, as well as other various forms of bodily harm
- Exercising to hurt oneself
- Stopping medication or starving with intent to cause harm
- Deliberate recklessness with intent to cause harm

SIB has been known to transcend gender, age, religion, and educational and income level. Children of divorced or separated parents; people who have undergone traumatic childhood experiences such as emotional, physical, and sexual abuse; and men and women with gay, lesbian, or bisexual orientation are particularly susceptible to SIB.[45] In addition, eating disorders and substance abuse can contribute to the incidence of SIB.

Self-injury and anorexia have a lot in common. Research has shown that 35% to 80% of people who self-injure also suffer from eating disorders. Afflicted persons use their bodies to work out psychological conflict and to obtain relief from overwhelming feelings of tension, anger, loneliness, emptiness, and self-hatred. Both behaviors are impulsive, secretive, ritualistic, and ridden with shame and guilt, and both involve attacks on the body and a disturbance in body image.[43]

Self-injury is viewed as a coping mechanism to help relieve unwanted emotions and painful memories, to punish oneself, and to get attention from others.[44] In essence, some adolescents and young adults may seek physical pain to distract themselves from emotional pain. Think of a high school student-athlete who may have just gotten into a heated argument with a teammate. This athlete may intentionally cut himself or herself to deal with anger from the argument. The pain from the self-inflicted wound instantly becomes the focus of attention for the athlete, helping to diminish the unwanted emotion of anger.

Many people who engage in SIB seek help from professionals or family and friends. As health care professionals, athletic trainers are well-positioned to intervene with self-injuring athletes. Athletic trainers should remember that not all SIB is considered abnormal. For example, piercings and tattoos can constitute self-injury; however, in this culture, various forms of piercings and tattoos are common trends.[43] When assessing the possibility of SIB, the athletic trainer should always consider the athlete's religious and cultural background in determining what is and what is not normal behavior.

Athletic trainers should be competent in the recognition and management of SIB. Several warning signs may assist at times when self-inflicted injury is not so obvious:[45]

- Sharp objects such as razor blades in the athlete's possession
- Unexplained frequent injuries such as scratches or burns
- The wearing of long sleeves or pants in warm weather
- Extreme mood swings
- Depression

Athletic trainers should consider themselves lucky to be entrusted with information about an athlete's destructive behavior. It is a positive sign when the athlete's abnormal behavior is no longer a secret. However, athletic trainers should always recognize their limitations in this role. They should express compassion, understanding, and support, and, most of all, they should listen to what the athlete has to say. Once SIB has been recognized and established, the primary role of the athletic trainer is to help the athlete get appropriate treatment. Clarify the importance of seeking the care of a mental health professional who has experience with SIB. Provide referral recommendations from an updated list. As with eating disorders, the athletic trainer may also offer to set up an appointment and accompany the athlete to the first session. The key is to get the athlete to seek care from the appropriate mental health professional. As part of helping the athlete, the athletic trainer may want to share some Web sites that have useful information. "Self-Abuse Finally Ends (SAFE) Alternatives" is one such site. This site has an information hotline and referral information for mental health professionals around the country. Another recommended site is "Secret Shame." This site features a wealth of information, excellent links, message boards, and chat rooms. Information regarding how to access this site is provided at the end of the chapter.

ROLE OF THE ATHLETIC TRAINER

Beyond their role in preventing and caring for injuries, athletic trainers also serve as educators, injury advisors, nutritionists, counselors, problem solvers, friends, and academic advisors.[46] Athletic trainers are in an ideal position to inform, educate, and assist with the psychosocial as well as the physiological ramifications of injury. Given their frequent contact with injured athletes and their wealth of knowledge regarding sports-related injury, athletic trainers are in the perfect position to train athletes to implement psychological intervention strategies (e.g., communication, self-talk, counseling, goal setting, imagery, relaxation techniques) to help prevent the occurrence of sports injuries, help the athlete adjust to injury, and facilitate rehabilitation.

Athletic trainers acknowledge the importance of psychological skills in the athletic training room, but many athletic trainers do not feel adequately trained to implement the interventions, nor do they perceive themselves to be adequately equipped to deal with some of the psychological aspects of recovery from injury. Therefore athletic trainers should receive specific training regarding this aspect of health care.

Psychosocial Intervention Strategies

Athletic trainers may implement psychological interventions with athletes to help prevent injury (stress-injury) and promote rehabilitation adherence. Several sport psychology interventions may be used during the rehabilitation process. Research has identified communication, goal setting, imagery, positive self-talk, and relaxation techniques as helpful skills for athletes to use both before and after injury. The goals of psychological intervention with injured athletes are to facilitate the rehabilitation process, maintain emotional equilibrium, mobilize coping resources, enhance mental readiness for return to sport, and promote self-efficacy.

It is important to realize that many athletes are skeptical about these interventions and dismiss them as "shrink stuff." When introducing psychological intervention strategies, athletic trainers should be careful to present the concept to athletes in a non-threatening manner. Athletes are accustomed to having a sense of control over their environment. Once injured, the athlete is placed in a position of dependency. The subsequent feelings of helplessness can be uncomfortable for someone who is accustomed to being in control. During rehabilitation and implementation of psychological interventions, the athletic trainer should make sure that the athlete has a role in the rehabilitation program. Helping the athlete maintain a sense of control during this period will facilitate both physical and psychological recovery.[47]

Communication and Education

Communication and education are simple, very straightforward intervention skills, but they are often overlooked. Athletic trainers interact with clients, various members of the sports medicine team, colleagues, coaches, and supervisors every day (Figure 22-6). Despite these frequent interactions, athletic trainers do not always possess good communication skills. Much of the language related to injury and rehabilitation is foreign to the injured athlete. Sports medicine practitioners often confuse their clients by using advanced medical terminology and providing only brief explanations that clients often simply do not understand. Such communication deficits may leave the injured athlete with unanswered questions or an inadequate understanding of treatment goals.

The first step in establishing good communication with a patient is to establish rapport. The greater the rapport between the athletic trainer and patient, the more effective the healing relationship will be. Rapport fosters trust, which is essential throughout the injury treatment and rehabilitation process. During this time, it is common for the patient to feel vulnerable because of pain, fear, and uncertainty. Trust helps reduce these anxious feelings; lack of trust will increase them.

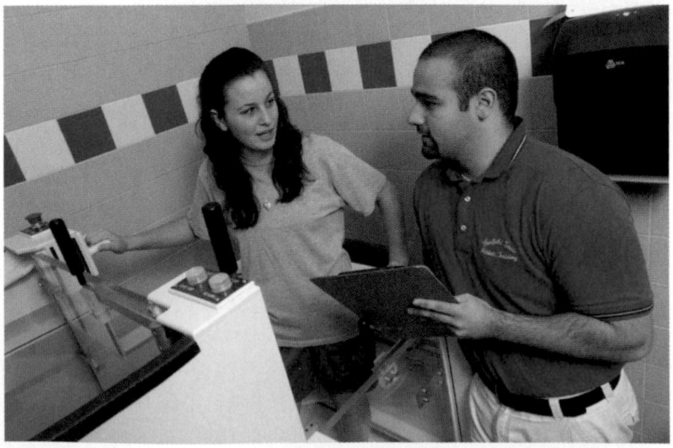

FIGURE 22-6 Communication is an essential component of any rehabilitation plan.

Listening is the most important part of the communication process.[48] It is also one of the hardest skills to learn. Do not just to listen to the words being said but also to the tone in which they are stated. Listen as well to what is not being said, and observe the client's body language. The following suggestions promote better listening skills:

- *Understand the problem before you try to fix it.* Listen carefully to what the patient has to say about his or her injuries. If you sense some emotional concerns, reinforce the person's feelings with a statement such as "You seem to be frustrated." Active listening skills such as paraphrasing or summarizing can help you uncover the emotional meaning of the injury.
- *Value the athlete's input.* If rehabilitation from injury is to be a collaborative process between athlete and athletic trainer, it is important to seek the athlete's input in a manner that communicates respect.
- *Check perceptions and get specifics.* Just because athletes who are injured do not ask you questions about their rehabilitation does not mean that they understand treatment goals, tasks, or exercise prescriptions. It is good practice to have them use concrete examples and specify how they intend to accomplish their treatment goals.
- *Listen for the "but."* Part of being a good listener is paying attention to the content and structure of what is being said. Take, for example, the following sentence: "Everything is going along great, but I know the season starts up real soon." In this example, the use of the "but" discounts the first half of the sentence and suggests that the athlete's most pressing concerns are related to his or her reentry to sports.[49]

Ensure a comfortable, non-threatening environment when communicating with the patient. Be receptive to their questions, and listen to their concerns and needs. Attempt to understand fully what the injury means to the athlete. For example, consider the patient with a torn anterior cruciate ligament. The athletic trainer may have rehabilitated such an injury 25 times. For the athletic trainer the injury may be routine, but for the involved patient this can be an extremely difficult time. Although the athletic trainer's natural tendency may be to focus on the physical aspects of recovery, it is important to address the athlete's psychosocial needs. Athletic

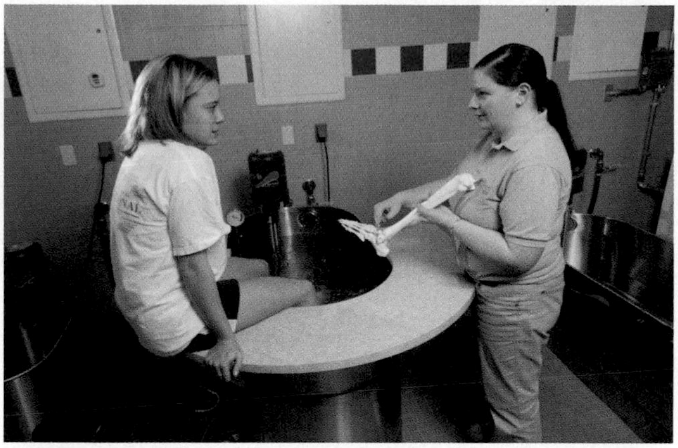

FIGURE 22-7 Educating the patient about the injury and subsequent rehabilitation encourages active participation during the rehabilitation process.

trainers should strive to talk to the client in the same way that they would like a health professional to communicate with them.

The primary goal of educating the individual is to help him or her understand in detail the injury and subsequent rehabilitation. This educational approach also encourages them to actively participate in the rehabilitation program (Figure 22-7).

Initially, the athletic trainer should provide information about the injury, proposed treatment, and expectations for recovery in terms that the client can understand. Athletic trainers should also convey a sense of how the injury will heal and provide specific information about methods of rehabilitation and how they will facilitate the client's recovery. Anatomical models, diagrams, video and computer graphics, and brochures all further this goal. Athletic trainers should explain the possibility of setbacks and plateaus while assuring the client that they will be there throughout rehabilitation. Lastly, athletic trainers should make sure that they have explained their expectations for the rehabilitation process and should ask what the client's expectations are as well.

Self-Talk

Self-talk is an important and omnipresent form of intrapersonal communication. Self-talk inevitably helps shape and predict a person's actions, and it can facilitate a positive approach to recovery from injury. The goal of self-talk in this context is to decrease negative self-talk, which can be detrimental to successful recovery. Positive self-talk can counteract dysfunctional thoughts by increasing one's awareness of inappropriate thoughts.[48]

A common intervention with self-talk is "thought stoppage." **Thought stoppage** is used with clients who have negative, self-defeating thoughts about their recovery. It helps clients become more aware of what they are thinking. The athletic trainer should ask the client to use a trigger word such as "stop" to interrupt negative thoughts. Injured athletes commonly have negative and irrational thoughts after sustaining an injury (e.g., "This is a terrible injury; there is no way I'll be able to play again; this ice will never help get rid of the swelling in my ankle; the athletic trainers don't know what they are doing"). Patients can be taught to control these thoughts and replace them with more positive and constructive thoughts. For example, "My leg is weak; I can't do anything!" could be replaced by "I will work hard and concentrate on each of my exercises to make it stronger!"[50]

An effective tool to determine whether a client engages in negative self-talk is to prescribe a self-talk diary. Do not tell the client specifically what you are looking for; simply ask him or her to keep a daily diary as part of the treatment and rehabilitation program. Have the client make daily entries regarding their treatment, how they are feeling, and so forth. After a few days, take a look at the diary to see whether any negative self-talk is evident. If so, point this out to the client and discuss the benefits of positive self-talk in the recovery from injury.

Counseling

Because athletic trainers typically spend extended periods of time with athletes under conditions that promote personal interaction and trust, they are in a position to provide counseling on a variety of issues. A study found that 79% of participating athletic trainers had found it necessary to counsel student-athletes about personal issues.[1,46] Because most athletic training programs do not have mental health professionals readily available, athletic trainers become the first point of contact for athletes who have psychosocial concerns that require attention (Box 22-7).

The Board of Certification's "Role Delineation Study for the Entry-Level Athletic Trainer" recognizes counseling as a relevant professional task. The National Athletic Trainers' Association's "Athletic Training Educational Competencies" supports this important area of professional preparation as well with a domain solely covering psychosocial intervention, referral competencies, and clinical proficiencies in which the entry-level athletic trainer must be competent and proficient.[51]

Who are counselors? This continues to be a controversial question in the helping professions. Credentialed or licensed counselors include school guidance and

self-talk a form of intrapersonal communication
thought stoppage technique used with clients who have negative, self-defeating thoughts about their recovery; helps clients become more aware of what they are thinking

BOX 22-7 Injury Education Guidelines

- Basic anatomy of the injured area
- Changes caused by injury
- Active and passive rehabilitation methods
- Mechanisms by which rehabilitation methods work
- Description of diagnostic and surgical procedures (if necessary)
- Potential problems with pain and inadequate coping mechanisms
- Differentiation of benign pain from dangerous pain
- Guidelines for independent use of modalities (e.g., heat, cold)
- Plan for progressing active rehabilitation (e.g., resistance training)
- Anticipated timetable for rehabilitation
- Possibility of treatment plateaus
- Purposes of medication with emphasis on consistent use as prescribed
- Potential side effects of medication with encouragement to report these to the physician
- Rationale for limits on daily physical activities during healing
- Guidelines for the use of braces, orthotic devices, or crutches
- Injury as a source of stress and a challenge to maintaining a positive attitude
- Rehabilitation as an active collaborative learning process
- Methods of assessing readiness for return to play
- Deciding when to hold back and when to go all-out
- Long-term maintenance and care of healing injury

From Heil J: A comprehensive approach to injury management. In Heil J, ed: *Psychology of sport injury,* Champaign, Ill, 1993, Human Kinetics.

BOX 22-8 Characteristics of the Effective Athletic Trainer Counselor/Helper

- *Has effective listening skills:* Allowing the athlete to talk and share useful information may be therapeutic in itself.
- *Is accessible:* Be available to the athlete when assistance is needed; demonstrate a willingness to take time to help the athlete.
- *Has a positive attitude:* Using both oral and body language, emphasize the positive elements of the injury or situation rather than focusing on the negative aspects.
- *Sets realistic goals using the athlete's input:* Realistic goal setting develops and implements both short-term and long-term goals.
- *Treats the athlete as an individual:* Approach the athlete with the understanding that no two individuals are alike.
- *Educates the athlete about the injury:* Provide a realistic and understandable explanation about the injury and what to expect regarding recovery.
- *Motivates the athlete:* Demonstrate empathy, not sympathy, by understanding the physical and emotional challenges the athlete is facing; provide encouragement.
- *Understands professional limitations:* Recognizing that the psychosocial problems are beyond his or her helping skills, the athletic trainer is willing to refer the athlete to an appropriate mental health care provider for more definitive care.

From Misasi SP, Kemler DS, Redmond CJ: Counseling skills and the athletic therapist, *Athl Ther Today* 3(1):35–38, 1998.

adjustment counselors, clinical psychologists, and psychiatrists. Athletic trainers, physical therapists, and other health care professionals are not credentialed counselors. Instead, they are de facto counselors because of their daily interactions with individuals who seek their assistance and guidance. It has been suggested that "helper" would be a more appropriate description. In this role, athletic trainers must respect their boundaries as "helpers" and rely on an established referral network of mental health professionals when referral is necessary.[52]

In addition to providing a trusting and accepting environment, athletic trainers must demonstrate suitable personal attributes that make them approachable and facilitate a good relationship with athletes (Box 22-8).

One of the ways in which athletic trainers become better counselors is through **attending.** *Attending* is defined as being aware of one's own nonverbal behavior as well as observing nonverbal behaviors and characteristics of the client. Attending requires the ability to focus one's energy, attention, and thoughts on another person. Important aspects of attending include physically facing the other person, maintaining eye contact and appropriate posture, and establishing rapport. Unconditional positive regard, or acceptance and warmth, is another important quality when counseling.[53]

Collaborative Goal Setting

Goal setting, an extremely popular psychological intervention strategy used by athletic trainers, is derived from a concept with which athletes are already comfortable and familiar because of their athletic experiences. "Goal setting can provide motivation and commitment, direct the athlete's attention to controllable factors, and help build confidence."[50] Goals motivate people to action, and goal setting has been shown to enhance rehabilitation adherence. Effective goal setting requires a systematic approach that can enhance the patient's commitment and motivation in several ways[54]:

- It clarifies each person's role in the rehabilitation process.
- It gives the athlete an active role both psychologically and physically in his or her rehabilitation.
- It helps the athlete understand the importance of the rehabilitation exercises.
- It provides optimal challenges.
- It gives the athlete a feeling of being back in control.

attending being aware of one's own nonverbal behavior as well as observing nonverbal behaviors and characteristics of the client

- It holds the athlete accountable for a given standard of performance.
- It increases the athlete's self-confidence.
- It breaks the rehabilitation process into manageable steps.
- It decreases anxiety by focusing on what needs to be done.

Box 22-9 provides a summary of guidelines for goal setting. To develop a goal setting plan, the athletic trainer may use a **goal ladder**. A goal ladder involves using small attainable steps to reach the goal.

Injured athletes often set long-term goals without focusing on what to do in the present. For example, a javelin thrower who had surgery for a torn ulnar collateral ligament might expect to miss a year of competition. When asked what goals he has set for himself, he might respond, "to return next season." This athlete must establish short-term goals through the use of a goal ladder that will lead to the long-term goal. On a related note, plateaus and setbacks occur because something is blocking the patient's progress. These roadblocks fall into the following four categories.[55]

1. *Lack of knowledge:* It is important to inform the client about the injury and the recovery process. Ensure that the client understands the rationale for treatment, the goals of rehabilitation, and the possible side-effects or sensations that may occur. By communicating this information to the client, the athletic trainer can minimize the impact of unnecessary surprises.

BOX 22-9 Summary of Guidelines for Goal Setting

- Goals should be meaningful to both the patient and the athletic trainer and established collaboratively to place the patient in an active role.
- Goals must be performance, not outcome, oriented.
- Goals should be stated in positive terms.
- Goals should be individualized for each patient.
- Goals must be specific, objective, and measurable.
- Goals should be accompanied by strategies for achievement.
- Goals must be challenging yet realistic. Do not set the patient up for failure.
- Goals should be process-oriented rather than outcome-oriented so that control over goal attainment rests with the patient.
- Establish short-term, and to a lesser extent, long-term goals.
- Goals should be few and prioritized.
- Goals should have a target date for completion.
- Goals must be recorded and monitored.
- Goals must hold the patient accountable.
- Goals must be reinforced or supported.
- Goals must be flexible, and modified as necessary.

Data from Wayda VK, Armenth-Brothers F, Boyce BA: Goal setting: a key to injury rehabilitation. *Athl Ther Today* 3(1):21–25, 1998.

2. *Lack of skill:* Do not assume that the patient is comfortable with the techniques being prescribed during the therapeutic exercise program. It is important for the athletic trainer to explain and demonstrate these techniques beforehand.
3. *Lack of risk-taking ability:* Some fear and anxiety is normal during recovery. For some injured athletes, however, fear of reinjury becomes a roadblock. These athletes are afraid to push themselves during rehabilitation, which prevents them from progressing through the recovery process. A frequently observed risk-taking roadblock occurs when an injury forces an athlete to ask for help. Many are uncomfortable about allowing themselves to be vulnerable. Talking about their fears or seeking medical advice is often quite difficult for such athletes.
4. *Lack of adequate social support:* Lack of social support can affect the injured athlete during recovery. This social support can come from family, friends, athletic trainers, coaches, teammates, or other athletes who have been through a similar injury experience.

Helping the patient understand these possible roadblocks facilitates a smoother transition through the recovery process.

Social Support

As previously mentioned, through skill and effort, athletes are accustomed to being in control. Once injured, the athlete is placed in an uncomfortable position of dependency. After incurring an injury that requires weeks or months of rehabilitation, the athlete may feel alienated from the team. The athlete may feel that the coaches no longer care, the teammates no longer have time to spend with him or her, and that all social opportunities revolve around rehabilitation. The athlete will be prone to loneliness and isolation during this period, which can negatively influence recovery.

During the injury and rehabilitation process, most athletes need support from those around them. Interactions with members of the sports medicine team, in addition to normal relationships with family, friends, teammates, and coaches, can provide the social support necessary for injured athletes to feel that they do not have to deal with the injury and rehabilitation alone. Athletic trainers are probably in the best position to provide the various forms of social support that athletes need during this difficult time. In addition to providing social support themselves, athletic trainers can encourage teammates, coaches, and other involved parties to support and encourage the injured athlete. For this reason,

goal ladder using small attainable steps to reach the goal athletic trainers should consider scheduling rehabilitation with the injured athlete when the team is present—in other words, at the usual prepractice or practice time.

Research supports the need for social support among individuals who suffer from health problems.[56] Pairing patients during rehabilitation or establishing an injury support group can be an invaluable aid to those recovering from injury. The support group should foster camaraderie, encouragement, and sharing of experiences to help injured athletes overcome feelings of apprehension and anxiety about the future. Being injured often leads to loneliness. Having the opportunity to interact with others who have recovered or are in the process of recovering from a similar injury can be extremely beneficial.

Imagery

Although it is a more advanced intervention for athletic trainers to use, **imagery** can be a very effective psychological intervention in conjunction with other modalities that facilitate recovery. Many people consider imagery and visualization to be the same. However, visualization uses only the visual sense, whereas imagery incorporates the use of all the senses to create or recreate an experience in the mind.[57] The senses relevant in imagery are visual (sight), auditory (hearing), olfactory (smell), tactile (touch), gustatory (taste), and kinesthetic (movement of body in space). By using all of the senses, a person who is using an image of the ocean to facilitate relaxation would be able to see the ocean, hear the ocean, feel the ocean breeze, and smell and taste the salt water.

Because athletes typically cannot participate in physical training while injured, imagery allows them to mentally practice skills and strategies during their recovery. Imagery can be used for rehabilitation rehearsal, healing imagery, performance rehearsal, relaxation, and emotional rehearsal. Mental practice of physical and performance skills may also be used in the imagery training. Imagery works best when the injured athlete believes that it will assist the healing process. One way to implement imagery is through the use of the following four-step process.[58]:

1. *Introduce imagery to the individual:* During this step, educate the client regarding what imagery is and how it can aid the healing process as an adjunct to the rehabilitation program. Providing examples of athletes who have used imagery successfully will help persuade the client that the intervention is efficacious.
2. *Evaluate the individual's imaging ability:* It is helpful if the client has some background training related to imagery. The client should be able to see, control, and vividly construct a mind-image.
3. *Assist the individual in developing basic imagery skills:* During this step, the client should work on improving the vividness, control, and self-perception of the images he or she creates. To enhance vividness, have the client practice a basic skill used in his or her sport. After the client masters this step, have the client practice with more complex images. To foster control, the client should expand from the previous skill and perform the skill with teammates and opponents. To enhance self-perception, the client should select a favorite performance and play this scenario over and over. As the client improves in the practice of these imagery techniques, he or she can progress to injury and rehabilitation imagery techniques.
4. *Provide tips on adjunctive use of imagery in rehabilitation programs:* Imagery in rehabilitation programs calls for athletic trainers to first educate the client regarding the details of the injury. This involves providing information to help the client understand what the injured part looks like and what it should look like as it heals. Augment your explanation with anatomical models, pictures, radiographs, and other relevant documentation. Then have the client create a mental picture of the injury, followed by an image of that injury being repaired. For example, the client may picture sprained ligaments reattaching to bone or increased blood flow to facilitate removal of waste products from a sprained ankle.

Relaxation Techniques

Interventions for lowering excessive physiological activity and enhancing concentration include relaxation techniques such as progressive muscle relaxation (PMR) and breathing exercises. These techniques help athletes release unnecessary muscle tension and calm the mind. The use of relaxation techniques teaches athletes how to relax their muscles, promoting a calm state. Relaxation techniques have been shown to decrease stress, decrease injury occurrence, and decrease time-loss after injury.[59]

Introduced by Jacobson, **progressive muscle relaxation** (PMR) is a form of relaxation that is often quite popular with athletes.[60] PMR involves the systematic tension and relaxation of muscle groups in an attempt to reduce anxiety associated with being injured. The client lies or sits in a comfortable position. The environment should be quiet and relaxing; some people find that relaxing music facilitates PMR. The client inhales and tenses a specific muscle group for approximately

imagery the ability to use all the senses to create or recreate an experience in the mind

progressive muscle relaxation the systematic tension and relaxation of muscle groups in an attempt to reduce anxiety associated with being injured

5 seconds, then exhales and releases the tension while focusing on relaxation. This is repeated for different muscle groups in a systematic fashion. The relaxation phase teaches an awareness of what absence of tension feels like and that it can be voluntarily induced. The basic premise is that by first concentrating on the contraction, or stressful feeling, the person can more thoroughly achieve the relaxation phase.

Diaphragmatic breathing, or belly breathing, is one of the easiest methods of relaxation. In this method, the emphasis of breathing is centered on the lower abdomen. Ask the athlete to take a deep belly breath and then fully exhale while focusing on the calming effect of the exhalation. Have the client concentrate on feeling the breath enter the body and finally leave it. Repeating a cue word (e.g., "relax," "calm," "focus") during the exhalation also helps.[57]

With regular practice, athletes can use these skills to help them relax and decrease their potential for injury, or reinjury, during stressful events and undesirable psychological states such as anxiety.

Determination for Referral to a Mental Health Practitioner

Because of their frequent contact with injured athletes, athletic trainers are in a unique position to monitor the athlete's physical and mental status and make timely referrals. Athletic trainers are often confronted with more than just injuries. Other reasons for referral may emerge, including stress, depression, anxiety, family and other relationship issues, physical or sexual abuse, academic difficulties, eating disorders, substance abuse, and self-injury. Athletic trainers obviously do not have the expertise to intervene, effectively manage, and assume primary treatment responsibilities for such individuals.[61,62]

Athletic trainers must know when to provide the counseling services themselves and when to refer an athlete to a mental health professional. The best way to make such decisions is to establish working relationships with local mental health specialists who can serve as consultants, practitioners, and in-service educators. Whether they are psychiatrists, psychologists, counselors, social workers, or guidance counselors, these specialists should have training in one or more of the typical problem areas and, if possible, an understanding of athletes and the sport experience. As consultants, mental health specialists can work with athletic trainers to help them assess athletes' psychological responses to injury. The athletic trainer and mental health specialists build a working alliance, establishing trust in each others' skills. For those who work in the collegiate setting, a good place to start establishing a referral network is the counseling center on campus. Athletic trainers who work in high schools should start with the school nurse and guidance counselors. Athletic trainers who work in clinical settings should form liaisons with referring physicians and other health care professionals in the community.[61,62]

SUMMARY

As health care providers, athletic trainers are central to the athlete's care from the onset of injury until the return to activity. Beyond the physical concerns of the athlete, athletic trainers must have, at minimum, a basic understanding of the psychosocial issues that affect athletes. Because of their frequent contact with injured athletes, athletic trainers are in a unique position to monitor athletes' physical and mental status and make timely referrals. For this reason, athletic trainers should establish working relationships with local mental health specialists who can serve as consultants, practitioners, and in-service educators. These consultants can help in the assessment of the psychosocial concerns covered in this chapter. In the most basic context, athletic trainers must have the ability to recognize when an athlete has a psychosocial issue that warrants referral. The rapport that the athletic trainer has developed with the athlete and an updated referral list are helpful tools in the rehabilitation process.

Revisiting The OPENING *Scenario*

Returning to the opening scenario, how do you account for Celeste's and Jacob's different reactions to their similar injuries? Did Wade spend more time communicating with and educating Celeste? Does Jacob have more stress in his life? Could Jacob have more negative perceptions of his injury than Celeste? Is it possible that Jacob does not get to play very much and considers his injury a more socially acceptable reason for not playing? Could Jacob feel alienated from his team and coach? Is Jacob more concerned about reinjury than Celeste? Is Celeste more resilient or hardy than Jacob? Does Celeste have a greater tolerance for pain and more effective social support? Does Celeste have greater coping skills? Does nutrition play a factor? How about alcohol abuse?

In general, any of these responses (and many more) could play a role in this scenario. The bottom line when treating an injured athlete is to look at the big picture; in many cases, the athletic trainer will be treating much more than just the injury.

The following comparison may help. When examining an injured athlete with anterior knee pain, the athletic trainer would also look at the foot and other structures to determine the treatment and rehabilitation plan. The athletic trainer would not focus on the knee alone. In the same context, are there any psychosocial or other variables (e.g., nutrition) that might play a role in the athlete's injury and recovery? If you were Wade, how would you approach Jacob to discuss his progress or lack thereof?

Issues & Ethics

Colleen, a 16-year-old world-class gymnast, sustains a major head and neck injury after losing her grip on the horizontal bar dismount and landing headfirst on the mats 10 feet below. Her injury will prevent her from practicing as well as competing in the Pan-Am Championships, which are scheduled for the following week. There is a possibility that this injury will terminate her gymnastics career. She is displaying outward signs of severe depression and antisocial behavior. She hardly speaks to anyone and refuses to respond to athletic trainer's questions about her feelings, adherence to her rehabilitation program, and her future plans. Colleen feels that her coaches have ceased to care about her, although they do. However, they are under tremendous pressure to prepare the other girls and elevate someone to replace Colleen in their competition next week.

What psychological or biopsychosocial responses could you expect Colleen to display? What coping strategies could you employ to help facilitate her recovery from this career-ending injury? What is your role as the athletic trainer with regard to her emotional stability?

Web Links

American Psychological Association Division 38 (Health Psychology): www.health-psych.org/
American Psychological Association Division 47 (Exercise and Sport Psychology): www.psyc.unt.edu/apadiv47
Association for the Advancement of Applied Sport Psychology: www.aaasponline.org
International Society of Sports Psychology (ISSP): www.issponline.org/
National Eating Disorders Association: www.nationaleatingdisorders.org
National Institute of Mental Health: www.nimh.nih.gov/healthinformation/index.cfm
National Mental Health Association: www.nmha.org
S.A.F.E. Alternatives (Self-Abuse Finally Ends): www.selfinjury.com
Secret Shame: www.palace.net/~llama/psych/injury.html

References

1. Larson GA, Starkey C, Zaichkowsky LD: Psychological aspects of athletic injuries as perceived by athletic trainers, *Sport Psychol* 10(1): 37–47, 1996.
2. Rotella RJ, Heyman SR: Stress, injury, and the psychological rehabilitation of athletes. In Williams J, editor: *Applied sport psychology*, Palo Alto, Calif, 1986, Mayfield.
3. Smith AM, Milliner EK: Injured athletes and the risk of suicide, *J Athl Train* 29(4): 337–341, 1994.
4. Andersen MB, Williams JM: A model of stress and athletic injury: prediction and prevention, *J Sport Exercise Psy* 10: 294–306, 1988.
5. Williams JM, Andersen MB: Psychosocial antecedents of sport injury: review and critique of the stress and injury model, *J Appl Sport Psychol* 10: 5–25, 1998.
6. Wiese-Bjornstal DM, Shaffer SM: Psychosocial dimensions of sport injury. In Ray R, Wiese-Bjornstal DM, editors: *Counseling in sports medicine*, Champaign, Ill, 1999, Human Kinetics.
7. Udry E, Andersen MB: Athletic injury and sport behavior. In Horn TS, editor: *Advances in sport psychology*, ed 2, Champaign, Ill, 2002, Human Kinetics.
8. Wiese-Bjornstal DM, Shaffer SM: Psychosocial dimensions of sport injury. In Ray R, Wiese-Bjornstal DM, editors: *Counseling in sports medicine*, Champaign, Ill 1999, Human Kinetics.
9. Williams JM, Scherzer CB: Injury risk and rehabilitation: psychological considerations. In Williams JM, editor: *Applied sport psychology: personal growth to peak performance*, ed 5, New York, 2006, McGraw Hill.
10. Johnson U: Psychological antecedents to injury and illness. In Kolt GS, Anderson MB, editors: *Psychology in the physical and manual therapies*, Philadelphia, 2004, Churchill Livingstone.
11. Smith RE, Smoll FL, Ptacek, JT: Conjunctive moderator variables in vulnerability and resiliency research: life stress, social support and coping skills, and adolescent sport injuries, *J Pers Soc Psychol*, 58(2): 360–369, 1990.
12. Williams JM, Tonymon P, Wadsworth WA: Relationship of stress to injury in intercollegiate volleyball, *J Human Stress*, 12: 38–43, 1986.
13. Hughes R, Coakley J: Positive deviance among athletes: the implications of overconformity to the sport ethic. In Yiannakis A, Melnick MJ, editors: *Contemporary issues in sociology of sport*, Rev ed., Champaign, Ill, 2001, Human Kinetics.
14. Safai P. Healing the body in the "culture of risk": examining the negotiation of treatment between sport medicine clinicians and injured athletes in Canadian intercollegiate sport, *Sociol Sport J* 20: 127–146, 2003.
15. Charlesworth H, Young K: Why English female university athletes play with pain: motivations and rationalizations. In Young K, editor: *Sporting bodies, damaged selves: sociological studies of sports-related injury,* Boston, 2004, Elsevier.
16. Weinberg RS, Gould D: *Foundations of sport and exercise psychology*, ed 3, Champaign, Ill, 2003, Human Kinetics.
17. Otto J, Newhouse D: *Jim Otto: the pain of glory*, Champaign, Ill, 1999, Sports Publishing Inc.
18. Nixon HL II: Social pressure, social support, and help seeking for pain and injuries in college sports networks, *Journal of Sport & Social Issues*, 18(4): 340–355, 1994.
19. Rome J: *The Jim Rome sport radio talk show*, October 18, 2005. Premiere Radio Networks. http://www.jimrome.com/home.html. pp
20. Theberge N: "It's part of the game": physicality and the production of gender in women's hockey. In Yiannakis A, Melnick MJ, editors: *Contemporary issues in sociology of sport*, Rev ed. Champaign, Ill, 2001, Human Kinetics.
21. Tracey J: The emotional response to the injury and rehabilitation process, *J Appl Sport Psych* 15: 279–293, 2003.
22. Petitpas AJ: To grieve or not to grieve? *Athlet Ther Today* 1(4): 38, 1996.

23. Johnston LH, Carroll D: The context of emotional responses to athletic injury: qualitative analysis, *J Sport Rehabil* 7: 206–220, 1998.
24. Flint FA: Integrating sport psychology and sports medicine in research: the dilemmas, *J Appl Sport Psychol* 10: 83–102, 1998.
25. Smith R: Recognition, management, and referral of the injured athlete with psychological problems, *Athlet Ther Today* 3(1): 14–18, 1998.
26. Schwenz SJ: Psychology of injury and rehabilitation, *Athlet Ther Today* 6(1): 44–45, 2001.
27. Petitpas A, Danish SJ: Caring for injured athletes. In Murphy SM, editor: *Sport spychology interventions,* Champaign, Ill, 1995, Human Kinetics.
28. Wiese-Bjornstal DM et al: An integrated model of response to sport injury: psychological and sociological dynamics, *J Appl Sport Psychol* 10(1): 46–69, 1998.
29. Brewer BW, Andersen MB, Van Raalte JL: Psychological aspects of sports injury rehabilitation: toward a biopsychosocial approach. In Mostofsky DI, Zaichkowsky LD, editors: *Medical and psychological aspects of sport and exercise,* Morgantown, W. Va, 2002, Fitness Information Technology.
30. Brewer BW, Cornelius AE: Psychological factors in sports injury rehabilitation. In Frontera WR, editor: *Rehabilitation of sports injuries: scientific basis*, Malden, Mass, 2003, Blackwell.
31. Brewer BW: Psychology of sport injury rehabilitation. In Singer RN, Hausenblas HA, Janelle CM, editor: *Handbook of sport psychology*, ed 2, New York, 2001, John Wiley & Sons,
32. American Psychiatric Association: *Diagnostic and statistical manual of mental disorders*, ed 4, Washington, DC, 2000, American Psychiatric Association.
33. Vaughan JL, King KA, Cottrell RR: Collegiate athletic trainers' confidence in helping female athletes with eating disorders, *J Athl Train* 39(1): 71–76, 2004.
34. Goss J et al: Eating disorders. In Taylor J, Wilson GS, editors: *Applying sport psychology: four perspectives*, Champaign, Ill, 2005, Human Kinetics.
35. Thompson RA, Sherman RT: Athletes, athletic performance, and eating disorders: healthier alternatives, *J Soc Issues* 55(2): 317–337, 1999.
36. Petrie TA, Sherman RT: Recognizing and assisting athletes with eating disorders. In Ray R, Wiese-Bjornstal DM, editors: *Counseling in sports medicine*, Champaign, Ill, 1999, Human Kinetics.
37. Swoap RA, Murphy SM: Eating disorders and weight management in athletes. In Murphy SM, editor: *Sports psychology interventions*, Champaign, Ill, 1995, Human Kinetics.
38. Pfeiffer RP, Mangus BC: *Concepts of athletic training*, ed 4, Boston, Mass, 2005, Jones and Bartlett.
39. Andersen MB, Tod D: When to refer athletes for counseling or psychotherapy. In Williams JM, editor: *Applied sport psychology: personal growth to peak performance*, ed 5, New York, 2006, McGraw Hill.
40. Petrie TA: Eating disorders in sports. Presentation at the Annual Meeting and Clinical Symposia of the National Athletic Trainers' Association, 2004, Baltimore, Md.
41. Bacon VL et al: Substance abuse. In Taylor J, Wilson GS, editors: *Applying sport psychology: four perspectives*, Champaign, Ill, 2005, Human Kinetics.
42. Gleason DJ: Substance abuse. In Scuderi GR, McCann PD, editors: *Sports medicine: a comprehensive approach*, ed 2, Philadelphia, 2005, Mosby.
43. Austin L, Kortum J: Self-injury: the secret language of pain for teenagers, *Education* 124(3): 517–527, 2004.
44. Saltz G: Identifying kids who cut themselves to cope: more adolescents practicing self injury to get rid of stress and anxiety, *Today Show*. New York, NY: NBC News; Accessed October 5, 2005, from http://www.msnbc.msn.com/id/9593427/.
45. Skegg K: Self-harm, *Lancet* 366: 1471–1483, 2005.
46. Moulton MA, Molstad S, Turner A: The role of athletic trainers in counseling collegiate athletes, *J Athl Train* 32(2): 148–150, 1997.
47. Petipas AJ: What's in a name?, *Athlet Ther Today* 1(1): 27, 1996.
48. Warner MJ, Amato HK: The mind: an essential healing tool for rehabilitation, *Athlet Ther Today* 2(3): 37–41, 1997.
49. Petipas AJ: Listen while you work, *Athlet Ther Today* 3(3): 10–11, 1998.
50. Gordon S, Potter M, Hamer P: Periodized mental skills training, *Athlet Ther Today* 5(4): 49–50, 2000.
51. National Athletic Trainer's Association Board of Certification: *Role Delineation Study for the Entry-Level Certified Athletic Trainer*, ed 5, Omaha, Neb, 2004, NATA.
52. Misasi SP, Kemler DS, Redmond CJ: Counseling skills and the athletic therapist, *Athlet Ther Today* 3(1): 35–38, 1998.
53. Larson GA, Zaichkowsky LD, King E: Counseling skills for the athletic trainer. Workshop presented at the annual meeting of the Eastern Athletic Trainers Association. Boston, 1997.
54. Wayda VK, Armenth-Brothers F, Boyce BA: Goal setting: a key to injury rehabilitation, *Athlet Ther Today* 3(1): 21–25, 1998.
55. Petitpas AJ: Going for the goal, *Athlet Ther Today* 2(4): 30–31, 1997.
56. Barefield B, McCallister S: Social support in the athletic training room: athletes' expectations of staff and student athletic trainers, *J Athl Train* 32(4): 333–338, 1997.
57. Vealey RS, Greenleaf CA: Seeing is believing: understanding and using imagery in sport. In Williams JM, editor: *Applied sport psychology: personal growth to peak performance*, ed 5, New York, 2006, McGraw-Hill.
58. Richardson PA, Latuda LM: Therapeutic imagery and athletic injuries, *J Athl Train* 30(1): 10–12, 1995.
59. Kerr G, Goss J: The effects of a stress management program on injuries and stress levels, *J Appl Sport Psychol* 8(1): 109–117, 1996.
60. Jacobson E: *Progressive relaxation*, Chicago, Ill, 1938, University of Chicago Press.
61. Dolan MG: Getting help—before you need it, *Athlet Ther Today* 2(4): 37, 1997.
62. Petipas AJ: When to counsel and when to refer?, *Athlet Ther Today* 2(2): 20, 1997.
63. Brewer BW: Psychological aspects of rehabilitation. In Kolt GS, Andersen MB, editors: *Psychology in the physical and manual therapies*, Philadelphia, 2004, Churchill Livingstone.
64. Billingsley KD, Waehler CA, Hardin SI: Stability of optimism and choice of coping strategy. *Retrieval Motor Skills* 79:91–97,1993

23

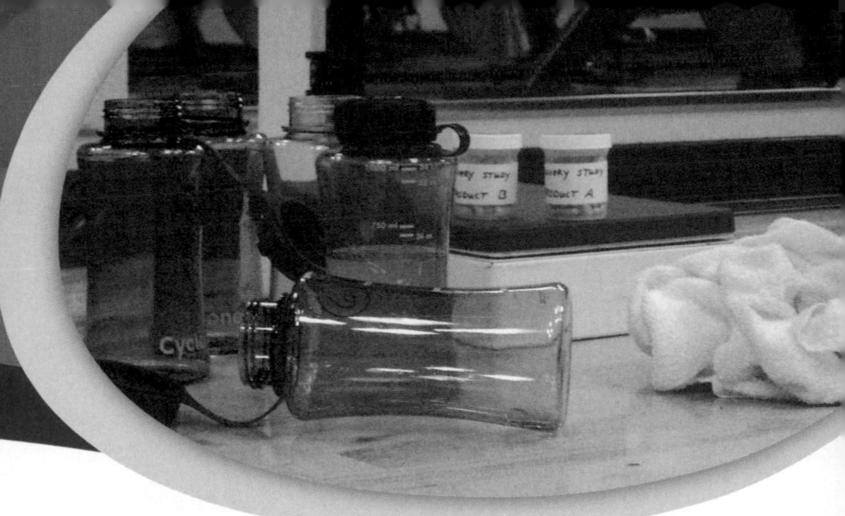

Pharmacology

THOMAS V. GOCKE III

Learning Goals

1. Know which pharmacological agents generally have an effect on athletes, regardless of their age or physical abilities.
2. Discuss pharmacokinetics and pharmacodynamics and how these concepts relate to the administration of drugs in the body.
3. Define common pharmacological terms.
4. Define *absorption, distribution, metabolism,* and *excretion* as they pertain to medication administration.
5. Identify the major classifications of medications that are commonly encountered by the athletic trainer.
6. Recognize appropriate recording systems, laws, and drug classification systems that affect the athletic trainer.
7. List the most common categories of medications used to treat both injuries and illnesses, and describe the basic function of each.

Most athletic trainers would agree that therapeutic rehabilitation and exercise, injury prevention and care, and anatomy and physiology are considered foundation courses in their education. Although this is true, the changing nature of health care and our population in general means that athletic trainers will be exposed to a greater variety of medical conditions as they treat the injuries of the physically active. As a result of healthier lifestyles and better technologies, people are living longer and sometimes living with complex conditions. Medications are a crucial factor in this trend because they help prevent further injury, alleviate pain, and manage chronic conditions. Understanding the way medications work and their effects on performance is an important part of an athletic trainer's role and a competency in which athletic trainers are expected to demonstrate proficiency. This chapter will provide a basic understanding of the way medications affect the control and alteration of disease processes and what this means for athletic trainers.

HISTORICAL PERSPECTIVES IN PHARMACOLOGY

Pharmacology is the study of interactions between chemical substances and living systems. If a substance has a therapeutic value, it is usually considered a pharmaceutical. The field of pharmacology is large and diverse. It includes the study of drug compositions and properties, drug interactions, toxicology, and, most important, medical applications. In addition to pharmacology's importance to medicine, the field is also a major economical and political force. The pharmaceutical industry is an important and complex field, with millions of dollars each year pouring into the research and development of new and better drugs. To protect the public and ensure quality standards, many government agencies exist to regulate the pharmaceutical industry.

Regulatory Agencies

In 1906, the Pure Food and Drug Act designated the **United States Pharmacopeia** (USP) and the National

United States Pharmacopeia the official public standards–setting authority for all over-the-counter medications, dietary supplements, and other health care products manufactured in the United States; USP

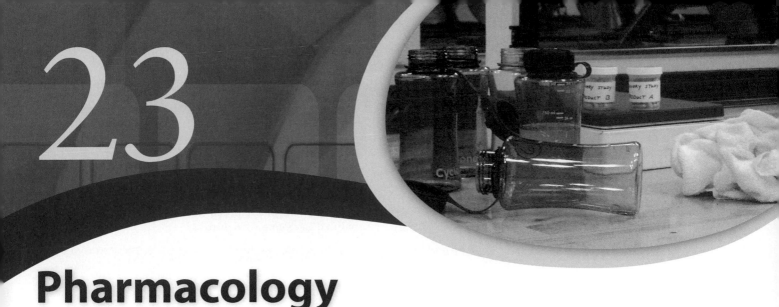

OPENING *Scenario*

The state volleyball championship is tomorrow, and Shannon, the best spiker on the team, goes to see the athletic trainer because of gastrointestinal distress. The athletic trainer learns that Shannon was advised to take a common antiinflammatory drug for a minor ankle injury that occasionally flares up during jumping activities. Her gastrointestinal distress is self-limiting, but she is concerned that the discomfort may affect her performance in the game. The athletic trainer checks with a physician and learns that there are medication alternatives for antiinflammatory disorders that might be less taxing on the gastrointestinal system. The athletic trainer also learns about various techniques that Shannon can employ to prevent medication-induced gastrointestinal distress.

Formulary (NF) as the official standard of drugs. This designation was updated in 1939 (and again in 1952) by the Federal Food, Drug and Cosmetic Act, which differentiated prescription and nonprescription medications and regulated the manner in which medications were dispensed. The Federal Food, Drug and Cosmetic Act is known today as the **Food and Drug Administration** (FDA). Today, the FDA is the main body that regulates pharmaceuticals. According to the FDA's mission statement, which is posted on the governmental Web site, the FDA is responsible for protecting the public health by ensuring the safety, efficacy, and security of human and veterinary drugs, biological products, medical devices, our nation's food supply, cosmetics, and products that emit radiation. The FDA is also responsible for advancing the public health by helping to speed innovations that make medicines and foods more effective, safer, and more affordable and helping the public get the accurate, science-based information they need to use medicines and foods to improve their health.[1] The specific federal agency that monitors medication *usage* is the Drug Enforcement Agency (DEA).

The USP is the official public standards–setting authority for all prescription and over-the-counter medicines, dietary supplements, and other health care products manufactured and sold in the United States. The USP sets standards for the quality of these products and works with health care providers to help them reach these standards. The USP's standards are also recognized and used in more than 130 countries. USP produces an annual formulary that gives the composition, description, method of preparation, and dosage for drugs. The book contains two separate official compendia: the USP and the NF.[2]

Nomenclature

Medications can be classified by their chemical, generic, or trade names. **Chemical names** are those names given to medications that specifically describe the compound that makes up the drug. A **generic name** is short so that chemists can quickly designate the molecule being discussed. A **trade name** is the designation given to a drug that helps the pharmaceutical company market the medication. Brand names and proprietary names are other ways to describe a trade name.

The official name is designated as an identifier that is recognized by the USP and the NF. For example, ciprofloxacin is a generic name for a drug whose trade name is Cipro. Similarly, many medications have similar sounding or spelled trade names but have completely different chemical names. This ambiguity has resulted in errors in the prescribing and filling of medication orders. Because such errors are a huge problem, athletic trainers should always remember to use the generic name when recording and ordering medicines if possible.

PHARMACODYNAMICS AND PHARMACOKINETICS

Pharmacology is divided into two areas: pharmacodynamics and pharmacokinetics. **Pharmacodynamics** is the study of the biochemical and physiological effects of drugs (Figure 23-1). In pharmacodynamics, many forms of potential actions can alter the cell membrane to allow medications to work. One of the main concepts is explained through pathways known as drug-receptor pathways. As the term implies, a drug will seek out specific receptor sites to attach itself to, and the attachment will in turn affect an action at the cellular level. This action may alter the cell function, causing an

Food and Drug Administration government agency that regulates pharmaceuticals; FDA

chemical name name given to a medication that specifically describes the compound that makes up the drug

generic name short name given to drug so that a chemist can quickly designate the molecule being discussed

trade name designation given to a drug that helps the pharmaceutical company market the medication; also known as brand name and proprietary name

pharmacodynamics the study of the biochemical and physiological effects of drugs

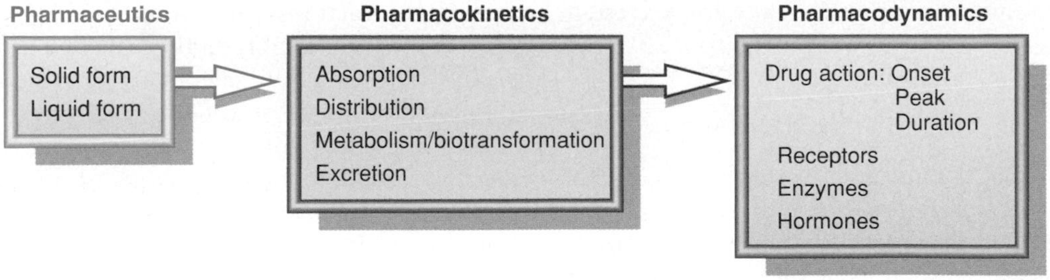

FIGURE 23-1 The three phases of drug action. (From Kee JL, Hayes ER, McCuiston LE: *Pharmacology: a nursing process approach,* ed 5, Figure 1-10, Philadelphia, 2006, Saunders/Elsevier.)

intended (or sometimes unintended) process in the body. Some medications, such as certain types of antibiotics, will alter the cell membrane to achieve their designated effects. Others will attach to enzyme molecules so that they can be transported across the cell membrane. This process prevents the drug from exerting any activity before it enters the cell. Once it has penetrated the cell membrane, it can begin its desired effect.

Pharmacokinetics is the study of what the body does with a drug and how these drug compounds are transported through the body. Specifically, pharmacokinetics explains how the body deals with drug absorption, distribution, metabolism, and excretion.

Absorption

Absorption is a process whereby a drug or medication is delivered into the bloodstream from its point of entry into the body. Many factors will have a positive or negative impact on how this medication is absorbed (e.g., the methods of drug administration, fat or water solubility, pH, drug dosage). A medication can be administered in many ways. Drugs administered in close proximity to the bloodstream (i.e., intravenously, intramuscularly, inhaled, or subcutaneously [under the skin]) will be absorbed more quickly and have a faster onset of action than will medications that are applied topically or taken orally. Environmental factors that have some effect on the skin or circulatory system (e.g., burns, hypotension, anemia) may cause delays in onset of action. Oral ingestion of medications relies on the absorption via the gastric mucosa and circulation. Although these medications take more time to reach the blood stream, their duration of action is usually longer and therefore the dosing requirements are less. A liquid preparation is absorbed more readily than the equivalent form in either tablet or powder configuration.

Gastric contents (e.g., food) can have either a positive or a negative effect on medication absorption. Medications are often prescribed to be taken with food or on an empty stomach. For example, if an athlete, such as Shannon from the opening scenario, takes an antiinflammatory medication such as ibuprofen (e.g., Advil, Motrin), she should take it with food to prevent gastrointestinal distress.

Next, the dosage of medication given, via any route, has an impact on absorption. A **loading dose** helps to quickly achieve a higher concentration of medication in the bloodstream. A loading dose is usually a one-time event; afterwards, a maintenance regimen is instituted to maintain the dosage in a therapeutic range until the desired effect has been achieved. A peak level is the point at which the highest concentration of drug has been absorbed. It is important to determine according to the drug dosage selected and the route of administration so that the drug dosage remains within its therapeutic range.

Distribution

Many factors affect the distribution of medications throughout the body. Some medications are moved by passive diffusion and others by active transport. **Passive diffusion** is simple and consists of one solution moving from a higher-concentration environment to a lower-concentration environment. Fat soluble (i.e., ionized) solutions pass through the cell membrane much better than nonfat soluble (i.e., nonionized) solutions. **Active transportation** occurs when a molecule attaches itself to another substance and is driven across the cell membrane.

Metabolism

Metabolism may be defined as biotransformation, which is the breakdown of a medication or drug into its inert forms. The liver is the body's primary detoxification organ. Substances pass through the liver, and the inactive

pharmacokinetics the study of what the body does to a drug and how these drug compounds are transported through the body

loading dose dose that helps achieve a higher concentration of medication in the bloodstream

passive diffusion process whereby one solution moves from a higher-concentration environment to a lower-concentration environment

active transportation occurs when a molecule attaches itself to another substance and is driven across the membrane drug forms are removed and made ready for excretion. Age and overall health and well-being have a direct influence on drug metabolism.

Excretion

Most inactive drug forms are excreted through the kidneys. Although the kidney is the primary route for elimination, the intestine and the perspiration, saliva, and mammary glands are also considered to be sources for medication by-product removal. Athletic trainers should always be concerned with their clients' renal function and general state of health because these factors greatly affect the elimination of medications from the body. A specific situation an athletic trainer may encounter is when an athlete is taking nonsteroidal antiinflammatory drugs (NSAIDs) for an overuse injury. The athlete may be older and have reduced renal function secondary to hypertension, may have lost the use of a kidney secondary to a trauma, or may have only one kidney as a result of a birth anomalies or previous donation.

MEDICATION FUNCTIONS

No matter how medications are administered, one of three things will happen: (1) the medication will have no effect; (2) the medication will produce the intended effect; or (3) the medication will produce an adverse effect (Figure 23-2). It is highly recommended that all athletic trainers be well-versed with the ill effects and potential allergic reactions of those medications commonly used by their facilities, their team physicians, or any physicians to whom clients are referred. Knowing how to handle allergic or adverse reactions to medications is very important. Every athletic trainer who deals with patients taking medications must know the intended effects of a pharmacological regimen in the treatment of injuries or medical conditions.

Intended Effects

Intended effects, sometimes called *therapeutic effects,* are those drug responses that are expected once a drug is administered. The body is affected by the drug's actions at the cellular level, which brings about a desired response to any given disease process. For example, a patient taking an NSAID could reasonably expect a reduction of the inflammation associated with tennis elbow. Likewise, a patient with strep throat could expect to have an infection eradicated after completing the prescribed course of antibiotics. These responses to medications are intended responses to the drug's actions. If the intended response is not achieved, the athletic trainer may need to consult a physician or re-evaluate the situation.

Adverse Effects

Adverse effects are drug actions that do not constitute an intended response by the body to a particular drug. Within the category of adverse effects, several

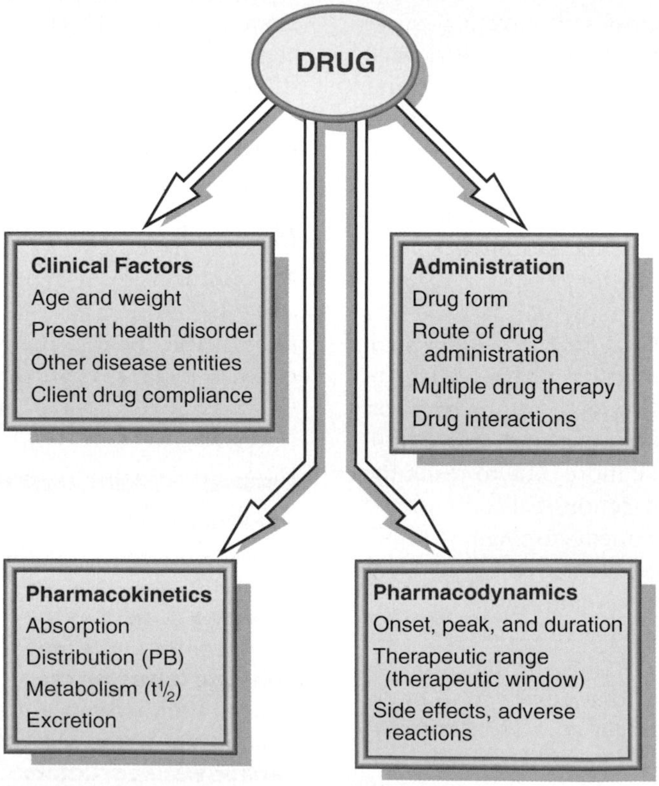

FIGURE 23-2 Determinants that affect drug therapy. (From Kee JL, Hayes ER, McCuiston LE: *Pharmacology: a nursing process approach,* ed 5, Figure 1-11, Philadelphia, 2006, Saunders/Elsevier.)

types of reactions can occur, ranging from mild to severe. These include idiosyncratic responses, drug allergies, anaphylactic reactions, drug tolerances, and drug interactions. Idiosyncratic reactions and drug reactions often overlap. **Idiosyncratic** means that some patients will react differently to medications than others will. If one member of a family is allergic to penicillin, it does not necessarily follow that all family members will also be allergic to this drug. Of course, the reverse is also true: It is possible that one family member may have a reaction to a medication in the absence of any family history or other information that would indicate the possibility of an adverse reaction.

Drug allergies can be severe and emerge immediately after administration, or they may occur after several doses of the medications. In an **allergic reaction**, the body develops an antigen-antibody reaction. The body is exposed to a compound and then develops an antibody against this compound. The next time the body recognizes this substance, it reacts as if it were foreign. These reactions can be mild, as in rashes, swelling, nausea, or diarrhea. More severe reactions include hives, respiratory difficulties, tachycardia, hypotension, and possibly even death. This extreme reaction to medications is referred to as an **anaphylactic reaction**. People have anaphylactic reactions to foods, insect stings, or any other substance to which their body has formed an antigen-antibody reaction. Once the athletic trainer has recognized that a potential anaphylactic reaction is evolving, he or she should take swift action to ensure the athlete's safety.

If the athletic trainer witnesses a severe response to medication, he or she should act quickly to treat the anaphylactic symptoms. These patients may need aggressive intravenous-fluid resuscitation, cardiopulmonary resuscitation (in extreme situations), antihistamine drugs, epinephrine, bronchodilator drugs, and steroids to help counteract the adverse effects. Although statistics vary, the number of deaths caused by anaphylactic reactions are estimated at approximately 1 per 10,000 cases. It is also believed that such cases may be underreported because the cause of death is sometimes attributed to other factors.[3]

Any client with an allergic reaction to any medication, food substance, or insect sting should have this allergy clearly documented in his or her permanent medical record. Adverse responses, although considered rare, must be thoroughly evaluated to investigate for potential drug class effects. For example, if enough people have a serious reaction, there may be a problem with the drug class, and in some cases the warning label may need to be revised or the drug recalled.

Points to Ponder
Have you noticed how many more people seem to have peanut allergies in recent years? Do you think the allergy has become more common or simply that more cases have been documented and publicized?

Idiosyncratic effects of medications are responses that are abnormal for the known pathways of action for any given drug. These can be a greater drug response, a lesser drug response, or a drug response that was not intended. A good example of idiosyncratic effects is in elderly patients who are receiving analgesics or pain killers after an operation. In most cases, pain medications help reduce pain and sedate or relax the patient. However, some older patients may become too relaxed and get more pain relief than was intended. Conversely, some patients may get no pain relief at all and become agitated.

Medication Interactions

Medication interactions are unintended effects between drugs. These reactions can have a synergistic effect and provide a greater response or an antagonistic response, which means that one of the drugs lessens the effect of the other drug. In most cases, this occurrence is unintended and often goes unnoticed by the clinician and the patient. An example of an antagonistic effect is a female patient taking antibiotics and oral contraceptives. The antibiotics can lessen the effects of the oral contraceptives in preventing pregnancy.

ADMINISTRATIVE ASPECTS OF MEDICATIONS

Liability

The athletic trainer must be aware of the overlapping liability and responsibility issues involved in the storage and administration of medications. Much discussion and investigation are necessary to ensure that the athletic training facility is in compliance with state and federal regulations regarding storage, packaging, dispensing, and administration of prescription medications. The DEA, state boards of medical examiners, and pharmacy boards have developed specific regulations that address

idiosyncratic quality whereby some patients react differently to medications than others
allergic reaction reaction whereby the body develops an antibody against a compound to which it is exposed
anaphylactic reaction sudden, severe, whole-body allergic reaction

these issues. Many colleges and universities and school districts have established policies and procedures that deal directly with issues pertaining to storage, packaging, dispensing, and the administration of prescription medications. Because state laws vary, it is extremely important that all athletic trainers be familiar with the specific policies of their organizations before considering the storage of medications in their facilities.

Although concerns about prescription and controlled substance medications are somewhat obvious, some athletic trainers might not consider over-the-counter (OTC) medications as posing a potential problem for their facilities. Although regulations for the storage, dispensing, and administration of OTC medications are not universally accepted, athletic trainers should follow the policies established by their school districts, colleges, or universities. If such a policy does not exist, the athletic trainer should develop one with the cooperation of the team physician(s) and the appropriate school officials (e.g., athletic director, principal, school district administrator, school nurse, student health service, pharmacist).

Record Keeping

Prescription Medications

Record keeping for prescription medications is a vital component in the administration responsibilities of athletic trainers. There is no clear-cut blueprint for record keeping. However, the more precise the information in the record is, the more likely it is to protect all parties. Medication records should be kept in two locations: a running medication log or inventory and each student-athlete's chart. The running medication log can be a professionally printed form or one that was created on a personal computer (Figure 23-3).

The medication log should be reviewed frequently, and all medication inventories should be completed on a regular basis. The team physician should have direct oversight over what medications are kept in the athletic training facility and is ultimately responsible for the storage, dispensing, and administration of medications. Ideally, a registered pharmacist should be involved in this process. Pharmacists are licensed by their respective states to supervise the storage, packaging, and dispensing of medications. Each record should be clearly legible and include the athlete's name, the date the medications were administered, the specific medication name (the generic or chemical name can be used), the amount administered, and the name of the responsible party. All entries should be co-signed by the team physician even if a pharmacist was present for dispensing. However, state and federal laws are specific as to who is licensed to dispense medications. Frequently, it is a licensed medical professional (i.e., MD, PA, NP) or a pharmacist. Therefore the best response to this situation is to have written protocols or guidelines that cover these situations. Athletic trainers should review the institution's policies before developing a position statement for their facilities. They should also enlist the advice of their team physicians and a pharmacist to ensure compliance with all state and federal regulations. By taking this approach, the athletic trainer will ensure the proper custodial care of medications kept in the facility.

As previously mentioned, medication information should also be recorded in the student athlete's chart or medical file. Doing so will help the athletic trainer or health care provider remember all medications being taken and avoid any possible drug interactions. Like the medication log, this record should include the date the medication was prescribed and dispensed, the amount administered, the medication name, and the person administering the medication.

Name	Date Administered	Medication	Dosage	Primary Complaint	Physician Signature
T. Brantley	05/03/07	Naprosyn	4 tabs: 375 mg Take 2 tabs every 12 hours	Knee pain	P. Brown, MD
S. Childs	05/15/07	Daypro	3 tabs: 1200 mg Take one daily	Shoulder pain, inflammation	S. Niergarth DO
M. Byrne	06/03/07	Albuterol	1 inhaler Administer 1 puff two times each day	Asthma	P. Brarr, MD

FIGURE 23-3 Sample prescription medication log.

Over-the-Counter Medications

Record keeping is just as important for OTC medications, but the information required is slightly different. Figure 23-4 provides an example of a medication log specific to OTC medications.

OTC medications are required by the FDA to meet certain labeling regulations (Box 23-1). The FDA requires that all medications carry this information regardless of packaging. Therefore if your facility buys OTC medications in bulk and repackages them in smaller unit doses, each unit-dose package label should include all information required by the FDA. An easy way to ensure labeling compliance is to purchase medications in prepackaged unit-doses with all the appropriate OTC labeling information included. Another option is to have the consulting pharmacist or student health service create unit-dose packages of medications with labels containing the appropriate information affixed to the package. Regardless of the method chosen, preplanning and a thorough knowledge of the rules, regulations, guidelines, and state laws will reduce the number of medication-related problems that occur in the athletic training facility.

MEDICATIONS USED TO TREAT INJURIES

The athletic trainer typically treats common injuries on the basis of the athlete's symptoms or complaints, which include pain, inflammation, and muscle spasms usually associated with musculoskeletal injuries such as fractures, dislocations, sprains, and strains. The athlete's signs and symptoms depend on whether the injury is acute or chronic. After the athletic trainer has completed the evaluation, he or she can select an appropriate medication.

Pain

Pain typically is the limiting factor in activity and performance. The athletic trainer's primary responsibility therefore lies in identifying the source of the pain and eliminating the pain or the perception of pain. Pain

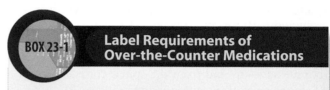

BOX 23-1 Label Requirements of Over-the-Counter Medications

1. Name of the medication or product
2. Company name
3. Package contents
4. Ingredients list
5. Listing of substances contained in this medication that have the potential for abuse
6. Warnings, precautions, and alerts
7. Directions for administration
8. Expiration date and lot number

Name	Date Administered	Medication	Dosage	Primary Complaint	Staff Member Signature
K. Whitfield	06/27/07	acetaminophen	1 pack: 2 tabs—325 mg	Headache	J. Geary, ATC
J. Wilson	07/22/07	ibuprofen	1 pack: 2 tabs—200 mg	Low back pain	J. Johnson, ATC
G. Miller	08/10/07	acetaminophen	1 pack: 2 tabs—325 mg	Headache	T. Bair, ATC
M. Harris	09/09/07	loratadine	1 tabs: 10 mg	Runny nose	L. Groover, ATC
S. Aldridge	11/10/07	phenylephrine	1 pack: 2 tabs—5 mg	Nasal congestion	M. Clanton, ATC

FIGURE 23-4 Sample over-the-counter medication log.

is generally treated with therapeutic modalities or medications and narcotic or non-narcotic analgesics.

Narcotic Analgesics

Narcotic analgesics are primarily derived from opium or opioid derivatives. Stimulation of the opioid receptors causes analgesia (removal of pain), sedation, and euphoria; if abused, it may cause hallucinations. Morphine, codeine, and oxycodone are opium-based medications. Drugs such as hydromorphone, hydrocodone, Talwin, meperidine, and fentanyl are all synthetic variations of opioid-based drugs (Table 23-1). Because these medications can produce euphoric sensations, the potential for abuse and addiction is high.

How they work: Narcotic analgesics work by depressing pain impulses, keeping pain receptors from transmitting messages to and from the spinal cord. This action decreases neurotransmitter activity.

Administration: Administration is through oral, subcutaneous, or intravenous methods.

Side effects: Some of the more common side effects of narcotic analgesic use are altered senses, mood alterations, dizziness, sedation, dyspepsia, nausea, vomiting, constipation, respiratory distress, and allergic reactions. To prevent accompanying gastrointestinal symptoms, narcotic analgesics should not be taken on an empty stomach. Ingesting these medications with food and a significant amount of clear liquids makes side effects less likely. Keeping the body hydrated, limiting the use of narcotic analgesics, and using a stool softener or laxative if necessary will help alleviate any associated constipation. The athletic trainer should always be watchful for drug-related skin rashes or hives. If a rash is evident or the athlete complains of itching, it is reasonable to discontinue that medication and consult a physician.

Contraindications: Common contraindications include acute bronchial asthma, upper airway obstruction, and use of alcohol and other central nervous system depressors.

Non-Narcotic Analgesics

The athletic trainer will most commonly come in contact with athletes using NSAIDs and nonopioids; such OTC medications are widely available. The most widely used non-narcotic analgesics are aspirin, acetaminophen, and ibuprofen. Because pain is often caused by inflammation, some of these medications also have antiinflammatory effects, which will be discussed in the next section.

How they work: Non-narcotic analgesics block pain without the negative side effects of drowsiness and possible addiction.

Administration: The method of administration is oral.

Side effects: Side effects include gastrointestinal distress and tinnitus (ringing of the ear).

Contraindications: Contraindications include gastrointestinal bleeding, bleeding disorders, and ulcers. These medications should not be used in children under 12 years of age.

Inflammation

The inflammatory cycle is the body's response mechanism to trauma and infection. Trauma can be classified as either acute or chronic (sometimes referred to as *repetitive/overuse-type injuries*). The inflammatory cycle begins after a trauma has occurred to the tissues and some form of tissue bleeding has commenced. The pressure associated with swelling causes an increase of pain secondary to pain receptors being stretched within the affected tissue. In general, antiinflammatory

narcotic analgesics drugs that depress pain impulses and prevent their transmission to the spinal cord; primarily derived from opium or opioid derivatives

TABLE 23-1 Narcotic Analgesics (Commonly Prescribed Medications)

Morphine (e.g., MS Contin: PO)	IM/PO/IV/PR	4–6 hr	Respiratory depression
Meperidine (e.g., Demerol)	IM/PO/IV/PR	4–6 hr	Constipation
Hydromorphone (e.g., Dilaudid)	IM/PO/IV/PR	4–6 hr	Central nervous system changes
Oxycodone (e.g., OxyContin, Percocet, Tylox)	Primarily oral	4–24 hr	Orthostatic hypotension
Hydrocodone (e.g., Vicodin, Norco, Lortab, Lorcet)	Primarily oral	4–6 hr	Nausea/vomiting
Propoxyphene (e.g., Darvocet, Darvon)	Oral	4–6 hr	Cholestasis
Codeine	Primarily oral: liquid suspension	4–6 hr	Rash/pruritus
			Anaphylactic reaction
			Dependency/abuse potential

*Narcotic analgesics are frequently combined with acetaminophen or ibuprofen for added pain relief.
IM, intramuscular; *PO*, oral; *IV*, intravenous; *PR*, rectal.

medications, corticosteroids, and NSAIDs are used to reduce the inflammation and associated pain.

Antiinflammatory Medications

Aspirin is an effective medication used to treat the symptoms of acute and chronic injuries. Although aspirin is used to help reduce and treat inflammation, it is also an anticoagulant and a pain reliever. Many athletes prefer newer and gentler forms of antiinflammatory medications to reduce inflammation.

How they work: Antiinflammatory medications block pain impulses in the central nervous system.

Administration: The predominant method of administration is oral.

Side effects: Possible side effects include gastrointestinal distress, prolonged bleeding time, and tinnitus.

Contraindications: The most common contraindications are gastrointestinal distress and bleeding, bleeding disorders, and ulcers. These medications should not be used in children younger than 12 years of age (Box 23-2).

Nonsteroidal Antiinflammatories

NSAIDs are used to reduce swelling and also act as analgesics to relieve pain and antipyretics to reduce fever. The most commonly used NSAIDs are ibuprofen (e.g., Motrin, Advil) and naproxen (e.g., Naproxen, Aleve), both widely available OTC medications. NSAIDs are also available by prescription.

How they work: NSAIDs are synthesized and released into the blood stream. They inhibit the effect of prostaglandin as it relates to the musculoskeletal system and inflammation.

Administration: Administration is oral, topical, or intravenous.

Side effects: Common side effects of NSAIDS are dyspepsia, gastric ulcers, gastrointestinal bleeding. Prolonged use of NSAIDs may have an adverse effect on renal function, leading to decreased urinary output, renal hypertension, and fluid retention (Box 23-3).

Contraindications: Athletes with a history of asthma-related illnesses and known hypersensitivities should be very cautious when taking NSAIDS, which can increase susceptibility to the sudden onset of catastrophic bronchospasm and other respiratory problems.

Box 23-4 summarizes the medications most commonly used to treat injuries.

Corticosteroids

Corticosteroids are naturally occurring substances that are found primarily in the adrenal glands. The adrenal hormones, glucocorticoids and mineralocorticoids, are responsible for regulating the effects of stress on the body, blood pressure, and blood glucose levels, as well as homeostasis, fat distribution, osteoporosis,

NSAIDs acronym for nonsteroidal antiinflammatory drugs

BOX 23-2 Reye's Syndrome

Reye's syndrome is a disease that can affect all organs of the body but primarily affects the liver and brain. It typically occurs in the winter months and has been reported among pediatric patients recovering from a viral illness. It has been reported specifically in those patients who were treated with aspirin for symptoms associated with the influenza or the varicella virus (i.e., chicken pox). Children between the ages of 4 and 12 years, with a peak age of 6 years, may be at increased risk for contracting this syndrome. If a pediatric patient is going to develop symptoms associated with Reye's syndrome, they will usually appear about a week after a viral illness.

Symptoms associated with Reye's syndrome include a history of a recent viral illness, persistent vomiting, brain dysfunction (e.g., drowsiness, fatigue, listlessness), irritability, aggressive or combative behavior, confusion, delirium, seizures, and coma.

Treatment primarily involves supportive care for suspected encephalitis, meningitis, and severe liver failure. A high level of suspicion for Reye's syndrome should be associated with the child who is recovering from a viral illness, who exhibits these symptoms, and who has been treated with aspirin-based products.

BOX 23-3 Generalized Adverse Reactions: NSAIDs

- Oral ulcers
- Esophagitis
- Exacerbation of hiatal hernia
- Gastric ulcer disease
- Bleeding in the upper gastrointestinal tract
- Fecal occult blood
- Hepatotoxicity
- Renal failure/insufficiency
- Tinnitus/vertigo
- Headaches
- Anemia/decreased platelet aggregation
- Bone healing alterations (animal studies)
- Urticaria, rashes, pruritus
- Stevens-Johnson syndrome (severe dermal reaction)
- Asthma/respiratory exacerbations

BOX 23-4 Medications Commonly Used to Treat Injury

Pain
Narcotic analgesics (e.g., morphine, codeine, oxycodone)
Non-narcotic analgesics (e.g., aspirin, acetaminophen [Tylenol], ibuprofen [Advil])

Inflammation
Antiinflammatory medications
Nonsteroidal antiinflammatory medications (e.g., ibuprofen [Advil], naproxen [Aleve])
Corticosteroids (e.g., cortisone, lidocaine, dexamethasone)

Muscle Spasm
Muscle relaxants (e.g., cyclobenzaprine [Flexeril], diazepam [Valium])

sexual function, and musculoskeletal development. These hormones can be naturally produced by the body or synthetically engineered for administration to correct adrenal gland deficiencies that may lead to disease. In the athletic population, corticosteroids are highly valuable in the treatment of acute, chronic, or rheumatological causes of inflammation. Corticosteroids are usually available by prescription. Common corticosteroids are cortisone, lidocaine, and dexamethasone.

How they work: Corticosteroids are synthesized and released into the blood stream. The corticosteroid medications help stimulate the body's ability to synthesize these naturally occurring substances. For temporary relief, corticosteroid use is beneficial.

Administration: Corticosteroids can be administered in several ways: oral ingestion, inhalation, or parenteral means. In the oral configuration, steroids are usually given in a tapering dose pack. The usual and customary length of treatment for athletic injuries is a 6- or 12-day dose pack. The dose pack is arranged so that the athlete takes a tapering dose of steroids each day until the course of medication has been completed.

Side effects: Some of the more notable adverse effects are dermal or subdermal skin changes, which can cause the skin to thin or change color. If injected directly into connective tissues, it can lead to tissue deterioration. In its worst-case scenario, this could lead to tendon ruptures.

Contraindications: Contraindications include liver, kidney, and heart diseases and diabetes.

Muscle Spasm

Muscle spasm is frequently seen as a result of musculoskeletal injuries. The pain-spasm-pain cycle is well-documented and can have a huge impact on the athlete's recovery after injury. Spasm of the musculoskeletal system results from the repetitive excitatory phase in the damaged muscle of connective tissue. Typically, athletic trainers will use modalities (e.g., e-stim, ultra-sound, manual muscle techniques) to help alleviate pain and spasm. Muscle relaxant medications may also be used to help alleviate pain and spasm. The medications that have typically been used as muscle relaxant agents are cyclobenzaprine (Flexeril), diazepam (Valium), carisoprodol (Soma), and methocarbamol (Robaxin).

How they work: It is believed that the transmission of neural impulse across the synapse is prolonged, which allows for muscle relaxation during a muscle spasm. Muscle relaxant agents will have a general effect on all the skeletal muscles and, to a limited extent, on gastric and vascular smooth muscle tissue as well.

Administration: Administration is usually oral, intravenous, or subcutaneous.

Side effects: The most notable of the side effects are lethargy, potential alteration of the central nervous system, dizziness, visual blurriness, anaphylactic reactions, skin reaction, gastric irritation, and headaches.

Contraindications: Common contraindications include hypersensitivity, cardiac dysfunction, glaucoma, and impaired liver function.

Points to Ponder
An athlete complains of an injury that is painful and is accompanied by swelling and muscle spasms in the surrounding tissues. Which medication do you choose, and how do you decide which symptom to prioritize?

MEDICATIONS USED TO TREAT MEDICAL CONDITIONS

The athletic trainer typically encounters athletes with general medical conditions that may or may not be preexisting. General medical conditions are treated on the basis of a medical diagnosis. The most common conditions include respiratory conditions, gastrointestinal conditions, skin conditions, and other specific conditions.

Respiratory Conditions

The athletic trainer will typically treat a variety of conditions, including upper respiratory ailments such as the common cold, flu, coughs, sinusitis, and asthma. Antibiotics, bronchodilator medications, common cold remedies, and antihistamine medications are the most common drug categories used to treat these conditions. Except for medications used to treat the common cold, most of the medications require a prescription.

Antibiotics

An **antibiotic** is simply a drug that kills or slows the growth of bacteria. Antibiotic medications are frequently prescribed to treat infections. Depending on the condition, physicians often prescribe antibiotics in an attempt to eliminate the infection and limit side effects. The antibiotic is selected to treat either a broad range of conditions or a specific condition. Common antibiotics are penicillin, tetracycline, macrolide, and sulfonamides.

How they work: Antibiotics either kill or slow the growth of bacteria.

Administration: Administration is either topical, oral, subcutaneous, or intravenous.

Side effects: Common side effects include gastrointestinal distress, rashes, and infection.

Contraindications: Contraindications include alcohol, sometimes dairy, oral contraceptives, and overexposure to sunlight. Because of the many classes of antibiotics, the athletic trainer should consult with the physician about any specific contraindications for the type of antibiotic prescribed.

Antiviral Agents

Athletic trainers often encounter athletes who are suffering from a nonlife-threatening viral illness such as influenza and herpes. Viral infections are sometimes more difficult to eradicate than bacterial infections are because the virus uses the body's host cells to replicate. Common antiviral medications include oseltamivir (Tamiflu), valacyclovir (Valtrex), and acyclovir (Zovirax).

How they work: Antiviral medications inhibit the replication process associated with the spread of viral infections. Simply stated, antiviral medications work by limiting or preventing the replication of the viral DNA and RNA. In so doing, they allow the host to mount a defense against the virus so that the body can heal. For these medications to be effective, they must be administered within 24 to 48 hours after symptoms first appear.

Administration: Administration is oral, topical, inhaled, or intravenous.

Side effects: Side effects include nausea, vomiting, headache, and kidney and liver toxicity.

Contraindications: The major contraindication is impaired renal or liver function.

Bronchodilator Medications

An athletic trainer will see many athletes who are affected by some form of asthma or other respiratory ailment. Exercise-induced asthma is the most prevalent respiratory problem in athletes. Additionally, the medical condition of asthma or reactive airway disease is becoming one of the most prevalent respiratory conditions in the world.[4,5] There are two types of bronchodilator medications: maintenance and rescue.

How they work: Bronchodilator medications work by relieving the constriction and reducing inflammation within the airways (Figure 23-5). The rescue inhalers stabilize the inflammation, and the maintenance inhalers relax the airway and raise the individual's tolerance to pulmonary stress.

Administration: Administration is oral or through a metered dose inhaler (Figure 23-6).

Side effects: Side effects include anxiety, irritation in the throat, and bronchospasm.

Contraindications: Contraindications to bronchodilator medications are glaucoma, tachycardia, and severe cardiac disease.

Common Cold Remedies

Runny nose, nasal congestion, sore throat, fever, cough, and generalized body aches are all frequent symptoms of the common cold. Although these symptoms may seem debilitating, they are usually nothing more than a nuisance. The viruses that make up the common cold are for the most part self-limiting. Therefore any medications that athletes take for these conditions are primarily for symptom relief and not necessarily to modify the disease state. Most of the medications for relief of common cold symptoms are sold as OTC drugs. Antihistamines, decongestants, and cough medications are all medications that combat cold symptoms.

Decongestants. **Decongestants** are meant to relieve those symptoms associated with blocked or restricted nasal passages. Specifically, the nasal mucosa becomes inflamed and the membranes swell, which impedes the passage of air and can contribute to headaches, dizziness, facial pain, hearing loss, and ear pain. The purpose of the decongestant is to relieve this congestion and allow normal air passage to resume. Decongestants are effective in relieving these symptoms, especially when they are used with antibiotics to clear up any associated bacterial infections. An example of a common decongest is pseudoephedrine (e.g., Sudafed).

How they work: Decongestants reduce inflammation in the swollen nasal mucosa.

Administration: Administration is oral and topical (i.e., nasal sprays and drops).

Side effects: Because most of these agents have some component of ephedrine, some adverse effects may result with prolonged use of these drugs. Dry mouth, dizziness, visual changes, nervousness, tachycardia, and rebound nasal congestion are some of the more common adverse effects noted with use of these agents.

antibiotic a drug that kills or slows the growth of bacteria

decongestants drugs used to relieve symptoms associated with blocked or restricted nasal passages

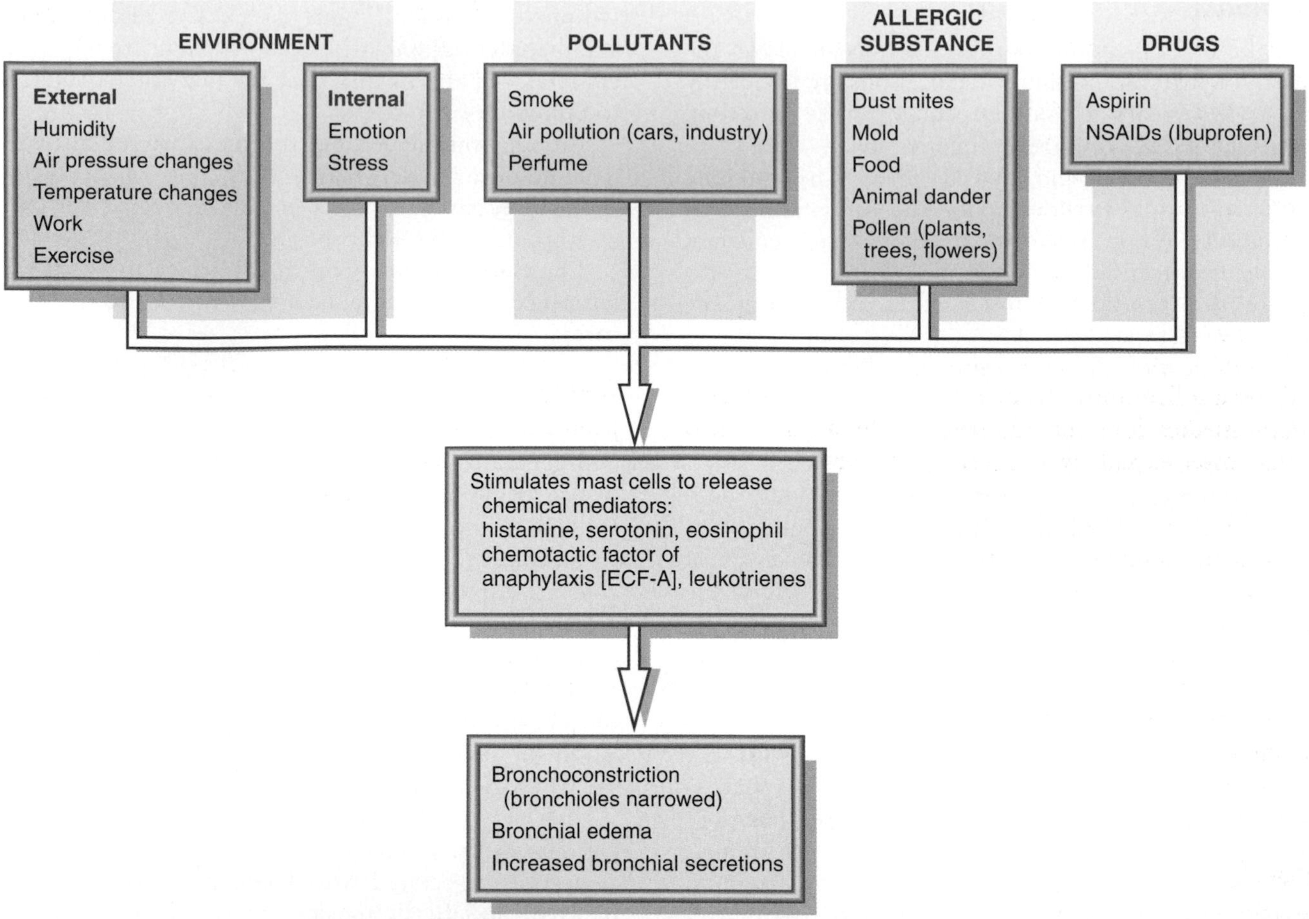

FIGURE 23-5 Factors contributing to bronchoconstriction. (From Kee JL, Hayes ER, McCuiston LE: *Pharmacology: a nursing process approach,* ed 5, Figure 39-2, Philadelphia, 2006, Saunders/Elsevier.)

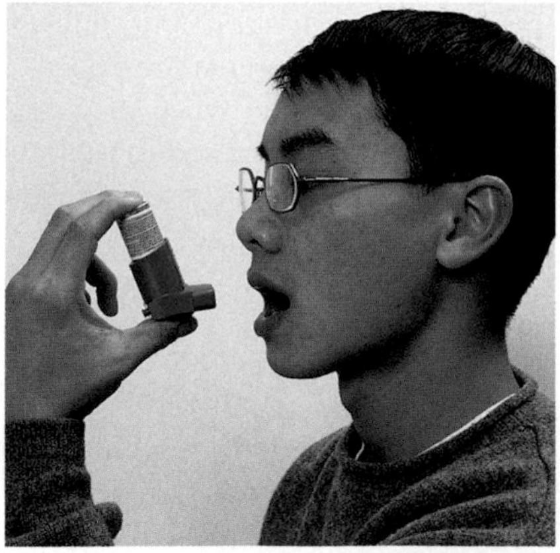

FIGURE 23-6 One technique for use of a metered-dose inhaler. The individual positions the mouthpiece 1 to 2 inches from the widely open mouth. This technique is considered the best way to deliver the medication without the use of a spacer. (From Perry AG, Potter PA: *Clinical nursing skills & techniques,* ed 6, Step 4d[2], p. 673, St Louis, 2006, Mosby/Elsevier).

Contraindications: Common contraindication to decongestants include cardiac disorders, urinary retention, glaucoma, and diabetes.

Cough Medications. Cough medicines either suppress a cough (antitussive agent) or work to expel mucus (expectorant). An example would be guaifenesin (e.g., Robitussin). Although guaifenesin is a cough expectorant, many common OTC medications, such as Robitussin, contain both an expectorant (guaifenesin) and a suppressant (e.g., dextromethorphan).

How they work: Antitussive agents work to suppress the cough reflex at either a local or a central site. Expectorants thin the mucus, making it easier to expel.

Administration: Administration is oral.

Side effects: Side effects are excitability, dry mouth, headache, drowsiness, and insomnia.

Contraindications: Contraindications are hypertension and decreased renal function.

Antihistamine Medications

The body reacts to bee stings, pollen, dust, animal dander, mold, foods, and other allergens by releasing histamines. Excessive amounts of histamines may increase body secretions, typically presenting as clear nasal discharge (i.e., rhinorrhea), swollen nasal membranes, and a secondary sore throat and cough resulting from postnasal drip. Common examples of antihistamine medications are diphenhydramine (e.g., Benadryl Allergy), brompheniramine (e.g., Dimetapp Allergy), and chlorpheniramine (e.g., Chlor-Trimeton Allergy).

How they work: Antihistamine drugs are antagonists to histamine release, meaning that they bind to the histamine receptor sites and prevent or inhibit further uptake or production of histamine.

Administration: Administration is oral, subcutaneous, intravenous, or topical.

Side effects: Side effects include drowsiness, dizziness, muscle weakness, gastrointestinal distress, and excitability.

Contraindications: Contraindications to antihistamine medications include acute asthma, glaucoma, cardiac disease, kidney disease, and hypertension.

Gastrointestinal Conditions

The athletic trainer typically treats a plethora of gastrointestinal ailments such as diarrhea, constipation, nausea, vomiting, heartburn, gastroesophageal reflux disease (GERD), and ulcers. Although most of these conditions are neither life-threatening nor permanently debilitating, they can cause the athlete much discomfort. Common medications for gastrointestinal ailments include antacids, antiemetics, laxatives, and antidiarrheals. Both OTC and prescription medications may be used.

Antacids

Antacids reduce the production of gastric acids and limit injuries of the gastric lining. Coupled with a reduction in food and liquid irritants, these medications help resolve the disease process. A typical antacid is calcium carbonate (e.g., Tums, Mylanta).

How they work: Antacids work by neutralizing gastrointestinal acid.

Administration: Administration is oral.

Side effects: Side effects are gastrointestinal distress and dehydration.

Contraindications: The major contraindication is kidney disease.

Antiemetics

Antiemetics are commonly used to treat nausea and vomiting. Examples of common antiemetics are promethazine (e.g., Phenergan) and phosphorated carbohydrate (e.g., Emetrol).

How they work: Antiemetics block one of the vomiting pathway and, in doing so, block the nerve impulse to vomit (Figure 23-7).

Administration: Administration is either oral, rectal, subcutaneous, or intravenous.

Side effects: Because there are a number of different classes of antiemetics, side effects vary depending on the medication. Common side effects include dizziness, drowsiness, blurred vision, dry mouth, and hypertension.

Contraindications: Contraindications vary by class and include glaucoma, shock, and seizure disorders.

Antidiarrheals and Laxatives

Diarrhea and constipation are usually self-limiting but can have an enormous effect on athletic activities. An example of a common antidiarrheal is Imodium.

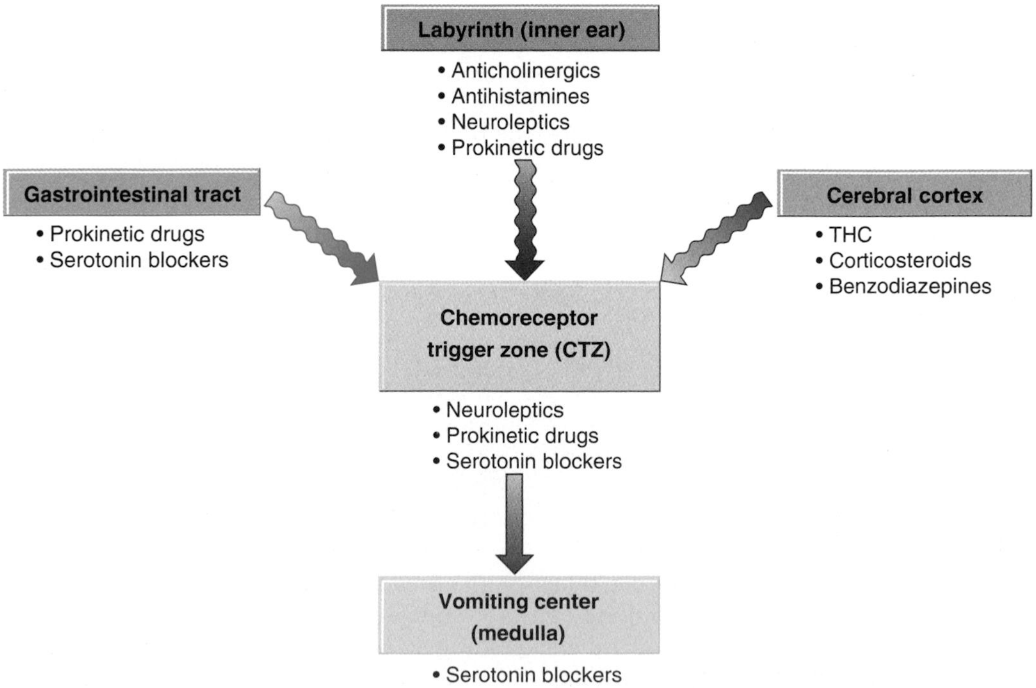

FIGURE 23-7 Sites of action of selected antinausea drugs. (From Lilley LL, Harrington S, Snyder JS: *Pharmacology and the nursing process,* ed 5, Figure 53-2, St Louis, 2007, Mosby/Elsevier.)

Examples of laxatives include salines such as Milk of Magnesia and stimulants such as Dulcolax.

How they work: Antidiarrheals work directly on the gastrointestinal muscles by decreasing muscular contractions and increasing water absorption from the digestive tract. The different categories of laxatives work in various ways, but all reduce the fluid in stool.

Administration: Administration is oral or rectal.

Side effects: Side effects of antidiarrheals include constipation, nausea, dry mouth, and abdominal pain. Side effects of laxatives include nausea, abdominal cramps, and diarrhea.

Contraindications: The most common contraindications of antidiarrheals is colitis. Contraindications for laxatives include gastrointestinal obstruction or perforation, colitis, abdominal pain, and fecal impaction.

Skin Disorders

The athletic trainer will typically treat several types of skin disorders, most of which are not serious medical conditions. Common skin conditions in the athletic setting can be categorized as fungal infections such as athlete's foot (tinea pedis), jock itch (tinea cruris), and tinea capitis (scalp ringworm). Typical medications used to treat these conditions are antifungal agents. Both OTC and prescription medications are available.

Antifungal Agents

Antifungal therapies are used to fight off a variety of yeasts or molds that emerge in the body. An example of a common antifungal medication is terbinafine (e.g., Lamisil).

How they work: To destroy the cell, antifungal agents infiltrate or bind to the fungal cell membrane.

Administration: Administration is either topical or oral.

Side effects: Side effects include nausea, vomiting, headache, gastrointestinal distress, skin rash, and hepatic toxicity.

Contraindications: Contraindication are renal or kidney disease.

Other Medical Conditions

Some common medical conditions that the athletic trainer may encounter do not fit into a specific category. However, they are important for the athletic trainer to understand because they require ongoing management that often includes medications.

Diabetes Medications

Diabetes mellitus is a chronic metabolic disorder that manifests in two ways. Type I results from the failure of the pancreas to produce insulin. Because an individual with type I diabetes does not produce enough insulin, he or she is dependent on supplemental insulin administration. Type II diabetes results from insulin resistance, wherein insulin secretion is inadequate to sustain normal metabolism. In other words, those who have type II diabetes produce insulin, but their bodies cannot use it effectively. This type of diabetes may be managed by diet and exercise, insulin, and other diabetic drugs. Common types of oral diabetes medications include sulfonylureas (e.g., Diabinese, Glucotrol), meglitinides (e.g., Prandin, Starlix), biguanides (e.g., Glucophage), thiazolidinediones (e.g., Avandia, Rezulin), and alpha-glucosidase inhibitors (e.g., Precose, Glyset).

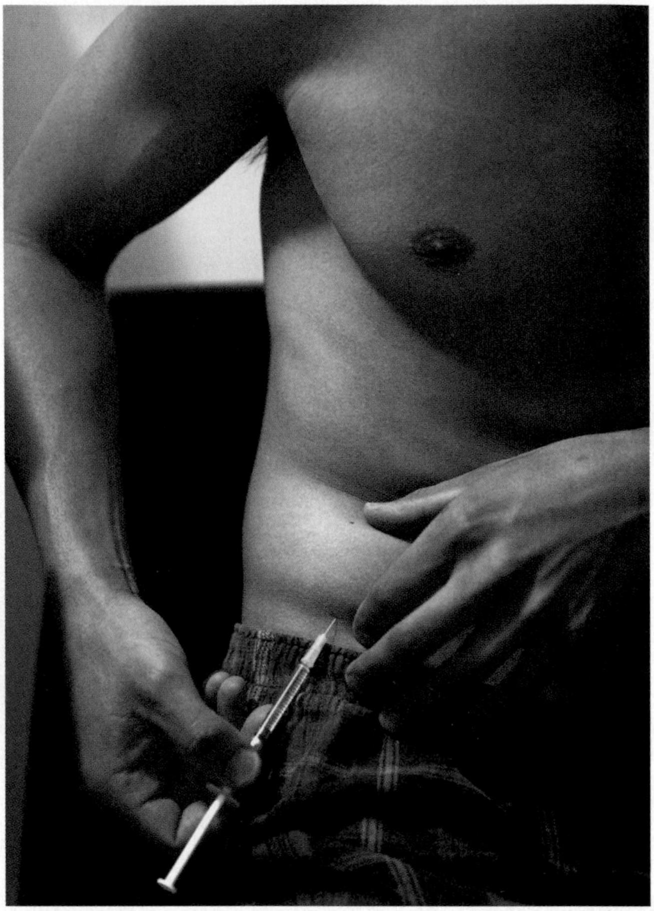

FIGURE 23-8 Man with diabetes injecting himself with insulin. (Credit: PhotoDisc.)

How they work: Medications for type I diabetes provide the individual with the necessary insulin for normal metabolical processes to occur. Medications for type II diabetes allow the body to properly metabolize and process available insulin.

Administration: Administration is oral, subcutaneous (Figures 23-8 and 23-9), intravenous, or inhaled.

Side effects: Side effects include headache, weakness, fatigue, poor vision, hunger, and nausea.

Contraindications: Contraindication for diabetes medication include active hypoglycemia and liver or kidney disease.

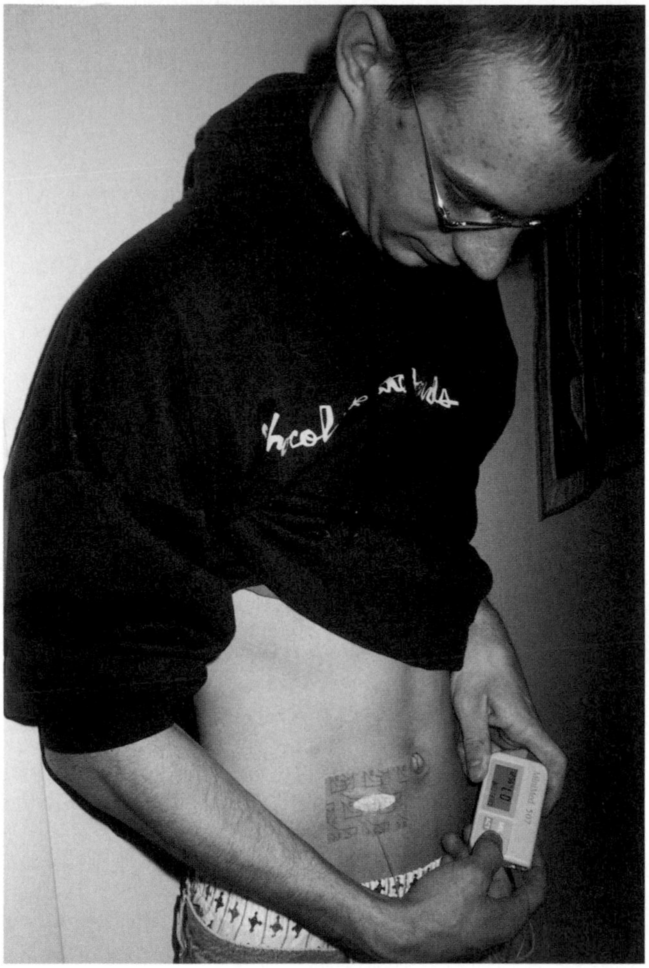

FIGURE 23-9 Insulin injection using an insulin pump. (From Peckenpaugh NJ: *Nutrition essentials and diet therapy,* ed 10, Figure 8-4, Philadelphia, 2007, Saunders.)

Antidepressants

Depression is one of the most common psychiatric disorders in the general population. Unfortunately, fewer than 50% of people with depression actually seek help. During a 1-year period, as many as 2.5% of children, 8.3% of adolescents, 5.8% of men, and 9.5% of women are affected by depression.[6,7] The primary pathophysiological response to depression is believed to be an alteration in the neurotransmitters serotonin and norepinephrine. Research shows that these two chemicals have a direct positive effect on treating depression. Many medications have been developed to improve the utilization or the availability of serotonin and norepinephrine in the brain so that they will have a positive effect on treating depression.[8,9]

Understanding the risk factors associated with depression is paramount to initiating an early treatment program. Those with a family history of mental illness or depression are at a higher risk for developing depression. Life stressors such as abuse, neglect, loss of a parent at an early age, loss of a child, or fertility problems are all risk factors contributing to depression. Substance and alcohol abuse are frequently associated with depression. Several classes of medication, both OTC and by prescription, are used to treat depression. Common OTC varieties include chamomile and St. John's wort. Examples of prescription medications include selective serotonin reuptake inhibitors (SSRIs; e.g., Prozac, Paxil, Zoloft), tricyclic antidepressants (TCAs; e.g., Elavil, Norpramin, Aventyl), heterocyclic antidepressants (e.g., Wellbutrin), monoamine oxidase inhibitors (e.g., Marplan, Parnate), and serotonin and norepinephrine reuptake inhibitors (e.g., Effexor, Cymbalta).

How they work: Antidepressants work in a number of ways, but all function as mood stabilizers. Various medications affect the production, utilization, and transportation of key neuron chemicals in the brain.

Administration: Administration is oral or intravenous.

Side effects: Side effects include gastrointestinal distress, dizziness, headache, sexual dysfunction, and changes in energy level.

Contraindications: Contraindications include cardiac disease, liver and kidney disease, and gastrointestinal distress.

Points to Ponder

Several athletes take medications for conditions that do not preclude their participation on the team. However, you notice that when the medication is taken, they display slightly lethargic behavior and at times seem a bit distracted and aloof. What is your role here, and what can you do to most effectively work with them and maintain their status on the team?

Antiepileptic Medications

Athletic trainers may occasionally encounter an athlete with epilepsy. The antiepileptic drugs are also known as anticonvulsants and are available only by prescription. Commonly prescribed medications include diazepam (e.g., Valium) and phenytoin (e.g., Dilantin).

How they work: Antiepileptic medications work by decreasing impulse transmission in the brain and the speed of neurotransmission.

Administration: Administration is oral, subcutaneous, or intravenous.

Side effects: Side effects include drowsiness, dizziness, gastrointestinal distress, and excitability

Contraindications: Contraindications for antiepileptic medications are liver and kidney disease, respiratory disease, and diabetes.

Box 23-5 summarizes the medications most commonly used to treat medical conditions.

BOX 23-5

Medications Used to Treat Common Medical Conditions

Respiratory Conditions

Antibiotics (e.g., penicillin, tetracycline, macrolide, sulfonamides)
Antiviral agents (e.g., oseltamivir [Tamiflu])
Bronchodilators (maintenance and rescue medications)
Common cold remedies
  Decongestants (e.g., pseudoephedrine [Sudafed])
  Cough medications (e.g., guaifenesin, dextromethorphan [Robitussin])
Antihistamine medications (e.g., diphenhydramine [Benadryl Allergy])

Gastrointestinal Conditions

Antacids (e.g., calcium carbonate [Tums])
Antiemetics (e.g., promethazine [Phenergan])
Antidiarrheals and laxatives (e.g., saline [Milk of Magnesia], stimulant [Dulcoax])

Skin Disorders

Antifungal agents (e.g., terbinafine [Lamisil])

Other Medical Conditions

Diabetes medications (e.g., insulin, sulfonylureas [Glucotrol])
Antidepressants (e.g., selective serotonin reuptake inhibitors [Prozac])
Antiepileptic medications (e.g., diazepam [Valium], phenytoin [Dilantin])

SUMMARY

Athletic trainers will be charged with caring for a variety of patients, with a variety of injuries, as the new millennium proceeds. The treatments provided may take on a new meaning as patients are living longer and health professionals are confronted with an ever-expanding list of medical problems. Therefore athletic trainers are advised to be familiar with all the medications used by the athletes under their care and the characteristic actions and side effects of these medications. Use of medications may make treatment decisions more complex and affect the care of athletes.

Revisiting the OPENING *Scenario*

Because Shannon was having difficulty tolerating the antiinflammatory medication given to alleviate the swelling in her ankle, the athletic trainer should look for other options that are less caustic to the gastrointestinal tract. Also, if she eats food or drinks milk with the medication, certain symptoms may be reduced. Having a working knowledge of both uses and side effects of medications gives the athletic trainer more treatment options. Another way to prevent or minimize side effects is to ask athletes whether they have ever been prescribed the intended drug and what their reactions and responses were. Knowing this in advance and choosing the best available medicinal plan from the outset may decrease delays in treatment and optimize healing time.

Issues & Ethics

As the newly hired assistant athletic trainer at your institution, a small college, one of your administrative assignments is drug testing of student-athletes. Apparently, very few tests over the years have been positive, and there is no real fear of problems occurring this year. However, during soccer season one of your best players tests positive for marijuana. You have heard rumors of a problem with this player, but this is her first failed test and only you and the testing lab know the results for now. The college drug testing policy states that any first-time positive drug test requires counseling and an immediate 2-week suspension of the athlete from all competition. You think this policy is fair and want to help the athlete with this problem, but the soccer team is deep into their season and is doing well against other teams in the conference for the first time in many years. A 2-week suspension means this player will miss four games, which will certainly hurt the team's chances of advancing in postseason play. Do you report the findings to the head athletic trainer and athletic director as dictated by the college testing policy, or do you delay the process until your team is playing nonconference games and the player's suspension will have a less dramatic effect on postseason play?

Web Links

All About Depression: www.allaboutdepression.com
American College of Clinical Pharmacy: www.accp.com/
American Diabetes Association: www.diabetes.org
American Pharmacists Association: www.aphanet.org
American Psychological Association: www.apa.org
American Psychiatric Association: www.psych.org
Epilepsy Foundation: www.epilepsyfoundation.org
Mental Health America: www.nmha.org
Pharmaceutical Research and Manufacturing of America: www.phrma.org/
Rx List (The Internet Drug List): www.rxlist.com
U.S. Food & Drug Administration: www.fda.gov
United States Pharmacopeia: http://www.usp.org/

References

1. Food and Drug Administration: *FDA's mission statement*, Rockville, Md, Author. Accessed June 15, 2007, 2007, from www.fda.gov/opacom/morechoices/mission.html.
2. U.S. Pharmacopeia: *About USP: an overview*, Rockville, Md, Author. Accessed June 15, 2007, from http://www.usp.org/aboutUSP/.

3. Leone R, et al: *Drug induced anaphylaxis: case/non-case study based on an Italian pharmacovigilance database, Drug Safety: An International Journal of Medical Toxicology and Drug Experience*, 28(6): 547–556, 2005.
4. Vargas PA, et al: System profiles and asthma control in school-aged children, *Annals of Allergy, Asthma & Immunology*, 96(6): 787–793, 2006.
5. Chen CH, Xirasagar S, Lin HC: Seasonality in adult asthma admissions, air pollutant levels, and climate: a population-based study, *The Journal of Asthma: Official Journal of the Association for the Care of Asthma* 43(4): 287–292, 2006.
6. Culpepper L, et al: Active management of depression and anxiety in primary care, *Journal of the American Academy of Physician Assistants, Supp* 1: 4–21, 2006.
7. World Health Organization: *The world health report 2001—mental health: new understanding, new hope*, Geneva, Switzerland, 2001, Author. Accessed June 15, 2007, from http://www.who.int/whr/2001/en/index.html.
8. Birmaher B, Ryan N, Williamson D: The NIMH diagnostic interview schedule for children, version 2.3 (disc 2.3): description, acceptability, prevalence rates, and performance in the MECA study, *Journal of the American Academy of Child and Adolescent Psychiatry*, 35(7): 865–877, 1996.
9. Wang JL, Patten SB: The moderating effects of coping strategies on major depression in the general population, *Canadian Journal of Psychiatry*, 47: 167–173, 2002.

Bibliography

Clayton BD, Stock YN: *Basic pharmacology for nurses*, ed 13, St Louis, 2004, Mosby.

Gladson B: *Pharmacology for physical therapists*, Philadelphia, 2006, Saunders/Elsevier.

Hopper T: *Mosby's pharmacy technician*, ed 2, Philadelphia, 2007, Saunders/Elsevier.

Kee JL, Hayes ER, McCuiston LE: *Pharmacology: a nursing process approach*, ed 5, Philadelphia, 2006, Saunders/Elsevier.

Lilley LL, Harrington S, Snyder JS: *Pharmacology and the nursing process*, ed 5, St Louis, 2007, Mosby/Elsevier.

The Merck manual of medical information, ed 2 (home edition), Whitehouse Station, NJ, 2003, Merck Research Laboratories.

Mosby's drug consult 2007, ed 17, St Louis, 2007, Mosby.

Mosby's drug consult for the health professions, St Louis, 2006, Mosby.

Skidmore-Roth L: *Mosby's 2008 nursing drug reference*, ed 21, St Louis, 2008, Mosby/Elsevier.

24

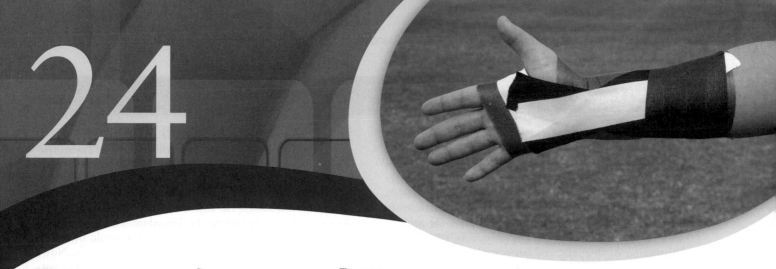

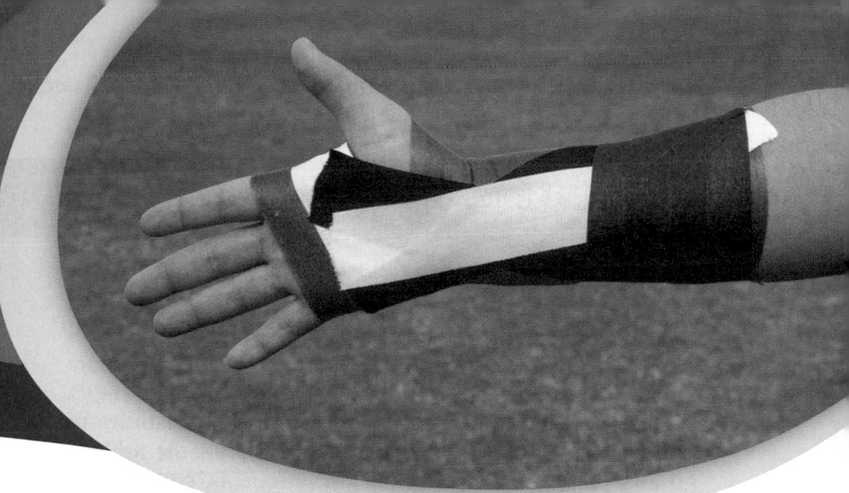

Prevention and Protection: Taping and Bracing

KAREN M. LEW AND SUE STANLEY-GREEN

Learning Goals

1. Identify and describe commonly used protective equipment required for participation in various sports.
2. Describe the steps necessary to properly fit commercial protective equipment.
3. Explain the benefits of taping as opposed to bracing.
4. Understand the principles of preventive and protective taping.
5. Choose the appropriate brace, wrap, or sleeve to protect the injured body part.

One of the most important jobs and biggest challenges for the athletic trainer is preventing the athlete from getting hurt. The athletic trainer can accomplish this task in a number of ways. The common prevention practices of taping, wrapping, and applying braces or other protective equipment are skills that most athletic trainers take pride in doing well. Taping and bracing is both an art and a science within the profession, requiring athletic trainers to use their skill and imagination to protect against injury.

In addition to proficiency in taping, wrapping, padding, and bracing, athletic trainers must have an extensive knowledge of equipment and supplies and the most effective techniques to use to prevent and protect injuries. It is necessary to know the rules of each sport and to be aware of what materials and braces are legal to use. Athletic trainers must be familiar with the latest research in injury prevention and protection to ensure that they are choosing, fitting, and using state-of-the art techniques.[1,2] Helmets and shoulder pads are examples of protective equipment that athletic trainers may be responsible for fitting in certain practice settings. Properly fitting equipment is imperative for injury prevention.

LIABILITY ISSUES

The athlete, athletic trainer, and coach all share in the responsibility of prevention and protection of athletic injuries. The athletic trainer and coach must know and follow the guidelines for proper equipment selection according to the rules and the organizations that govern the sport. The athlete must share in the responsibility and follow the rules by wearing the proper equipment to prevent or protect injuries. It is important to inspect any braces or equipment that an athlete may borrow, purchase independently, or bring from home. There is a tremendous amount of risk involved in equipment selection and potential fit, especially equipment that is not issued specifically by the coach, equipment manager, or athletic trainer. For example, if the equipment is not used exactly as the manufacture specifies and an injury occurs, there could be a question of **liability**.

liability legal responsibility for the harm caused to another person provide support in a way similar to that of ankle taping. The athlete may choose from a variety of braces, ranging from lace-up models to rigid stirrups with hinges (Figure 24-5). Certain shoes are even designed with ankle braces already enclosed. For schools with a limited budget, braces may prove to be more economical than taping. A pair of ankle braces should last for the entire season, whereas it may cost up to several dollars to tape each ankle for a practice or game. Taping also is more time consuming. However, when personnel and budget constraints are not issues, taping is still considered the gold standard for ankle injury prevention.

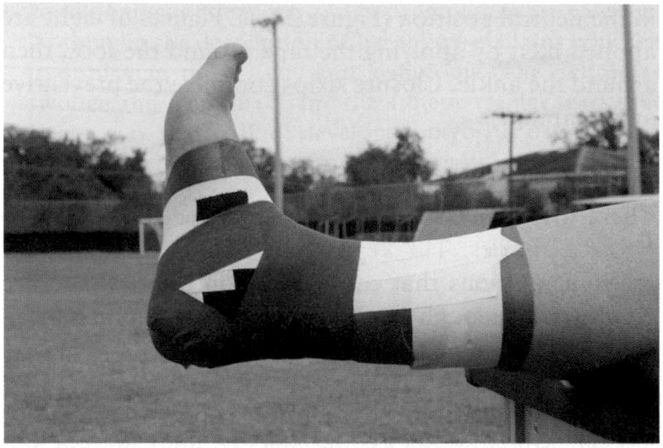

FIGURE 24-4 Heel locks and figures of eight are applied to stabilize the ankle joint.

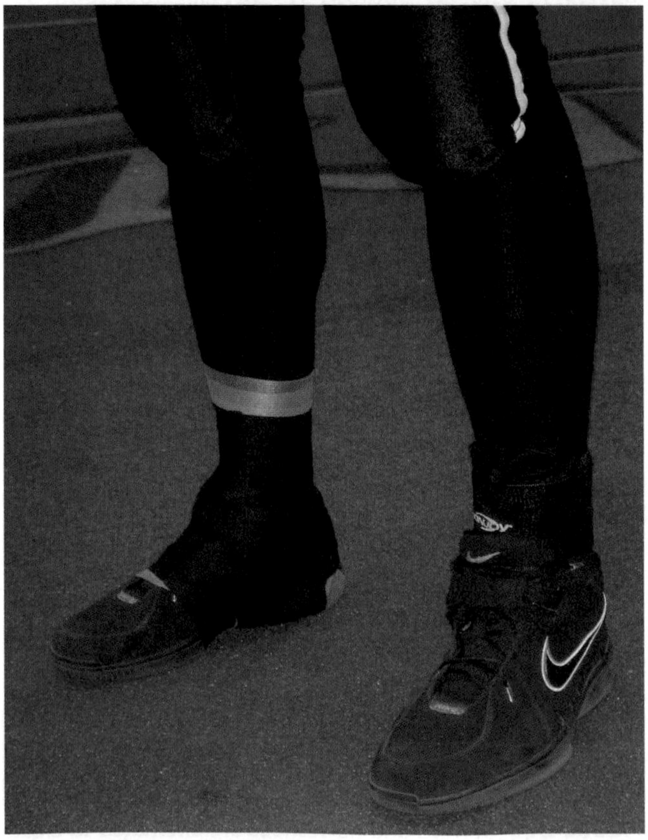

FIGURE 24-5 An ankle brace may be chosen instead of ankle taping on the basis of function, cost, or personal preference.

Knee Braces

Athletic trainers, physicians, and coaches all are challenged to devise ways to prevent potentially season-ending knee injuries. In the mid-1980s, it became popular to wear lateral knee braces to prevent a lateral blow or clip to the knee from injuring the medial collateral ligament. Some research showed that a number of knee injuries were prevented or the severity of the injury was reduced, but conflicting studies showed that the braces may have caused other injuries.[3,4] Today the controversy continues. Many athletic trainers and coaches at the collegiate and professional levels still encourage their athletes to wear knee braces to prevent injuries. The braces range from simple off-the-shelf knee sleeves with lateral support to custom knee braces originally designed for anterior cruciate injuries. These braces may cost more than $1000 each. Even with the expensive custom braces, knee injures still can occur (Figure 24-6).

Neck Braces

The main reason to use preventive taping or bracing is to limit a body part's range of motion. Because of excessive

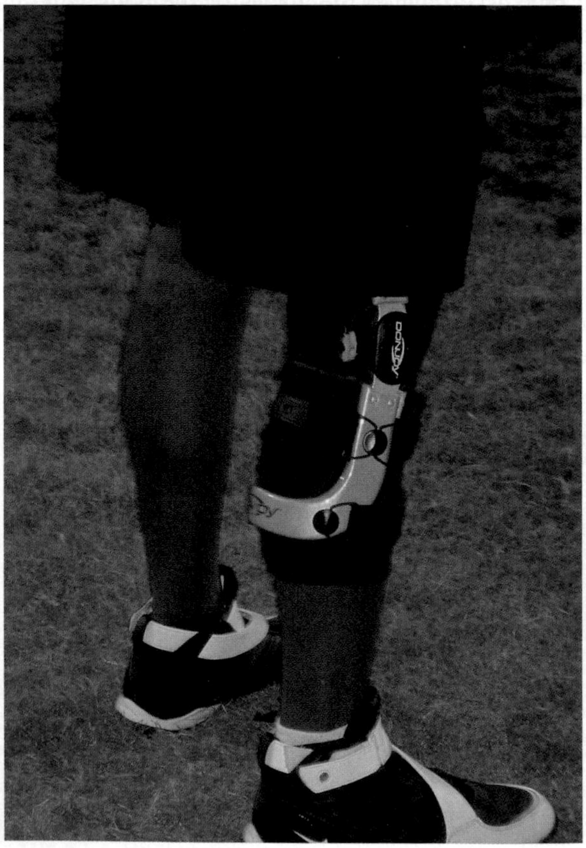

FIGURE 24-6 A knee brace may be used after injury or surgery for support and added confidence.

lateral motion or extension of the neck, a cervical brace or neck collar is commonly used to prevent excessive motion in contact sports such as football. A common injury that occurs from that excessive motion is a brachial plexus stretch, more commonly called a *burner* or *stinger*. This injury is caused by the head being forced in a lateral direction while the shoulder is depressed. The signs and symptoms of the brachial plexus stretch include radiating pain, burning, and numbness down the arm. The injury is usually transient, but recurrent burners or stingers can cause permanent nerve damage, resulting in loss of sensation or strength. The purpose of neck collars is to prevent recurrence of brachial plexus injuries. Many types of neck collars on the market today are very effective. The appropriate collar should be chosen for the best possible fit and function depending on the position and the sport.

Taping Versus Bracing

Athletic trainers have used taping and bracing techniques to treat athletic conditions and injuries for many years. Not surprisingly, the trends and ideas regarding taping and bracing have changed significantly. The availability of braces and the changes in construction and development have caused an increase in brace usage. Braces are now being made for all body parts in a variety of shapes, sizes, and colors. Research is also continuously being conducted to support the use of bracing versus taping.

The common argument against taping is the quick loss of **tensile strength** of the tape. Recently, is has been argued that although tape may lose some of its tensile strength, it still helps prevent against excess range of motion. The cost is also a consideration when deciding whether to use a brace or tape. Athletic trainers usually prefer one over the other, depending on the body part, the injury's severity, the type of activity required of the athlete, and the level of performance. With so many varieties of tape and braces available, there is something for everyone. When deciding what to use, the athletic trainer should also consider the athlete's preferences.

INJURY PROTECTION

After an injury occurs, often the body part needs some additional protection or support to prevent re-injury. Taping, bracing, or protective equipment can be used to limit the motion of a joint, support soft tissue, or provide additional padding to protect the injury until it heals completely.

Protective Taping

Protective taping is based on the same principles as preventive taping. The body part should be positioned to prevent the movement that caused the injury. For example, for a hyperextension elbow injury, the elbow should be positioned in slight flexion. The supportive strips would hold the elbow in a position to keep it from hyperextending again. Additional strips should be applied for increased support, and stronger elastic tape may be used to keep the tape job from loosening during activity. It is important to remember that taping must allow the athlete to perform the skills required for the specific sport. The taping must be functional as well as protective.

The following sections provide examples of common protective taping. They all adhere to the basic taping principles, but they may be modified for individual athletes and their unique needs. Reference may be made to taping techniques that describe how the tape is applied, such as figure 8s, half-figure 8s, Cs, anchors, stirrups, and horseshoes. These terms describe the shape that is made with the tape and help the athletic trainer visualize how the tape should look when it is applied correctly to the body part.

Arch Taping

Rationale: Arch taping is primarily used to support the longitudinal arch in the case of a sprain or other chronic condition that may be caused by overuse. The arch is the base for all weight-bearing activities. If the arch is not adequately supported, injuries may occur at various sites on the body. Shin splints are chronic injuries that cause pain in the anterior or lateral shin area. Often, taping the arch provides some relief for this aggravating condition. Plantar fasciitis is an inflammation of the sheath on the bottom of the foot. Arch taping may provide relief for plantar fasciitis and allow the athlete to perform with decreased pain.

Method: One of the methods for arch taping is to place an anchor across the ball of the foot, then use half figures of eight to "X" the longitudinal arch. Four to six "Xs" are used to fill in the arch area. Straight strips are applied from the heel area to the ball of the foot, with the strips pulled firmly into the arch. The arch taping may be finished or closed with elastic tape (Figure 24-7).

Great Toe Taping

Rationale: The metatarsophalangeal joint of the great toe is a joint that commonly becomes inflamed. Injuries that occur at this joint are caused by improperly fitted shoes, a bunion, or from the stop-and-go action of certain sports such as soccer. One chronic condition of this joint is called "turf toe." Turf toe is a very painful condition that may keep an athlete from participation. The athlete may be more comfortable if the toe is taped to prevent excessive and painful movement.

tensile strength the force required to pull something to the point at which it breaks or tears

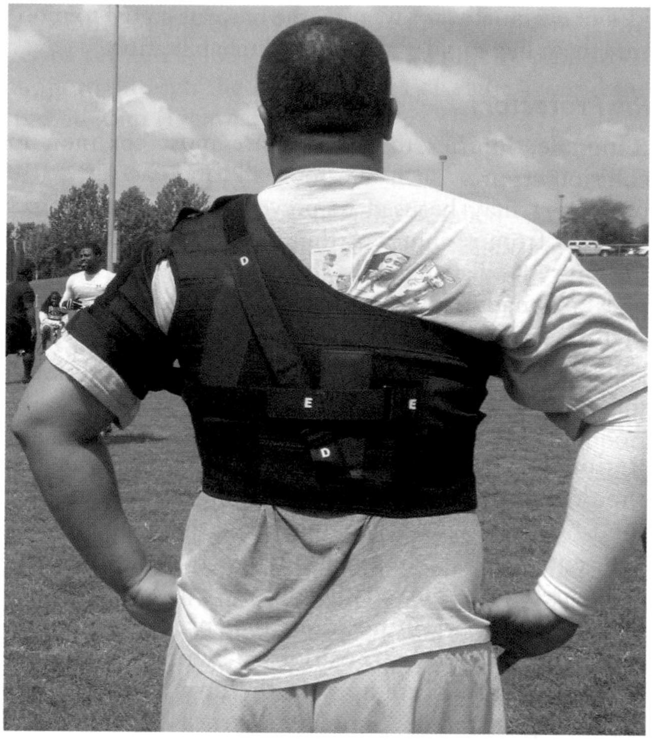

FIGURE 24-17 A shoulder harness helps limit arm abduction and external rotation, movements that can make an athlete who has previously dislocated or subluxed the shoulder vulnerable to re-injury .

ATHLETIC PROTECTIVE EQUIPMENT

The purpose of protective equipment is to decrease the risk of injury and provide protection during a contact or collision sport. When equipment is selected, fitted, and used as intended, it should help prevent the athlete from incurring injuries associated with a particular sport. Protective equipment is determined by the sport and its specific rules and guidelines. Football is the first sport that comes to mind during discussions of protective equipment, but hockey, lacrosse, field hockey, soccer, and many other sports also depend on specific equipment to protect athletes from injuries (Box 24-1).

BOX 24-1 Factors That Must be Considered in Athletic Equipment Design

- Areas prone to injury
- Transfer or dispersing area of impact
- Friction reduction
- Absorption of energy
- Limiting of movement or range of motion
- Addition of mass to the individual area

The benefits of appropriate and properly fitted equipment are numerous. In a collision sport, an increase in the impact area allows the extrinsic force to be absorbed and dispersed throughout the area to decrease potential for injury. The forces that the body must absorb vary, but with appropriate protection the risk and/or severity of the injury may be reduced or even eliminated. The transfer of the impact area to another body part may allow the body to further absorb the impact without complications. Another requirement for well-fitting equipment is its capacity to limit the relative motion. By acting as a block or a stopping point in the range of motion, the equipment prevents the joint from moving beyond its normal range, which could result in injury. Other benefits that athletic equipment can provide include reducing friction between contacting surfaces and even protecting the body from dirt and harmful agents.

Selecting Athletic Equipment

Several factors are involved in equipment selection. The equipment must conform to the rules of the sport and allow the athlete to perform the skills of the sport without restriction. Likewise, the athlete wearing the equipment must be comfortable and feel confident that his or her performance will not be hindered; if this is not the case, the athlete will be less likely to wear or use the equipment. For example, if a sprinter is prescribed a clunky **orthotic** that adds weight to her shoe, she may risk injury rather than run in a shoe that could take seconds off her time. It is imperative that the athlete use the comfortable and functional equipment that conforms with the rules of the sport and prevents or protects against common injuries.

Considerations for Equipment Sizing and Selection

Selecting and fitting athletic equipment is a group activity with shared responsibility. The coach, athletic trainer, and equipment manager should discuss the demands of the sport and its associated risks, the various positions within the sport, the strength of the athletes, and the forces that will be produced during contact. The athlete's age and physical development are also factors in choosing and fitting equipment. Every athlete involved in a given sport does not wear equipment of the same size. The ages of the athletes on one team may be consistent, but the heights and weights of those athletes may vary tremendously (Figure 24-18). There is a degree of risk involved in all athletic participation but

orthotic a device that fits in a shoe and is designed to correct problems with the foot

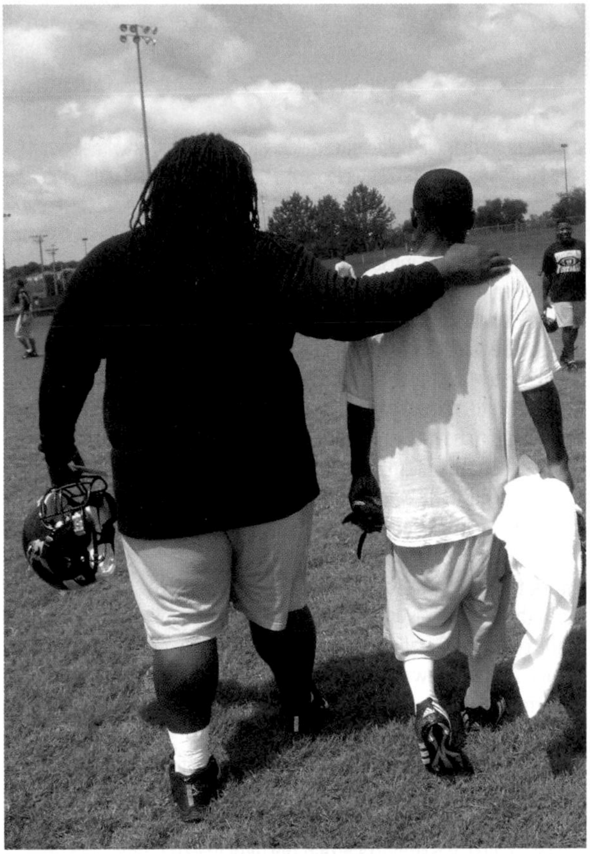

FIGURE 24-18 The heights and weights of similar-age athletes on one team may vary tremendously, and these factors must be considered during equipment selection.

every effort must be made to ensure that all athletes are protected by appropriate and properly fitted equipment. Budgets are often tight in athletics, but the safety of the athlete cannot be compromised by inadequate, improperly fitted, or outdated equipment.

Points to Ponder
Who has the final word in protective equipment selection and fitting?

Specific Types of Protective Equipment

Almost every sport has different requirements or recommendations for protective equipment. Certain equipment is designed to prevent injuries, and other types are intended to protect the body part after an injury occurs. Common rules for decisions about equipment include choosing the appropriate, approved equipment and ensuring that it is in good condition, fits properly, and is worn consistently.

Helmets and Headgear

All sports that require helmets or headgear have specific standards that are established specifically for these items. Helmets are required to meet or exceed the standards established by National Operating Committee on Standards for Athletic Equipment (NOCSAE). They must meet the standards of the Canadian Standards Association (CSA), the Hockey Equipment Certification Council (HECC), and the American Society of Testing and Materials (ASTM).

Although helmets are usually associated with football, they are often required in a variety of other sports, including baseball, softball, ice hockey, field hockey, boxing, and lacrosse. The purpose of the helmet in all sports-related activities is to protect the brain and other related structures from direct impact by deflecting the forces and decreasing the potential for serious injury. If an athlete has a history of head injury, he or she should be encouraged or required to wear a helmet.

Helmets are constructed from high-density materials, which are used in the outer shell and padding. The high-density padding is composed of polycarbonate, thermoplastic, and plastic materials. When fitting helmets, the athletic trainer should inspect the helmets to make sure that they have not been altered, that the materials have not been compromised, and that all hardware is in good condition. It is important that all athletes wearing helmets be properly fitted by a coach or athletic trainer experienced in equipment fitting (Box 24-2).

A warning label is placed on all helmets that are approved by NOCSAE. The warning gives specific cautions and directions regarding the use of the helmet. Before the first practice, the warning should be read and explained to the athletes and, if the athletes are minors, to their parents. The athletes and their parents should have the opportunity to ask questions about the risks of the sport and should sign a waiver confirming that they understand and accept the potential risks. This warning is of the utmost importance to ensure that athletes and parents have been properly warned about the risks of their specific sport (Box 24-3).

In addition to helmets, other equipment is designed to protect the head, face, and neck. Wrestling is an example of a sport in which ear guards are worn as part of the required uniform. A protective ear guard must be worn whenever active wrestling takes place. The purpose of the ear guard is to prevent friction to the ear that causes a condition called *cauliflower ear*. The only time the ear guard or protective head gear is not required is during passive drills or the warm-up period. Fencing is an example of a sport that requires a face guard to protect against sharp objects and other threats. Additional examples of sports in which such equipment is worn include hockey, lacrosse, baseball, and softball. Players in these sports may also use a throat protector, which is attached to the helmet.

BOX 24-4 Shoulder Pad Fitting

- The width of the shoulder is measured to determine the proper size of pads.
- The inside shoulder pad should cover the tip of the shoulder in a direct line with the lateral aspect of the shoulder.
- The epaulets and cups should cover the deltoid muscle and allow movements required by the athlete's specific position.
- The neck opening must allow the athlete to raise the arm overhead but not allow the pad to slide back and forth.
- If a split-clavicle shoulder pad is used, the channel for the top of the shoulder must be in the proper position.
- Straps underneath the arm must hold the pads firmly in place but not in such a way that they constrict soft tissue. A collar and drop-down pads may be added to provide more protection.

taping, bracing, and equipment. Athletic trainers should be proactive and lobby for rule changes that may be necessary to prevent injuries or better protect injuries after they occur. Athletic trainers must work with athletes, coaches, equipment managers, and equipment companies to design and develop the best materials and equipment possible.

Revisiting the OPENING *Scenario*

Logan needs better protection of her deltoid to prevent further injury. New shoulder pads are not a budgetary option, but a smaller deltoid pad that can be wrapped in place will solve the problem. The athletic trainer can create a pad for this purpose, and inexpensive commercially made pads are also available. With this pad in place, Logan's risk of further injury to this area is significantly decreased. After a few days of treatment with therapeutic modalities, Logan's arm is no longer swollen and the discoloration is nearly gone. The risk of myositis ossificans is no longer a major concern. Logan is able to complete the season with full motion of her arm and compete at her highest level.

Issues & Ethics

You are the host athletic trainer for a football game. The visiting team does not have an athletic trainer. The star running back for the visiting team sprains his ankle. After evaluating the athlete, you determine that he has a first-degree ankle sprain and give him the option to return play after taping. You have the choice of applying a basic ankle taping or one with additional support to better protect his ankle and prevent further injury. The game is close. Which one would you choose?

The women's soccer team is playing for the conference championship. Your star player has just returned after having suffered an anterior cruciate ligament injury, and her orthopedic surgeon has required that she wear a custom knee brace. Your player had the brace on during warm-ups, but just as the game starts, you notice that she is not wearing her brace. This is the first time she has played without the brace, and she is going against her doctor's orders. What do you do?

Web Links

Athletic Equipment Managers Association: www.aema1.com
National Association of Intercollegiate Athletics: www.naia.org
National Collegiate Athletic Association: www.ncaa.org
National Federation of State High School Associations: www.nfhs.org
National Institute for Sports Science and Safety: www.nisss.org
National Junior College Athletic Association: www.njcaa.org
National Operating Committee on Safety for Athletic Equipment: www.nocsae.com
Riddell Sports Equipment: www.riddell.com
SGMA International: www.sportlink.com

References

1. Board of Certification: *Role delineation study,* ed 5, Omaha, Neb, 2006, Author.
2. National Athletic Trainers' Association: *Athletic training educational competencies,* ed 4, Dallas, 2006, Author.
3. Paulos LE, Drawbert JP, France P, Rosenberg TD: Lateral knee braces in football: do they prevent injury? *Phys Sportsmed* 14: 119–126, 1986.
4. Grace TG, Skipper BJ, Newberry JC, et al: Prophylactic knee braces and injury to the lower extremity, *J Bone Joint Surg [Am]* 70A: 422–427, 1988.
5. Committee on Competitive Safeguards and Medical Aspects of Sports: *Position regarding eye protection in women's lacrosse,* Indianapolis, 2000 (June), National Collegiate Athletic Association.
6. Honsik KA: Emergency treatment of dentoalveolar trauma: essential tips for treating active patients, *The Physician and Sports Medicine* [online] 32(9): 1, 2004. Accessed June 7, 2007, from www.physsportsmed.com/issues/2004/0904/honsik.htm.

APPENDIX A

NATA Code of Ethics

PREAMBLE

The National Athletic Trainers' Association Code of Ethics states the principles of ethical behavior that should be followed in the practice of athletic training. It is intended to establish and maintain high standards and professionalism for the athletic training profession.

The principles do not cover every situation encountered by the practicing athletic trainer, but are representative of the spirit with which athletic trainers should make decisions. The principles are written generally; the circumstances of a situation will determine the interpretation and application of a given principle and of the Code as a whole. When a conflict exists between the Code and the law, the law prevails.

PRINCIPLE 1:

Members shall respect the rights, welfare and dignity of all.

1.1 Members shall not discriminate against any legally protected class.

1.2 Members shall be committed to providing competent care.

1.3 Members shall preserve the confidentiality of privileged information and shall not release such information to a third party not involved in the patient's care without a release unless required by law.

PRINCIPLE 2:

Members shall comply with the laws and regulations governing the practice of athletic training.

2.1 Members shall comply with applicable local, state, and federal laws and institutional guidelines.

2.2 Members shall be familiar with and abide by all National Athletic Trainers' Association standards, rules and regulations.

2.3 Members shall report illegal or unethical practices related to athletic training to the appropriate person or authority.

2.4 Members shall avoid substance abuse and, when necessary, seek rehabilitation for chemical dependency.

PRINCIPLE 3:

Members shall maintain and promote high standards in their provision of services.

3.1 Members shall not misrepresent, either directly or indirectly, their skills, training, professional credentials, identity or services.

3.2 Members shall provide only those services for which they are qualified through education or experience and which are allowed by their practice acts and other pertinent regulation.

3.3 Members shall provide services, make referrals, and seek compensation only for those services that are necessary.

3.4 Members shall recognize the need for continuing education and participate in educational activities that enhance their skills and knowledge.

3.5 Members shall educate those whom they supervise in the practice of athletic training about the Code of Ethics and stress the importance of adherence.

3.6 Members who are researchers or educators should maintain and promote ethical conduct in research and educational activities.

From National Athletic Trainers' Association: *NATA code of ethics*, Dallas, 2005 (September 28), Author.

Index

PRINCIPLE 4:

Members shall not engage in conduct that could be construed as a conflict of interest or that reflects negatively on the profession.

4.1 Members should conduct themselves personally and professionally in a manner that does not compromise their professional responsibilities or the practice of athletic training.

4.2 National Athletic Trainers' Association current or past volunteer leaders shall not use the NATA logo in the endorsement of products or services or exploit their affiliation with the NATA in a manner that reflects badly upon the profession.

4.3 Members shall not place financial gain above the patient's welfare and shall not participate in any arrangement that exploits the patient.

4.4 Members shall not, through direct or indirect means, use information obtained in the course of the practice of athletic training to try to influence the score or outcome of an athletic event, or attempt to induce financial gain through gambling.

APPENDIX B

National Athletic Trainers' Association

MEMBERSHIP STANDARDS AND SANCTIONS

I. Membership Standards

By joining the NATA, the member is agreeing to:

A. Abide by the NATA Bylaws, policies and procedures, Code of Ethics, membership standards and other rules and regulations, and demonstrate compliance when asked.

B. Avoid improper or unauthorized use of the trademarks ATC, C.A.T., the NATA logo or its companion marks.

i. To discontinue immediately and correct at his/her own expense any misuse of these marks.

ii. That if such activities do not cease immediately upon notification, NATA shall be entitled to obtain injunctive relief, damages, costs and attorney's fees.

C. Submit complete and accurate membership data and other information requested.

D. Felons convicted for crimes related to minors, health care, athletics or education are ineligible for membership application until one year after the exhaustion of appeals, completion of sentence or parole, whichever is later. This includes but is not limited to felonies of a sexual nature; threatened or actual use of a weapon or violence; and the prohibited sale, distribution of or possession with intent to distribute controlled substances. Also included in this prohibition are convictions where an athletic trainer has used his or her position improperly to influence, or try to influence, the score or outcome of an athletic event, or in connection with gambling activity.

II. Membership Sanctions

When joining NATA, a member assumes certain obligations and responsibilities. Sanctions may be imposed if a member does not properly fulfill those responsibilities.

A. Grounds for Sanctions

A member may be subject to sanctions set forth below if s/he:

i. Submits fraudulent information or in any other way attempts to improperly obtain NATA membership.

ii. Misrepresents membership or certification status, or other professional qualifications or credentials.

iii. Is convicted of a felony for the crimes described in §I D. of the Membership Standards or others.

iv. Commits serious or repeated violations of NATA bylaws, policies and procedures, Code of Ethics, rules, regulations and standards.

v. Is subject to license, certification, or registration revocation or suspension by a state athletic training regulatory agency.

B. Sanctions

i. Sanctions for violations of any membership standard shall be reasonable.

ii. Sanctions may include: denial of eligibility, cancellation, non-renewal and suspension of membership; public censure; and/or private reprimand.

iii. In cases where sanctions are imposed, the earliest that reconsideration could occur is one year from the date of the final ruling, a court decision, or completion of sentence or parole, whichever is later.

From National Athletic Trainers' Association: *National Athletic Trainers' Association membership standards and sanctions*, Dallas, 2005 (September 28), Author.

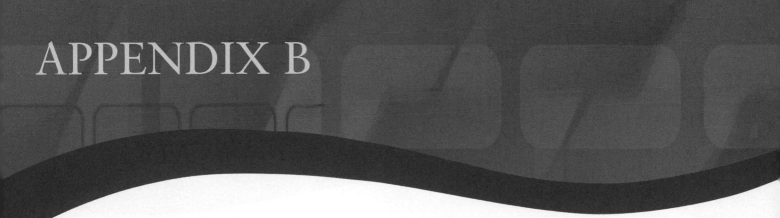

APPENDIX C

Official Statement from the National Athletic Trainers' Association

ON COMMUNITY-ACQUIRED MRSA INFECTIONS (CA-MRSA)

In an effort to educate the public about the potential risks of the emergence of community-acquired methicillin-resistant staphylococcus infection (CA-MRSA), the National Athletic Trainers' Association (NATA) recommends that health care personnel and physically active participants take appropriate precautions with suspicious lesions and talk with a physician.

According to the Centers for Disease Control and Prevention (CDC), approximately 25% to 30% of the population is colonized in the nose with *Staphylococcus aureus*, often referred to as "staph" and approximately 1% of the population is colonized with MRSA[1].

Cases have developed from person-to-person contact, shared towels, soaps, improperly treated whirlpools, and equipment (mats, pads, surfaces, etc). Staph or CA-MRSA infections usually manifest as skin infections, such as pimples, pustules and boils, which present as red, swollen, painful, or have pus or other drainage. Without proper referral and care, more serious infections may cause pneumonia, bloodstream infections, or surgical would infections.

Maintaining good hygiene and avoiding contact with drainage from skin lesions are the best methods for prevention.

Proper prevention and management recommendations may include, but are not limited to:

1. Keep hands clean by washing thoroughly with soap and warm water or using an alcohol-based hand sanitizer routinely.
2. Encourage immediate showering following activity.
3. Avoid whirlpools or common tubs with open wounds, scrapes or scratches.
4. Avoid sharing towels, razors, and daily athletic gear.
5. Properly wash athletic gear and towels after each use.
6. Maintain clean facilities and equipment.
7. Inform or refer to appropriate health care personnel for all active skin lesions and lesions that do not respond to initial therapy.
8. Administer or seek proper first aid.
9. Encourage health care personnel to seek bacterial cultures to establish a diagnosis.
10. Care and cover skin lesions appropriately before participation.

---

[1] CA-MRSA Information for the Public. Centers for Disease Control and Prevention. Available on-line at: www.cdc.gov/ncidod/hip/aresist/ca_mrsa_public.htm

From National Athletic Trainers' Association: *Official statement from the National Athletic Trainers' Association on community-acquired MRSA infections (CA-MRSA)*, Dallas, 2005 (March 1), Author.

APPENDIX D

Official Statement from the National Athletic Trainers' Association

ON COMMOTIO CORDIS

According to the U.S. Commotio Cordis Registry, since 1998, 130 athletes have died from blunt force injury to the heart (*Commotio Cordis*). Of those, 70 were children ages 4-18, according to the Heart Center at TUFTS New England Medical Center.

In an effort to educate the public about the potential risks physically active youth can face, the National Athletic Trainers' Association (NATA) Age-Specific Task Force recommends that parents and coaches take proactive steps to protect their athletes against *Commotio Cordis*.

Commotio Cordis is caused by a blow to the chest (directly over the heart) that occurs between heart contractions. The blunt force causes a lethal abnormal heart rhythm.

The following suggestions can help prevent *Commotio Cordis* and keep young athletes safe.

- Encourage all coaches and officials to become trained in cardiopulmonary resuscitation (CPR), automatic external defibrillator (AED) use, and first aid.
- Establish an emergency action plan at all athletic venues. Parents, coaches, and officials should be involved in these plans. (NATA's Position Statement on Emergency Planning in Athletics—www.nata.org/publicinformation/files/emergencyplanning.pdf—is a useful resource.)
- Use all-purpose sports chest protectors during practices and games. *(Note: NATA recommends continued research in this area because current information is limited. However, use of properly fitted, quality chest protectors are recommended to reduce the risk of injury to the athlete.)*
- Ensure all protective equipment fits properly and is used as intended by the manufacturer.
- Teach athletes how to protect themselves against chest injuries.
- Maintain an even and clean playing surface.

Links

To learn more about *Commotio Cordis,* and how you can protect your child from this type of injury, go to:

www.momsteam.com
www.teamsofangels.org
www.la12.org/articles/commotio_cordis.htm
www.tufts-nemc.org/medicine/card/commotiocordis.htm
www.emedicine.com/ped/topic3019.htm
www.usabaseball.com/commotio_cordis.html
www.ncbi.nlm.nih.gov/entrez/query.fcgi?cmd=Retrieve&db=PubMed&dopt=Abstract&list_uids=21872311

From National Athletic Trainers' Association: *Official statement from the National Athletic Trainers' Association on commotio cordis*, Dallas, 2004 (May), Author.

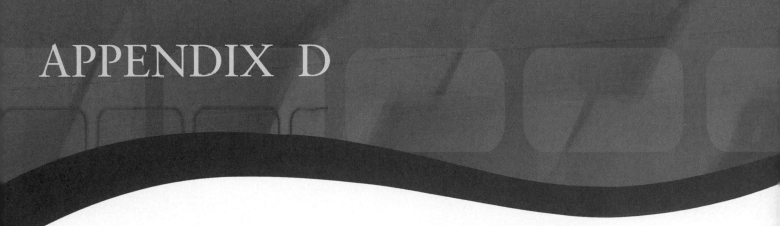

Disclaimer: The NATA publishes its position statements as a service to promote the awareness of certain issues to its members. The information contained in the position statement is neither exhaustive nor exclusive to all circumstances or individuals. Variables such as institutional human resource guidelines, state or federal statutes, rules, or regulations, as well as regional environmental conditions, may impact the relevance and implementation of these recommendations. The NATA advises its members and others to carefully and independently consider each of the recommendations (including the applicability of same to any particular circumstance or individual). The position statement should not be relied upon as an independent basis for care, but rather as a resource available to NATA members or others. Moreover, no opinion is expressed herein regarding the quality of care that adheres to or differs from NATA's position statements. The NATA reserves the right to rescind or modify its position statements at any time."

APPENDIX E

Body Mass Index Table

Body Mass Index Table

	Normal						Overweight					Obese										Extreme Obesity														
BMI	**19**	**20**	**21**	**22**	**23**	**24**	**25**	**26**	**27**	**28**	**29**	**30**	**31**	**32**	**33**	**34**	**35**	**36**	**37**	**38**	**39**	**40**	**41**	**42**	**43**	**44**	**45**	**46**	**47**	**48**	**49**	**50**	**51**	**52**	**53**	**54**
Height (inches)												**Body Weight (pounds)**																								
58	91	96	100	105	110	115	119	124	129	134	138	143	148	153	158	162	167	172	177	181	186	191	196	201	205	210	215	220	224	229	234	239	244	248	253	258
59	94	99	104	109	114	119	124	128	133	138	143	148	153	158	163	168	173	178	183	188	193	198	203	208	212	217	222	227	232	237	242	247	252	257	262	267
60	97	102	107	112	118	123	128	133	138	143	148	153	158	163	168	174	179	184	189	194	199	204	209	215	220	225	230	235	240	245	250	255	261	266	271	276
61	100	106	111	116	122	127	132	137	143	148	153	158	164	169	174	180	185	190	195	201	206	211	217	222	227	232	238	243	248	254	259	264	269	275	280	285
62	104	109	115	120	126	131	136	142	147	153	158	164	169	175	180	186	191	196	202	207	213	218	224	229	235	240	246	251	256	262	267	273	278	284	289	295
63	107	113	118	124	130	135	141	146	152	158	163	169	175	180	186	191	197	203	208	214	220	225	231	237	242	248	254	259	265	270	278	282	287	293	299	304
64	110	116	122	128	134	140	145	151	157	163	169	174	180	186	192	197	204	209	215	221	227	232	238	244	250	256	262	267	273	279	285	291	296	302	308	314
65	114	120	126	132	138	144	150	156	162	168	174	180	186	192	198	204	210	216	222	228	234	240	246	252	258	264	270	276	282	288	294	300	306	312	318	324
66	118	124	130	136	142	148	155	161	167	173	179	186	192	198	204	210	216	223	229	235	241	247	253	260	266	272	278	284	291	297	303	309	315	322	328	334
67	121	127	134	140	146	153	159	166	172	178	185	191	198	204	211	217	223	230	236	242	249	255	261	268	274	280	287	293	299	306	312	319	325	331	338	344
68	125	131	138	144	151	158	164	171	177	184	190	197	203	210	216	223	230	236	243	249	256	262	269	276	282	289	295	302	308	315	322	328	335	341	348	354
69	128	135	142	149	155	162	169	176	182	189	196	203	209	216	223	230	236	243	250	257	263	270	277	284	291	297	304	311	318	324	331	338	345	351	358	365
70	132	139	146	153	160	167	174	181	188	195	202	209	216	222	229	236	243	250	257	264	271	278	285	292	299	306	313	320	327	334	341	348	355	362	369	376
71	136	143	150	157	165	172	179	186	193	200	208	215	222	229	236	243	250	257	265	272	279	286	293	301	308	315	322	329	338	343	351	358	365	372	379	386
72	140	147	154	162	169	177	184	191	199	206	213	221	228	235	242	250	258	265	272	279	287	294	302	309	316	324	331	338	346	353	361	368	375	383	390	397
73	144	151	159	166	174	182	189	197	204	212	219	227	235	242	250	257	265	272	280	288	295	302	310	318	325	333	340	348	355	363	371	378	386	393	401	408
74	148	155	163	171	179	186	194	202	210	218	225	233	241	249	256	264	272	280	287	295	303	311	319	326	334	342	350	358	365	373	381	389	396	404	412	420
75	152	160	168	176	184	192	200	208	216	224	232	240	248	256	264	272	279	287	295	303	311	319	327	335	343	351	359	367	375	383	391	399	407	415	423	431
76	156	164	172	180	189	197	205	213	221	230	238	246	254	263	271	279	287	295	304	312	320	328	336	344	353	361	369	377	385	394	402	410	418	426	435	443

Data from National Heart Lung and Blood Institute/National Institute of Diabetes and Digestive and Kidney Diseases: *Clinical guidelines on the identification, evaluation, and treatment of overweight and obesity in adults: The evidence report*, Bethesda, Md, 1998, Authors.

Glossary

CHAPTER KEY TERMS

ABC acronym used in primary assessment (airway, breathing, circulation)
abduction movement away from the midline of the body
abrasion an injury that occurs when the skin is scraped against a rough surface
acclimatization process by which the body gradually adjusts from one environment to another
Achilles tendonitis chronic condition in which the Achilles tendon becomes irritated and inflamed from repetitive jumping, running, or friction (as from a shoe)
acoustic spectrum range of frequencies involving mechanical vibrations or sound waves that can travel only through certain mediums
active range of motion (AROM) movement possible when an individual actively moves a joint
active transportation process that occurs when a molecule attaches itself to another substance and is driven across the membrane
acute injuries injuries that have occurred in the preceding 24 to 48 hours
acute describes a rapid onset
adduction movement toward the midline of the body
agonists primary movers
allergic reaction reaction whereby the body develops an antibody against a compound to which it is exposed
amenorrhea an absence of the menstrual cycle; delayed menarche; also the absence of menstrual periods
amino acids the building blocks of protein; there are nine essential ones
anabolic steroids chemical derivatives of testosterone used to increase muscle mass, which helps improve strength and power
analgesic medication taken to relieve pain
anaphylactic shock severe reaction to a stimulus (allergen) such as a bee sting, medication, or food
anchors the first tape strips applied during taping
anecdotal research research that is based on experiences
angular motion movement that occurs when a body segment, the entire body, or an object moves about a fixed axis
anisocoria unequal pupil size, usually indicating neurological damage to the eye or brain
anorexia athletica a subclinical eating disorder syndrome characterized by disordered eating and compulsive exercising
antagonists muscles opposing the agonists
anterior in front of something else; toward the front
anterograde amnesia amnesia in which events after the injury are not remembered
anterolateral impingement syndrome soft tissue impingement of the anterolateral gutter resulting from synovial hypertrophy and fibrotic scar tissue
antibiotic a drug that kills or slows the growth of bacteria
antipyretic fever-reducing medication
antitussive a cough suppressant
aponeurosis a tough, broad, fibrous sheet of connective tissue serving as a means to connect bone and muscle to bone
apophyseal avulsion fracture fracture in which a forceful muscle contraction causes the tendon to pull off a fragment of the pelvis; associated with adolescent athletes
appendicular skeleton all the bones that form the upper and lower extremities (arms and legs); referring to an appendage or limb
approximate the injury bring the edges of an injured structure close together
arrhythmia abnormal heart rhythm occurring when the normal electrical patterns of the heart become disrupted
arthralgia joint pain
arthrokinematics movement of the joint surfaces, such as rolls, slides, and glides
assumption of risk informed decision based on knowledge and information regarding the dangers involved, as in a decision to participate in athletics
asthma a chronic disease in which the respiratory system becomes inflamed and constricts as a result of external triggers; also known as reactive airway disease
asymmetrical irregular or uneven
athlete-exposures the number of times every athlete on a team has the opportunity to either practice or compete

attending being aware of one's own nonverbal behavior as well as observing nonverbal behaviors and characteristics of the client

attenuated tissue elongation or stretching

automatic external defibrillator (AED) a device that uses a controlled and externally applied electrical current to restart a heart that has stopped beating or to regulate a suddenly irregular heartbeat

avascular necrosis bone death due to loss of blood flow to an area

avulsion a wound in which a portion of the tissue is torn away

axial loading a vertical compressive load placed on the top of the head that transmits through the cervical spine

axial skeleton all the bones that form the trunk and serve as an axis for the attachment of extremities

axilla anatomical term for armpit

bacteriostatic not conducive to growth of bacteria

Bankart lesion detachment of the capsule from the labrum or the labrum from the glenoid fossa

basal metabolic rate the amount of energy in calories needed on a daily basis when the body is at rest

Bennett's fracture dislocation occurring at the carpometacarpal (CMC) joint near the base of the thumb

bioenergetic analysis a physical analysis that looks at activity from an energy system utilization standpoint

biohazards bodily specimens or conditions that pose harm to humans

biomechanical analysis a physical analysis that determines how and why movements occur through linear and angular observations

Board of Certification (BOC) a certification program incorporated in 1989 for entry-level athletic trainers intended to provide standards for entry into the profession; also sets recertification standards for certified athletic trainers

board of directors organization within NATA made up of the 10 district directors; also included are NATA's president, vice president, and secretary/treasurer

body mass index measure in which body weight is divided by height

bony Bankart actual avulsion of the glenoid fossa bony surface

boutonnière deformity rupture of the extensor tendon on the dorsal side of the finger

boxer's fracture a fracture to the fifth metacarpal bone

bradycardia slow pulse rate (<60 bpm)

break test a test designed to break the athlete of a particular position

buddy-taped taping one body part with another (as in two fingers) to create stability

burner injury in which the cervical nerve is pinched

bursitis inflammatory condition of the bursa (in and around the shoulder)

calcaneal apophysitis inflammatory condition of the apophysis in which the heel bone (calcaneus) is subjected to traction forces; most common in athletes between the ages of 8 and 13 years.

calorie energy intake in the form of food substances

carbohydrates organic compounds that contain carbon (C), hydrogen (H), and oxygen (O) molecules to form ($C_6H_{12}O_6$)

cardiopulmonary resuscitation (CPR) procedure used to support and maintain breathing in an emergency

catastrophic injury career-ending type of injury that usually requires advanced medical care for the rest of the individual's life; not a life-threatening, but rather a life-altering, event

cauda equina distal end of the spinal cord along the spinal cord canal in the vertebral column; so named because it resembles a horse's tail

cervical myelopathy disorder that involves compressive forces on the spine, likely caused by multiple factors; the most serious condition of cervical spondylosis

chalazion lesion similar to a stye but occurring proximally farther on the eyelid

chemical name name given to a medication that specifically describes the compound that makes up the drug

chilblains cold-related irritation of the skin resulting from prolonged and constant exposure to cold air or moisture; usually affecting the fingers and toes

chronic injuries injuries that have persisted for longer than 2 or 3 weeks

chronic describes a long progression

circadian dysrhythmia condition commonly known as jet lag in which the body is placed under physiological stress after crossing multiple time zones

circumduction movement in a circular direction

clonus sudden, reflexive twitches

closure straps in taping, the final strips used to hold all the underlying tape layers in place

coagulation clotting, or changing blood from a liquid to a solid state

Colles' fracture a fracture to the distal aspect of the radius

commission doing something that is incorrect or inappropriate in a situation

commotio cordis disturbance of the heart rhythm caused by a blunt, nonpenetrating impact to the chest

community-associated methicillin-resistant *Staphylococcus aureus* (CA-MRSA) a community-acquired bacterial infection ("super bug"); difficult to treat because of its resistance to a strong cousin of penicillin

compartment syndrome condition characterized by increased pressure within the compartment; restricts blood supply to nearby muscles and involves increased pressure in any of the compartments

complex carbohydrates chains of two or more sugar molecules

concave a type of curve rounded inward like a bowl

concussion injury sustained from either a direct blow or an indirect force

conduction the transfer of heat through physical contact

condyle rounded prominence at the end of a bone that facilitates articulation with another bone

congenital describes a characteristic present at birth and not caused by an injury or traumatic event

conjunctivitis highly contagious bacterial infection of the posterior eyelid lining

constriction process by which something becomes smaller in diameter

contractile quality of contraction in tissue

contraindications modalities or exercises that should not be performed on the basis of a particular diagnosis

contralateral opposite

contrecoup injury a severe blow that creates a whiplashlike mechanism in the brain wherein the brain shifts and collides with the cranium; a rebound effect from the coup impact that affects the side of the head opposite to the side on which the impact was made
contusion a wound that causes bleeding in the tissue but does not break the skin
convection the transfer of heat from the body by the circulation of a medium (e.g., wind, water current)
core temperature the internal temperature of the body
corporate sponsors businesses that serve as funding sources for an organization by paying an agreed-upon fee to the organization for a certain amount of publicity
coup injury a direct blow that causes the brain to shift from its normal position in the skull and cerebrospinal fluid toward the point at which contact was made
coxa saltans snapping hip syndrome
cranium the skull
crepitus crackling sensation ("crunchies") noted with movement of an area indicating damage (e.g., dislocation, fracture) to the underlying tissue
cryotherapy family of modalities that primarily induces vasodilation; examples include cold packs, ice massage, ice immersion, cold sprays, mechanical cooling systems, and cold whirlpools
culture of risk unquestioned tolerance of pain and injury for those who accept the potentially negative (risky) consequences of sports participation
cystitis bladder infections
de Quervain's syndrome stress injury occurring when the sheath or tunnel surrounding the thumb tendons becomes irritated or inflamed
decongestants drugs used to relieve symptoms associated with blocked or restricted nasal passages
deep vein thrombosis blood clot in a major vein, often in the leg; life-threatening condition
dehydration a state in which the body is low on water
dental avulsion traumatic dislodging of a tooth from its socket
dermatomes structures that identify skin sensations from the nerve root
dermis the middle layer of the skin
diabetes mellitus a disorder of the body's ability to properly metabolize carbohydrates
diagnosis the end result of the evaluation specifically identifying the exact cause of the injury or illness
diastasis a disunion between two adjoining bones or a complete disarticulation of a nonmobile joint
diastolic blood pressure the force exerted by the volume of blood on the artery walls when the heart is not actively contracting
Dietary Reference Intake framework of nutrient standards that has replaced the old RDAs (Recommended Daily Allowances)
differential diagnosis a list of diagnoses considered after an evaluation
dilation process by which something becomes larger in diameter
diplopia medical term for double vision
disordered eating pattern of eating behavior that can negatively affect an athlete's performance and potentially lead to an eating disorder
displaced a fracture that separates into two pieces
distal farther away from the body's midline or center relative to another landmark
dorsiflexion upward movement by the distal segment; used to describe motion in the toes or ankle
dynamometer device for measuring muscle strength
eating disorder pattern of eating behavior that is no longer under personal control and causes significant adverse changes in psychological, social, or physical functioning
ecchymosis bruising or discoloration resulting from direct trauma
Education Council organization that represents NATA in all educational matters; facilitates continuous quality improvement in entry-level, graduate, and continuing athletic training education; and coordinates the delivery of educational programming for the profession of athletic training
elastic wrap stretchy substance used as an alternative to adhesive tape to provide support without constricting the muscle
electrical stimulating currents (ESTIM) group of modalities that have a physiological effect at any point between positioned electrodes; examples include high-voltage pulsed stimulation (HVPS), transcutaneous electrical nerve stimulation (TENS), interferential stimulation (IF), neuromuscular electrical stimulation (NMES), iontophoresis, and microcurrent electrical stimulation (MENS)
electrolytes minerals in the blood that are important for the regulation of the amount of water in the body, blood pH, muscle action, and other important functions
electromagnetic spectrum range of radiation frequencies that primarily involves radiant energy produced by moving electrons that can travel through either space or a vacuum
electromyography in patient care, a test used to determine whether a person's muscle weakness is caused by a disease within the muscle or by a problem in the nerve supplying the muscle
emergency action plan (EAP) a written emergency plan identifying key personnel, equipment, and communications involved in order to safely address all possible emergencies
empirical research research that is based on documented observations and experimental designs
energy balance caloric balance; when energy intake from food and fluids equals energy expenditure
energy expenditure the sum of all energy expended as basal metabolism, the thermic effect of food, and any voluntary physical activity
epicondyle rounded projection at the end of a bone and the center of a condyle that serves as an attachment point for tendons and ligaments
epicondylitis inflammation of the epicondyles of the humerus
epidermis the outer protective layer of the skin
epidural hematoma usually an arterial bleed into the epidural space of the brain
EpiPen preloaded syringe used to administer an emergency dose of epinephrine
epistaxis medical term for a nosebleed
ergogenic aid a product that is work-enhancing; potentially improves performance
erythematous reddish
evaluation a systematic process that enables the athletic trainer to determine what is wrong with the injured person

evaporation the dissipation of heat from the body through conversion of water to vapor
eversion a turning out (turning laterally)
executive director individual in charge of leading the day-to-day operations of the NATA organization
extensible describes a tissue that elongates in response to repeated tension
extension straightening of a joint; increase in its angle
external (lateral) rotation movement in which the anterior surface of the distal segment moves away from the midline of the body
extravasation the movement of fluid from a physiological space (e.g., a blood vessel or intracapsular joint space) into surrounding tissues
extrinsic muscles muscles that originate in the leg and proceed down to attach on some aspect of the foot
facet joints articulations between the two levels of the respective vertebrae
Family Education Rights and Privacy Act a provision that protects athletes' medical records; also known as the Buckley Amendment
fats lipids
febrile possession of a fever
fiber an indigestible complex carbohydrate
fibroplasia formation of granulation, or fibrous tissue, in healing
fibrous joint a type of joint allowing little or no motion
figures of eight strips of tape applied around the foot, then around the ankle, to resemble the number 8
flexibility movement through an available range allowed at a joint by the tissues external to that joint (muscles, tendons, fascia)
flexion bending of a joint; decrease in the angle
fluorescein material that glows under certain types of lights
folliculitis an infection of the base of a hair follicle
Food and Drug Administration (FDA) government agency that regulates pharmaceuticals
FOOSH acronym for falling on an outstretched hand
foramen magnum large opening at the bottom of the skull where the spinal cord exits
foramina anatomical holes or openings in a bone; usually used as passageways for nerves or blood vessels
fossa a shallow, broad, round depression on a bone that serves as a base of articulation for the head or rounded surface of another bone in the same joint
fracture an injury to a bone; a traumatic break
frostbite potentially severe cold-related injury resulting from ice crystals that form in and around the cells of tissue exposed to cold air and humidity for prolonged periods
frostnip cold-related injury describing a mild form of frostbite to the ears, nose, cheeks, chin, fingers, or toes
functional bracing bracing designed to provide stability for an unstable joint
furuncle a progression of the follicle infection into an abscess
gait pattern technique of walking
gamekeeper's thumb injury to the ulnar collateral ligament of the metacarpophalangeal joint of the thumb; also called skier's thumb
ganglion cyst soft tissue tumor commonly located on the dorsal side of the wrist
generic name short name given to drug so that a chemist can quickly designate the molecule being discussed
goal ladder using small attainable steps to reach the goal
goniometer an apparatus to measure joint movements and angles
grade I ankle sprain stretching or disruption in the integrity of the ligament
grade II ankle sprain partial tearing of the ligament
grade III ankle sprain complete tearing of the ligament
gunstock deformity an elbow with a varus angle instead of a valgus angle
hallux valgus deformity of the first metatarsophalangeal joint involving lateral angulation of the great toe
hangman's fracture bilateral traumatic spondylolisthesis of the pars interarticularis; fracture at the axis (C2 vertebra)
Hank's solution a special commercially available pH-balanced liquid made for storage of avulsed teeth; prevents cell death of the periodontal ligament tissue during transport for dental treatment
Health Insurance Portability and Accountability Act (HIPAA) federal legislation designed to ensure the confidentiality of electronically transmitted records and of oral and written communication contained in medical records
heat cramps heat-related painful muscle contractions that often involve the calf or abdomen
heat exhaustion heat-related condition characterized by excessive sweating and dehydration
heat index scale used to predict the level of heat stress placed on the body during activity in a given temperature and humidity
heat stroke heat-related medical emergency resulting from the body's inability to efficiently remove excess heat
heat syncope heat-related fainting; also known as heat collapse
heel locks strips of tape applied in both directions during ankle taping to support ligaments of the ankle and "lock" the ankle into a neutral position
hemarthrosis condition in which blood is within the joint
hematoma a contusion that is very swollen and discolored
hematoma auris "cauliflower ear"; localized inflammation of the external ear resulting from repeated blunt force trauma
hemi prefix that indicates half of something
hemothorax condition occurring when blood enters the pleural cavity and prevents inflation of the lung
herniated bulging usually due to excessive pressure or force on one side
Hill-Sachs lesion osteochondral compression fracture on the posterior surface of the humeral head; associated with a dislocation of the glenohumeral joint
hip pointer a bruise to the soft tissue overlying the iliac crest
Hoffman's sign reflex test finding that indicates the presence or absence of corticospinal problems
HOPS/HIPS acronym used to guide secondary assessment (history, observation/inspection, palpation, stress)
humidity amount of water vapor in the air
hyaline cartilage smooth, shiny cartilage that allows one bone to glide smoothly over another
hydration the amount of water that the body contains at any given moment
hyperglycemia abnormally high circulating blood sugar (glucose)

hypermotility excessive motion in a joint that can result in injury and instability
hyperthermia abnormal increase in core body temperature
hypertrophy increase in size
hyphema a pooling of blood in the anterior chamber of the eye secondary to blunt force trauma
hypodermis the subcutaneous layer that lies under the dermis
hypoglycemia abnormally low circulating blood sugar (glucose)
hypothermia abnormally low core body temperature
hypovolemic shock a state of shock that follows large amounts of blood loss
idiosyncratic quality whereby some patients react differently to medications than others
ilia plural of *ilium*
iliotibial band (ITB) syndrome chronic syndrome responsible for lateral knee pain in triathletes, cyclists, and distance runners characterized by weak hip abductors and knee flexors and extensors and a tight ITB/tensor fascia latae (TFL) complex
imagery the ability to use all the senses to create or recreate an experience in the mind
impetigo an oozing lesion sometimes accompanied by large blisters that may be caused by the bacteria *Staphylococcus* or *Streptococcus*
inert noncontractile tissues
inferior under or beneath
influenza a viral infection typically referred to as flu; much more serious than the common cold
inguinal hernias weakening of the abdominal wall
injury management a comprehensive approach to providing care to an individual that includes immediate care and treatment of the current injury while providing pertinent education to prevent further or future injuries from occurring
in-line stabilization method used to ensure that no movement occurs at the head, cervical spine, and shoulder in an athlete with suspected head and cervical injury
instability excessive movement
integument the skin of the human body
internal (medial) rotation movement in which the anterior surface of the distal segment moves toward the midline of the body
interosseous membrane thin fibrous tissue separating bones at the joint
interstitial space space between elements
intertrigo inflammation caused by folds of skin rubbing together
intrathecal term used in reference to the interior of the trunk, usually indicating the cavity that contains the internal organs and the thoracic and lumbar spinal regions
intrinsic muscles muscles that start and end (originate and insert) within the foot, without extending to the ankle or lower leg
inversion a turning in (turning medially)
iontophoresis modality that combines a low-dose electrical current with an ionized medication to introduce treatment
ipsilateral same side
isokinetic exercise resistance training that involves a device with a fixed speed and allows for varying resistances through a predetermined range of motion
isometric exercise resistance training that does not involve moving the involved body part
isotonic exercise resistance training performed with either concentric or eccentric contractions, causing movement of the limb
jaundice yellowing
Jefferson fracture fracture to the ring of the C1 vertebra; typically involves minimal neurological deficit
jersey finger injury to the flexor digitorum profundus tendon that sometimes occurs when an athlete uses a flexed finger to grab the jersey of another athlete
keloids raised formations of fibrous scar tissue; caused by excessive scarring
keratinocytes cells that produce a protein called keratin that provides the waterproofing capacities of the body
keratosis the formation of calluses
kinesthesia the ability to perceive joint motion or movement
kyphosis spinal abnormality characterized by an exaggerated forward head appearance and an excessively forward-flexed thoracic spine
laceration trauma in a smaller or more restricted area that results in jagged edges around the wound
Langerhans cells cells that ingest foreign, or antigenic, particles to prevent allergic reactions
lateral away from the midline or center of the body (outer aspect) relative to another landmark
lateral ankle sprain injury to the lateral ankle region induced through inversion forces
laxity asymptomatic movement within a joint
Legg-Calve-Perthes disease a loss of blood supply to the femoral epiphysis causing loss of bone mass and avascular necrosis
lesion an injury to the skin
liability legal responsibility for the harm caused to another person
linear motion movement that occurs when all points within a body or object move at the same time and over the same distance
loading dose dose that helps achieve a higher concentration of medication in the bloodstream
longitudinal occurring along the midline of a bone
long-term goals goals that are designed to be met at any point from 4 weeks to several months and even years
lordosis spinal abnormality characterized by an exaggerated lumbar curve, or arched back
lordotic position position in which the spine is naturally aligned and the vertebrae form a curve anteriorly, or toward the front of the body; term "sway-back" usually describing an excessive spinal curve in this direction
macronutrients the nutrients that collectively provide most of the body's energy: carbohydrates, proteins, and fats
macrophages phagocytes involved in later phases of inflammation; cells that release chemical mediators in response to hypoxia
macrotrauma a larger lesion caused by a single large force
malaise nonspecific feeling of discomfort or being ill
malleolus the distal end or knob of the tibia or fibula recognized as the ankle
mallet finger injury in which the extensor tendon of the finger is avulsed at the tendinous attachment
margination initial response of platelets in early phase of inflammation

mechanism of injury (MOI) the "why" and "how" of an injury
medial toward the midline or center of the body (inner aspect) relative to another landmark
medial ankle sprain injury to the medial ankle region induced through eversion forces
melanocytes cells that release a pigment that provides the myriad of skin tones
menisci cartilaginous structures that lie between the femur and the tibia and fibula; provide shock absorption and stability to the knee
metabolism normal working processes of the body systems
metatarsalgia tenderness and burning within the metatarsal region
metered-dose inhaler device used to deliver medication to the respiratory system during an asthmatic attack
micronutrients substances necessary to the body in small amounts: vitamins and minerals
microtrauma very small lesion caused by small amounts of force over time
monocytes phagocytes involved in later phases of inflammation; cells that aid in coagulation and phagocytosis
monounsaturated fatty acid a fatty acid with one double bond available
muscular endurance the ability to perform repeated muscular contractions over a period of time
muscular power the ability to produce a large amount of force in a relatively short period of time
muscular strength the ability to generate force against a resistance
myalgia muscle pain
myocardial infarction a heart attack resulting from a lack of blood supply to a portion of the heart
myositis ossificans inflammation of muscle tissue marked by ossification of the intramuscular fascia; repeated trauma to the same injured area that causes an advanced form of hematoma with calcification
myotome specific muscle controlled by a given nerve; muscle weakness possibly indicating injury to the nerve controlling that particular muscle; areas that identify the motor function of the muscle from a nerve root
narcotic analgesics drugs that depress pain impulses and prevent their transmission to the spinal cord; primarily derived from opium or opioid derivatives
National Athletic Trainers' Association (NATA) based in Dallas, Texas, the membership association for certified athletic trainers and others who support the athletic training profession
negligence failure to provide the standard of care that would otherwise have been deemed appropriate for that particular circumstance
Neoprene sleeve device similar to elastic wrap used to compress a body part but made out of a material that helps the body retain heat
nephrolithiasis formation of kidney stones
neurapraxia cessation of nerve function through a complete tearing of the neurological tissue
neuroma small area of inflammation that forms around a nerve
neuromuscular control the motor response to kinesthetic (sensory) input
neutrophils white blood cells that destroy bacteria during inflammation; "smart bombs" of inflammation
nonunion failure of two pieces of bone to heal together
NSAIDs acronym for nonsteroidal antiinflammatory drugs
nystagmus "dancing eyes"; a symptom of eye injury in which the globe moves erratically, appearing to bounce or shake when following an object moving across the field of vision; abnormal eye movements, possibly jerking or jumping
olecranon bursitis inflammation of the bursa that sits behind the elbow (olecranon bursa)
oligomenorrhea irregular or very light menstrual cycles
omission lack of action by an athletic trainer to take appropriate and necessary steps to render care
onychia an infection that occurs at the nail bed
ophthalmoscope instrument used to view the interior of the eye
OPIM abbreviation defined by the Occupational Safety and Health Administration (OSHA) as all human body fluids and unfixed tissues, excluding intact skin (other potentially infectious materials)
orthotic a device that fits in a shoe and is designed to correct problems with the foot
Osgood-Schlatter disease a common cause of knee pain in young athletes that causes swelling, pain, and tenderness just below the knee, over the shin bone; occurs mostly in boys who are having a growth spurt during their preteen or teenage years
osmophobia intense discomfort, even to the point of nausea, during exposure to intense smells
osteitis pubis inflammation of the pubic symphysis and surrounding muscle insertions
osteoblast cell responsible for bone formation
osteochondritis a piece of articular cartilage and underlying bone that has been dislodged from its origin
osteoclast bone cell that removes bone tissue
osteokinematics classic movements of bones, such as flexion and extension
osteoporosis disease in which the bones become abnormally thin, porous, and subject to fracture
otitis externa infection of the lining of the auditory canal distal to the tympanic membrane (eardrum); commonly known as "swimmer's ear"
otitis media infection in the middle ear, between the eardrum and inner ear; usually a complication of an upper respiratory infection in which the eustachian tube is blocked
otoscope instrument used to view the interior of the ear
Ottawa ankle rules a clinical model designed to assist with the diagnosis and management of suspected ankle fractures
Ottawa knee rule specifies that if the individual exhibits any of the following five conditions, a radiograph should be obtained; age 55 years or older; tenderness at the head of the fibula; isolated tenderness of the patella; inability to flex the knee to 90 degrees; and an inability to bear weight for four steps immediately and in the examination room regardless of limping
palpated felt or noticed through touch
paronychia an infection that happens in the nail fold, mostly the side nail fold
passive diffusion process whereby one solution moves from a higher-concentration environment to a lower-concentration environment
passive range of motion (PROM) movement possible when another person moves an individual's joint

patellar tendinopathy overuse injury commonly called "jumper's knee" in which the patellar tendon becomes inflamed and may tear or degenerate; common cause of pain in the inferior knee region

pathology the study of the nature, causes, and development of abnormal conditions involving changes in structure and function

pathomechanics the unique combination of external forces and joint displacements that produce an injury

periodization a method to facilitate progress toward conditioning and rehabilitation goals that involves manipulating exercise variables to achieve certain performance goals at certain times

peristalsis the undulating contraction and relaxation of the smooth muscles in the gastrointestinal tract that aid in digestion and transportation of food through the system

personal protective equipment (PPE) articles such as gloves, masks, and eyewear designed to protect health care personnel from disease or infection

phagocytosis the process of ingestion and digestion of solid substances by other cells

pharmacodynamics the study of the biochemical and physiological effects of drugs

pharmacokinetics the study of what the body does to a drug and how these drug compounds are transported through the body

phonophobia literally "fear of sound"; refers to intense ear discomfort during exposure to loud noise

photophobia literally "fear of light"; refers to intense eye discomfort during exposure to bright light

piriformis syndrome irritation or compression of the piriformis muscle or the sciatic nerve

Pittsburgh knee rule recommends obtaining a radiograph for patients with a recent fall or blunt trauma, those who are younger than 12 years of age or older than 50 years, and those who are unable to take at least four weight-bearing steps in the emergency department

plantar fasciitis painful condition caused by excessive wear and strain on the plantar fascia of the foot

plantar flexion downward motion by the distal segment; used to describe motion in the toes or the ankle

plyometrics reactive training that stimulates changes in the neuromuscular system, enhancing the ability of the muscle groups to respond more quickly and powerfully to slight and rapid changes in muscle length

pneumothorax an emergency condition occurring when air leaks into the pleural cavity located between the lining of the chest wall and the covering of the lungs

pocket mask hand-held device containing a one-way valve that is used to perform rescue breaths

policies written rules used to guide the decision-making process or a course of action

political action committee (PAC) a committee formed by business, labor, or other special-interest groups to raise money and make contributions to the campaigns of political candidates whom they support

polyunsaturated fatty acid a fatty acid with two or more double bonds

popliteal area behind the knee, generally between the hamstring tendon insertions, where knee flexion occurs

popliteal angle widely used means of assessing hamstring length

positive deviance overconformity to the goals and norms of sport

posterior behind something else; toward the back

post-traumatic amnesia amnesia suffered after any concussive injury in which the ability to remember is altered

postural neutral position the functional position; a neutral posture

posture the means of supporting one's own body weight while sitting, standing, or walking

preparticipation physical examination (PPE) document used to determine an individual's capacity to undertake the intended physical activity involved in athletics

pressure point a location where the artery is close to the skin surface or overlies a bone (e.g., brachial artery on medial upper arm, femoral artery on anterior hip)

prewrap protective covering for the skin used to prevent skin burns, rashes, or cuts from taping

PRICES acronym for the appropriate treatment path (participation, rest, ice, compression, elevation, and stabilization)

principle of overload fundamental law describing a stimulus that continuously overloads the muscles and soft tissues, causing them to become stronger

procedures documented steps taken to adhere to a policy

Professional Education Committee organization responsible for issues pertaining to precertification education; also a resource for existing and developing accredited programs at the undergraduate and graduate level

progressive muscle relaxation the systematic tension and relaxation of muscle groups in an attempt to reduce anxiety associated with being injured

pronation combination of movements resulting in the rolling-in movement of the foot as it lands on the ground

prophylactic bracing type of bracing intended to prevent or reduce the severity of injuries

proprioception awareness of a joint relative to the rest of the body and the environment surrounding it

proprioceptive describes information sent to the brain concerning body position and muscle tension; used to maintain balance and coordination

proteins amino acids that assist with enzymes, antibodies, and the transportation of key substances such as oxygen, vitamins, and minerals to the cells

proximal closer to the midline or center of the body relative to another landmark

puncture a serious wound resulting in a small hole caused by a sharp object

putrescible subject to decomposition by microorganisms that produce a foul odor

radiation the transfer of heat from a source to an object without direct contact or assistance from a current

range of motion the specific movement provided at a joint by the joint structures (ligaments, joint capsules, cartilage, bones)

reflex a predictable, involuntary, neurological response to a stimulus

regulation a process that provides laws to define expected professional behaviors as well as methods to address unacceptable behaviors

rehabilitation adherence committing to and following through with a rehabilitation program

rehabilitation bracing a type of bracing that allows protected controlled motion during exercises and rehabilitation

release of medical information form paper restricting the type of medical information that is provided to the public outside of the athlete and family

retinaculum tight, tough connective tissue that keeps the patella from sliding laterally or medially

retrograde amnesia amnesia in which events preceding the injury are not remembered

roid rage sudden outbursts of aggressive and violent behavior that is often uncontrollable and is caused by steroid misuse

Role Delineation Study (RDS) a job analysis performed by the Board of Certification every 5 years to formulate the blueprint for the certification examination

sacralization an abnormality in which the last lumbar vertebra, L5, is fused with the sacrum

SAID principle fundamental law stating that any human structure will adapt accordingly over time to stressors and overloads; acronym stands for "specific adaptations to imposed demands"

scaphoid navicular fracture break in the carpal bone on the thumb side of the wrist

scoliosis an abnormal lateral curvature of the spine

self-injurious behavior a voluntary, deliberate, repetitive, impulsive, nonlethal harming of one's body

self-talk a form of intrapersonal communication

shell temperature the temperature of the body's skin

short-term goals goals that are designed to be met within four to eight visits or within 2 to 4 weeks

shortwave diathermy modality that introduces a high-frequency current into the tissues to produce deep heating

simple carbohydrates substances composed of simple sugars, which are glucose, fructose and galactose; commonly considered empty calories

Sinding-Larsen-Johansson syndrome inflammation of the knee cap

sinus tarsi syndrome clinical syndrome of the opening on the outside of the foot between the ankle and heel; causes pain and restricts movement

sinuses air cavities found in the bones of the head

skin sulcus a dimpling of the skin indicating a gap in the integrity of the soft tissue being tested

sling psychrometer device used to measure air temperature and humidity

slipped capital femoral epiphysis condition in which the head of the femur slides out of its socket; associated mainly with adolescent boys

Smith's fracture (reverse Colles') a fracture to the distal aspect of the radius that displaces to the palmar aspect

Snellen chart vision assessment tool containing a series of characters arranged in rows

SOAP note acronym for documentation in an evaluation (subjective, objective, assessment, plan)

spearing a football tackle in which the tackler uses the helmet (including face mask) to butt or ram an opponent

specificity-based program a conditioning and rehabilitation program that replicates the activity in which the individual participates

spica a wrapping technique involving a figure applied around two body parts

spina bifida occulta congenital defect in which the laminae at L5 or S1 fail to develop, resulting in an exposed posterior spinal cord

spinal stenosis condition in which one or more areas in the spine narrow, putting pressure on the spinal cord or the roots of the branching nerves; can be congenital or result from trauma

splint rigid or formable device used to immobilize a body part when a fracture or dislocation is suspected

spondylolisthesis condition occurring in bilateral spondylolysis in which the cracked vertebrae slip forward onto the vertebrae below; commonly known as "Scotty dog has lost his head"

spondylolysis crack in the pars interarticularis of the lumbar vertebrae; commonly known as "Scotty dog with a collar"; can be congenital or result from trunk extensions performed in the course of athletics

sports hernias weakening of the muscles or tendons of the lower abdominal wall

stenosis a narrowing of a passageway, often the vertebral or intervertebral foramina in the cervical and lumbar areas

stinger upper trunk injury to the brachial plexus

stress-strain curve concept illustrating how connective tissue adapts to physical stress

stye also known as a *hordeolum;* staphylococcus infection of the eyelid at the eyelash line that occurs from blockage of the area's oil glands

subdural hematoma injury that occurs when a cerebral blood vessel tears

subtalar sling ankle taping procedure that helps restrict ankle movement

superficial closer to the skin's surface of the body; farther away from the layer of tissue near the bone and closer to the skin

superior above or on top

supination movement of the foot and ankle that allows the food and ankle to become a rigid lever to enhance the pushing-off motion of the foot from the ground

surgical fasciotomy surgery to cut away the fascia to remove tension or pressure

symmetrical equal in size and shape

symptomatically term used to describe a method in which symptoms are treated rather than the cause of an injury; designed to restore function

syncope fainting

syndesmotic ankle sprain injury to the high, lateral ankle region induced through direct contact and external rotation of the foot

synovial joint a type of joint allowing some degree of free movement

systolic blood pressure the pressure of blood into the arteries resulting from ventricular contractions

tachycardia rapid pulse rate (>100bpm)

tarsal tunnel syndrome condition in which the posterior tibial nerve is compressed within the tarsal canal, causing pain and burning

tensile strength the force required to pull something to the point at which it breaks or tears

The First Aider a classic athletic training publication written and published by the Cramer brothers after they traveled with the U.S. Olympics Team in 1932 and had the opportunity to learn different techniques to care for injured athletes; still in print today

therapeutic exercises exercises that are used in a preventive or prescriptive manner to either prevent injury or to rehabilitate an injury
therapeutic modality any type of device, mechanical or manual, that aids in the healing process of an injury or illness
therapeutic rehabilitation program plan of care combining modalities with conditioning and rehabilitative exercises
thermoregulatory describes an involuntary system of the body that controls heating and cooling
thermotherapy family of modalities that primarily induces vasodilation; examples include hydrocollator packs, paraffin baths, warm whirlpools, infrared lamps, and fluidotherapy
thoracic outlet syndrome (TOS) collection of signs and symptoms that are attributed to compression of the neurovascular bundle at the thoracic inlet
thought stoppage technique used with clients who have negative, self-defeating thoughts about their recovery; helps clients become more aware of what they are thinking
tinea corporis more commonly known as ringworm; spread by direct contact with infected skin; often results in variation in skin color
tinea cruris an infection of the groin frequently referred to as "jock itch"; commonly characterized by red patches that itch, blister, and ooze
tinea pedis athlete's foot; infection characterized by patterned scaling and macerated skin between the toes
tinea unguium an infection of the nails characterized by discoloration and sometimes by scaling and nail destruction
tinnitus ringing in the ears
torsional brain injury injury that results from a severe blow to the head that causes the head to rotate on impact
tort an intentional or unintentional civil wrong
torticollis nontraumatic muscle strain caused by incorrect positioning or cold draft; commonly called *wryneck*
trade name designation given to a drug that helps the pharmaceutical company market the medication; also known as *brand name* and *proprietary name*
trauma bag kit containing all the emergency equipment
triage process by which care is prioritized according to the severity of injury or illness in those seeking treatment
trigger finger stress injury caused by repetitive gripping action with flexed fingers
trochanteric bursitis inflammatory condition that manifests as an aching pain over the lateral aspect of the hip
tuberosity a normal outgrowth or bump on a bone
turf toe sprain of the first metatarsophalangeal joint; common in football athletes playing on artificial turf
United States Pharmacopeia the official public standards–setting authority for all over-the-counter medications, dietary supplements, and other health care products manufactured in the United States
valgus movement movement in which the distal segment is forced inward, toward the midline of the body
varus movement movement in which the distal segment is forced outwardly, away from the midline of the body
vascular limbus system fine network of small blood vessels in the outer layers of the eye
vasoactive causing constriction or dilation of blood vessels
vasodilation opening or widening of a blood vessel
verrucae warts caused by the human papillomavirus (HPV)
vicarious liability perceived wrongdoing of an individual who is acting on behalf of an institution
Volkmann's ischemic contracture a complication resulting from a displaced fracture that puts pressure on the brachial artery and inhibits circulation; an emergency situation
wet bulb globe temperature (WBGT) describes a device used to assess relative heat stress
wind chill scale used to predict the level of cold stress placed on the body during activity in a given temperature and wind speed

ANATOMICAL TERMINOLOGY

abductor pollicis longus muscle located along the thumb-side of the forearm that serves to flex and radially deviate the wrist as well as abduct and flex the thumb
Achilles tendon union of the muscles in the calf region of the leg that form a common tendon at the back of the heel serving to plantar flex the foot primarily
acromioclavicular joint union of the acromion process of the scapula (shoulder blade) and the distal clavicle (collar bone); commonly called the *AC joint*
acromioclavicular ligament connective tissue joining the acromion of the scapula to the clavicle
adductor muscles muscles of the hip that serve to move the leg toward the midline of the body
ala large, projecting winglike part of a bone
anconeus muscle that extends from the lateral epicondyle of the humerus to the lateral aspect of the olecranon process of the ulna and serves primarily to stabilize the elbow during extension and also to pronate the forearm
annular ligament ligament that encircles the head of the radius in the forearm, forming a tight sling that allows the radius to rotate inside as the forearm pronates and supinates
annulus fibrosus outer dense covering of the intervertebral disk
anterior longitudinal ligament dense band of ligamentous tissue extending along the front (anterior) surface of the vertebra
anterior shoulder girdle muscles controlling the motion and stability of the shoulder girdle (clavicle and scapula) that attach at the front, or anterior portion, of this area, including the pectoralis major, pectoralis minor, and subclavius muscles
aponeurosis a tough, broad, fibrous sheet of connective tissue serving as a means to connect bone and muscle to bone
arachnoid covering middle layer of the three levels of membranes covering the brain and spinal cord, so called because of its weblike appearance
articular disk a cartilaginous bundle of tissue that serves to separate two bones that move against each other as in the temporomandibular joint (TMJ)
auditory ossicles very small bones of the ear that transfer sound wave energy from the middle ear to the inner ear, specifically the malleus (hammer), incus (anvil), and stapes (stirrup)
auricle outer part of the ear, seen on the outside of the head serving as the entry point of sound waves into the auditory canal
biceps muscle group in the front of the upper arm that serves primarily to flex the elbow; so called because it has two origins, or heads, and one common insertion; also called biceps brachii

bicuspids one of the two teeth with two points, situated between the canines and the molars
brachialis muscle that extends from the lower (distal) humerus to the coronoid process of the ulna and serves to flex the elbow
brachial plexus network of related nerves, or a plexus, that control sensation and motion in the arm, including the nerve roots C5-T1 and extending from the neck and across the shoulder down the arm to the fingers
brachioradialis muscle extending from the distal humerus to the distal radius serving to flex the elbow and assist with supination and pronation of the forearm
brainstem the part of the brain that connects the medulla oblongata to the spinal cord
buccinator muscles broad muscles that form the wall of the cheek
calcaneus heel bone
capitate one of the carpal bones, found in the distal row and palpated at the base of the third metacarpal
capitulum point on the humerus that articulates with the radius
carpal tunnel wide circular anatomical formation made by the bones of the hand near the wrist as well as the transverse ligament connecting the top of the two sides and enclosing an array of nerves and blood vessels that extend from the forearm into the hand
carpals bone of the hand between the wrist and the fingers
carrying angle normal alignment of the arm at the elbow wherein the arm is slightly abducted when the elbow is fully extended
cauda equina the distal end of the spinal cord that has the appearance of a horse's tail
cerebellum small section of neurological tissue at the posterior base of the brain
cerumen ear wax that serves to protect the delicate tissue of the auditory canal
ceruminous glands glands that produce protective ear wax in the auditory canal
cilia very fine hairlike structures that serve to filter an area or that may actually be very small nerve endings that pass along information about the local surroundings to the brain via the sense organs
clavicle collar bone
clear lens transparent, nearly spherelike body in the eye that helps focus the light entering the eye onto the retina
coccyx collection of fused spinal vertebrae at the base of the spine, also known as the *tailbone*
cochlea coiled organ in the inner ear that processes mechanical energy from sound waves and converts them to neurological impulses that are sent to the brain for processing
conjunctiva clear lining of the eyelids that also covers the sclera, or front white part of the eye
conus medullaris the tapering area of the spinal cord at the lumbar level of the spine
coracoacromial ligaments connective tissue bands that extend from the coracoid process of the scapula to the acromion of the clavicle
coracobrachialis muscle that extends from the coracoid process of the scapula to the midshaft of the humerus and serves to flex and adduct the shoulder
coracoid process tuberosity of the scapula that serves as an attachment site for muscles and ligaments
corrugator muscle in the face that assists with wrinkling the skin of the forehead and drawing the eyebrows closer together
costal cartilage any of the elastic cartilage bands that connect the ends of the ribs to the sternum
costotransverse joints area where the ribs join the transverse process of the vertebrae
costovertebral related to the point where the ribs join the vertebral body
cranium the part of the skull that encases the brain
cribriform plate heavily perforated section of the ethmoid bone through which parts of the olfactory (smell) nerves pass on their way to the brain from the nose
cruciate ligaments crossing ligaments in the knee that connect the tibia to the femur
cuboid outermost of the distal row of tarsal bones in the foot that, along with the cuneiforms, forms the transverse arch of the foot
cuneiforms group of three bones that, along with the cuboid, form the transverse arch of the foot
cuspids the relatively long pointed teeth, also known as *canines*
deltoid muscle at the outer aspect of the shoulder that serves primarily to abduct the arm
dentin a dense material similar to bone that composes the bulk of a tooth
diaphragm partition of muscle separating the chest cavity from the abdominal cavity
diencephalon a subdivision of the forebrain
distal radioulnar joint articulation of the radius and ulna at the wrist
dura mater highly vascular outermost layer of protective membranes that cover the brain and spinal cord
erector spinae muscles group of muscles that primarily extend parallel to the lumbar spine
ethmoid bone of the skull that forms part of the wall of the nose and orbits
eustachian tube pathway connecting the middle ear to the throat that serves to equalize air pressure on both sides of the eardrum (tympanic membrane)
extensor carpi radialis brevis muscle extending from the lateral epicondyle of the humerus to the base of the third metacarpal that serves to extend and radially deviate the wrist
extensor carpi radialis longus muscle extending from the lateral epicondyle of the humerus to the base of the second metacarpal that serves to extend and radially deviate the wrist
extensor carpi ulnaris muscle with two heads that extends from the lateral epicondyle of the humerus and posterior ulna to the base of the fifth metacarpal that serves to extend and ulnarly deviate the wrist
extensor digiti minimi muscle extending from the lateral epicondyle of the humerus to the extensor tendons of the proximal phalanges that assists with extension of the fingers
extensor digitorum muscle that extends from the lateral condyle of the humerus to the dorsum of the hand and serves primarily to extend the fingers
extensor digitorum longus muscle in the lower leg that extends from the lateral proximal tibia to the phalanges that serves to extend the toes and assists with dorsiflexion and eversion of the ankle

extensor hallucis longus muscle that extends from the proximal tibia to the distal hallux (big toe) that serves to extend the hallux and assists with dorsiflexion of the ankle

extensor indicis muscle in the forearm that extends from the distal ulna to the base of the index finger and serves to extend the index finger

extensor pollicis brevis shorter branch of a divided muscle in the forearm that extends from the distal radius and ulna to the base of the thumb and serves to extend and abduct the thumb

extensor pollicis longus longer branch of a divided muscle in the forearm that extends from the distal ulna to the base of the thumb and serves to extend and abduct the thumb

external oblique muscles abdominal muscle group forming the lateral walls of the abdominal cavity

external rotators muscles of the rotator cuff in the shoulder that turn the humerus outward or laterally

facet joints points of articulation of one spinal vertebra with the one below (inferior) to it

false ribs the five most inferior or lower ribs that do not connect directly to the sternum but may or may not connect to a shared expanse of cartilage

femur thigh bone, extending from the hip joint to the knee joint

fibula bone along the outer (lateral) aspect of the lower leg extending from the knee joint to the ankle joint parallel to the tibia

fibularis brevis muscle extending from the lower lateral fibula to the lateral base of the fifth metatarsal that is primarily responsible for eversion of the foot

fibularis longus muscle extending from the upper lateral surface of the fibula and tibia to the underside of the lateral medial cuneiform and first metatarsal that is primarily responsible for eversion and plantar flexion of the foot

flexor carpi radialis muscle extending from the medial epicondyle of the humerus to the anterior surface of the second and third metacarpal that is responsible primarily for flexion of the wrist and assisting with abduction of the wrist and flexion of the elbow

flexor carpi ulnaris muscle extending from the medial epicondyle of the humerus to the palmar surface of the hamate and base of the fifth metacarpal, primarily responsible for flexion of the wrist and assisting with adduction of the wrist and flexion of the elbow

flexor digitorum longus muscle extending from the middle third of the posterior tibia to the base of the distal phalanges of the toes that is primarily responsible for flexing the four lesser toes and assisting mildly with ankle plantar flexion and inversion

flexor digitorum profundus muscle extending from the proximal ulna to the base of the distal phalanges of the four fingers; primarily responsible for flexion of the four fingers at the interphalangeal joints and assisting somewhat with wrist flexion

flexor digitorum superficialis muscle extending from the medial epicondyle of the humerus, medial ulna, and medial radius to the middle phalanx of each of the four fingers; primarily responsible for flexion of the fingers at the metacarpophalangeal joint and assisting mildly with wrist flexion

flexor hallucis longus longer of the two branches of the flexor hallucis muscle, extending from the posterior fibula and interosseous membrane of the lower leg to the plantar aspect of the distal phalanx of the big toe (hallucis); responsible for flexion of the big toe as well as assisting with plantar flexion of the ankle

flexor pollicis muscle that extends from several attachments on the carpals to the base of the thumb and is responsible for flexion of the thumb

floating ribs the two lowest, or most inferior, of the false ribs that do not connect to any other structure distally

frontal bone bone forming the front of the face above the eyes, or the forehead region

frontalis a muscle of the forehead

gastrocnemius largest of the muscles of the calf region at the back (posterior) of the lower leg, extending from just above the knee to the back of the heel, where it forms part of the Achilles tendon

glenohumeral joint articulation of the humerus with the scapula at the glenoid fossa

glenohumeral muscles any of the group of muscles that cause the humerus to move in the glenoid fossa of the scapula

globe the sphere of the eye

gluteal muscles muscles of the posterior hip region; also known as the *buttocks*

gracilis muscle extending from the front edge of the pubis to the medial anterior edge of the tibia, primarily responsible for adduction and internal rotation of the hip and flexion of the knee

gray matter another term for the neurological tissue of the brain

greater tubercle enlarged lateral area of the proximal humerus

hamate one of the carpal bones located at the base of the fourth metacarpal

hamstrings group of three muscles at the back (posterior) of the upper leg serving primarily to flex the knee and extend the hip

humeroradial joint articulation of the humerus and radius bones at the elbow

humero-ulnar joint articulation of the humerus and ulna bones at the elbow

humerus upper arm bone, extending from the shoulder joint to the elbow joint

hyoid bone a U-shaped bone that is located between the base of the tongue and the larynx and serves as support for the tongue and an attachment point for several of the swallowing muscles; the only bone in the body that does not directly articulate with another bone

hypothenar muscles enlarged area of the palm, primarily composed of muscle, located in line with the fifth finger

iliocostalis muscles group of superficial muscles that control motion of the upper spine and neck

iliopsoas union of the iliacus and psoas muscles that forms a common muscle extending from the anterior aspect of the lower thoracic vertebrae, lumbar vertebrae, and sacrum to the lesser trochanter of the tibia; primarily responsible for hip flexion and external rotation of the hip

incisors any of the eight cutting teeth located between the canine teeth, including four on the upper row and four on the lower row of teeth

incus middle of the three ossicles of the ear that serves to transmit sound waves to the inner ear; also known as the *anvil*

infraspinatus one of the four rotator cuff muscles extending from the medial aspect of the infraspinous fossa of the scapula to the greater tubercle of the humerus; primarily responsible for external rotation of the humerus

intercostals the structures, such as muscles or cartilage, located between the ribs

internal oblique muscles group of abdominal muscles extending from the edges of the lower ribs to the superior crest of the ilium; when the left and right sides act together, they serve to flex the trunk, and when the sides act individually, they act to laterally flex or rotate the trunk

interossei related to the space between two long parallel bones as in the forearm or lower leg

interphalangeal joints articulations of bones in the fingers

interspinous spanning from one spinous process of a vertebra to another

intertransverse ligaments connective tissue that spans from one transverse process of a vertebra to another

intervertebral disk shock-absorbing, gel-filled ring of cartilaginous tissue located between the vertebrae

intervertebral joint any of the articulations of one spinal vertebra with another

iris the colored ring of muscle in the front of the eye

Kiesselbach's area area of concentrated blood vessels in the face located just behind the upper lip that supply a tremendous amount of blood to the nose

lacrimal bones small thin bone making up part of the orbital wall and through which pass the lacrimal ducts

lacrimal gland tissue that secretes tears in the eyes

latissimus dorsi a muscle of the lower part of the back that extends from a broad aponeurosis attached to the spinous process of the vertebrae of the lower back and the crest of the ilium to the bicipital groove of the humerus, and is primarily responsible for extending, adducting and internally rotating the arm, as well as retracting the shoulders.

lesser tubercle enlarged medial area of the proximal humerus, smaller than the greater tubercle

levator scapulae muscle that extends from the upper four cervical vertebrae to the medial border of the scapula and is primarily responsible for elevating the medial scapula

ligamentum flavum somewhat elastic ligamentous tissue connecting the laminae of adjacent vertebrae that serves to limit flexion of the spine

lipids fats

longissimus muscle general name of the group of muscles extending along the posterior spine from the base of the skull to the transverse processes of many of the cervical and thoracic vertebrae

longus longer section of a muscle divided into at least two parts

lumbricals group of four intrinsic muscles of the plantar aspect of the foot that serve to maintain the arch and flex the toes

lunate one of the proximal carpal bones, located between the scaphoid bone and the triquetral bone

malleus outermost of the ossicles of the ear that serves to transmit sound waves to the inner ear; also known as the *hammer*

mandible lower jaw bone

manubrium upper section of the sternum

masseter muscle used for chewing

maxilla upper jaw bone

maxillae plural of *maxilla*

medulla oblongata part of the posterior brain that leads to the spinal cord and houses the control centers for many involuntary functions of the body

meninges any of the three protective linings that cover the brain and spinal cord

menisci plural of meniscus; the shock absorbing cartilage located between the tibia and femur in the knee

metacarpals any of the group of five bones that extend from the carpals to the phalanges in the hand

metacarpophalangeal joints any of the articulations of the metacarpal bones with the proximal phalanges in the hand

metatarsals any of the group of five bones that extend from the tarsals to the phalanges in the foot

metatarsophalangeal (MTP) joints any of the articulations of the metatarsal bones with the proximal phalanges in the foot

midbrain middle section of the brain

molars the group of teeth with rounded or flattened surfaces in the posterior of the mouth that are used for grinding food

motor nerves nerves that cause movement in an area rather than sensation

multifidus group of muscles present along the entire spine; most developed in the lumbar spine and are primarily responsible for extension of the trunk and neck, laterally flexing and rotating the spine, and anteriorly tilting the pelvis

nares nostrils

nasal bones bones of the nose

nasion the small projection where the nasal bones articulate with the frontal bone

navicular bone in the medial foot located at the top of the metatarsal arch

nucleus pulposus inner gel-filled area of the vertebral disk

oblique eye muscles muscles controlling diagonal eye motion

obturator externus muscle that extends from the anterior sacrum and posterior ischium to the greater trochanter of femur and are primarily responsible for external rotation of the hip

occipital bone bone located at posterior aspect of the skull

occipitalis posterior section of the occipitofrontalis muscle that is primarily responsible for moving the scalp

oculi related to the eye

olecranon fossa depressed area at the distal humerus that articulates with the olecranon of the ulna in the elbow joint

optic nerve nerve that transmits information from the eye to the brain

orbicularis either of the circular muscles that are responsible for closing a major opening such as the mouth or the eye

orbicularis oris circular muscle underlying the eyelid that closes the eyes when contracted

orbit bony wall of the opening in the skull for the eye

outer ear auricle; the part of the ear seen on the outside of the head

palantine bones either of the L-shaped bones that form part of the hard palate and the nasal cavity

palmaris longus muscle extending from the medial epicondyle of the humerus to the palmar aspects of the second through fifth metacarpals through an aponeurosis; primarily responsible for flexion of the wrist and assisting mildly with flexion of the elbow

parietal either of the two bones forming most of the superiolateral aspects of the skull joining each other at the sagittal suture line and joining the frontal bone at the coronal suture line

patella sesamoid bone commonly referred to as the kneecap that is embedded in the underside of the quadriceps tendon

patellofemoral joint articulation of the undersurface of the kneecap with the upper surface of the patellar groove of the femur

pectineus muscle extending from the anterior pubis to an area near the lesser trochanter of the femur that is primarily responsible for flexion, adduction, and internal rotation of the hip

pectoralis major broad muscle extending from the medial half of the clavicle and medial sternum to the proximal humerus near the lesser tubercle; depending on which fibers of the muscle are active, primarily responsible for internal rotation, horizontal adduction, and flexion and extension of the shoulder

pectoralis minor muscle extending from the anterior surfaces of the third through fifth ribs to the coracoid process of the scapula; primarily responsible for protraction, downward rotation, and depression of the scapula

pelvis region of the body between the lower spine and the hips

phalanges the fingers or toes and the bones that comprise them

phrenic nerve nerve that exits the spinal cord in the cervical spine and innervates the diaphragm and pericardium

pia mater highly vascular innermost layer of the three meninges of the brain and spinal cord

pisiform one of the bones located on the medial side of the proximal row of carpals in the hand, articulating with the triquetrum

plantaris small muscle consisting of a small belly and long tendon that extends from the distal lateral femur to the calcaneus, where it becomes part of the Achilles tendon and assists in knee flexion and ankle plantar flexion

pons middle section of the brain stem that regulates many involuntary actions such as breathing

popliteus small triangular muscle at the posterior knee that extends from the proximal posterior tibia upward to the lateral femoral condyle and serves to unlock the knee by rotating the femur on the tibia when the knee is fully extended

posterior longitudinal ligament long band of connective tissue extending along the posterior surfaces of the vertebral bodies and vertebral disks, lining the anterior spinal cord canal

posterior shoulder girdle muscles muscles controlling the motion and stability of the shoulder girdle (clavicle and scapula) that attach at the back, or posterior portion, of this area, which includes the trapezius, levator scapulae, and rotator cuff

pronator quadratus muscle extending from the anterior distal ulna to the anterior distal radius and primarily responsible for pronation of the forearm

pronator teres muscle extending from the medial distal humerus to the central lateral radius and primarily responsible for pronation of the forearm and assisting with flexion of the elbow

proximal radioulnar joint articulation of the ulna and the radius in the proximal forearm near the elbow

proximal tibiofibular joint articulation of the tibia and fibula in the proximal lower leg, near the knee joint

pterygoid muscles group of muscles that are primarily responsible for elevating the mandible to close the mouth

pulp inner section of a tooth

pupil the dark circle at the center of the iris of the eye; actually an opening in the front of the eye that allows light to enter the interior of the eye

quadratus lumborums muscle extending from the posterior iliac crest to the lower border of the twelfth rib and transverse processes of the first through fourth lumbar vertebrae; primarily responsible for lateral flexion of the trunk, as well as overall lumbar spine and pelvis stabilization

quadriceps group of four muscles in the thigh that serve primarily to extend the knee and flex the hip

radial collateral ligament ligament connecting the radius to the humerus in the elbow

radial deviation movement of the hand in the frontal plane laterally toward the radius

radius bone in the forearm, extending from the elbow to the wrist

rectus abdominis muscle extending from the crest of the pubis to the cartilage of ribs five through seven and the xiphoid process; primarily responsible for trunk flexion and assisting with lateral trunk flexion and trunk rotation

rectus eye muscles group of muscles located superiorly, inferiorly, medially, and laterally on the eye that control motion of the eye in each of these respective directions when acting individually or, when working with other muscles, serve to move the eye in a diagonal motion

retina area of neurological tissue at the back of the eye where light images are focused as they are processed and passed to the brain for interpretation

retinaculum band of connective tissue that serves to hold muscles and tendons in place, especially as they cross a very movable joint

rhomboid major muscle extending from the spinous processes of thoracic vertebrae two through five to the medial border of the scapula; primarily responsible for retracting or adducting the scapula and also elevating the scapula

rhomboid minor muscle extending from the spinous processes of cervical vertebra seven and thoracic vertebra one to the medial border of the scapula; primarily responsible for retracting or adducting the scapula and also elevating the scapula

rotators muscles that turn the hip or shoulder inward and outward in the transverse plane

sacrum section of fused vertebrae at the distal spine where it articulates with the pelvis

sartorius muscle in the front of the thigh extending from the anterior superior iliac spine to the proximal anteromedial tibia as part of the pes anserine tendon; primarily responsible for hip flexion, hip abduction, and knee flexion

scaphoid one of the bones of the proximal row of carpals in the hand, articulating with the trapezium, in line with the first metacarpal and palpated in the "anatomical snuffbox"

scapula bone commonly referred to as the *shoulder blade*

sclera white layer of the front of the eye seen around the iris

semicircular canals structures in the ear that are responsible for interpreting head position and assisting in balance

sensory nerves nerves that process information regarding sensation rather than movement

septum a dividing wall, as in the separating wall of the nostrils in the nose

serratus anterior muscle extending from the anterolateral aspects of ribs one through nine to the anterior medial border of the scapula; primarily responsible for upwardly rotating and abducting, or protracting, the scapula

sesamoids any of the small ("sesame seed"–shaped) bones embedded in a tendon as it crosses a joint to provide a mechanical advantage to that tendon in moving the limb or appendage, such as the patella embedded in the quadriceps tendon

soleus one of the muscles in the calf that forms part of the Achilles tendon

sphenoid bones one of the bones of the anterior skull that forms most of the floor of the cranial vault and the sides of the orbits

spinalis muscles part of the erector spinae group of muscles extending from the spinous processes of the upper cervical and thoracic vertebrae to the spinous processes of the lower thoracic and lumbar vertebrae; primarily responsible for trunk and neck as well as rotating the cervical spine

spinous processes easily palpated projections of bone that extend posteriorly from the vertebrae

stapes innermost of the ossicles of the ear that serves to transmit sound waves to the inner ear; also known as the stirrup

sternoclavicular joint articulation of the sternum with the clavicle in the front of the chest

sternum bone in the front of the ribcage commonly referred to as the *breastbone*

subclavius muscle muscle extending from the superior aspect of the first rib to the inferior aspect of the clavicle; primarily responsible for stabilization of the sternoclavicular joint

subscapularis one of the four rotator cuff muscles extending from the entire subscapular fossa to the lesser tubercle of the humerus; primarily responsible for internal rotation, adduction, and extension of the glenohumeral joint

subtalar joint articulation of the talus with the tibia and fibula

supercilii muscle muscle group located in the upper face responsible for wrinkling the skin of the forehead and drawing the eyebrows closer together; also known as the *corrugator muscle*

superior orbital fissure opening in the sphenoid bone of the skull through which nerves and blood vessels pass to and from the orbit

supinator muscle extending from the lateral epicondyle of the humerus and posterior ulna to the proximal radius; primarily responsible for supination of the forearm

supraspinatus one of the four rotator cuff muscles extending from the posterior scapula on the supraspinous fossa to the greater tubercle of the humerus; primarily responsible for assisting in abduction of the humerus and stabilization of the humerus in the glenoid fossa of the scapula

supraspinous ligaments band of connective tissue that extends from the spinous process of one vertebra to the spinous process of the vertebra inferior to it

talocalcaneonavicular joint articulation of the talus, calcaneus, and navicular bones in the foot

talocrural joint another name for the ankle joint

talus most proximal of the tarsal bones, located directly under, or inferior to, the tibiofibular articulation and above, or superior to, the calcaneus

tarsometatarsal joints any of the articulations of the tarsals with the metatarsals in the foot

temporal bones either of the bones that form the upper and superior sides of the skull

temporalis large fan-shaped muscle on the side of the skull extending from the temporal bone to the coronoid process of the mandible; primarily responsible for elevating the mandible (closing the mouth)

temporomandibular joint (TMJ) articulation of the mandible (lower jawbone) with the skull

tensor fasciae latae muscle extending from the anterior iliac crest down the lateral thigh about a quarter of the distance to the knee, where it becomes a dense tendon, the iliotibial band, and ends at Gerdy's tubercle on the proximal lateral tibia; primarily responsible for abduction, rotation, and flexion of the hip as well as mildly assisting with flexion of the knee

teres major muscle extending from the lateral border of the scapula to the proximal humerus, inferior to the rotator cuff attachments; primarily responsible for internal rotation, extension, and adduction of the glenohumeral joint

teres minor one of the four rotator cuff muscles extending from the posterior lateral border of the scapula to the greater tubercle of the humerus; primarily responsible for external rotation and extension and assisting with horizontal abduction of the glenohumeral joint

thenar muscles the prominent group of muscles at the base of the thumb, which control several motions of the hand, including opposition

thoracic cage the area created by the sternum, ribs, and spine; also known as the *rib cage*

tibia bone along the inner (medial) aspect of the lower leg extending from the knee joint to the ankle joint parallel to the fibula

tibialis anterior muscle extending from the lateral surface of the tibia and interosseous membrane to the medial cuneiform and first metatarsal; primarily responsible for dorsiflexion of the ankle, inversion of the foot, and support of the medial arch of the foot

tibialis posterior muscle extending from the posterior tibia, fibula, and interosseous membrane to the navicular and medial cuneiform; primarily responsible for inversion and plantar flexion of the foot and support of the medial arch of the foot

tibiofemoral joint part of the knee joint composed of the articulation of the tibia with the femur

transverse (mid) tarsal joint term given to the talocalcaneonavicular and calcaneocuboid joints in the ankle, where many of the movements of the ankle take place

transverse processes lateral projections of bone from each side of the vertebral bodies and serving as a point for muscle and ligament attachment

transversus abdominis deep abdominal muscle extending from the thoracolumbar fascia, iliac crest, and lower ribs horizontally to the pubis and linea alba; primarily responsible for compressing the abdomen

trapezium a bone in the distal row of carpals at the base of the thumb

trapezius muscle extending from the occipital bone of the skull and spinous processes of the lower cervical vertebrae and upper thoracic vertebrae outward to the lateral clavicle, acromion, and spine of the scapula; primarily responsible for glenohumeral abduction as well as rotation and elevation of the scapula

trapezoid a bone in the distal row of carpals at the base of the index finger

triceps muscle group at the back (posterior) of the upper arm that serves primarily to extend the elbow and extend the shoulder

triquetrum the pyramid-shaped bone in the proximal row of carpals that is located between the lunate and pisiform bones

trochlea anatomical structure resembling a pulley on the distal humerus, where it articulates with the ulna

true ribs any of the seven pairs of ribs that connect directly to the sternum through individual cartilaginous attachments

tympanic membrane the eardrum

ulna medial bone of the forearm extending from the elbow joint to the wrist joints

ulnar collateral ligament connective tissue extending from the medial humerus to the medial ulna

ulnar deviation movement of the wrist medially in the frontal plane

vestibulocochlear nerve cranial nerve with two divisions, vestibular and cochlear, which process information regarding balance and hearing respectively

vestibulocochlear system neurological structures that process balance and hearing information and pass this information to the brain for interpretation

vomer bone in the skull that is located on the midline of the sphenoid and forms part of the nasal septum

xiphoid process extension of cartilage at the distal end of the sternum

zygomatic bones cheekbones

zygomaticus major muscle extending from the posterior zygomatic bone to the skin at the corner of the mouth that is primarily responsible for drawing the corner of the mouth upward and laterally (as in smiling)

SPECIAL TESTS TERMINOLOGY

90/90 straight leg raise test with the client in a supine position and the uninvolved leg flat on the table, flex the involved hip to 90 degrees and then passively extend the knee into extension until end range or a firm end-feel is felt; this test is used to measure and assess hamstring length

AC posterior shear test with the client seated and the examiner sitting beside the involved arm, place the front hand slightly medial to the distal clavicle while the posterior hand is placed on the posterior lateral border of the acromion and provide a posterior shearing force along the anterior clavicle; pain, replication of symptoms (and/or a lack of symptoms) or excessive mobility indicates a positive AC posterior shear test for AC joint trauma

active compression test have the client abduct the shoulder to 90 degrees and horizontally adduct approximately 15 degrees, then manually internally rotate the shoulder as far as possible and apply an inferior force to the distal forearm; pain deep in the shoulder in this position indicates a positive active compression test for a SLAP lesion, whereas pain felt on the top of the shoulder indicates trauma to the AC joint

Adson maneuver have the client actively rotate the head to the involved side while taking a deep breath, then passively extend and externally rotate the shoulder while assessing the radial pulse; a diminished pulse or replication of symptoms indicates a positive Adson maneuver for thoracic outlet syndrome

alar ligament stress test with the client seated, stand to the client's side and palpate the spinous process of C2 while slightly passively side bending the head; abnormal movement of the spinous process not kicking to the opposite side indicates a positive alar ligament stress test for alar ligament trauma and whiplash

Allen test passively move the client's shoulder to 100 degrees of abduction and 90 degrees of elbow flexion while palpating the radial pulse, then ask the client to rotate the cervical spine away from the side being tested; a diminished pulse and return of symptoms indicates a positive Allen test for thoracic outlet syndrome

anterior drawer test performed on the knee, ankle or shoulder; pull the tibia and fibula forward underneath the femur, or pull the calcaneus forward underneath the lower leg, or pull the humerus medially and anteriorly in an oblique plane; the femur, lower leg and scapula are stabilized—the appearance of a skin sulcus along the joint line or marked anterior translation indicates a positive anterior drawer for the respective ligaments

apprehension test with the client supine, stand at the client's side and move his or her shoulder and elbow both to 90 degrees of flexion with your outside hand holding the client's elbow; with your inside hand, stabilize the anterior shoulder while you externally rotate the client's shoulder with your opposite hand; pain or apprehension indicates a positive apprehension test for glenohumeral instability

Bakody's test place the involved upper extremity on top of the client's head; a significant reduction of symptoms indicates a positive Bakody's test for cervical disk lesions

balance and reach test with the client standing, have the client reach forward three times with one leg as far as possible, touching the floor with his or her heel (the majority of the client's body weight should be on the standing leg); measure the maximum distance, and calculate 80% by placing a mark on the floor; have the client perform as many heel touches as possible beyond the 80% mark with each leg in 30 seconds; a deficit in heel touches on the involved side indicates a positive balance and reach test for patellofemoral pain

bowstring test with the client supine and the hip and knee flexed to 90 degrees, passively extend the knee while palpating the popliteal fossa to compress the sciatic nerve; once pain occurs, slightly flex the knee and compress the sciatic nerve again while maintaining the same hip position; radiating pain down the leg with passive knee extension and pain in the popliteal fossa with compression indicate a positive bowstring test for sciatic nerve irritation and lower lumbar spine trauma

brachial plexus stretch test with the client seated or standing, passively flex the cervical spine by laterally placing your hand on the involved shoulder to stabilize it and moving the head away from that shoulder; pain and tingling along the neck and possibly down the arm of the stabilized side indicate a positive brachial plexus stretch test for brachial plexus stretch; pain and tingling along the nonstabilized side indicate a positive brachial plexus stretch test for brachial plexus compression

brachial plexus tension test with the client seated or standing, ask the client to abduct, then externally rotate his or her arms until symptoms are replicated, and then ask the client to lower the arms to a point where the symptoms disappear; hold the client's arms in this position while the client flexes both elbows, and place the client's hands behind the head;

replication of symptoms in this final position indicates a positive brachial plexus tension test for cervical nerve root injury or brachial plexus injury

C1-C2 stress testing with the client supine, stand at the client's head, place your right hand on the transverse process and arch of C1 and the occiput, and place your left hand on the transverse process and arch of C2; provide a lateral shear to C1 and the occiput while stabilizing C2; do this to both sides; reverse this, and stabilize C1 while providing a lateral shear to C2 on both sides; replication of symptoms or excessive movement indicates a positive C1-C2 stress test for lateral instability of the atlanto-axial joint (C1-C2) and whiplash

cervical compression test with the client seated and looking forward, press gently down on the head, creating an axial load on the cervical spine; pain in the neck and radiating pain down one or both arms indicate a positive cervical compression test for damage to the cervical vertebral disks

cervical distraction test with the client supine, stand at the client's head and grasp his or her chin and occiput, allowing for minimal flexion to comfort, then gradually apply a distraction force of approximately 0 to 15 kilograms; relief or reduction of symptoms indicates a positive cervical distraction test for cervical disk lesions

compression and distraction test with the client supine, stand at the client's head and cup the occiput in one hand while stabilizing the cervical spine with the other hand near base of the neck; apply a traction-compression-traction force; pain with compression indicates a positive cervical compression test for vertebral body fracture, disk herniation, vertebral end plate fracture, acute arthritis or joint inflammation of the facet joint, or nerve root irritation; pain with distraction indicates a positive cervical distraction test for spinal ligament tear, tear or inflammation of the annulus fibrosus, muscle spasm, large disk herniation, or dural irritability

compression test placing your hands on both sides of the injured body part, apply a compressive force along the length of the injured area; starting distal and working in a proximal direction, apply gentle then progressively more pressure; pinpoint pain in the injured area and/or crepitus may indicate a fracture (also called long bone compression test)

coracoid impingement test with the elbow flexed to 90 degrees, flex the shoulder to 90 degrees and have the client gently internally rotate the shoulder; medial pain indicates a positive coracoid impingement test for trauma to the long head of the biceps or subscapularis, whereas lateral pain indicates trauma to the supraspinatus ligament

costoclavicular test with the client in an exaggerated military position (standing with shoulder blades retracted and depressed, or at attention), assess the radial pulse for 1 minute; an alteration of the pulse or replication of symptoms indicates a positive costoclavicular test for thoracic outlet syndrome

crank test with the client supine, passively flex the client's shoulder to 150 to 160 degrees in the scapular plane, then manually apply a compressive force along the axis of the humerus while internally and externally rotating the shoulder; pain, clicking, clunking, or pseudolocking indicates a positive crank test for a torn labrum

Ely's test with the client prone, passively flex his or her knee; flexion of the same side hip coming off of the plinth indicates a positive Ely's test for tight rectus femoris

Fairbank test apply a straight lateral glide to the patella in full knee extension with the client in a supine position; an urge to contract the quadriceps to prevent a perceived patellar subluxation or dislocation indicates a positive Fairbank test for patellar dislocation

Feagan test with the client seated passively, abduct his or her shoulder to 90 (or 45) degrees and perform the sulcus sign test with the fingers of both your hands interlocked on the superior portion of their shoulder; excessive inferior translation indicates a positive Feagan test for multidirectional laxity of the shoulder

Finkelstein's test with the client seated and his or her thumb flexed into the palm of the hand, ask the client to close the fist over the thumb and ulnarly deviate the wrist; pain indicates a positive Finkelstein's test for DeQuervain's syndrome

fulcrum test with the client sitting on a plinth, position one of your arms under his or her thigh while you apply gentle pressure to the dorsum on the knee; start distally and work proximally, repeating the test several times; replication of symptoms or sharp pain indicates a positive fulcrum test for femoral stress fracture

Hawkins-Kennedy impingement test with the elbow flexed to 90 degrees, flex the shoulder to 90 degrees in the scapular plane and have the client gently internally rotate his or her shoulder; pain indicates a positive Hawkins-Kennedy impingement test for trauma to the supraspinatus

hip log roll with the client supine, stabilize the pelvis at the anterior iliac crest while moving the femur into internal and external rotation; pain or the inability to roll and glide the femoral head indicates a positive hip log roll test for hip fracture or dislocation

hip scouring test with the client supine and the hip and knee in 90 degrees flexion, apply a downward pressure on the knee while internally and externally rotating the hip; increased pain in the hip with rotation indicates a positive hip scouring test for hip joint pathology

Homan test with the leg in full extension, elevate the leg from the hip and passively move the ankle into dorsiflexion; pain in the calf indicates a positive Homan test for deep vein thrombosis

hop test ask the client to hop on the involved leg; replication of symptoms indicates a positive hop test for femoral stress fracture

Jefferson fracture test with the client supine, stand at his or her head and palpate both transverse processes of C1, then stabilize one side and provide a medial force in the opposite direction on the other side; a soft end-feel or replication of symptoms indicates a positive Jefferson fracture test for disruption in the ring of the atlas and whiplash

Kleiger test with the client seated, hold the lower leg stationary with one hand while holding the involved foot on the medial aspect and rotate it laterally with your other hand; pain along the deltoid ligament indicates injury to the involved ligament, a medial ankle sprain (MAS), or syndesmotic ankle sprain

Lachman's test hold the client's knee in approximately 20 degrees of flexion while you stabilize the thigh and grasp just above the knee with your outside hand; with your other hand, grasp just below the medial aspect of the knee; while the outer hand stabilizes the thigh, the inner hand draws the tibia anteriorly on the femur; anterior translation on the femur compared with the uninvolved side indicates a positive Lachman's test for anterior cruciate ligament injury

Lasegue's test with the client supine, keep the knee extended and move the hip into internal rotation and adduction, then ask the client to slowly flex the hip, bringing the leg toward the head until tightness is felt in the hamstring; reposition the leg in slight hip flexion where no tightness or pain is felt, and dorsiflex the foot; pain felt at 30 degrees indicates a positive Lasegue's test for disk involvement, whereas no replication of pain indicates tight hamstrings (also known as the *straight leg raise test)*

Lateral step-down test with the client standing on the involved leg in full knee extension on the edge of a 20 centimeter step and his or her hands on the waist while the opposite leg is hanging down toward the floor in extension, have the client squat down, allowing the opposite foot to touch the floor, and return to the standing start position; repeat this five times, if possible; this functional test is used to assess the quality of movement in the lower extremity

McMurray test with the client supine, grasp his or her knee with your proximal hand and his or her foot and ankle with your distal hand; provide a varus stress to the knee while internally rotating the tibia on the femur, moving the knee in and out of flexion, and also provide a valgus stress to the knee while externally rotating the tibia on the femur moving the knee in and out of flexion; numerous symptoms indicate a positive McMurray test for meniscal lesions, including clicking, snapping, popping, locking, and pain in the lateral or medial joint lines

modified Thomas test with the client sitting on the edge of the plinth, have the client roll back while holding both knees to the chest; next, have the client continue to hold the uninvolved leg while you slowly lower the involved leg towards the plinth; this test is used to measure and assess iliopsoas, quadriceps, and iliotibial band length

Neer impingement test grasp the client's arm at the elbow, and passively move the shoulder into end range flexion; then apply a gentle passive overpressure; replication of symptoms or pain indicates a positive Neer's impingement test for trauma to the supraspinatus or long head of the biceps

Ober's test with the client lying on the uninvolved side and the hips and knees slightly flexed, passively abduct and extend the upper leg (involved leg), allowing the iliotibial band to cross over the greater trochanter; inability of the leg to lower back to or beyond midline and/or pain indicates a positive Ober's test for iliotibial band tightness

partial sit-up test with the client supine and his or her knees flexed to 90 degrees, place your hand behind the client's head and have the client contract the lower abdominals to perform a partial sit-up; pain with contraction or the inability to perform a partial sit-up indicates a positive partial sit-up test for an avulsion fracture at the pelvis

passive straight leg raise test with the client supine and the uninvolved leg flat on the table, the involved leg is passively flexed until end range or a firm end-feel is felt; this test is used to measure and assess hamstring length

patellar tendon palpation palpate the insertion of the patellar tendon on the inferior pole of the patella; pain indicates a positive patellar tendon palpation test for patellar tendonitis or tendinopathy

Patrick's or Faber's test with the client supine and the foot of the affected leg lying across the opposite knee, assess the height of the knee in relation to the opposite leg; the inability of the knee to drop below the unaffected leg or touch the plinth indicates a positive Patrick's or Faber's test for hip joint pathology

Phalen's test with the client either standing or sitting and the client's wrist passively flexed, apply overpressure in flexion to the wrist for at least 1 minute; tingling or numbness that radiates into the hand and into the second through fourth digits indicates a positive Phalen's test for carpal tunnel syndrome

piano key test stand in front of the seated client, and apply an inferior force to the distal end of the clavicle; pain or an excessive rebound translation once the force is removed indicates a positive piano key test for AC joint instability

piriformis test with the client in a side-lying position, uninvolved side on the plinth, flex the involved hip to 60 degrees with the knee flexed as well; stabilize the hip, and manually internally rotate the femur; pain with internal rotation indicates a positive piriformis test for piriformis tightness or sciatic nerve impingement

posterior drawer test similar to the anterior drawer test for the knee or shoulder; position the client supine with the hips at 45 degrees and the knees at 80 degrees, and wrap your fingers around the proximal tibia while giving a posterior force to the proximal tibia with your thumbs; an increase in translation compared with the uninvolved side or a soft end-feel indicates a positive posterior drawer test for the posterior cruciate ligament (PCL); with the client seated, pull the humerus laterally and posterior in an oblique plane while the scapula is stabilized; the appearance of a skin sulcus along the joint line or marked posterior translation indicates a positive posterior drawer for posterior shoulder instability

recurvatum test passively extend the knee while the client relaxes in a supine position, then apply overpressure at end range extension; medial or lateral joint line pain indicates a positive recurvatum test for the meniscus

resisted knee extension with the knee in full extension, ask the client to perform resisted knee extension; replication of symptoms indicates a positive resisted knee extension test for patellar tendonitis or tendinopathy

Roo test have the client abduct his or her shoulders 90 degrees and move into external rotation; then ask the client to slowly open and close the hands for up to 3 minutes; replication of symptoms, especially unilaterally, indicates a positive Roo test for thoracic outlet syndrome

Scapular compression test with the patient either sitting or standing, tap the scapular spine; a painful response is positive for a scapular fracture

shoulder depression test with the client seated laterally, flex his or her head to one side while applying a downward pressure to the opposite shoulder; increased pain indicates a positive shoulder depression test for irritation or compression of the cervical or brachial plexus nerve roots

slump test this seven-position test is performed with the client seated; pain persisting throughout the seven positions or any increase in pain indicates a positive slump test for peroneal nerve injury

Spurling's test with the client seated and looking forward, place the cervical spine in slight lateral flexion as you apply a gentle downward pressure on the top of the head (this can be performed in cervical extension as well); tingling pain down the arm of the side receiving the stretch indicates a positive Spurling's test for cervical disk trauma or brachial plexus nerve root irritation

squeeze test manually compress the fibula toward the tibia at the midpoint of the calf; distal lower leg pain indicates a positive squeeze test for syndesmotic ankle sprain

star-excursion balance test (SEBT) have the client perform the eight-position lower extremity reaching tasks; any inconsistency between the involved and uninvolved extremities indicates limitations in functional dynamic balance

step-up test with the client in a supine position with his or her knees flexed to approximately 80 degrees and the hips at 45 degrees, place your thumb pads on the distal femoral condyles and your respective interphalangeal joints on the tibial plateaus; an absence of the standard 1-centimeter anterior tibial condyle "step" indicates a positive step-up test for posterior cruciate ligament (PCL) rupture

stork test with the client standing on one leg with hands on the waist, have the client move into back extension while you observe the client's movements and provide assistance for balance from behind; significant pin-point pain indicates a positive stork test for posterior vertebral fracture (spondylolysis or spondylolisthesis)

sulcus sign test with the client seated, stabilize the involved shoulder with one hand and gently apply an inferior traction force with the other hand; a shallow depression above the humeral head just below the acromion indicates a positive sulcus sign test for multidirectional laxity of the shoulder

talar tilt test manually induce inversion of the calcaneus with the foot in either a neutral position or 10 degrees of dorsiflexion; a palpable click or noticeable pain or movement distinctly exaggerated compared with the uninvolved side indicates a positive talar tilt for the calcaneofibular ligament (CFL), a lateral ankle sprain (LAS), or a medial ankle sprain (MAS)

tap or percussion test tap the skin and bone surrounding the injured body part with your index finger, checking for pinpoint pain, radiating pain, or crepitus may indicate a fracture

Thomas test for this two-part test, have the client assume a supine position and first assess the lumbar curve; next, have the client flex one knee and pull it to the chest; excessive lordosis in the first position and lifting of the opposite leg off the plinth in the second position indicate a positive Thomas test for tight hip flexors; abduction without the leg rising off the plinth in the second position indicates a positive Thomas test for tight iliotibial band

Thompson test squeeze the calf midbelly as the client lies prone with his or her feet off the edge of the plinth; the absence of plantar flexion or reduced plantar flexion compared with the uninvolved side indicates a positive Thompson test for Achilles tendon rupture

tibial sag test with the client in a supine position with the knees flexed to approximately 80 degrees and the hips at 45 degrees, visually inspect the position of the tibias; an unusual sag on the involved side indicates a positive tibial sag test for the posterior cruciate ligament (PCL)

Tinel's test with the client seated and his or her elbow flexed to 75 degrees and the forearm supinated, tap the groove between the olecranon process and the medial epicondyle of the humerus; tingling or radiating pain into the forearm and hand into the fourth and fifth digits indicates a positive Tinel test for trauma to the ulnar nerve or carpal tunnel syndrome

transverse ligament stress test with the client supine, stand at his or her head and palpate the bilateral lamina of C1 and the occiput as well as C2; lift the head and C1 while ventrally maintaining a neutral head position; a soft end feel, muscle spasm, dizziness, paresthesia of the lip, face, or limb, nystagmus, or a lump sensation in the throat indicate a positive transverse ligament stress test for trauma to the transverse ligament and whiplash

Trendelenburg test position yourself behind the client, and have the client stand; ask the client to transfer his or her weight and stand on one leg while you observe the movement of the posterior iliac crest of the nonweight-bearing leg; dropping of the nonweight-bearing posterior iliac crest indicates a positive Trendelenburg test for weak gluteus medius

valgus stress test of the finger with the client seated and the elbow flexed to 90 degrees with the forearm pronated and the wrist and fingers in neutral, grasp the finger distal and proximal to the injured joint and then gently apply a valgus force to the medial aspect of the injured joint; pain or laxity indicates a positive valgus stress test of the finger for trauma to the ulnar (medial) collateral ligament

valgus stress test of the elbow with the client standing or seated and the elbow flexed to 20 degrees and the forearm supinated, use one of your hands as a fulcrum at the lateral elbow joint to apply a valgus force to the medial aspect of the elbow while your other hand pulls the forearm/wrist toward you; pain or laxity indicates a positive valgus stress test of the elbow for trauma to the ulnar (medial) collateral ligament

valgus stress test of the knee with the client supine and the knee in either full extension or 30 degrees of flexion, grasp the medial side of the foot with your distal hand and apply a varus force while providing a fulcrum on the medial aspect of the client's knee with either your proximal hand or thigh; a lateral joint opening greater than the uninvolved side with a soft end-feel indicates a positive varus stress test for the lateral collateral ligament (LCL)

valgus stress test of the wrist with the client seated and the elbow flexed to 90 degrees and the forearm pronated with the wrist and fingers in neutral, grasp the distal forearm with one of your hands while applying a valgus force with your other hand to the medial side of the client's wrist by pulling the hand toward the thumb side; pain or laxity indicates a positive valgus stress test of the wrist for trauma to the ulnar (medial) collateral ligament

Valsalva maneuver with the client seated and his or her legs hanging off the table, have the client inhale deeply and forcefully exhale; pain in the low back or down the legs indicates a positive Valsalva maneuver test for herniated disk

varus stress test of the elbow with the client standing or seated and his or her elbow flexed to 20 degrees and the forearm supinated, use one of your hands as a fulcrum at the medial elbow joint to apply a varus force to the lateral aspect of the elbow while your other hand pulls the forearm/wrist toward you; pain or laxity indicates a positive varus stress test of the elbow for trauma to the radial (lateral) collateral ligament

varus stress test of the finger with the client seated and the elbow flexed to 90 degrees with the forearm pronated and the wrist and fingers in neutral, grasp the finger distal and proximal to the injured joint, then gently apply a varus force to the lateral aspect of the injured joint; pain or laxity indicates a positive varus stress test of the finger for trauma to the radial (lateral) collateral ligament

varus stress test of the knee with the client supine and the knee in either full extension or 30 degrees of flexion, grasp the lateral side of the foot with your distal hand and apply a valgus force while providing a fulcrum on the lateral aspect of the client's knee with either your proximal hand or thigh; a medial joint opening greater than the uninvolved side with a soft end-feel indicates a positive valgus stress test for the medial collateral ligament (MCL)

varus stress test of the wrist with the client seated and the elbow flexed to 90 degrees and the forearm pronated with the wrist and fingers in neutral, grasp the distal forearm with one of your hands while applying a varus force with your other hand to the lateral side of the client's wrist by pulling the hand toward his or her pinky side; pain or laxity indicates a positive varus stress test of the wrist for trauma to the radial (lateral) collateral ligament

Watson's test with the client seated and resting his or her elbow on the plinth in forearm pronation, passively move the wrist into extension and ulnar deviation, then manually force the distal scaphoid dorsally while passively moving the wrist into flexion and radial deviation; shifting of the scaphoid and lunate that causes pain indicates a positive Watson's test for an unstable wrist and trauma to the scapholunate ligament complex

well-leg straight leg raise test perform the Lasegue's test on the uninvolved side; pain on the involved side indicates a positive well-leg straight leg raise test for severe disk injury

Wright test passively move the client's shoulder into full flexion and external rotation while palpating the radial artery, then have the client take a deep breath and rotate or extend the cervical spine; a change in pulse or reduction in symptoms indicates a positive Wright test for thoracic outlet syndrome

C

E

F

N

T

U

V

FRENCH XVIIIth CENTURY PAINTINGS

WILDENSTEIN

NINETEEN EAST SIXTY-FOURTH STREET, NEW YORK

The XVIII *Century—a time of greatness and accomplishment in every field of artistic endeavor—has often been recognized as the most typically French of all the centuries of French art. In this period France witnessed an extraordinary wealth of artistic production, and French painting succeeded in reaching one of its most perfect, most admirable expressions.*

A surprisingly large and brilliant galaxy of highly gifted and industrious painters contributed to an equal flowering of all genres. Hardly ever before had portrait painting been represented by so impressive a lineage of masters. While sharing in a long and noble tradition, they all showed, in the interpretation of the human face and personality, an urge for intimacy, a search for individuality and a growing sense of truth, constantly served by an increasing virtuosity of the brush, the pencil and the rediscovered pastel.

Still life, filled with a deep poetic feeling, was endowed with universal grandeur. Genre painting was carried forward from the placid dignity of the Le Nains to the emotional dynamism in which Romanticism was to bask. Landscape, as an independent subject, gained a new atmospheric and spacial treatment. It attained unequalled fascination in the century's favorite child, the "Fête Galante," displaying endless and enchanting concerts of color and light, of love and pleasure, of games and pastoral delight, of theatre and Italian comedy, of the most luxurious marriage between a rejoicing nature and a gay and carefree humanity sometimes tinged with a dash of melancholy.

All this, however, did not prevent XVIII *Century painting from reflecting to a supreme degree the eminently French qualities of measure, balance and soundness. A miracle of unity was achieved in that art between delicate grace and frank sensuousness, glittering charm and sharp wit, lightness of conception and carefully planned composition, spontaneity of spirit and powerful consciousness of the necessary underlying structure. Above all, the pictorial creations of the time exuded, and still do, that peculiar type of harmony which reveals and proclaims true greatness in a work of art.*

Those who are only superficially acquainted with French painting of the XVIII *Century often indulge in the thought that charm is both the distinctive and paramount characteristic of that art. But its most striking feature is that such an amazing image of the "douceur de vivre" was achieved through a determined and relentless struggle against all the technical hardships of the art process. In that century of tradition and individual genius, novelty was never pursued at the expense of the noble lessons of the past; never did freedom or variety, in the high ideals of the* XVIII *Century painters, take the place of work, professional integrity and technical skill.*

That explains, perhaps, why French artists of the XVIII *Century were in demand all over the world in their own time; why royal courts and men of the most refined taste of the century entrusted them with the decoration and embellishment of their palaces and castles; why their works today are more than ever called upon to adorn and enrich our homes and our lives; and why they are a part of the most precious art patrimony of modern nations and are proudly treasured as such in the museums and public collections of every civilized country.*

G. W.

PRINTED IN THE UNITED STATES OF AMERICA

WILDENSTEIN & COMPANY, since its foundation in Paris in 1875, has been known for its specialization in French eighteenth century painting. The firm was also largely responsible for the growth of the popularity of this period both in Europe and America. The scope of WILDENSTEIN & COMPANY widened with years and by the 1900's the gallery was handling pictures, sculpture and works of art of all schools from fourteenth century primitives to contemporary European and American artists. A steady expansion began at the start of the present century when WILDENSTEIN & COMPANY assumed some of its present international character. In addition to the Paris establishment at 57 Rue La Boetie, the New York gallery was opened in 1902 and moved to its present location at 19 East 64 Street fifteen years ago. In 1925 a London gallery was established in the Nelson Historical House at 147 New Bond Street, and finally, the Buenos Aires gallery, at Florida 914, was opened in 1940.

For seventy-three years the firm's activities have been extremely varied. It has loaned paintings to thousands of exhibitions here and abroad and has gained renown for its acquisitions of famous private collections, among which were the Foulc Collection of Italian and French Renaissance painting and works of art; the Rodolphe Kann, of Dutch art, and the Oscar Schmitz and Fayet Collections of French Impressionists. The house numbers among its clients the world's outstanding private collectors and has placed pictures in every museum of importance from the Louvre to the Melbourne Museum in Australia.

Since it was opened, the New York Gallery alone has arranged over two hundred exhibitions of importance. Among them were: El Greco, French Seventeenth Century Art, Italian Masterpieces from Giotto to Tintoretto, and a series of comprehensive shows devoted to great French Masters of the eighteenth and nineteenth centuries, such as Fragonard, Chardin, Hubert Robert, Delacroix, Corot, Toulouse-Lautrec, Pissarro, Monet, Gauguin, Van Gogh, Cezanne, Manet, as well as exhibitions of American artists, –Winslow Homer and Mary Cassatt.

It is again in the tradition of Wildenstein exhibitions that this select group of Masterpieces of French Eighteenth Century Painting is being presented to both the collectors and the art-loving public.

For generations the American collector of discrimination has considered French eighteenth century painting as an indispensable item in any representative private or public collection. WILDENSTEIN & COMPANY is proud to be able to say that many of the important eighteenth century paintings in this country have passed through their hands and are now in American Museums. A partial list of these works and the Museums in which they hang follows:

BALTIMORE, MD.	Chardin	*La Joueuse d'Osselets* (Jacobs Coll.)
BALTIMORE MUSEUM OF ART	Fragonard	*Rest on the Flight to Egypt* (Jacobs Coll.)
	Greuze	*Marquise de Besons* (Jacobs Coll.)
	La Tour	*Portrait of the Chevalier de Jars* (Jacobs Coll.)
	Nattier	*Baronne Rigolay d'Ogny* (Jacobs Coll.)
	Hubert Robert	*The Terrace* (Jacobs Coll.)
	Hubert Robert	*The Roman Garden* (Jacobs Coll.)
	Vigée-Lebrun	*Portrait of Princess Galitzyne* (Jacobs Coll.)
THE WALTERS ART GALLERY	Hubert Robert	*Italian Villa*
BUFFALO, N. Y.		
ALBRIGHT ART GALLERY	David	*Portrait of Desmaisons*
BOSTON, MASS.		
MUSEUM OF FINE ARTS	Fragonard	*La Bonne Mère* (Robert T. Paine II Coll.)
CAMBRIDGE, MASS.	Chardin	*L'Aveugle de Quinze Vingt* (Winthrop Coll.)
FOGG MUSEUM OF ART	Fragonard	*Fanchon* (Winthrop Coll.)
	Lancret	*Portrait of Monsieur Gaignat* (Winthrop Coll.)
	Lancret	*Portrait of Madame Gaignat* (Winthrop Coll.)
	Largillière	*Portrait of Norbert Roettiers* (Winthrop Coll.)
	Largillière	*Madame Norbert Roettiers* (Winthrop Coll.)
	La Tour	*Monsieur Garnier d'Isles* (Winthrop Coll.)
	La Tour	*Portrait of Monsieur Julienne* (Winthrop Coll.)
CHICAGO, ILL.		
THE ART INSTITUTE OF CHICAGO	Chardin	*La Nappe Blanche*
CINCINNATI, OHIO		
THE CINCINNATI ART MUSEUM	Fragonard	*La Lettre* (Hanna Coll.)

CLEVELAND, OHIO THE CLEVELAND MUSEUM OF ART	David	*La Citoyenne Crouzet* (Rogers Coll.)
	Drouais	*La Marquise d'Aiguirandes* (Severance Coll.)
	Fragonard	*Evariste* (Rogers Coll.)
	Lancret	*Déclaration d'Amour* (Prentiss Coll.)
	Nattier	*Madame de Pompadour as Diana* (Severance Coll.)
DETROIT, MICH. DETROIT INSTITUTE OF ARTS	Boucher	*Birth of Venus* (Whitcomb Coll.)
	Nattier	*Madame Sophie de France as a Vestal Virgin*
HARTFORD, CONN. WADSWORTH ATHENAEUM	Chardin	*Le Poulet*
	David	*Les Licteurs apportant à Brutus les corps de ses fils*
	Greuze	*La Paresseuse*
	Largillière	*The Artist and his Family*
	Hubert Robert	*Camille Desmoulin in his Prison*
KANSAS CITY, MO. THE WILLIAM ROCKHILL NELSON GALLERY OF ART	Boilly	*Game of Checkers*
	Chardin	*The Bubble Blowers*
	David	*Portrait of a Young Boy*
	Pater	*L'Accord Parfait*
LOS ANGELES, CALIF. LOS ANGELES COUNTY MUSEUM	Boucher	*Les Confidences Pastorales*
	Fragonard	*L'Hiver*
	Greuze	*L'Amitié* (Hearst Coll.)
	Greuze	*Portrait of Madame Guimard* (Hearst Coll.)
MINNEAPOLIS, MINN. MINNEAPOLIS INSTITUTE OF ART	Hubert Robert	*Le Pont Rustique*
	Drouais	*Portrait of the Comte de Cheverny*
NEW YORK, N. Y. FRICK COLLECTION	Boucher	*Madame Boucher*
	Chardin	*La Serinette*
	Chardin	*Still-Life*
	David	*Portrait of Comtesse Daru*
	Boucher	*Decorative Panels from the Château de Crécy*
METROPOLITAN MUSEUM OF ART	Boucher	*Bergère endormie* (Bache Coll.)
	David	*Charlotte du Val D'Ognes* (Fletcher Coll.)
	Drouais	*Marquise de Villemonble* (Bache Coll.)
	Drouais	*The Son of President Desvieux* (Bache Coll.)
	Drouais	*Madame Favart* (Fletcher Coll.)
	Fragonard	*Le Billet Doux* (Bache Coll.)
	Fragonard	*The Cascade* (Bache Coll.)
	Fragonard	*The Shady Grove* (Bache Coll.)
	Largillière	*Marie-Marguerite Lambert de Torigny*
	Nattier	*Madame de Marsollier and her Daughter* (Schuette Coll.)
	Nattier	*Princesse de Condé as Diana* (Rogers Coll.)
	Hubert Robert	*Portico of a Country Mansion* (Hewitt Coll.)
	Hubert Robert	*Return of the Cattle* (Hewitt Coll.)
	Vigée-Lebrun	*Portrait of Emanuel de Crussol* (Bache Coll.)
	Watteau	*Le Mezzetin*

NORTHAMPTON, MASS.		
THE SMITH COLLEGE MUSEUM OF ART	Rigaud	*Portrait of the Duc d'Estrées*
SAN FRANCISCO, CALIF.		
PALACE OF THE LEGION OF HONOR	Fragonard	*Education of the Virgin*
	Greuze	*Citoyen Dubard*
ST. LOUIS, MO.		
CITY ART MUSEUM OF ST. LOUIS	Chardin	*Le Gobelet d'Argent*
	Vigée-Lebrun	*Portrait of her Brother*
WASHINGTON, D. C.		
CORCORAN GALLERY OF ART	Boucher	*La Musique* (Clark Coll.)
PHILLIPS MEMORIAL GALLERY	Chardin	*Still-Life*
NATIONAL GALLERY OF ART	Boucher	*Madame Bergeret* (Kress Coll.)
	Boucher	*Allegory of Music*
	Boucher	*Allegory of Painting*
	Chardin	*Still-Life, Pheasants and Hares* (Kress Coll.)
	Chardin	*Boy Blowing Bubbles* (Simpson Coll.)
	Chardin	*Monsieur Jeaurat* (Chester Dale Coll.)
	Chardin	*Still-Life* (Chester Dale Coll.)
	Chardin	*Portrait of an Old Woman* (Kress Coll.)
	Fragonard	*The Visit to the Nursery* (Kress Coll.)
	Fragonard	*A Game of Hot Cockles* (Kress Coll.)
	Fragonard	*A Game of Horse and Rider* (Kress Coll.)
	Fragonard	*L'Amour et la Folie* (Simpson Coll.)
	Greuze	*M. de la Live de Jully* (Kress Coll.)
	Lancret	*Picnic after the Hunt* (Kress Coll.)
	Nattier	*Madame de Caumartin as Hebe* (Kress Coll.)
	Rigaud	*Portrait of President Hébert* (Kress Coll.)
	Hubert Robert	*Ponte Solario* (Kress Coll.)
	Pater	*Conversation Galante* (Kress Coll.)
	Van Loo	*La Lanterne Magique* (Schuette Coll.)
	Van Loo	*Les Bulles de Savon* (Schuette Coll.)
	Vigée-Lebrun	*Marquise de Laborde* (Kress Coll.)
	Watteau	*Italian Comedians* (Kress Coll.)
	Watteau	*Portrait of Jeanne Rose Guyonne Benozzi known as "Sylvia"* (Kress Coll.)

TABLE OF CONTENTS

29.	Le Moine, M.	*Portrait of the Princesse de Lamballe*
30.	Le Moine, F.	*Hunting picnic*
31.	Lépicié	*La famille du menuisier*
32.	Mercier	*La promenade* or *L'heureuse rencontre*
33.	Nattier	*Portrait of Madame Elizabeth, Duchess of Parma*
34.	Nattier	*Portrait of the Comtesse de la Porte*
35.	Oudry	*Dog and swan*
36.	Pater	*Ladies bathing, with the statue of Neptune*
37.	Pater	*Ladies bathing, with the statue of Venus*
38.	Perronneau	*Portrait of Madame Miron*
39.	Prud'hon	*Portrait of Madame Barbier-Walbonne*
40.	Robert	*Fountain in a Roman villa*
41.	Robert	*Interior of a Roman temple with figures*
42.	Roslin	*Portrait of Madame Boucher*
43.	Schall	*Le portrait chéri*
44.	Tocqué	*Portrait of Pierre Jéliotte as Apollo*
45.	Trinquesse	*Portrait of an unknown lady*
46.	de Troy	*Fête aux Porcherons*
47.	Vallayer-Coster	*Portrait of Madame Saint-Huberty*
48.	Van Loo	*Portrait of Madame de Tencin holding a cat*
49.	Vestier	*Portrait of M. de Sarette; Portrait of Mme. de Sarette*
50.	Vigée-Lebrun	*Portrait of the Princesse Youssoupoff*
51.	Vigée-Lebrun	*Portrait of Madame Adelaide*
52.	Vincent	*Portrait of a child knitting*
53.	Watteau	*Ceres* or *Summer*
54.	Watteau	*Pleasures of summer*
55.	Watteau	*Alliance of Music and Comedy*
56.	Watteau	*Promenade sur les remparts*

PORTRAIT OF THE MARQUISE DE SAINTE-MAURE

BY

J.-A.-J. AVED

1702-1766

J.-A.-J. AVED

1702-1766

Born of Flemish parents, probably at Douai and brought up in Amsterdam where his father was a doctor. First, a pupil of Bernard Picart, a French engraver living in Holland. In 1721 went to Paris where he studied under A. S. Belle and worked with Chardin who became an intimate friend. Accepted by the Academy in 1731, elected a member in 1734 and appointed a counsellor in 1744. He exhibited regularly in the Salon until 1759. His work is in many ways closely related to the Dutch, and he developed a very personal kind of synthesis between the Dutch and the French painting of the period.

Portrait of the Marquise de Sainte-Maure

canvas: 95¾ x 70⅜ inches

Signed and dated: *Aved 1743*.

Aved painted many portraits "à la turque" besides the portrait of Mehemet Effendi, Ambassador of the Sultan, which made his reputation in the Salon of 1742. The present picture shows the Marquise de Sainte-Maure in a somewhat classical pose leaning against a pedestal and vase of an antique style. She is imagined as standing in the garden of a seraglio along the banks of the Bosphorous; the dome and minarets of a mosque are silhouetted against the horizon. The Marquise was the former Marie de Guérin, daughter of Pierre Guérin and Louise de Mirande; she married Louis de Sainte-Maure in 1739.

References: *Collection de livrets des anciennes expositions,* Paris, x, Salon de 1743, p. 24, no. 73; Paris, Musée des arts decoratifs, *Exposition de la turquerie au XVIIIe siècle,* May-Oct., 1911, p. 27, no. 19; J.-L. Vaudoyer, "L'Orientalisme en Europe au xviiie siècle," *Gazette des Beaux-Arts,* 1911, ii, ill. opp. p. 102, p. 101-102, "One can only prove it a little by mentioning the large standing portrait of the Marquise de Sainte-Maure-Montausier by Aved which, less well known than the *Pasha*, was, with the drawings of Liotard, responsible for the success of these 'turqueries' . . . It is with the impression of this magisterial work that we wish to end this rapid study . . ."; G. Wildenstein, *Le peintre Aved,* 1922, ii, p. 124, no. 96, ill. opp. p. 102, i, p. 64-65, "The public is able to judge easily the talent of Aved in this exotic genre. The most beautiful Turkish portrait of our painter appeared in the Salon of 1743. It was that of the Marquise de Sainte-Maure.";

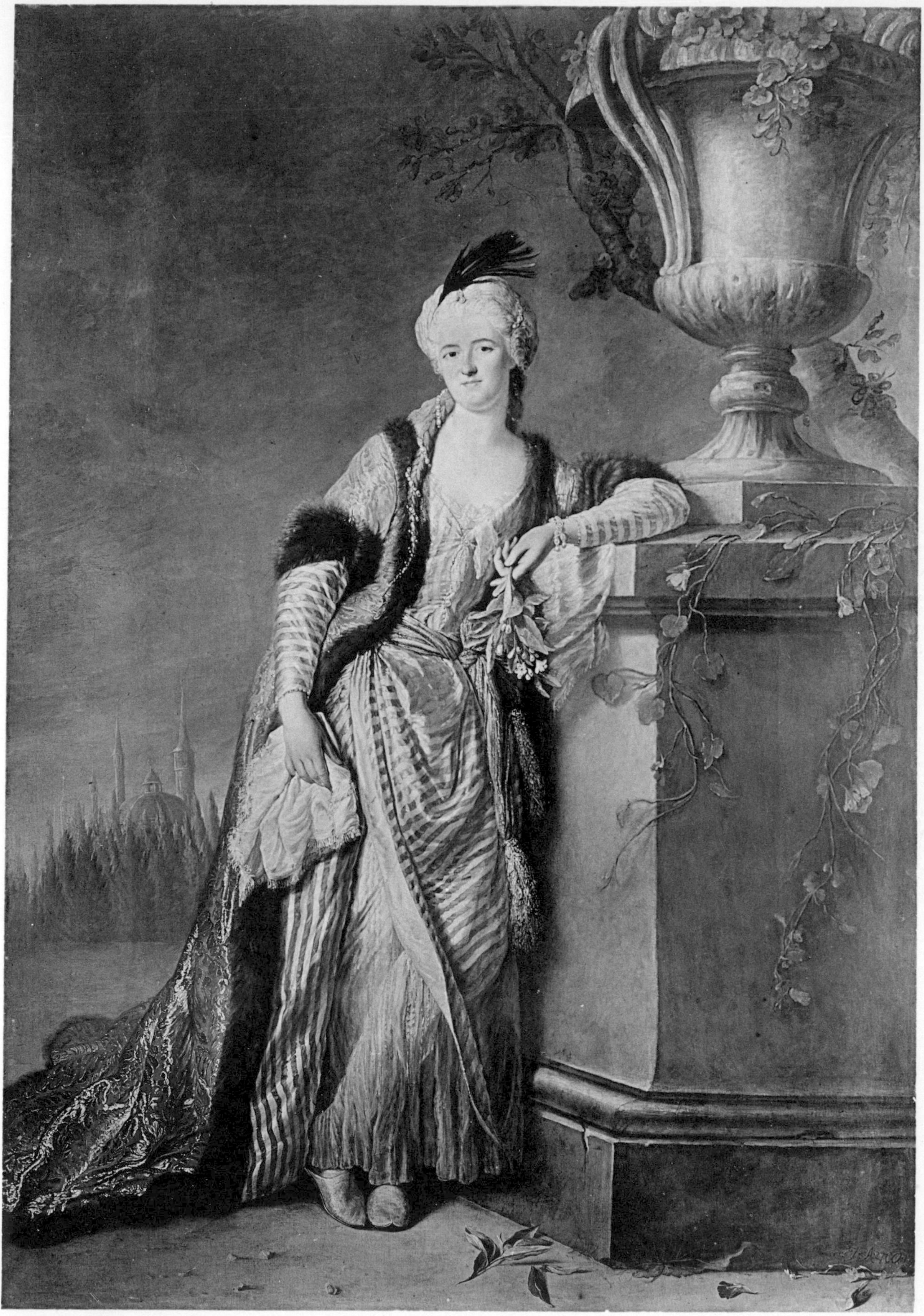

Paris, Gazette des Beaux-Arts, *Le siècle de Louis XV vu par les artistes,* 1934, p. 59, no. 140; S. Rocheblave, *French painting of the 18th century,* 1937, p. 19, no. 28, ill.

Exhibited: 1743, Paris, Salon; 1911, Paris, Musée des arts decoratifs; 1934, Paris, Gazette des Beaux-Arts.

Collections: Marquis de Saint-Maurice Montcalm, Hotel Pozzo di Borgo, Paris.

L'HEUREUSE FECONDITE

BY

FRANÇOIS BOUCHER

1703-1770

FRANÇOIS BOUCHER

1703-1770

A thorough Parisian, he lived in the city all his life except for occasional trips to Beauvais and one journey to Italy with Carle Van Loo, 1727-1731. First studied with his father, Nicolas Boucher, a painter and engraver, and then with François Le Moine who greatly influenced him although Boucher himself denied this. Became a member of the Academy in 1734 and rose through all the ranks to Director in 1765. First painter of the King and a great favorite of Madame de Pompadour. Through the influence of his friend, Oudry, he received many commissions for tapestry designs, and on Oudry's death in 1755, he became Inspector of the Gobelins factory. An industrious worker, he earned quite a good living and accumulated a valuable collection of drawings.

L'heureuse fécondité

canvas, oval: 25½ x 21¼ inches

Signed and dated lower right: *F. Boucher 1764.*

Engraved by R. Gaillard.

In a sheltered nook in a park a young woman is seated, her hat beside her on the ground. A cupid leans against her and with an arrow pierces the egg she holds in her left hand so that a chicken appears. With her right hand the girl points to the hen who is sitting on her nest. At her feet is a dog. Two cupids in the upper left are emptying a vase from which a small waterfall descends gently towards the central group.

References: G. Kahn, *Boucher* (L'Art et le beau), n.d., ill. opp. p. 42 (engraving); *Choix de tableaux gravés d'après François Boucher,* n.d., pl. 66 (engraving); A. Michel, *François Boucher,* n.d., p. 81, no. 1460, p. 165; *Bulletin des Beaux-Arts,* "Liste des pièces gravées par et d'après François Boucher," 2nd year, 1884-1885, suppl. p. 24.

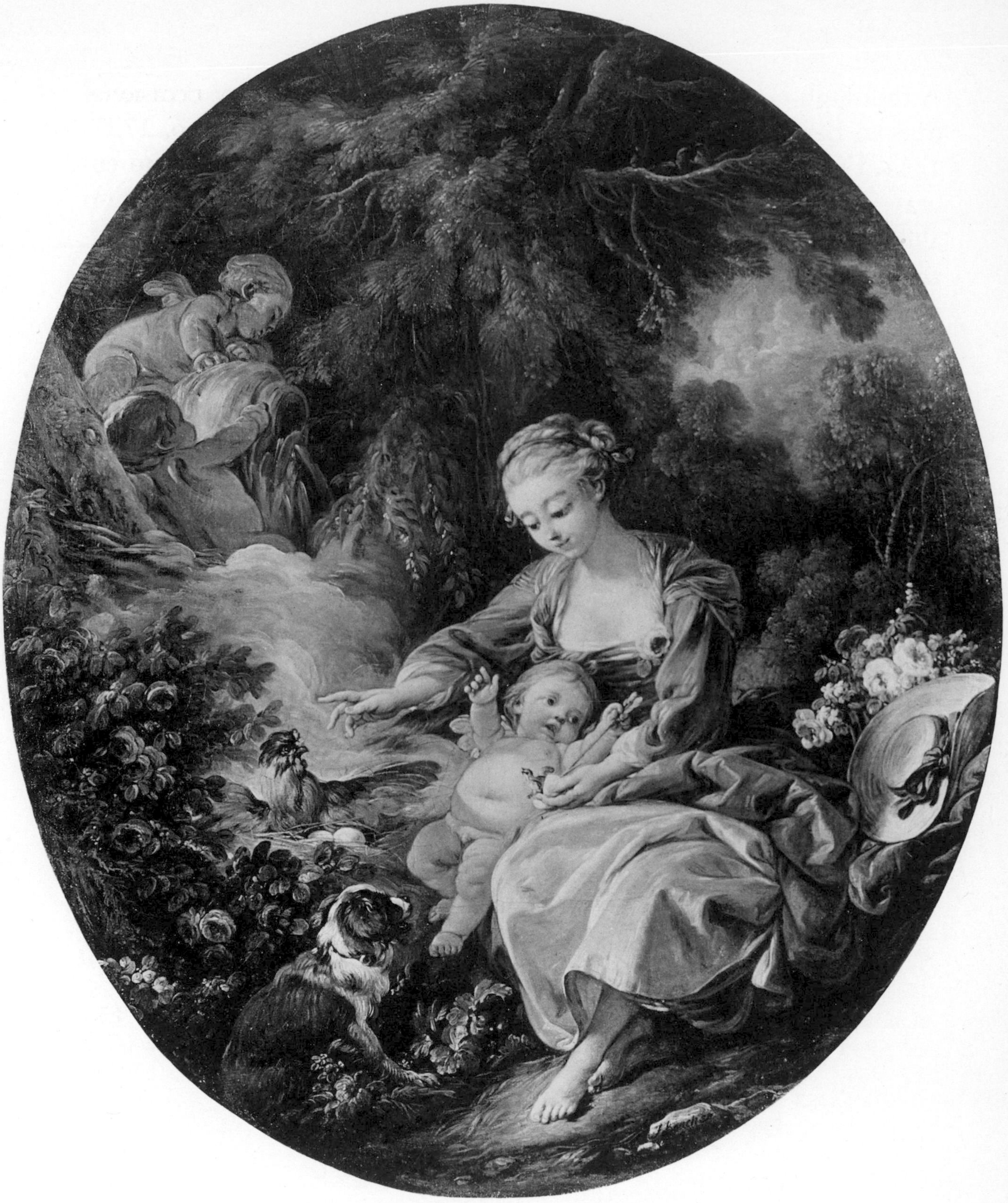

MERCURY CONFIDING THE YOUNG BACCHUS TO THE NYMPHS

BY

FRANÇOIS BOUCHER

1703-1770

FRANÇOIS BOUCHER

1703-1770

A thorough Parisian, he lived in the city all his life except for occasional trips to Beauvais and one journey to Italy with Carle Van Loo, 1727-1731. First studied with his father, Nicolas Boucher, a painter and engraver, and then with François Le Moine who influenced him greatly although Boucher himself denied this. Became a member of the Academy in 1734 and rose through all the ranks to Director in 1765. First painter of the King and a great favorite of Madame de Pompadour. Through the influence of his friend, Oudry, he received many commissions for tapestry designs, and on Oudry's death in 1755, he became Inspector of the Gobelins factory. An industrious worker, he earned quite a good living and accumulated a valuable collection of drawings.

Mercury confiding the young Bacchus to the Nymphs

canvas: 23½ x 29 inches

According to Lucian, Bacchus, the son of Jupiter and Semele, was carried by Mercury immediately after his birth, to the nymphs of Nysa. In this illustration of the scene, five nymphs surround the infant Bacchus while Mercury hovers above. Two more nymphs are lightly indicated in the left background. This picture is a study for the one in the Wallace collection which was bought by Lord Hertford at the Paul Périer sale in 1843.

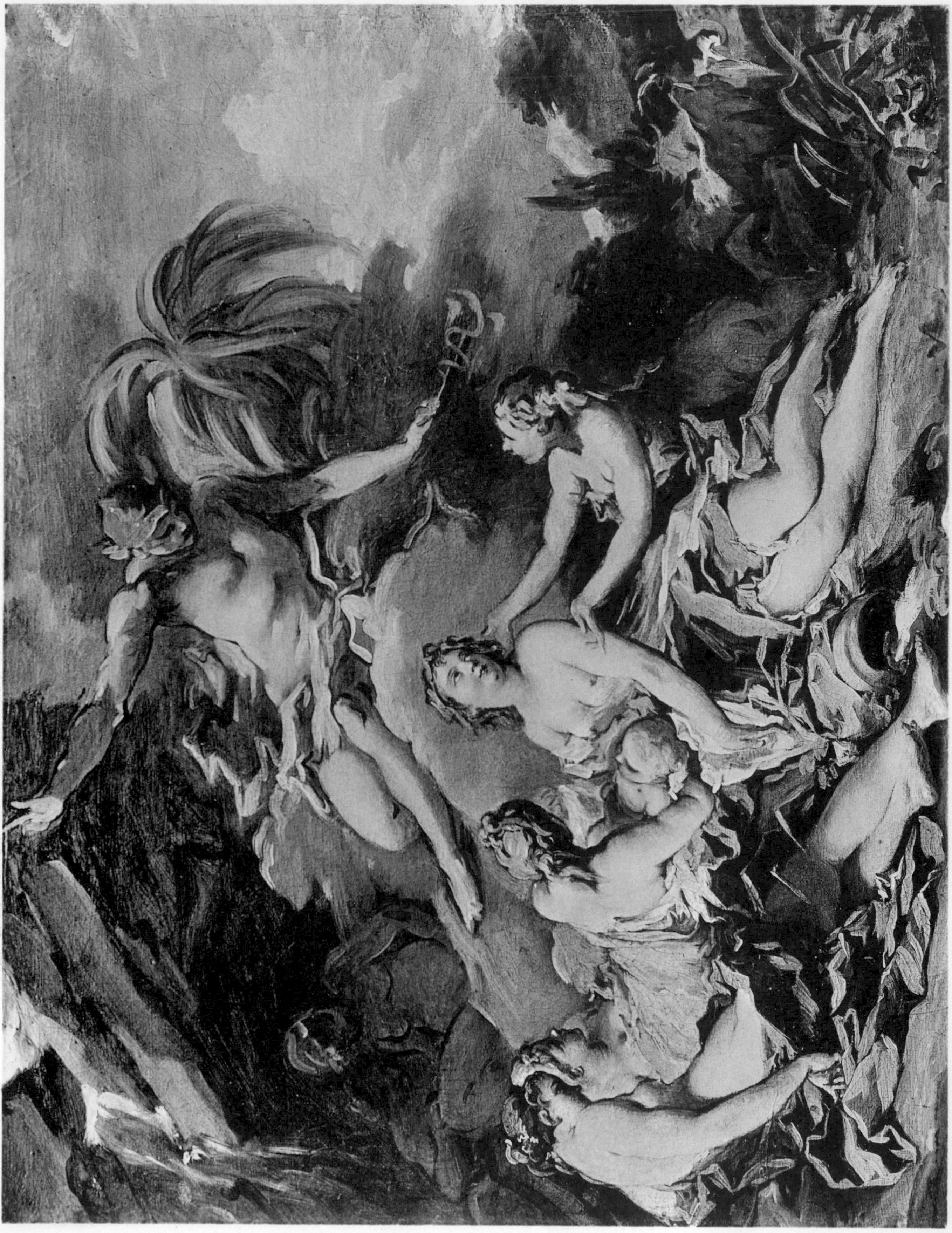

LE SOIR OR LA DAME ALLANT AU BAL

BY

FRANÇOIS BOUCHER

1703-1770

FRANÇOIS BOUCHER

1703-1770

A thorough Parisian, he lived in the city all his life except for occasional trips to Beauvais and one journey to Italy with Carle Van Loo, 1727-1731. First studied with his father, Nicolas Boucher, a painter and engraver, and then with François Le Moine who influenced him greatly although Boucher himself denied this. Became a member of the Academy in 1734 and rose through all the ranks to Director in 1765. First painter of the King and a great favorite of Madame de Pompadour. Through the influence of his friend, Oudry, he received many commissions for tapestry designs, and on Oudry's death in 1755, he became Inspector of the Gobelins factory. An industrious worker, he earned quite a good living and accumulated a valuable collection of drawings.

Le Soir OR *La dame allant au bal*

canvas: 28¾ x 23 inches

Signed and dated lower right: *F. Boucher 1734.*

Engraved by Petit.

A half-length figure of a blond girl in a slate-colored dress, holding a mask in her right hand. On her head she wears a small blue cap with a feather and around her neck a piece of blue ribbon. A red drapery falls from the right corner and billows around her.

References: A. Michel, *Boucher,* n.d., p. 169; London, Christie, Manson & Woods, *Novar sale,* June 1, 1878, p. 5, no. 16; London, Christie, Manson & Woods, *John White sale,* Mar 28, 1903, p. 11, no. 52; H. MacFall, *Boucher,* 1908, p. 155.

Collections: Novar (Hugh A. J. Munroe); J. Posno; John White; Otto Beit; Mrs. Arthur Bull, Tewin Waters, Welwyn.

LE CHIEN BARBET

BY

J.-B.-S. CHARDIN

1699-1779

J.-B.-S. CHARDIN

1699-1779

Chardin's entire life was spent in Paris in the region of St. Germain des Près. Little is known of his youth except that he was born on the Rue de Seine and was the son of a cabinet maker and woodcarver. A pupil of Pierre-Jacques Caze and of Noël Nicolas Coypel, he was admitted to the Academy in 1728 and exhibited regularly at the Salon thereafter. His paintings of domestic scenes and still lifes were much appreciated by his contemporaries and his technical innovation – the juxtaposition rather than the blending of colors – aroused great interest. In 1734 he was appointed a counsellor and in 1755, Treasurer of the Academy. Chardin is generally conceded to be the greatest exponent of the realistic trend of the 18th century.

Le chien barbet

canvas: 75½ x 53½ inches

Signed and dated on the lower part of the stone pedestal: *J. S. Chardin 1730.*

A monumental still life composed of souvenirs of the hunt: a duck and a rabbit, a gun and a hunting horn, and a dog, arranged against a background of a vase on a pedestal.

References: Paris, *Vente Aved,* Nov. 24, 1766, p. 50-51, no. 131; Paris, *Vente P * * * (Passalagna),* Mar. 18-19, 1853, p. 24, no. 112; E. & J. de Goncourt, *L'Art du XVIIIe siècle,* 1906, 1, p. 186: "In 1770, at the second sale of the painter Aved, the friend of Chardin . . ."; G. Wildenstein, *Le peintre Aved,* 1922, p. 155, no. 131; New York, Wildenstein & Co., *Exhibition Chardin,* 1926, no. 5, ill.; Chicago, Art Institute, *Paintings by Chardin,* Feb. 3-Mar. 8, 1927, no. 5; G. Wildenstein, *Chardin,* 1933, ill. pl. LII, no. 68, p. 206, no. 677; Hartford, Wadsworth Atheneum, *The painters of still life,* Jan. 25-Feb. 15, 1938, no. 52, ill.; *Art News,* Aug., 1941, 40, p. 23, ill., "Its wonderful naturalism and compositional rhythms go so far ahead of its conventional souvenir de la chasse subject that it seems a prophecy of Courbet rather than a reminiscence of Snyders."; E. Goldschmidt, *J.-B.-S. Chardin,* 1945, fig. 17, opp. p. 70 (detail).

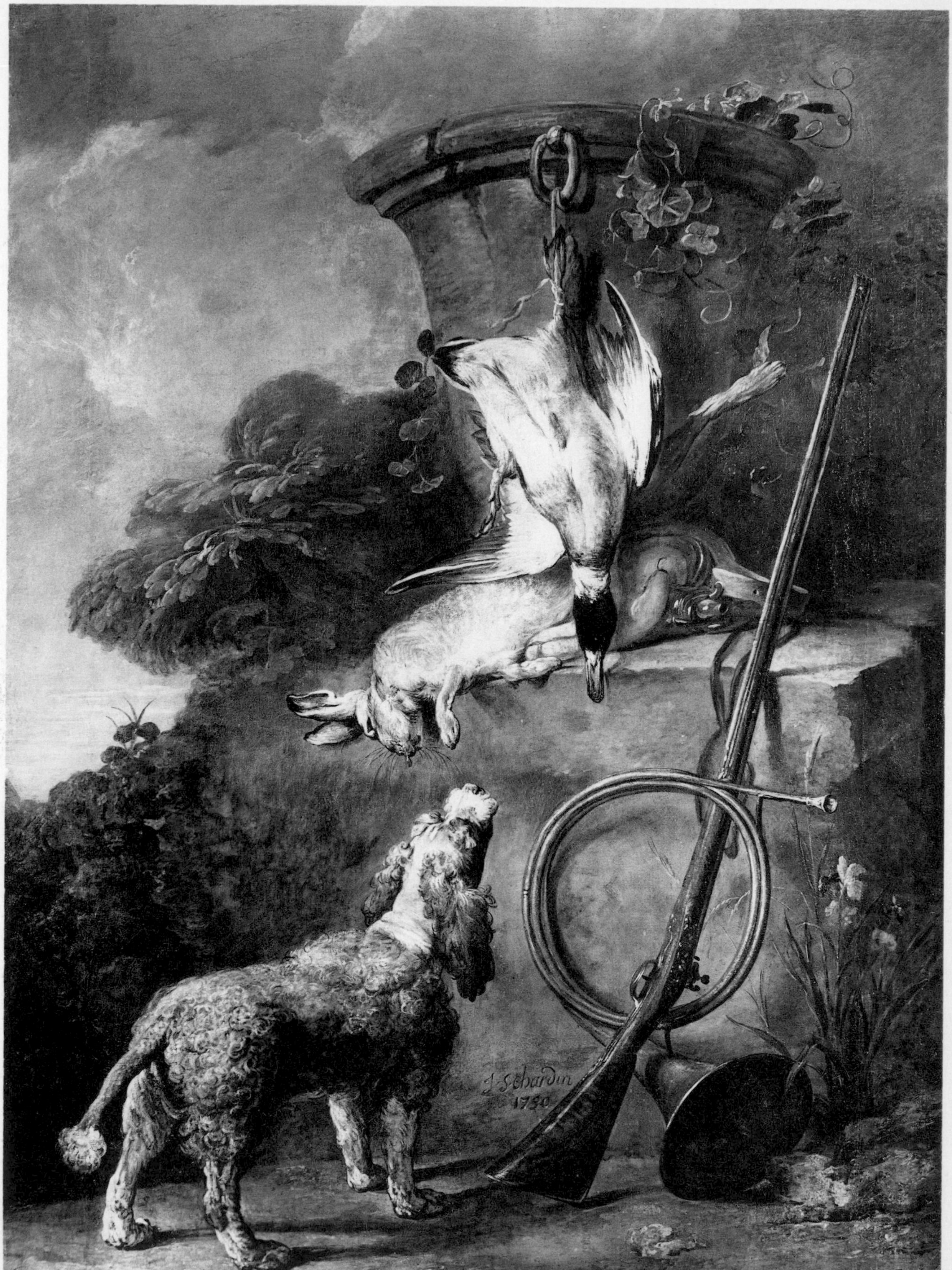
J. S. chardin
1730

Exhibited: 1926, New York, Wildenstein & Co.; 1927, Chicago, Art Institute; 1935, Wilmington, Society of Fine Arts; 1938, Hartford, Wadsworth Atheneum; 1941, New York, Wildenstein & Co.

Collections: J. A. J. Aved; Passalagna ?; Russian collection until 1918.

LE LAPIN ET LA GIBECIERE

BY

J.-B.-S. CHARDIN

1699-1779

J.-B.-S. CHARDIN

1699-1779

Chardin's entire life was spent in Paris in the region of St. Germain des Près. Little is known of his youth except that he was born on the Rue de Seine and was the son of a cabinet maker and woodcarver. A pupil of Pierre-Jacques Caze and of Noël Nicolas Coypel, he was admitted to the Academy in 1728 and exhibited regularly at the Salon thereafter. His paintings of domestic scenes and still lifes were much appreciated by his contemporaries and his technical innovation – the juxtaposition rather than the blending of colors – aroused great interest. In 1734 he was appointed a counsellor and in 1755, Treasurer of the Academy. Chardin is generally conceded to be the greatest exponent of the realistic trend of the 18th century.

Le lapin et la gibecière

canvas: 28¾ x 23½ inches

A simple but beautifully constructed and impressively painted still life composed of only a few objects: a rabbit, a powder flask, a game bag and an apple. Each article is placed with an almost mathematical precision, a quality which must have appealed to Cézanne who admired and frequently imitated this type of painting by Chardin.

References: New York, Wildenstein & Co., *Exhibition Chardin,* 1926, no. 8, ill.; Chicago, Art Institute, *Paintings by Chardin,* Feb. 3-Mar. 8, 1927, no. 8; G. Wildenstein, *Chardin,* 1933, fig. 76, p. 209, no. 709; New York, World's Fair, *Masterpieces of Art,* May-Oct., 1940, no. 195, p. 133, ill. p. 131.

Exhibited: 1926, New York, Wildenstein & Co.; 1927, Chicago, Art Institute; 1940, New York, World's Fair.

Collections: Comte Siry, Paris; Comte Aubarey, Paris.

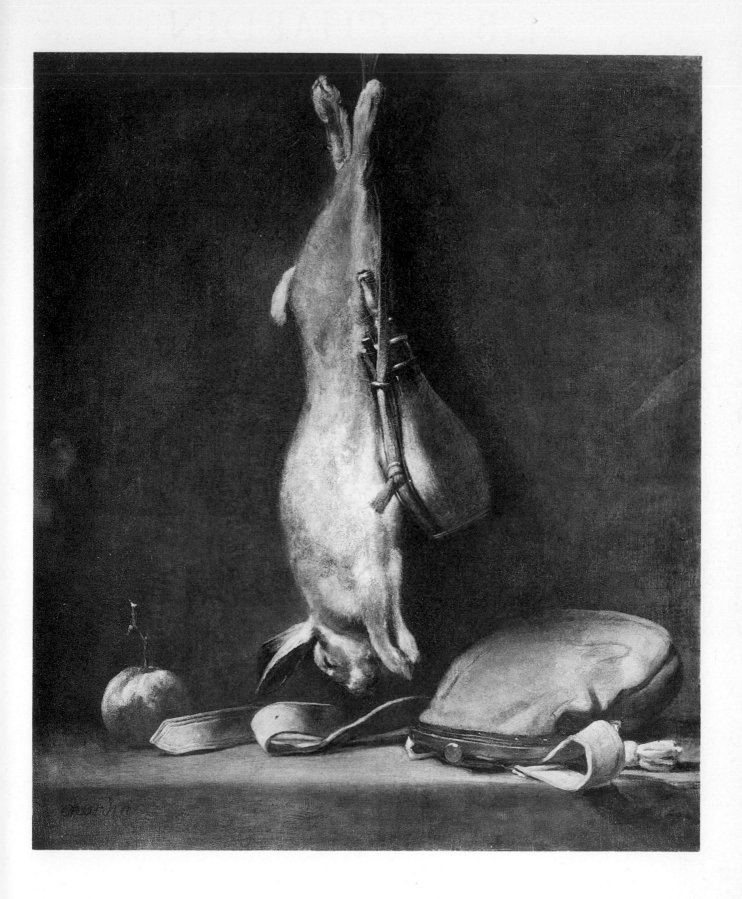

PORTRAIT OF A BOY

BY

J.-B.-S. CHARDIN

1699-1779

J.-B.-S. CHARDIN

1699-1779

Chardin's entire life was spent in Paris in the region of St. Germain des Près. Little is known of his youth except that he was born on the Rue de Seine and was the son of a cabinet maker and woodcarver. A pupil of Pierre-Jacques Caze and of Noël Nicolas Coypel, he was admitted to the Academy in 1728 and exhibited regularly at the Salon thereafter. His paintings of domestic scenes and still lifes were much appreciated by his contemporaries and his technical innovation – the juxtaposition rather than the blending of colors – aroused great interest. In 1734 he was appointed a counsellor and in 1755, Treasurer of the Academy. Chardin is generally conceded to be the greatest exponent of the realistic trend of the 18th century.

Portrait of a boy

canvas: 16¼ x 13 inches

One of Chardin's relatively few portrait studies which illustrates the new current of realism in the 18th century by its casual pose and costume and by its detailed study of the person. Chardin's natural gifts made him admirably equipped as a portraitist, but his contemporaries preferred him as a painter of still life and genre, and it was not until the 19th century, specifically with the Goncourts, that his excellence in this métier was understood and appreciated.

References: New York, Wildenstein & Co., *The child through four centuries,* Mar. 1-28, 1945, no. 11, ill.

Exhibited: 1945, New York, Wildenstein & Co.

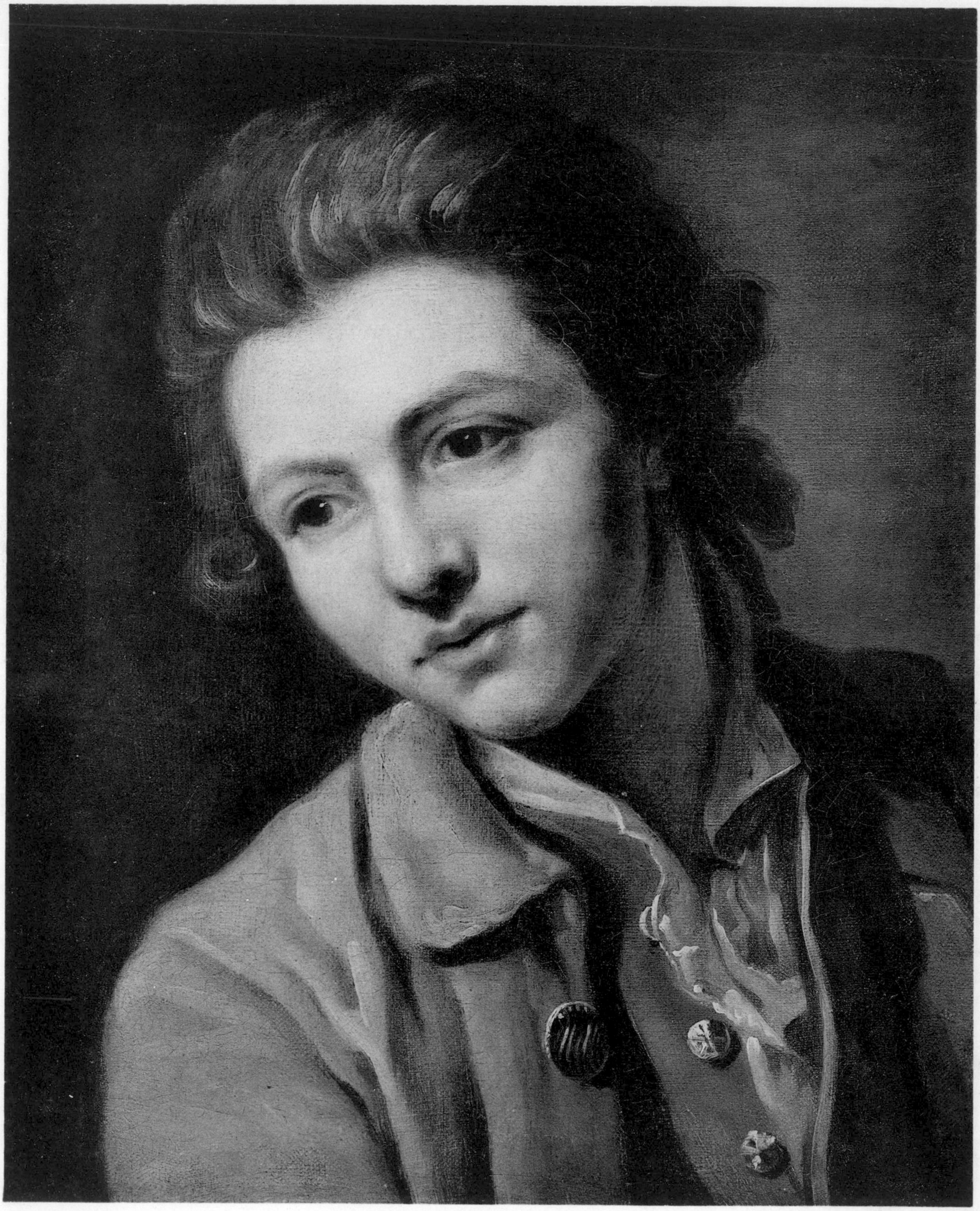

PORTRAIT OF THE ARTIST'S SON, JULES

BY

JACQUES-LOUIS DAVID

1748-1825

JACQUES-LOUIS DAVID

1748-1825

Born in Paris and studied first under Vien on the advice of Boucher, a distant relative. In 1774 he won the Prix de Rome and from 1775 to 1780 travelled in Italy where the study of archaeology was in great favour. Accepted by the Academy in 1783, and again in Rome in 1784. On his return to Paris, he became the most fashionable painter of the day and later, under the Directoire, his status was similar to that of Lebrun under Louis XIV. An enthusiastic Republican and follower of Robespierre, he was twice imprisoned. Although he had said, after Robespierre's fall, that he would never again have anything to do with man, only with principles, he became an ardent admirer of Napoleon and the Emperor's favorite painter. Died in Brussels where he was living in exile after the return of the Bourbons.

Portrait of the artist's son, Jules

canvas: 15½ x 13⅛ inches

A portrait of Charles-Louis-Jules David, the son of David and his wife, the former Marguerite Charlotte Pecoul. He was born in 1783 in Paris and in 1815 accompanied his father in exile to Brussels. In 1816 he went to Greece and from this time until 1820 he taught, first at Chio and then at Smyrne. Returned to France where he taught Greek literature at the Faculté des lettres de Paris. Published several books on the Greek language in addition to his famous biography of his father. Died in Paris in 1854. The present portrait appears to have been painted when he was about five years old.

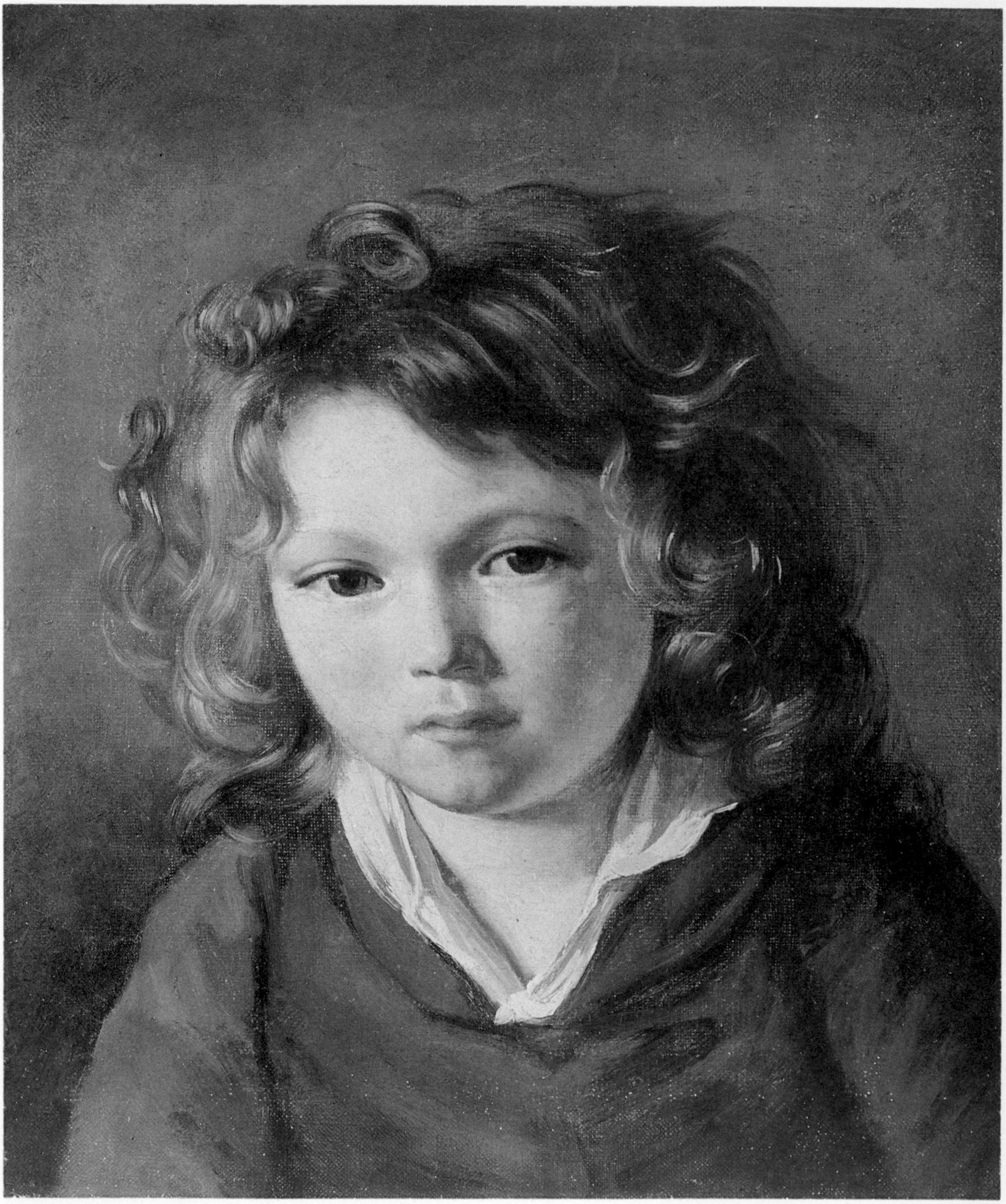

PORTRAIT OF MADAME BURON

BY

JACQUES-LOUIS DAVID

1748-1825

JACQUES-LOUIS DAVID

1748-1825

Born in Paris and studied first under Vien on the advice of Boucher, a distant relative. In 1774 he won the Prix de Rome and from 1775 to 1780 travelled in Italy where the study of archaeology was in great favour. Accepted by the Academy in 1783, and again in Rome in 1784. On his return to Paris, he became the most fashionable painter of the day and later, under the Directoire, his status was similar to that of Lebrun under Louis XIV. An enthusiastic Republican and follower of Robespierre, he was twice imprisoned. Although he had said, after Robespierre's fall, that he would never again have anything to do with man, only with principles, he became an ardent admirer of Napoleon and the Emperor's favorite painter. Died in Brussels where he was living in exile after the return of the Bourbons.

Portrait of Madame Buron

canvas: 25¾ x 21½ inches

Signed and dated over left shoulder: *J. L. David 1769.*

A half-length figure seated in an armchair before a small table on which she rests her arms. In her left hand she holds an open book and with her right she shades her eyes. An early portrait of David's aunt, already exhibiting those qualities which make David one of the greatest portraitists of all time, but still completely within the 18th century tradition.

References: J. J. David, *Le peintre Louis David,* 1880, I, pp. 7, 631; Paris, *Vente Regnault,* June 22, 1905, p. 8, no. 2, ill. pl. opp. p. 8; Paris, Palais des beaux-arts, *Exposition David et ses élèves,* Apr. 7-June 9, 1913, p. 14, no. 2; R. Cantinelli, *Jacques-Louis David,* 1930, p. 99, no. 3, p. 8, "Cited by Miel as dating among the earliest studies of David, 1766-1775."; K. Holma, *David, son évolution et son style,* 1940, p. 124, no. 2, pp. 21, 111, "These canvases (M. & Mme Buron) are studied with an attention which fortells the penetration of the individual's character, later so remarkable in the painter."; New York, Wildenstein & Co., *Fashion in headdress,* Apr. 27-

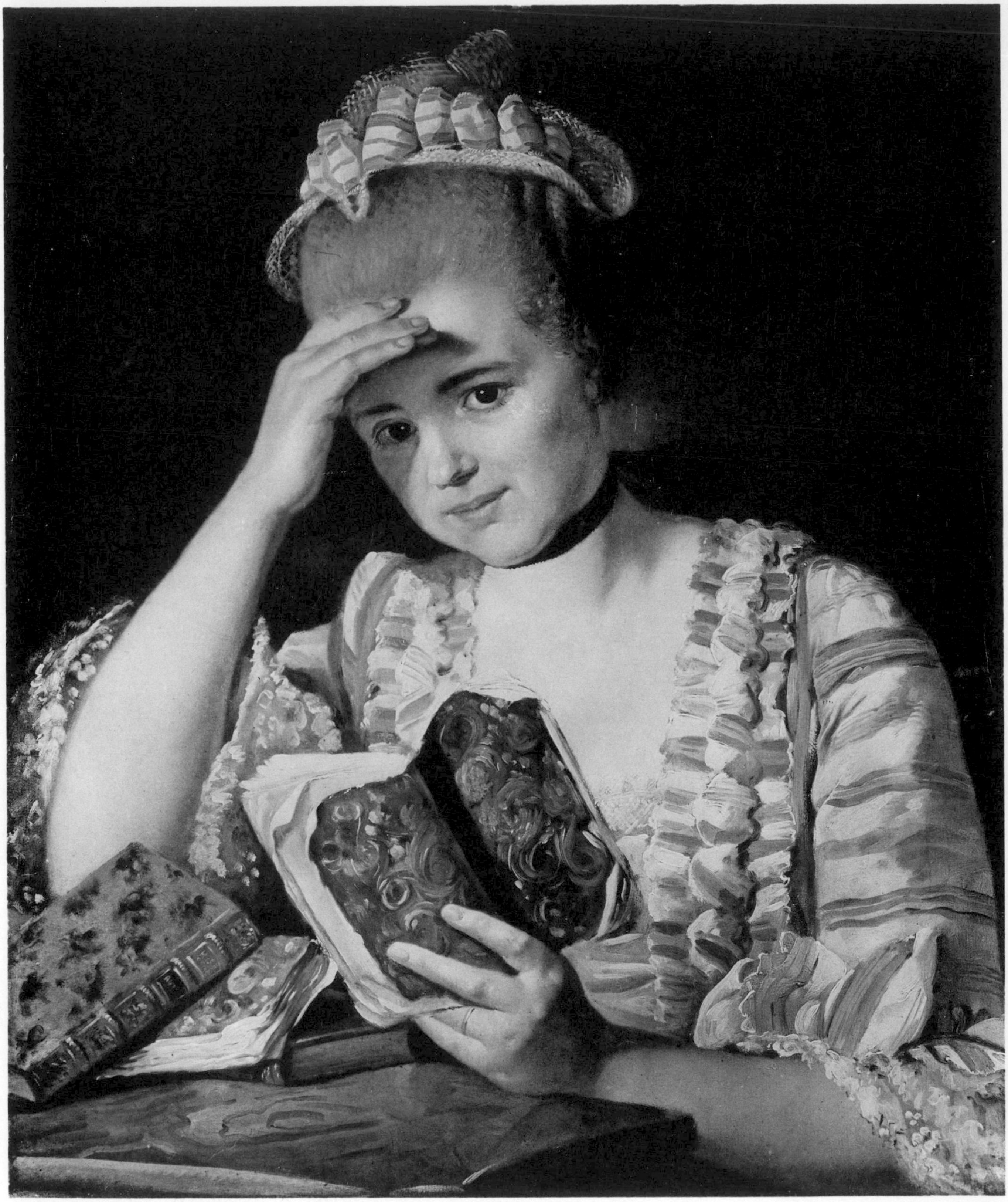

May 27, 1943, fig. 73, no. 53; Toledo, Museum of Art, Nov.-Dec., 1946, Toronto, Art Gallery, Jan.-Feb., 1947, *Spirit of modern France,* no. 10.

Exhibited: 1913, Paris, Palais des beaux-arts; 1943, New York, Wildenstein & Co.; 1946, Toledo, Art Museum; 1947, Toronto, Art Gallery.

Collections: M. Regnault, in Paris until 1925 (A member of the family of David).

PORTRAIT OF THE DUC DE BERRY AND THE COMTE DE PROVENCE AS CHILDREN

BY

FRANÇOIS-HUBERT DROUAIS

1727-1775

FRANÇOIS-HUBERT DROUAIS

1727-1775

The most eminent member of a family of artists, the son of the fashionable portraitist and miniaturist, Hubert Drouais (1699-1769). Pupil of his father and later of Carle Van Loo, Natoire and Boucher. Famous as a painter of children and also very popular at the Court where he produced several portraits of Madame de Pompadour and Madame Dubarry. His son, Germain-Jean, was also a painter and became a pupil of David.

Portrait of the Duc de Berry and the Comte de Provence as children

canvas: 37½ x 50 inches

Signed and dated on the stone pedestal: *Drouais le fils 1757.*

The Duc de Berry and the Comte de Provence became Louis XVI and Louis XVIII respectively. This portrait was commissioned in 1756 by Monsieur le Dauphin and Madame la Dauphine, son and daughter-in-law of Louis XV, and was completed in April 1757.

References: *Collection des livrets des anciennes expositions,* Salon de 1757, p. 25, no. 105; "Observations sur les tableaux exposés au Louvre, par MM. de l'Académie royale de peinture & de sculpture," *Mercure de France,* Oct. 1757, 2nd part, p. 166, "M. Drouais le fils shows much talent and facility in the different portraits which he exhibited. That in which the Duc de Berry is represented holding some fruits and the Comte de Provence playing with a dog, has carried away all the votes."; E. Bellier de la Chavignerie & L. Auvray, *Dictionnaire général des artistes de l'école française,* 1882, I, p. 448; F. Engerand, *Inventaire des tableaux commandés et achetés par la direction des bâtiments du Roi,* 1901, p. 166-167; P. Dorbec, "Les Drouais," *Revue de l'art,* XVII, 1905, p. 53; C. Gabillot, "Les trois Drouais," *Gazette des Beaux-Arts,* XXXIV, 1905, p. 387-388, "It is superfluous to say that the first picture (the Duc de Berry & the Comte de Provence) was particularly carefully painted by Drouais; it was a great success and brought immediately to its author other portrait commissions in the circle of the royal

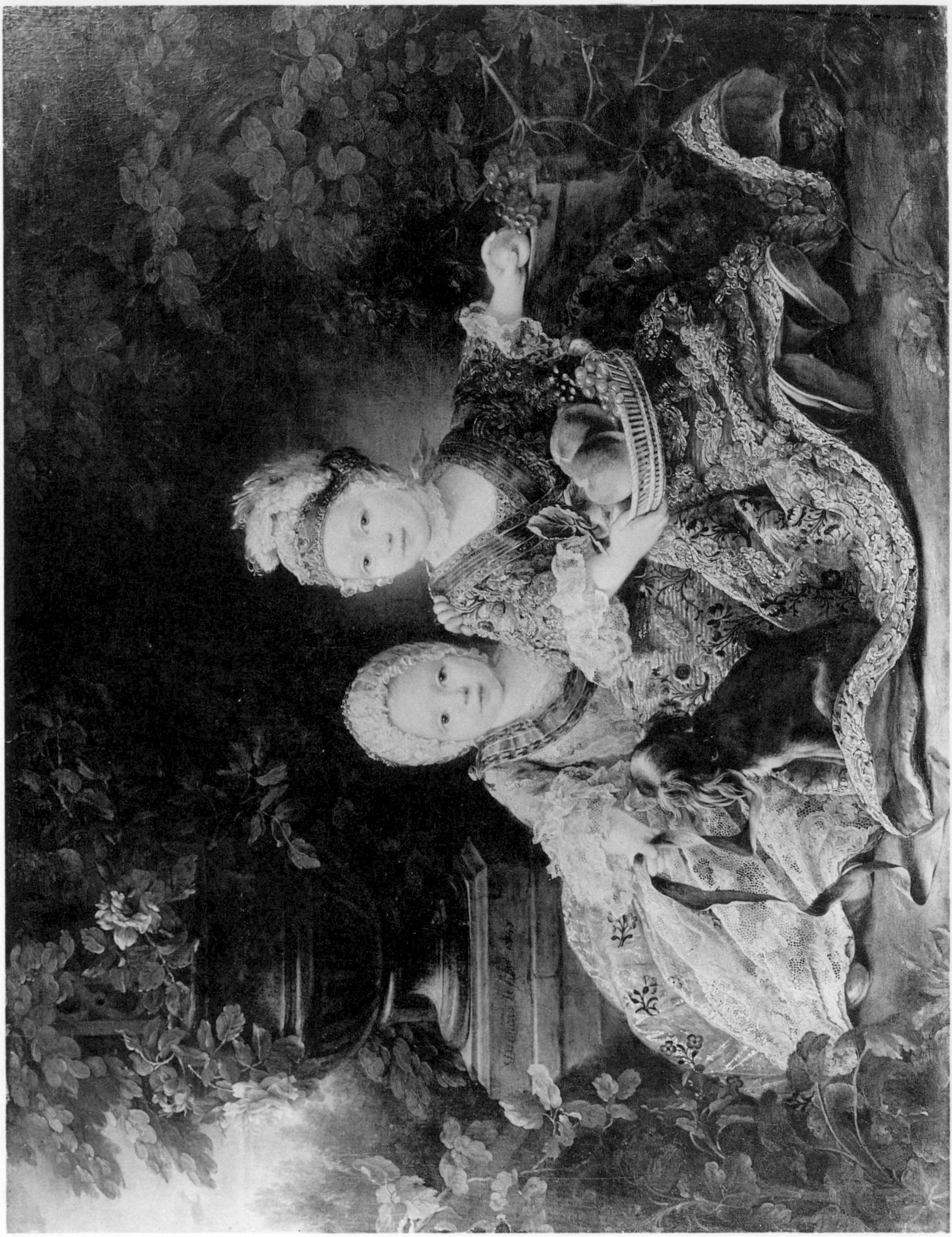

family."; H. Vollmer, "François-Hubert Drouais," *Thieme-Becker,* IX, 1913, p. 577; L. Réau, *Histoire de la peinture française au XVIIIe siècle,* 1925, I, p. 72; G. Wildenstein, *La peinture française au XVIIIe siècle,* 1937, fig. 8; New York, Wildenstein & Co., *Great tradition of French painting,* June-Oct. 1939, no. 21; *Art News,* 41, Apr. 1, 1942, p. 25, ill.; *Pictures on exhibit,* 5, Mar. 1942, p. 7, ill.; New York, Wildenstein & Co., *French revolution,* Dec. 1943, no. 30, ill.; Toledo, Museum of Art, Nov.-Dec., 1946, Toronto, Art Gallery, Jan.-Feb. 1947, *Spirit of modern France,* no. 3.

Exhibited: 1757, Paris, Salon; 1939, New York, Wildenstein & Co.; 1943, New York, Wildenstein & Co.; 1946, Toledo, Museum of Art; 1947, Toronto, Art Gallery.

Collections: Monsieur le Dauphin & Madame la Dauphine, (sold probably in Versailles during the Revolution); Burdett-Coutts, England.

PORTRAIT OF JEANNE-
ADELAIDE D'ANGOT

BY

FRANÇOIS-HUBERT DROUAIS

1727-1775

FRANÇOIS-HUBERT DROUAIS

1727-1775

The most eminent member of a family of artists, the son of the fashionable portraitist and miniaturist, Hubert Drouais (1699-1769). Pupil of his father and later of Carle Van Loo, Natoire and Boucher. Famous as a painter of children and also very popular at the Court where he produced several portraits of Madame de Pompadour and Madame Dubarry. His son, Germain-Jean, was also a painter and became a pupil of David.

Portrait of Jeanne-Adelaide d'Angot

canvas oval: 28¾ x 23¼ inches

Signed and dated: *Drouais, 1772.*

A portrait of Jeanne-Adelaide d'Angot, later Madame de la Motte de Cheney, as a child. She is clothed in a striped dress elaborately trimmed with lace and bows, and is leaning against a chair, part of which is visible in the left-hand corner of the canvas. With her left hand she holds a cat whom she has dressed in a lace bonnet and with her right she tries to persuade the cat to admire his reflection in a mirror.

References: C. Gabillot, *Les trois Drouais,* ill. p. 33 & frontispiece, p. 84, p. 64, "In 1772, Drouais painted four portraits belonging to M. the Marquis de Frotté"; *Art News* 44, Mar. 1-15, 1945, p. 15, ill.; New York, Wildenstein & Co., *The child through four centuries,* Mar. 1-28, 1945, no. 14, ill.; *Art News,* 44, Feb., 1946, p. 20, ill.

Exhibited: 1945, New York, Wildenstein & Co.

Collections: Remained always in the family of Mlle d'Angot, her last descendent being the Marquis de Frotté, Château de Couterne.

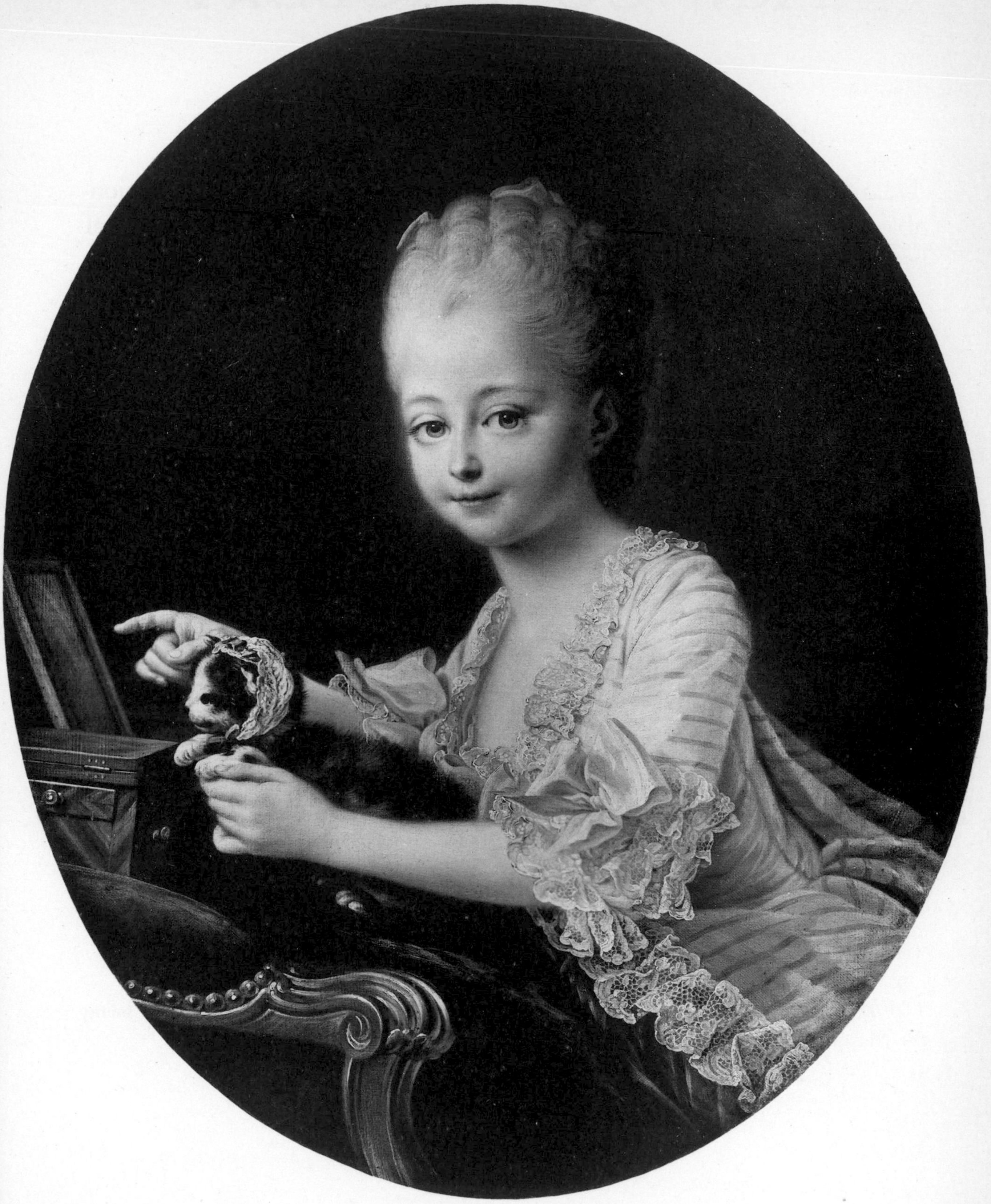

PRESUMED PORTRAIT OF
ANDRE DUPRE DE BILLY

BY

JOSEPH-SIFREDE DUPLESSIS

1725-1802

JOSEPH-SIFREDE DUPLESSIS

1725-1802

First taught by his father and then by the Carthusian monk, J. G. Imbert. At the age of twenty, went to Rome where he studied under Pierre Subleyras. Stayed four years to 1749 and in 1752 went to Paris. Accepted by the Academy in 1769 and made a counsellor in 1780. In 1792 returned to Genoa for a short stay. Almost exclusively a portraitist, and a competitor of Aved, Roslin and Tocqué.

Presumed Portrait of André Dupré de Billy

canvas: 57¾ x 44¾ inches

Knee-length portrait, seated in an armchair and facing the spectator. His left hand rests on some papers which are lying on the corner of a table and his right hand holds a goose quill pen. In the background is a chimney with a mirror in a Louis XVI frame, some candelabras, a porphyry vase and a wall clock. A cup and a sugar bowl are placed on the end of the mantlepiece.

References: New York, Wildenstein & Co., *Portraits of the French 18th century,* 1923, no. 5, ill.; J. Belleudy, *J. S. Duplessis,* 1913, p. 340-341; San Francisco, Museum of Art, *Loan exhibition of paintings by old masters,* 1920, no. 94, ill.

Exhibited: 1923, New York, Wildenstein & Co.; 1920, San Francisco, Museum of Art.

Collections: Comte d'Arjuzon.

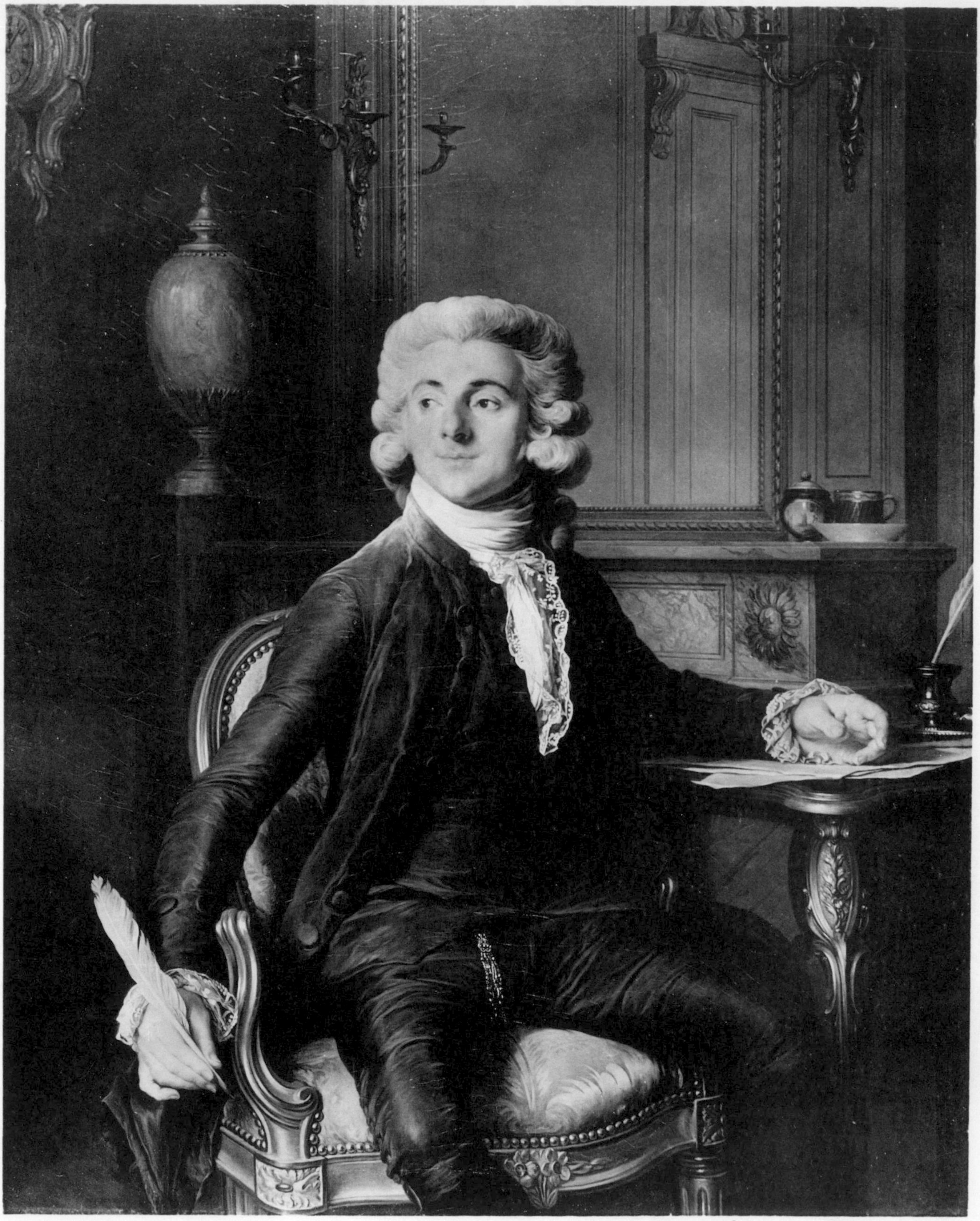

LES AMOURS OR LE PRINTEMPS

BY

JEAN-HONORE FRAGONARD

1732-1806

JEAN-HONORE FRAGONARD

1732-1806

Born at Grasse, the son of a glovemaker, he came to Paris in 1750 where he studied under Chardin for six months and under Boucher for an even shorter period. In 1752 he won the Prix de Rome but did not leave for Italy until 1756, meanwhile attending the Ecole Royale des Elèves Protégés, directed by Carle Van Loo. In Italy, besides travelling to Venice and Naples, he lived for a year at the Villa d'Este with Hubert Robert. Here he studied particularly Cortona and Tiepolo, both of whom helped him to develop the astonishing virtuosity and decorativeness of his mature style. In 1765 he was accepted as a member of the Academy, and when he returned from his second journey to Italy, Austria and Germany in 1773, he was given rooms at the Louvre. The Revolution, however, destroyed his popularity, and although he was protected by David, he was nearly forgotten at the time of his death.

Les Amours OR *Le Printemps*

canvas, oval: 30 x 34¼ inches

In the center of the canvas, two little cupids with short wings, surrounded by roses. The figure to the left holds open with both hands a book of music and that to the right rests his left hand on his companion's shoulder. They are encircled by doves flying in the sky.

References: Paris, Galerie Georges Petit, *Vente M. le comte Daupias de Lisbonne,* May 14-15, 1892, No. 12, ill.

Collections: Comte Daupias de Lisbonne; Miss Burns, London; Marquise of Harcourt, London.

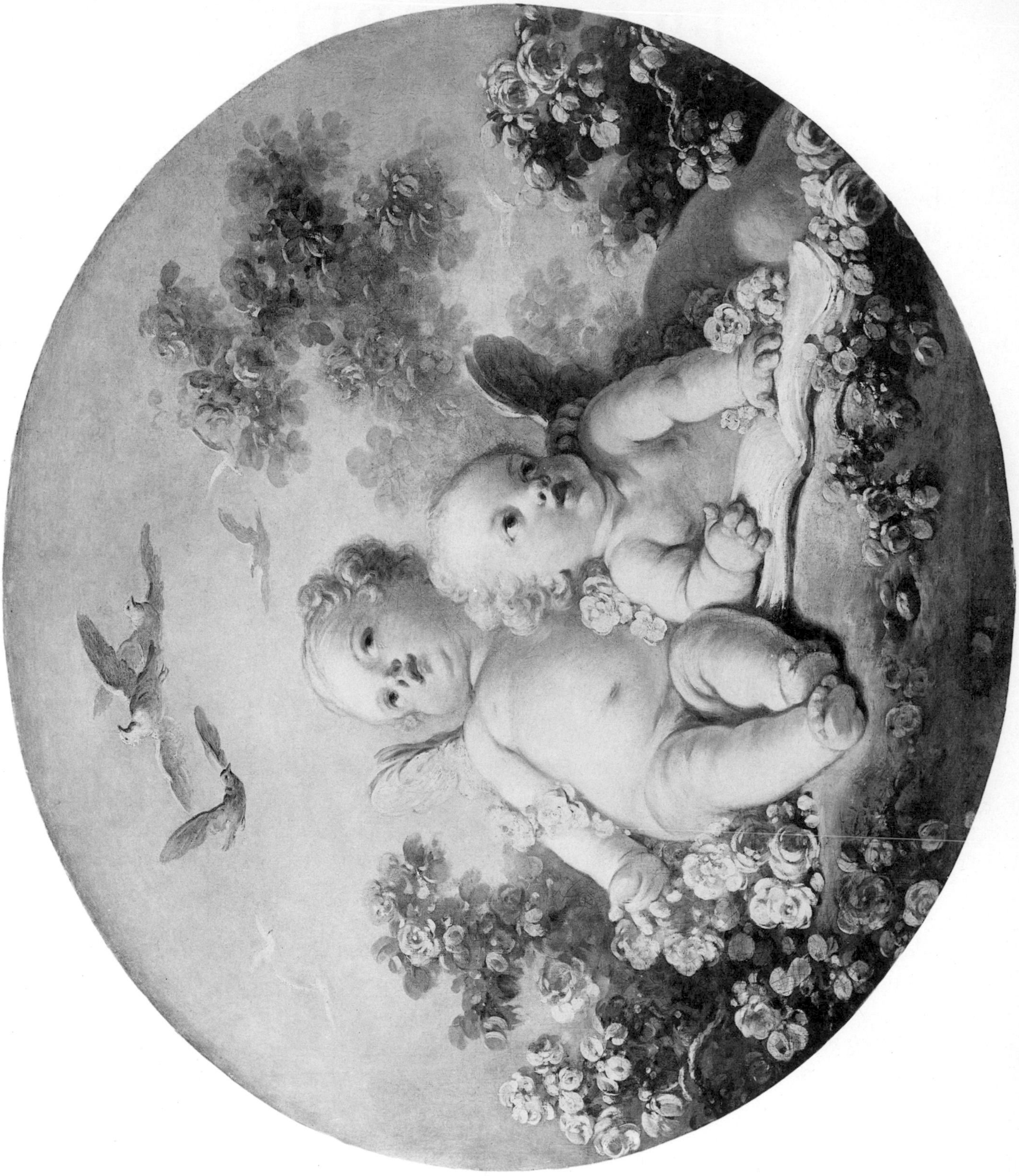

MADEMOISELLE COLOMBE EN AMOUR

BY

JEAN-HONORE FRAGONARD

1732-1806

JEAN-HONORE FRAGONARD

1732-1806

Born at Grasse, the son of a glovemaker, he came to Paris in 1750 where he studied under Chardin for six months and under Boucher for an even shorter period. In 1752 he won the Prix de Rome but did not leave for Italy until 1756, meanwhile attending the Ecole Royale des Elèves Protégés, directed by Carle Van Loo. In Italy, besides travelling to Venice and Naples, he lived for a year at the Villa d'Este with Hubert Robert. Here he studied particularly Cortona and Tiepolo, both of whom helped him to develop the astonishing virtuosity and decorativeness of his mature style. In 1765 he was accepted as a member of the Academy, and when he returned from his second journey to Italy, Austria and Germany in 1773, he was given rooms at the Louvre. The Revolution, however, destroyed his popularity, and although he was protected by David, he was nearly forgotten at the time of his death.

Mademoiselle Colombe en Amour

canvas, oval: 21⅝ x 17¾ inches

An allegorical portrait of one of the famous so-called Colombe sisters, Marie Madeleine Riggieri, born in Venice, December 15, 1760. She and her sister were taken to Paris by their father, a travelling musician, in their early youth, and both had successful careers in the Comédie Italienne. Marie Madeleine made her debut as a dancer in 1771 and performed as a singer from 1776 to 1792. She died in Versailles on the fourth of February, 1841.

Collections: Barlow Webb, England.

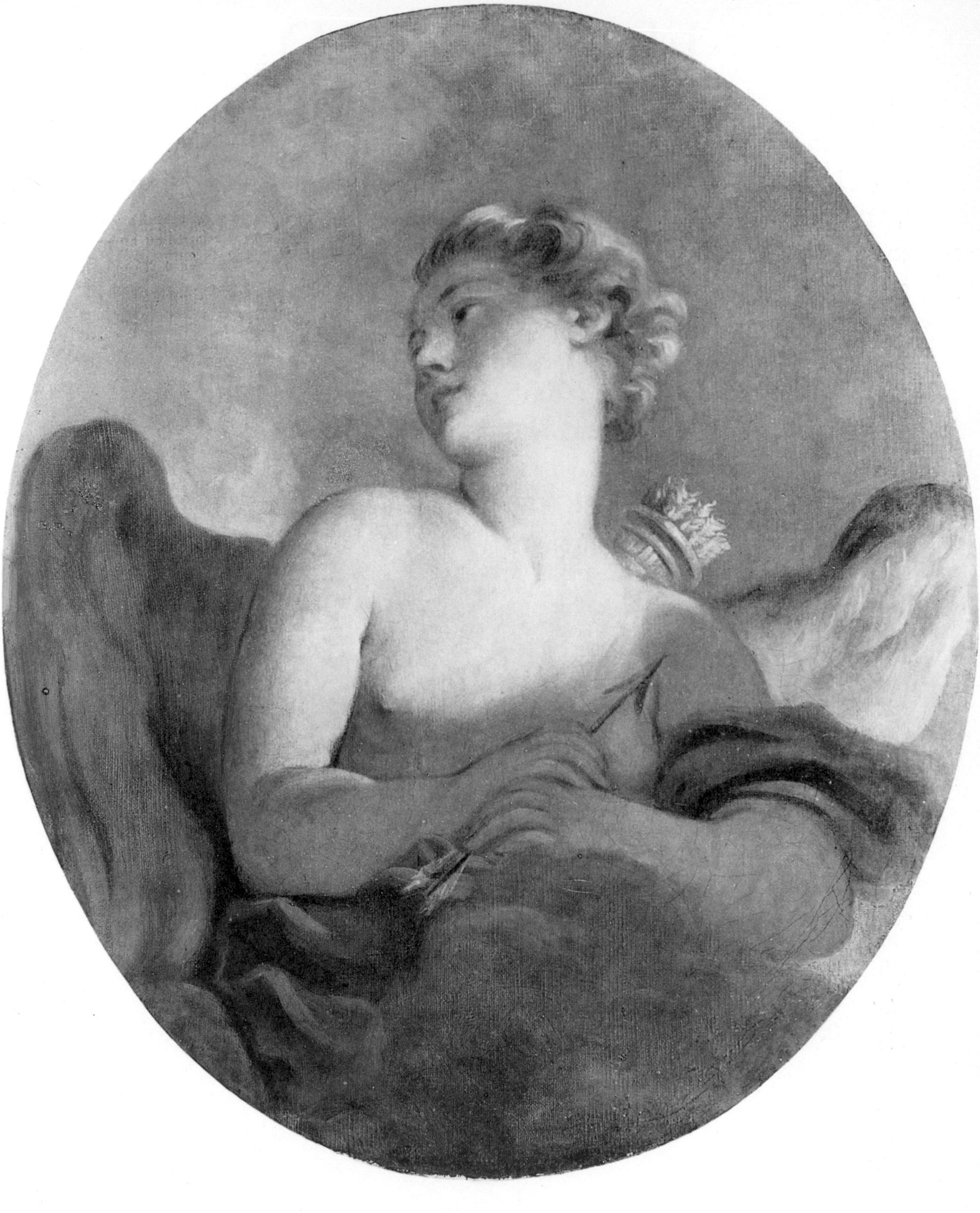

LE PONT DE BOIS

BY

JEAN-HONORE FRAGONARD

1732-1806

JEAN-HONORE FRAGONARD

1732-1806

Born at Grasse, the son of a glovemaker, he came to Paris in 1750 where he studied under Chardin for six months and under Boucher for an even shorter period. In 1752 he won the Prix de Rome but did not leave for Italy until 1756, meanwhile attending the Ecole Royale des Elèves Protégés, directed by Carle Van Loo. In Italy, besides travelling to Venice and Naples, he lived for a year at the Villa d'Este with Hubert Robert. Here he studied particularly Cortona and Tiepolo, both of whom helped him to develop the astonishing virtuosity and decorativeness of his mature style. In 1765 he was accepted as a member of the Academy, and when he returned from his second journey to Italy, Austria and Germany in 1773, he was given rooms at the Louvre. The Revolution, however, destroyed his popularity, and although he was protected by David, he was nearly forgotten at the time of his death.

Le pont de bois

canvas: 24⅜ x 32½ inches

Near a waterfall and under a tent suspended from two trees, a group of women and children are washing clothes. One child points towards the right where a shepherd is guiding his cattle across a rustic bridge.

References: Paris, *Vente M. S.,* Feb. 16, 1861, p. 9-10, no. 16; Paris, *Vente Otto Mundler,* Nov. 27, 1871, p. 4, no. 6; Paris, Hotel Drouot, *Vente X,* May 20-21, 1873, p. 7, no. 15; Paris, *Vente Beurnonville,* 1881, p. 40, no. 63; R. Portalis, *Honoré Fragonard,* 1889, p. 285; P. de Nolhac, *J. H. Fragonard,* 1906, p. 138; Paris, Musée des arts decoratifs, *Exposition d'oeuvres de J.-H. Fragonard,* June 7-July 10, 1921, p. 32, no. 75; *Art News,* Mar. 16, 1929, 27, p. 2, ill., "The smaller 'Pont de Bois' is of a much rarer type, an easel picture in which Fragonard exhibits the full range of his virtuosity."; New York, Wildenstein & Co., *French 18th century paintings,* Mar.-Apr. 1929, no. 18; *Art Digest,* Mar. 15, 1931, 5, p. 32, ill.; *Art News,*

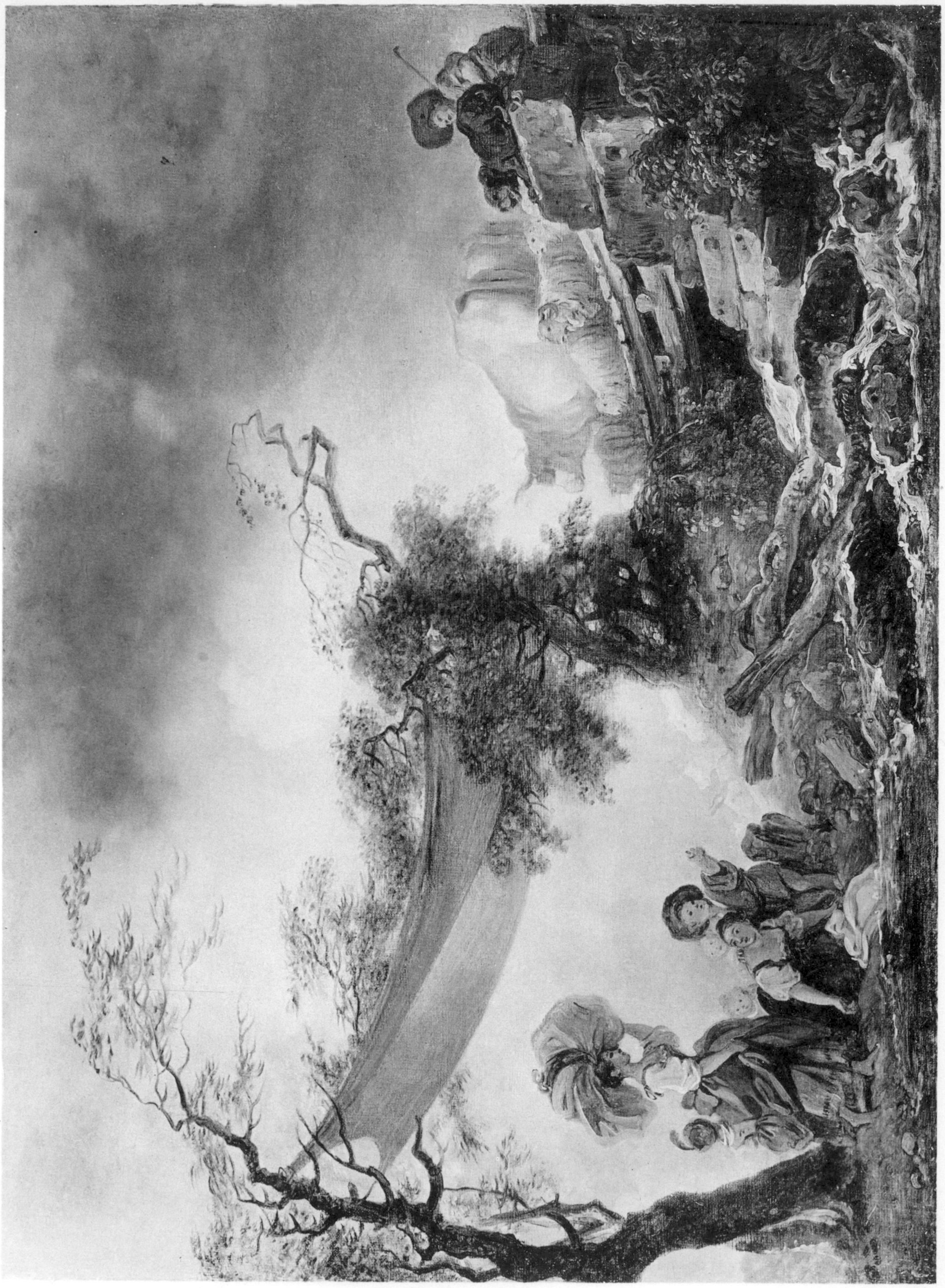

Mar. 14, 1931, 29, p. 5, ill.; New York, American Art Association—Anderson Galleries, *Old and modern masters in the New York art market,* Mar. 15-Apr. 4, 1931; C. Burroughs, "Letter from New York," *Apollo,* 13, May 1931, p. 314, ill., "Among the French paintings one of the most enjoyable is Fragonard's 'Le Pont de Bois'. This illustrates the elegance of the French 18th century in a delightful pastoral vein. . ."

Exhibited: 1921, Paris, Musée des arts decoratifs; 1929, New York, Wildenstein & Co.; 1931, New York, American Art Galleries.

Collections: M. S.; Otto Mundler; Beurnonville; Duc de Castries; Vicomte Emmanuel d'Harcourt, Paris.

LES DELICES MATERNELLES

BY

JEAN-HONORE FRAGONARD

1732-1806

JEAN-HONORE FRAGONARD

1732-1806

Born at Grasse, the son of a glovemaker, he came to Paris in 1750 where he studied under Chardin for six months and under Boucher for an even shorter period. In 1752 he won the Prix de Rome but did not leave for Italy until 1756, meanwhile attending the Ecole Royale des Elèves Protégés, directed by Carle Van Loo. In Italy, besides travelling to Venice and Naples, he lived for a year at the Villa d'Este with Hubert Robert. Here he studied particularly Cortona and Tiepolo, both of whom helped him to develop the astonishing virtuosity and decorativeness of his mature style. In 1765 he was accepted as a member of the Academy, and when he returned from his second journey to Italy, Austria and Germany in 1773, he was given rooms at the Louvre. The Revolution, however, destroyed his popularity, and although he was protected by David, he was nearly forgotten at the time of his death.

Les délices maternelles

canvas: 57 x 38½ inches

One of Fragonard's most charming family scenes, of which he painted a great number after his marriage in 1769. A young mother, assisted by her older child, wheels her baby through a garden where M. René Mauray discerns the strong though thoroughly assimilated influence of Rubens.

References: *Beauty from Bulbs* (Sheepers), frontispiece; R. Mauray, "Les 'scènes familiales' de Fragonard," *Revue de l'art,* Mar., 1925, ill. p. 159, pp. 159-160, 161-162, 163-164, "And thanks to that intelligent pilfering, does not that grand decoration of the *Délices maternelles,* the most important of the 'scènes familiales', become one of the most convincing? If Diderot had been cleverly solicited to draw a moral, what a verse of touching courage would he not have written to his friend Grimm."; New York, Wilden-

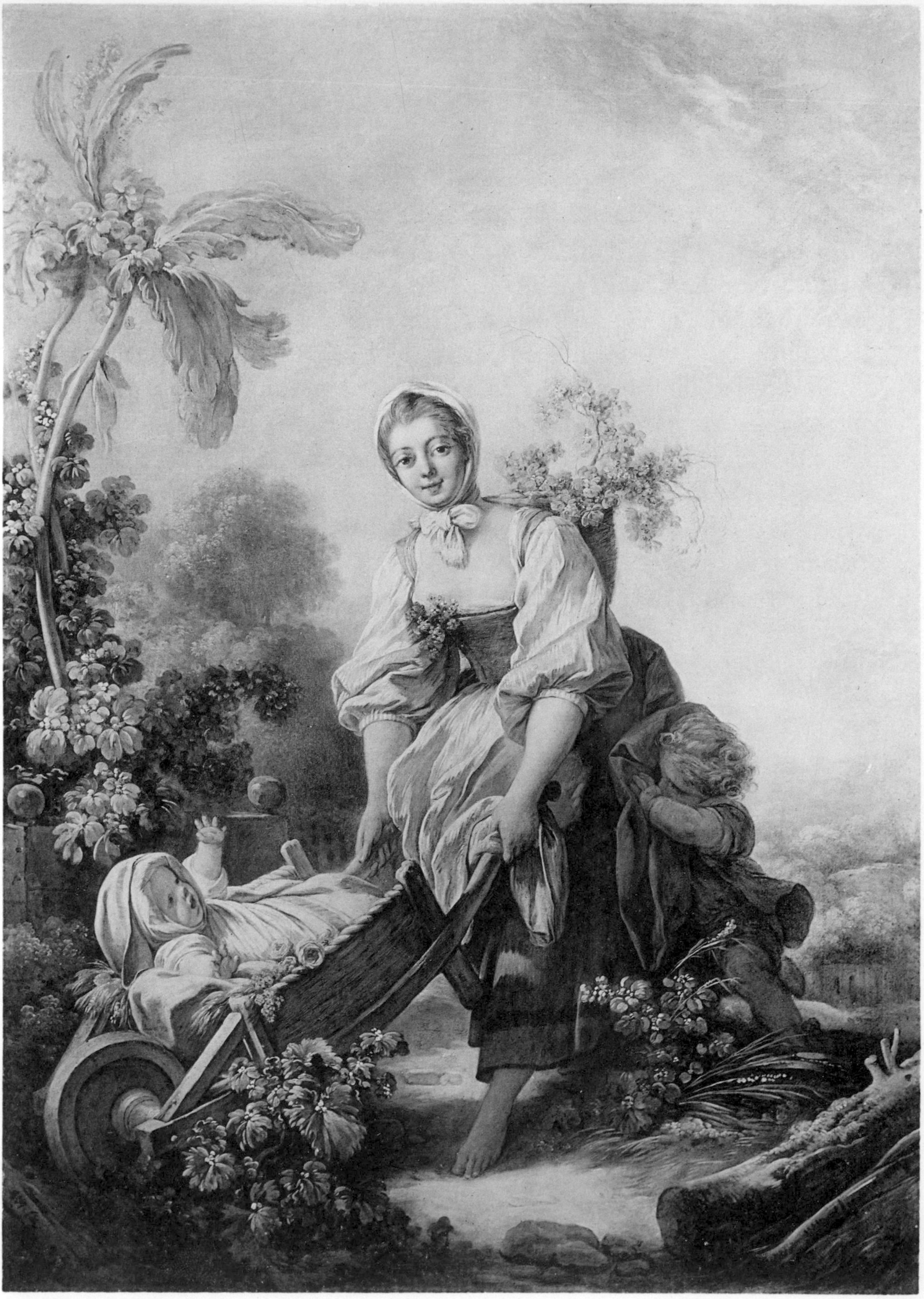

stein & Co., *French 18th century paintings,* Mar.-Apr., 1929, no. 19; Los Angeles, Museum of Art, *Five centuries of European painting,* Dec., 1933, no. 34, ill.

Exhibited: 1929, New York, Wildenstein & Co.; 1933, Los Angeles, Museum of Art; 1935, Wilmington, Society of Fine Arts.

Collections: Comte de Malleray, Versailles; Baron de Rothschild, Paris.

PORTRAIT OF THE ARTIST'S DAUGHTER, ROSALIE

BY

JEAN-HONORE FRAGONARD

1732-1806

JEAN-HONORE FRAGONARD

1732-1806

Born at Grasse, the son of a glovemaker, he came to Paris in 1750 where he studied under Chardin for six months and under Boucher for an even shorter period. In 1752 he won the Prix de Rome but did not leave for Italy until 1756, meanwhile attending the Ecole Royale des Elèves Protégés, directed by Carle Van Loo. In Italy, besides travelling to Venice and Naples, he lived for a year at the Villa d'Este with Hubert Robert. Here he studied particularly Cortona and Tiepolo, both of whom helped him to develop the astonishing virtuosity and decorativeness of his mature style. In 1765 he was accepted as a member of the Academy, and when he returned from his second journey to Italy, Austria and Germany in 1773, he was given rooms at the Louvre. The Revolution, however, destroyed his popularity, and although he was protected by David, he was nearly forgotten at the time of his death.

Portrait of the artist's daughter, Rosalie

canvas, oval: 23 x 20 inches

Bust-length portrait of the painter's daughter at about the age of fourteen. Her head and eyes are turned slightly to the right and she holds a dove with her right hand. Rosalie was the first child of Fragonard and Marie-Anne Gérard, who were married in 1769. She was born in 1770 and died when she was eighteen.

Collections: Madame d'Orbigny Bernon; Mademoiselle de la Gonterie.

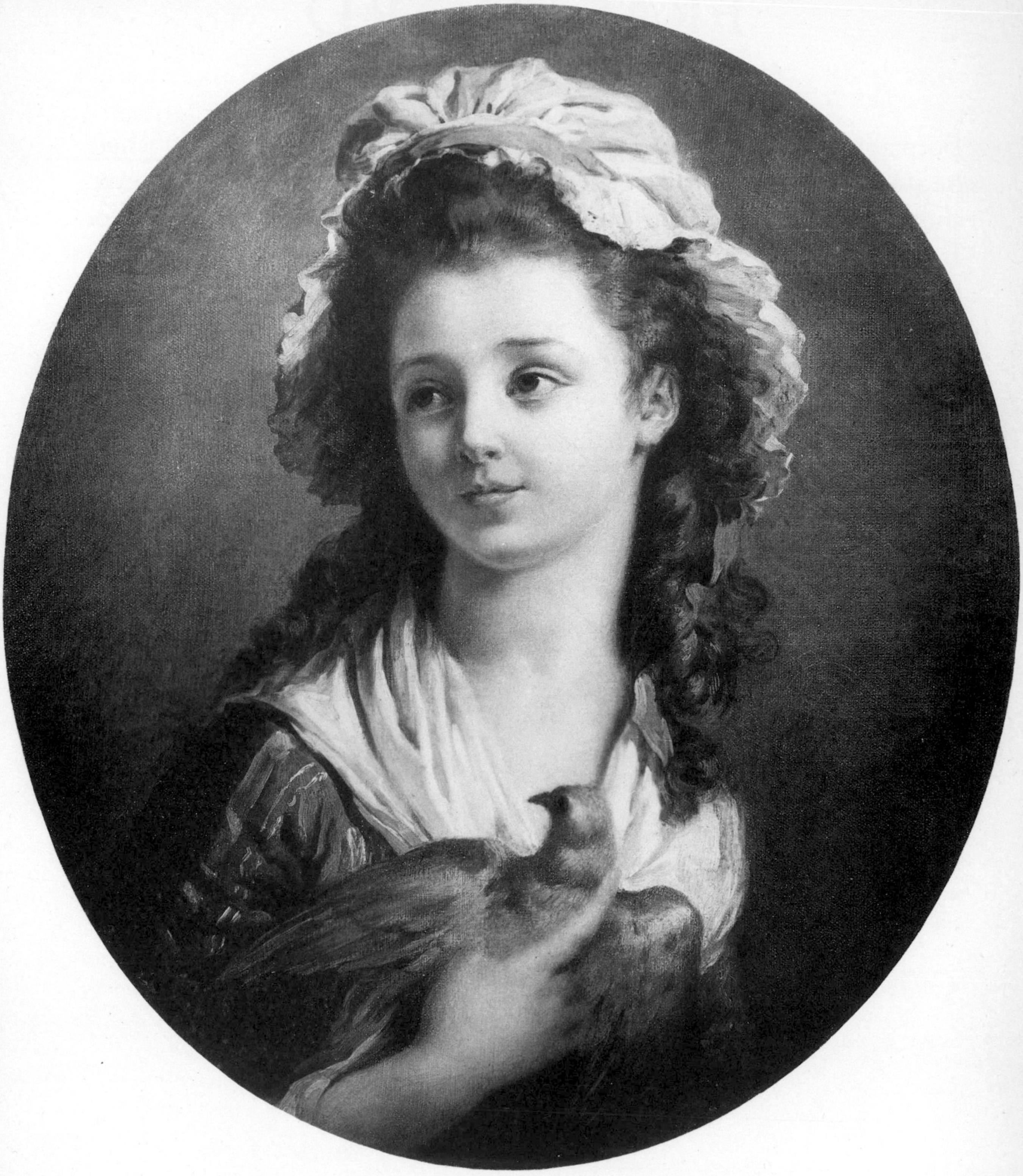

THE GUITAR TUNER

BY

JEAN-BAPTISTE GREUZE

1725-1805

JEAN-BAPTISTE GREUZE

1725-1805

The son of an architect, born in Tournus. Went to Lyon to study under Charles Grandon and then to Paris where he took a course at the Royal Academy under the direction of Natoire. In 1767 accepted by the Academy as a genre painter for the painting of the *Emperor Severus reproaching Caracalla,* which disappointed him as he had hoped to be received as a history painter. Became very popular after the exhibition of 1755 and was highly praised by Diderot for the morality of his paintings and for his marvelous technique.

The guitar tuner

panel: 23½ x 19¼ inches

Engraved by Pierre-Etienne Moitte.

One of a series of pictures painted by Greuze shortly after his return from Italy in 1755. It represents a bird catcher seated on a wooden bench tuning his guitar, after returning from his work. His head is turned towards the spectator so that his ear is near the strings, and his right hand is raised to adjust the pegs. On the wall, the floor and the table in front of him are scattered the tools of his trade: a bird cage, wooden decoys, etc.

References: *Collection des livrets des anciennes expositions,* Salon de 1757, p. 26, no. 115; J. Martin, *Catalogue raisonné de l'oeuvre peint et dessiné de Jean-Baptiste Greuze,* n.d., pp. 10, no. 115, 111; C. Mauclair, *Jean-Baptiste Greuze,* n.d., pp. 39, 41, "In 1757 Greuze exhibited at the Salon an important series of works inspired by his trip to Italy. . . . And finally that Italian series was closed by a bird catcher who tunes his guitar after returning from the hunt."; Baltimore, Museum of Art, *Musical instruments and their portrayal in art,* Apr. 26-June 2, 1946, p. 14, no. 42.

Exhibited: 1757, Paris, Salon; 1874, Paris; 1946, Baltimore, Museum of Art.

Collections: M. Boyer de Fonscolombe, Aix-en-Provence; Branicki.

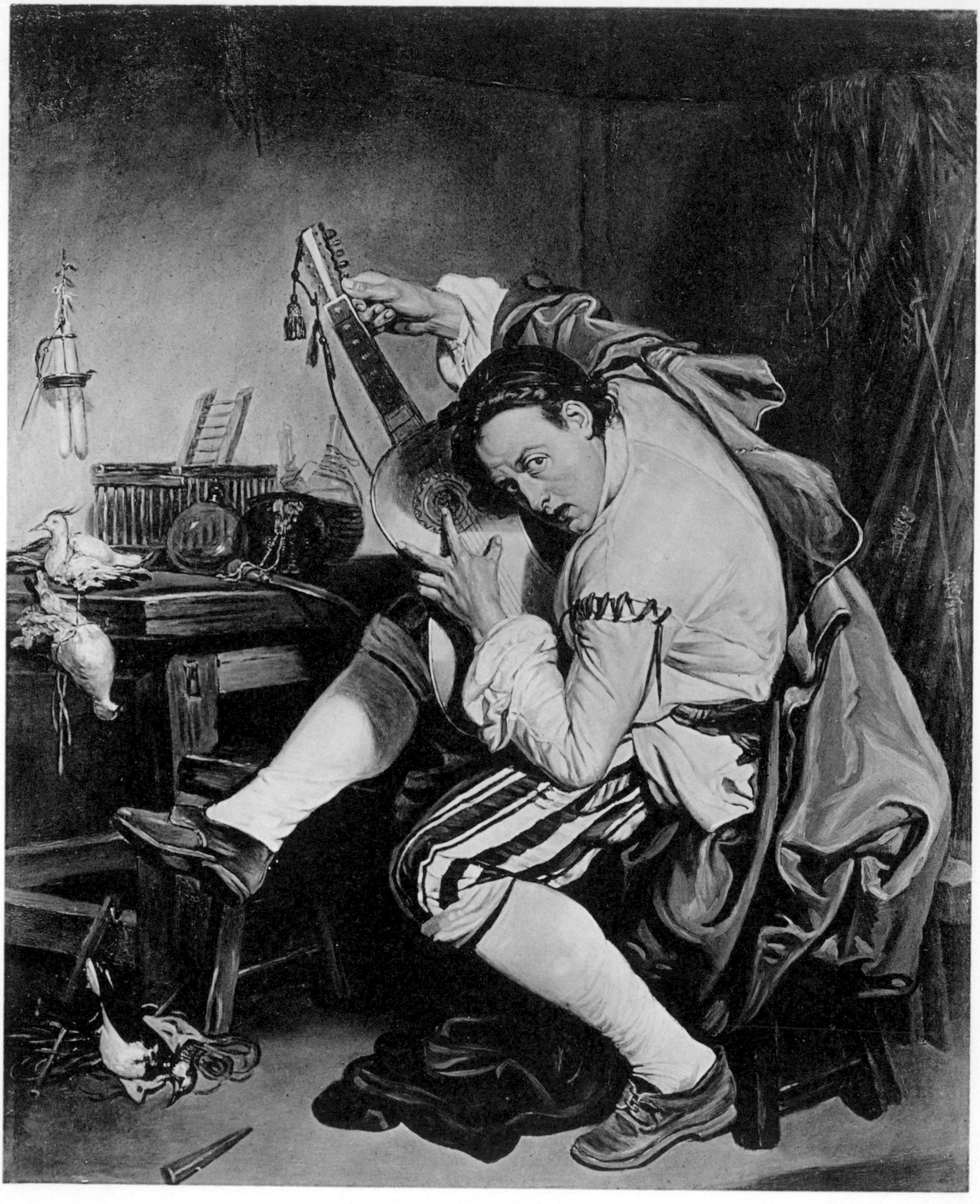

THE DREAMER

BY

JEAN-BAPTISTE GREUZE

1725-1805

JEAN-BAPTISTE GREUZE

1725-1805

The son of an architect, born in Tournus. Went to Lyon to study under Charles Grandon and then to Paris where he took a course at the Royal Academy under the direction of Natoire. In 1767 accepted by the Academy as a genre painter for the painting of the *Emperor Severus reproaching Caracalla,* which disappointed him as he had hoped to be received as a history painter. Became very popular after the exhibition of 1755 and was highly praised by Diderot for the morality of his paintings and for his marvelous technique.

The dreamer

canvas: 15¾ x 12¾ inches

Bust-length portrait study of a young girl reclining against a chair of which only a portion of the tapestried back is visible. Her head is turned slightly to the left and is covered with a transparent veil, the ends falling down over her nude shoulders.

References: Cincinnati, Art Museum, *Exhibition of French paintings of the 18th and early 19th centuries,* Oct. 2-Nov. 7, 1937, no. 10.

Exhibited: 1937, Cincinnati, Art Museum.

Collections: Prince Dietrichstein, Vienna.

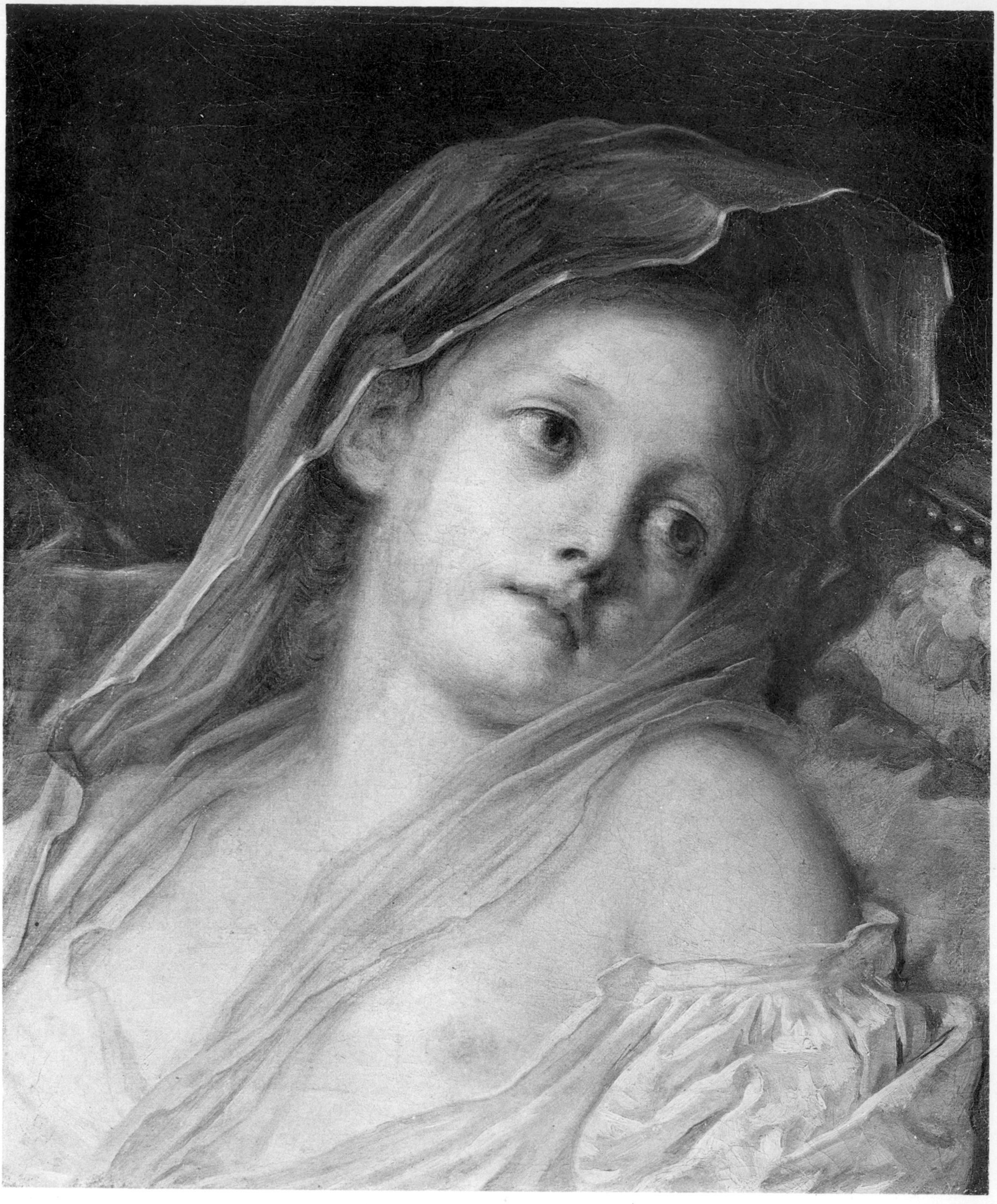

PORTRAIT OF M. DESAIN DE SAINT-GOBERT

BY

JEAN-BAPTISTE GREUZE

1725-1805

JEAN-BAPTISTE GREUZE

1725-1805

The son of an architect, born in Tournus. Went to Lyon to study under Charles Grandon and then to Paris where he took a course at the Royal Academy under the direction of Natoire. In 1767 accepted by the Academy as a genre painter for the painting of the *Emperor Severus reproaching Caracalla,* which disappointed him as he had hoped to be received as a history painter. Became very popular after the exhibition of 1755 and was highly praised by Diderot for the morality of his paintings and for his marvelous technique.

Portrait of M. Desain de Saint-Gobert

canvas: 26 x 21 3/4 inches

Waist-length portrait, seated with his left arm resting on the back of the chair. A handwritten label by M. Desain de St. Gobert states that this portrait of him by M. Greuze was finished the 27th of Vendemiaire 1797 after nineteen sittings and was sent to him the 1st of Nivôse of the same year. A complete record of his sittings for Greuze is also included among the documents. Until recently, the painting has been in the family of M. Desain de St. Gobert.

References: Lafenestre, "Exposition retrospective de Reims," *L'Art,* VI, 1876, p. 262, "Among the numerous pieces which we would like to see again we add to those which we have already mentioned a beautiful portrait of *Desain* by J. B. Greuze, completely authentique and finely executed, belonging to Madame Mora."

Exhibited: 1876, Reims.

Collections: M. Desain de Saint-Gobert; Mme. Prevoteau Desain (sister); Mme Mora-Prevoteau (niece of Desain); M. Edmond Mora; Mme de Joncières-Bailly and Mme Stochet-Bailly; M. Augustin de Joncières.

PASTORALE

BY

JEAN-BAPTISTE HUET

1745-1811

JEAN-BAPTISTE HUET

1745-1811

Son of the animal painter, Nicolas Huet. After studying drawing with C. Renou, became the pupil of J.-B. Leprince and worked also with Boucher and Ch. Dagomer. Accepted by the Academy in 1768, elected a member in 1769 and exhibited continually until 1802. Extremely successful from the time of his debut, an excellent engraver as well as painter and draughtsman. Also connected with the factories of both Gobelin and Beauvais tapestries.

Pastorale

canvas: 25½ x 31½ inches

Engraved by Demarteau in color.

To the right, a shepherd seated on the ground holding a bird's nest. Behind him a cow and a hay loft on which a small boy is reclining. A shepherdess stands next to them, her dog and her flock of goats surrounding her. To the left, a tree and a distant landscape view.

References: C. Gabillot, *Les Huet,* 1892, p. 170; Paris, Bagatelle, *Le XVIIIe siècle aux champs,* June 6-July 7, 1929, no. 32; Hartford, Wadsworth Atheneum, *Retrospective exhibition of landscape painting,* Jan. 20-Feb. 9, 1931, no. 66, ill.; Toledo, Museum of Art, *French furnishings of the 18th century,* Dec. 3-31, 1933, no. 29; Los Angeles, Museum of Art, *European paintings by old and modern masters,* June 13-Aug. 5, 1934, no. 11; S. Rocheblave, *French painting in the XVIII century,* 1937, pl. 72; Buenos Aires, Wildenstein & Co., *Pinturas francesas del siglo XVIII,* June, 1947, no. 10.

Exhibited: 1929, Paris, Bagatelle; 1931, Hartford, Wadsworth Atheneum; 1931, New York, Union League Club; 1933, Toledo, Museum of Art; 1934, Los Angeles, Museum of Art; 1935, Wilmington Society of Fine Arts; 1947, Buenos Aires, Wildenstein & Co.

Collections: Dr. de Payenneville.

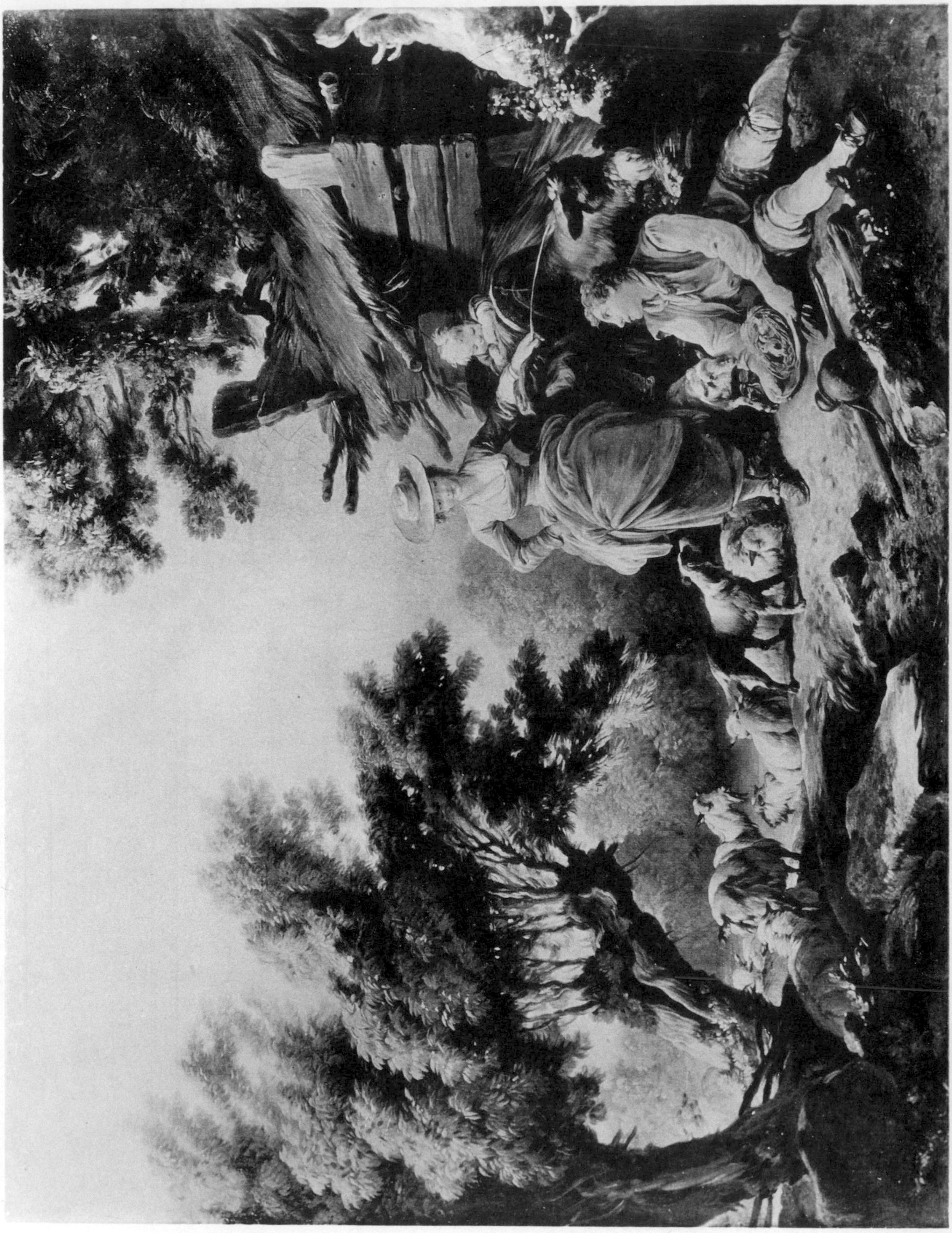

PORTRAIT OF
THE COMTESSE DE SELVE

BY

ADELAIDE LABILLE-GUIARD

1749-1803

ADELAIDE LABILLE-GUIARD

1749-1803

A portrait painter and pastellist, she was born in Paris. Received in the Academy the 31st of May 1783 at the same time as Madame Vigée-Lebrun. Exhibited at the Salon continuously from 1783 to 1800. Died in Paris the 3rd of April 1803.

Portrait of the Comtesse de Selve

canvas: 35½ x 28⅜ inches

Signed and dated left center: *Labille Guiard 1787.*

Knee-length portrait of the comtesse seated before a table at the right of the canvas. Her left elbow is resting on it and with her right hand she turns a page of the music book which is placed on top. She is dressed in a grey-blue velvet gown trimmed with lace and a large velvet toque with an ostrich feather.

References: *Collection des livrets des anciennes expositions,* Salon de 1787, no. 117; R. Portalis, "Adelaide Labille-Guiard," *Gazette des Beaux-Arts,* 1902, p. 111, ill., p. 110, "At the moment when Mme Guiard painted her the Comtesse de Selve was a young woman of perhaps 28 or 30 years, with high color and an animated and witty physiognomy."; Paris, Hotel des Négociants, *Femmes peintres du XVIIIe siècle,* May 14-June 6, 1926, p. 39, no. 52, p. 54, no. 110; Paris, Galerie Georges Petit, *Vente Madame de Polès,* June 22-24, 1927, no. 18, pl. XIX; Amsterdam, Frederick Muller & Cie, *Vente F. J. E. Horstmann,* Nov. 19-21, 1929, no. 27, ill.; *Art News,* 29, Mar. 14, 1931, p. 19, ill.; *Social Calendar,* Mar. 16, 1931, n.p., ill.; New York, American Art Association-Anderson Galleries, *Old and modern masters in the New York art market,* Mar. 15-Apr. 4, 1931, no. 115; New York, Union League Club, *18th century French paintings,* Apr. 9-15, 1931, no. 24; *Arts and decorations,* Feb., 1932, p. 36, ill.; Toledo, Museum of Art, *French furnishings of the 18th century,* Dec. 3-31, 1933, no. 28; Los Angeles, Museum, *European paintings by old and modern masters,* June 13-Aug. 5, 1934, no. 9; New York, Wildenstein & Co., *Fashion in headdress,* Apr. 27-May 27, 1943, no. 62, ill.; *Art News,* 42, May 15-31, 1943, p. 10, ill.

Exhibited: 1787, Paris, Salon; 1926, Paris, Hotel des Négociants; 1931, New York, American Art Association, Anderson Galleries; 1931, New York, Union League Club; 1933, Toledo, Museum of Art; 1934, Los Angeles, Museum of Art; 1943, New York, Wildenstein & Co.

Collections: Madame de Polès, Paris; F. J. E. Horstmann, Amsterdam.

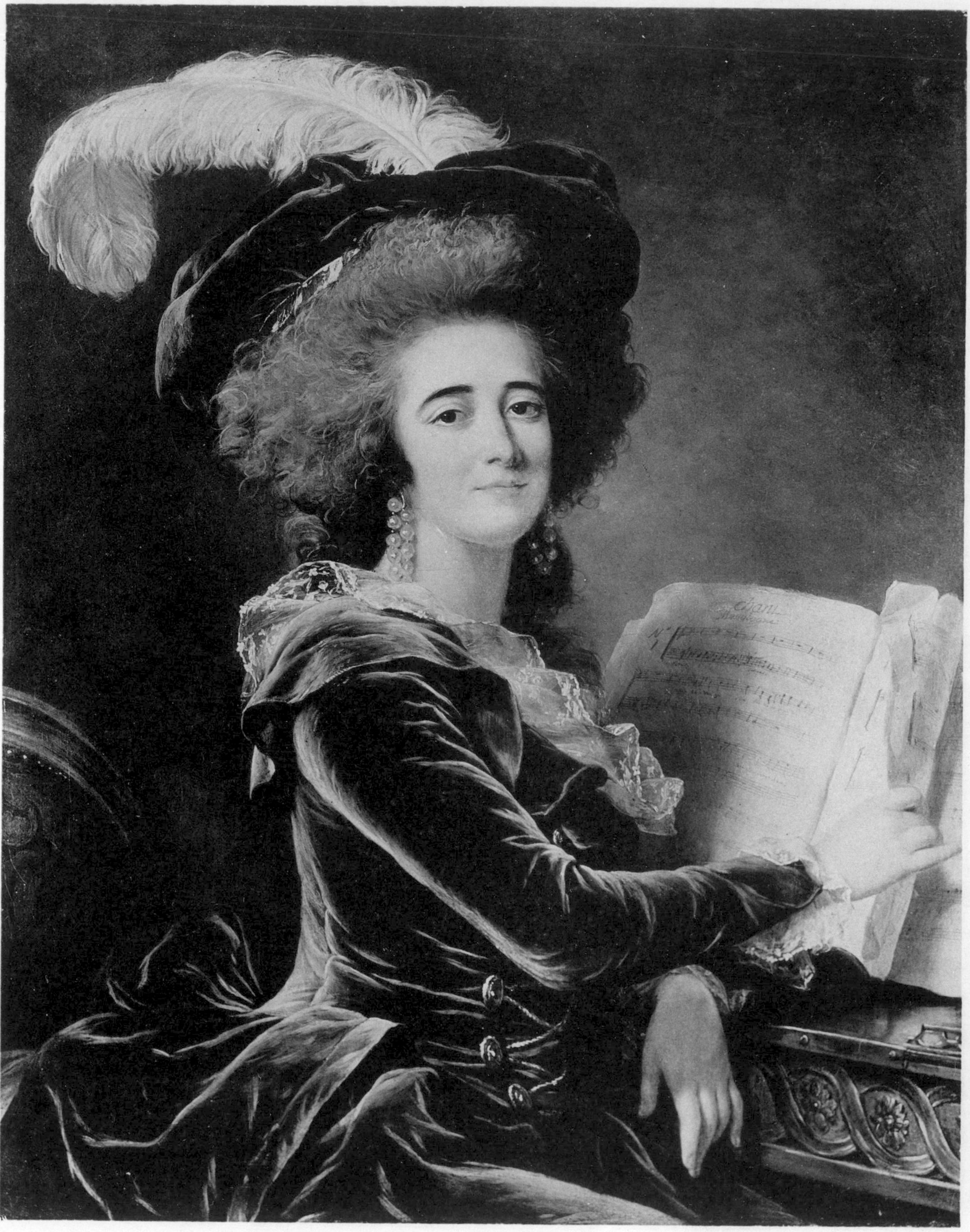

PORTRAIT OF A YOUNG BOY

BY

L.-J.-F. LAGRENEE

1724-1805

L.-J.-F. LAGRENÉE

1724-1805

Pupil of Carle Van Loo, won the Prix de Rome in 1749 and spent three years in Italy. Accepted by the Academy in 1755 and quickly became popular. In 1760, Empress Elizabeth of Russia named him her "premier peintre" and invited him to St. Petersburg where he was made Director of the Academy of Beaux-Arts. Returned to Paris after three years, but in 1781 went to Rome for six years as the Director of the Ecole de Rome. In Paris was given a pension and an apartment in the Louvre and in 1804 was appointed "Conservateur des musées." Many of his paintings have been engraved and he himself made several interesting etchings.

Portrait of a young boy

canvas: 12¾ x 16 inches

A bust-length study of a nude child with curly blond hair and blue eyes. The background is composed of a draped green curtain which the boy holds with his right hand. In front of him are two more pieces of drapery, one yellow and one white.

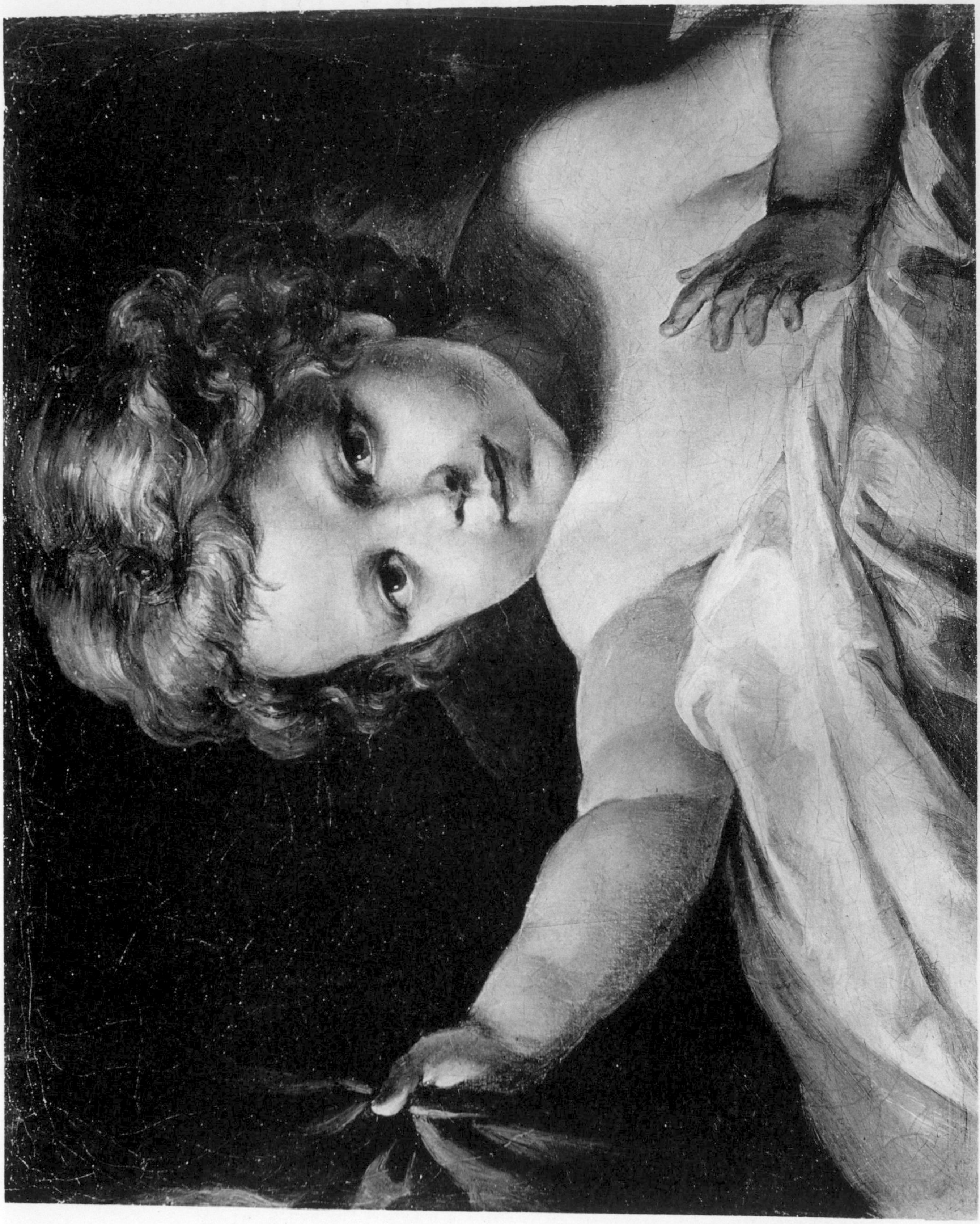

LE JEU DE PIED-DE-BOEUF

BY

NICOLAS LANCRET

1690-1745

NICOLAS LANCRET

1690-1745

Studied first with Pierre d'Ulin, a professor at the Academy and then, from 1712-1713, worked in the studio of Claude Gillot where he met the painter who was to become his real master, Antoine Watteau. Rejected by the Academy in 1711 as a history painter but admitted in 1719 as a "peintre dans le genre de Watteau." An assiduous worker and an expert technician, he became extremely successful and universally celebrated for his "fêtes galantes."

Le jeu de pied-de-boeuf

canvas: 32 x 42 inches

A group of two young women and one young man, seated on a grassy mound, play *pied-de-boeuf,* a popular 18th century game. The central composition is beautifully framed by a large tree on either side of the canvas. Painted in 1742-1743 as a *dessus de porte* for the Marquise de la Tournelle. Pendant to no. 25.

References: J. J. Guiffray, *Nicolas Lancret suivi de l'Eloge de Lancret par Ballot de Sovot,* n.d., pp. 37, 43; Paris, *Vente Granet,* 1853; Amiens, *Exposition rétrospective d'Amiens,* Aug.-Sept. 1866, no. 101; G. Wildenstein, *Nicolas Lancret,* 1924, p. 97, no. 406, p. 66.

Exhibited: 1866, Amiens.

Collections: Marquise de la Tournelle, Palais de Versailles; M. Granet, Paris; Duc de Vicence.

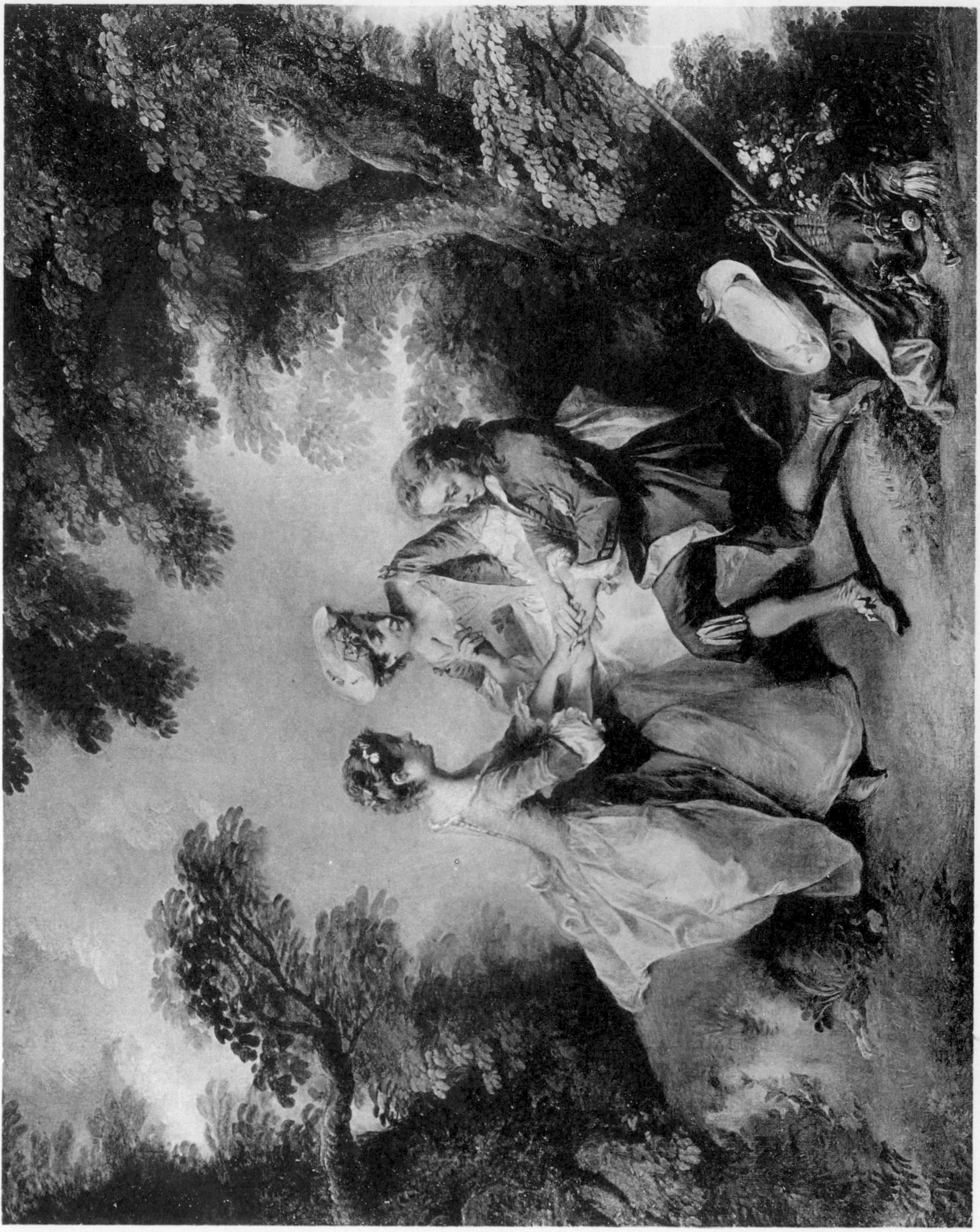

LA SERENADE

BY

NICOLAS LANCRET

1690-1745

NICOLAS LANCRET

1690-1745

Studied first with Pierre d'Ulin, a professor at the Academy and then, from 1712-1713, worked in the studio of Claude Gillot where he met the painter who was to become his real master, Antoine Watteau. Rejected by the Academy in 1711 as a history painter but admitted in 1719 as a "peintre dans le genre de Watteau." An assiduous worker and an expert technician, he became extremely successful and universally celebrated for his "fêtes galantes."

La sérénade

canvas: 32 x 42 inches

On a stone bench beneath a large tree, three young women are seated watching a young man who stands to their left and plays a mandolin. To their right, partly hidden by the trunk of a tree, another musician serenades them with a bagpipe. Painted in 1742-1743 as a *dessus de porte* for the Marquise de la Tournelle. Pendant to no. 24.

References: J. J. Guiffrey, *Nicolas Lancret suivi de l'Eloge de Lancret par Ballot de Sovot,* n.d., pp. 37, 43; Paris, *Vente Granet,* 1853; Amiens, *Exposition rétrospective d'Amiens,* Aug.-Sept. 1866, no. 100; G. Wildenstein, *Nicolas Lancret,* 1924, p. 97, no. 405, p. 66.

Exhibited: 1866, Amiens.

Collections: Marquise de la Tournelle, Palais de Versailles; M. Granet, Paris; Duc de Vicence.

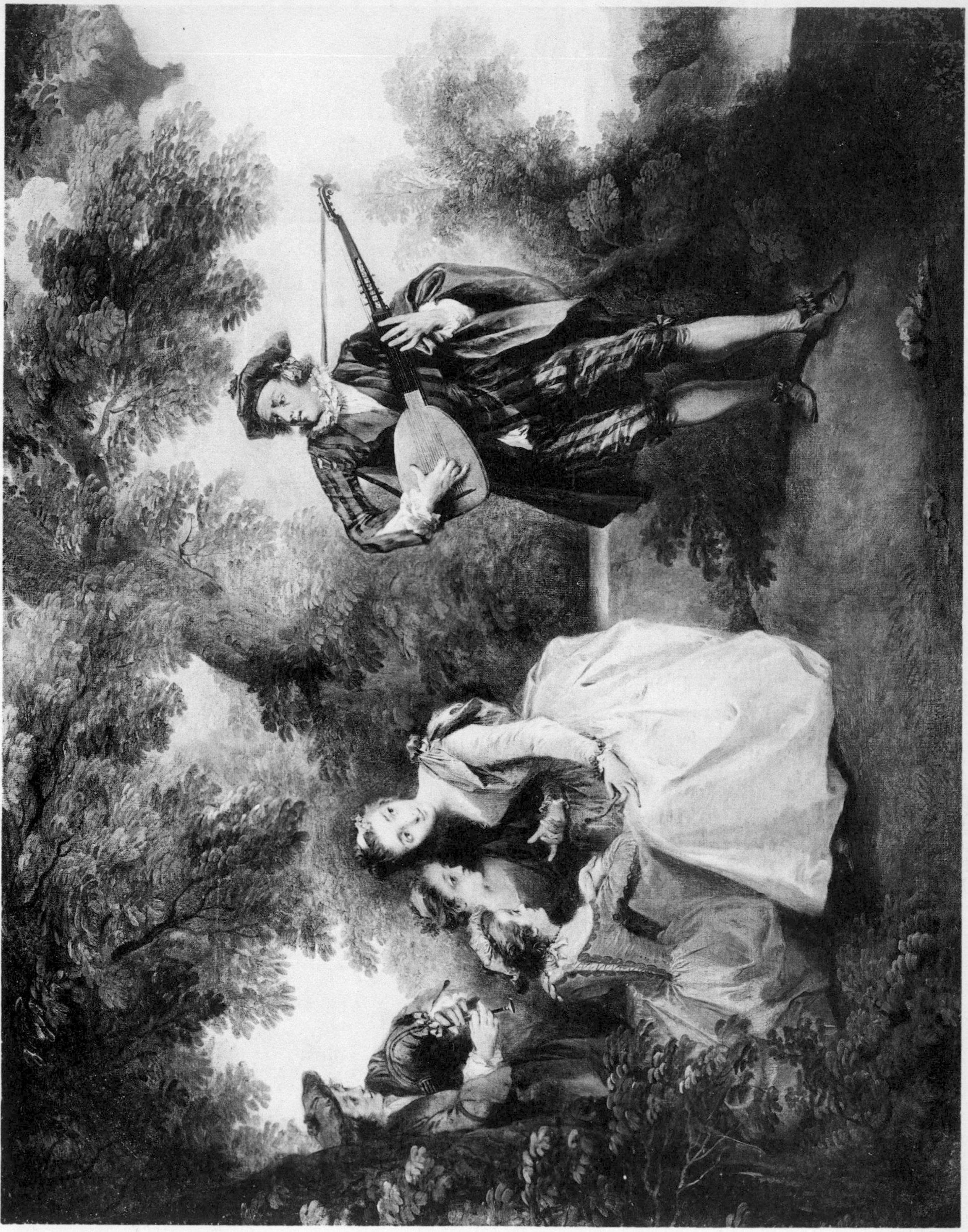

LES AMOURS DU BOCAGE
OR
L'OISELEUR

BY

NICOLAS LANCRET

1690-1745

NICOLAS LANCRET

1690-1745

Studied first with Pierre d'Ulin, a professor at the Academy and then, from 1712-1713, worked in the studio of Claude Gillot where he met the painter who was to become his real master, Antoine Watteau. Rejected by the Academy in 1711 as a history painter but admitted in 1719 as a "peintre dans le genre de Watteau." An assiduous worker and an expert technician, he became extremely successful and universally celebrated for his "fêtes galantes."

Les amours du bocage OR *L'Oiseleur*

canvas: 17½ x 19 inches

Engraved by Larmessin in 1736.

A shepherd seated near a tree holds a bird cage on his lap. A young girl sitting at his left offers food to the bird, and at his right, another girl with a shepherd's crook and three sheep watches the incident.

References: C. Phillips, *Masterpieces of French art in the 18th century,* n.d., pl. II, p. 11, "In 'Les Amours du Bocage'—so brilliantly engraved by Nicolas de Larmessin—Lancret is all himself."; P. Seidel, *Friedrich der Grosse und die französische Malerei seiner Zeit,* n.d., pl. f.p. 48, p. 46, p. 69, no. 5; P. Seidel, *Gemälde alter Meister im Besitze seiner Majestät des deutschen Kaisers und Königs von Preussen,* n.d., p. 199, no. 47, p. 152; M. Osterreich, *Description de tout l'intérieur des deux palais de Sans-Souci, de ceux de Potsdam et de Charlottenbourg,* 1773, p. 33, no. 80, 9; L. Dussieux, *Les artistes français à l'étranger,* 1876, p. 221; E. Bocher, *Les gravures françaises du XVIIIe siècle,* Nicolas Lancret, IV, 1877, p. 80, no. 80, p. 9, no. 8; Dilke, *French painters of the 18th century,* 1899, ill. p. 106, pp. 91, 105; P. Seidel, *Die Kunstsammlung Friedrichs des Grossen auf der Pariser Weltausstellung,* 1900, ill. p. 56, p. 39, no. 12; P. Seidel, *Des collections . . . appartenant à sa majesté l'Empereur d'Allemagne,* 1900, ill. p. 37, p. 98, no. 53; L. de Fourcaud, "Potsdam à Paris," *Revue de l'art,* Oct. 10, 1900, 8, p. 272; J. Staley, *Watteau and his school,* 1902, ill. opp. p. 26, p. 137; J. J. Foster, *French art from Watteau to Prud'hon,* I, pl. XLIX, p. 152, "The great Frederick loved Lancret's pictures and bought many of them."; P. de Nolhac, "L'Art français en Allemagne ce qui peut revenir," *Les Arts,* 1919, no. 173, ill. p. 14, p. 28; P. Seidel, *Friedrich der Grosse und die bildende Kunst,* 1924, ill. p. 190;

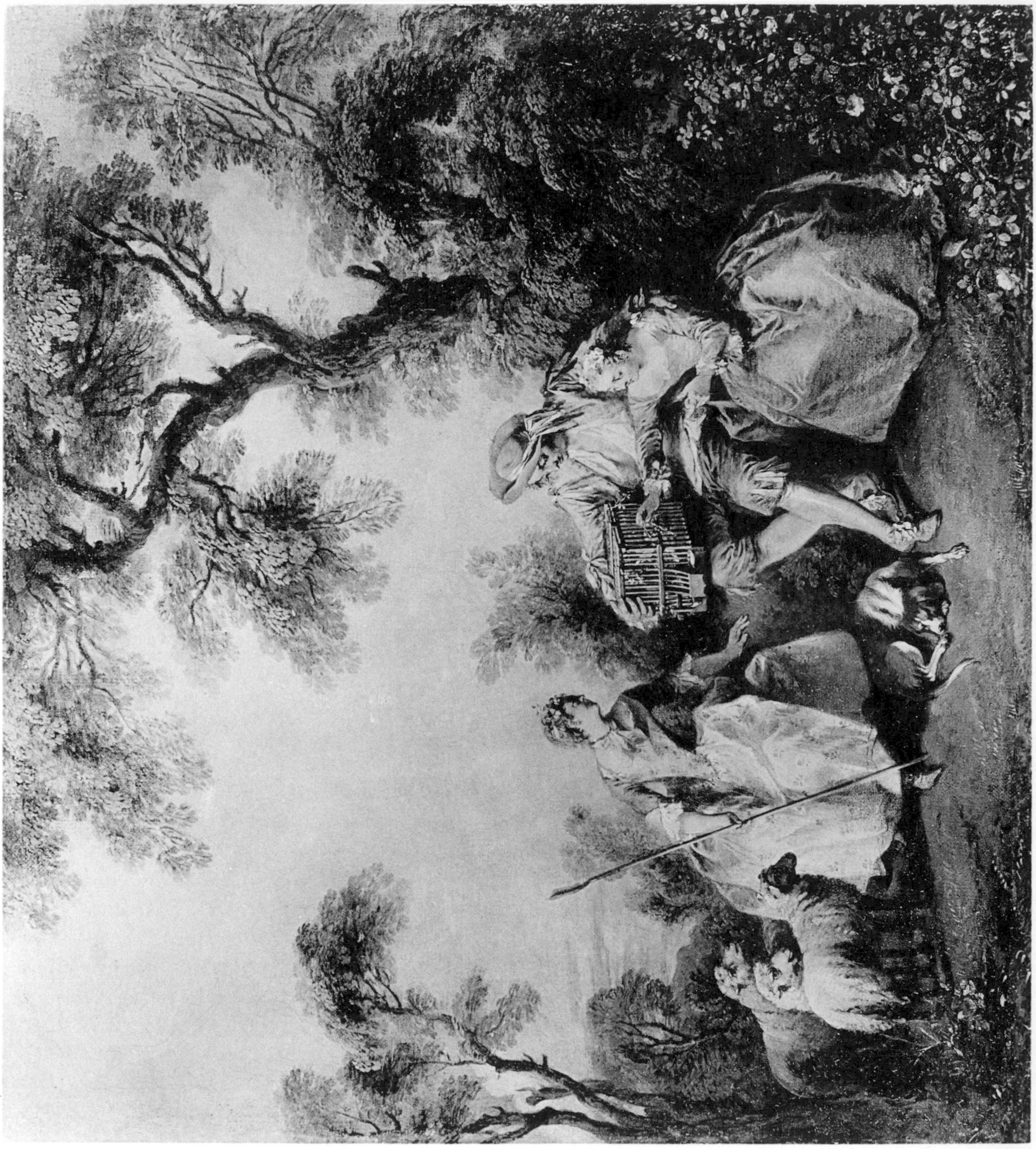

G. Wildenstein, *Nicolas Lancret,* 1924, pl. III, p. 100, no. 455; Thieme-Becker, *Allgemeines Lexikon der bildenden Künstler,* 1928, 22, p. 287; Chicago, Art Institute, *Century of progress,* June 1-Nov. 1, 1933, p. 34, no. 219; Hartford, Wadsworth Atheneum, *Loan exhibition in honor of the opening of the Avery Memorial,* 1934, no. 29; San Francisco, Palace of the Legion of Honor, *Exhibition of French painting,* 1934, pp. 38-39, no. 40; W. King, "A Lancret subject in English porcelain," *Apollo,* Jan. 1935, ill. fig. IV, p. 32, pp. 31-32.

Exhibited: 1739, Paris, Salon (?); 1900, Paris; 1933, Chicago, Art Institute; 1934, San Francisco, Palace of the Legion of Honor; 1934, Hartford, Wadsworth Atheneum.

Collections: Frederick II of Prussia; Kings of Prussia, New Palace, Potsdam to 1923.

PORTRAIT OF THE COMTESSE DE COURBOUZON

BY

NICOLAS LARGILLIERE

1656-1746

NICOLAS LARGILLIERE

1656-1746

A Parisian who spent his youth in Antwerp where his father was a merchant and where he himself received an excellent technical training in the studio of Antoni Goubeau. In 1674 he was in London studying under Peter Lely but four years later was forced to leave because of religious persecution. Accepted by the Academy in 1683 with a portrait of Lebrun and returned to London in 1685 to work at the court of Charles II. Enormously popular and executed many commissions for Parisian society and for prominent middle class families. Rigaud's greatest rival and really more influential than he in the future development of portraiture both in France and in England.

Portrait of the Comtesse de Courbouzon

canvas: 54¼ x 41½ inches

A formal allegorical portrait of the countess standing against a background of trees and sky. She is accompanied by a semi-nude small boy placed in the lower left-hand corner of the composition and partly hidden by the voluminous drapery of the countess' skirt. In her raised right hand she holds a carnation.

References: G. Pascal, *Largillière,* 1928, p. 75, no. 190, pl. xv; Paris, Petit Palais, *Exposition Largillière,* 1928, p. 35, no. 89; *Pantheon,* July, 1928, p. 377, ill.; New York, Wildenstein & Co., *French 18th century paintings,* Mar.-Apr., 1929, no. 2; New York, Union League Club, *18th century French paintings,* Apr. 9-15, 1931, no. 25; Los Angeles, *Five centuries of European painting,* Dec., 1933, no. 21.

Exhibited: 1928, Paris, Petit Palais; 1929, New York, Wildenstein & Co.; 1931, New York, Union League Club; 1933, Los Angeles, Museum.

Collections: Family of the Comtesse de Courbouzon.

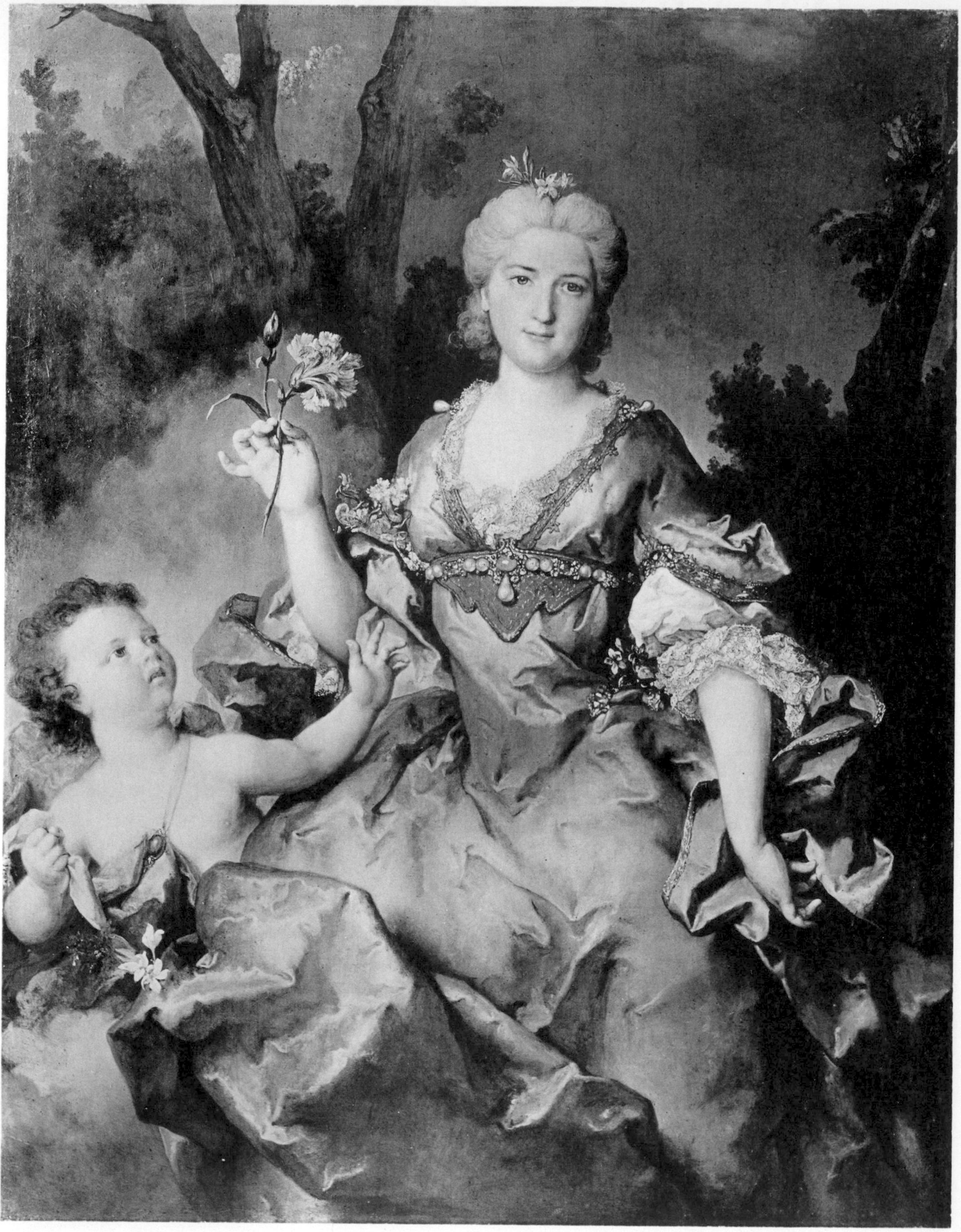

PORTRAIT OF VOLTAIRE

BY

MAURICE-QUENTIN DE LA TOUR

1704-1788

MAURICE-QUENTIN DE LA TOUR

1704-1788

The most famous practitioner of pastel, a medium which had been popularized by Rosalba Carriera, a Venetian artist who came to Paris about 1720. Little information about his youth except that he left St. Quentin early to go to Paris where the engraver Tardieu took charge of him and placed him in the studio of Jacques Spoëde. Later, he probably worked with Claude Dupouch and Jean Restout. Elected to the Academy in 1746 and in 1778 founded a school of drawing in his birthplace of St. Quentin. Died in 1788.

Portrait of Voltaire

pastel on blue paper: 20⅜ x 7⅛ inches

Engraved by Jules de Goncourt.

One of the famous masks by La Tour, a study for a pastel portrait of the writer (François-Marie Arouet, called Voltaire, 1694-1778) which has been lost since the 18th century.

References: M. Tourneau, *La Tour,* n.d., p. 9, ill., p. 31; L. de Fourcaud, "Le pastel et les pastellistes français au XVIIIe siècle," *Revue de l'art,* XXIV, 1908, p. 125, ill., p. 126, "The oldest study of the master . . . was the masque of Voltaire.[2] (2. Belonging to M. Emile Strauss). One cannot doubt that the portrait of the philosopher is before 1731."; L. Roger-Miles, *Cent pastels,* 1908, pl. opp. p. 40, p. 40; Paris, Galerie Georges Petit, *Exhibition de cent pastels,* May 18-June 10, 1908, p. 22, no. 52; M. Tourneaux, "L'exposition des cent pastels," *Gazette des Beaux-Arts,* 1908, II, p. 9; L. Dumont-Wilden, *Le portrait en France,* 1909, p. 210; L. M. Richter, "Voltaire painted by Latour," *Connoisseur,* Aug. 1919, LIV, p. 207; Paris Hotel Jean Charpentier, *Exposition de pastels français du XVIIe et du XVIIIe siècle,* May 23-June 26, 1927, p. 18, no. 29; E. Dacier & P. R. de Limay, *Pastels français des XVII et XVIII siècles,* 1927, pl. XXIII, fig. 32, p. 54, no. 32; Paris, Galerie Georges Petit, *Vente Emile Straus,* June 3-4, 1929, no. 73, ill.; P. de Nolhac, *La vie et l'oeuvre de Maurice Quentin de la Tour,* 1930, pl. opp. p. 34 (in color), p. 126; Paris, Bibliotèque

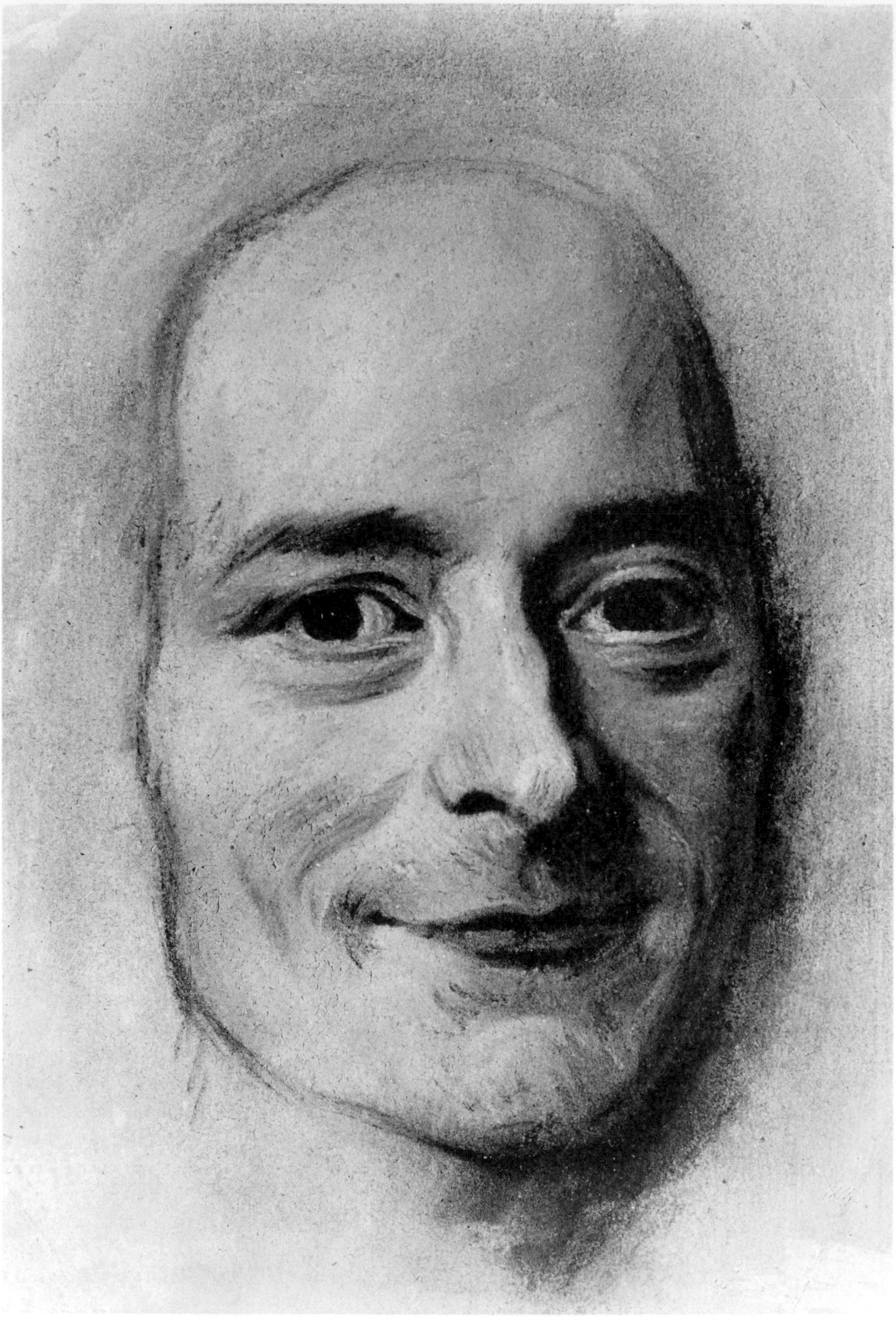

nationale, *L'encyclopédie et les encyclopédistes,* 1932, ill. opp. p. 40, no. 388; *Fine Arts,* Nov., 1932, 19, p. 24, ill.; A Leroy, *Maurice-Quentin de la Tour,* 1933, pl. 30, p. 70, no. 30, p. 24, "Happily there exists a very beautiful study for a portrait slightly before that of 1736, engraved by Jules de Goncourt. Having passed through the collections of Marcille and Jules Strauss it belongs today to M. Wildenstein."; Paris, "Gazette des Beaux-Arts," *Le siècle de Louis XV vu par les artistes,* 1934, p. 67, no. 171; Pennsylvania Museum of Art and Phillips Memorial Gallery, *Problems in portraiture,* Oct. 16-Nov. 18, Dec. 6-Jan. 3, 1937-1938, p. 13, ill.; *Renaissance de l'art,* 20, Mar., 1937, p. 29, ill.; *Magazine of Art,* 30, suppl., Nov., 1937, p. 13, ill.; A. Besnard & G. Wildenstein, *La Tour,* 1938, fig. 39, pl. XXVI, no. 525; New York, Wildenstein & Co., *French revolution,* Dec., 1943, no. 45, ill.; *Art Digest,* 18, Dec. 1, 1943, p. 10, ill.; New York, Wildenstein & Co., *French pastels from Clouet to Degas,* Feb. 9-Mar. 2, 1944, no. 52; Toledo, Museum of Art, Nov.-Dec., 1946, Toronto, The Art Gallery of Toronto, Jan.-Feb., 1947, *Spirit of modern France,* no. 6.

Exhibited: 1908, Paris, Galerie Georges Petit; 1927, Paris, Hotel Jean Charpentier; 1932, Paris, Bibliotèque Nationale; 1934, Paris "Gazette des Beaux-Arts;" 1937; Philadelphia, Museum of Art; 1938, Washington, Phillips Memorial Gallery; 1943, New York, Wildenstein & Co.; 1944, New York, Wildenstein & Co.; 1946, Toledo, Museum of Art; 1947, Toronto, The Art Gallery of Toronto.

Collections: Jules de Goncourt; Emile Straus.

PORTRAIT OF
THE PRINCESSE DE LAMBALLE

BY

MARIE-VICTOIRE LE MOINE

1754-1820

MARIE-VICTOIRE LE MOINE

1754-1820

Painter of genre scenes, portraits and miniatures, a pupil of Ménageot and Madame Vigée-Lebrun. From 1779 to 1785 she exhibited at the Salon de la Correspondance and from 1796 to 1814 at the Salon.

Portrait of the Princesse de Lamballe

canvas, oval: 24½ x 19½ inches

Signed and dated lower left: *Vic.re*
Le moine
1779

Marie Thêrèse Louise de Savoie-Carignan was born in Turin on September 8, 1749, the fourth daughter of Louis Victor de Savoie-Carignan and Christine Henriette de Hesse-Rhinfelds-Rothembourg. Married in 1767 to the son of the Duc de Penthièvre, Louis Alexandre Stanislas de Bourbon, the Prince de Lamballe, who died a few months later. After the death of Marie Leczinska, there was some question of marrying her to Louis XV, but because of court intrigue she was not chosen. When the Dauphin married Marie-Antoinette she reappeared at court and became very close to the Queen. She was made "Surintendante de la maison" and was involved in many court activities during the revolution. She was killed in the September massacres of 1792.

References: E. B. de Chavignerie & L. Auvray, *Dictionnaire général des artistes de l'école français,* 1882, I, p. 998; L. Benoist, "Les ventes," *Beaux-arts,* IV, 1936, p. 336, ill.; Thieme-Becker, *Allgemeines Lexikon der bildenden Künstler,* 1939, XXIII, p. 34; New York, Wildenstein & Co., *The French revolution,* Dec. 1943, p. 23, no. 27.

Exhibited: 1779, Paris, Salon de la Correspondance; 1943, New York Wildenstein & Co.

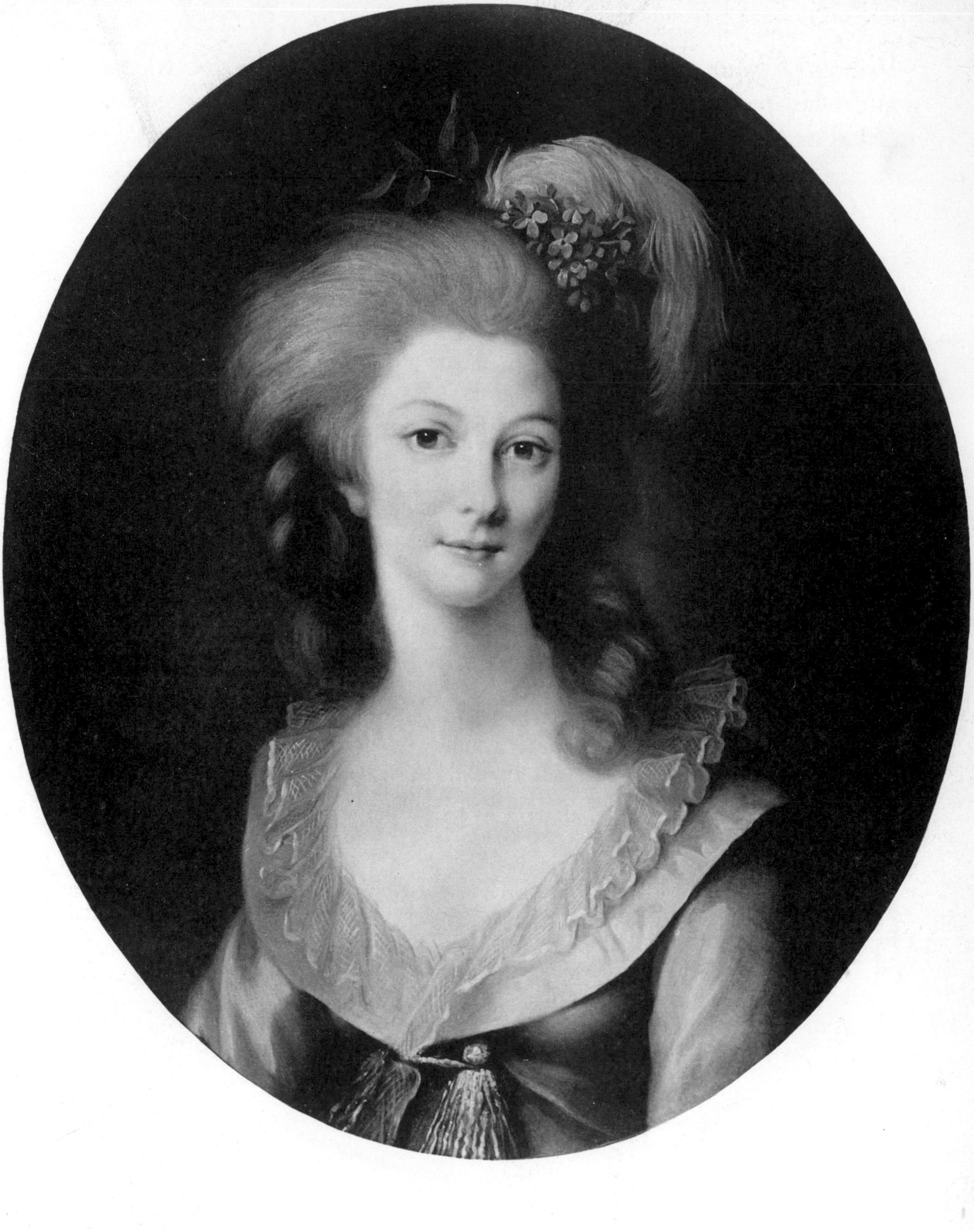

HUNTING PICNIC

BY

FRANÇOIS LE MOINE

1688-1737

FRANÇOIS LE MOINE

1688-1737

Studied first with his stepfather, Robert Tourniéres, then with D. Galloche (1701) and J.-P. Cazes. Elected a member of the Academy in 1718 and won the Prix de Rome in 1711 but did not go to Italy until 1723. It was here that his real training took place particularly in his study of the Venetian school. Known as *Le Moine du plafond* since he was famous for his ceiling decorations, his masterpiece being the Salon d'Hercule at Versailles completed in 1736. In the same year was appointed official painter to the King, but in 1737 committed suicide because of psychological difficulties. Natoire and Boucher were his most important pupils.

Hunting Picnic

canvas: 88 x 73 inches

Signed and dated on rock at right: *F. Le Moine 1723.*

In a small clearing between an old mill on one side and several large trees on the other a group of ladies and gentlemen returned from a hunt, have stopped to rest. In the left foreground six of them are refreshing themselves with a glass of wine. Beside them on the ground is some food, a bottle of wine and some dead game. To the right, one man is looking for something in a bag on the back of a white horse while another, seated and still holding his gun, watches him. Next to them are two hunting dogs. In the middle ground are several more figures: a man on horseback and another helping a lady to dismount. Further back, three people — a man, a woman and a child—are crossing a rustic bridge. An extensive and richly painted landscape stretches into the distance.

Collections: Lord Rosebery.

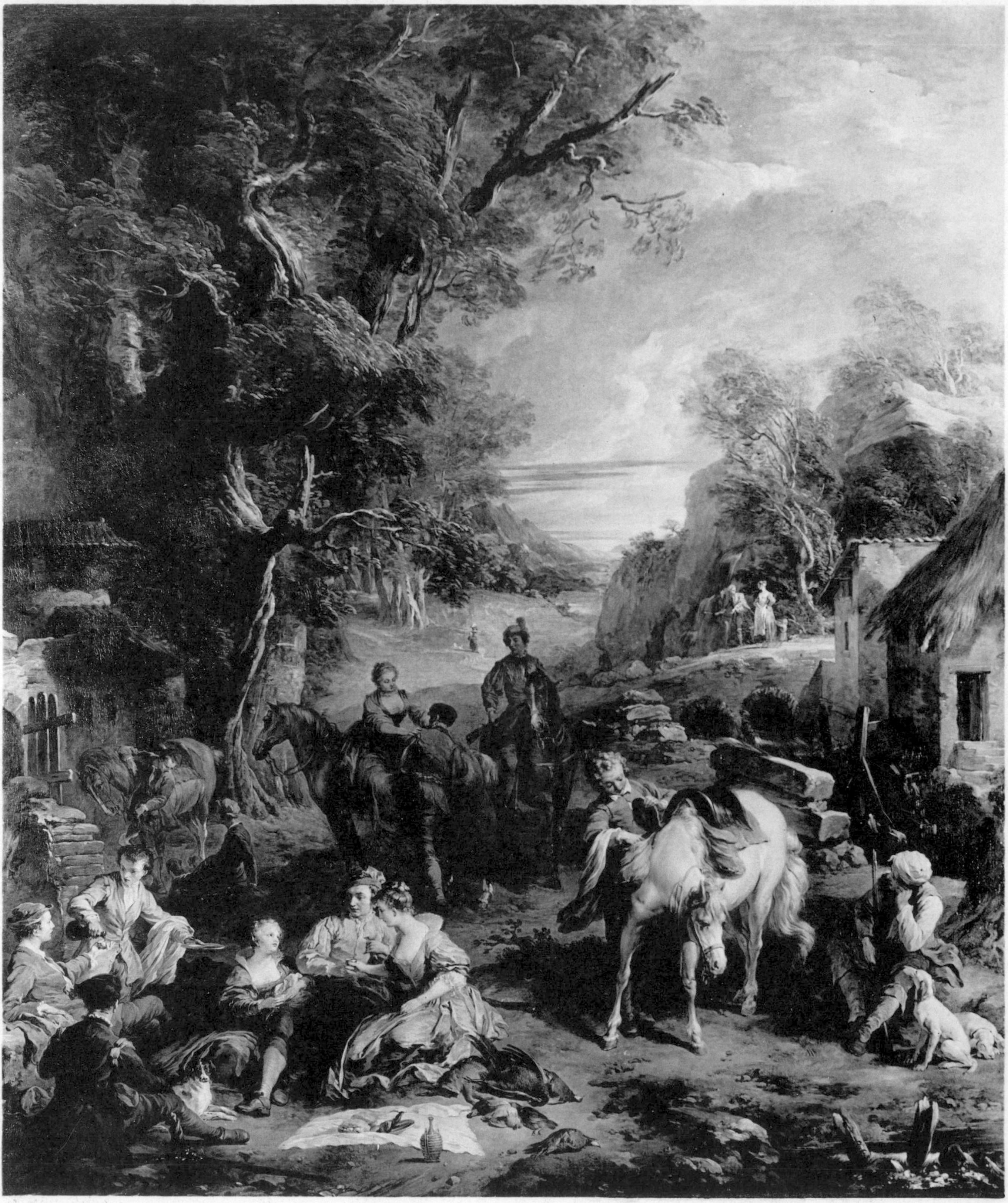

LA FAMILLE DU MENUISIER

BY

M.-N.-B. LEPICIE

1735-1784

M.-N.-B. LÉPICIÉ

1735-1784

His father and first teacher was Bernard François Lépicié, the engraver. Studied later with Carle Van Loo, but little influenced by him and more closely related to Chardin in his painting of domestic scenes. Elected a member of the Academy in 1769 and became professor in 1779. Very popular with his contemporaries after the Salon of 1767. Teacher of Carle Vernet.

La famille du menuisier

canvas: 19¼ x 24⅜ inches

Signed lower right: *Lépiciè.*

Engraved by Hémery, 1777; Le Bas.

An interior scene where a carpenter works surrounded by his family. His wife sits next to his work table and both he and she watch the figures in the foreground—the grandmother who is teaching her granddaughter to read. To the left are two small boys and in the right background an older man with his back turned. Mentioned in Lépicié's will and cited by the critic of the *Mercure de France* when it was exhibited at the Salon of 1775.

References: Paris, Hotel Drouot, *Vente M. Boittelle,* Apr. 24-25, 1866, p. 35, no. 77; London, *Exposition internationale,* May 1871, p. 36, no. 433; P. Gaston-Dreyfus, "Une dernière volonté de Nicolas-Bernard Lépicié," *Bulletin de l'histoire de l'art français,* 1910, pp. 25-30, 31-32, "*La famille du menuisier* of Lépicié, which has the same title as a celebrated picture by Rembrandt, is a charming canvas of a remarkable harmony and fineness of touch."; P. Gaston-Dreyfus, *Catalogue raisonné de l'oeuvre peint et dessiné de Nicolas-Bernard Lépicié,* 1923, ill. opp. p. 76 (Le Bas engraving), p. 77, no. 179; F. Ingersoll-Smouse, "Nicolas-Bernard Lépicié," *Revue de l'art,* 50, Dec. 1926, p. 295, ill., pp. 293-296, "Finally, three important works are connected with that same year 1774, so fruitful in the work of Lépicié; the too famous *Atelier d'un menuisier. . .*"

Exhibited: 1871, London.

Collections: Niece of Lépicié; M. Boittelle; Baronne d'Erlanger, Paris.

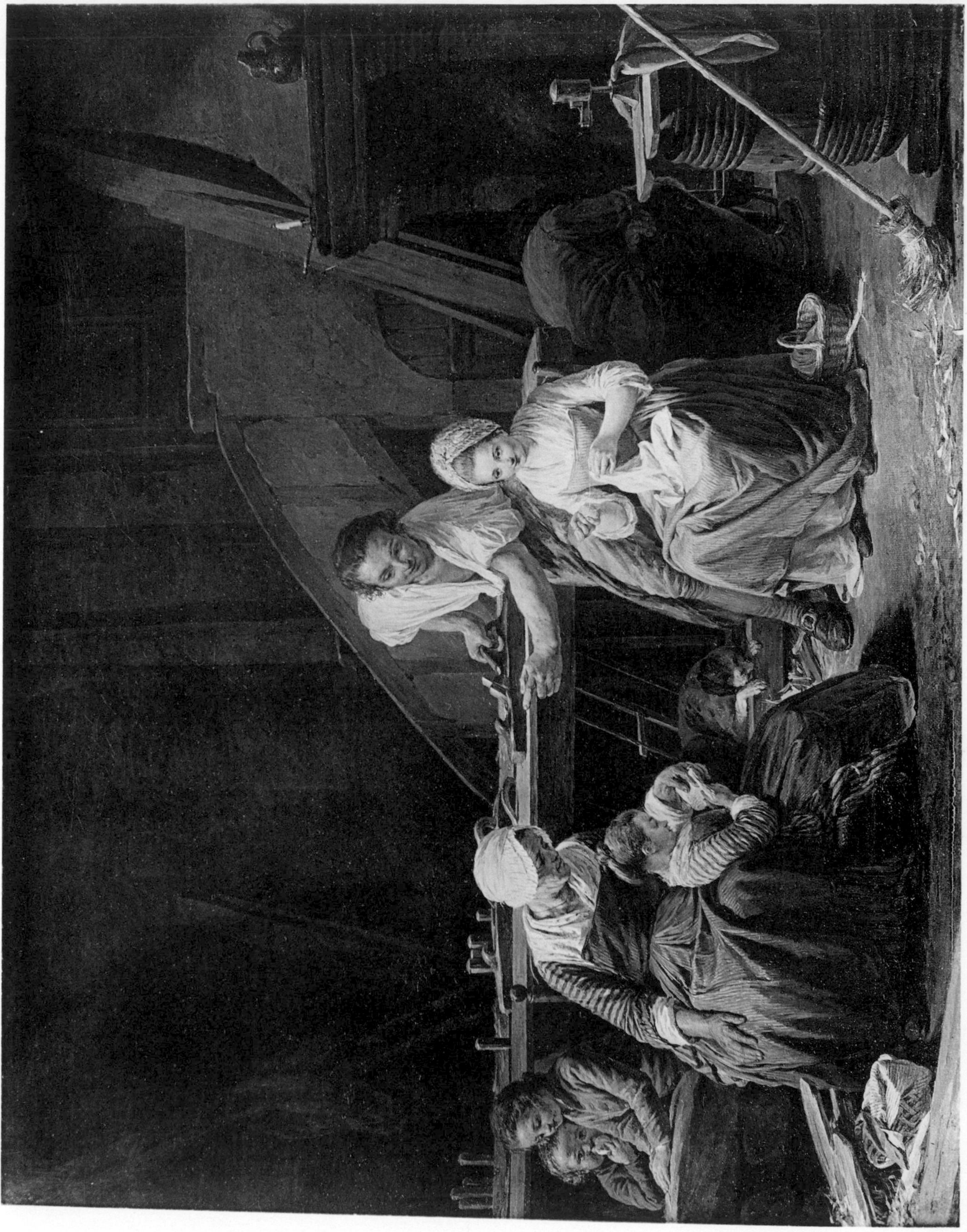

LA PROMENADE OR L'HEUREUSE RENCONTRE

BY

PHILIPPE MERCIER

1689-1760

PHILIPPE MERCIER

1689-1760

Born in Berlin of French parents who had fled to Germany after the Edict of Nantes had been revoked. Began his studying under Antoine Pesne, court painter of the King of Prussia, and then travelled to Italy and France where he seems to have been most impressed by Watteau's work. Returned to Germany in 1720 and was patronized by the son of George II who invited him to London. Lived for quite a while in England and did several portraits of the royal family, but painted mostly "fêtes galantes" which became very popular. Despite his German birth and his almost continuous life abroad, his paintings are so French that they have frequently been attributed to Watteau.

La promenade OR *L'heureuse rencontre*

canvas: 14¼ x 12 inches

Engraved by Mercier, Lalauze.

A young man and woman walking in a park. In the left background, a woman reclining against a tree trunk and sleeping, and in the right, two seated figures. Attributed to Watteau until an engraving with the inscription *P. Mercier Pinxit et Sculp.* betrayed its true author.

References: P. Mantz, "Watteau," *Gazette des Beaux-Arts,* Mar., 1890, I, ill. opp. p. 226, p. 227; P. Mantz, *Antoine Watteau,* 1892, ill. opp. p. 184, pp. 179-180; L. Roger-Miles, *Cent chefs-d'oeuvre des collections françaises et étrangères,* 1892, ill. p. 61, p. 153, no. 27, p. 60, "*La Scène champêtre, la Romance, le Bain* of Pater, *les Amusements de la campagne* of Lancret and Watteau's *L'Heureuse rencontre* are not elegant modernized allegories like Pater's *Le Colin-Maillard;* they are genre paintings which give us a faithful image of the tastes and pleasures of the period."; E. Dacier & A. Vuaflart, *Jean de Jullienne et les graveurs de Watteau,* 1922, III, p. 142; R. Rey, *Quelques satellites de Watteau,* 1931, pp. 68, 77, 78; K. T. Parker, "Mercier, Angélis & de Bar," *Old master drawings,* Dec., 1932, ill. p. 37, pp.36-38, "Mercier's best known pictures in the Watteau style are the so-called *Escamoteur* in the Louvre and M. Wildenstein's *Heureuse rencontre* (otherwise *La Promenade*), formerly the property

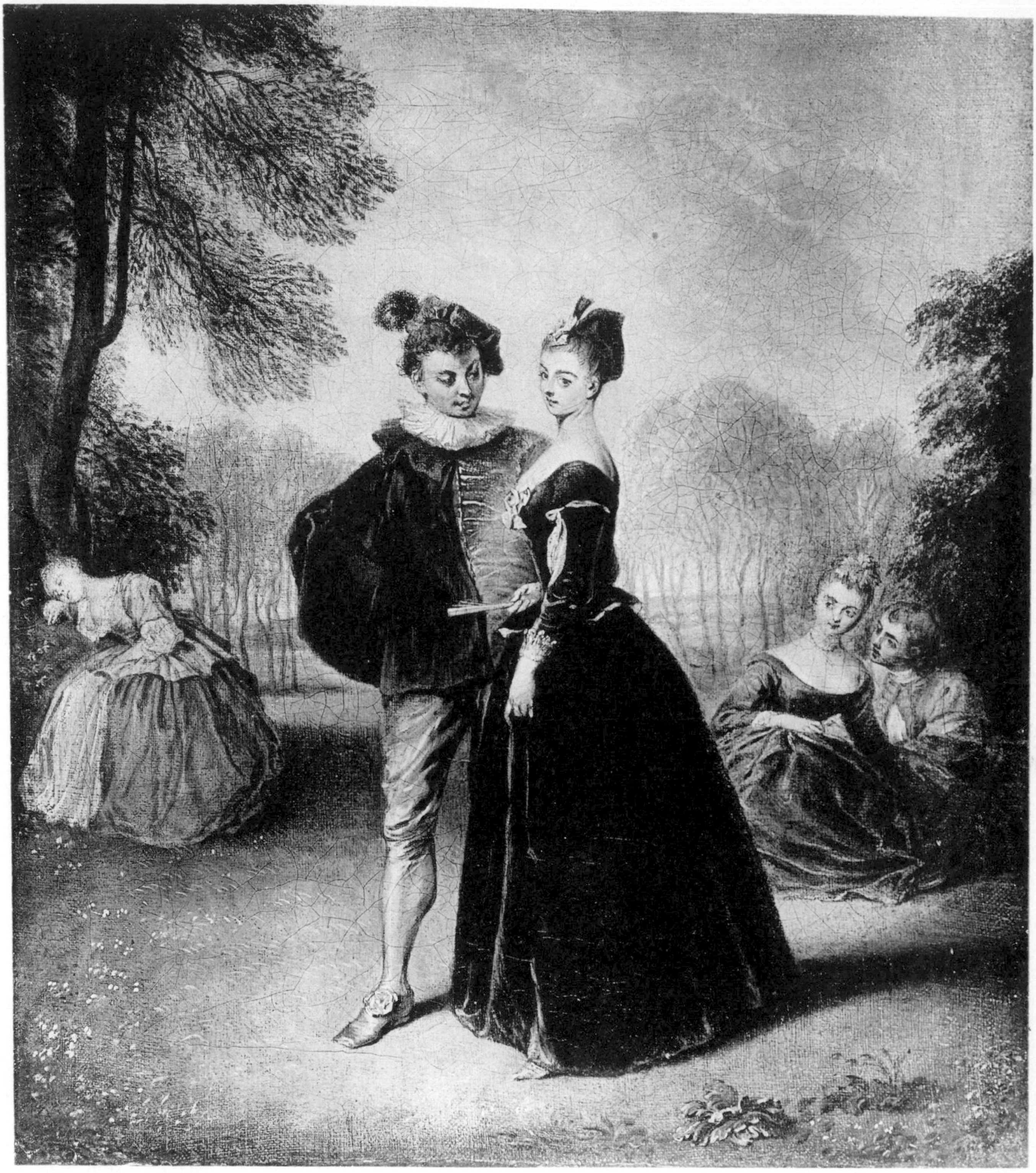

of M. Marcel Bernstein."; London, Wildenstein & Co., *Watteau and his contemporaries*, 1936, no. 14.

Exhibited: 1892, Paris; 1936, London, Wildenstein & Co.

Collections: Marcel Bernstein, Paris.

PORTRAIT OF MADAME ELIZABETH,
DUCHESS OF PARMA

BY

JEAN-MARC NATTIER

1685-1766

JEAN-MARC NATTIER

1685-1766

Born in Paris, his father, mother and elder brother were all artists. Accepted by the Academy in 1715 and elected a member in 1718. Began as an historical painter but later specialized in portraits and became one of the most fashionable portraitists of the court, particularly renowned for his representations of women. Except for one trip to Holland in 1715 where he painted the Czar and Czarina of Russia, remained in Paris despite invitations from Rome and Russia.

Portrait of Madame Elizabeth, Duchess of Parma

canvas, oval: 33 x 27 inches

Signed and dated center right: *Nattier P^{xt} 1754.*

Bust portrait of the princess in formal court dress with an ermine-lined cape around her shoulders. The head is a study after nature which Nattier made for the full-length portrait of Madame Infante ordered by the King. Madame Elizabeth was the eldest daughter of Louis XV and in 1739 married Philippe, the Prince of Spain, who later became the Duke of Parma. The portrait was finished in 1754 at the request of the Duke of Parma and sent to him in Italy.

References: New York, Rockefeller Center, Maison Française, Gallery for French Art, *Exhibition of famous women of French history,* May 8-30, no. 41; P. de Nolhac, *Jean-Marc Nattier,* 1910, p. 84, "These precious studies made after nature, where the way in which Nattier saw and interpreted his august models is more revealed than in the formal portraits, have suffered different fates. . . That of Madame Infante in court dress was given to the Duke of Parma, who paid 1,800 livres for its completion."; *New York Times,* Mar. 17, 1929, ill.; Springfield, Museum of Fine Arts, *Opening Exhibition,* Oct. 7-Nov. 2, 1933, p. 26, no. 60; New York, Wildenstein & Co., *Four centuries of portraits,* Sept., 1945, no. 32.

Exhibited: New York, Rockefeller Center, Maison Française, Gallery for French Art; 1929, New York, Wildenstein & Co.; 1933, Springfield, Museum of Art; 1945, New York, Wildenstein & Co.

Collections: Dukes of Parma.

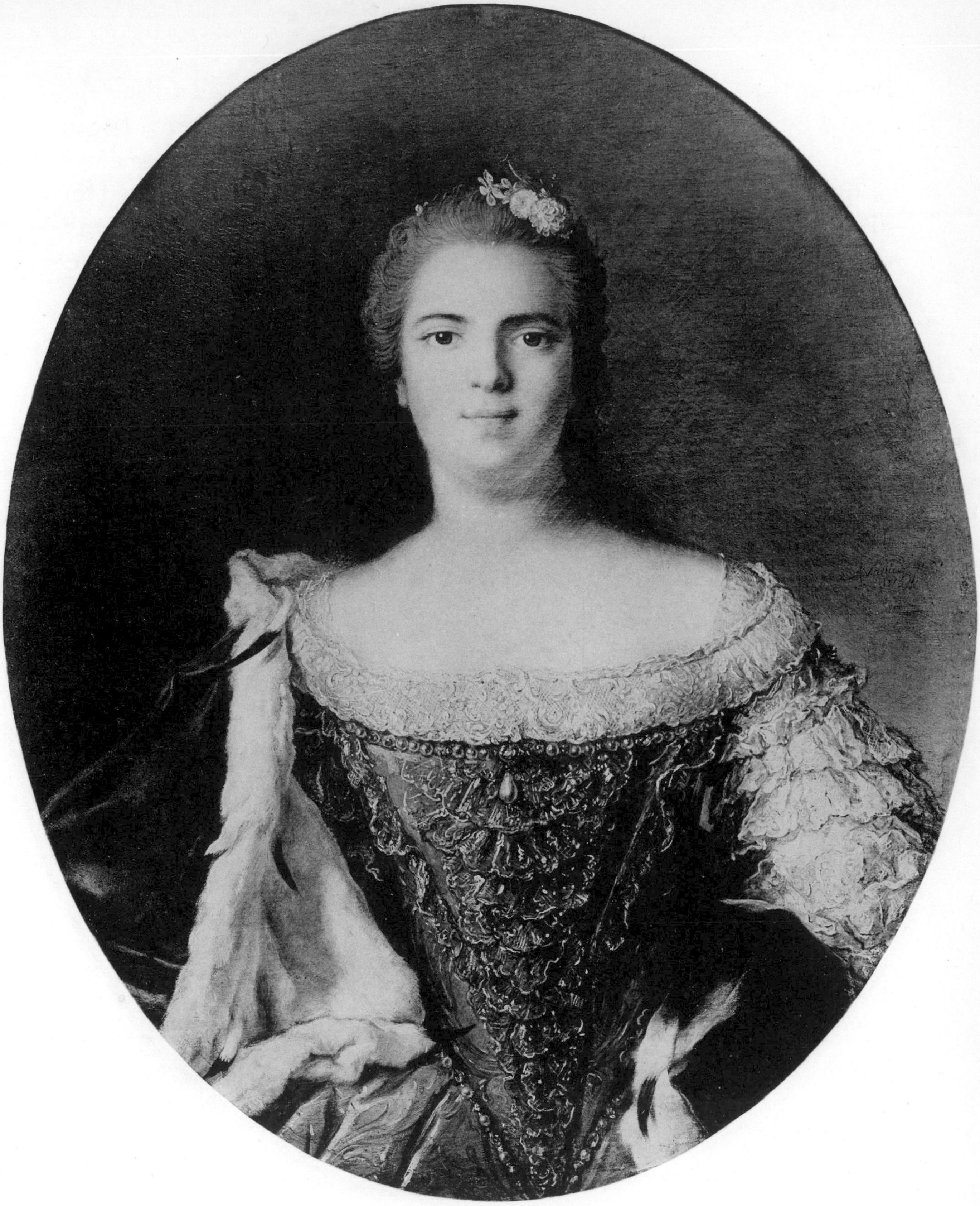

PORTRAIT OF
THE COMTESSE DE LA PORTE

BY

JEAN-MARC NATTIER

1685-1766

JEAN-MARC NATTIER

1685-1766

Born in Paris, his father, mother and elder brother were all artists. Accepted by the Academy in 1715 and elected a member in 1718. Began as an historical painter but later specialized in portraits and became one of the most fashionable portraitists of the court, particularly renowned for his representations of women. Except for one trip to Holland in 1715 where he painted the Czar and Czarina of Russia, remained in Paris despite invitations from Rome and Russia.

Portrait of the Comtesse de la Porte

canvas: 31¼ x 25 inches

Signed and dated left center: *Nattier pinxit 1754.*

Half-length portrait, standing, full face. Wearing a white satin embroidered dress and a blue scarf which is draped from her left shoulder and fastened with a jewel at her waist. Hair powdered and ornamented with flowers.

References: W. Bode, *Gemäldesammlung des Herrn Rudolf Kann in Paris,* 1900, pl. 90; E. Michel, "La galerie de M. Rodolphe Kann," *Gazette des Beaux-Arts,* June, 1901, p. 503-504, "Unposed and unprepared, the two half-length portraits of a young man and a young woman executed by Nattier in 1756, give a good idea of the natural distinction . . . of these brilliant scions of a great family, carrying with ease the multiple seductions of birth, youth and fortune. Nattier has not forced this. Beneath his apparent and legitimate facility, one sees quickly, in the sureness of the composition, in the dexterity of the brush, in the freshness of the coloring, that he understood profoundly his medium and that he had not usurped the position of official painter which he occupied at the French court."; A. Marguillier, "La collection de M. Rodolphe Kann," *Les Arts,* Mar., 1903, p. 4, ill.; *Catalogue de la collection Rodolphe Kann; Tableaux,* II, 1907, no. 152, pl. opp. p. 62.

Collections: Rodolphe Kann, Paris; Sir Ernest Cassel; Lady Louis Mountbatten (daughter of Sir Ernest Cassel).

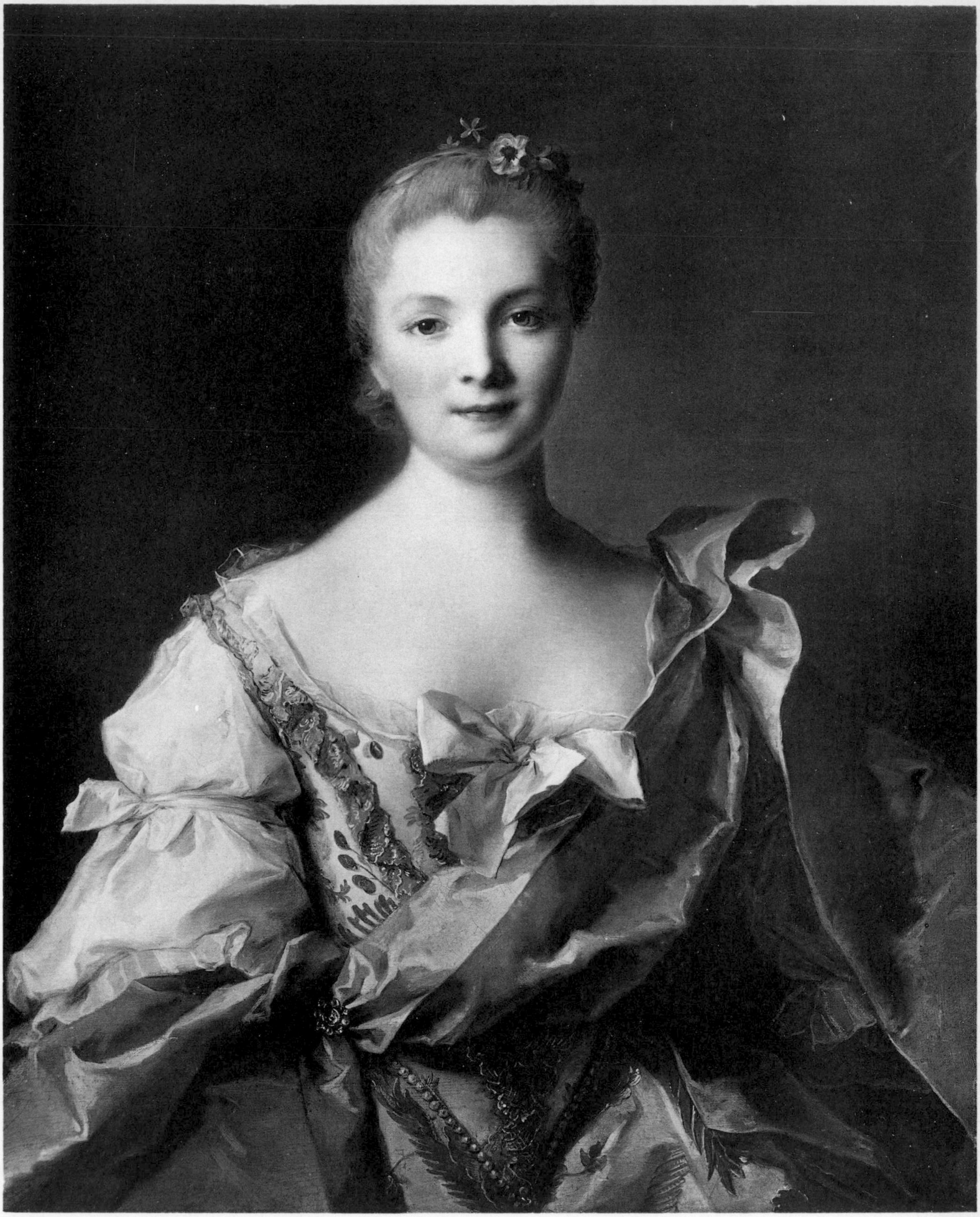

DOG AND SWAN

BY

JEAN-BAPTISTE OUDRY

1686-1755

JEAN-BAPTISTE OUDRY

1686-1755

Taught first by his father Jacques Oudry, a picture dealer and portrait painter, and then by Largillière who became very fond of him and treated him like a son. Because of his talent, his diligence and the protection of the Duc d'Antin, he quickly rose to a high position. Accepted by the Academy in 1717, became a member in 1719 and was made court painter of Louis XV. In 1726 was appointed a designer at the Beauvais tapestry factory and thereafter became Director of the Beauvais works and Inspector General of the Gobelins in Paris. Known chiefly for his genre paintings of animals and still lifes, and influenced in this both by Desportes and by the Flemish painters, Rubens and Snyders.

Dog and swan

canvas: 82 x 70 inches

Signed and dated lower right: *J. B. Oudry 1745.*

In the lower left hand corner, a ferocious dog running with his jaws open and his ears laid back on his head. The swan, at the right, with wings spread and beak open, turns to face his attacker. The background is composed of finely painted grasses, a stone wall and architectural details, and on the left of the canvas, a tree trunk. A typical example of Oudry's large animal scenes.

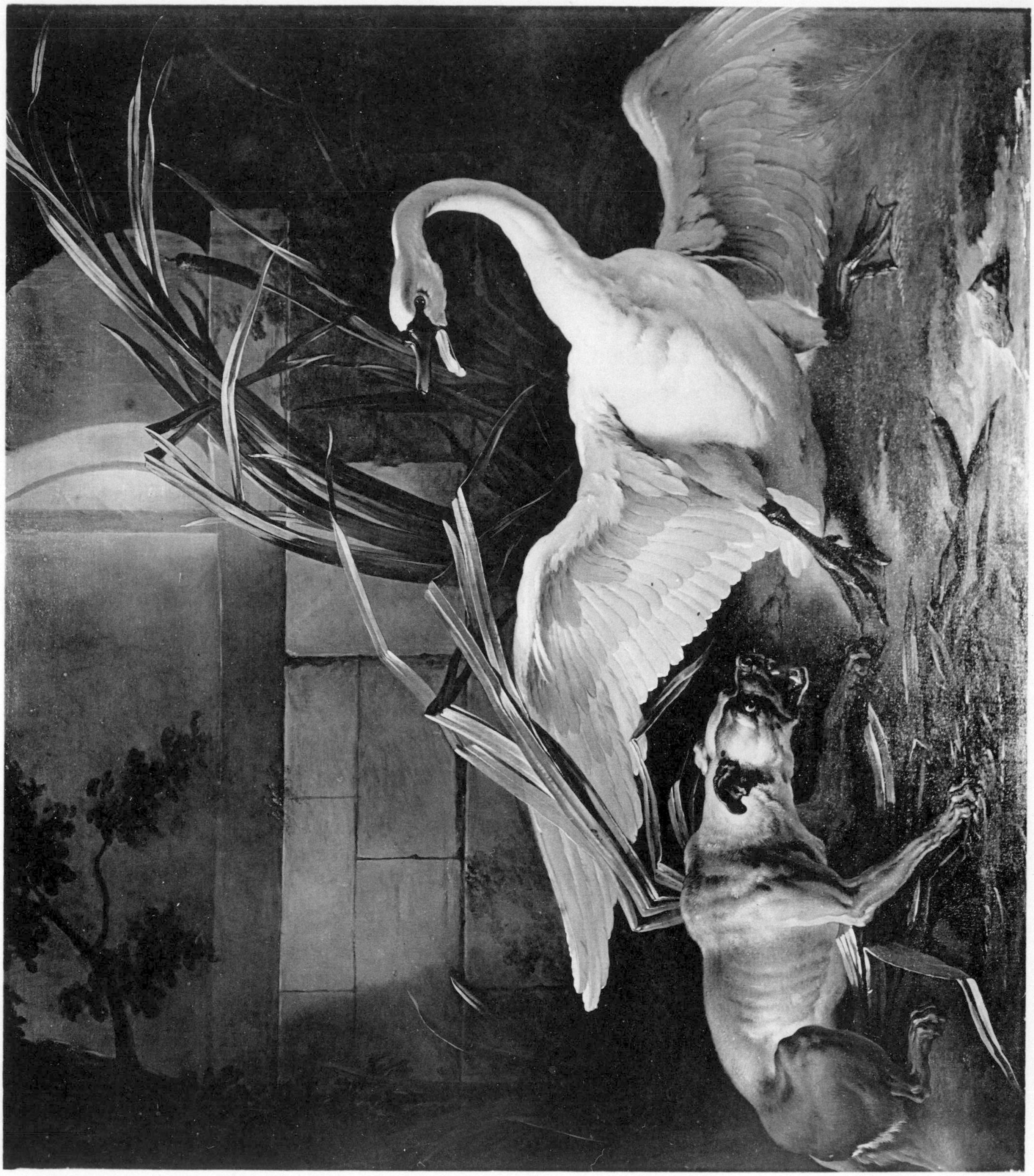

LADIES BATHING, WITH THE STATUE OF NEPTUNE

BY

J.-B.-J. PATER

1695-1736

J.-B.-J. PATER

1695-1736

Born in Valenciennes, his father was a sculptor and a friend of Watteau's family. Sent to Paris to study under Watteau but was not accepted as a pupil by him because of a quarrel. Shortly before Watteau's death, the two artists became reconciled and for a brief period Pater benefited by the instruction of the older master. Elected to the Academy in 1728, he died at the age of forty-one reputedly from overwork. With Lancret, he is considered the most important follower of Watteau.

Ladies bathing, with the statue of Neptune

canvas: 19⅞ x 23⅞ inches

A composition of fourteen figures in and on the banks of a river at the corner of a garden overshadowed by trees. Ten are ladies of whom three are in the pool; the others are either preparing for the bath or have just emerged. In the left background a statue of Neptune and in the right, a distant landscape view of a building with a tower. Pendant to No. 37.

References: T. Ward & W. Roberts, *Pictures in the collection of J. Pierpont Morgan, Princess Gate and Dover House,* 1907, v, no number, ill., "One of the most important of Pater's many versions of this subject is now in the National Gallery of Scotland, and another version is in the Wallace collection (No. 426)."; F. Ingersoll-Smouse, *Pater,* 1928, ill. p. 152, no. 95, p. 63, no. 323; *Bulletin of the Metropolitan Museum of Art,* Nov., 1935, xxx, p. 206; New York, Metropolitan Museum of Art, *French painting and sculpture of the XVIII century,* Nov. 6, 1935-Jan. 5, 1936, no. 9, ill.

Exhibited: 1935-1936, New York, Metropolitan Museum of Art.

Collections: Martin Colhaghi; Rodolphe Kann, Paris; J. Pierpont Morgan, New York.

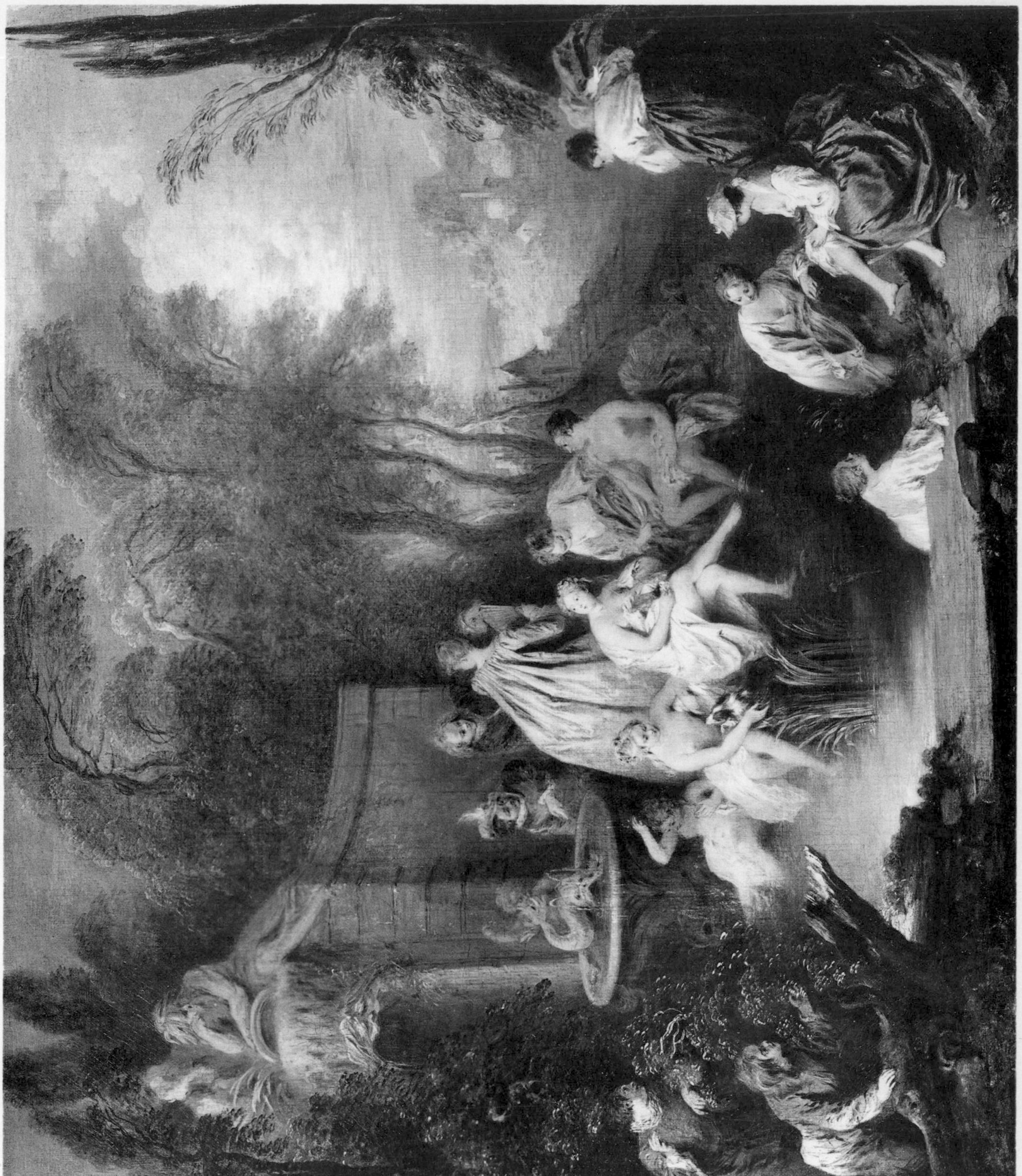

LADIES BATHING, WITH THE STATUE OF VENUS

BY

J.-B.-J. PATER

1695-1736

J.-B.-J. PATER

1695-1736

Born in Valenciennes, his father was a sculptor and a friend of Watteau's family. Sent to Paris to study under Watteau but was not accepted as a pupil by him because of a quarrel. Shortly before Watteau's death, the two artists became reconciled and for a brief period Pater benefited by the instruction of the older master. Elected to the Academy in 1728, he died at the age of forty-one reputedly from overwork. With Lancret, he is considered the most important follower of Watteau.

Ladies bathing, with the statue of Venus

canvas: 19⅞ x 23⅞ inches

A composition of fourteen figures by a stream, in the shadow of a tall overhanging tree. Three ladies are bathing, one is sitting on the bank dressing, and another is conversing with a cavalier who is playing a guitar. In the right background, a statue of Venus and in the left, a distant landscape view of a church and several cottages. Pendant to No. 36.

References: T. Ward & W. Roberts, *Pictures in the collection of J. Pierpont Morgan, Princess Gate and Dover House,* 1907, v, no number, ill., "One of the most important of Pater's many versions of this subject is now in the National Gallery of Scotland, and another version is in the Wallace collection (No. 426)."; F. Ingersoll-Smouse, *Pater,* 1928, ill. p. 152, no. 96, p. 63, no. 325; *Bulletin of the Metropolitan Museum of Art,* Nov., 1935, xxx, p. 206; New York, Metropolitan Museum of Art, *French painting and sculpture of the XVIII century,* Nov. 6, 1935-Jan. 5, 1936, no. 8, ill.

Exhibited: 1935-1936, New York, Metropolitan Museum of Art.

Collections: Martin Colhaghi; Rodolphe Kann, Paris; J. Pierpont Morgan, New York.

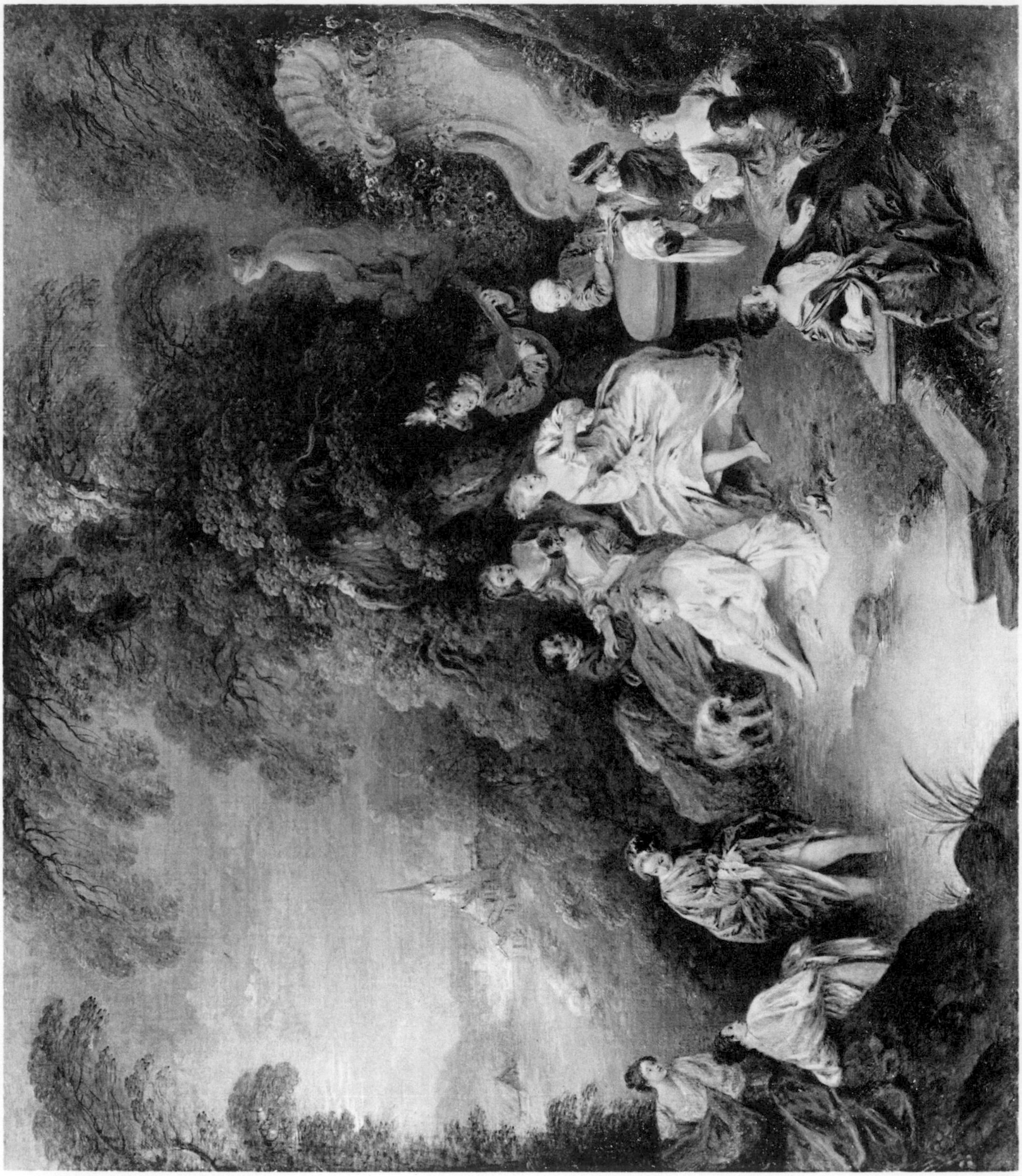

PORTRAIT OF MADAME MIRON

BY

JEAN-BAPTISTE PERRONNEAU

1715-1783

JEAN-BAPTISTE PERRONNEAU

1715-1783

First training was in copper plate engraving under Laurent Cars and did some engravings after Boucher, Van Loo and Natoire, but better known for his portraits, particularly in pastel. A pupil of Natoire and Drouais the Elder. Elected a member of the Academy in 1753 for his portraits of the painter Oudry and the sculptor Lambert Adam, and exhibited frequently in the Salon thereafter. Travelled a great deal in France, Italy and Holland, and died in Amsterdam.

Portrait of Madame Miron

canvas: 25½ x 21 inches

Signed and dated upper right: *Perronneau 1771.*

Bust-length portrait turned to the right, looking at the spectator. Dressed in a pink gown with pink and white bows and a black lace shawl. She wears a small white lace cap on her powdered hair. Probably a member of the Miron family of Spanish origin, several members of which distinguished themselves in medicine and law.

References: L. Vaillat & Ratouis de Limay, *Perronneau,* p. 227; Paris, Galerie Georges Petit, *Vente collection Degas,* Mar. 26-27, 1918, no. 4, ill.; London, Christie's, *Sir Edmund Davis sale,* July 7, 1939, p. 26, no. 124.

Collections: Edgar Degas, Paris; Sir Edmund Davis, Paris.

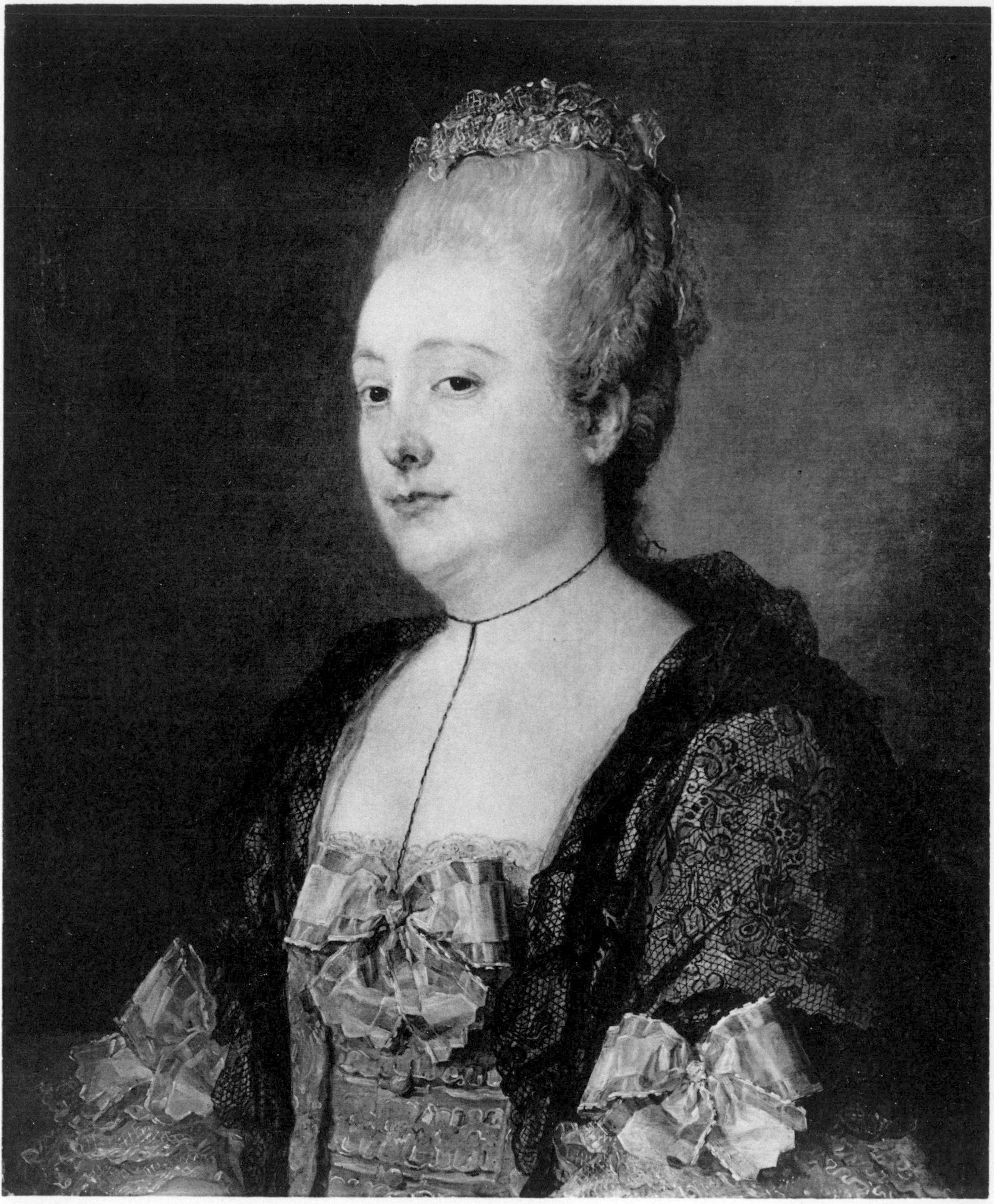

PORTRAIT OF
MADAME BARBIER-WALBONNE

BY

PIERRE-PAUL PRUD'HON

1738-1823

PIERRE-PAUL PRUD'HON

1738-1823

Born at Cluny and brought up partly by Benedictine monks as he was an orphan. Studied first at Dijon under Desvoges and then in Paris under Jean-Baptiste Pierre. In 1874 won a Burgundian prize which enabled him to study in Rome for three years. Here he was particularly influenced by Leonardo, Raphael and Correggio, as well as by the baroque painters. An admirer of David and a Jacobin during the revolution, but not very active in political events. Died in Paris in 1823.

Portrait of Madame Barbier-Walbonne

canvas: 21¾ x 18¼ inches

Waist-length, three quarters to the left with the head turned almost full face. Her dark hair falls in curls on her forehead and cheeks and is dressed high in back. Her crossed hands rest on a table which protrudes into the left hand corner of the canvas. She wears a white dress and a rose colored scarf. The wife of Jacques-Luc Barbier-Walbonne, a portraitist and painter of historical scenes who was born in 1769 and died in 1860 and was a pupil of David.

References: Paris, Bagatelle, *Portraits de femmes sous les trois Républiques,* 1909, no. 163, ill.; G. Mourey, "Exposition rétrospective de portraits de femmes sous les trois républiques," *Les Arts,* July, 1909, p. 30, ill., p. 28; C. Saunier, "Les dessins de Prud'hon," *Renaissance de l'art français,* May, 1922, p. 306, ill.; Paris, Petit Palais, *Exposition Prud'hon,* May-June, 1922, no. 45 New York, Wildenstein & Co., *Exposition Prud'hon,* Nov., 1922, no. 10; J. Guiffrey, "L'oeuvre de Pierre-Paul Prud'hon," *Archives de l'art français,* n.p. XIII, 1924, p. 154, no. 415; Buffalo, Albright Art Gallery, *19th century French art,* Nov. 1-30, 1932, no. 48, pl. III; New York, World's Fair, *Masterpieces of Art,* May-Oct., 1940, no. 234, ill.; New York, Wildenstein & Co., *Fashion in headdress,* Apr. 27-May 27, 1943, no. 74; New York, Wildenstein & Co., *French revolution,* Dec., 1943, no. 56.

Exhibited: 1909, Paris, Bagatelle; 1922, Paris Petit Palais; 1922, New York, Wildenstein & Co.; 1932, Buffalo, Albright Art Gallery; 1940, New York, World's Fair; 1943, New York, Wildenstein & Co.

Collections: Alphonse Kann, Paris.

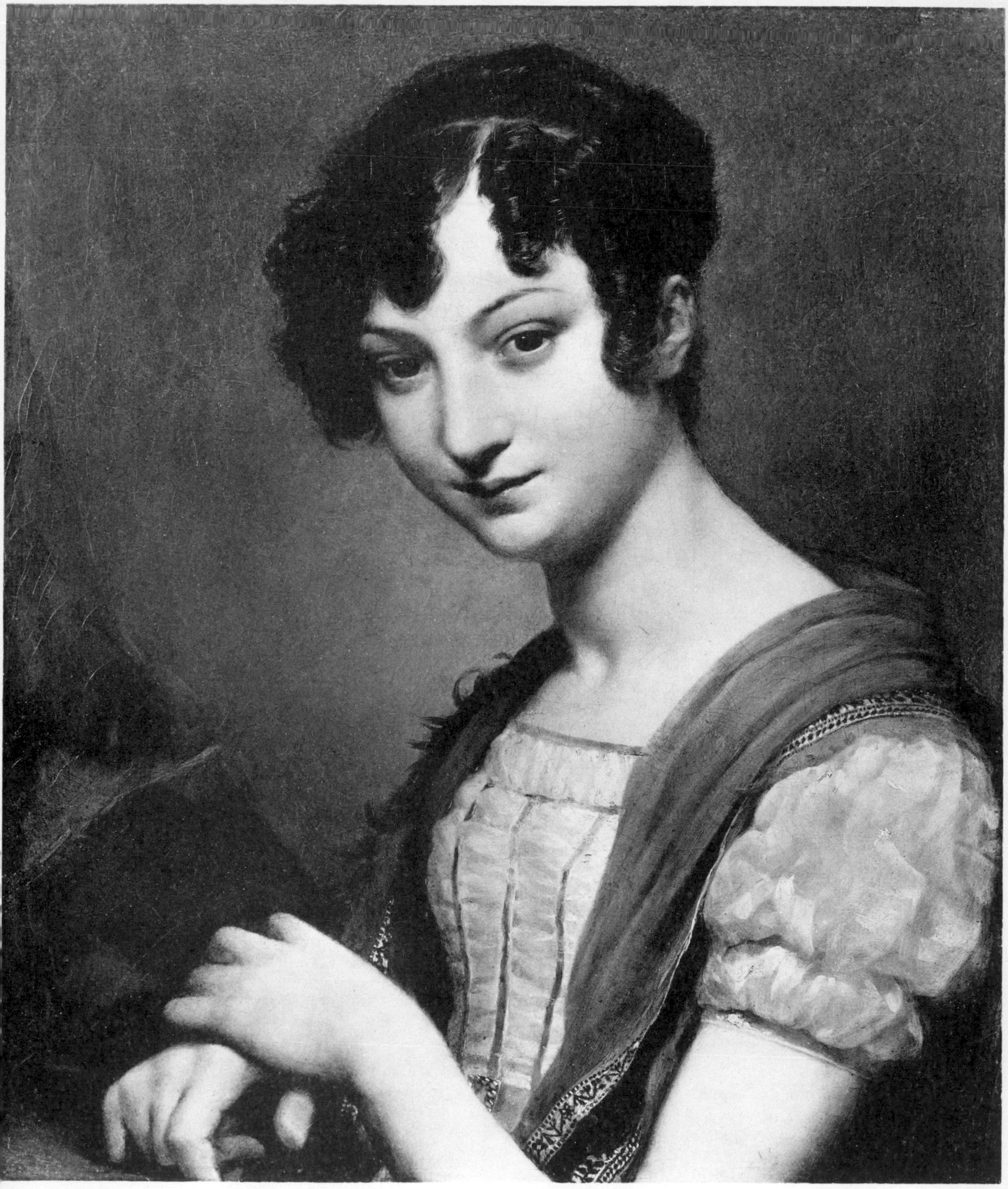

FOUNTAIN IN A ROMAN VILLA

BY

HUBERT ROBERT

1733-1808

HUBERT ROBERT

1733-1808

Began his artistic career working under the sculptor, Slodtz, but in 1754, thanks to the patronage of the Duc de Choiseul, went to Rome. Lived for a while with the Abbé de Saint-Non and Fragonard at the Villa d'Este in Tivoli. In addition to following the archaeological discoveries then being made, he studied especially Pannini and Piranesi. In 1765 returned to Paris with many sketches which he used in his later paintings. A member of the Academy in 1776. During the revolution was imprisoned from 1793-1794 and worked diligently in Saint-Lazare. Appointed Custodian of the Louvre under the Directoire, but in 1806 was forced by Napoleon to leave his studio in the Louvre.

Fountain in a Roman villa

canvas: 22 x 29¾ inches

A fountain in the center of a basin, surrounded by a semi-circular wall which is decorated with niches and statues. In the background, a waterfall enters the basin through one of the niches, and around the edge of the basin groups of women are washing clothes. In the right foreground three laundresses are working in a smaller pool of water which is filled by a fountain from a lion's mouth; in the left foreground a woman is walking with a child.

References: Paris, Galerie Georges Petit, *Vente Groult,* June 21-22, 1920, no. 101, ill.

Collections: Camille Groult.

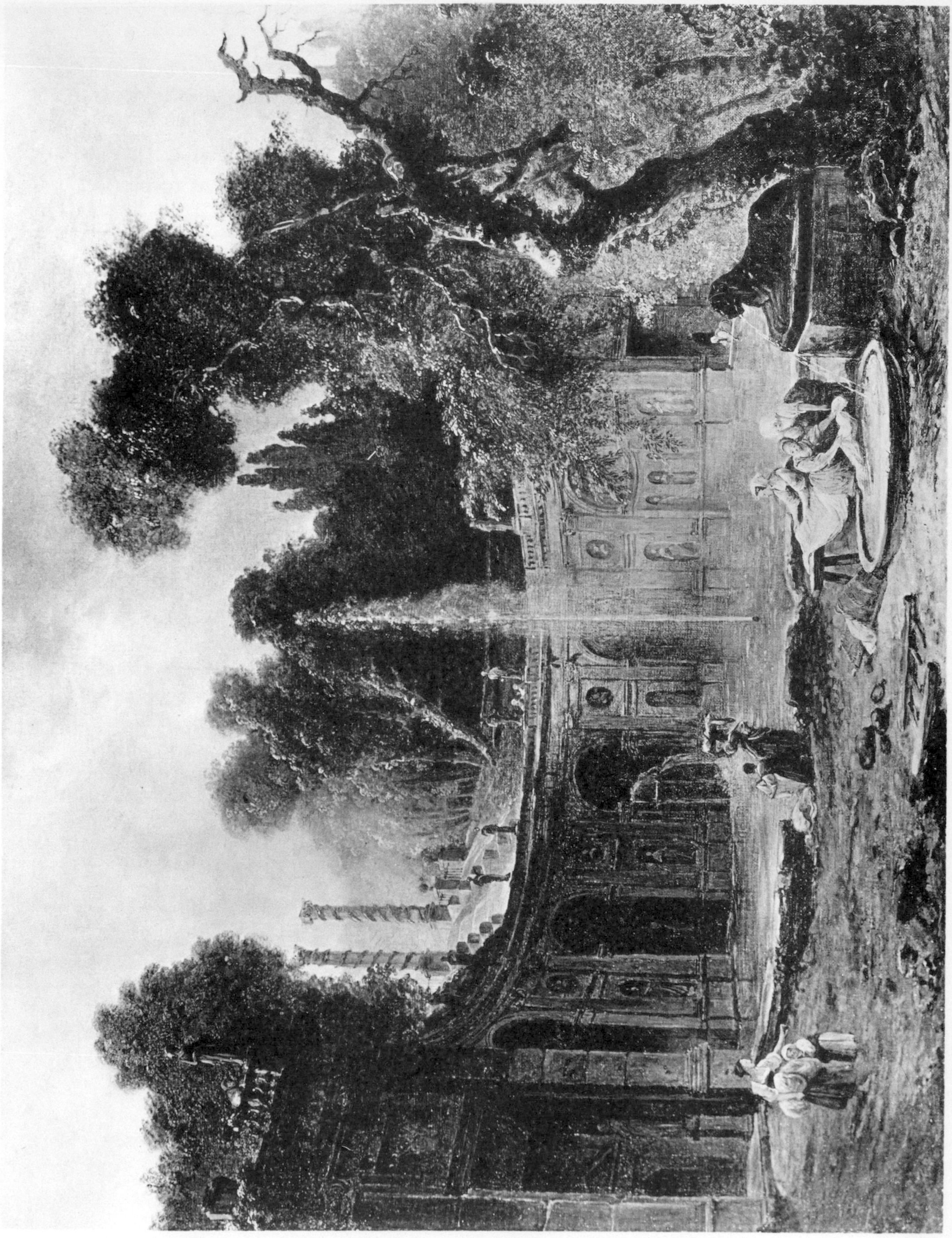

INTERIOR OF A ROMAN TEMPLE WITH FIGURES

BY

HUBERT ROBERT

1733-1808

HUBERT ROBERT

1733-1808

Began his artistic career working under the sculptor, Slodtz, but in 1754, thanks to the patronage of the Duc de Choiseul, went to Rome. Lived for a while with the Abbé de Saint-Non and Fragonard at the Villa d'Este in Tivoli. In addition to following the archaeological discoveries then being made, he studied especially Pannini and Piranesi. In 1765 returned to Paris with many sketches which he used in his later paintings. A member of the Academy in 1776. During the revolution was imprisoned from 1793-1794 and worked diligently in Saint-Lazare. Appointed Custodian of the Louvre under the Directoire, but in 1806 was forced by Napoleon to leave his studio in the Louvre.

Interior of a Roman temple with figures

canvas: 44 x 57 inches

View of the interior of a circular temple. The walls and the dome are decorated with mosaics and coffering and the open court is surrounded by a colonnade. The exterior wall contains niches which are filled with statues. In the center is a large sculptured fountain and at each group of columns are three fountains: two in the form of lions and one in the form of a mask. The temple is enlivened with small figures engaged in various activities. In the mid foreground, two women accompanied by a dog stop to converse; to the left, a seated man is drawing. A good example of Robert's use of archaeological research.

References: New York, Parke-Bernet galleries, *Mrs. Cooper Hewitt sale,* Apr. 3-6, 1935, p. 120, no. 618, ill.

Collections: Mrs. Lucy W. Hewitt.

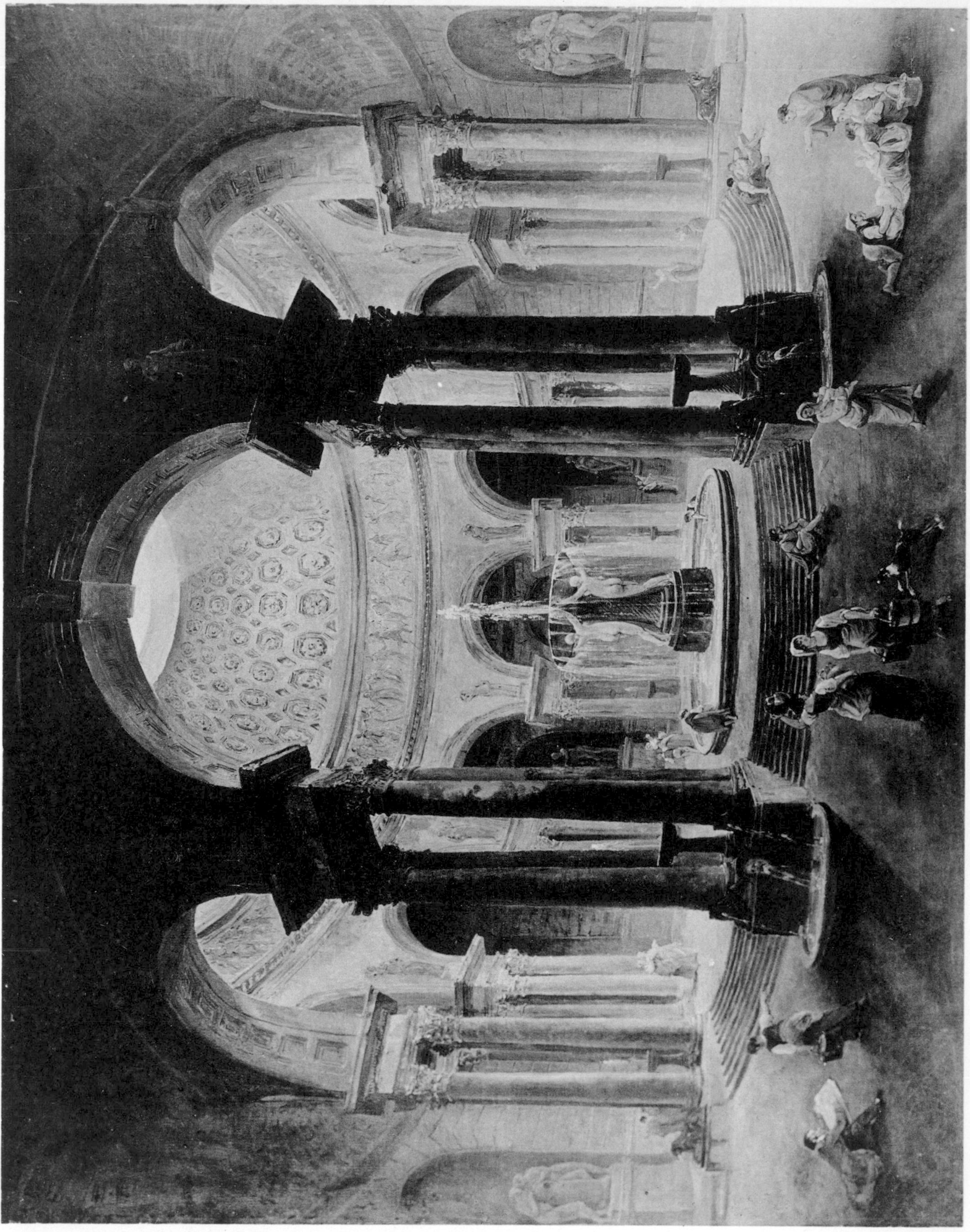

PORTRAIT OF MADAME BOUCHER

BY

ALEXANDER ROSLIN

1718-1793

ALEXANDER ROSLIN

1718-1793

Born in Malmoe, Sweden. Studied in the school of Georg Engelh. Schröders in Stockholm from 1736 to 1739, and then worked in his studio for two more years. In 1741 he was in Gothenburg and in 1747, travelled to Italy–Venice, Bologne, Florence and Naples where he remained for sixteen months in 1748 and 1749. Back in Paris, was accepted by the Academy in 1753. Married a young artist, Marie-Suzanne Giboust in 1770 and after her death in 1772 went to Sweden and then Russia. Returned to Paris and lived in the Louvre from 1788 until his death.

Portrait of Madame Boucher

canvas, oval: 25½ x 21½ inches

Signed and dated center right: *Roslin le Suedois 1761.*

Marie-Jeanne Buseau who became the wife of the painter François Boucher in 1733, when she was seventeen. The mother of his three children: Juste Nathan, an architect, and two daughters who married his favorite pupils, Baudoin and Deshayes. Jeanne Boucher probably worked in his studio although only one etching with her signature is known. She was a celebrated beauty and frequently served as the painter's model. Pendant to the portrait of Boucher in the Versailles Museum.

References: *Collection des livrets des Manciennes expositions,* Salon de 1761, no. 72; *Catalogue du salon de 1761,* illustrated by Saint-Aubin, p. 20; D. Diderot, *Oeuvres* complètes, 1876, x, Salon de 1761, p. 136, "One finds, however, that the painter has made progress since the last Salon, and the Portrait of Boucher and that of his still beautiful wife have been highly praised."; H. MacFall, *Boucher,* 1908, p. 27, "In 1761, when she was forty-five, Roslin painted the dainty creature whom even Diderot, the man of growls, confesses to be 'always beautiful'."; Paris, Galerie Georges Petit, *Vente Léon Michel-Lévy,* June 18, 1925, no. 152, ill.; San Francisco, California Palace of the Legion of Honor, *French painting from the 15th century to the present day,* June 8-July 8, 1934, no. 54; Cincinnati, Art Museum, *French paintings of the 18th and early 19th centuries,* Oct. 2-Nov. 7, 1937, no. 18; New York, Wildenstein & Co., *Fashion in headdress,* Apr. 27-May 27, 1943, no. 49.

Exhibited: 1761, Paris, Salon; 1934, San Francisco, California Palace of the Legion of Honor; 1937, Cincinnati, Art Museum; 1943, New York, Wildenstein & Co.

Collections: Léon Michel-Lévy.

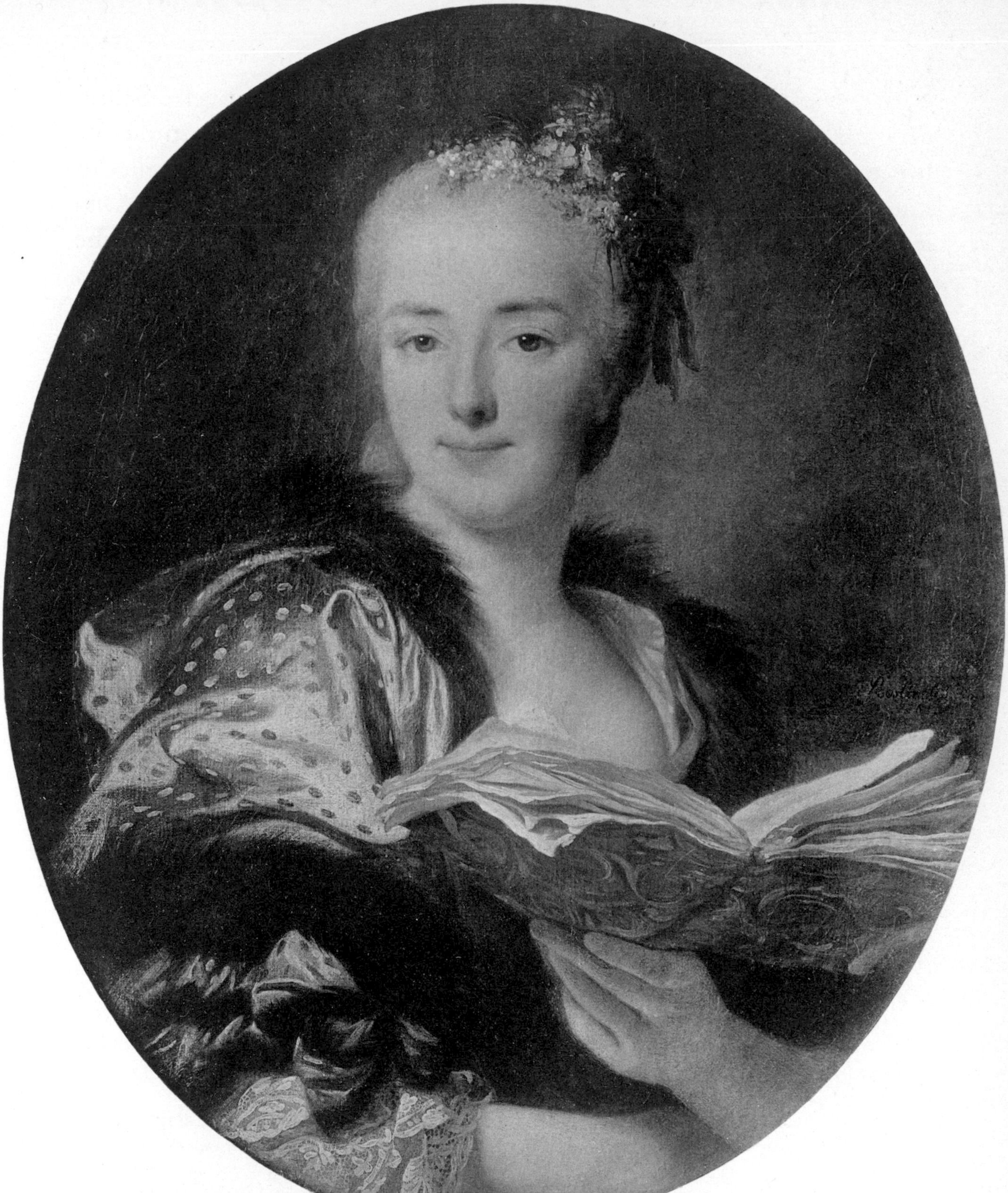

LE PORTRAIT CHERI

BY

JEAN-FREDERIC SCHALL

1752-1825

JEAN-FREDERIC SCHALL

1752-1825

Born in Strasbourg, educated in the studio of Pierre and Henri Haldenwanger and then in the public drawing school of Strasbourg. Went to Paris with a letter of introduction to the engraver, Wille, and after studying with François Casanova, entered the school of the Royal Academy under the protection of Brenet, in 1772. Worked also with Lépicié from 1776 to 1779. Has been confused with Michel-Ange Challe. An imitator of Fragonard, his work and some of the engravings after his canvases are much in demand.

Le portrait chéri

panel: 11⅝ x 9 inches

Engraved by Bonnet.

A young woman seated on a couch in a boudoir hung with blue brocade and decorated with an oval picture of a nymph surprised by a satyr. In her right hand she holds a letter and in her left hand a medallion which she is lifting to her lips. Dressed in a pink gown and a straw hat with roses. To her left, a table with a box and some flowers, and at her feet a small dog. A curtain is draped from the upper left hand corner and falls over a cushion on the end of the couch.

References: Paris, Galerie Georges Petit, *Vente Madame de Polès,* June 22-24, 1927, no. 24, ill.; A. Girodié, *Un peintre de fêtes galantes, Jean-Frédéric Schall,* 1927, pp. 8, 18, 62, 68, 71, "In the same collection of Georges Wildenstein we cite several more important works of Schall which we knew too late to mention in the proper place in our book . . . et *Le Portrait chéri,* de l'ancienne collection de Madame de Polès . . ."

Collections: Madame de Polès.

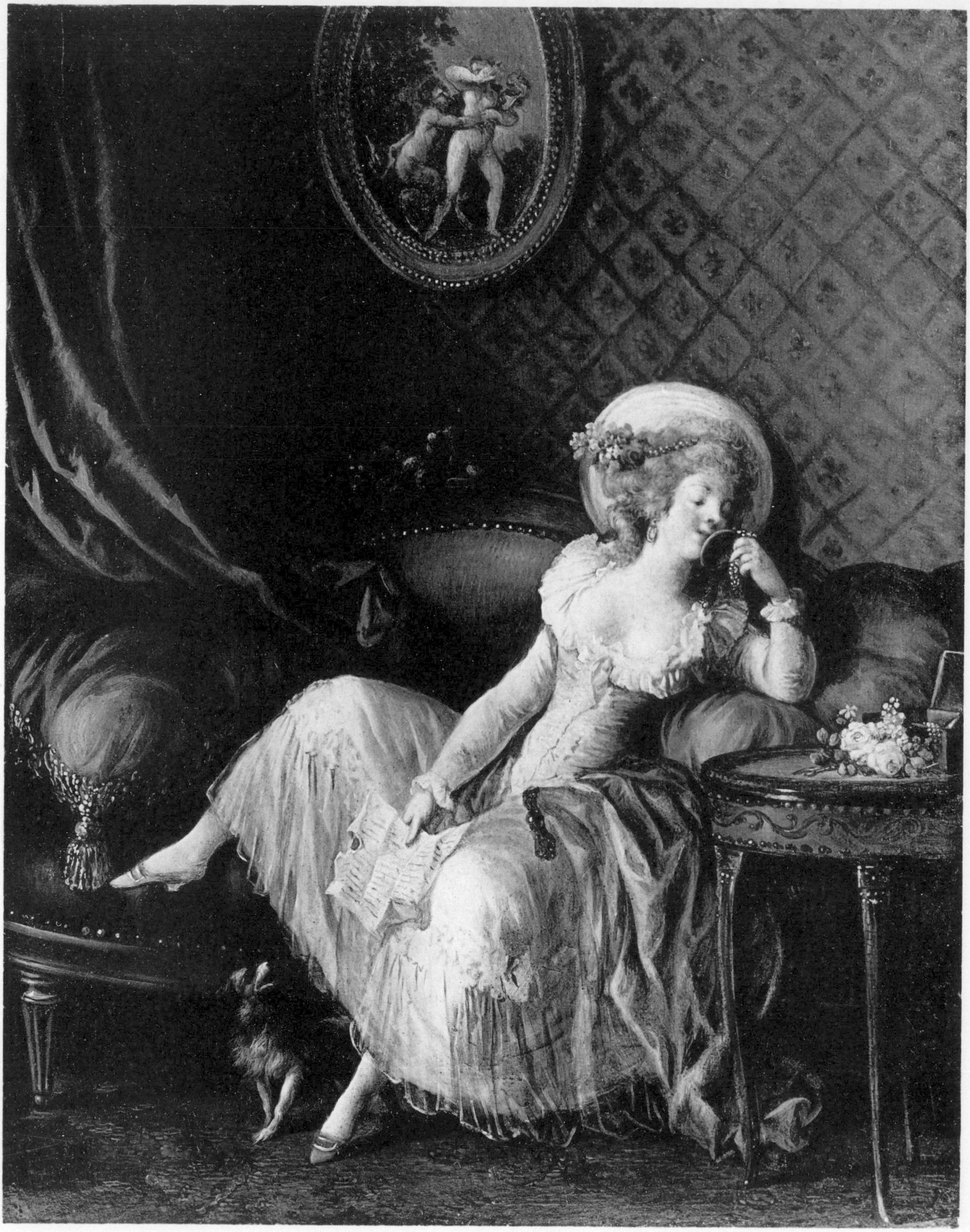

PORTRAIT OF PIERRE JELIOTTE AS APOLLO

BY

LOUIS TOCQUE

1698-1772

LOUIS TOCQUE

1698-1772

First training from Nicolas Bertin. Married Nattier's eldest daughter and therefore closely connected with that painter as well as a friend of Chardin, Aved and Boucher. Elected a member of the Academy in 1734 for his portraits of Galloche and the sculptor, Jean-Louis Lemoyne. Was successful very early in his career and travelled a great deal executing many important commissions. Called to Russia by the Empress Elizabeth in 1757; in 1759 and again in 1769, in Denmark where he did portraits of the King and Queen. His work so impressed people in Russia and Scandinavia that twenty Russians and nine Danes registered at the Academy after his visit. In Paris, painted many court portraits and, with Largillière, the most popular portraitist of the wealthy bourgeoisie.

Portrait of Pierre Jéliotte as Apollo

canvas: 35½ x 28¾ inches

Signed and dated lower right: *L. Tocqué p. 1755.*

Engraved by Louis Jacques Cathelin.

Pierre Jéliotte or Jélyotte, the famous French singer, was born in Lasseube (Basses-Pyrenées) on April 13, 1713. He studied for a few years at the Cathedral in Toulouse learning to play several instruments, but was soon called to Paris. From the time of his debut at the age of twenty he was one of the most justly popular singers of the Paris opera, playing roles in all the main operas by Rameau, Mouret, Mondonville and others. In 1755 this portrait of him was painted to celebrate his retirement. He was also a composer of some note writing the lyrics for a musical comedy by La Noue as well as several songs. In 1775 he returned to the country of his birth where he died on September 12, 1797.

References: *Nouveau Larousse Illustré,* ill. under Jéliotte (detail of head); *Collection des livrets des anciennes expositions,* Salon de 1755, no. 53; Pau, *Catalogue de l'exposition de Pau,* 1891, pl. XXI, p. 69; R. Portalis & H. Beraldi, *Les graveurs du XVIIIe siècle,* 1892, I, p. 331, no. 32; P. Mantz, "Louis Tocqué," *Gazette des Beaux-*

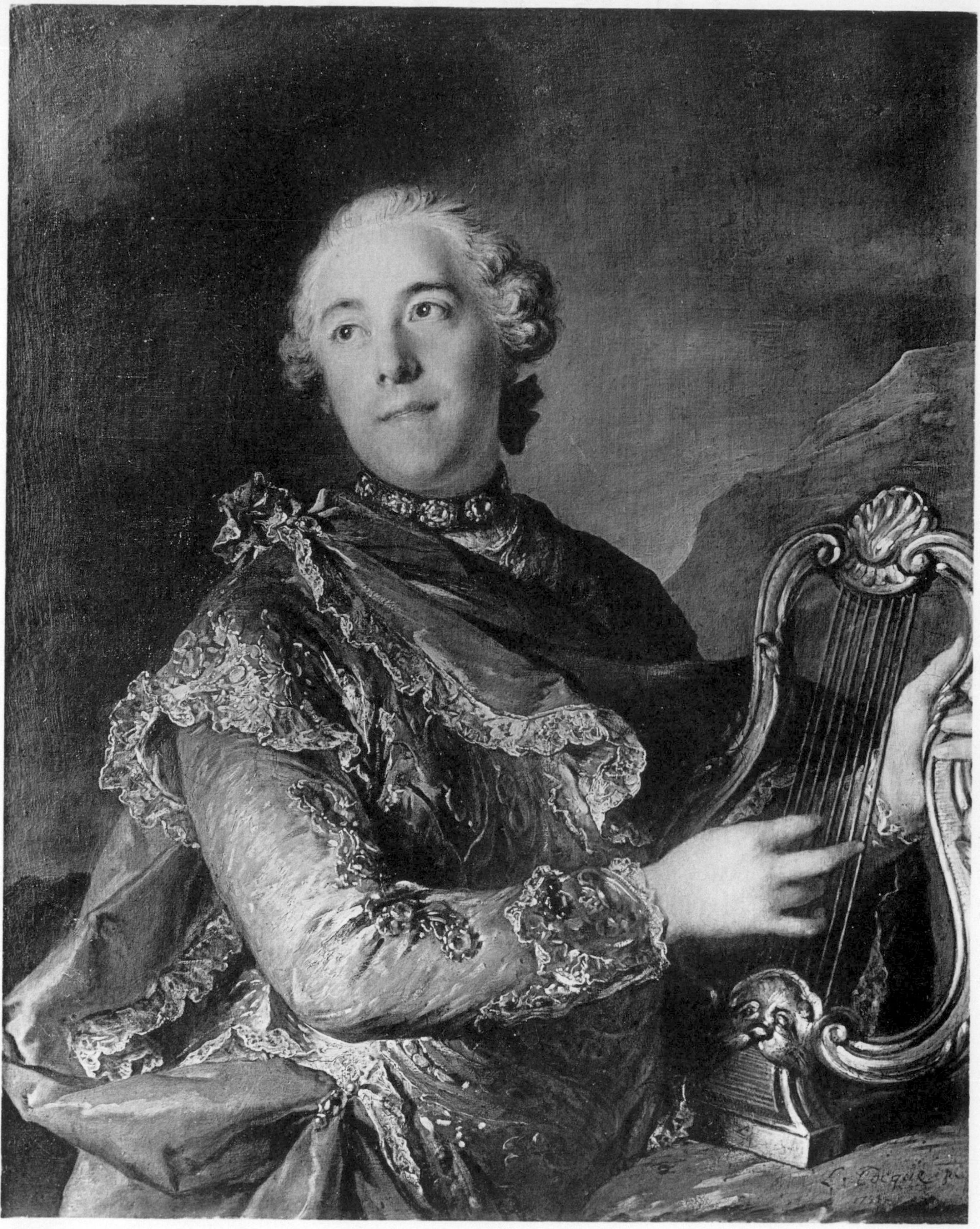

Arts, 1894, II, pp. 464-465; P. Dorbec, "Louis Tocqué," *Gazette des Beaux-Arts,* 1909, II, p. 458; J. J. Foster, *French art from Watteau to Prud'hon,* 1905-1917, II, p. 122; A. Doria, *Louis Tocqué,* 1929, no. 144, fig. 55, p. 113; P. Schommer, "Musée Carnavalet, exposition du théâtre au XVIIe et au XVIIIe siècles," *Bulletin des musées de France,* I, Apr. 1929, p. 77, ill.; Paris, Musée Carnavalet, *Le théâtre à Paris, XVIIe-XVIIIe siècle,* Mar. 19-May 4, 1929, p. 18, no. 67, ill.; Paris, "Gazette des Beaux-Arts," *Le siècle Louis XV vu par les artistes,* 1934, p. 73, no. 193; S. Rocheblave, *French painting of the 18th century,* 1937, no. 22, ill.; G. Wildenstein, *La peinture française au XVIIIe siècle,* 1937, no. 29, ill.

Exhibited: 1775, Paris, Salon; 1891, Pau; 1929, Paris, Musée Carnavalet; 1934, Paris, "Gazette des Beaux-Arts."

Collections: Pierre de Manco (nephew of Jéliotte); Madame Théophile de Navailles (Born Manco); Lamotte d'Incamps (cousin of de Navailles); Mimaud, Pau.

PORTRAIT OF AN UNKNOWN LADY

BY

LOUIS-ROLLAND TRINQUESSE

c. 1746-1800

LOUIS-ROLLAND TRINQUESSE

c. 1746-1800

Was a pupil at the school of the Royal Academy in 1758 under the protection of Halle. Tradition says that he also studied under Largillière but this seems impossible since Largillière died in 1746, too early for Trinquesse to have been working. In 1767 went to Le Hague and was appointed a master of the painters' guild in that city. Returned to Paris where he was known for his portraits and particularly for his genre paintings.

Portrait of an unknown lady

canvas, oval: 28½ x 23⅞ inches

Signed and dated above corsage at left: L. R. Trinquesse F., 1785.

A charming half length portrait of a young woman seen in profile with her head full face, turned towards the left. Her fair curly hair falls down her back and on her head she wears a large grey hat. A corsage of flowers decorates the front of her dress.

References: London, Wildenstein & Co., *Women of France in the 18th century,* Apr.-May 1938, no. 20; *Illustrated London News,* Christmas number, 1938, p. 25, ill. (in color); London, Wildenstein & Co., *Woman and her background in 18th century France,* June 1946, p. 8, no. 13; D. Sutton, "French paintings of the 18th and 19th centuries," *Burlington Magazine,* 88, July 1946, pl. A, p. 178, "In this exhibition, the charm and coquetry of eighteenth century woman . . . are best seen in Louis Trinquesse's delicious signed and dated *Portrait of an Unknown Lady* (Plate A) . . . Here woman is depicted not as the mysterious creature of the Romantic movement, that 'Femme fatale' who can already be discerned in Prud'hon's portraits, but as the offspring of a pleasure loving century which practised what it preached, and applied rationalism in life as well as in thought."

Exhibited: 1938, London, Wildenstein & Co.; 1946, London, Wildenstein & Co.

Collections: Madame Louis Burat.

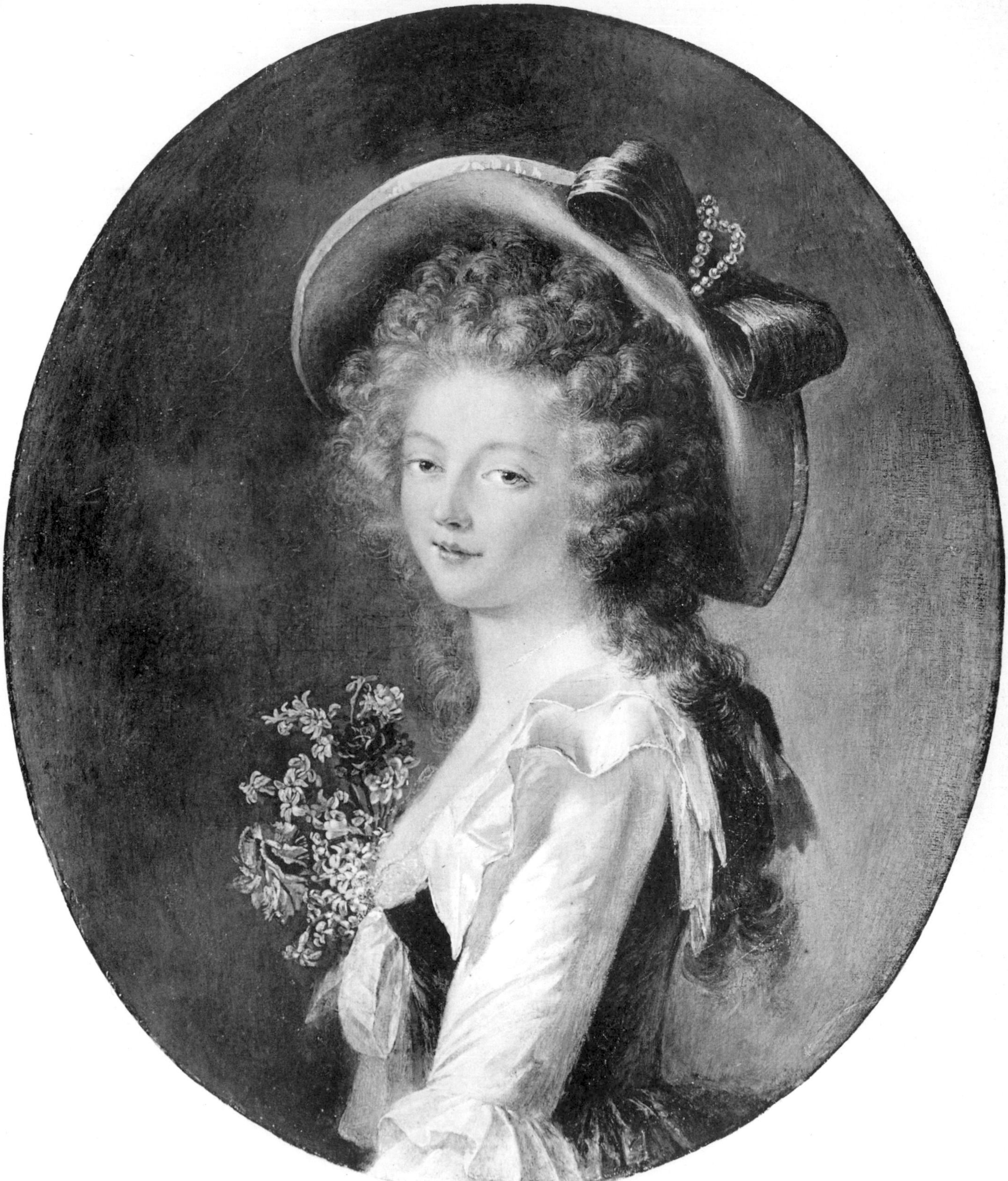

FETE AUX PORCHERONS

BY

JEAN-FRANÇOIS DE TROY

1679-1752

JEAN-FRANÇOIS DE TROY

1679-1752

Son of the portrait painter, François de Troy, and Jeanne Colette. Pupil of his father before attending the School of the Royal Academy. Sent to Italy by his father and stayed six years, partly studying at the Academy in Rome and partly travelling. Returned to Paris, accepted by the Academy in 1708 and was soon much in demand executing many decorations for royal residences and churches in Paris. Also painted portraits and other easel pictures which are usually superior to his decorations. In addition, did cartoons for tapestry, the best known being the History of Esther (1738-1742). Appointed professor at the Academy in 1719 and Director of the Academy in Rome in 1738. Died in Rome.

Fête aux Porcherons

canvas: 35½ x 46 inches

A crowd of ladies and gentlemen scattered throughout the landscape enjoying themselves at the famous amusement area of Les Porcherons. This section of Paris which today is occupied by the church of La Trinité near the intersection of the Rue Saint-Lazare and the Rue Clichy, was nearly open country in the 18th century and quite a journey from the center of town. It became very fashionable for society people to go there, particularly on Sundays, and to frequent the equally famous cabaret, Tambour-Royal, run by Ramponneau. A comic opera was written by Thomas Sauvage and Albert Grisar in 1850 to commemorate the gaiety of those Sunday afternoons.

Collections: Baron M. de Rothschild.

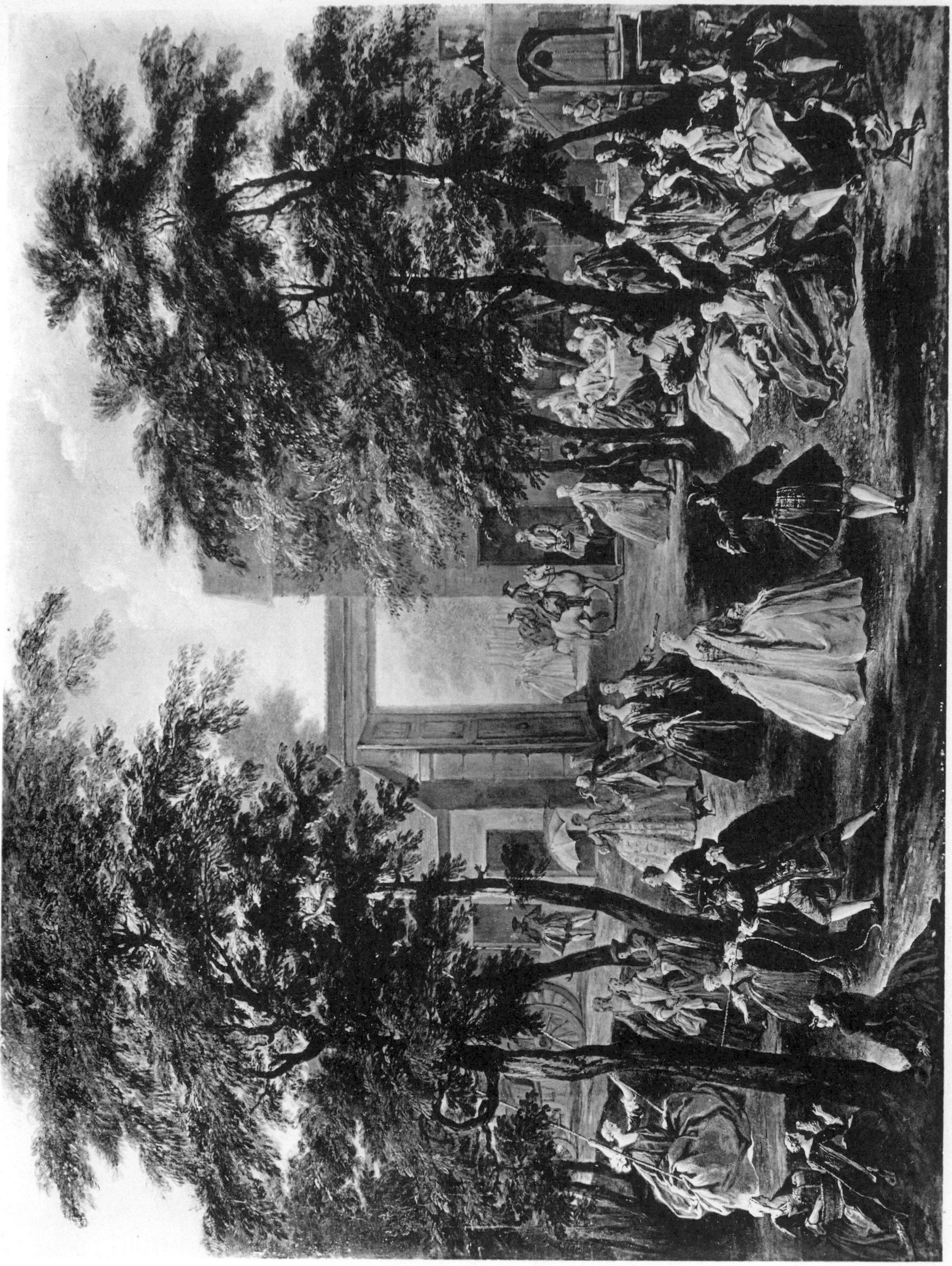

PORTRAIT OF
MADAME SAINT-HUBERTY

BY

ANNE VALLAYER-COSTER

1744-1818

ANNE VALLAYER-COSTER

1744-1818

Daughter of a jewelry merchant, Joseph Vallayer. Elected a member of the Academy in 1770 and exhibited in the Salon from 1771 until just before her death in 1818. Married in 1781 to a lawyer, Coster. Painted portraits and still life, the latter being close to Chardin. Highly praised by Diderot.

Portrait of Madame Saint-Huberty

canvas: 57⅜ x 40 inches

Anne Antoinette Cecile Clavel, called Madame Saint-Huberty, was a celebrated singer and actress of the Paris opera. She was born in Strasbourg in 1756 and received most of her musical education in Germany and Poland. In 1777 she made her debut in a small role of Gluck's *Armide;* Gluck himself noticed her talent and prophesied her future success. The role of Dido in Piccinni's opera, in which she is represented here, was her most famous portrayal. Towards 1789 she abandoned opera and travelled to Lausanne, Vienna and Gratz with her husband, the Count d'Entraigues, who was a member of the Constituent Assembly. He was also a secret Russian agent and shortly after, they went to London where he was commissioned to give the secret terms of the Peace of Tilsitt to the English minister. Here, in a country house near London, they were both assassinated by one of their servants.

References: *Collection des livrets des anciennes expositions,* Salon de 1785, no. 58; E. de Goncourt, *Madame Saint-Huberty,* 1882, pp. 9, 253; London, Wildenstein & Co., *Women of France in the 18th century,* Apr.-May, 1938, no. 21.

Exhibited: 1785, Paris, Salon; 1938, London, Wildenstein & Co.

Collections: Collection of Esternay Castle, France; Madame de Cuny.

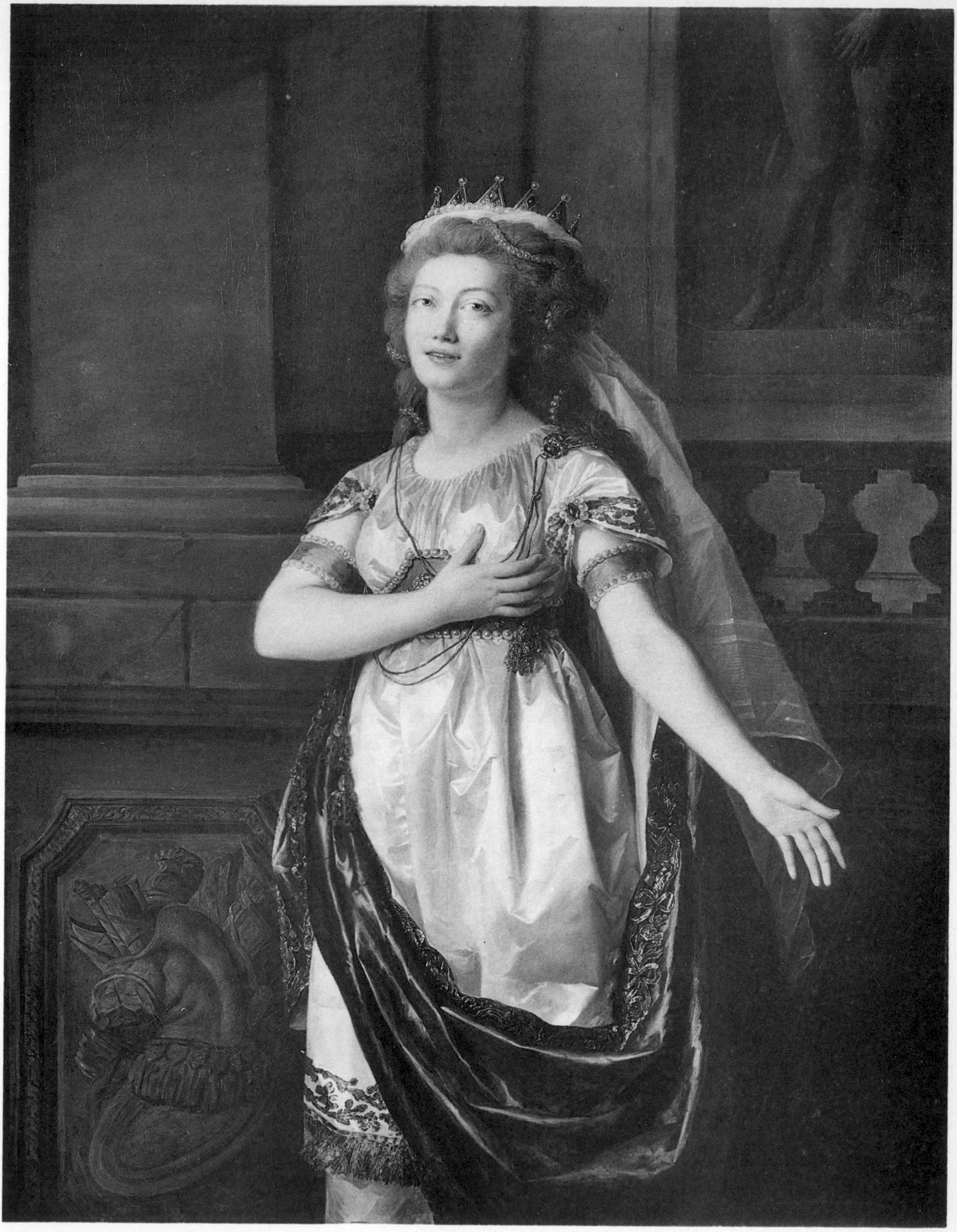

PORTRAIT OF MADAME DE TENCIN HOLDING A CAT

BY

CARLE VAN LOO

1705-1765

CARLE VAN LOO

1705-1765

Second son of Louis Van Loo, a painter of Flemish origin, born at Nice. Instructed by his brother Jean-Baptiste whom he accompanied in 1714 to Rome and in 1720 to Paris. Studied under Benedetto Luti in Rome and learned sculpture in both wood and stone in Legros' studio. In 1724 won the Grand Prix and returned to Rome with his two nephews and Boucher; in 1735 elected a member of the Academy. An extremely able technician, he could work in all mediums–oil, fresco, etc.–, and received many court commissions. Named 'Premier peintre du roi' in 1762 and Director of the Academy in 1763.

Portrait of Madame de Tencin holding a cat

canvas: 36 x 29 inches

Signed and dated lower left: *Van Loo 1736.*

Born in 1680 in Grenoble, Madame de Tencin was celebrated for both her intrigues and her Salon. At an early age she was placed by her parents in a nunnery, but that life did not suit her and her brother, the Abbé de Tencin, obtained her release. From this time on she was involved in a succession of political intrigues and love affairs culminating in the death of one of her lovers, Lafresnaye, who either killed himself or was shot by her. She was suspected and put in the Bastille in 1726, but her powerful friends soon freed her. The second half of her life was more peaceful and she concentrated on gathering around her the writers and scholars of the day and on developing her famous salon. With the aid of her nephews she wrote several books before her death in 1758.

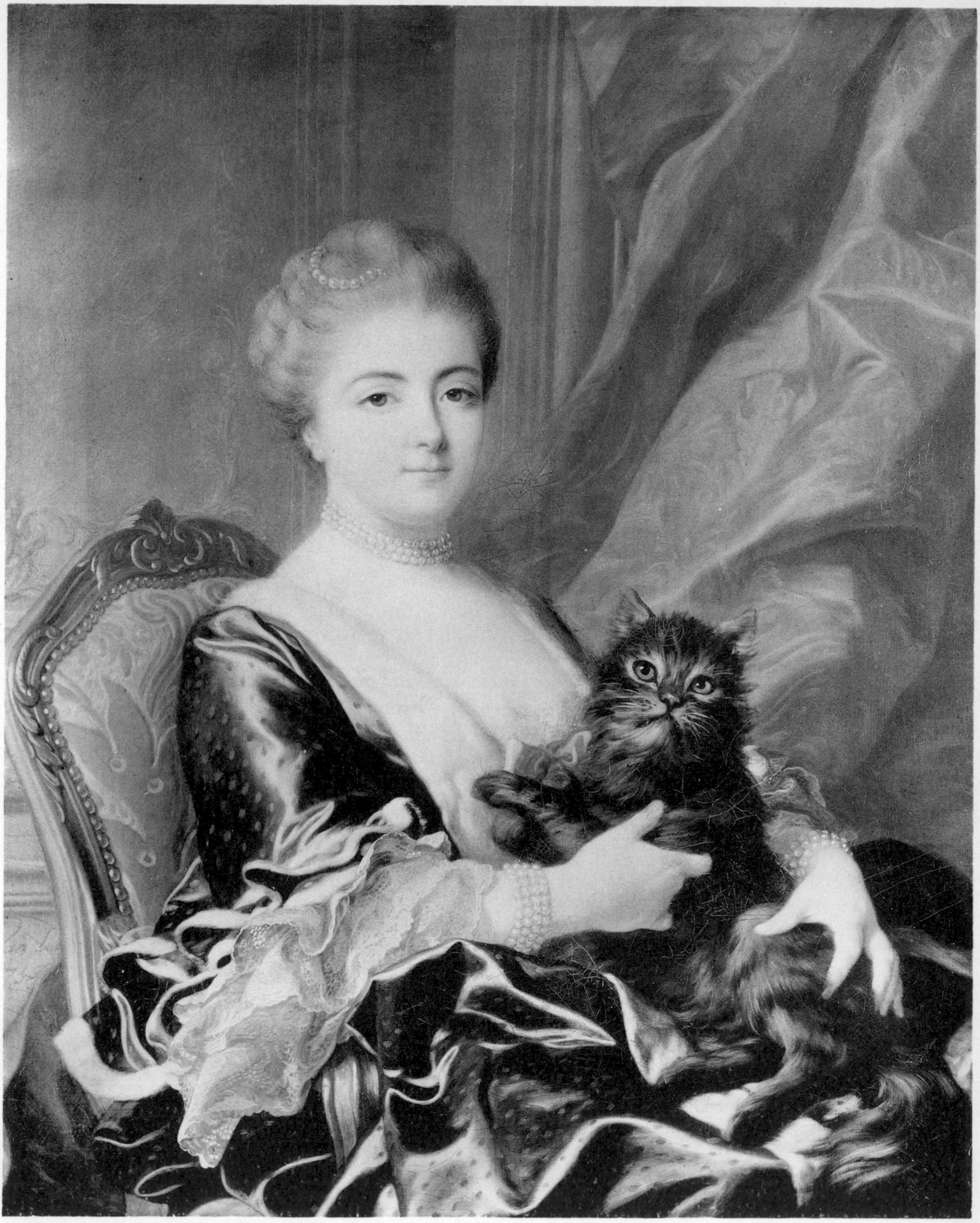

PORTRAIT OF MONSIEUR DE SARETTE
PORTRAIT OF MADAME DE SARETTE

BY

ANTOINE VESTIER

1740-1824

ANTOINE VESTIER

1740-1824

Born in Avallon and worked for the Parisian enamelist, Antoine Révérend, whose daughter, Marie-Anne, he married in 1764. Studied under Jean-Baptiste Pierre and travelled in Holland and England in the 1770's. Accepted by the Academy in 1785 and elected a member in 1787. Towards 1789 began to abandon the painting of miniatures, but his portraits show the effects of his early training.

Portrait of Monsieur de Sarette

Portrait of Madame de Sarette

canvas: 32¼ x 26 inches each

Signed and dated left center: *Vestier pinxit 1788* (M. de Sarette).

Signed and dated lower left: *Vestier pt 1791* (Mme de Sarette).

Two half-length portraits-pendants. M. de Sarette, seated in a red upholstered arm chair and facing towards the right, is holding a cello, his fingers across the strings as if he had just stopped playing. He wears a grey-blue suit with narrow stripes, and lace at his throat and wrists. His wife, dressed in a blue striped dress with a pink sash and a white kerchief, is seated in a similar chair and faces in the opposite direction. She leans her right arm on the piano and in her left hand she holds a sheet of music. Both are looking towards the spectator.

References: New York, Wildenstein & Co., *French 18th century paintings,* Mar.-Apr., 1929, nos. 1 & 3.

Exhibited: 1929, New York, Wildenstein & Co.

Collections: Comte de Buisseret, Brussels.

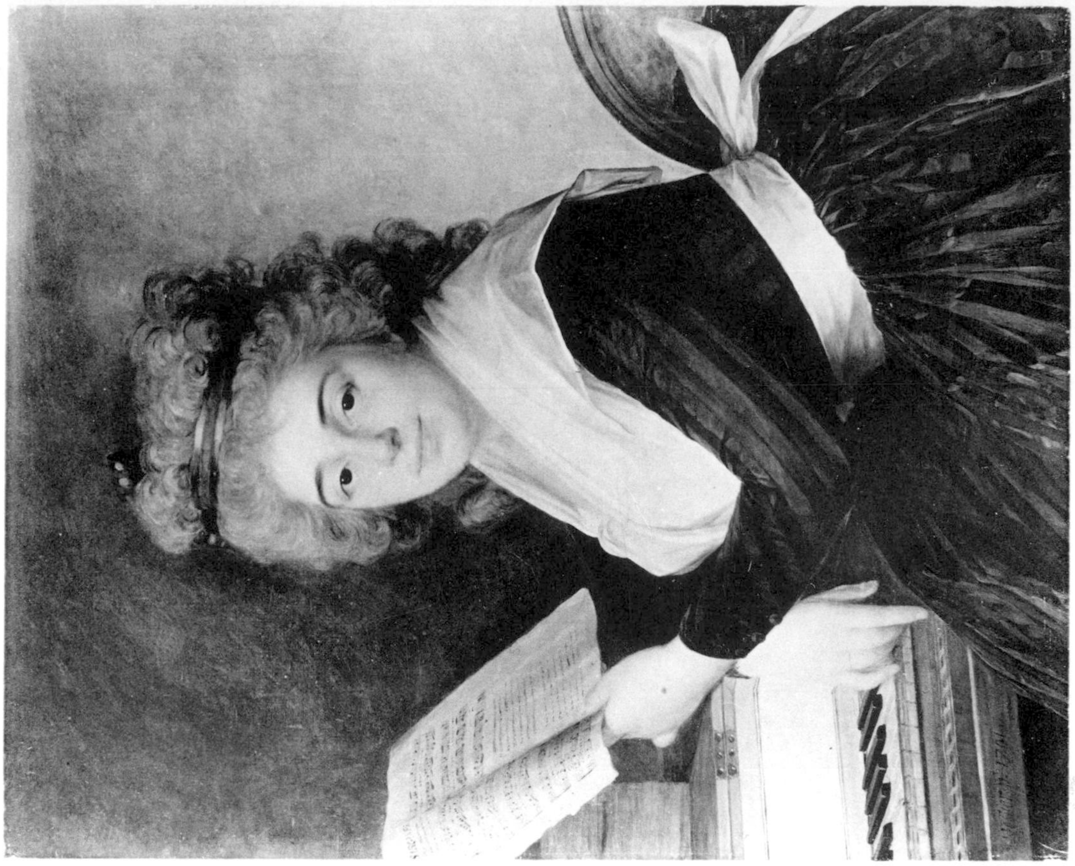

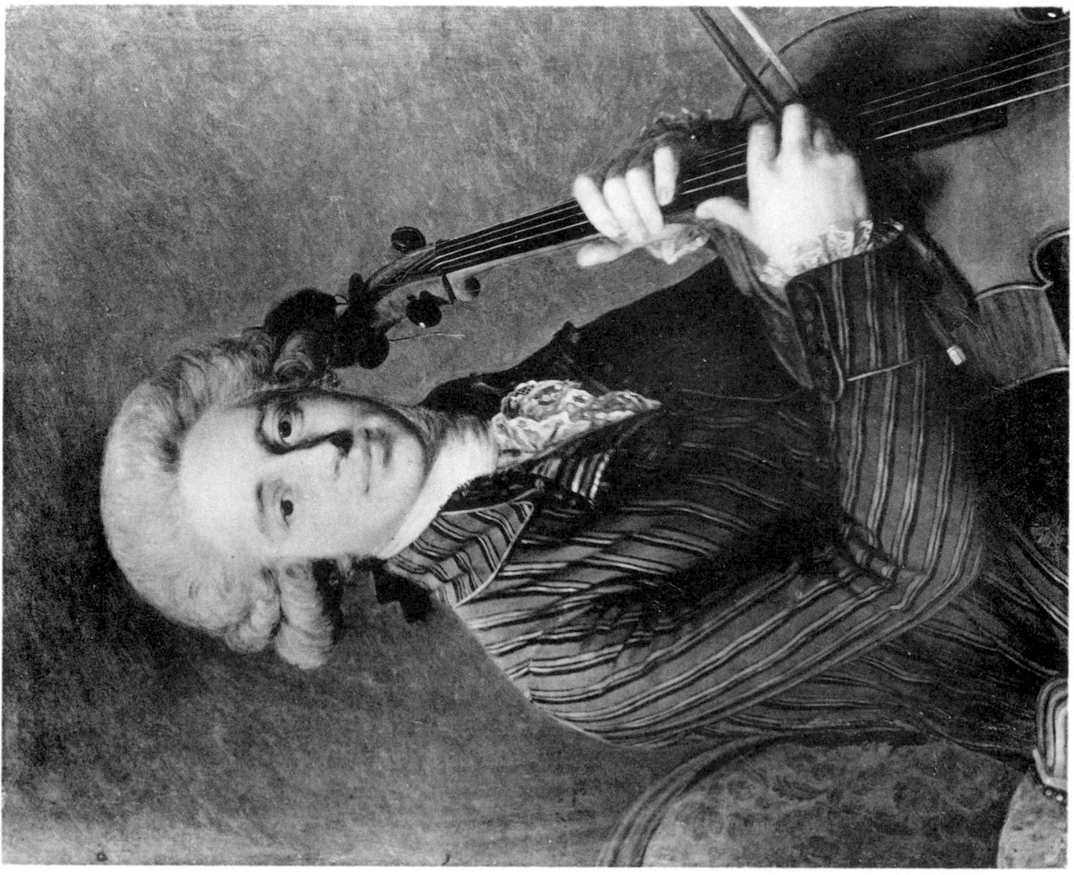

LOUISE ELISABETH VIGEE-LEBRUN

1755-1842

First training from her father, Louis Vigée, the portrait painter; later also studied with Greuze. A member of the Academy in 1783, she became Marie Antoinette's favorite painter and until the revolution, was busy in Paris executing many important court portraits. At the beginning of the revolution fled to Italy–Turin, Florence, Rome and Naples –and then to St. Petersburg where she stayed for six years painting for Paul I, Alexandre I and the Empress Catherine. Returned to Paris the winter of 1801, but went to England for three years and also visited Holland and Switzerland before settling finally in Paris.

Portrait of Princesse Youssoupoff

canvas: 55½ x 41 inches

Signed and dated on the tree trunk: *L. E. Vigée Le Brun 1797 à St. Petersbourg.*

Princesse Youssoupoff, the daughter of a noble of Smolensk, Basile Andréewitch Engelhardt, was born in 1769. In 1785 she married Lieutenant General M. S. Potemkine who was twenty-five years older than she and who died in six years. She became the Princesse Youssoupoff in 1793 but the marriage was not a happy one and resulted in a separation. The princess retired to the country and gathered around her a circle of artists, among them Pushkin. She died in 1841 and was buried in the monastery of Alexander Nevsky. This portrait was painted during Madame Vigée-Lebrun's visit to St. Petersburg. The monogram on the tree trunk, C.S., stands for the name of Princesse Youssoupoff's sister.

References: Nikolai Mikhailovitch, *Portraits Russes des XVIII et XIX siècles,* I, no. 10, ill.; *Catalogue de la collection Youssoupoff,* p. 96, no. 1920; L. E. Vigée-Lebrun, *Souvenirs de Mme. Vigée-Lebrun,* 1869, II, p. 371; St. Petersburg, Taurida Palace, *Exhibition of historical Russian portraits,* 1905, no. 257; *Khudozhestvennyia sokrovishcha Rosii* (Trésors d'art en Russie), 1906, VI, no. 144, ill.; P. de Nolhac, *Madame Vigée-Lebrun,* 1908, ill. opp. p. 160, pp. 112, 162; W. H. Helm, *Vigée-Lebrun, her life, works and friendships,* 1915, p. 225; A. Blum, *Madame Vigée-Lebrun,* 1919, pp. 71, 102; New York, Wildenstein & Co., *Fashion in headdress,* Apr. 27-May 27, 1943, no. 68.

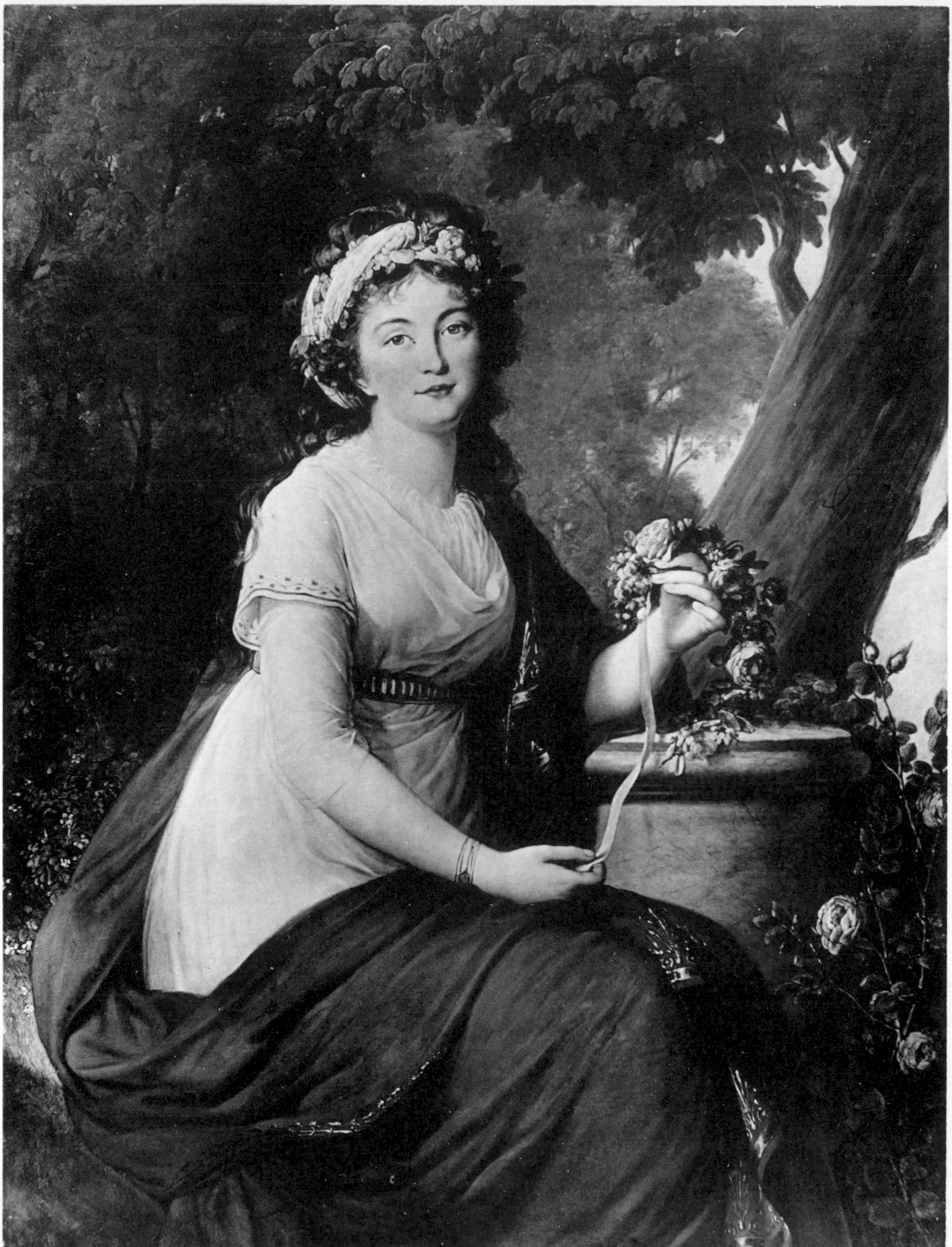

Exhibited: 1905, St. Petersburg, Taurida Palace; 1943, New York, Wildenstein & Co.

Collections: Prince Felix Felixovitch Youssoupoff

PORTRAIT OF MADAME ADELAIDE

BY

LOUISE ELISABETH VIGEE-LEBRUN

1755-1842

LOUISE ELISABETH VIGEE-LEBRUN

1755-1842

First training from her father, Louis Vigée, the portrait painter; later also studied with Greuze. A member of the Academy in 1783, she became Marie Antoinette's favorite painter and until the revolution, was busy in Paris executing many important court portraits. At the beginning of the revolution fled to Italy –Turin, Florence, Rome and Naples –and then to St. Petersburg where she stayed for six years painting for Paul I, Alexandre I and the Empress Catherine. Returned to Paris the winter of 1801, but went to England for three years and also visited Holland and Switzerland before settling finally in Paris.

Portrait of Madame Adélaïde

canvas: 30⅜ x 25½ inches

Signed and dated lower right: *E. Vigée-Lebrun, Rome 1791.*

Madame Adélaïde, eldest daughter of Louis XV and Marie Leczinska, was born in 1732. At the time of the revolution she and her sister, Victoire, fled to Italy living first in Rome where they met Madame Vigée-Lebrun, and then in Naples. When the French invaded Italy they moved to Trieste where both died, Adélaïde in 1800 and Victoire in the previous year.

References: W. H. Helm, *Vigée-Lebrun, her life, works and friendships,* 1915, p. 185.

Collections: Comtesse de Behague.

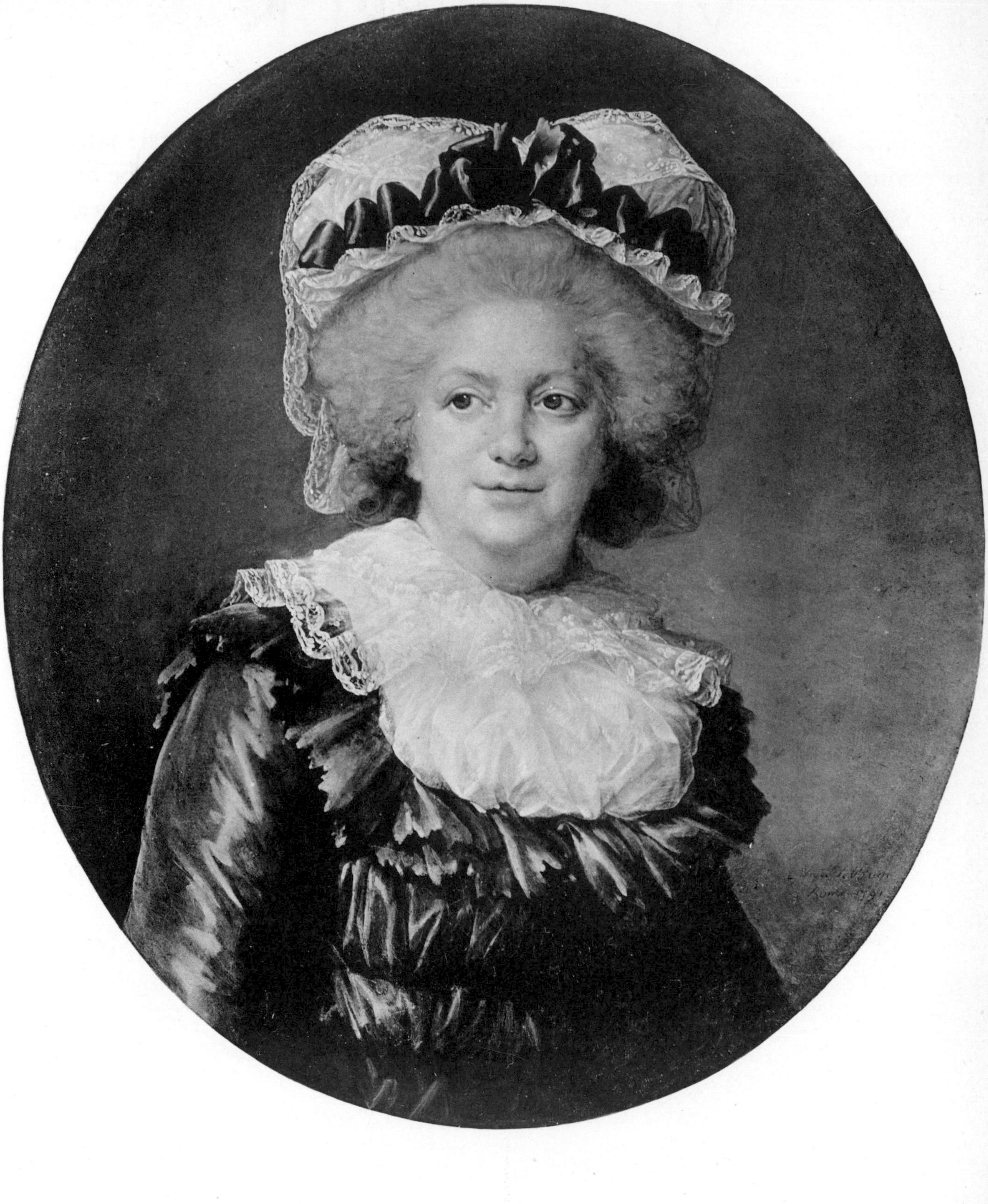

PORTRAIT OF A CHILD KNITTING

BY

FRANÇOIS-ANDRE VINCENT

1746-1816

FRANÇOIS-ANDRE VINCENT

c. 1746-1816

Son and pupil of the miniaturist, François-Elie Vincent. His father had intended him to be a banker but was persuaded to allow him to study in the Academy school under Vien. In 1767 won the first prize and spent three years in Rome at the Academy then directed by Natoire. Elected a member of the Academy in 1782 and from 1777 to 1801 exhibited continuously at the Salon. In 1792 appointed a professor at the Royal Academy. A very successful artist and a rival of David in his historical painting. Married his pupil, Adelaide Labille-Guiard.

Portrait of a child knitting

canvas: 21¾ x 19¼ inches

Signed and dated lower left: *F. A. Vincent 1792.*

A half-length figure of a young girl seated on a chair facing left. She wears a short-sleeved green dress with white cuffs and a white kerchief. Around her throat is a red necklace and her somewhat dishevelled black hair is tied back with a red ribbon. She looks away from her work towards the spectator but her fingers are busy knitting a cream colored sock. Grey background.

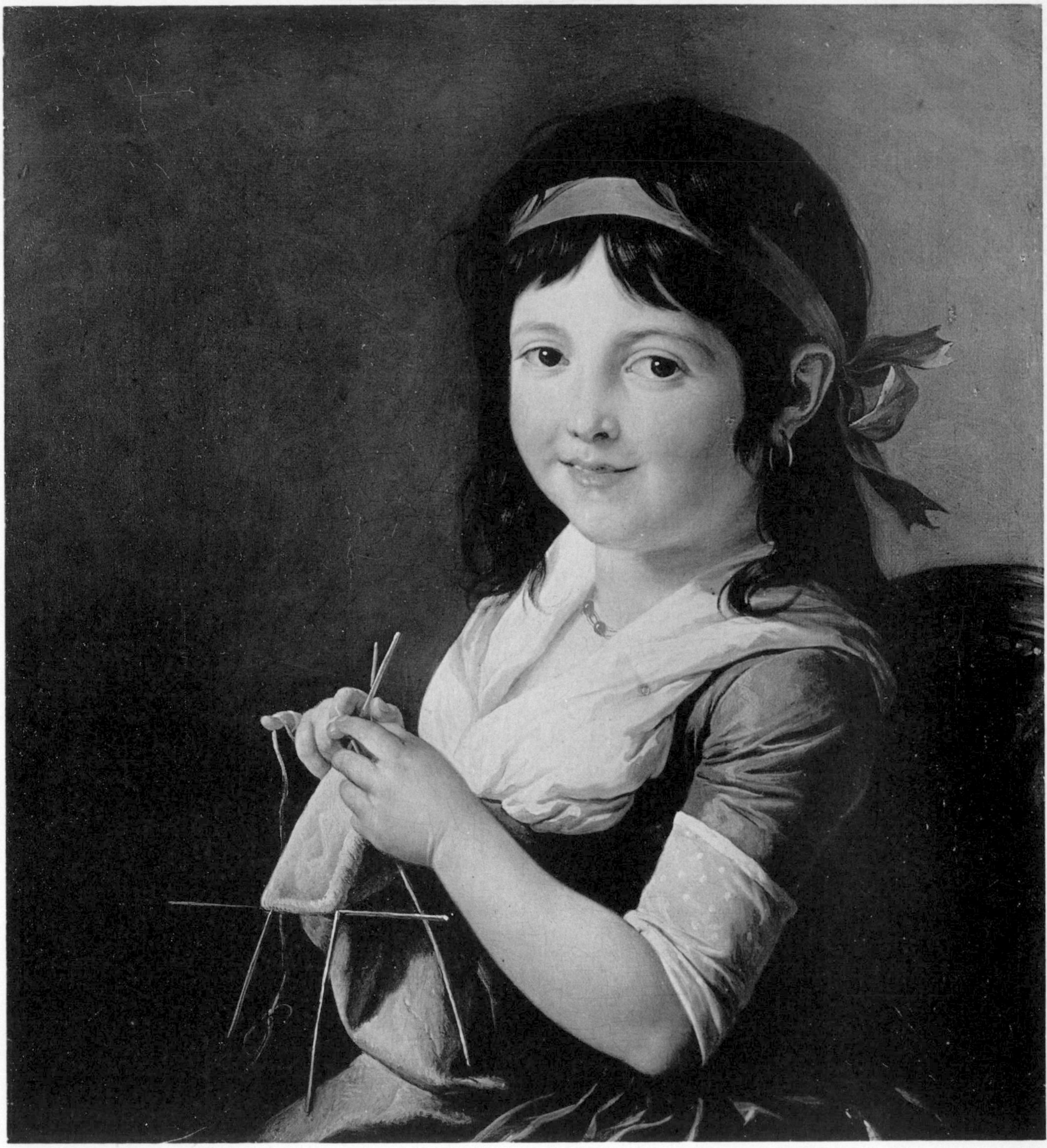

CERES OR SUMMER

BY

ANTOINE WATTEAU

1684-1721

ANTOINE WATTEAU

1684-1721

Born in Valenciennes which had only become part of France in 1668, but which had always been within the sphere of French culture. Came to Paris in 1702 as an assistant to a painter from Valenciennes who made decorations for the Paris opera. From 1705 to 1708 studied with Gillot, and then worked with Claude Audran, official painter of stage settings at the Opera and Conservator of the Luxembourg; here he had the opportunity to study Rubens who influenced him greatly. Stayed in Valenciennes from 1709 to 1711; returned to Paris and lived for some time with Pierre Crozat, the financier, whose magnificent collection of drawings was invaluable to the young artist. In 1720 went to London to consult the celebrated Dr. Mead on his consumption but the disease was already too far advanced for treatment and he came back to France where he died in 1721.

Ceres or *Summer*

canvas, oval: 54½ x 49½ inches

Engraved by J. Renard du Bos, Desplaces, Fessard, Audran.

One of a series of the four seasons painted about 1711 for Crozat's dining room. Ceres, wearing a white robe with a pink cloak is seated on the clouds holding a sickle in her left hand and resting her right arm on a lion's back. On her blond hair is a wreath of wheat, cornflowers and poppies. A nymph and a cherub carrying sheaves of wheat are seen on the right and in the left foreground, Cancer, the summer Zodiac sign.

References: V. Josz, *Antoine Watteau,* n.d., pp. 74, 75-76; Paris, *Vente Choiseul,* Dec. 18, 1786, p. 5, no. 3; Paris, *Vente Lebrun,* Apr. 11, 1791, pp. 103-104, no. 204; E. de Goncourt, *Catalogue raisonné de l'oeuvre . . . d'Antoine Watteau,* 1875, pp. 50-51, no. 47; E. & J. de Goncourt, *L'Art du XVIIIe siècle,* 1, 1880, p. 56; P. Mantz, *Antoine Watteau,* 1892, pp. 65-66, Paris, *Sedelmeyer* Galleries, *Second hundred paintings by old masters,* 1895, no. 71, ill.; London, Arundel Club, *Arundel Portfolio,* 1906, no. 13, ill.; London, Grafton Galleries, *National loan exhibition,* Oct.-Jan., 1909-1910, p. 147, no. 95; London, Christie, Manson & Woods, *Sir Lionel Phillips sale,* Apr. 25, 1913, no. 72, ill.; Paris, Galerie Georges Petit, *H. Michel-Lévy sale,*

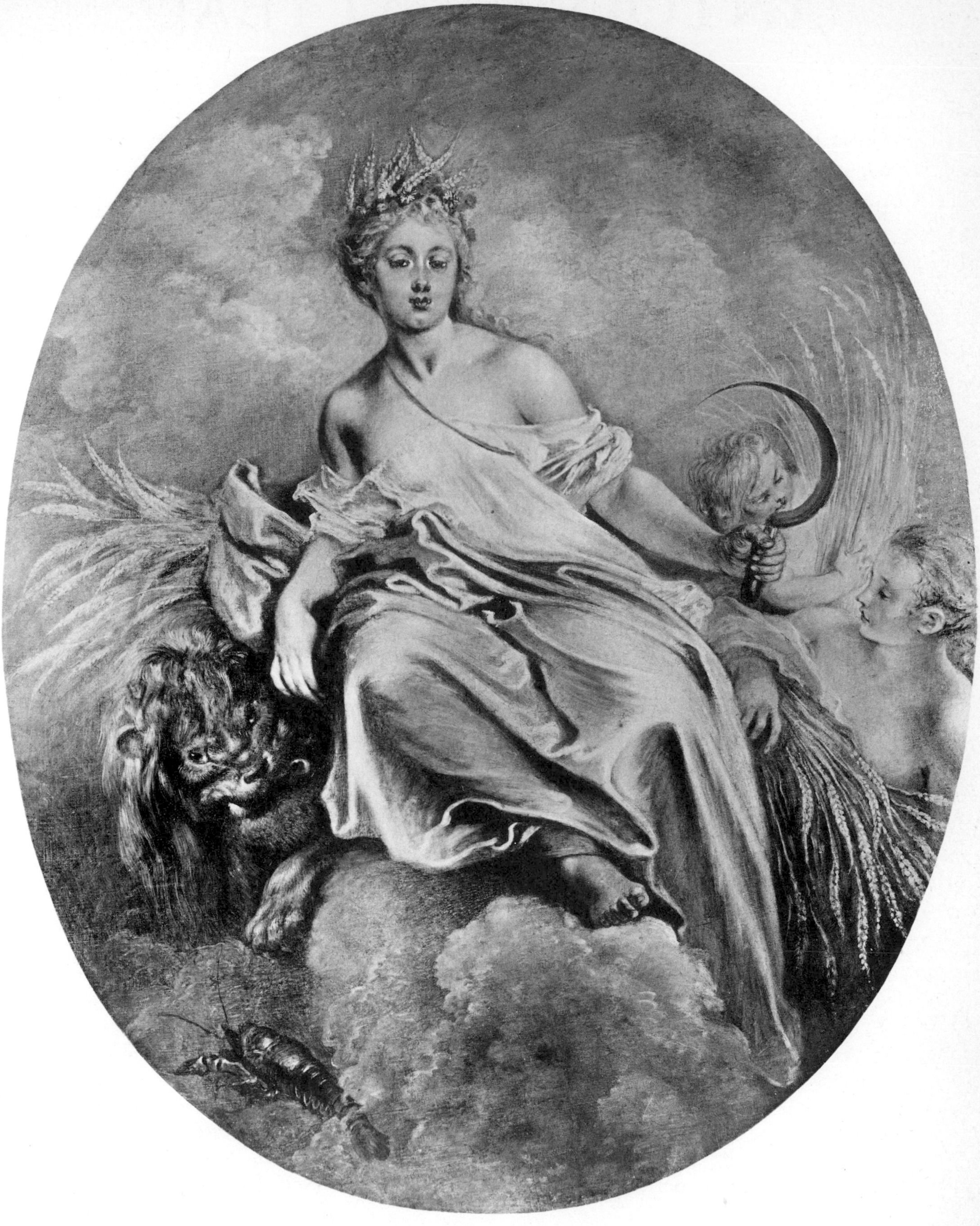

May 12, 13, 1919, no. 28, ill.; E. Pilon, *Watteau et son école,* 1921, pp. 118, 119-120; E. Dacier & A. Vuaflart, *Jean de Jullienne et les graveurs de Watteau,* 1922, IV, no. 106, ill. (du Bos engraving), III, pp. 50-51, no. 106; London, Wildenstein & Co., *Watteau and his contemporaries,* 1936, no. 27; S. Rocheblave, *French painting of the 18th century,* 1937, no. 10, ill.; *Burlington Magazine,* 73, Dec. 1938, pl. XVII, supplement; Thieme-Becker, *Allgemeines Lexikon der bildenden Künstler,* XXXV, 1942, p. 193.

Exhibited: 1910, London, Grafton Galleries; 1936, London, Wildenstein & Co.

Collections: Pierre Crozat (1661-1740); L. F. Crozat (nephew of Pierre); Duc de Choiseul — 1786; Le Brun — 1791; Novar; Charles Sedelmeyer — 1895; Sir Lionel Phillips, London — 1913; Henry Michel-Lévy, Paris; Léon Michel-Lévy; Charles-Louis Dreyfus, Paris.

PLEASURES OF SUMMER

BY

ANTOINE WATTEAU

1684-1721

ANTOINE WATTEAU

1684-1721

Born in Valenciennes which had only become part of France in 1668, but which had always been within the sphere of French culture. Came to Paris in 1702 as an assistant to a painter from Valenciennes who made decorations for the Paris opera. From 1705 to 1708 studied with Gillot, and then worked with Claude Audran, official painter of stage settings at the Opera and Conservator of the Luxembourg; here he had the opportunity to study Rubens who influenced him greatly. Stayed in Valenciennes from 1709 to 1711; returned to Paris and lived for some time with Pierre Crozat, the financier, whose magnificent collection of drawings was invaluable to the young artist. In 1720 went to London to consult the celebrated Dr. Mead on his consumption but the disease was already too far advanced for treatment and he came back to France where he died in 1721.

Pleasures of summer

canvas: 9¼ x 13¼ inches

Engraved by Jacques de Favannes.

In the foreground five figures are resting, one reclining with his back to the spectator. They are seated in the shade of large trees and near a waterfall at the left. In the center, a break in the trees allows one to see a view of some harvesters in the background.

References: V. Josz, *Antoine Watteau,* n.d., p. 136, note 1; Paris, *Vente Saint,* May 4, 1846, p. 14, no. 72; E. & J. de Goncourt, *Catalogue raisonné de l'oeuvre . . . d'Antoine Watteau,* 1875, p. 98, no. 99; J. W. Mollet, *Antoine Watteau,* 1883, p. 66, no. 99; E. & J. de Goncourt, *L'Art du XVIIIe siècle,* 1906, I, p. 75; E. Dacier & A. Vuaflart, *Jean de Jullienne et les graveurs de Watteau,* 1922, III, no. 132 ill. (engraving), p. 67, no. 132; Detroit, Institute of Arts, *Fourth loan exhibition of old masters,* Dec. 2-20, 1926, no. 55; *Art News,* "Landscape art in the Hartford Museum show," Jan. 31, 1931, p. 13, ill.; Hartford, Wadsworth Atheneum, *Retrospective exhibition of landscape painting,* Jan. 20-Feb. 9, 1931, no. 82, ill.; New York, Union League Club, *18th century French paintings,* Apr. 9-15, 1931, no. 2.

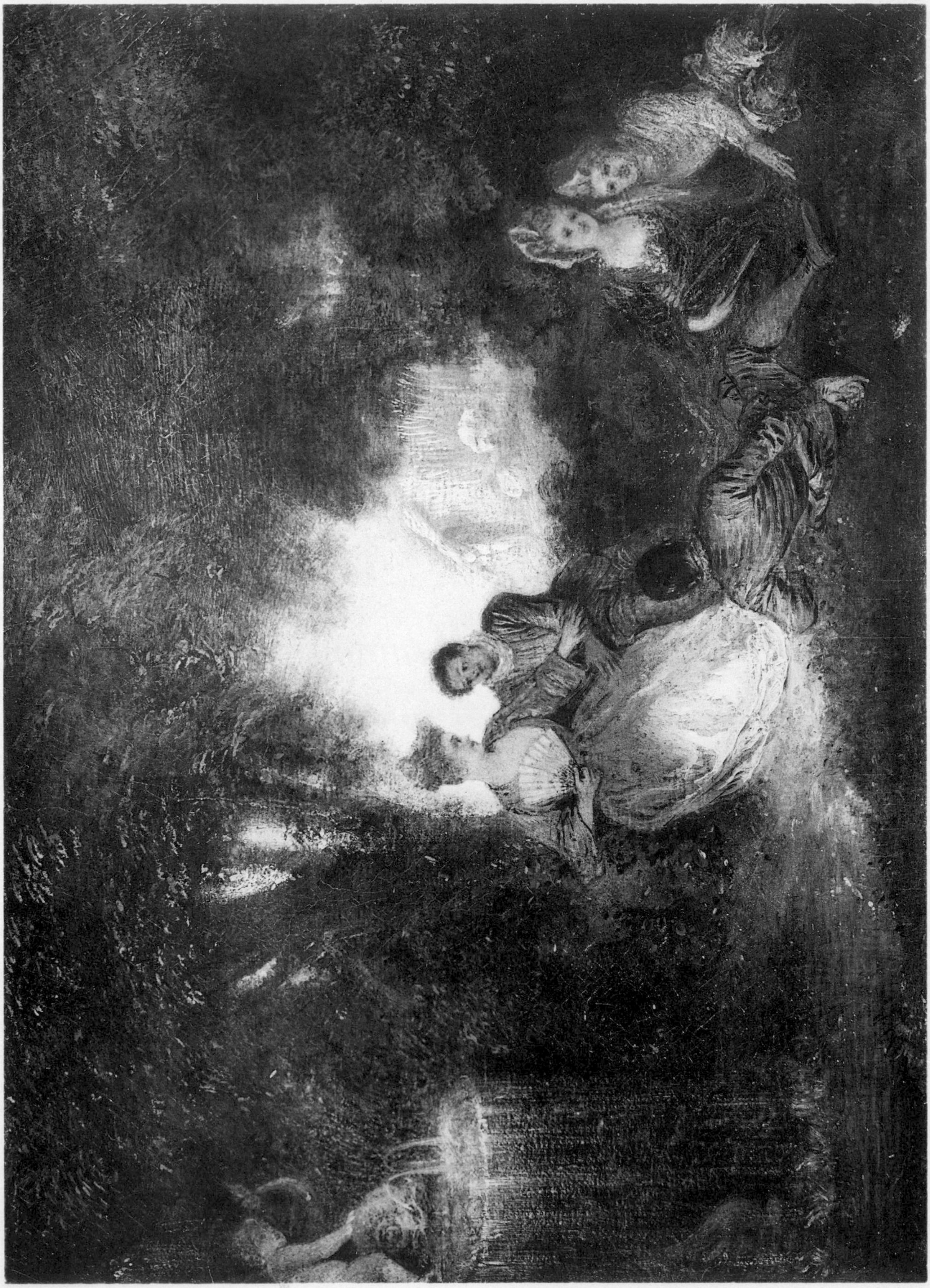

Exhibited: 1926, Detroit, Institute of Arts; 1931, New York, Union League Club; 1931, Hartford, Wadsworth Atheneum; 1933, Los Angeles, Museum.

Collections: Saint, Paris; Private collection in England; Mrs. John W. Simpson, New York.

ALLIANCE OF MUSIC AND COMEDY

BY

ANTOINE WATTEAU

1684-1721

ANTOINE WATTEAU

1684-1721

Born in Valenciennes which had only become part of France in 1668, but which had always been within the sphere of French culture. Came to Paris in 1702 as an assistant to a painter from Valenciennes who made decorations for the Paris opera. From 1705 to 1708 studied with Gillot, and then worked with Claude Audran, official painter of stage settings at the Opera and Conservator of the Luxembourg; here he had the opportunity to study Rubens who influenced him greatly. Stayed in Valenciennes from 1709 to 1711; returned to Paris and lived for some time with Pierre Crozat, the financier, whose magnificent collection of drawings was invaluable to the young artist. In 1720 went to London to consult the celebrated Dr. Mead on his consumption but the disease was already too far advanced for treatment and he came back to France where he died in 1721.

Alliance of Music and Comedy

canvas: 25⅝ x 20⅞ inches

Engraved by Jean Moyreau.

Allegorical painting arranged according to the principals of heraldry. On the face of the shield, a mask of comedy, a G clef, a tenor clef, a flat and a sharp. Above the shield, a bust of harlequin with a laurel wreath over his head, and surrounding it, a circle of instruments, masks and scores. Thalia, the Comic muse, contemplating a mask, stands to the left, and Euterpe, the Musical muse, holding a lyre, to the right. Probably made as a signboard—Louis de Fourcaud has proposed a sign for a music shop and Dacier & Vuaflart have suggested one for a small theatre.

References: V. Josz, *Antoine Watteau,* n.d., p. 88, note 2; Paris, *Vente Saint,* May 4, 1846, no. 66; Paris, *Vente Barroilhet,* Mar. 10, 1872, no. 20; E. de Goncourt, *Catalogue raisonné de l'oeuvre . . . d'Antoine Watteau,* 1875, p. 63, no. 63; E. & J. de Goncourt, *L'Art du XVIIIe siècle,* I, 1880, p. 56; P. Mantz, *Antoine Watteau,* 1892, p. 28; R. Portalis & H. Beraldi, *Les graveurs du XVIIIe siècle,* II, 1892, p. 219 (engraving); G. Schéfer, "Le portraits dans l'oeuvre de Watteau," *Gazette des Beaux-Arts,* XLII, 1896, p. 188; A. Rosenberg, *Antoine Watteau,* 1896,

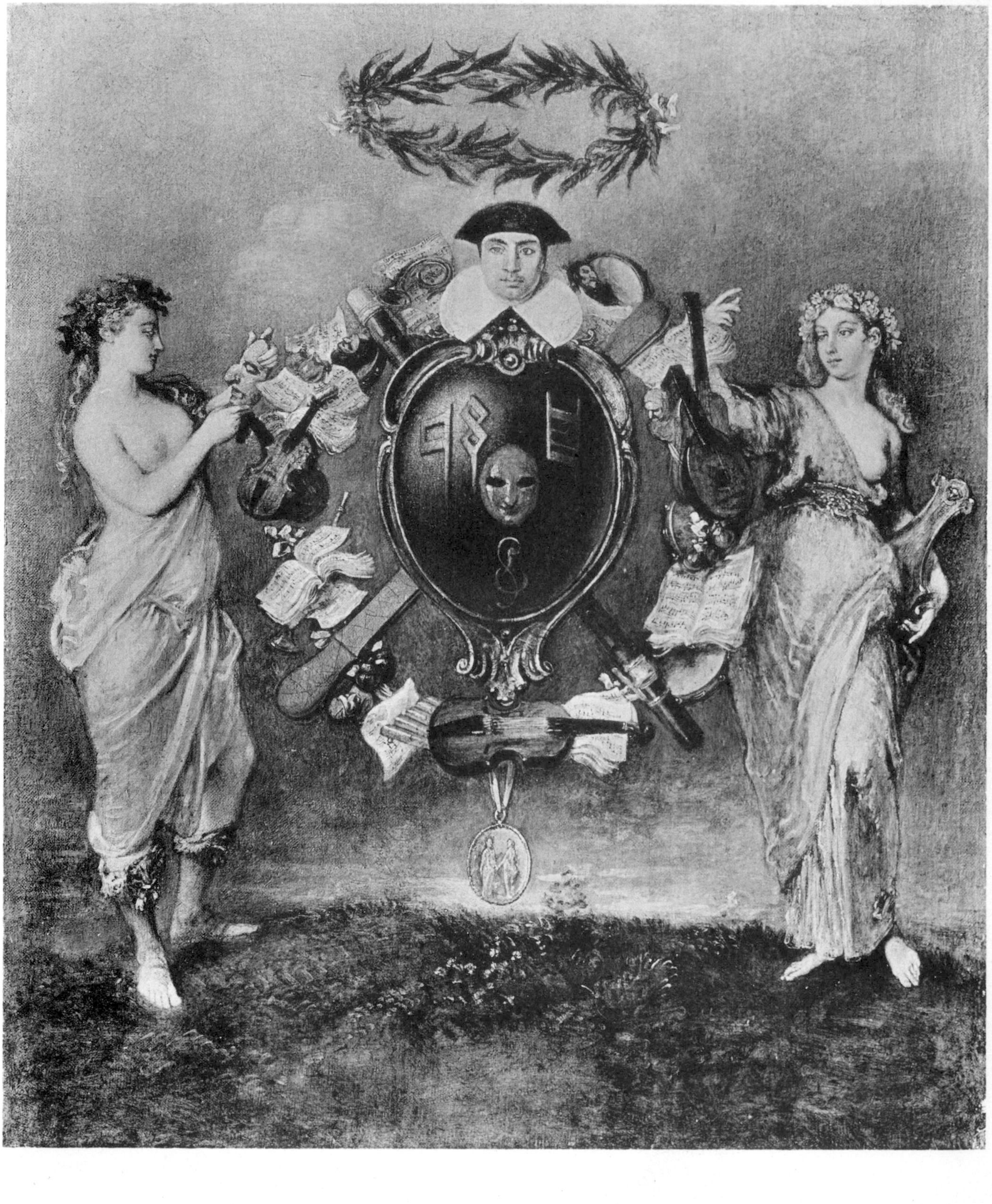

p. 9, ill. (engraving); L. de Fourcaud, "Antoine Watteau; peintre d'arabesques," *Revue de l'art,* XXV, 1909, p. 133; E. Pilon, *Watteau et son école,* 1912, pp. 130-131; Paris, Galerie Georges Petit, *Vente Michel-Lévy,* May 12, 1919, no. 39; E. Dacier & A. Vuaflart, *Jean de Jullienne et les graveurs de Watteau,* 1922, IV, pl. 39 (engraving), III, p. 24, no. 39, II, p. 33, I, pp. 61-63, 260; Paris, Galerie Jean Charpentier, *Exposition de la musique et de la danse,* 1923, no. 159; Paris, Musée Carnavalet, *Le théâtre à Paris, XVIIe et XVIIIe siècles,* Mar. 19-May 4, 1929, no. 81; G. Barker, *Antoine Watteau,* 1939, p. 184; New York, New School for Social Research, *Loan exhibition of paintings,* Mar. 3-17, 1946, no. 19.

Exhibited: 1923, Paris; 1929, Paris, Musée Carnavalet; 1946, New York, New School for Social Research.

Collections: Saint, Paris; Barroilhet, Paris; Léon Michel-Lévy, Paris.

PROMENADE SUR LES REMPARTS

BY

ANTOINE WATTEAU

1684-1721

ANTOINE WATTEAU

1684-1721

Born in Valenciennes which had only become part of France in 1668, but which had always been within the sphere of French culture. Came to Paris in 1702 as an assistant to a painter from Valenciennes who made decorations for the Paris opera. From 1705 to 1708 studied with Gillot, and then worked with Claude Audran, official painter of stage settings at the Opera and Conservator of the Luxembourg; here he had the opportunity to study Rubens who influenced him greatly. Stayed in Valenciennes from 1709 to 1711; returned to Paris and lived for some time with Pierre Crozat, the financier, whose magnificent collection of drawings was invaluable to the young artist. In 1720 went to London to consult the celebrated Dr. Mead on his consumption but the disease was already too far advanced for treatment and he came back to France where he died in 1721.

Promenade sur les remparts

canvas: 18¼ x 21¾ inches

Engraved by Aubert in 1732.

Twenty-six figures spread through the foreground of a landscape which has been thought to be the view Watteau saw from his window in Crozat's house. Recent opinion, however, denies this and says that the landscape is entirely imaginary, vaguely Italian in style. Perhaps he was inspired by one of Crozat's innumerable Italian drawings or perhaps, as Pilon suggests, it is the ramparts of Vauban at Valenciennes that he had in mind.

References: *L'Oeuvre d'Antoine Watteau . . . gravé par les soins de M. de Julienne,* n.d., n.p., ill. (Aubert engraving); V. Josz, *Antoine Watteau,* n.d., pp. 134-135; E. de Goncourt, *Catalogue raisonné de l'oeuvre . . . d'Antoine Watteau,* 1875, pp. 141-142, no. 157; E. Pilon, *Watteau et son école,* 1912, p. 78; E. & J. de Goncourt, *L'Art du XVIIIe siècle,* 1918, I, p. 87; L. Gillet, *Watteau,* 1921, p. 60; E. Dacier & A. Vuaflart, *Jean de Jullienne et les graveurs de Watteau au XVIIIe siècle,* 1922, III, pl. 113 (Aubert engraving), p. 54, no. 113; E. Hildebrandt, *Antoine Watteau,* 1922, p. 166, ill. (Aubert engraving), p. 167; Los Angeles, Museum, *Five centuries of European painting,* Dec., 1933, no. 22; Cincinnati, Art Museum, *French paintings of*

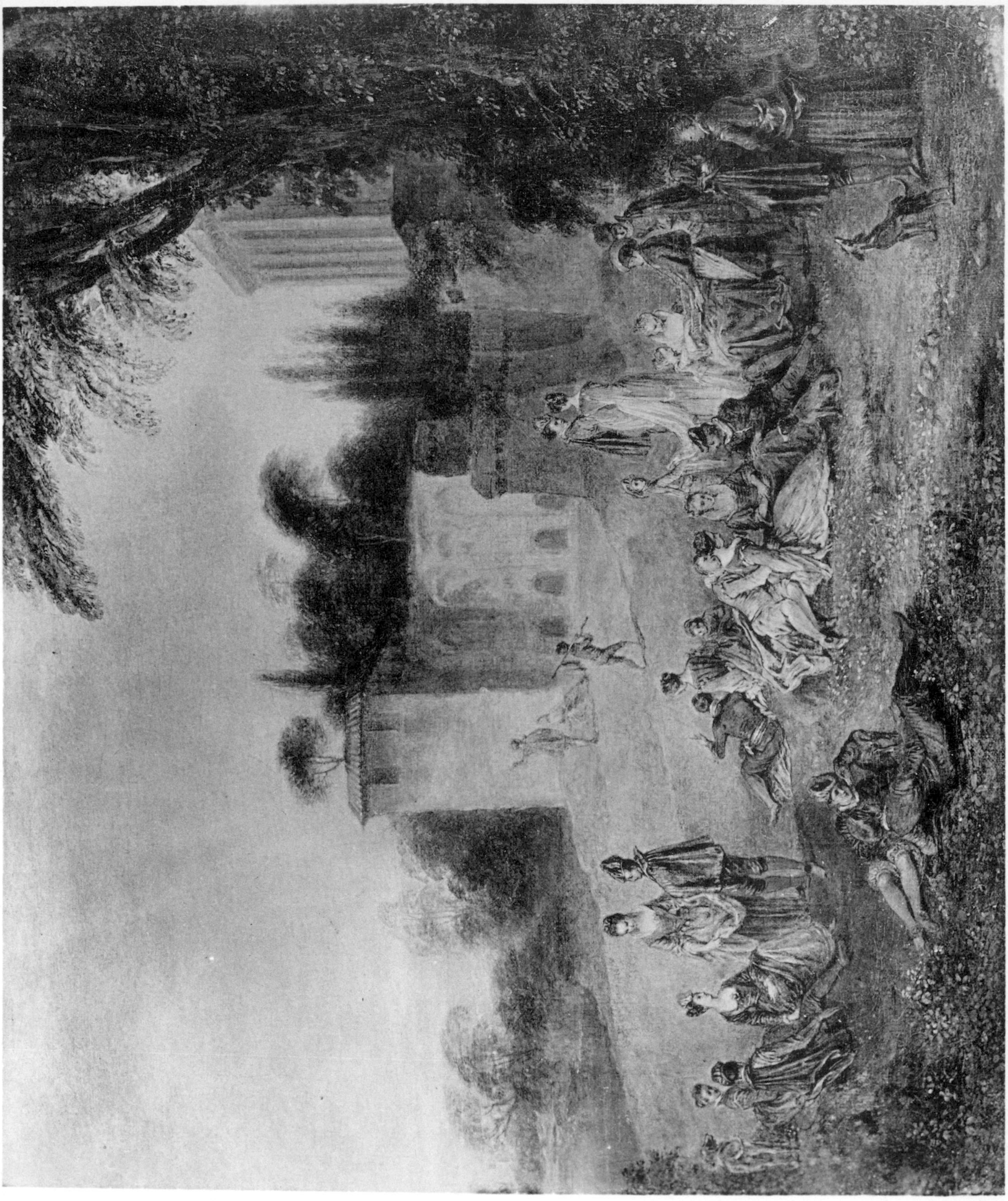

the 18th and early 19th centuries, Oct. 2-Nov. 7, 1937, no. 21; G. Barker, *Antoine Watteau,* 1939, p. 52.

Exhibited: 1933, Los Angeles, Museum; 1937, Cincinnati, Art Museum.

Collections: M. de Julienne, until 1756; Private Spanish collection; Madame de Charnisey.